ACUTE CARDIOVASCULAR MANAGEMENT

Edited by **ALLEN K. REAM,** M.D.

Associate Professor of Anesthesia
Director, Institute of Engineering Design in Medicine
Stanford University School of Medicine
Stanford, California

and **RICHARD P. FOGDALL,** M.D.

Associate Professor of Anesthesia
Associate Director, Cardiovascular Anesthesia
Stanford University School of Medicine
Stanford, California

with 21 additional authors

ACUTE CARDIOVASCULAR MANAGEMENT

Anesthesia and Intensive Care

J. B. Lippincott Company
Philadelphia

London   Mexico City   New York   St. Louis   São Paulo   Sydney

Sponsoring Editor: Richard Winters
Manuscript Editor: Don Shenkle
Art Director: Maria S. Karkucinski
Designer: Ronald Dorfman
Production Supervisor: N. Carol Kerr
Production Assistant: Charlene Catlett Squibb
Compositor: Ruttle, Shaw & Wetherill, Inc.
Printer/Binder: Halliday Lithograph

The authors and publishers have exerted every effort to ensure
that drug selection and dosage set forth in this text are in accord
with current recommendations and practice at the time of publication. However, in view of ongoing research, changes in government regulations, and the constant flow of information relating to
drug therapy and drug reactions, the reader is urged to check the
package insert for each drug for any change in indications and
dosage and for added warnings and precautions. This is particularly important when the recommended agent is a new or infrequently employed drug.

3 5 6 4 2

PRINTED IN THE UNITED STATES OF AMERICA

Library of Congress Cataloging in Publication Data
Main entry under title:

Acute cardiovascular management.

Includes index.
1. Cardiovascular system—Surgery.
2. Anesthesia.   3. Cardiovascular system—Diseases
—Treatment.   4. Critical care medicine.
I. Ream, Allen K.   II. Fogdall, Richard P.
RD597.A27   617'.41   81-19279
ISBN 0-397-50438-1   AACR2

To every physician
with the need to help patients
and the desire to understand effective methods

Contents ///

Contributors

John R. Ammon, M.D.
Attending Anesthesiologist
St. John Hospital
Detroit, Michigan
Clinical Instructor
Department of Anesthesia
Wayne State University

Ronald A. Dritz, M.D.
Department of Anesthesia
Alta Bates Hospital
Berkeley, California

Norig Ellison, M.D.
Associate Professor
Department of Anesthesia
Hospital of the University of Pennsylvania and
*   Children's Hospital of Philadelphia*
Philadelphia, Pennsylvania

Michael A. Flynn, M.B., Ch.B.
Assistant Professor of Anesthesia
Stanford University School of Medicine
Stanford, California

Richard P. Fogdall, M.D.
Associate Professor of Anesthesia
Associate Director, Cardiovascular Anesthesia
Stanford University School of Medicine
Stanford, California

Robert E. Fowles, M.D.
Assistant Professor of Medicine
Division of Cardiology
Stanford University School of Medicine
Stanford, California

J. Kent Garman, M.D.
Associate Professor
Chief, Cardiovascular Anesthesia
Stanford University School of Medicine
Stanford, California

Jerry C. Griffin, M.D.
Assistant Professor of Cardiology
Baylor Cardiology Associates
Methodist Hospital
Houston, Texas

Alvin Hackel, M.D.
Associate Professor of Clinical Anesthesia and
*   Clinical Pediatrics*
Stanford University School of Medicine
Stanford, California

Mark Hilberman, M.D.
972 Mears Court
Stanford, California

Carl C. Hug, Jr., M.D., Ph.D.
Professor and Associate Director
Division of Cardiothoracic Anesthesia
Department of Anesthesia
Emory University School of Medicine
Atlanta, Georgia

Joel A. Kaplan, M.D.
Professor and Director
Division of Cardiothoracic Anesthesia
Department of Anesthesia
Emory University School of Medicine
Atlanta, Georgia

Chris H. Kehler, M.D.
Assistant Professor
Department of Anesthesia
Health Sciences Center
Winnipeg, Manitoba

James C. Loomis, M.D.
Assistant Professor of Anesthesia and Pediatrics
Stanford University School of Medicine
Stanford, California

William New, Jr., M.D., Ph.D.
Clinical Assistant Professor of Anesthesia
Stanford University School of Medicine
Stanford, California

Peer M. Portner, Ph.D.
President
Director of Research
Novacor Medical Corporation
Oakland, California

Allen K. Ream, M.D.
Associate Professor of Anesthesia
Director, Institute of Engineering Design in Medicine
Stanford University School of Medicine
Stanford, California

Bruce A. Reitz, M.D.
Professor of Surgery
Cardiac Surgeon In Charge
Johns Hopkins Hospital
Baltimore, Maryland

Robert N. Sladen, M.B., Ch.B.
Assistant Professor of Anesthesia
Associate Medical Director, Intensive Care Unit
Stanford University School of Medicine
Stanford, California

Theodore H. Stanley, M.D.
Professor of Anesthesiology
Department of Anesthesiology
University of Utah Medical Center
Salt Lake City, Utah

Susan Prince Watson, M.D.
Associate Professor of Anesthesia and Child Health and Development
Children's Hospital
National Medical Center and George Washington University School of Medicine
Washington, D.C.

Donald C. Watson, M.D.
Associate Cardiovascular Surgeon
Department of Child Health and Development
Children's Hospital
National Medical Center
Assistant Professor of Surgery
George Washington University School of Medicine
Washington, D.C.

Philip H. Wells, M.D.
Fellow, Cardiothoracic Anesthesia
Department of Anesthesia
Emory University School of Medicine
Atlanta, Georgia

Preface

THE ACUTE MANAGEMENT of the cardiovascular patient has followed two intellectual pathways, depending on whether or not the patient required surgery. These pathways are now converging, as results improve and clinical experience is integrated with basic knowledge.

While many roots of this book draw from surgical experience, the subject is the acutely unstable cardiovascular patient. Our central clinical examples are drawn from patients undergoing aggressive therapy because it is most instructive, but the lessons are broadly applicable.

This book is written for the clinician. Its goal is to enhance the quality of medical practice by collecting known principles, many of which are not widely discussed in the general medical literature. Yet we are equally determined, when possible, to present a scientific basis for medical care and to separate habitual approaches from those proven better than available alternatives.

To this end, a substantial part of the book deals with basic principles. The remainder deals with their applications. In each instance, we have endeavored to tie basic principles closely to clinical practice. However, we have not attempted to duplicate material in basic texts, certain basic material widely and well discussed elsewhere (as blood gas analysis), or to include material which has uncertain clinical application. The text is written to be a complete basic clinical reference on the subject; additional areas are addressed by references to further reading.

We have endeavored to avoid the problems of a multiauthor text. One of us has worked closely with the author(s) of each chapter. Considerable effort has been expended to assure that each major topic is covered once, completely and concisely. Our only deliberate exception is a succinct recapitulation of the most critical concerns, in the clinical chapters of sections four and five, to assure that clinical summations are complete. We hope that the reader will find that the book reads like a single author text, with the exception that the special skills and interests of our authors are not obscured.

Much of the material is new, and much more appears new, because of organization or original publication in obscure places. These observations apply particularly to the basic concepts of section one, the presentation of congenital anomalies, and the discussion of cardiac transplantation, hypothermia, oxygenators, and the artificial heart. We hope that the reader will give equal attention to the more familiar subjects; new material and rarely discussed but important relationships are found in every chapter.

Finally, we would like to share with you, the reader, our excitement and professional satisfaction in working in a field of medicine where progress has been of such broad application, and so rapid, stimulating, and effective.

ALLEN K. REAM, M.D.
RICHARD P. FOGDALL, M.D.

Acknowledgments ///

THIS EFFORT TO document and improve a rapidly emerging discipline depended upon the contributions of an extraordinary number of people.

In particular, we would like to thank our authors, who have labored not only over their own contributions, but in many instances have reviewed substantial portions of other chapters, adding ideas and insights.

Inspiration and support for a formidable task has come from many quarters. We thank Lew Reines, former Editor-in-Chief of Lippincott Medical Books, for his unwavering support during the phases of planning and early writing. Stuart Freeman, Lisa Biello, Richard Winters, Don Shenkle, and their colleagues have continued to demonstrate the professionalism of this organization.

Our students, residents, fellows, and faculty have generously given time and demonstrated interest. And many workers from other major centers have provided a significant supplement to our knowledge of divergent practices and discussion of techniques which appear to have more than regional value or interest.

We owe a particular debt to our Stanford colleagues Norman Shumway, Chairman of the Department of Cardiovascular Surgery, C. Philip Larson, Jr., Chairman of the Department of Anesthesia, and J. Kent Garman, Chief of Cardiac Anesthesia, for their support of an environment which demands excellence while permitting discussion of weaknesses, and which has nurtured mutual respect.

We thank Professor Joh. Spierdijk for the opportunity for Dr. Ream to practice Cardiovascular Anesthesia at the University of Leiden, the Netherlands, and to observe and discuss European medical practices.

We thank those who served as reviewers for their time and painstaking efforts. In particular we thank Ad von Binen, David Bolton, Norbert DeBruin, John Howse, C. Philip Larson Jr., Jon Mark, Jay Mason, Doug Merrill, David Ruderman, N. Ty Smith, Roderick Thomson, and Janet Wyner.

A special contribution was the material provided by Dr. Leslie Rendell–Baker enhancing the history of cardiopulmonary bypass presented in Chapter 14.

The art of Stephanie Williams, with assistance from Barbara Haynes, has left a special mark on our work. The cover tracing was contributed by Robert Fowles.

The secretarial and administrative effort was a major task. In particular we gratefully acknowledge the work of Adena Goodart, Ruth Schimke, Barbara Ybarra, Virginia Duncan, Gail Christie, Norma Garcia, Kathy Westlake, Betty Hampton, Louise Carlstrand, and Susan Ahlering.

Finally, we acknowledge a special debt to our wives and families, whose support has made this effort possible and to whom the thousands of hours reserved for this effort can never be repaid adequately.

Part I / GENERAL CONCEPTS

1

General Considerations

ALLEN K. REAM
RICHARD P. FOGDALL

Although the essential role of the heart in body function was appreciated before the beginning of recorded history, it has proven difficult to separate subjective views from repeatable observations. It is somehow demeaning to consider an organ representing the essence of life, and even of heroic attributes, as a physical object, subject to natural laws and frailties. From this perspective, Harvey's work, defining the distribution and sequence of blood flow, was of profound import.[1] It altered our view of ourselves, making an essential body function less mysterious, more understandable, and accessible to intervention. The account of the anxiety associated with early treatment of penetrating wounds of the heart illustrates how this conceptual difficulty has affected the development of open-heart surgery.[2] It is startling to realize that while underlying techniques have developed slowly, the present concepts of acute care are less than 15 years old. And the sorting of subjective from objective views continues, as evidenced by the strong public interest in the artificial heart and heart and lung transplantation.

The literature reveals the effects of this recent rapid development. The determinants of disease remain unclear,[3-6] though mortality and morbidity associated with heart disease have begun to decline.[7] But the techniques associated with acute management have undergone rapid progress in both the medical and surgical arenas.[8-13] The principal development has been therapeutic understanding; facilities for care were already available at the beginning of this 15-year period.[14]

Because of this rapid growth, the literature is often obscure. Much detailed material has been written by cardiologists about patients with terminal diseases not susceptible to surgical correction. The literature of the coronary care unit tends to be highly specialized, with particular emphasis on arrhythmias and evolution of disease related only to acute myocardial infarction. The internist who wishes to read about surgical management is therefore often frustrated. Until recently the best centers taught a comprehensive pattern through apprenticeship and many of the most useful concepts are scattered in original papers. Many of the most interesting recent developments, such as in basic physiology, hypothermia, oxygenators, and assist devices, are published in journals and reports not easily accessible to the practicing clinician. Few recent publications in the surgical literature address these questions in a broad and quantitative manner. Habits learned in one context are sometimes painfully inappropriate in another: for example, the transition from salt deprivation of the patient in chronic congestive failure to more appropriate salt loading during cardiovascular surgery and intensive care.

A major stimulus for the creation of this book was the recognition that the acute management of the cardiovascular patient is a maturing specialty. The techniques of successful centers are becoming more and more alike. Justification of management is more often based on demonstrated basic principles than on extensive personal experience. For these reasons, it is now possible to describe the basic clinical principles of management that are becoming widely accepted.

We have noted also a teaching phenomenon of considerable importance. In teaching, one rarely explains a therapeutic response on the basis of a principle which has been only recently accepted. But management has changed dramatically in the last ten years. The difference appears to lie in the fact that with increasing skill and experience, therapeutic decisions are made on the basis of multiple factors, rather than on a perceived single cause and effect relationship. (See the discussion of the effects of narcotics on acute pulmonary edema in Chap. 2 and the account

of the patient requiring defibrillation in Chap. 16 for specific examples.) Although in theory all of the information required to make these connections is in the original literature, this approach to learning is inadequate in practice. However, these relationships are better understood if studied in traditional form before caring for patients on the wards, in the operating room, or in an intensive surgical or coronary care unit.

Yet another incentive is the broad relevance of these skills to parallel activities. Although few of the anesthesia residents at Stanford plan to specialize in cardiovascular anesthesia, they indicate uniformly that the experience has enhanced their basic skills. The occasional cardiologist who rotates through cardiovascular surgery likewise develops a significantly enhanced sense of professional competence. And, at Stanford, the residents and students participating in cardiac intensive care are divided between anesthesia and medicine. (The surgical students interact with the same group of residents during their surgical rotation.) The rotation to intensive care has been one of the most popular in the medical school curriculum.

The reasons for this interest are not difficult to appreciate. The cardiovascular patient represents an unusual professional opportunity and challenge. His problems are common to many patients, though he is more demanding. The time response is short, which enhances "feedback" on therapeutic maneuvers. Because of rapidly burgeoning professional skills, intervention is often heroic, permitting an ethical glimpse of physiologic mechanisms otherwise perceived only indirectly. Because drug mechanisms are increasingly well defined, this patient is often the appropriate object of multiple drug therapy, requiring enhanced pharmacologic skill and monitoring.

In addition, the acute cardiovascular patient warrants a special category in his own right. At least two Americans each minute suffer a heart attack. Diseases of the heart are still the leading cause of death in this country, although the incidence is finally declining. Even the numbers for relatively esoteric applications can be impressive; more than 50,000 Americans a year may be candidates for cardiac-assist devices, and cardiac transplantation has now achieved a survival rate equal to that of unrelated kidney transplantation.

Finally, in skilled hands, the relative risks associated with acute interventions have declined. For example, the overall perioperative mortality for coronary artery revascularization at Stanford is now well below one percent, a result associated with adequate factual knowledge and experience, and the availability of essential resources.

As might be expected from these biases, the book is not subdivided on the basis of the anatomic lesions that may be encountered. Rather it is divided on the basis of specific skills that must be mastered and the physiologic insults that the patient must endure. Differences in management are identified where appropriate, in context, so that similarities in care and general principles are not obscured by repetitive detail. Because the literature associated with acute management in the coronary care unit is well developed, we have not considered this as a separate topic, though comparison with the literature demonstrates that the associated specialized concerns have been addressed.[15] Considerable effort has been expended to provide a balanced presentation.

The exposition is ecumenical. Although many authors are from the Stanford medical community, regular contact with other centers and the contributions of other authors suggest that the principles espoused are generally accepted. We have required that the basis of all clinical recommendations be clear—whether securely based on scientific fact, clinical experience, or the author's personal bias (in order of decreasing clinical value).

The book is divided into eight sections, each considering a basic area of knowledge. Outlines precede each chapter, and an index is provided to assure rapid location of desired specialized material. The method of referencing is intended to encourage further reading. We are aware that many of the concepts central to effective clinical performance are difficult, partly because supporting information is not always included in the standard medical curriculum. A special effort has been made to supplement vital concepts visually and to provide additional information for the interested reader.

Section one is an introduction to the general concepts that the cardiac intensivist must understand fully. Each chapter presumes prior reading in medical school level texts and provides a summary of the pertinent information, with emphasis on concepts which have direct clinical application. Glossaries are provided for the chapters dealing with significant specialized vocabulary and bibliographic references are provided for those desiring further preparation or detail. Concepts that are not associated in other basic texts are brought together here and illustrated by examples and figures.

Chapter 2 provides a review of cardiovascular physiology, with emphasis on cardiac supply and demand problems, distribution of blood flow, systemic concepts, and selected clinical examples.

Chapter 3 provides a unique clinical introduction to the electromechanics of myocardial cellular function and develops a direct relationship between physiologic concepts and clinically observable behavior.

Chapter 4 is a review of the quantitative means of assessing cardiovascular function before surgery, with special emphasis on cardiovacular catheterization. This work is especially enlightening on normal values, the problems and risks of preoperative evaluation, and the analysis and use of these data in acute patient management.

Chapter 5 provides a review of the concepts of quantitative assessment as applied to continuous monitoring. Rather than recite a list of possible measurements, the focus is on determining what needs to be measured, how to measure and present it, and how to use it.

Section two summarizes the phenomena surrounding the electrical activity of the heart. Although these seem often to represent a mysterious set of events, a direct and organized approach removes much of the mystery.

In Chapter 6, the basic concepts of electrocardiographic (ECG) monitoring and interpretation are reviewed. The identification, severity, and treatment of abnormal events are discussed and further reading is suggested. The treatment of arrhythmias receives special consideration.

Chapter 7 provides an unusually complete discussion of pacemakers, examining the newest technology, indications for use, management during insertion, avoidance of complications, and subsequent management.

Chapter 8 is a discussion of the new technique of intraoperative cardiac mapping—the electrophysiologic identification of abnormal tissue that is the origin of arrhythmias—and the subsequent surgical treatment. The multiple hazards involved in identifying, provoking, and excising this abnormal tissue are discussed.

Section three is a summary of the pharmacologic agents used in acute cardiovascular management. A separate chapter on antiarrhythmic agents is not included because, under conditions permitting surgical intervention, more effective therapies are usually available. These drugs are discussed in Chapters 6 and 16.

Chapter 9 is a review of the anesthetic agents, with details on cardiovascular effects, specialized techniques, new drugs, and expanded usage of conventional drugs.

Chapter 10 provides discussions of muscle relaxants and antagonists, with special attention to cardiovascular effects, dose requirements, and clinical implications.

Chapter 11 is an examination of adrenergic receptor function, and the inotropic agonists and antagonists and their place in cardiovascular management. This is an area in which clinical progress and the concepts of effective management have matured markedly in recent years.

The aggressive and specific use of vasodilators is one of the most significant recent advances in acute cardiovascular care. Chapter 12 is a review of these drugs, emphasizing therapeutic indications in the cardiovascular

patient. A departure from conventional discussions is the one on the separation of effects on preload and afterload. Because, in the cardiovascular patient, preload is usually therapeutically constrained to a specified value, the interactions can be separated in discussion, making appropriate management easier to understand and implement, even though the effects must be merged in practice.

Section four is a collection of the practical considerations associated with adult cardiovascular surgery, providing a link with the basic relationships previously discussed.

Chapter 13 is a review of the events of the prebypass period, including preoperative evaluation, induction of anesthesia, and intraoperative management.

Chapter 14 is an examination of cardiopulmonary bypass, with special emphasis on technical considerations, physiologic abnormalities, controversies over optimal care, and goals of therapy.

The concepts of postbypass management—the transition to the "corrected" state—are reviewed in Chapter 15. Flow charts are provided to guide management.

Chapter 16 is a primer on postoperative cardiovascular and respiratory intensive care, which specifically focuses on the patient undergoing cardiopulmonary bypass.

Chapter 17 is a review of the special perioperative and surgical requirements of the patient undergoing cardiac transplantation. This unique population is described with reference to the largest and longest duration series of patients undergoing this treatment.

Section five includes considerations of the practical aspects of managing the pediatric patient with cardiovascular disease.

Chapter 18 provides discussions of the pathophysiology of the typical pediatric patient, with special attention to congenital cardiovascular lesions. A complete set of new drawings has been created to illustrate the concepts and to provide a connection between topologic relationships, relative chamber size and muscle mass, hemodynamics, and catheterization data.

Chapter 19 includes considerations of the

preoperative and intraoperative management problems peculiar to the pediatric patient with cardiovascular disease.

Chapter 20 is a primer on the burgeoning specialty of postoperative cardiovascular pediatric intensive care.

Section six is a collection of the specialized clinical considerations for patients with significant cardiovascular disease undergoing surgery for noncardiac problems. The chapters do not repeat the basic material in the preceding adult and pediatric sections, but identify the major considerations and the appropriate methods of dealing with them.

Chapter 21 is a review of the management of the patient undergoing general surgery.

The patient undergoing aortic vascular surgery is discussed in Chapter 22.

Chapter 23 is an examination of the special problems of the patient undergoing carotid artery surgery.

Section seven is a review of the specialized skills, of which everyone involved in the acute care of the cardiovascular patient must be aware and which the cardiovascular intensivist must master.

Chapter 24 provides a review of the practical aspects of coagulation mechanisms, including clinical decisions and therapy.

The special problem of renal function, the most common serious complication of the cardiovascular patient not involving the heart, are considered in Chapter 25.

Chapter 26 is a review of the clinical management of hypothermia, a technique which is being rediscovered with new appreciation and aggressive application.

Chapter 27 is a discussion of the burgeoning field of cardiac-assist devices and the artificial heart. The era of artificial organs has arrived.

Finally, section eight is an examination of the problem of educating medical professionals in the acute care of the cardiovascular patient. Both the existing programs and their goals, and the broader question of clinical competence, a fitting subject to complete our discussion, are reviewed in Chapter 28.

While the organization of the book is intended to encourage sequential reading,

those with substantial clinical experience may prefer a different approach. The practicing cardiovascular anesthesiologist may want to read clinical sections four and five to learn how closely his own perceptions parallel those of the authors. Similarly, the cardiovascular surgeon who plans to assume primary responsibility for his patients will find progress easier after reviewing the clinical sections and then relating the material to his own experiences.

The pediatrician will have a special interest in section five and the chapters dealing with hypothermia and pharmacologic agents. There are now increasing numbers of pediatric patients who require pacemaker support, and it is likely that other "adult" therapies will be applied more frequently to these pediatric patients.

It seems likely that the internist will be interested first in section two, the electrical activity of the heart, and the two chapters (16 and 20) discussing postoperative care. However, the editors feel that all of the included material is useful and relevant. The era of the preoperative medical consultation which advised "avoid hypoxia and hypotension" has passed, although this advice is still preferred by internists in training.[16] It is now more common to request a preanesthetic medical consultation to establish preoperative management and problems than to request advice regarding intraoperative management when cardiovascular anesthesia is contemplated. Too few internists presently understand the nature of intraoperative stresses and techniques because of the natural separation of specialties. Preoperative management is more effective and efficient when the intraoperative events are better understood. The overlap between the specialties is increasing, as assist devices and therapeutic modalities, such as coronary angioplasty, are being applied in medical settings. And some concepts, first aggressively applied in the surgical setting, are now being accepted in the medical literature. The bond of common interest appears quite strong.

Some of the most difficult concepts contained in the entire book are found in section one, but the editors have made a diligent effort to include only material of direct clinical relevance. Both the editors and the contributing authors feel strongly that it is not possible to provide optimal cardiovascular care by memorizing formulas, no matter how complex. The clinician must have a clear idea of the underlying processes, in order to respond appropriately and to recognize when a reliable habit is a liability. (For particularly graphic examples, see the chapters on hypothermia and cardiac transplantation.) Equally, many egregious errors appear to arise from a failure to distinguish between situations requiring differing therapies, such as excessive blood volume as opposed to excessive vascular tone. For these reasons, it is hoped that every serious reader will master the material in section one. The editors' promise is twofold: to make every effort to exclude clinically irrelevant material and to make difficult concepts as clear as presently possible.

Often the newcomer to this field is perplexed by the proliferation of terms and the insistence on distinctions which appear unnecessary. But precision of control is related to precision of understanding. The Eskimo is reputed to have more than 35 words describing the material most people call snow because these distinctions affect decisions and the quality of life. In the same way, the clinician who does not distinguish between afterload and systemic vascular resistance, who uses a single narrow measure (*e.g.*, the rate-pressure-product or diastolic perfusion pressure) to assess myocardial status, who does not understand the difference between delay and response time in monitoring, or who feels that decreasing blood pressure by the use of halothane, trimethaphan, nitroprusside, or nitroglycerin is equally appropriate, cannot hope to be fully effective. Distinctions that lead to differing therapeutic approaches are useful and they have therefore been included.

This book is written to provide the basic information necessary for intelligent management decisions even when unforeseen combinations arise. When a theory improves practice, it provides a particularly satisfying intellectual experience. It also satisfies the goals of every motivated clinician.

REFERENCES

1. Harvey, W: An Anatomical Disputation Concerning the Movement of the Heart and Blood in Living Creatures (1578). Whitteridge G (trans): Oxford, Blackwell, 1976
2. Johnson, SL: The History of Cardiac Surgery 1896–1955. Baltimore, Johns Hopkins Press, 1970
3. Steinberg D: Research related to underlying mechanisms in atherosclerosis. Circulation 60:1559–1565, 1979
4. Mann GV: Diet heart: end of an era. N Engl J Med 297:644–650, 1977
5. Stamler J: Research related to risk factors. Circulation 60:1575–1586, 1979
6. Dustan HP: Research related to the underlying mechanisms in hypertension. Circulation 60:1566–1568, 1979
7. Levy RI: Progress toward prevention of cardiovascular disease. Circulation 60:1555–1559, 1979
8. Haywood LJ, Scheinman MM: Key references: coronary care. Circulation 60:715–716, 1979
9. Harrison DC: Research related to noninvasive instrumentation. Circulation 60:1569–1574, 1979
10. Mundth ED, Austen WG: Surgical measures for coronary heart disease. I. N Engl J Med 293:13–19, 1975; II. New Engl J Med 293:75–80, 1975; III. New Engl J Med 293:124–130, 1975
11. Connolly JE: The history of coronary artery surgery. J Thorac Cardiovasc Surg 76:733–744, 1978
12. Miller DW Jr: The Practice of Coronary Artery Bypass Surgery. New York, Plenum, 1977
13. Kouchoukos NT: Key references: coronary bypass surgery. Circulation 60:960–962, 1979
14. Crocetti AF: Cardiac diagnostic and surgical facilities in the United States. Public Health Rep 80:1035–1053, 1965
15. Haywood LJ, Scheinman MM: Key references: coronary care. Circulation 60:715–716, 1979
16. Keown KK: Anesthesia for surgery of the heart. Springfield Charles C Thomas, 1963, pp 16–17

2

Cardiovascular Physiology: Application to Clinical Problems

ALLEN K. REAM

INTRODUCTION

An understanding of the basic concepts of cardiovascular physiology is essential for effective patient management. Unfortunately, the concepts are relatively new and the terminology is confusing. Two kinds of problems are common: (1) a proliferation of terms with similar meanings and (2) the use of terms with imprecise or multiple inconsistent definitions. To deal with the former, we have selected the term with the most useful application and, to handle the latter, we add precision and show why the distinctions are of practical importance. Our precision in management can be no better than our precision in understanding the underlying physiologic process.

This approach permits most clinical situations to be explained using a limited number of powerful physiologic concepts. Fewer memorized arbitrary rules are necessary, which should lead to more consistent and effective clinical practice.

The clinician's goal in cardiovascular management is to resolve a fundamental conflict. It is necessary to increase demand on the myocardium sufficiently to assure adequate systemic perfusion, but also to limit demand sufficiently to avoid myocardial injury. This problem may be broken into two parts: (1) myocardial energy requirements (how much work the heart can safely do under given conditions and how this limit changes with conditions) and (2) heart-systemic relationships (how to match the heart and body to maximize perfusion while minimizing cardiac stress).

The goal is to provide concepts basic to clinical needs. Each section of the chapter contains a discussion of the basic findings, the underlying physiology, and a summary oriented to clinical application. A glossary of terms is provided at the end of the chapter, keyed to the text and original papers, to help sort out the overlapping terms found in the supporting literature. The chapter ends with a summary of concepts with examples of general value. Applications continue in subsequent chapters. More material is included in this chapter than can be assimilated in a single reading; it is hoped that the reader will agree that the unifying concepts presented here are less intimidating than the descriptions used in the original literature and of great practical value.[1-3]

ENERGY BALANCE IN THE MYOCARDIUM

One might think that the safest course in protecting the heart would be to demand minimum work consistent with adequate systemic perfusion. However, available information does not support this view. So long as the limits of mechanical work which cardiac muscle can safely perform are not exceeded, increasing work does not appear to increase risk of injury, if adequate oxygen and metabolic fuel are also available. In other words, up to a functional maximum, energy demand can be safely increased if energy supply is adequate.

Interestingly, the rules appear to be the same for the "classic" failing heart. A number of studies of isolated papillary muscle and samples from failing myocardium suggest that none of the steps in generation, storage, or utilization of energy cause impaired function.[4, 5] Below maximum capacity, failing myocardium performs just as effectively as normal myocardium, if it is not ischemic. In practical circumstances, oxygen is usually the limiting metabolic substrate and failure follows tissue hypoxia.

Thus, the best definition of the safety margin of the myocardium is the ratio of energy supply to energy demand, not absolute demand nor actual myocardial work. The ratio is more useful than the difference between supply and demand. First, it eliminates units, permitting clinical interpretation of relative changes. Secondly, it seems intuitively more reasonable to express the safety margin as a fraction of current work, rather than as an absolute value. (We tend to alter our work load with reference to the work already performed.) We will first examine the determinants of energy consumption by the heart, then the sources of supply, and finally a clinically useful ratio.

A common way of thinking of the sources of energy requirements for the human heart is presented in Table 2-1. Here, the requirements are divided into four groups: basal, activation, tension development, and actual work. While the data are interesting (note how little energy goes into actual work), they are not particularly useful for clinical management. What we require is a subdivision of energy requirements that relates them to factors which we can measure or control.

A practical way to think about the energy requirements of the heart is to divide them into two groups: *extrinsic* and *intrinsic*. *Extrinsic* factors are those which are determined by interaction between the heart and the body; *intrinsic* factors are those which are influenced by the functioning of the myocardium. In each case we use oxygen consumption as the measurement of energy demand because it is normally the limiting factor. The reader should bear in mind, however, that in some unusual situations (as with severe hypoglycemia) another metabolic substrate may be the limiting factor.

MYOCARDIAL OXYGEN DEMAND

Extrinsic Work of the Heart

Extrinsic work of the heart is the work performed in pumping blood. Classic physics would suggest that the *work* done by the heart is equal to force multiplied by distance

Table 2-1. Resting Myocardial Oxygen Consumption in Man

	ACTUAL*	PERCENT OF TOTAL
Basal	1.75	20%
Activation		
without Ca^{++}	0.04	
Ca^{++} component	substantial	25%
Tension Development	4.0	50%
Mechanical Work	small	5%
Total Resting Oxygen Consumption	8.5	100%

*ml oxygen/100 g tissue-minute

Note:

1. Tension corresponds to extrinsic factors (preload, afterload)
2. Ca^{++} corresponds primarily to intrinsic factors (contractility)
3. These two factors comprise 75% of the oxygen consumption of the heart in the resting state.
4. These two factors account for virtually all of the increase in $M\dot{V}_{O_2}$ above baseline. (It will be shown that changes with heart rate can be included in these two categories.)

(Braunwald E, Ross JR Jr, Sonnenblick EH: Mechanisms of Contraction of the Normal and Failing Heart, 2nd ed. Boston, Little, Brown and Co., 1976, pp. 171–177)

or, in the case of hemodynamics, pressure multiplied by flow and time. *Power* is equal to work per unit time—the rate at which work is performed. The *efficiency* of the heart is the ratio of energy supplied to mechanical energy produced. Assuming that efficiency is constant, fuel or oxygen consumption in cubic centimeters per minute (for a given fuel) will be directly proportional to the power transmitted to the moving blood by the heart.

Unfortunately, the heart does not appear to work in this fashion. The oxygen consumption of the heart does not vary in a simple way with the work done. To say it differently, the efficiency of the heart varies considerably, depending on how its mechanical work is performed. In 1936, Gollwitzer–Meier showed that if cardiac work is increased by increasing arterial resistance, the energy cost is greater than when a similar increase is produced by augmenting venous return.[6, 7] Sarnoff quantified this concept in 1958[8] (Fig. 2-1). Studying a series of isolated dog hearts, he related the mechanical work done by the heart to the oxygen consumption of the heart. In Table 2-2A, his data is presented for the basal state and two states in which work was increased by increasing pressure or flow. These results have been normalized to show the increase in oxygen consumption when work was doubled by either doubling pressure or flow. To say the least, the results are not intuitively obvious. He demonstrated that doubling cardiac work, by increasing the pressure into which the heart pumped, doubled oxygen consumption (up by 102%), but doubling work by doubling flow increased oxygen consumption by less than one tenth (up 8%) (Table 2-2B).

These data correlated with studies of isolated papillary muscle in which it was shown that the oxygen consumption of the muscle was related to the tension developed in the muscle during active contraction multiplied by the duration of active contraction. That is, in the intact heart, increasing aortic root pressure with constant flow would increase wall tension, but increasing flow into the aortic root with the same pressure would not, except for a small increase in wall tension caused by increased ventricular size at the beginning of systole, associated with increased stroke volume. Thus, isolated papillary muscle studies predicted Sarnoff's findings in the isolated heart.

Sarnoff proposed that a clinical measure (referred to as the tension-time index [TTI]) be used, which was the product of mean pressure during systole and the duration of systole as measured in the left ventricle. A careful examination of subsequent papers

Table 2.2. Sarnoff's work. *A:* Actual data. *B:* Normalized data.

	P	F	W	$M\dot{V}_{O_2}$	
BASELINE	1	1	1	1	
↑ PRESSURE	2.75	1	2.75	2.78	A
↑ FLOW	1	7.96	7.96	1.53	

	P	F	W	$M\dot{V}_{O_2}$	
BASELINE	1	1	1	1	
↑ PRESSURE	2	1	2	2.0	B
↑ FLOW	1	2	2	1.1	

Fig. 2-1. Sarnoff's work: $M\dot{V}O_2$ versus pressure and flow. Isolated dog hearts were studied in a preparation in which contractility presumably did not change. The change in myocardial oxygen consumption is presented (1) with a change in the rate of work by increasing mean aortic pressure while flow is held constant. Doubling the rate of work in this way almost exactly doubles oxygen consumption. (2) with a change in the rate of work by increasing flow while mean aortic pressure is held constant. The increase in oxygen consumption is minimal, and preload almost certainly increases. (Modified from Sarnoff SJ et al: Am J Physiol 192:148, 1958)

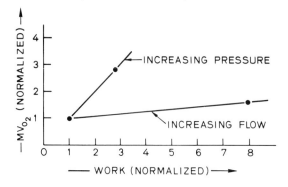

discussing the tension-time index reveals variations in the precise definition of the clinical measurement. These are summarized in the list below. The most common clinical definition currently employed is the average pressure during ejection in the root of the aorta multiplied by the duration of systole in the aorta (*i.e,* when the aortic valve is open). Notice that this interval begins later than the ejection period (ignoring the isometric contraction phase of the left ventricle) and continues after the period of active contraction. Other pressures may be used for measurement convenience, such as that in the radial artery.

An alternate measure frequently proposed by investigators presumes that oxygen consumption is related to the peak systolic pressure achieved during ejection.[9, 10] Sarnoff also addressed this issue in his original paper by using a resonance chamber to change the peak systolic pressure and observing the change in oxygen consumption. He was able to construct a variety of experimental situations in which the product of mean pressure

A summary of the clinically employed definitions of the TTI. All other definitions stem from the last definition. The first definition is the clinical measure proposed by Sarnoff.[8]

1. The product of mean aortic root pressure during aortic systole (the time when the aortic valve is open) and the duration of aortic systole.
2. Alternative 1: The product of peak aortic root pressure and the duration of aortic systole.
3. Alternative 2: The product of a peripherally measured pressure (used as in definition 1) and the duration of aortic systole as estimated from the measured pressure.
4. Alternative 3: The product of a peripherally measured peak pressure (used as in definition 2) and the duration of aortic systole as estimated from the measured pressure.
5. The product of tension produced and the duration of tension, summed over the period of active contraction of a myocardial fiber. This product can be mathematically related to pressure in the intact ventricle by estimating ventricular wall thickness, and using the Law of Laplace.

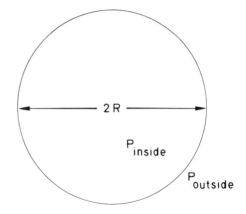

$$P = P_{inside} - P_{outside}$$
$$T = \text{WALL TENSION} \implies T = \left(\frac{R}{2}\right)P$$
$$R = \text{RADIUS OF SPHERE}$$

and duration did correlate with oxygen consumption, but peak systolic pressure did not. Despite this data, the concept of clinically monitoring extrinsic determinants of oxygen consumption using peak systolic pressure persists. While the difference between Sarnoff's calculation of TTI and the cruder indicator using peak systolic pressure may be small in many practical situations, there is good reason not to use peak pressure under typical conditions. The resonances involved in measuring pressure with a catheter can substantially alter the peak pressure reported at the monitoring instrument relative to what the heart actually encounters, particularly if a peripherally measured pressure is used. It is therefore not surprising that the correlation of peripherally and centrally measured pressure is improved when mean, rather than peak pressure, is used.[11] Thus, peak pressure is less useful and practical than Sarnoff's original proposal, using mean systolic pressure and duration.

One must consider a hidden assumption in order to use the TTI to assess the influence of external factors on myocardial oxygen con-

Definition of TTI:

1. fiber

$$TTI_{fiber} = \int_{\substack{\text{time of}\\\text{active}\\\text{contraction}}} T\,dt$$

2. intact heart

$$TTI_{clinical} = \int_{\substack{\text{ejection}\\\text{time}}} P\,dt$$

3. relationship

$$TTI_{fiber} \approx (TTI_{clinical}) \times \left(\frac{R}{2}\right)$$

This simple relation does not take wall thickness into account

Fig. 2-2. Relation between isolated muscle and clinical TTI. A graphic summary of the relation between the clinical measure of TTI and the underlying work on the isolated papillary muscle stretched linearly.

sumption. The original work was performed on a muscle stretched out linearly. In the intact heart, the muscle is curved into a roughly spherical shape. By the Law of Laplace, as illustrated in Figure 2-2, the tension

---

Assumptions Underlying the Generalization of Isolated Papillary Muscle Studies to the Intact Heart

1. Mean tension in an isolated papillary muscle, multiplied by the duration of active contraction, is linearly related to oxygen consumption.
2. The same relation holds for muscle taken elsewhere in the ventricular myocardium.
3. The left ventricle is approximately spherical.
4. Changes in ventricular wall thickness may be ignored.
5. The radius of the left ventricle does not change.
6. Multiplying mean aortic root pressure while the aortic valve is open by the duration of this interval gives essentially the same result as multiplying mean left ventricular pressure during active contraction by the duration of active contraction.

---

in the muscle fiber in the wall of the heart can be related to the pressure in the heart, assuming that the chamber is roughly spherical. This assumption is reasonable under normal conditions.[12] The Law of Laplace substitutes pressure (multiplied by half the radius) for tension in the equation relating oxygen consumption to cardiac work. (This factor of R/2 is a constant, but only if the radius does not change. This was approximately the case in Sarnoff's study.) If the heart dilates, the radius increases and the actual wall tension will increase for the same intraventricular pressure. Thus, these studies suggest that in the dilating heart, oxygen consumption will rise, even though the clinical TTI does not change. The true TTI of a single fiber in the wall of the heart would change, as noted in the list below.

The original work on the relation of TTI to myocardial oxygen consumption was independently corroborated.[13-15] Of all the work on myocardial energetics, it has proven to be the most reproducible and consistent. Sarnoff's report has not yet been seriously challenged. However, although hundreds of papers have been published in the intervening years, using the TTI in assessment of myocardial function, the number of experimenters measuring oxygen consumption and re-

lating it to the TTI remains small because of the exquisite experimental effort required for such studies.

The relation of the TTI to a well-known index, the rate-pressure product (RPP), does not seem to be widely appreciated. First known as the index of cardiac effort,[16] it was christened the RPP by Robinson, who reported that in patients with a history of angina, angina would consistently appear when the product of peak systolic pressure and heart rate exeeded an experimentally determined threshold, different for each patient.[17] Not so widely appreciated is that this result was true only if the duration of ejection did not `change. If it did, the reliable threshold was the product of rate, peak systolic pressure, and the duration of ejection—in other words, the TTI. Robinson did not suggest this modification to his equation because he wanted a measure that was convenient and noninvasive. There is little excuse for not using the TTI in its place in invasive monitoring, if the measurement is automated.

The important point to remember is tnat the tension-time relationship describes oxygen consumption relative to mechanical work performed by the heart. If this relationship is taken into account, additional information about mechanical work is not required. For example, if the TTI is held constant, changes in the mechanical work done by the heart do not alter myocardial oxygen consumption significantly.[18]

The principal difficulty in using the TTI is that the same term is used to describe performance at the isolated muscle and at the intact heart levels. Changes in the clinical TTI accurately reflect changes in oxygen consumption only if the diameter of the heart has not changed or if the change is taken into account in calculation of the index. It is also essential that the TTI be expressed per minute, not per beat. As noted in the following discussion, only in this form is comparison with the other determinants of energy balance straightforward. For this reason, the TTI is always expressed per minute in this book, unless otherwise noted.

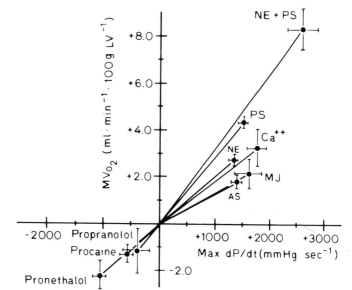

Fig. 2-3. Relation between maximal intraventricular dP/dt and MVO₂. Each point represents the average of a series of experiments with the associated standard error. *AS:* acetyl-strophanthidin, *Ca:* calcium, *NE:* norepinephrine, *PS:* paired electrical stimulation. (Braunwald E: Trans Assoc Am Physicians 84:63, 1971)

Intrinsic Work of the Heart

Contractility. It appears that the first direct evidence that the contractile state of the heart affected oxygen consumption was a report by Sonnenblick in 1965 in which he showed a rise in oxygen consumption with a decrease in TTI during inotropic stimulation.[19] The inotropic state of the heart has been referred to as "contractility." In general, contractility is said to increase when the rate of active contraction or force developed during active contraction is increased while extrinsic factors (muscle loading or length) remain the same.

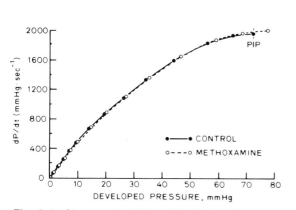

Fig. 2-4. Change in dP/dt with afterload. The relation between left ventricular *dP/dt* and developed isovolumic pressure at 5 msec intervals throughout isovolumic systole in the control period and during methoxamine. (Braunwald E: Trans Assoc Am Physicians 84:63, 1971)

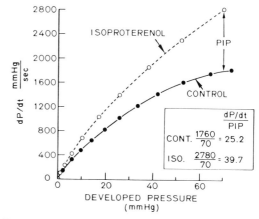

Fig. 2-5. Change in DP/dt with contractility. Effects on the relation between developed pressure and left ventricular *dP/dt* of augmenting contractility with isoproterenol while heart rate, aortic pressure, and stroke volume were maintained constant. (Braunwald E: Trans Assoc Am Physicians 84:63, 1971)

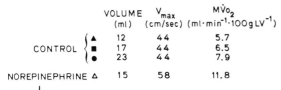

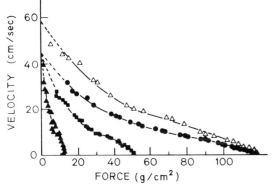

Fig. 2-6. Illustration of V_{max} calculated from whole-heart studies. Left ventricular element force-velocity relationships. *Velocity:* contractile element velocity; *force:* force/unit area; V_{max}: intercept on the ordinate. *closed symbols:* effect of varying ventricular volume at a constant V_{max}; *open symbols:* effect of increasing V_{max} with norepinephrine. Values of V_{max} are estimates and not absolute values. (Graham TP et al: J Clin Invest 47:375, 1968)

It is important to realize that contractility is not a quantitative term. In the following discussion, many specific measurements which have been studied in an attempt to quantify changes in contractility and the associated changes in myocardial oxygen consumption are examined. In this book, the word *contractility* describes all intrinsic factors affecting myocardial oxygen consumption, beyond basal requirements.

In practical terms, contractility is increased by certain drugs, such as epinephrine and isoproterenol, by increasing heart rate, and by sympathetic stimulation, and is decreased by drugs such as propranolol. In the data shown in Figure 2-3, the correlation between oxygen consumption and inotropic agents is clearly demonstrated.[20] Also shown in this figure is a measure which appeared to correlate with the inotropic effect: the maximum rate of rise of pressure in the ventricle, referred to as *maximum dP/dt* or, often, *dP/dt.*

An exciting development was the suggestion that *dP/dt,* measured during isovolumic contraction, was virtually independent of extrinsic factors influencing myocardial oxygen consumption, changing only slightly with changes in *preload:* the pressure in the ven-

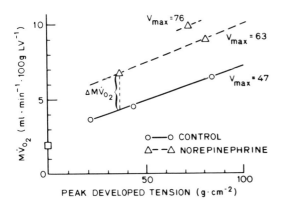

Fig. 2-7. $M\dot{V}O_2$ versus peak developed tension for two values of contractility. *Closed circles:* increasing tension at a constant V_{max}; *open triangles:* observations during norepinephrine infusion; *open square:* MVO_2 with potassium chloride arrest. The change in MVO_2 with norepinephrine at a constant tension was obtained by interpolation when tension was not precisely matched, as illustrated here by the *dotted vertical line.* These data suggest that oxygen consumption varies with changes in peak tension when V_{max} is constant. (Graham TP et al: J Clin Invest 47:375, 1968)

tricle just before contraction begins.[21] This was demonstrated in a series of studies shown in the next two figures. In Figure 2-4, the curve for *dP/dt* in the control state was compared with that in the state when methoxamine was given, substantially altering *afterload:* the pressure in the ventricle just after the aortic valve opens. Note that the two curves lie precisely on top of each other. In Figure 2-5, the control state is compared with the effects of isoproterenol. In this case, the entire curve is shifted upwards, and it is presumed that the increase in dP/dt is an indication of the increase in contractility.

This result was particularly encouraging because studies in isolated heart muscle suggested that separating intrinsic and extrinsic factors would be a difficult task. Separate measurements are valuable because separate approaches are required to clinically control intrinsic and extrinsic factors. The actual force and velocity of shortening for a given myocardial fiber was known to vary with its resting length or, alternatively, the resting load because this determines resting length. However, the velocity of contraction (V_{ce}) as measured in the isolated muscle did appear to offer a consistent property. When the contractile velocity was measured for a given muscle fiber, the extrapolated value at zero force changed very little if the contractile state of the muscle did not change, even if the applied force were changed. Or, expressed conversely, if an inotropic agent were given, the extrapolated velocity at zero force substantially increased. This velocity at zero force, which must be calculated, was entitled V_{max}.[22, 23]

This result, a stable value of V_{max} when contractility did not change, suggested that while the measured value of *dP/dt* and V_{ce} might vary with extrinsic factors, such as the tension at the start of contraction, and intrinsic factors, such as the contractility, the calculated value of V_{max} was dependent only upon changes in contractility.

Using the Law of Laplace and the experimentally derived curve relating velocity to muscle length in the isolated muscle prepa-

ration, a formula could be derived permitting calculation of V_{ce} using measurements on the intact heart during the period of isometric contraction. Then simplifying assumptions permit reducing the number of terms in the equation. This process is summarized below.[24, 25] The final form of the equation is *(dP/dt)/PK,* where *K* is a constant.

Because the discussion usually revolves around relative changes, the *K* is sometimes

---

Origin of the Formula for Calculation of Vce During Isometric Contraction From Measurement of *dP/dt* in the Intact Heart

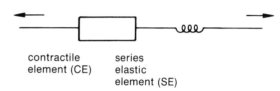

contractile element (CE)

series elastic element (SE)

1. The assumed muscle model is
   T = tension
   t = time
   K,C = constants
   L = length
   V_{ce} = velocity of contraction of contractile element

2. From experimental data, the following formula is suggested:
   $$dT/dL = KT + C$$

3. Because $V_{ce} \triangleq dL/dt$,
   Then $(dT/dt)/T = V_{ce}(KT + C)/T$

4. The Law of Laplace can be used, presuming a spherical shape of radius *R*, to relate wall tension *T* to transmural pressure *P* in the intact ventricle:
   $$T = (R/2)P$$

5. Combining (3) and (4) gives
   $(1/P)(dP/dt) = V_{ce}(K + 2C/RP)$
   Or $V_{ce} = (dP/dt)R/(RKP + 2C)$
   If we presume $RKP \gg 2c$ (true only if *P* is large enough),
   Then: $V_{ce} = (dP/dt)(1/KP)$
   Note that this formula requires *dP/dt* to be divided by *P*.
   (Modified from Taylor RR: Cardiovasc Res 4:429, 1970, using assumptions from Mirsky I: Biophysical J 9:189, 1969)

discarded, although values of from 28 to 32 have been used in the literature to calculate a presumed actual value for V_{ce}.[26, 27] One can then plot V_{ce} during the isometric phase of a contraction and extrapolate to V_{max}. An example of such an extrapolation from an early paper, shown in Figure 2-6, suggests agreement with the conclusion based on isolated muscle studies that V_{max} changes only with a change in contractility. Figure 2-7, from the same paper, shows that oxygen consumption varied with peak tension when V_{max} was held constant.

Disagreement exists regarding the pressure which should be used in the equation.[28] Some suggest *developed pressure* (ventricular pressure minus end diastolic pressure),[29] others believe that the *total pressure* (ventricular pressure) is better.[30] While each side refers the argument to the muscle model, the motivation for refinement is to make the equation more sensitive to clinically observable changes.

The approach is illustrated in Figure 2-8 in which left ventricular pressure versus calculated V_{ce} is shown for a heart in which the aortic valve is not allowed to open. The calculated contractile velocity is initially low as the heart changes shape and becomes more spherical; it then rises to a maximum and decays as the pressure in the ventricle con-

tinues to rise. Note that at no time does the curve approach the value of V_{max}. V_{max} must be calculated by extrapolation.

Unfortunately, early studies showed that while the data just cited were very encouraging, actual changes in V_{max} were not very reliable and correlations were not very successful. Thus a whole series of alternate measurements were evaluated. These included the peak measured velocity (V_{pm}),[31] and the velocity at given pressures, such as V_{40}.[32, 33] Because of the poor correlation between these measures and other evidence of changes in the inotropic state, a number of empiric modifications were then made to these formulas. Often, these changes were not related to the underlying muscle model.

Thus, the use of V_{max} measurements in clinical medicine has become uncertain because the origins of the cited equations are obscure, and the clinical correlation of calculated measures with other clinical evidence of inotropic changes is weak. It is not surprising that most clinicians, while accepting the concept of contractility and agreeing that *dP/dt* does increase when inotropic agents are administered, have difficulty using this information to manage their patients more effectively.

Some of the reasons why V_{max} is not an effective quantitative clinical tool in its pres-

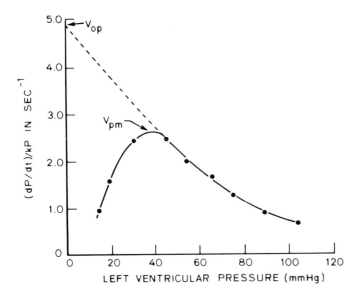

Fig. 2-8. Illustration of V_{pm}. Force-velocity relation based on pressure analysis. V_{op} (or V_{max}) represents the theoretical maximum velocity of shortening of the contractile element at zero load obtained by extrapolation. V_{pm} represents the physiologic maximum velocity of shortening as observed from the curve. (Mirsky I: Am J Cardiol 27:359, 1971)

ent state of development are now briefly analyzed. Questions and uncertainties go all the way back to the original measurements.

Pollack and coworkers have suggested that the original muscle model of Hill, shown in Figure 2-9, is not correct for cardiac muscle. They demonstrated that the calculated properties of the elastic element depend on its history. Unlike a spring, the elastic force is not simply defined by the stretched length of the elastic element (Fig. 2-10). The failure to identify a histologic equivalent of an elastic element in cardiac muscle is also consistent with these results. Therefore, the reason for choosing the form of extrapolation to V_{max} is removed, making it an empirical calculation. This data also suggests that V_{max} is sensitive to changes in fiber length under certain conditions, as well as to contractility.[35] The discrepancies between the data and simpler models may be due to inertial forces not taken into account, as suggested by Teplick and implied by models using d^2P/dt^2, but this remains to be demonstrated.[36]

Yet another concern is the way information is obtained in studying isolated cardiac muscle. Many studies used isometric contractions, which are not truly "clinical" because heart shape changes during the "isometric" phase, or quick-release studies, which alter V_{max} and which may not be generalizable to the normal physiologic state.[37, 38]

Another problem is the generalization of isolated muscle activity to the intact heart. The curve at lower pressure is not trustworthy. The derivation of V_{ce} clinically requires dropping of the constant C. This is a valid assumption only when the pressure is large. Secondly, at low pressures, the ventricle is changing shape and the relation of pressure and contractile element velocity is not reliably given by the formula, even with the extra constant. Thirdly, the modified equation is much more sensitive to errors in measurement at smaller values of P. Thus, the evidence suggests that values of dP/dt associated with P less than a threshold value which may exceed the value at which peak measured dP/dt occurs have little clinical utility.

These arguments suggest that dP/dt at a

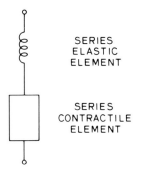

Fig. 2-9. Hill model of cardiac muscle.

Fig. 2-10. Force-length curves of series of elastic element (SEC). The Hill model of muscle consists of a contractile component in series with an elastic component. In this figure, force-length curves for the SEC are shown, calculated from data obtained from quick-release studies at various times during the cardiac cycle. The lack of superimposability indicates that the SEC force-length curve differs at different times during the contraction. Similar differences were found in all cardiac muscles. (Pollack GH et al: Circ Res 31:569, 1972)

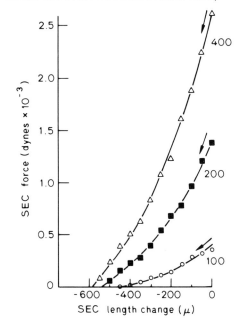

pressure well above that associated with V_{pm} should be used to assess contractility (see Fig. 2-8). But in the clinical situation, the value at higher pressure is not always usable because once the aortic valve opens and contraction is not isometric, the assumptions used in the equation are not valid. Hence, the calculation of a velocity reflecting changes in contractility cannot be made over a wide range of extrinsic effects on the heart because dP/dt at a pressure above that attained before the aortic valve opends is then required.

If only midrange pressures are used, from above the peak at 40 to 50 torr to a maximum of 80 torr, the extrapolation back to V_{max} depends on curve fitting to a very short segment of curve. Arguments exist as to whether the curve fit should be linear,[39] exponential,[40] or hyperbolic.[41] Each alternative yields a different result. All of these considerations severely limit the accuracy that can be obtained in calculating V_{max} from a clinical intraventricular pressure measurement.[42]

Additional problems must be considered. The original curve was derived over a change in cardiac muscle length not exceeding 12 percent of its resting length.[43] In the failing heart, this limitation is likely to be violated.

Those who have attempted to overcome these problems and make useful clinical measurements have noted that the changes in these indices with changes in inotropic state rarely exceeded 10 percent of the basal value of the velocity measure being employed.[44] Yet the standard deviation in measurements of V_{ce} even in the best studies, is a minimum of 6 percent. Because two standard deviations are necessary to show significance, the entire range of change in contractility is approximately equal to the resolution of the measurement technique.[45] Small wonder then that it was difficult to show a statistically significant change in contracility by using a narrowly selected part of the dP/dt curve, even when the patients were clinically abnormal.[46-49] When the difficulty in measuring left ventricular pressure clinically is considered, it is understandable that the measurement is often discussed but rarely used quantitatively in clinical practice.

What can be learned from the concept of measurement of contractility? Inotropic stimulants increase and myocardial depressants decrease myocardial oxygen consumption. Overall considerations of mycardial oxygen demand can be related to the specific contribution of inotropic changes. However, the promise of increased accuracy and specificity from utilization of V_{max} or its analogs, rather than average dP/dt during ejection, has not been borne out. Contractility is a useful clinical concept, but the most appropriate means of measurement is probably $\Delta P/\Delta t$ over the whole time of contraction, rather than an instantaneous or extrapolated value. The discussion of the concept of contractility is completed in the next section.

Heart Rate. In addition to contractility, one other intrinsic determinant of myocardial oxygen consumption is often mentioned: heart rate. In this section, the effects of heart rate on oxygen consumption are examined. Available information suggests that it is not a separate effect. With a change in heart rate, the associated changes in TTI and contractility per minute specify the resulting change in myocardial oxygen consumption.

While the change in oxygen consumption with changing heart rate has been known for many years, agreement on the nature of the relationship has been slow to develop. A major contribution was made in 1956 by Laurent and coworkers in reporting a quantitative relationship between heart rate, work per unit time (or power), and oxygen consumption.[50] This result is shown in Figure 2-11 and may be summarized by two conclusions:

1. For a fixed power level, oxygen consumption increases when heart rate increases.
2. The percentage increase in oxygen consumption when power is tripled at high heart rate is the same as at low heart rate. In other words, because of (1), increasing the work load is also more expensive when the heart rate is higher.

Laurent reported marginally adequate experimental correlation with these conclusions

($r = 0.81$) and, because he studied both pressure and flow mediated changes in mechanical work, these results appear broadly applicable. The problem with this approach is that it leaves rate as a separate entity, not clearly related to other intrinsic and extrinsic factors. Moreover, the data are not consistent with the previous discussion when examined carefully; oxygen consumption can be changed with a fixed heart rate and external work load by altering the relationship of contractility and TTI. Their description does not permit this result.

Another approach appears to offer greater precision. Under ordinary clinical conditions, when heart rate increases, myocardial oxygen consumption must also increase because of necessary changes in TTI and contractility.

The following hypothetical experiment should be considered. The heart rate is increased while preload, afterload, and mean systolic pressure are held constant (*i.e.,* the external determinants of the TTI are not permitted to change). Then, if the TTI is held constant, contractility must increase, and if contractility is held constant, the TTI must increase. This result is summarized below. This is the clinical situation most often desired by the anesthesiologist who seeks to maintain preload to keep the heart on the most effective part of the Starling curve and

to maintain afterload to maintain body perfusion. Under these circumstances, increasing heart rate must increase oxygen consumption by increasing TTI, contractility, or both.

This leads to an interesting question. It seems intuitively clear that the change in ox-

Calculation of TTI and dP/dt With Changing Heart Rate

Assume that mean aortic root pressure and stroke volume are constant.
Then if

1. Myocardial wall tension/minute is held constant

   $$t_s \times HR = \text{constant} \qquad t_s = \text{duration of systole}$$
   $$HR = \text{heart rate}$$

   And as HR increases, t_s must shorten.
   Result: dP/dt per minute must increase with increasing heart rate.

Or if

2. dP/dt per minute is held constant, HR/t_s is constant and t_s increases as HR increases.
   Result: $TTI/minute$ must increase with increasing heart rate.

We therefore conclude that when heart rate increases with constant aortic root pressure and stroke volume, contractility per minute, wall tension (per minute), or both must increase.

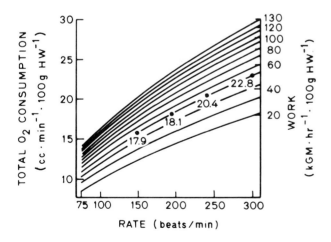

Fig. 2-11. Heart rate versus MVO$_2$ for different work loads. Graph of calculated lines of constant cardiac work per time (power), relating total myocardial oxygen consumption to heart rate. The points show the experimental data. Oxygen consumption increases with heart rate. The percentage increases in oxygen consumption at any fixed heart rate is fixed for a given percentage increase in heart work per unit time. (Laurent D et al: Am J Physiol 185:355, 1956)

ygen demand with a change in heart rate is coupled in some way to changes in TTI, contractility, or both. But is this the whole story or is there some other mysterious effect of heart rate on oxygen consumption? Available information indicates that, for clinical purposes, there is not.

This can be shown in the following way. If a variable is uniquely determined by other variables, as myocardial oxygen consumption is by contractility and TTI, then over a reasonable range of values, a regression equation can be written to express this relationship. The correlation coefficient is a measure of how well the results correlate with actual experiment. While no experimenter has yet reported the results in just this way, the data from reported experiments can be used to test this result. The author has done this for the data reported by Boerth,[51] summarized below. A regression for myocardial oxygen consumption using TTI and contractility results in a correlation coefficient of $r = 0.90$. When heart rate is added as a separate term, the correlation coefficient increases to $r = 0.92$, a trivial improvement. The change in r is a measure of the information added with heart rate. The added information is not significant.

The insignificant improvement in the correlation coefficient r indicates that clinical assessment of myocardial oxygen consumption requires consideration of only three factors: (1) basal oxygen consumption, (2) TTI, and (3) contractility as measured by dP/dt. This conclusion is reinforced by the fact that, although the correlation coefficient improved slightly with the inclusion of heart rate, the uncertainty in determination of the correlation coefficient increased. Note that heart rate must be used to calculate the other terms; tension-time and contractility are expressed per minute, not per beat.

These data also correlate with the recent studies of Weber, showing a linear correlation between the integral of systolic force and $M\dot{V}_{O_2}$ for any given contractile state, and a linear correlation between dF/dt and $M\dot{V}_{O_2}$ for a given value of systolic force.[52] Thus we conclude that changes in contractility and TTI define the changes in myocardial oxygen consumption with heart rate.

Why is this a more useful way of looking at the effects of heart rate than the earlier view suggested by Laurent?

As Langer has pointed out, Bowditch described in 1871 "the progressive increase in contractile tension developed by heart tissue upon an abrupt increment in the frequency of contraction."[53] With increasing contractility, the duration of active contraction shortens. This shortening with heart rate has been recognized for many years and is roughly linear.[54–56]

Thus, an increase in heart rate shortens the duration of ejection per beat as a consequence of the increased contractibility per beat.[57] Increasing the heart rate also increases the duration of ejection per minute, increasing the systolic wall tension per minute, so that oxygen demand increases by both extrinsic and intrinsic pathways. Afterload does not ordinarily alter this result until the heart is overdilated or, as noted below, until time in diastole per minute is significantly reduced.

We thus are left with two general conclusions regarding heart rate: (1) myocardial oxygen demand increases with heart rate under ordinary conditions and (2) if TTI and contractility are taken into account, heart rate

---

Relation of $M\dot{V}_{O_2}$ to Basal Rate and Extrinsic and Intrinsic States

1. $M\dot{V}_{O_2} = a_0 + a_1(\text{TTI/minute})^*$
   $+ a_2(dP/dt\text{-minute})\dagger$

   $r = 0.90$

2. $M\dot{V}_{O_2} = b_0 + b_1(\text{TTI/minute})$
   $+ b_2(dP/dt\text{-minute}) + b_3(HR)$

   $r = 0.92$

* Here, peak pressure was used to calculate TTI. Other data suggests using mean pressure during active contraction would slightly improve the correlation. Note: TTI/minute = TTI/beat × Heart Rate.

† Here, maximum dP/dt was used. Other data suggests $K \Delta P/\Delta t$ is an acceptable substitute. Note: dP/dt per minute = dP/dt per beat × Heart Rate.

has *no* significant additional effect on myocardial oxygen consumption.

An Overview of Clinical Determinants of Oxygen Demand

The most accurate description available to the clinician of the determinants of oxygen demand is summarized in Table 2-3, and consists of an equation with three terms. The first is a constant, representing basal requirements under clinical conditions. The second varies with heart wall tension and is an expression of extrinsic factors, or useful mechanical work. The third varies with the rate of rise of left ventricular pressure during systole, and reflects the intrinsic state of the heart, or contractility. All three are useful clinical concepts.

In order to provide perspective, Table 2-3 also shows the common descriptive terms used to describe the determinants of myocardial energy consumption and their relation to this equation. Table 2-4 summarizes the origin of these concepts in simplified form. The

work was originally performed on isolated heart (usually papillary) muscle. Early extrapolation was to per-beat results in the intact

Table 2-3. The Suggested Mathematical Relation for the Clinical Determinants of Myocardial Oxygen Consumption

Clinical relation: $\dot{M}VO_2 = a_0 + a_1 TTI + a_2 \dfrac{dP}{dt}$

The terms in the equation correspond to three clinical concepts: basal, extrinsic, and intrinsic. Note that heart rate is a special case. When TTI and *dP/dt* are expressed per minute (per beat × heart rate), a separate term for heart rate is not required. Note also that this equation does not explicitly represent heart size; for the equation to be valid, heart size must be fixed, or the term a_1 must change with heart size.

	EXTRINSIC	INTRINSIC
Wall tension	X	
Rate of contraction		X
Heart rate	X	X
Rate-pressure product	X	
TTI	X	
Afterload	X	
Preload	X	
Heart size	X	
dP/dt		X
Stroke volume	X	X

Table 2-4. Evolution of Terms for TTI and Contractility

		ISOLATED MUSCLE	INTACT HEART Per Beat	INTACT HEART Per Minute
Extrinsic	(Tension-Time Index)	$\int_{contraction}(tension)dt$ TTI	$\int_{systole}Pdt^*$ original "clinical TTI"	$HR \times \int_{systole}Pdt^*$ true "clinical TTI"
Intrinsic	("Contractility")	V_{max}	dP/dt or dP/dt/P "clinical"	$HR \times \dfrac{dP}{dt}$ or $HR \times \dfrac{\Delta P}{\Delta t}$ "clinical"
Intrinsic	Basal	$\dot{M}V_{O_2}$ (/min)	rarely used	$\dot{M}V_{O_2}$/min

*Must correct for heart size (law of LaPlace)

heart. The most useful expression, and that used in this book, is the result per minute, to correlate with oxygen consumption.

The following points must be remembered to use these results effectively. First, expressing the energy requirements in this way leaves no significant additional effect of heart rate. Secondly, the clinical assessment of contractility appears to be just as accurate with a simple estimate of dP/dt as with the more complex estimates of V_{ce} during the isometric phase, or V_{max}. Thirdly, the relation for TTI in the intact heart, as expressed in Table 2-3, presumes no change in heart size. A correction must be applied when heart size changes, or the relation is no longer valid.

The energy supply is now examined in order to complete the story.

MYOCARDIAL OXYGEN SUPPLY

This section is an examination of the oxygen supply of the heart and the ratio of supply to demand—the preferred method of estimating myocardial reserve.

The blood supply to the wall of the heart comes through the coronary arteries, which originate in the coronary sinuses just distal to the aortic valve. The majority of this sup-

ply returns to the circulation through the coronary sinus, which empties into the right atrium. Unfortunately, some flow also returns directly to the left atrium and ventricle (thebesian flow). The circulatory patterns are summarized in Figure 2-12.

This means that studies of myocardial oxygen extraction which require samples of mixed venous blood are difficult to obtain

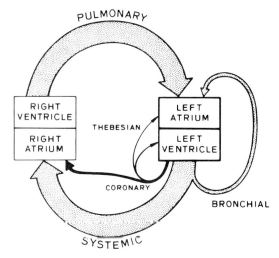

Fig. 2-12. Major anatomic pathways of blood flow.

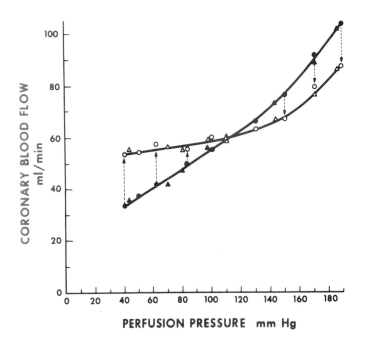

PERFUSION PRESSURE mm Hg

Fig. 2-13. Autoregulation of coronary blood flow. Data is from the beating dog heart. The point where the curves cross represents the control steady-state pressure and flow. A sudden, sustained change in perfusion pressure caused an abrupt change in flow represented by the *closed symbols* (transient flow). The *open symbols* represent the steady state flows obtained at each perfusion pressure. The points represented by *triangles* were obtained after blockade of cardiac prostaglandin synthesis with indomethacin. (Rubio R, Berne RM: Regulation of coronary blood flow. Prog Cardiovasc Dis 43:105, 1975)

and limited in accuracy because sampling venous flow can be done clinically only through cannulation of the coronary sinus. The first quantitative studies in humans were not performed until 1949.[58] One can also examine flow by probes around selected branches of the coronary vasculature, but one must then destructively sample after the experiment to determine the mass of muscle supplied, a technique which is suitable only in animal studies. It is evident that there are many factors that make precise measurement difficult.

It has been well-known for many years that coronary sinus oxygen content is consistently low, typically around 25 percent. Only recently, however, has the concept of coronary autoregulation been widely accepted, despite early reports.[59] A typical study shows how coronary flow remains constant with constant demand and changing perfusion pressure (Fig. 2-13). Similarly, reducing demand reduces flow at constant perfusion pressure. While studies have concentrated on the left heart, the right behaves similarly.[60]

The factors affecting supply are (1) supply, or arterial oxygen content, as affected by pulmonary and hemodynamic factors, and hemoglobin type and content; (2) flow, as affected by available perfusion pressure and coronary vascular resistance; and (3) distribution of flow by redistribution from nonexchanging to exchanging vessels, and redistribution by recruitment of exchanging channels.[61] This is a useful classification because each category relates to a different clinical approach.

Oxygen content of the blood is dealt with elsewhere (see Chap. 16 on postoperative care of the cardiac patient). The concept of flow is examined first and, later in this chapter, available information on the clinical management of distribution of blood flow is discussed.

Many early studies attempted to assess coronary blood flow in order to estimate changes in oxygen supply. With recognition of the role of coronary autoregulation, [62, 63] studies shifted to impairing autoregulation to assess changes in maximal flow, an approach fraught with experimental difficulties.[64]

However, in recent years a different approach has developed, based on the measurement of pressure instead of flow. This shift is of tremendous practical significance; the pertinent pressures can be monitored clinically, while the pertinent flows cannot.

Assessment of coronary oxygen supply by measurement of pressure depends on the following assumptions:

1. Assuming effective local coronary autoregulation, then the essential measurement is maximum possible oxygen supply. This is true because, with autoregulation, the heart can increase supply up to the maximum as necessary, without any extracardiac response.[65] Conversely, in patients with ischemic heart disease, resting flow may be normal while vasodilators do not increase flow; it is maximal.[66]

2. Because coronary artery inlet flow occurs only when perfusion pressure is greater than intraventricular pressure, maximum possible flow is estimated as proportional to the area between the aortic root pressure and left ventricular (left atrial) pressure during diastole (*i.e.*, perfusion pressure during the period of coronary flow).

3. Assuming that the maximum work the heart can perform without injury is the maximum possible with fully aerobic metabolism, then below this limit the safety margin of the heart is determined by the maximum oxygen supply available relative to demand, or the ratio of supply to demand.

Buckberg tested this hypothesis in an ingenious way.[67] He defined the diastolic perfusion index (DPI; or the diastolic perfusion time index DPTI) as the integral of the difference between aortic root and left ventricular pressure during diastole. Then he examined the ratio of supply to demand (DPI/TTI; now referred to as the endocardial viability ratio, or EVR) *with the inotropic state unaltered*, and varied both supply and demand (by changing afterload and pacing with a crushed sinoatrial [SA] node). He also measured the change in the ratio of endocardial to epicardial blood flow (Fig. 2-14).[68]

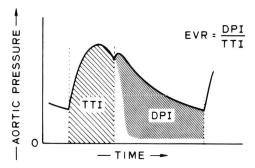

$$EVR = \frac{DPI}{TTI}$$

Fig. 2-14. The EVR. The area under the aortic pressure curve used for calculation of TTI and DPI is shown schematically.

His results are summarized in Figure 2-15. The ratio of endocardial to epicardial flow remained above 0.8 until the viability ratio fell below a value of approximately 0.8, then it also fell. These data suggest that the EVR is a useful predictor of the safety margin in perfusion reserve when contractility does not change.

The presumption that a falling ratio of endocardial/epicardial perfusion represents ischemia rests on a number of considerations:

1. The value remained constant until the viability ratio fell below a specific threshold.
2. Understanding of local tissue perfusion suggests that local ischemia produces local vasodilation. Available evidence suggests that myocardial tissue throughout the left ventricle has roughly the same oxygen requirements. Thus, a changing ratio suggests ischemia, in the absence of any agent which would preferentially increase flow in already adequately perfused areas.
3. The endocardium may be expected to be ischemic first with failing blood supply because it is there that the pressure in the left ventricle interferes most with coronary flow. Clinical data supports this; in patients who die after cardiopulmonary bypass, up to 90 percent are reported to have subendocardial necrosis.[69] Preferential endocardial flow deprivation during bypass with fibrillation has also been reported.[70] The gradient is thought to be larger with left ventricular hypertrophy.[71]
4. Restoring the viability ratio to a higher

value resulted in demonstrated reactive hyperemia, with a payback of approximately 350 percent, but only when the viability ratio exceeded 1.0.[72]
5. S–T segment changes in the ECG correlated with the fall in endocardial/epicardial flow ratios.[72]

This work was first performed with fixed oxygen content. The same results apply for the viability ratio multiplied by arterial oxygen content when content is varied.[72]

A laboratory example of the increased resolution of the technique is shown in Figure 2-16. It is clear that the use of the ratio makes significant differences far more evident than the use of single components of myocardial oxygen supply or demand.

Available studies suggest equivalent value in clinical application. Bregman demonstrated that the viability ratio correlated with identification of patients who required intraaortic balloon support after cardiopulmonary bypass.[73] The clinical threshold was 0.8. The correlation between the viability ratio and patient survival after termination of intra-aortic balloon support was even greater.

The measurement is also attractive because it is clinically feasible. There is good correlation between central and peripheral values when mean systolic pressure ($r = 0.96$) rather than peak systolic pressure ($r = 0.92$) is used in the calculation of the TTI,[74] and good correlation between $\Delta P/\Delta t$ measured centrally and peripherally.[75]

ENERGY BALANCE: A SUMMARY

The best single value presently known for assessing the safety margin of the myocardium is the EVR or the estimated ratio of oxygen supply to oxygen demand. The discussion of demand suggests that this estimator could be improved by adding basal oxygen requirement and contractility to the denominator (giving the demand/supply ratio, or D/SR) because the viability ratio includes only extrinsic factors (the TTI). A disadvantage is the difficulty of measurement and calculation because additional information is required.

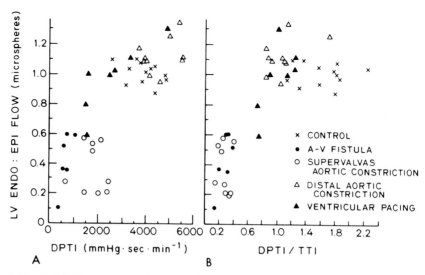

Fig. 2-15. DPI/TTI versus endocardial/epicardial flow. Flow per gram of tissue of left ventricular subendocardial to subepicardial blood flow measured by microspheres is plotted against DPI (*A*) and DPI/TTI (*B*) measured when the microspheres were injected. (Buckberg GD et al: Circ Res 30:67, 1972)

Fig. 2-16. An example of the increased discrimination of the EVR. *A.* TTI. *B.* DPI. *C.* EVR in relation to heart rate for the three states. A study in a calf of human size of the effect of a left ventricular assist system (LVAS), which pumps blood from the left ventricle to the thoracic aorta in parallel with the ejection of blood from the ventricle through the aortic valve. *Open circles:* LVAS off; *diamonds:* LVAS operating in asynchronous mode; *crosses:* LVAS operating in synchronous mode.
Argument between investigators has existed for some time as to whether synchronous operation of this assist device confers significant physiologic advantage. The small differences in TTI and DPI taken alone are not impressive, but doubling the EVR is clearly significant, and consistent with recent clinical studies (See Chap. 27.)
In this case, synchronous assistance improved both demand (by reducing it) and supply (by increasing it), so that either measurement suggested the probability of clinical improvement. However, how would one predict the viability ratio from one of these two when the other was moving in the opposite direction? The use of isolated measurements to predict patient status is valid only if other determinants do not change. Unfortunately, when one changes myocardial oxygen supply or demand, the other almost always changes also.

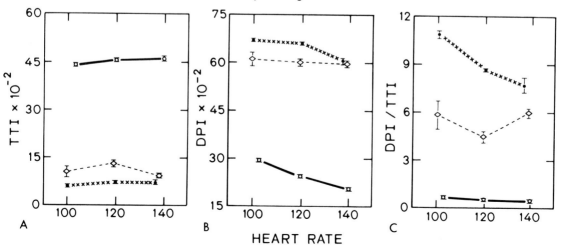

HEART RATE

CAPILLARIES

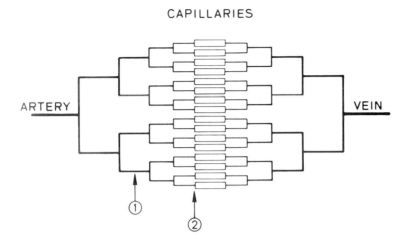

ARTERY

VEIN

① ②

Fig. 2-17. Schematic diagram of systemic vascular system. A functional representation of the concepts discussed in the test. (1) The ganglionic or systemic level. (2) The precapillary or local level.

The difficulty of measurement is a major influence in the selection of clinical measures of myocardial safety. For example, the RPP has been widely used to assess myocardial reserve. Yet, as shown above, it is a crude estimator of the TTI only. Recent work has underscored the limited clinical utility of the concept alone,[76] and its enhanced value when combined with dP/dt.[77] However, it is easy to measure.

However, during major surgery or intensive care, the decision seems clear. The viability ratio offers superior precision in patient management and therefore facilitates superior care. As monitoring equipment becomes available which will facilitate this measurement, it is likely to become far more common. It also seems likely that the denominator will be expanded to included basal and intrinsic determinants of myocardial oxygen consumption, the demand/supply ratio (D/SR), though clinical studies to document this presumption have not yet been reported.

PRESSURE, FLOW AND THE DISTRIBUTION OF BLOOD FLOW

While the previous discussion of myocardial oxygen supply presumed an understanding of the relationship of blood pressure and flow, many of the nuances that have direct value in clinical practice have been neglected. In this section, the basic concepts of pressure, flow, and distribution of blood flow are examined.

The basic relationship is defined by the analog of Ohm's law, and is best expressed as

$$Resistance = Pressure \: / \: Flow$$

where pressure and flow are mean values. Pulsatile pressure appears to be of value in assisting in the continual reopening of capillary channels (discussed in Chap. 14 on cardiopulmonary bypass). However, convenience is the major reason for the historic emphasis on measurement of systolic and diastolic pressures in preference to mean pressure (see Chap. 5 on monitoring).

Systemic perfusion always begins in a major arterial vessel, first descending through a hierarchy of smaller vessels to the capillary level, where exchange of oxygen, nutrients, and wastes occurs, then ascending through another hierarchy of vessels to a major vein. This is represented schematically in Figure 2-17, demonstrating three key attributes. First, as the vessels become smaller in diameter, their aggregate cross-sectional area increases. Secondly, as the vessels become smaller, their number increases. Thirdly, as a permitted consequence of these attributes, the flow resistance at each level before regulatory activities are included is believed to be roughly equal.

Available data also permits a simplistic view of the level of regulation. On the arterial side, central regulation is largely controlled through the tone of the larger arterial vessels,

CAPILLARIES

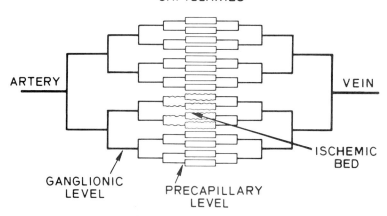

Fig. 2-18. Responses of the systemic vascular system. A schematic illustration of the differing results of vasodilation at the ganglionic and precapillary levels, given constant arterial supply pressure and an area of local ischemia.

1. Ganglionic vasodilation
    a. Flow resistance to the precapillary level decreases.
    b. Well-perfused capillary beds autoregulate to keep tissue flow constant
    c. Perfusion pressure at the precapillary level increases.
    d. Flow through the fully dilated ischemic bed increases.
2. Precapillary vasodilation
    a. Flow in well-perfused capillary bed increases.
    b. Precapillary perfusion pressure decreases.
    c. Flow through the fully dilated ischemic bed decreases.

Table 2.5. Differing Results of Vasodilation at Ganglionic and Precapillary Levels

SUPPLY PRESSURE	VASODILATION		PRECAPILLARY PRESSURE	FLOW TO ISCHEMIC BED
	Ganglionic	Precapillary		
Constant	+	0	↑	↑
	0	+	↓	↓

schematically represented in Figure 2-17 by the first *arrow*. The major effect of central control of vasomotor tone appears to be redistribution of blood flow among different vascular beds (both within and between organs). For convenience in discussion, this shall be referred to as the *middle artery, systemic*, or *ganglionic level*.

Local regulation is effected through the precapillary arteriole and sphincter, shown by the second *arrow* in Figure 2-17. The major effect of local autoregulation appears to be control of the metabolic environment, with vasodilation in response to ischemic drives,

though the nature of the relationship between hypoxia, hypercarbia and changes in pH in effecting control is still under discussion. Studies of many capillary beds show that after a period of perfusion, they close off, in effect accepting flow only when metabolic requirements dictate. This site is referred to as as the *local* or *precapillary level*.

The effect of regulation on the venous system is less clear. The historical view has been that change in central venous tone is significant. More recent data suggest (but do not prove) that many of these effects can be accounted for by capillary pooling. As noted in the summary discussion at the end of this chapter, the distinction is not of great practical importance, unless tissue oxygen reserve during low flow or cardiac arrest is considered.

How do these relationships affect physiologic function?

1. The primary site of regulation of flow in tissue with adequate perfusion pressure at required flow is at the precapillary sphincter.[78] This is nicely demonstrated by looking at the run-off portion of the aortic pressure wave. Careful examination shows that the extrapolated pressure decays to roughly 30 torr, the estimated value of perfusion pressure at the precapillary sphincter. When perfusion is not adequate, it decays to venous pressure, suggesting that the precapillary sphincter can no longer autoregulate.[79]

2. The effect of reducing total vascular resistance by agents acting at the precapillary level is significantly different than that achieved by agents acting at the ganglionic level, as represented in Figure 2-18 and Table 2-5.

These concepts are well illustrated by a practical comparison of the effects of nitroglycerin and nitroprusside (See also Chap. 11). Available data strongly indicates that the major arterial site of action of nitroprusside is at the precapillary or local level,[80] whereas for nitroglycerin it is at the middle artery or systemic level, improving collateral flow.[81]

Thus, nitroprusside is more effective as a sole agent in lowering blood pressure because it acts at the primary site of vascular resistance. However, studies suggest that when the two agents are compared with arterial pressure controlled to the same value and in equipotent doses (as determined by change in vascular resistance), nitroglycerin confers greater protection against myocardial ischemia. This is logical because the difference in primary site of action suggests that nitroprusside lowers pressure at the precapillary level by increasing flow through nonischemic tissue (overriding metabolic auto-

regulation), while nitroglycerin reduces flow resistance upstream of the site of local metabolic autoregulation, increasing the perfusion pressure available to ischemic tissue, which is already maximally vasodilated at the precapillary level.* Studies not demonstrating differences usually did not provoke ischemia.[82]

Similarly, the serial action of the drugs suggests an explanation for the clinical observation that, when used together, resistance falls more than with either used alone. Chlorpromazine HCl (Thorazine), another "ganglionic" drug, used with nitroprusside is suggested in Chapter 15 to overcome nitroprusside "resistance."

The rational reasons for the more common use of nitroprusside intraoperatively and in the unstable postoperative patient lie in the clinical value of a rapid response with change in the rate of administration, and the preserved capacity to reduce afterload (and hence myocardial oxygen demand), not in the false presumption of equivalent protection against ischemia.

These data also suggest an explanation for some of the confusing data observed in studies of myocardial perfusion. The rise in coronary sinus saturation with significant stress, observed by many early investigators, was not an argument against coronary autoregulation, but rather evidence of its failure to compensate adequately when the deficits are primarily subendocardial, such as when demand exceeds supply. Similarly, vasodilator therapy, which increases coronary sinus saturation, may not be beneficial because the rise may be at the expense of ischemic tissue. And administration of drugs such as nitroprusside may dramatically alter the numerical threshold of safety for the EVR because of the likely microvascular shunting through

---

* Studies of the effects of varying arterial carbon dioxide tension suggest the same interpretation (See Chap. 26). Hypercapnia increases cerebral blood flow, but there is no evidence that it increases cerebral protection. The available data suggest that hypercapnia acts by direct precapillary vasodilation, coupled with adrenergically mediated middle artery or ganglionic vasoconstriction, a combination just demonstrated to be undesirable.

healthy myocardium. Evaluation of vasodilator effects on the myocardium is complex because both supply, as noted above, and demand, through reduction in afterload, are altered.[83]

The physiologic response to ischemia is instructive. When flow is restored to an ischemic local area of myocardium, a period of "reactive hyperemia" ensues. During this period, flow to the recovering tissue is significantly higher than during equilibrium. Interestingly, this difference is quantitatively consistent; the excess of flow during this period is roughly three times the flow lost during the period of ischemia.[84] Calculation suggests that this is a reasonable value to permit wash-out of accumulated ischemic byproducts.

This result has important clinical implications. More flow, and hence more myocardial stress, is required to recover fully from a period of ischemia than to avoid it. In effect this is not solely because of the ischemic insult, but also because, unless supply is increased in excess of that which was lost during ischemia, the insult persists. Of course, payback (washout) requirements can also be reduced by reducing oxygen demand.[85]

Investigators who are sensitive to this concern have substituted measurement of serum lactate, or more simply, the decrease in HCO_3^- from the control value obtained with a blood gas determination, for venous saturation. Lactate is ordinarily produced only with tissue hypoxia, although the exceptions may be clinically important, such as with nitroprusside toxicity. However, under the rapidly changing conditions that prevail during surgery or early in the intensive care unit, the change in blood level may be misleading. An acutely rising serum lactate level may correlate with progressive ischemia (patient deterioration) or improved perfusion of ischemic tissue (patient improvement).

Finally, application of the concepts of middle artery and precapillary vasoregulation as described above must be tempered in organs where shunting without metabolite exchange is an important physiologic mechanism. The most obvious example, of course, is the skin.

However, it does not appear that this concern invalidates the concepts just presented.

There is little to add about venous capacitance effects. While real, these effects are expressed primarily through changes in central venous pressure or preload and are of lesser clinical subtlety because

1. Except in acute congestive failure, properly a rare intraoperative event, it is more appropriate for the anesthetist to manage preload by fluid management (infusion, diuresis, and so on) than with vasoactive drugs.
2. Normal anesthetic practice echoes the discussion of Starling's Law (see next section) and constrains preload to an optimal value for the individual patient. Thus, changes in preload with administration of vasoactive drugs must usually be corrected, not accepted.
3. The remaining and most valuable application of vasoactive drugs is management of the arterial system, as discussed above—control of vascular resistance and distribution of blood flow.

THE HEART AS A PUMP

Means of evaluating the performance of the heart that relate the demands on it to its own needs have been previously considered. The factors that influence the performance of the heart relative to the body's needs are now examined; these are the factors that determine its effectiveness as a pump. First, discussion considers how well the pump is working and whether further demands are tolerated, and then the energy balance, muscle mass, and other factors that determine performance and reserves.

While much of the groundwork had been laid by Frank,[86] the classical exposition of myocardial pumping performance was presented by Starling in the Linacre Lecture of 1915.[87] Unfortunately, much confusion persists about precisely what "Starling's Law" is and when it is valid.

Precisely, Starling stated, "Within physiological limits, the larger the volume of the

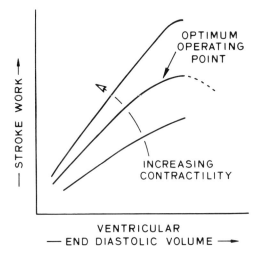

Fig. 2-19. Starling's Law.

1. The abcissa is end diastolic volume, not end diastolic pressure.
2. The ordinate is stroke work, not stroke volume or cardiac output.
3. Using the curve requires the assumption that contractility is constant; the slope of the curve varies with contractility.
4. The slope is always positive in the clinically useful range.
5. The concept of the curve bending downward to the right stems from isolated muscle studies, where it is valid. In the intact heart, this part of the curve does not exist.
6. Optimal efficiency appears near the maximum value of stroke work.

heart, the greater are the energy of its contraction and the amount of chemical change at each contraction."[87] This concept is generally accepted in modern terms to be equivalent to a linear relation between left atrial filling pressure and stroke work, good only over a given range, as schematically depicted in Figure 2-19. The slope of the line is determined by the contractile state of the heart, and the maximum energy correlates with the myocardial fiber length at which maximum contractile force and maximum efficiency in pumping blood are achieved. The location of the line is determined by myocardial contractility (*i.e.*, contractility is presumed constant while one remains on a given Starling curve).

Unfortunately, in developing this relation,

Starling was influenced by the curve for isolated skeletal muscle, which shows a "folding over" of the curve when the length is greater than the value associated with maximum force of contraction. Thus, it became common in clinical circles to discuss the function of a failing heart (as in congestive failure) in terms of the "descending limb of the Starling curve." It is now known that, for practical purposes, the descending limb does not exist. When the filling pressure associated with maximally effective contraction is exceeded, the heart cannot return after each beat to the previous end diastolic volume,* the chamber enlarges, stretches to the point where myocardial injury occurs, and the contractility of the heart is diminished. If a stable state is subsequently reached, it must then be on the ascending portion of another function curve, not on the descending portion of the original curve, as originally implied.

Despite this misunderstanding, the value of the concept in understanding and correcting heart-caused problems of perfusion is enormous. In the remainder of this section, the subtleties of interpretation, which make the concept more useful, but limit its application, are examined.

Despite documentation in the literature, many have incorrectly presented the concept as relating ventricular filling pressure to *stroke volume* or cardiac output (rather than stroke work).[88] While these relations are also often true, the exceptions are of clinical importance. With certain function curves, increasing afterload with filling pressure can ablate any significant increase in stroke volume, even though Starling's Law applies. Thus, Starling's Law does not reliably relate stroke volume and filling pressure, unless afterload is fixed.

---

* That is, because of the descending slope, any failure on a given beat to eject sufficient blood to return to the same end diastolic volume increases the required work on the next beat, just to stay even. But here the heart can do less work with increased end diastolic pressure, and the heart dilates further with the next beat. Conversely, if the heart shrinks slightly on one beat, it will contract more forcefully on the next beat, ensuring that it shrinks until reaching the point where the slope of the curve is no longer negative.

Cardiac output is influenced by both stroke volume and heart rate. But, as noted previously, a change in heart rate is nearly always accompanied by a change in contractility, (*i.e.*, a move to another Starling curve). Thus, relating filling pressure to cardiac output violates one of the insights of the Starling relation, by obscuring the difference between movement along one curve and movement to another curve.

Finally, the relation between the clinical measure of *end diastolic pressure* and Starling's measure of *end diastolic volume* is altered in many patients with compromised myocardial function. The classical assumption was that the two are reliably related, permitting substitution of pressure for volume in the relation. The relation is not linear, and the Law of Laplace magnifies the nonlinearity. But the major problem lies elsewhere: in the assumption that compliance is a reproducible value as a function of chamber size.

In the situations in which one is most interested in using Starling's Law for patient management, *compliance* is not fixed. A common example is the need for high left ventricular filling pressures to assure adequate cardiac output immediately after terminating cardiopulmonary bypass. Direct observation confirms that the heart is not filling adequately unless this is done; the explanation seems clearly related to the preceding period of ischemia with hypothermia, the consequent edema, and the associated decrease in ventricular compliance. In a relatively healthy heart, the rate of recovery is so rapid that filling pressure must be reduced a few hours later to avoid myocardial distention and injury. Recent work supports these conclusions.[89]

Chronic factors that alter ventricular compliance include left ventricular hypertrophy and infiltrative cardiomyopathy. Acute changes often relate to myocardial injury, which appears to act by tissue edema.[90] One important factor which is not often discussed is the effect of right heart function on left ventricular compliance. It appears likely, for example, that vasodilators enhance cardiac output partly by increasing left ventricular compliance through a reduction in right heart pressures.[91]

All of these considerations suggest a very succinct and useful clinical formulation of Starling's Law. The useful fact is the slope of the Starling curve at the *operating point* (where the patient currently lies). If the slope is steeply upward, then the heart will do more work, and work more efficiently, if filling pressure is increased. If increasing filling pressure rapidly decreases the slope, the point of maximum efficiency is near. If the slope is barely positive, a further increase in filling pressure is contraindicated because it must result in an unstable state, which is likely to cause myocardial injury.

Because the optimal locus for myocardial efficiency always falls on the same portion of the curve (whether the heart is athletic, normal, or compromised), this location is desirable in the failing heart, irrespective of other factors. Thus, the rational first step in therapy for the failing heart is to move function to this point on the curve, maximizing systemic support relative to myocardial demand.

A Summary of Starling's Law

Original definition
   Within physiologic limits, increasing end diastolic volume increases stroke work.
Working definition
   Increasing end-diastolic pressure (preload) increases stroke work to a maximum value.
Limitations of concept

1. In many important clinical situations, ventricular compliance, and hence, the relation between end diastolic volume and pressure, is not constant.
2. At a fixed end diastolic volume, stroke volume changes with afterload.
3. The curve is undefinable for an end diastolic volume greater than that associated with maximum work, and the heart should never operate in that region. Injury results, and the heart will move to a different operating curve.
4. A change in cardiac output may be caused by moving on the curve or moving to a different curve.

Clinical Utility
   To optimize pumping performance, and efficiency, for a given contractility, filling pressure should be adjusted to just below that for maximum stroke work. Filling pressure must *never* be increased to where the slope is almost zero.

One can then alter afterload, contractility, and heart rate, while controlling preload to achieve the best state for patient recovery.

This point was first "brought home" to the author in 1970, when a government supported study of cardiogenic shock was initiated, and it became necessary to write a common protocol. Review with a number of centers in the United States revealed mortality figures for this entity ranging from 50 to 95 percent. When a common protocol was developed, which required as part of the diagnosis failure of patient response after titration to adequate left ventricular preload, mortality was uniformly greater than 95 percent. That is, optimization of patient status using the Starling curve improved patients in whom cardiac failure was not the entire problem. When these improved patients were excluded from the study population, the grim prognosis of cardiogenic shock was uniformly demonstrated in the remainder.

In teaching this concept, many encourage the inexperienced clinician to draw the function curve for the managed patient. The experienced clinician quickly achieves the same result by noting the degree of response to altered filling pressure, and increasing filling pressure to the point of diminishing return.

Other estimates of the adequacy of pump function have been suggested in recent years. In our clinical experience, the ejection fraction is a very useful preoperative estimate of myocardial pump reserve. Values above 0.6 suggest excellent reserve; values below 0.4 imply serious compromise. However, the interpretation rests on the assumption that cardiac function has been optimized. As noted in Figure 2-20, ejection fraction changes significantly with afterload, and this effect must be taken into account.[92]

A recently identified measure, the ratio of end diastolic pressure and volume, appears to have considerable promise.[93] The measure appears to be independent of preload and afterload, and to reflect changes in compliance. It is sensitive to changes in contractility and must be scaled to the size of the patient. The measurement currently requires fluoroscopic or ultrasound techniques. Yet it appears to have promise in monitoring pump reserve and effectiveness.

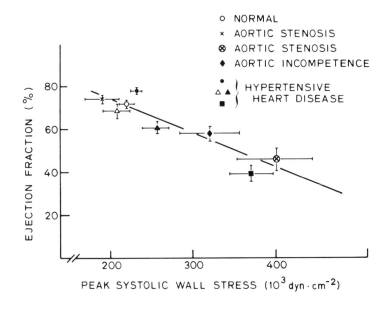

○ NORMAL
× AORTIC STENOSIS
⊗ AORTIC STENOSIS
♦ AORTIC INCOMPETENCE

● △ ▲ ■ } HYPERTENSIVE HEART DISEASE

Fig. 2-20. Relation between peak left ventricular wall stress and ejection fraction. There is a decrease in ejection fraction with increasing afterload. (Strauer BE: AM J Cardiol 44:730, 1979)

HEART-SYSTEMIC RELATIONSHIPS

In this final section, we examine the entire cardiovascular system. Much behavior of practical interest is the result of system interactions and is not obvious from isolated behavior. First, an outline of system characteristics are provided and then selected practical illustrations are considered.

The interrelationship of the important components of the cardiovascular system are shown in Figure 2-21. The outputs of the heart are stroke volume, heart rate, and *dP/ dt*. The inputs to the heart are afterload and preload. Heart and vascular responses can be modified by humoral (largely catechola-

mines) and neural (vagal and sympathetic) pathways. Thus, while the system's behavior can be amazingly complex, the number of key functional elements and inputs and outputs are small, permitting an understandable approach to system behavior. The essential element in analysis is a recognition of the concept of a control loop. The presence of control loops permits the system to be largely self-adjusting and to exhibit characteristic behavior.

Similarly, the goals of the control system can be thought of in amazingly simple terms. Assuming that the goals are (1) to assure blood flow adequate for body needs, (2) to assure that cardiac demands are less than energy supply and maximum work capacity,

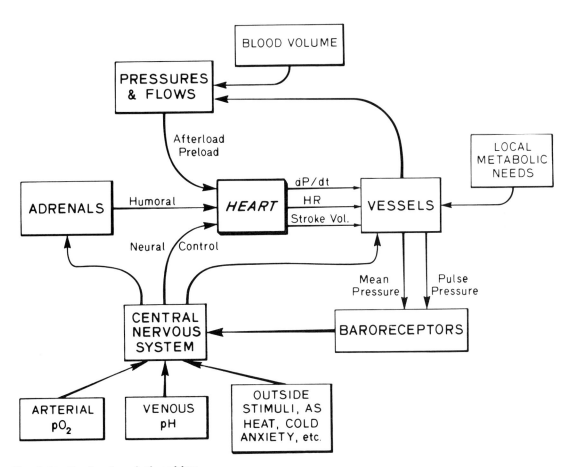

Fig. 2-21. Systemic relationships.

and (3) that results must be accomplished in the most energy-efficient manner, then most control law behavior can be predicted with surprising accuracy. "Good" physician management should emulate these goals.

A logical approach to analysis is to look first at the loop directly affected by the intervention and to predict the response. Then the responses of the other loops may be predicted, based on this information.

The reader is referred to Chapter 5 for a more detailed discussion of loop behavior.

EXAMPLES

1. *Systematic approach.* The key to sorting out this kind of process is the systematic approach, in which one variable at a time is varied, and the physician has predetermined criteria as to whether he is moving in the right direction. Cause and effect are associated. The most nearly infallible method for ensuring that a therapeutic intervention is appropriate is to observe whether improvement occurs. In hemodynamic therapy, inadequate observation is a guarantee of disaster.

   A classic example is the use of inotropic agents with an acutely failing heart. While usually a rational therapy, the results can be catastrophic if the cause is high output failure, aortic stenosis, or hypoxia. In particular, while the danger of using inotropic agents in idiopathic hypertrophic subaortic stenosis is widely appreciated, this appreciation often does not carry over to classic aortic stenosis, even though symptoms may already be more dramatic at rest. Attention to patient response will identify the error early.

2. Remember that most *results can have more than one cause;* one tends to remember a single cause for each clinical difficulty. There is no problem with beginning with a single cause, particularly if it is the most likely alternative. But once initial therapy has begun, the alternatives must be sequentially examined and ruled in or out.

An example is the treatment of acute congestive heart failure with morphine sulfate. Every clinician who has employed this approach can testify to the frequently dramatic response. Yet at least four mechanisms exist, each with a different therapeutic end point: (1) oxygen demand is reduced because the patient is less restless; (2) preload is reduced by vasodilation, reducing cardiac oxygen consumption and pulmonary vascular pressures; (3) anxiety is reduced by reducing perceived discomfort, without changing the underlying illness; and (4) the narcotic-induced shift in ventilatory drive removes the perception of hypoxia, reducing minute ventilation and oxygen supply and increasing carbon dioxide tension which decreases tissue pH. These four mechanisms produce respectively positive, no, and negative improvement in patient status. All four mechanisms are active and each could dominate under appropriate circumstances. The clinician who titrates to a desired response is more likely to achieve the desired effect than one who treats by a predetermined dose.

3. *Use all available information.* Background information, when coupled with the formal work-up frequently clarifies an uncertain diagnosis. For example, careful evaluation of a patient previously well-managed yields valuable information not evident in the catheterization data. A classic example is the differentiation between the patients who do best with propranolol and those responding best to nitroglycerin. The patient preferring propranolol typically has myocardial reserve, with angina appearing during exercise or stress, rather than at rest. A beta blocker limits his activities, reducing peak demand. When queried as to the effectiveness of propranolol, the patient will often say, "Well, I don't have chest pain any more, but I sure get tired climbing stairs."

   The patient doing best with nitroglycerin usually has little reserve. The drug improves supply relative to demand and is more likely to relieve the patient with angina at rest. When this patient attempts to climb stairs, angina stops him before fatigue is noted.

If one is reassured that the trial of therapies was adequate, this differentiation suggests differentiated anesthetic management.

4. Use the relationship between blood volume and vasomotor tone. The body has no volume receptors; all of the effects of changing blood volume are expressed through the blood pressure. Functionally, hypovolemia represents a disparity between the volume of the vascular space (*blood volume*) and the volume associated with adequate pressures (*vascular volume*). This distinction is important because we can adjust them independently, as shown in Table 2-6. The usual clinical approach is to provide correction in two steps: (1) bringing pressure toward normal by adjusting the vascular volume (*e.g.,* giving a vasopressor after hemorrhage and (b) adjusting blood volume toward the normal range (*e.g.,* by transfusion).

One must ultimately be sure the 'blood volume' is adequate because the alternative is inadequate presence of nutrients at the capillary level. A simple rule of thumb is that if pressure is normal but cardiac output is depressed, blood volume is below the optimal value.

5. *Retain physiologic responses* when possible. Homeostatic assistance to physician therapy increases patient safety. An example is the now widespread use of salt solutions (Ringer's or normal saline) in preference to free water (Dextrose 5% in H_2O) in transfusion of cardiac patients during surgery. The stress of surgery increases antidiuretic hormone (ADH) secretion, preventing production of dilute urine. The extra salt preserves renal excretory capacity, preserving a natural response to fluid overload.

In early open heart surgery, failure to appreciate these concerns led to difficulty. A natural reluctance to transfuse, particularly to provide adequate salts, appears to have stemmed from appreciation of the appropriate medical therapy of salt depletion (to reduce preload and afterload in the failing heart) in the patient with volume overload. Consequently, diminished blood volume was associated with increased vascular instability, particularly during post surgical warming.

Similarly, edema is not an absolute contraindication to fluid infusion necessary for adequate blood volume. There are basically two deleterious effects of edema: (1) increased pressure in a closed space, such as the brain; and (2) increased nutrient diffusion pathway, such

Table 2-6. Blood Volume Versus Vascular Volume

		PRESSURE	
		Increase	Decrease
VOLUME	Blood	Transfusion	Third space Hemorrhage Diuresis Insensible loss
	Vascular	Vasoconstrictors	Vasodilators

Major concepts
1. Assessment is usually made by measured pressures. This approach requires many assumptions.
2. First therapy usually effects vascular volume because this approach is faster and easier.
3. Blood volume must also be optimized for tissue protection.
Goals
1. Normal intravascular blood volume.
2. Avoid the dangerous complications of edema. (But optimal therapy may not avoid edema.)

as in the lungs. Both are relative and must be balanced against the general requirement of tissue perfusion.

6. *Low blood pressure can be due to either systemic or cardiac derangements.* Systemic difficulties fall under the balance between blood and vascular volume discussed above. The most common cause of cardiac failure is a failure of contractility, but other causes must not be forgotten. The acute differential diagnosis of pericardial tamponade versus primary myocardial failure can be exquisitely difficult in the postoperative period if the pleural membranes are intact.

7. *The presumed "obvious" relationship between pressure and flow does not always hold.* For example, tilting the hypotensive patient head down (Trendelenburg's position) does not increase cardiac output if the patient is sufficiently hypovolemic, even though central arterial pressure increases.[94]

8. *Inotropic agents always increase myocardial oxygen consumption.* The classic beneficial effects of digitalis in congestive heart failure are consistent with this observation. Increased contractility increases ejection, ultimately reducing end diastolic volume. This reduces wall tension during contraction, reducing oxygen demand more than the inotropic agent increased it, a net beneficial effect.[95]

    It is for this reason that patients with severe cardiac disease are more vulnerable to digitalis toxicity. In this case, the inotropic effect is not adequate, and clinical experience shows improvement with higher doses because of the associated reduction in heart rate and oxygen demand. But reduction of heart rate is an early sign of toxicity.

    This concept also indicates when digitalis is not helpful. The patient without an enlarged heart or in high output failure (such as in normals with pericardial tamponade or thyrotoxicosis) can be expected to exhibit increased myocardial oxygen consumption after administration of digitalis.

9. Adequate *patient control is easier when beginning from a stable baseline,* rather than the untreated state. This lesson must be learned with each new drug. Students are no longer taught that the stabilized patient on antihypertensive drugs or propranolol must have them withdrawn before surgery, but the instinct to abruptly substitute a familiar anesthetic approach remains. Substitution may be entirely appropriate, but it should occur smoothly, and slowly enough to be under complete control.

10. *Heroic measures do not represent a departure from routine principles,* but rather an intensive application of them. The sequential approach to therapeutic changes is even more important. Assumptions must be rechecked and secondary drug effects reviewed for undesirable effects. Each intervention must be convincingly associated with beneficial changes.

SUMMARY

In the management of a typical problem, certain principles are surprisingly consistent:

1. The problem is usually a disparity between body needs and cardiovascular performance.

2. Because myocardial efficiency varies with the position on the Starling curve, end diastolic volume should be optimized. It should be remembered that
    a. this means adjustment of preload (filling pressure)
    b. Starling's law refers to end diastolic volume. The physician must be sure to consider whether ventricular compliance is normal.
    c. heart rate, afterload, and heart size are not yet optimized

3. Obvious and urgent inadequacies in cardiac function should be treated as soon as possible (*e.g.*, arrhythmias, hypovolemia). A common pathway for dysfunction is hypoxia, and oxygen alone is often of exceptional value.

4. Aortic pressure (afterload) should be normalized, both to assure control of myocardial oxygen demand (not too high) and adequate perfusion (not too low). A low pressure may require inotropic agents; high pressure usually requires vasodilation, and inotropic depression if pulse pressure is excessive.

5. Blood and vascular volume must be brought into balance. The normotensive, hypovolemic patient with cardiovascular disease is at unnecessary risk in many anesthetic situations.

6. The contractile state of the heart should be optimized consistent with systemic needs and the constraints of disease. A low heart rate and inotropic depression reduce oxygen demand. However, maximizing the EVR or, better, the D/SR is a more rational means of providing cardiac protection than minimizing cardiac work. As in the hyperdynamic patient (See Chap. 16), increasing cardiac work is not always appropriate.

The cardiovascular system is complex in appearance and behavior, but can usually be managed with ease, if a systematic approach is developed. In this way, very simple concepts yield dramatic results when applied with sufficient care. The concepts of myocardial energy balance, Starling's Law, distribution of blood flow, and closed-loop control systems are particularly helpful.

GLOSSARY

afterload. Pressure in the ventricle just as the aortic valve opens in systole. This clinical definition is simply related to the definition in isolated muscle studies (tension immediately after contraction begins), if end-diastolic heart size does not change. *Not* systemic resistance.

blood volume. As used in this book, intravascular fluid status is the balance between the fluid contents of the blood vessels (*blood volume*) and the volume of the vascular space associated with acceptable arterial and venous pressures (*"vascular volume"*). There is also *absolute* blood volume (actual blood volume) and *functional* blood volume (the balance between blood and vascular volume). Separation of these concepts is essential for clinical effectiveness.

contractility. The intrinsic contractile state of the heart, measured by changes in force and rate of contraction (*dP/dt*). It is often conceptually useful to think of *dP/dt* per beat. But in comparing contractility with myocardial oxygen consumption, contractility per minute must always be used.

coronary reserve. The ratio of coronary vascular resistance resting to maximally dilated.[92]

demand/supply ratio (D/SR). A definition proposed by the author to account for all of the major determinants of supply and demand. Similar to the EVR, except that the estimate of myocardial oxygen demand includes basal and inotropic requirements.

developed pressure. The pressure in the left ventricle during contraction minus the end diastolic pressure.

diastole. The part of the heart cycle not spent in systole.

diastolic perfusion index (DPI or DPTI). The area between the curves of aortic root pressure and left ventricular pressure during ventricular diastole—an estimate of coronary flow with maximum coronary artery dilation.[67] Also known as diastolic pressure-time index.

efficiency. Work *out* divided by the energy *in*; maximum possible is 1.0 (or 100%).

ejection fraction. The ratio of stroke volume to end diastolic volume of the left ventricle.

endocardial viability ratio (EVR). The ratio of DPI to TTI—an estimate of myocardial oxygen supply relative to demand when contractility and arterial oxygen content do not change. In customary use of this index, mean rather than peak systolic pressure is used to calculate TTI. Also the ratio is dimensionless; per beat or per minute values may be used so long as one is consistent.[68]

extrinsic factors. Used in this chapter to refer to factors outside of the heart which influence cardiac function.

force. That agent which, when applied to a free body, causes it to move. The basic quantity. Often confused with tension and stress.

index of cardiac effort. See rate-pressure product. Early name proposed by Katz.[16]

inotrope. A drug which affects the contractility of the heart.

intrinsic factors. Used in this chapter to refer to factors within the heart that influence cardiac function.

law of Laplace. For *spheres*, transmural pressure equals twice the wall tension divided by the radius. For *tubes*, transmural pressure equals the wall tension divided by the radius. Because of the Law of Laplace, changes in heart size change the true TTI even though the pressure (and hence clinical TTI) does not change.

left ventricular ejection time (LVET). The period when the aortic valve is open.

oxygen demand. Refers to oxygen required by specific tissue, in this context, usually the heart. The literature is confusing because demand is given per beat and per time. Because supply is usually per time and is conceptually more convenient, all data are expressed per time in this chapter unless otherwise indicated.

oxygen supply. Usually the limiting metabolic substrate used presumptively in this chapter.

Preejection period (PEP). From onset of the QRS complex to opening of the aortic valve.

power. Work per unit time; work divided by time. Usually expressed as watts (joules per second) by all noncardiologists. The mechanical power of an adult human heart with minimal activity is approximately one watt.

preload. The pressure in the ventricle just before contraction begins. Note that this clinical definition is simply related to the definition used in isolated muscle studies (the tension just before active contraction), only if end diastolic heart size is stable.

Q–S2. PEP plus LVET.

rate-pressure product (RPP). The product of heart rate and peak systolic pressure—an estimate of myocardial oxygen demand. The RPP improves as an estimator of work tolerance when multiplied by ejection time; it is then the TTI. An earlier name is the index of cardiac effort.

resistance. Calculated as the ratio of mean pressure to mean flow. The preferable units are dyne-sec/cm^5. Also used are torr-min/liter or Wood units. Multiply Wood units by 79.7 to convert to dyne-sec/cm^5. There are two terms to define the level of resistance: *ganglionic* (or middle artery or systemic) refers to changes in the larger arteries and *precapillary* (or local) refers to changes near the level of the precapillary sphincter.

Starling's Law. Original statement: the larger the volume of the heart, the greater is the energy of its contraction (Fig. 2-19). The relationships between preload, stroke volume, and cardiac output do not always follow the Starling curve

because of changes in ventricular compliance, afterload, contractility, and heart rate.

systolic time intervals (STI). Measures which can be obtained noninvasively, typically by using phonocardiogram, ECG, and arterial pulsation, such as $Q-S_2$, PEP, LVET.

stress. Force in a material (such as the wall of the heart) divided by the area over which it is applied; force divided by area. *See* force, tension.

stroke volume. The volume of blood pumped with each contraction of the heart.

systole. Originally the time during the cardiac cycle when the heart is contracting. Alternative definitions: the time when the left ventricle is contracting (ventricular systole), the time when the aortic valve is open (aortic systole), the time when the aortic valve is open and the heart is contracting, and all of the preceding using an arterial waveform from a peripheral artery. These definitions are not always interchangeable in calculating cardiac indices.

tension. In a strand, such as papillary muscle, the force applied; in a membrane, such as the wall of the heart, force applied divided by the distance perpendicular to the force along which it is applied.

tension-time index (TTI). Original definition: the product of average force of contraction and duration of contraction in isolated papillary muscle (units of force multiplied by time). Clinical definition: the product of average left ventricular pressure during systole and the duration of systole in the intact heart (units of pressure multiplied by time). In this book, unless otherwise specified, TTI is the clinical definition, and is expressed per minute, not per beat.[8] Clinical TTI is related to isolated muscle TTI by the diameter and wall thickness of the ventricle.

triple index: The product of the RPP and pulmonary capillary wedge pressure. In effect, this index modifies the RPP by taking into account the effect of the Law of Laplace on myocardial oxygen demand. *See* Rate pressure product.

V_{ce}**.** Derived from velocity of the contractile element in the model of isolated heart muscle. Often used in clinical literature to describe calculated value. The clinical units of measurement are inconsistent dimensionally with the units employed in isolated papillary muscle studies.

V_{max}**.** A calculated value, never measured directly. Originally the velocity of contraction of a muscle fiber with zero load. Often used to describe the analogous condition in the intact heart, sometimes corrected to the same units, often not, and using many different formulas.

V_{pm}. The measured maximum value of V_{ce}, as calculated from intact ventricle pressure measurements. Not the same as V_{max}.

V_{40}. The contractile velocity for intact ventricle, calculated at a given pressure, here, for example, 40 torr.

work. The total amount of energy expended. Equal to force multiplied by distance. The preferable unit is the joule. There are 0.74 foot-pounds per joule.

REFERENCES

GENERAL REFERENCES

1. Graham TP, Covell JW, Sonnenblick EH et al: Control of myocardial oxygen consumption: relative influence of contractile state and tension development. J Clin Invest 47:375–385, 1968

2. Braunwald E, Ross JR Jr, Sonnenblick EH: Mechanisms of contraction of the normal and failing heart, 2nd ed. Boston, Little, Brown & Co, 1976

3. Gibbs CL: Cardiac energetics. Physiol Rev 58:174-254, 1978

ENERGY BALANCE IN THE MYOCARDIUM

4. Pool PE, Chandler BM, Spann JF Jr et al: Mechanochemistry of cardiac muscle. IV. Utilization of high energy phosphates in experimental heart failure in cats. Circ Res 24:313–320, 1969

5. Braunwald E: Mechanics and energetics of the normal and failing heart. Trans Assoc Am Physicians 84:63–94, 1971

6. Gollwitzer–Meier K, Kramer K, Kruger E: Der gaswechsel des suffizienten und insuffizienten warmblutterherzens. Pfluegers Arch 237:68–92, 1936

7. Gollwitzer–Meier K, Kruger E: Herzenergetik und strophanthinwirkung bei verschiedenen formen der experimentellen herzinsuffizienz. Pfluegers Arch 238:251–278, 1936

8. Sarnoff SJ, Braunwald E, Welch GH Jr et al: Hemodynamic determinants of oxygen consumption of the heart with special reference to the tension-time index. Am J Physiol 192:148–156, 1958

9. Monroe RG: Myocardial oxygen consumption during ventricular contraction and relaxation. Circ Res 14:294–300, 1964

10. Gibbs, CL: Cardiac Energetics. In Langer GA and Brady RJ The Mammalian Myocardium, New York, Wiley, 1974

11. Oliveras RA, Boucher CA, Haycraft GL et al: Myocardial oxygen supply-demand ratio: a validation of peripherally versus centrally determined values. Chest 75:693–696, 1979

12. Mirsky I: Left ventricular stresses in the intact human heart. Biophys J 9:189–208, 1969

13. Rodbard S, Williams F, Williams C: The spherical dynamics of the heart (myocardial tension, consumption, coronary blood flow and efficiency). Am Heart J 57:348–360, 1959

14. McDonald RH: Developed tension: a major determinant of myocardial oxygen consumption. Am J Physiol 210:351–356, 1966

15. Coleman HN, Sonneblick EH, Braunwald E: Myocardial oxygen consumption associated with external work: the Fenn effect. Am J Physiol 217:291–296, 1969

16. Katz LN, Feinberg H: The relation of cardiac effort to myocardial oxygen consumption and coronary flow. Circ Res 6:656–669, 1958

17. Robinson BF: Relation of heart rate and systolic blood pressure to the onset of pain in angina pectoris. Circulation 35:1073–1083, 1967

18. Braunwald E: The determinants of myocardial oxygen consumption. Physiologist 12:65–93, 1969

19. Sonnenblick EH, Ross J Jr, Covell JW et al: Velocity of contraction as a determinant of myocardial oxygen consumption. Am J Physiol 209:919–927, 1965

20. Braunwald E: Mechanics and energetics of the normal and failing heart. Trans Assoc Am Physicians 84:63–94, 1971

21. Mason DT, Braunwald E, Covell JW et al: Assessment of cardiac contractility. Circulation 44:47–58, 1971

22. Burns JW, Covell JW, Ross J Jr: Mechanics of isotonic left ventricular contractions. Am J Physiol 224:725–732, 1973

23. Sonnenblick EH: Force-velocity relations in mammalian heart muscle. Am J Physiol 202:931–939, 1962

24. Sonnenblick EH, Parmley WW, Urschel CW: The contractile state of the heart as expressed by force-velocity relations. Am J Cardiol 23:488–503, 1969

25. Taylor RR: Theoretical analysis of the iso-volumic phase of left ventricular contraction in terms of cardiac muscle mechanics. Cardiovasc Res 4:429–435, 1970

26. Parmley WW, Sonnenblick EH: Series elasticity in heart muscle: its relation to contractile element velocity and proposed muscle models. Circ Res 20:112–123, 1967

27. Mason DT, Spann JF, Zelis R: Quantification of the contractile state of the intact human heart. Am J Cardiol 26:248–257, 1970

28. Mirsky I, Parmley WW: Force-velocity studies in isolated and intact heart muscle. In Mirsky D et al (eds): Cardiac Mechanics, New York, Wiley, 1974

29. Davidson DM, Covell JW, Malloch CI et al: Factors influencing indices of left ventricle contractility in the conscious dog. Cardiovas Res 8:299–312, 1974

30. Mehmel HC, Krayenbuehl HP, Wirz P: Isovolumic contraction dynamics in man according to two different muscle models. J Appl Physiol 33:409–414, 1972

31. Mirsky I, Ellison RC, Hugenholtz PG: Assessment of myocardial contractility in children and young adults from ventricular pressure recordings. Am J Cardiol 27:359–367, 1971

32. Falsetti HL, Mates RE, Greene DG et al: V_{max} as an index of contractile state in man. Circulation 43:467–479, 1971

33. Davidson DM, Covell JW, Malloch CR et al: Factors influencing indice's of left ventricle contractility in the conscious dog. Cardiovas Res 8:299–312, 1974

34. Pollack GH, Huntsman LL, Verdugo P: Cardiac muscle models: an overetension of series elasticity. Circ Res 31:569–579, 1972

35. Pollack GH: Maximum velocity as an index of contractility in cardiac muscle. Circ Res 26:111–127, 1970

36. Teplick R: Personal Communication.

37. Pollack GH, Huntsman LL, Verdugo P: Cardiac muscle models: an overextension of series elasticity. Circ Res 31:569–579, 1972

38. Huntsman LL, Nichols GL: Determination of segment length in the isolated cardiac muscle preparation. Annual Conference Engineering in Medicine and Biology (ACEMB) Proceedings 29:270, 1976

39. Mason DT, Spann JF, Zelis R: Quantification of the contractile state of the intact human heart. Am J Cardiol 26:248–257, 1970

40. Kreulen TH, Bove AA, McDonough MT et al:

The evaluation of left ventricular function in man. Circulation 51:677–688, 1975

41. Hill AV: The heat of shortening and the dynamic constants of muscle. Proc R Soc London [Biol] 126:136–195, 1938

42. Steinberg RB, Katona PG, Hung JC et al: On line digital computation of V_{max} from intraventricular pressure. Proceedings: Alliance for Engineering in Medicine and Biology 18:127, 1976

43. Brutsaert DL, Sonnenblick EH: Cardiac muscle mechanics in the evaluation of myocardial contractility and pump function: problems, concepts, and directions. Prog Cardiovasc Dis 16:337–361, 1973

44. Van Den Bos GC, Elizinga G, Westerhof N et al: Problems in the use of indices of myocardial contractility. Cardiovasc Res 7:834–848, 1973

45. Kreulen TH, Bove AA, McDonough MT et al: The evaluation of left ventricular function in man. Circulation 51:677–688, 1975

46. Nejad NS, Klein MD, Mirsky I et al: Assessment of myocardial contractility from ventricular pressure recordings. Cardiovasc Res 5:15–23, 1971

47. Wolk MJ, Keefe JF, Bing OHL et al: Estimation of V_{max} in auxotonic systoles from the rate of relative Increase of Isovolumic pressure. J Clin Invest 50:1276–1285, 1971

48. Falsetti HL, Mates RE, Greene DG et al: V_{max} as an index of contractile state in man. Circulation 43:467–479, 1971

49. Krayenbuehl HP, Rutishauser W, Wirz P et al: High-fidelity left ventricular pressure measurements for the assessment of cardiac contractility in man. Am J Cardiol 31:415–427, 1973

50. Laurent D, Bolene–Williams C, Williams FL, Katz LN: Effects of heart rate on coronary flow and cardiac oxygen consumption. Am J Physiol 185:355–364, 1956

51. Boerth RC, Covell JW, Pool PE: Increased myocardial oxygen consumption and contractile state associated with increased heart rate in dogs. Circ Res 24:725–734, 1969

52. Weber KT, Janicki JS: Interdependence of cardiac function, coronary flow and oxygen extraction. Am J Physiol 235:H784–793, 1978

53. Langer GA: The intrinsic control of myocardial contraction-ionic factors. N Engl J Med 285:1065–1071, 1971

54. Wallace AG, Mitchell JH, Skinner NS, Sarnoff

SJ: Duration of the phases of left ventricular systole. Circ Res 12:611–619, 1963

55. Mitchell JH, Wallace AG, Skinner NS Jr: Intrinsic effects of heart rate on left ventricular performance. Am J Physiol 205:41–48, 1963

56. Boerth RC, Covell JW, Pool PE: Increased myocardial oxygen consumption and contractile state associated with increased heart rate in dogs. Circ Res 24:725–734, 1969

57. Braunwald E, Sarnoff SJ, Stainsby WN: Determinants of duration and mean rate of ventricular ejection. Circ Res 6:319–325, 1958

58. Bing RJ, Hammond MM, Handelsman JC et al: The measurement of coronary blood flow, oxygen consumption and efficiency of the left ventricle in man. Am Heart J 38:1–24, 1949

59. Shaw RF, Mosher P, Ross J Jr et al: Physiologic principles of coronary perfusion. J Thorac Cardiovasc Surg 44:608–616, 1962

60. Manohar M, Bisgard GE, Bullard V et al: Myocardial perfusion and function during acute right ventricular systolic hypertension. Am J Physiol 235:H628–H636, 1978

61. Weber KT, Janicki JS: The metabolic demand and oxygen supply of the heart: physiologic and clinical considerations. Am J Cardiol 44:722–729, 1979

62. Braunwald E, Sarnoff SJ, Case RB et al: Hemodynamic determinants of coronary flow: effect of changes in aortic pressure and cardiac output on the relationship between myocardial oxygen consumption and coronary flow. Am J Physiol 192:157–163, 1958

63. Shaw RF, Mosher P, Ross J Jr et al: Physiologic principles of coronary perfusion. J Thorac Cardiovasc Surg 44:608–616, 1962

64. Bacaner MB, Lioy F, Visscher MB: Coronary blood flow, oxygen delivery rate and cardiac performance. J Physiol 216:111–127, 1971

65. Harden WR, Barlow CH, Simson MB, Harken AH: Temporal relation between onset of cell anoxia and ischemic contractile failure. Am J Cardiol 44:741–746, 1979

66. Gorlin R, Brachfeld N, MacLeod C et al: Effect of nitroglycerin on the coronary circulation in patients with coronary artery disease or increased left ventricular work. Circulation 19:705–718, 1959

67. Buckberg GD, Fixler, DE, Archie JP, Hoffman JIE: Experimental subendocardial ischemia in dogs with normal coronary arteries. Circ Res 30:67–81, 1972

68. Philips PA, Bregman D: Intraoperative application of intraaortic balloon counterpulsation determined by clinical monitoring of the endocardial viability ratio. Ann Thorac Surg 23:45–51, 1977

69. Buckberg GD: Left ventricular subendocardial necrosis. Ann Thorac Surg 24:379–393, 1977

70. Kleinman LH, Wechsler AS: Pressure-flow characteristics of the coronary collateral circulation during cardiopulmonary bypass: effects of ventricular fibrillation. Circulation 58:233–239, 1978

71. Neill WA, Fluri–Lundeen JH: Myocardial oxygen supply in left ventricular hypertrophy and coronary heart disease. Am J Cardiol 44:747–783, 1979

72. Brazier J, Cooper N, Buckberg G: The adequacy of subendocardial oxygen delivery. The interaction of flow, arterial oxygen content and myocardial oxygen need. Circulation 49:968–977, 1974

73. Philips PA, Bregman D: Intraoperative application of intraaortic balloon counterpulsation determined by clinical monitoring of the endocardial viability ratio. Ann Thorac Surg 23:45–51, 1977

74. Oliveros RA, Boucher CA, Haycraft GL et al: Myocardial oxygen supply-demand ratio: a validation of peripherally versus centrally determined values. Chest 75:693–696, 1979

75. Diamond, G, Forrester JS, Chatterjee K, Wegner S, Swan HJC: Mean electromechanical Δ P/Δ T: an indirect index of the peak rate of rise of left ventricular pressure. Am J Cardiol 30:338–342, 1972

76. Kissin I, Reves JG, Mardis M: Is the rate-pressure product a misleading guide? Anesthesiology 52:373–374, 1980

77. Wilkinson PL, Moyers JR, Ports T et al: Rate-pressure product and myocardial oxygen consumption during surgery for coronary artery bypass. Circulation 60:I-170–173, 1979

PRESSURE, FLOW, AND THE DISTRIBUTION OF BLOOD FLOW

78. Feldstein ML, Henquell L, Honig CR: Frequency analysis of coronary intercapillary distances: site of capillary control. Am J Physiol 235:H321–325, 1978

79. Jackman AP and Green JF: Arterial pressure-flow relationships in the anesthetized dog. Ann Biomed Eng 5:384–394, 1977

80. Longnecker DE, Creasy RA, Ross DC: A microvascular site of action of sodium nitroprusside in striated muscle of the rat. Anesthesiology 50:111–117, 1979

81. Winbury MM, Howe BR, Hefner MA: Effect of nitrates and other coronary dilators on large and small coronary vessels: a hypothesis for the mechanism of action of nitrates. J Pharmacal Exp Therapeut 168:70–95, 1969

82. Kerber RE, Martins JB, Marcus ML: Effect of acute ischemia, nitroglycerin and nitroprusside on regional myocardial thickening, stress and perfusion: experimental echocardiographic studies. Circulation 60:121–129, 1979

83. Kaplan JA, Jones EL: Vasodilator therapy during coronary artery surgery. J Thor Cardiovasc Surg 77:301–309, 1979

84. Brazier J, Cooper N, Buckberg G: The adequacy of subendocardial oxygen delivery. The interaction of flow, arterial oxygen content and myocardial oxygen need. Circulation 49:968–977, 1974

85. Maroko PR, Kjekshus JK, Sobel BE et al: Factors influencing infarct size following experimental coronary artery occlusions. Circulation 43:67–82, 1971

THE HEART AS A PUMP

86. Frank O: Zür dynamik des herzmuskels. Ztschr Biol 32:370–437, 1895

87. Starling EH: The Linacre Lecture on the Law of the Heart. London, Longmans, Green & Co, 1918

88. Sarnoff SJ, Berglund E: Ventricular function. I. Starling's law of the heart studied by means of simultaneous right and left ventricular function curves in the dog. Circulation 9:707–718, 1954

89. Parker JO, Case RB: Normal left ventricular function. Circulation 60:4–12, 1979

90. Grossman, W, McLaurin LP: Diastolic properties of the left ventricle. Ann Intern Med 84:316–326, 1976

91. Glantz SA, Parmley WW: Factors which affect the diastolic pressure-volume curve. Circ Res 42:171–180, 1978

92. Strauer BE: Myocardial oxygen consumption in chronic heart disease: role of wall stress, hypertrophy and coronary reserve. Am J Cardiol 44:730–740, 1979

93. Sagawa K: The ventricular pressure-volume diagram revisited. Circ Res 43:677–687, 1978

HEART-SYSTEMIC RELATIONSHIPS

94. Sibbald WJ, Paterson NAM, Holliday RL et al: The Trendelenburg position: hemodynamic effects in hypotensive and normotensive patients. Crit Care Med 7:218–224, 1979

95. Covell JW, Braunwald E, Ross J Jr et al: Studies on digitalis. XVI. Effects on myocardial oxygen consumption. J Clin Invest 45:1535–1542, 1966

3

Cellular Mechanisms: A Clinical View

WILLIAM NEW, JR

INTRODUCTION

Muscle physiologists understand heart muscle physiology reasonably well. Many doctors and medical students do not. One reason is that most muscle physiologists in their original and review articles write for other muscle physiologists and not for doctors or medical students. This is *not* a chapter for muscle physiologists; it is written for doctors and medicals students. Like the tutorial lectures for anesthesia residents upon which it is based, it has only one purpose: to map out in simple words and diagrams these central aspects of heart muscle physiology that are fundamental to critical care.

Other chapters in this book consider cardiovascular anesthesia and critical care at the organ, system, or integrated patient level. This chapter views a single myocardial cell. All electrical and mechanical behavior of the heart originates from actions and interactions of ions moving through heart cells. Any physical or pharmacologic maneuvers that affect cardiac electromechanical performance can ultimately be explained in terms of altered ionic movements. A conceptual grasp of cellular ionic flows is thus the most fundamental clinical basis for interpreting myocardial performance and initiating (or terminating!) therapy.

Medicine is generally taught in a linear format:

Physiology→Pathophysiology→Pharmacology→Clinical Sciences→Clinical Art

One learns everything about one level before going on to the next level. This sequence is logical. One can proceed in an orderly manner, starting from first principles. From

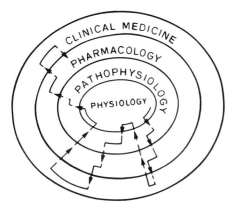

Fig. 3-1. The onion structure of medical learning.

a teacher's perspective, it has the added advantage that each section can be delivered relatively independently of the material in other sections. Life is easier for example, if one doesn't have to muddy the conceptual purity of a sodium pump in the cell membrane with the pragmatics of digitalis-toxic rhythms seen that day in the operating room. On the other hand, a medical student who sees firsthand an effective therapy, which is designed upon the first principles of a sodium pump, will remember sodium pumps forever. One learns principles more completely when the practical applications are clear.

For this reason, the author prefers to remap the linear form above into concentric layers, into an "onion" (see Fig. 3-1). Teaching proceeds by moving from an inner layer to successive outer layers until one subtopic is completed; one then returns to the core to start another. This system has two distinct advantages beyond facilitating student understanding: first, one can stop after any single topic is discussed and have a relatively complete science-to-practice grasp of it; and second, one can build each topic upon those previously covered, if order is carefully considered. The order chosen to present the ionic underpinnings of cardiac electromechanical behavior has been selected with this in mind; one can stop at any point and have learned clinically useful concepts, or one can

continue to build toward a more complete understanding.

This chapter leads to the following general conclusions:

1. All electrical and mechanical activity of the heart (and other muscles, for that matter) is determined at the cellular level by the concentrations, flows, and interactions of ions.
2. Calcium is an ubiquitous ion of central importance.
3. Electromechanical behavior of the heart can be modified (for better or for worse) by physiochemical influences on ions, and
4. Cardiac anesthesia and intensive care can be usefully conceptualized as the beneficial control of ionic behavior, especially that of calcium.

References are provided for further reading.[1-6]

GENERAL CONCEPTS

ENVIRONMENT

Heart cells are surrounded by extracellular fluid that contains over ten types of ions (Table 3-1). The most prevalent extracellular cations (positive charges) are, in descending order of concentration, sodium (Na^+), potassium (K^+), calcium (Ca^{++}) and magnesium (Mg^{++}). The flows and accumulations of Na^+, K^+, and Ca^{++} are the primary active determinants of cardiac electromechanical behavior. By contrast, anions (negative charges) play a relatively minor, passive role, distributing themselves in such a way as to maintain local electroneutrality, that is, to maintain essentially equal numbers of negative charges and positive charges in each neighborhood. The most prevalent extracellular anions are (in order) chloride (Cl^-) and bicarbonate (HCO_3^-).

The same cations and anions appear inside heart cells within the cytoplasm but at considerably different concentration levels (see Table 3-1). Potassium is the most prevalent cation inside the cell at a concentration roughly 30-fold greater than outside. Intracellular sodium and calcium are a small fraction of their outside concentrations. There is a much higher concentration of protein in cytoplasm than in plasma. Intracellular proteins are negatively charged (*i.e.,* anions) at the neutral pH levels ($\approx$ 7.0) found inside cells. These immobile proteins plus intracellular phosphate (PO_4^-) provide nearly all the negative charge required for electroneutrality. Thus relatively little chloride and bicarbonate need be present.

Figure 3–2 graphically illustrates the concentration differences outside to inside across the cell membrane for sodium, potassium, calcium, and chloride. It is clear that calcium has the steepest transmembrane gradient with roughly a 10,000-fold difference in concentration from outside to inside. As will be seen, this means that Ca^{++} is trying to enter the cell with far greater relative force than any other ion.

IONIC MOVEMENTS

There are two forces that move ions in solution: *diffusion,* which forces ions down a concentration gradient; and *drift,* which forces ions down an electrical gradient. Diffusion and drift forces operate independently from each other because concentration and electrical fields are independent physical phenomena. Both forces, however, will be felt by an ion simultaneously situated in *both* a concentration gradient and an electrical gradient. The forces may augment each other, resist each other, or operate perpendicular to each other, depending upon the relative direction of the concentration and electrical gradients, respectively. Ionic movement will proceed in the direction of the vector sum of the two forces. Actually there is a third type of movement—*bulk* movement—that occurs as the entire solution moves *en masse* hydraulically, such as down a blood vessel. Drift only affects electrically charged particles (viz, ions); diffusion and bulk flow affect both charged and uncharged particles. It is noteworthy that ions moving by bulk flow through a *magnetic* field will separate slightly, positive

Table 3-1. Ion Concentrations (mmol/l)

	EXTRACELLULAR	INTRACELLULAR
Na^+	140	10
K^+	4	150
Ca^{++}	3 (unbound)	10^{-6} (unbound)
Mg^{++}	1	26 (bound)
HCO_3^-	30	10
Cl^-	105	3
PO_4^-	2	100
Protein	1	65

(Modified from Diem K, Lentner C (eds): Scientific Tables, 7th ed. Basel, Switzerland, Ciba–Geigy, 1970, pp. 523, 565)

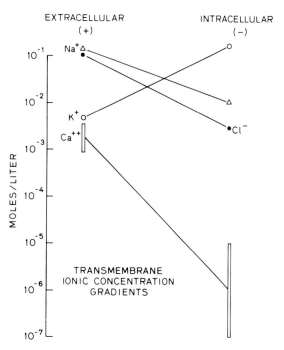

Fig. 3-2. Transmembrane ionic concentration gradients.

charges moving to one side of the flow, negative charges to the other. This sets up an electrical potential difference proportional to flow velocity. Electromagnetic flowmeters to measure blood flow in vessels work on this principle.

If the ion finds itself in a position where drift and diffusion forces are exactly equal in magnitude and exactly opposite in direction, the forces cancel each other and the ion stops moving. The ion is still moving *randomly* by thermal agitation but with no *net* movement

48 /// GENERAL CONCEPTS

in any direction over time. This means that the diffusion gradient is exactly opposite in direction and equal in magnitude to the electrical gradient. In this position, the ion is said to be in *equilibrium;* it will stay in this position until there is unequal change in either the electrical or concentration gradient or both that creates a new net force on the ion.

IONIC EQUILIBRIA

Generally speaking there are the same number of cations and anions in the neighborhood (electroneutrality). If cations move to a less concentrated area by diffusion, an equal number of anions will accompany them to maintain electroneutrality. But assume now that a semipermeable barrier has been erected through which cations can pass but anions cannot. If cations move through this barrier to a less concentrated area, anions cannot follow and soon there will be surplus positive charge in the less concentrated area caused by the unaccompanied cations. There will be concomitant surplus negative charge on the other side of the barrier where there is a pile-up of anions left behind by the moving cations. As more and more cations move, there will be ever greater charge difference across the barrier, creating an ever growing electric field. The positive cations are attracted backward by the trapped negative anions. This attraction gets greater and greater as cation diffusion continues. A point is finally reached when the electrical attraction force pulling the cations back through the barrier (drift) exactly equals the diffusion force pushing the cations over to the less concentrated area. At this moment, ion flow stops and equilibrium exists.

The electrical field set up by the separation of even a small number of cation-anion pairs is quite intense. Thus, only very few cations have to cross the barrier unaccompanied by anions before equilibrium is established. (In heart cells, "very few" turns out to be roughly a 10^{-6} of 1% imbalance between cations and anions!) Potassium cations can pass relatively easily through the membrane. Most intracellular anions, particularly proteins,

cannot pass through the membrane. Thus, the equilibrium situation just described indeed takes place with the inside of the cell (having anion surplus), being negative in electrical potential with respect to the outside of the cell. With physical chemistry legerdemain one can show that the magnitude E_K of this electrical potential is proportional to the difference between the logarithm of inside potassium concentration $[K]_i$ and the (lesser) logarithm of outside concentration $[K]_o$.

$$E_K \propto \log [K]_i - \log [K]_o$$

At body temperature, the proportionality constant equals roughly -60 mv per log unit, hence

$$E_K = -60 \text{ mv} \times \log \frac{[K]_i}{[K]_o}$$

where the minus sign indicates that the inside negative with respect to outside. This equation is termed the *Nernst equation* and the equilibrium condition it describes between drift and diffusion is known as the *Nernst equilibrium.*

From Table 3-1, it can be seen that the intracellular concentration of potassium $[K]_i$ is 150 mmol/l and the extracellular potassium concentration $[K]_o$ is 4 mmol/l. Thus, one would expect to find the inside of a heart cell electrically negative with respect to the outside with a voltage difference of

$$E_K = -60 \text{ mv} \times \log \frac{150}{4}$$
$$\approx -90 \text{ mv}.$$

This is very close to that ordinarily observed if the cell is impaled with a microelectrode to measure the inside voltage. Note that an *increase* in extracellular potassium level (*e.g.,* hyperkalemia) or a *decrease* in intracellular potassium (*e.g.,* after hypothermic cardiac arrest) will *decrease* the magnitude of this transmembrane voltage. This can profoundly alter the sensitivity of the heart to electrical excitability.

SEMIPERMEABLE MEMBRANES

It is clear that only two conditions are necessary to create a Nernst equilibrium voltage: first, a semipermeable membrane through which one or more ions cannot pass; and second, a concentration difference between the two sides of the membrane for an ion that can, and thus will, move freely through the membrane. These two conditions are provided by heart cells. However, there are four additional properties that influence intracellular ion concentrations, and thus transmembrane voltage, in a clinically significant way.

1. The membrane is flexible and freely permeable to water; therefore, heart cells can shrink or swell slightly as water exits or enters. This property means that osmotic equilibrium exists between the inside and outside of cells. As water moves in, the intracellular concentrations (viz, potassium) are decreased; this dilution will typically decrease the transmembrane voltage.

2. The membrane is slightly permeable to sodium and calcium cations; their relatively high outside concentrations and the negative intracellular voltage both create driving forces that "leak" these ions into the cell. There is both a sodium pump and a calcium pump to "mop up" these leaks. Without these metabolically driven pumps in operation (*e.g.*, during hypothermic cardiac arrest), the sodium and calcium levels inside the cell will slowly rise. Every sodium ion that comes in allows a potassium ion to leak out without any net change in electrical charge (one charge in for one charge out). In time, potassium leaking out and sodium/calcium leaking in would destroy the cation concentration gradients across the membrane and the cell would cease to function electromechanically (*e.g.*, stone heart). If sodium leaks in faster than potassium leaks out, the typical situation, there will then be a net influx of ions; water following these ions into the cell to maintain osmotic equilibrium will cause the cell to swell temporarily (cardiac edema) unless osmotically active solute that cannot enter the cell is added to the extracellular milieu to "pull" water back out (*e.g.*, mannitol).

3. Glucose can enter heart cell, in the presence of the hormones insulin and epinephrine. This increases the solute level intracellularly and accordingly water enters the cell to maintain osmotic equilibrium. Water influx dilutes the intracellular potassium concentration. As shall be shown shortly, this decrease in $[K]_i$ stimulates a sodium-potassium exchange mechanism within the cell membrane (the sodium pump) to transport potassium ions from outside to inside the cell. The overall effect is that intracellular potassium content rises and the extracellular concentration falls. Simultaneous administration of insulin and glucose is a well-known clinical treatment for hyperkalemia. It is also an effective method to increase previously depleted intracellular potassium levels so long as supplemental potassium is given concurrently to prevent hypokalemia. (*e.g.*, cardioplegia solutions).

4. Finally, hydrogen ion can leak into the cell when extracellular acidosis occurs. In a manner comparable to a sodium leak, hydrogen ion influx allows potassium to leak out of the cell, one charge in for one charge out. As a consequence, the intracellular potassium level drops and extracellular potassium rises. Conversely, an extracellular alkalosis (low hydrogen ion concentration) causes hydrogen ions to leave the cell and be replaced by potassium ions entering the cell. In this case, intracellular potassium rises and extracellular potassium falls. This coordinated change of serum potassium concentration with blood pH means that the normal value of potassium depends entirely on the acid-base status of the patient.

One major conclusion should be apparent from the discussion so far. The ratio of intracellular to extracellular potassium level, and thus transmembrane voltage, is affected by multiple influences. These include acid-base balance, osmotically active solutes, metabolic activity and insulin/glucose levels. Therefore a simple determination of serum potassium level is a poor indicator of either intracellular potassium status and/or transmembrane electrical voltage, in the absence of a clinical history and other laboratory data.

HEART MUSCLE

CELL STRUCTURE

There is more to a cell than its membrane. There is a complexity of structure both within the cell and around the cell (Fig. 3-3). Heart cells are generally quite elongated and clustered tightly together in rope-like strands. Each cell generally makes an electrically conductive physical connection (a *nexus*) with two or more neighbors. The overall result is an electrical network, which conducts an electrical stimulus from cell to cell to cell.

Some cells (*e.g.*, Purkinje cells) are especially well configured for rapid electrical conduction (*e.g.*, large diameter, very tightly packed strands, low-resistance connections, relatively smooth membrane) and they form a network over the endocardium to distribute an electrical impulse rapidly (1–4 m/sec) throughout the ventricular muscle mass. Ordinary muscle fibers, whose chief role is mechanical contraction, conduct noticeably more slowly (0.3–0.4 m/sec) because they have deep transverse tube-like clefts (T-tubules) to conduct electrical stimuli deep within the cell. These clefts increase substantially the amount of membrane that must be excited electrically and thus slow down the rate of spread of an electrical impulse (see Figs. 3-3 and 3-4).

By contrast, certain other cells in the atrial junction portion of the atrioventricular node that conduct electrical impulses from the atrium to the His bundle and Purkinje network below are especially well configured for slow electrical conduction. They are small in diameter, have few high-resistance connections, and have a convoluted cell surface with disproportionately large membrane area. They have sluggish electrical excitability for reasons that are discussed. Conduction speed here is less than 0.1 m/second. As would be expected, most of the difficulty one might experience in successfully conducting an impulse from the sinus pacemaker to the ventricles occurs in the AV node region.

Despite these particular specializations for electrical conduction, all myocardial cells share certain common structures. The first is a cell membrane that exhibits *ion selectivity*, the name that electrophysiologists give to that property of semipermeable membranes which allows them to pass ions of a given element group in the periodic chemical table with greater or lesser facility ordered in a certain characteristic sequence. For example, there appear to be channels or pores through heart cell membranes which allow potassium ions to pass easily but through which sodium ions pass with great difficulty. That is, the potassium permeability (P_K) is far greater than the sodium permeability (P_{Na}), although *both* ions can in fact pass through this particular type of pore. If one tests *in vitro* salt solutions containing other so-called alkali metal ions, one discovers that *all* members of this periodic group (K, Rb, Cs, Na, and Li) will in fact pass through the membrane with the permeability sequence:

$$P_K > P_{Rb} > P_{Cs} > P_{Na} > P_{Li}.$$

This is the permeability sequence for a giant nerve fiber, where these experiments can be run relatively easily. The sequence for heart cells is probably the same.

The important point here is not the particular order of the sequence, but simply that there *is* a sequence. Some ions species pass through the membrane pores more easily than others of the same family, but they all can pass.

The exact mechanism by which the membrane effects this selectivity is unknown. One theory is that there are receptor sites (mouths of pores?) surrounded by a highly charged ring-like molecular structure through which cations fit with variable difficulty, depending on their radius, that is, the radius of the hydration cloud all cations drag along with them in solution. The visual image of a tube-like pore which passes spherical ions of one size selectively and largely rejects others is intuitively appealing. This is the graphic representation shown in Figure 3-4.

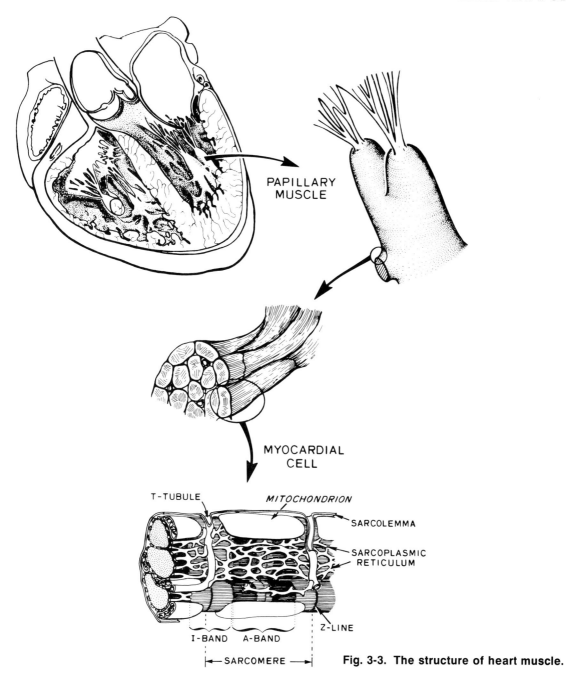

PAPILLARY
MUSCLE

MYOCARDIAL
CELL

T-TUBULE

MITOCHONDRION

SARCOLEMMA

SARCOPLASMIC
RETICULUM

Z-LINE

I-BAND   A-BAND

SARCOMERE

Fig. 3-3. The structure of heart muscle.

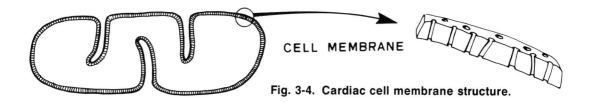

CELL MEMBRANE

Fig. 3-4. Cardiac cell membrane structure.

MEMBRANE CONDUCTANCE

There exist at least three types of cation channels or *pores* in the membrane: one that passes potassium ions, another that passes sodium ions, and a third that passes calcium ions. In fact, there may be several distinguishable types of potassium channels, all operative in parallel at different opening-closing rates during a heart beat. As shall be seen shortly, the sodium channel opens with lightning speed if the membrane voltage rises to a certain threshold point and thereby allows sodium ions to rush into the cell. But it quickly shuts off, restricting the sodium inrush to a brief burst. By contrast, the calcium channel opens slowly and closes slowly, allowing calcium ions to enter the cell as a slow inward current following the sodium burst.

Despite this confusing array of dynamic behavior, each ion channel obeys the laws of diffusion and drift. The law of diffusion is

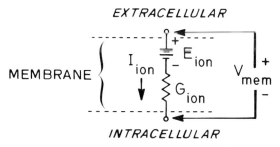

EXTRACELLULAR

MEMBRANE

INTRACELLULAR

Fig. 3-5. An electrical analog of the voltage-current relation across a cell membrane for a single ion. $I_{ion} \propto (V_{mem} - E_{ion})$

easy to obey. An extremely small number of ions actually passes through the membrane, a fraction too minute to have any detectable effect on either intracellular or extracellular concentrations of the ion. Thus the concentration gradient remains virtually constant and the diffusion force is constant.

The drift force, however, is directly related to the electrical voltage gradient across the membrane. As shown earlier, if this transmembrane voltage was made to exactly equal the Nernst equilibrium potential then drift force exactly canceled diffusion force and ion movement stopped dead. If the transmembrane voltage is increased even higher than the Nernst potential, thereby creating a more intense electric field, ions will flow backward, uphill against the concentration gradient but downhill with the more powerful electrical gradient. Drift force here is greater than the diffusion force. The greater the membrane voltage is increased over the Nernst equilibrium point, the proportionately greater will be this backward flow.

Conversely, if the membrane voltage is slightly less than the Nernst equilibrium potential, diffusion is still greater than drift and a trickle of forward ion flow continues. As the membrane voltage is made progressively less and less, the drift force resisting diffusion becomes less and less, hence the forward ion flow becomes proportionately greater and greater.

Flow of electrically charged ions constitutes an electrical current. As was just shown

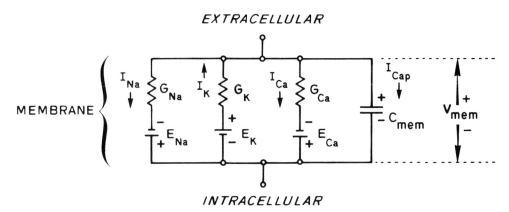

EXTRACELLULAR

MEMBRANE

INTRACELLULAR

Fig. 3-6. The electrical analog for multiple ions.

above, net membrane ionic current flow (I_{ion}) is proportional to the difference between the membrane voltage (V_{mem}) and the Nernst equilibrium potential for that type of ion (E_{ion}), that is,

$$I_{ion} \propto (V_{mem} - E_{ion})$$

Electrical engineers recognize that many electrical conductors behave in this manner; current flow is proportional to the voltage driving that current. This proportionality can be schematically represented therefore by an electrical conductance (G_{ion}) and a battery (E_{ion}) as shown in Figure 3-5. Algebraically, the proportionality constant is the value of the electrical conductance G_{ion}:

$$I_{ion} \triangleq G_{ion} (V_{mem} - E_{ion})$$

This is a nice shorthand representation of channels or pores. Every ion channel can be individually modeled as an electrical conductance through which that ion flows across the membrane. The value of each conductance *changes with time* during a heart beat. This change is closely related to the transmembrane voltage. If the battery-conductance pair for each ion is connected with the others, there is a good overall electrical model to describe the total ionic flow through heart cell membranes (Fig. 3-6).

An electrically equivalent model that combines all individual ion conductances into one equivalent conductance G_{eq} and all the Nernst batteries into one equivalent battery E_{eq} can be drawn for simplicity. Electrical engineers call this a *Thevenin equivalent circuit* (Fig. 3-7).

Note in passing the capacitor (C_{mem}). Capacitors store electrical charge (Q) proportional to the voltage (V) applied to them: $Q = C \times V$. In other words, C is the proportionality constant between the number of cations that are separated by diffusion from their anions to set up the *Nernst equilibrium* and the voltage across the membrane when the equilibrium is established. This is the *Nernst equilibrium potential.* The measured value of C_{mem} is approximately 10^{-6} farad/cm² of membrane area (1 farad $\triangleq$ 1 coulomb charge/1 volt potential).

Every time the voltage changes across the membrane (during an action potential, for example), the amount of stored charge Q on C_{mem} must change proportionately. It takes time to charge up or discharge C_{mem}; this limits the rate at which the membrane voltage (V_{mem}) can change. If a cell has a disproportionately large amount of surface membrane all convoluted and folded (i.e., large membrane capacitance), there will be a pronounced slowing down of electrical activity and the cell will require that a disproportionately large electrical charge be delivered to it by neighbors to stimulate activity. This is characteristic of cells in the atrial junction portion of the atrioventricular (AV) node and partially explains the slow conduction and high probability of blocked spread of the descending pacemaker impulse in that area.

If $Q = C \times V$, then, differentiating with respect to time, $\delta Q/\delta t = C \times \delta V/\delta t$. But, by definition, I (current flow; amperes) $\triangleq \delta Q/\delta t$ (coulombs per second). Thus the current (I_{cap}) charging the membrane capacitor (C_{mem}) is $I_{cap} = C_{mem} \times \delta V_{mem}/\delta t$. The faster one wants to change the membrane voltage, the greater the current required to charge C_{mem}. The current is limited by the speed of movement of ions in solution; thus there is a limit to the rate at which C_{mem} can be charged and a limit to the rate of change of membrane voltage.

Fig. 3-7. The simplified electrical analog for multiple ions.

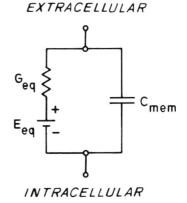

CELL-TO-CELL CONDUCTION

It was pointed out previously that heart cells make electrically conductive physical connections with their neighbors and in so doing create a large cell-to-cell network through which electrical stimuli can pass easily. This network property is unique to cardiac muscle and some smooth muscle (*e.g.,* uterus, gut) where electrical activity occurring in one part can automatically spread throughout, causing an accompanying wave of mechanical contraction. Thus, if one cell group contracts, the whole organ will normally contract (all-or-nothing behavior). Skeletal muscle cells, by contrast, do *not* make electrical connection with their neighbors. An electrical stimulation in one cell stays in that one cell.

To make a group of skeletal muscle cells contract, it is necessary to stimulate the nerve going to that group. Nerve endings on each individual cell will release transmitter substance to stimulate that individual cell. No nerves are needed to stimulate heart cells into contraction. The heart will beat even if removed from the body and virtually any piece of heart muscle can beat slowly by itself.

The cell-to-cell connection is termed a *nexus* (Latin: a bond or link). Its structure appears to be a circular fusion of membranes from adjoining cells with a honeycomb-like array in the center. Through this array can pass very small molecules from one cell to the other. Experiments show that large molecules cannot pass. The nexus conducts electrical current well because small ions pass unimpeded.

If the transmembrane voltage in one cell is greater (*e.g.,* 100mv) than the voltage in a neighboring cell (80 mv, for example), there is then a voltage difference across the nexus connecting them (here, 20 mv). This voltage difference will cause a current to flow (ions moving by drift in the electric field created) from the higher voltage to the lower voltage. Such a current tends to drain off the extra voltage in the first cell and charge up the second cell. Thus the 100 mv in the first will drop toward 90 mv and the voltage in the second will rise toward 90 mv. Current will stop flowing when there is no longer a voltage difference across the nexus. The speed with which this drain-off/charge-up process proceeds depends on the membrane capacitance in each cell and the small resistance to electrical flow offered by the nexus; the smaller the capacitance and the smaller this resistance, or both, the faster the speed with which the membrane voltages "relax" toward the equilibrium value of 90 mv.

The nexus connection represents an internal connection between cells through which current runs *intracellularly* from the membrane of one cell to the membrane of a second. To complete the electrical current, the current returns *extracellularly* from the membrane of the second cell to the first. Figure 3-8 illustrates this circular current flow around the electrical circuit. The extracellular return path has an extremely low electrical resistance because there is a relatively large amount of interstitial fluid around the cell and thus a large electrical conductor to carry the return current. The only exception is when cells are packed extremely tightly together (such as in a Purkinje fiber), excluding virtually all extracellular space between cells in the inner core. In this case, it is the outermost cells that carry much of the electrical activity. The effect is to make the fiber function like a very large diameter single cell; it conducts an electrical stimulus very quickly, analogous to the rapid conduction in a large diameter nerve fiber.

Conduction along a muscle strand from cell to cell is analogous to conduction along an electrical transmission cable. Using the simple conductance-battery model for each cell and connecting them with an intracellular current conduction path (R_i) through the nexus connections and an extracellular return conduction path (R_e), a circuit for the cable can be drawn as shown in Figure 3-9.

As shall be shown shortly, an electrical impulse in this cable is regenerated in each cell by the firing of an action potential. Without this regeneration, the impulse would die out within a millimeter or so along the cable unless an alternate regenerative pathway for electrical conduction around that area were

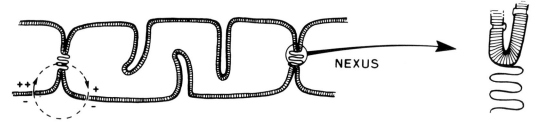

Fig. 3-8. The nexus connection between cells.

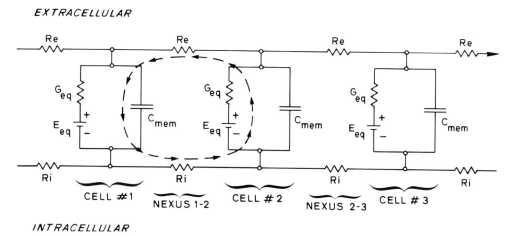

Fig. 3-9. An electrical cable analog for transmission of the action potential between cells.

stimulated. Alternate pathways are generally available in both the atria and ventricles since *every* muscle cell has the ability to conduct and regenerate an electrical impulse. Only within the AV node and bundle of His is there a shortage of alternative paths because of the relatively small total width (viz, 1 mm) of that pathway; this is another reason why the AV node is a common site for blockage of conduction.

If a sizeable piece of myocardium fails to function (*e.g.,* postinfarction), there can be a noticeable disturbance of the normal electrical conduction pattern as the impulse travels around this site. This is usually evident clinically by a change in the ECG, especially if the nonfunctioning area involved a major conduction path such as the interventricular septum or a large Purkinje bundle. Sequential changes will be seen as the nonfunction-

ing area continues to expand. However, once the infarcted area dies and becomes disconnected from the surrounding viable tissue, there should be no additional ECG changes.

There is an additional period of weeks until the dead myocardium is well replaced by scar. Until that time the infarction is mechanically weak and may stretch or rupture during ventricular contraction. A stable ECG is thus an unreliable indicator of the *mechanical* status of the infarction.

The process of cells dying is important clinically because this is the period of electrical instability, when arrhythmias and conduction defects are frequently life-threatening. If blood supply is cut off from a group of cells, no oxygen or nutrients arrive to support metabolism. As intracellular energy stores are depleted, the intracellular ion pumps that mop up sodium and calcium leaks run out of fuel and stop. Potassium leaks out; sodium and calcium leak into the cell. The transmembrane voltage decreases and eventually becomes zero, making it impossible for the cell to regenerate an incoming impulse with an action potential. As the calcium level rises the cell contracts for reasons about to be explained. But, more importantly, the high internal calcium level seals off the electrical connection of the nexus so that there is no longer an electrical conduction path to the adjoining cells.

The mechanism by which high calcium levels ($> 10^{-5}$ mmol/l) cause nexus disconnection is unknown but is literally life-saving. Until the dying cells are electrically disconnected from the adjoining normal tissue, they act as a current drain on the good cells. This drain increases as the membrane voltage on the dying cells decreases. The Nernst "batteries" in the good cells try without success to charge the dying cells by passing current through the nexus. Unless the nexus connection is broken, this drain would eventually exhaust the good cells and they too would die. This process would eventually kill a much larger area than the original infarction. In sealing off the nexus connections, the rising calcium levels in the dying cells literally seal their own doom but in so doing save their neighbors. The final common irreversible pathway to cell death, for all types of cells studied, is a rising intracellular calcium level.

There is a therapeutic moral to this story. When a cell is well supplied with oxygen and nutrients and the mop-up ion pumps are functioning well, raising intracellular calcium slightly (for example, by administering intravenous calcium chloride) makes the cells contract more strongly. This generally raises cardiac output slightly which in turn usually improves myocardial perfusion. If the cells were marginally perfused initially, this action can dramatically improve cardiac function, at least temporarily. On the other hand, this same calcium chloride tonic can be lethal if administered to a cell whose mop-up pumps are not working, for example, in a cold standstill heart. If the heart shows regular *electrical* activity (indicating reasonably good membrane voltages and functioning ion pumps), calcium can probably be administered safely to improve *mechanical* contractility. But if the heart does not have a regular electrical beat, one should beware of administering calcium. It can make matters worse by killing possibly viable cells. The general rule for resuscitation of the heart is to establish a good *electrical* rhythm first; *then* try to improve mechanical contraction. Good coronary artery perfusion is required for both. This should be ensured at the outset by cardiac massage, open or closed chest, depending on the situation. If in doubt, one should massage until a good *steady* electrical rhythm is established. Massage can do little harm and much good.

ACTION POTENTIALS

It was noted earlier that various ion channels in the cell membrane open and close during a heart beat and, moreover, that this behavior can be described as variations in electrical conductances. Recall, too, that both sodium and calcium ions want to enter the cell, forced by diffusion and drift. And when the cell is at rest, recall that potassium is nearly at Nernst equilibrium; the diffusion force that pushes potassium ions out of the cell is essentially balanced by drift force pulling them back. This situation prevails when the heart is temporarily at rest, relaxed, in diastole. Thus the *resting potential* for the membrane voltage is nearly equal to the Nernst equilibrium voltage.

For reasons not understood, the potassium conductance in atrial heart cells slowly starts to decrease while in this state. That is, the potassium channel starts to close. This process is accelerated by β-catecholamines (*e.g.*, epinephrine, isoproterenol, ephedrine) and slowed by acetylcholine.

Acetylcholine in fact increases the potassium conductance substantially. Therefore it takes much longer for the closing-off process to reduce the conductance to the point where an action potential starts. Other choline drugs, such as the muscle relaxant succinylcholine, can have a similar slowing effect in large doses.

As the potassium conductance (G_K) shuts

off, sodium continues to leak in, bringing positive charge into the cell. This positive charge influx makes the transmembrane voltage drift up positively from the −80 mv resting potential, while the ever-shrinking potassium conductance makes the Nernst equilibrium for potassium progressively less a determinant of membrane voltage.

As the membrane voltage rises to −65 mv, an exceedingly interesting phenomenon is observed: the sodium conductance (G_{Na}) starts to *increase* (i.e., the sodium channel opens up further). This allows sodium to flow into the cell more easily and makes the membrane voltage rise more quickly. It appears that the sodium conductance is exquisitely sensitive to the membrane voltage, increasing dramatically as the membrane voltage goes above −65 mv, the threshold for this behavior.

This can be demonstrated by voltage-clamp experiments in which the membrane voltage is electronically measured and precisely controlled to follow a prescribed voltage pattern. The current required to hold the membrane at the prescribed voltage is exactly equal to the membrane current. When the membrane voltage is stepped from resting potential to −65 mv the first trace of a sodium inward current is seen. As steps are made from resting potential to −60 mv and higher, this current increases very quickly, so quickly that electronic control is frequently difficult.

The result is clear; an explosive burst of sodium enters the cell through a conductance that becomes extremely high as the transmembrane voltage shoots up to approximately 20 mv or more. If no other ion conductances had influence, the membrane voltage would approach 60 mv, the Nernst equilibrium potential for sodium.* Two things prevent this from happening.

First of all, the sodium channel shuts off nearly as quickly as it turns on. If only this shutoff occurred, the membrane voltage would not change drastically from the 20 mv

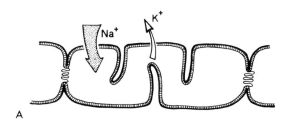
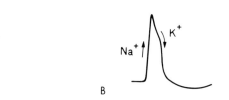

Fig. 3-10. A, B. The action potential.

region; the positive charges on the membrane capacitor would hold the voltage at this level. But a second action occurs; the potassium channel turns back on slowly. This permits a few positive charges (potassium) to leave the cell, thus discharging the membrane capacitor. The potassium conductance continues to grow and the cell thus returns to its beginning state, with a resting potential near the Nernst equilibrium for potassium. The membrane voltage has made a full cycle, shooting up positively from the resting potential as the sodium burst rushes in, then sliding back as the potassium conductance turns back on, allowing the positive charge brought in by the sodium to leave again as an equivalent number of potassium ions leak out (Fig. 3-10). This whole cycle, up and back, which generates an electrical pulse, is called an *action potential*.

In a short time, the potassium conductance will once again start to decrease, beginning another cycle, another heartbeat. Once again, β-catecholamine will speed up this decrease and acetylcholine will delay this decrease. Thus it is clear that catecholamine will shorten the interval between heartbeats and thereby increase the heart rate. Conversely acetylcholine will increase the interval and thus slow the heart rate.

Very rapid heart rates are possible (150–200/minute) when circulating β-catechola-

$$*E_{Na} = 60 \text{ mv} \times \log ([Na]_o/[Na]_i)$$
$$= 60 \text{ mv} \times \log (140 \text{ mmol}/14\text{mmol})$$
$$= 60 \text{ mv} \times \log 10$$
$$= 60 \text{ mv}$$

mine levels are high, either from endogenous (epinephrine during fight/flight response) or exogenous (intravenous inotropic support) sources.

The diastolic resting period becomes very short indeed. Unfortunately, it is only during this diastolic interval, when the myocardium relaxes, that the coronary vessels are perfused. Thus the blood supply to the heart is compromised and it is understandable that angina can develop in this situation. But catecholamines have another effect which helps compensate for this problem: they increase the rate at which the potassium channel turns on again to bring the membrane voltage back to resting potential after the sodium burst. Thus in addition to increasing heart rate, catecholamines shorten the duration of the action potential and systole. This tends to keep the ratio of diastolic coronary perfusion time to systolic contraction time more evenly matched over a wide range of heart rates. As shall be seen shortly, β-catecholamine has another important effect: to increase the calcium flow into the cell during this shortened systole. This calcium increases the contractile force of the heart even though the duration of force (because systole is shorter) is less. Thus the work output of the heart (contractile force × contractions per minute) increases substantially in the presence of catecholamine.

Acetylcholine increases the potassium conductance. Thus it not only slows the diastolic phase of the heart beat, but also shortens the systolic phase because with an increased potassium conductance the return to resting potential is faster after the sodium burst. Acetylcholine cannot be administered intravenously because the cholinesterase in the blood stream breaks it down immediately. But it can be given indirectly; vagal nerve stimulation, such as with carotid sinus massage, causes acetylcholine to be released from the nerve endings onto the sinus node, the portion of the heart that sets the rate for the rest to follow. Effective vagal stimulation can slow the heart noticeably. An alternative method is to administer a cholinesterase inhibitor such as edrophonium. This allows acetylcholine to build up with normal activity

at the vagal nerve endings, without being destroyed, and thereby slows the heart rate.

The reverse is also true. Drugs that block the effects of β-catecholamines (*e.g.,* propranolol) slow heart rate and lengthen the action potential duration and systole. Drugs that block the effect of acetylcholine (*e.g.,* atropine) speed the heart rate and lengthen the action potential. Note that unlike catecholamines, atropine increases the heart rate without a compensatory shortening of systole. The diastolic perfusion time is measurably shorter for a given heart rate after atropine administration than after catecholamine administration. This means that blood supply to the heart can be unduly compromised. Angina during atropine-caused tachycardia is frequently seen in coronary patients. This difference between atropine and β-catecholamine for treatment of bradycardia should be kept in mind, particularly for coronary patients.

SPECIFIC IONS

SODIUM PUMP

Each action potential produces a minute increase in intercellular sodium content and a correspondingly minute loss of intercellular potassium content. The change in ionic concentration with one action potential is far too small to measure. However, after several thousand action potentials there would be a noticeable reduction in $[K]_i$, which would lower the Nernst equilibrium potential and thus the transmembrane resting potential. If the process continued, eventually no action potential would fire even if the cell were electrically stimulated quite vigorously. Why?

The explosive turning on of the sodium conductance depends upon the membrane voltage. Roughly speaking, the more negative the resting potential, the faster the sodium conductance turns on. The less negative the resting potential, the more sluggish will be the turn-on of sodium conductance. Because either a decrease in $[K]_i$ and an increase in $[K]_o$ or both will lower the Nernst equilibrium potential (and resting potential), these conditions make the turn-on of G_{Na} very sluggish. Indeed, if the resting potential rises above the sodium threshold voltage (about -65mv), no action potential at all can be elicited.

There is a relatively narrow voltage range below the sodium threshold (-70mv) where the sodium conductance can still fire, albeit sluggishly, and where the magnitude of stimulus (5 mv) to reach threshold is small. In this region, the cell is hypersensitive to any disturbance and ectopic generation of action potentials in this area is probable and potentially lethal. This is the cause of ectopic beats seen briefly after myocardial infarction before the dying cells with low resting potentials are sealed off from good tissue.

By good fortune, there is a molecular mechanism, the sodium pump, within the cell membrane that effectively pumps *out* of the cell sodium which has come in from action potentials and simultaneously pumps back *in* to the cell potassium roughly equal to the amount that left (Fig. 3-11). This pump restores the transmembrane concentration gradients for potassium (thereby restoring the resting potential) and sodium back to original levels. It requires energy to run because it has to push each ion against its concentration gradient. The ATPase enzyme in this exchange pump is sensitive to intracellular sodium and extracellular potassium; an increase in either will activate the enzyme and make the pump run faster. There is some evidence that if $[Na]_i$ activates the pump, slightly more sodium will be carried out per potassium ion in the cell than is normally found. If $[K]_o$ is the activating factor, the pump carries more potassium in per sodium ion out than the normal (see Fig. 3-11).

If precisely one sodium ion goes out for each potassium ion in there is no net change in electrical charge within the cell. Any deviation from this 1:1 ratio will cause a change in electrical charge and thus a change in the membrane voltage. There are several ways to reversibly turn off this pump experimentally (*e.g.*, hypothermia, glycosides). All seem to cause a small concomitant reduction in resting potential. This implies that operation of the sodium pump augments the resting potential and suggests that there is not a 1:1 exchange ratio, but rather that more positive charge (sodium) is pumped out of the cell than is pumped in (potassium). The normal ratio seems to be more likely 3:2 (sodium out:potassium in) with deviations depending on whether intracellular sodium or extracellular potassium is the dominant activating factor.

Notice especially that glycosides (*e.g.*, digitalis) make the sodium pump run slower whereas elevated extracellular potassium makes the pump run faster. In other words, high blood potassium levels antagonize the effect of digitalis. This is well-known clinically. Partial inhibition of the sodium pump is the basic mechanism by which digitalis renders its clinical effects, both beneficial (increased contractility, decreased AV conduction) and detrimental (ectopic beats and electrical irritability).

Partial inhibition of the sodium pump means that the intracellular concentration of sodium will be abnormally high and that of potassium abnormally low. It should be remembered that the lowered resting potential associated with low $[K]_i$ slows excitation of the sodium conductance. Under these conditions, the AV node, which is normally slow and hard to stimulate, responds poorly to a rapid atrial input of action potentials. At best,

Fig. 3-11. The sodium pump.

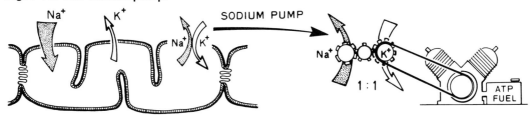

it may generate an action potential every other atrial impulse, or perhaps every third impulse, depending on the atrial rate. The rest of the atrial impulses are effectively blocked from reaching the ventricles. The greater the digitalis level, the lower the resting potential, the less responsive the AV node, and the slower the ventricular response to a high atrial rate.

Also, if the resting potential is reduced, the voltage difference between resting potential and excitation threshold for G_{Na} is smaller; thus the self-cycling pacemaker cells in the atrium spend less time in diastole before starting a new cycle, increasing the cycling rate. Episodes of atrial tachycardia are commonly seen with high digitalis doses. Atrial tachycardia with AV block is the mark of excessive digitalis. Low resting potentials cause ectopic beats and hypersensitivity to stimulation (irritability) after myocardial infarction; low resting potentials from excessive digitalis inhibition of the sodium pump cause the same ectopic beats and irritability.

The well-known electrical effects of digitalis can be explained on the basis of the digitalis-produced decreased intracellular *potassium* level. However, the mechanical effect, increased contractility, is caused by the digitalis-produced increased intracellular *sodium* level. There are anionic binding sites on the intracellular side of the cell membrane that attract both calcium and sodium cations, which mutually compete to occupy these sites. Under normal conditions the majority of sites are occupied by calcium. However, when the intracellular sodium level rises after digitalis administration, sodium ions displace some of the calcium ions from membrane binding. This increase in cytoplasmic calcium level leads, as will be shown shortly, to greater contractile force. Thus, despite its electrical perils, digitalis is a clinically useful way to augment contractility and cardiac output.

CALCIUM INFLUX

There is one more ion to consider in addition to sodium and potassium: calcium, the ion species directly responsible for activating mechanical contraction. Calcium also has some prominent electrical effects, both direct (caused by the flow of calcium itself) and indirect (caused by calcium's influence on the flow of sodium and potassium). Indeed it is these indirect influences on other ions that makes experimental elucidation of calcium action difficult at best. Only sodium and potassium are involved in the action potentials of nerves; moreover the flow of each is entirely independent of the other. This is the so-called *independence principle* that permits the concentration and flow of each ion species to be manipulated without fear that the flow of the other ion will be influenced. Obviously this simplifies sorting out the behavior of each ion, and was an insight that led Hodgkin and Huxley to Nobel prize-winning experiments defining exactly how a nerve action potential takes place.

The fact that ions interact and influence each other in muscle, as well as the vastly increased multicellular architectural complexity in muscle, makes sorting out such matters much less straightforward in muscle than in nerve. As a result, what is presented here cannot be considered fact, but only a "best-guess," synthesized from informed sources that is probably 90 percent correct. (If only we knew *which* 10% were in error!)

Starting with direct flows of calcium, there is a "family resemblance" between sodium and calcium. Both are cations with high extracellular concentrations, both trying to get into the cell, both being forced by diffusion and drift, and both competing for the same internal membrane sites. It should not seem surprising therefore that the calcium conductance behaves similarly to the sodium conductance; there is a threshold voltage (-20 mv) at which the calcium conductance will turn on and allow calcium to rush into the cell. This calcium conductance, like G_{Na}, is voltage sensitive; the more positive the membrane voltage rises above threshold the greater the conductance and the faster the calcium inrush.

Perhaps "rush in" would be better termed "stroll in." The calcium channel turns on and off much more slowly than the lightning-fast sodium channel, and peak calcium current flow is noticeably less than the rapid sodium current. Nevertheless, the total amount of charge brought into the cell by the slow inward calcium current[7, 8] is comparable to the amount brought in by the rapid sodium current. The calcium inflow is more spread out during the action potential. The effect of this slow inward current is to create a plateau on the top of the action potential, extending until the potassium efflux (which eventually will take the cell back to resting potential) grows great enough to exceed the calcium influx. At this point, the membrane voltage starts down from the plateau fairly rapidly. The transition from plateau back to resting potential can be sharp because the slow calcium conductance is turning off at the same time that the slower potassium conductance is turning on. Two slows can make a fast. The result is that an action potential in heart muscle where the calcium influx is relatively high (*i.e.,* ventricle) has a somewhat "boxy" look: extremely fast upstroke (*phase 0*) caused by brief sodium inrush; a flatter plateau (*phase 2*) caused by the slow action calcium inward current; and then a moderately quick slide back to resting potential (*phase 3*) as the slow inward current turns off and simultaneously the repolarizing outward potassium current turns on.

Most of the slow inward current is calcium. There may be some sodium coming in through this slow channel. Experiments indicate that the slow channel has less selectivity between ions than the rapid channel, which is quite selective for sodium compared

to calcium. Apparently lithium can also travel through the rapid channel, but even at the high lithium blood levels therapeutically achieved in psychiatric patients, there is no noticeable clinical effect on the heart.

Oftentimes the rapid sodium inrush is completely finished before the slower calcium inward current gets underway. This results in a slight positive overshoot (*phase 1*) before the plateau starts (Fig. 3-12).

There exist a number of pharmacologic agents that can block the rapid and slow channels individually. These have proven useful tools to electrophysiologists trying to sort out the individual ion currents. Some of these agents are used clinically. Local anesthetics (procaine, for example) tend to make the sodium conductance less sensitive and harder to turn on at its threshold voltage. The effect is to reduce irritability. Procainamide and xylocaine are the two most common drugs of this local anesthetic type used clinically for treatment of cardiac irritability.

Similarly there are drugs that block the slow inward current without any effect on the rapid sodium inrush. These include verapamil and nifedipine,[9, 10] both introduced relatively recently to clinical practice (see Chap. 26). The net effect is to block the calcium inward current and thereby largely inhibit contraction, especially in vascular smooth muscle cells. In these cells, there is little if any sodium inrush; all the inward current is carried by calcium, although the outward current is still potassium. The action potentials in such cells are slow but associated with a mechanical contraction. Blocking

Fig. 3-12. The influence of calcium on the action potential.

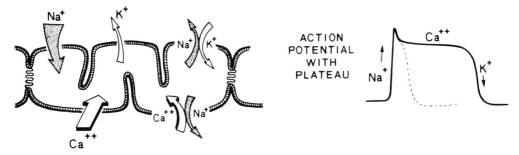

the slow inward current with verapamil stops these slow action potentials and corresponding contractions if the dose is high enough. Coronary artery vascular smooth muscle (among others) appears to operate on this slow action potential mechanism and can develop a significant maintained contraction (a spasm), which may lethally reduce blood flow to the myocardium. Treatment with slow inward current blockers can offer life-saving relief from angina in this situation.

Some older frequently used drugs also partially block the calcium slow inward current by reducing calcium conductance (G_{Ca}). These include both thiopental[11] and halothane,[12] high doses of which cause well-known drops in contractility and peripheral vascular resistance and occasionally AV block, all predominantly the effect of reduced calcium inflow to the cells. These effects may be desirable or undesirable, depending on the clinical situation. In general they can be reversed, at least temporarily, by intravenous bolus administration of calcium chloride (5–10 mg/kg).

The sluggish cells in the AV node also have this characteristic: a meager sodium inrush and primary dependence on the calcium slow inward current to initiate an action potential. This explains the relative sluggishness with which AV node cells operate. It also explains why local anesthetics (*e.g.*, xylocaine) that retard rapid sodium currents have little effect on AV conduction. AV block, however, is a real risk of treatment with verapamil or comparable calcium-blocking drugs. And calcium administration can encourage AV conduction for better (improve high-grade heart block) or for worse (increase ventricular rate in atrial fibrillation).

Increasing extracellular calcium concentration increases calcium's slow inward current by augmenting the diffusion force driving calcium into the cell. Another way to increase the calcium slow inward current without changing the concentration gradient is by increasing the G_{Ca}. Catecholamines do exactly this. They increase G_{Ca} so that more calcium flows into the cell at any given extracellular calcium level. Both catecholamines and aug-

mented extracellular calcium increase the *rate* of inflow, not the duration.

In fact, catecholamine shortens the action potential by increasing the repolarizing potassium conductance. This shortens the *phase 2* plateau and in effect shortens the duration of the slow inward current slightly. As discussed below, enhanced calcium influx itself shortens the action potential.

Thus administration of either β-catecholamine or calcium ion enhances the action potential upstroke and conduction in the AV node. Their use together is rational therapy for heart block.

One should stress the word *together.*[13] Catecholamine augments the diffusion flow inward from whatever extracellular calcium concentration exists. However, if the extracellular calcium concentration is extremely low (typically iatrogenic) then there is almost nothing to augment. The administration of catecholamine in the presence of severe hypocalcemia will still accelerate heart rate and shorten systole (potassium conductance effects), but will not significantly improve contractility or AV conduction (calcium conductance effects). To achieve the latter requires concurrent administration of calcium ion.

Most calcium carried in the blood stream is bound to albumin. There is comparatively little ionized calcium (the active form for cellular use). If a large bolus injection of deionized albumin (salt-poor albumin) is suddenly administered intravenously, there is a measurable reduction in ionized calcium as it binds to the new albumin. A similar effect occurs with massive transfusions of citrated blood. Both can cause a drop in cardiac contractility and blood pressure. Concurrent administration of sufficient calcium ion avoids this drop.

So much for the direct flows of calcium into the cell. Calcium also affects the flows of sodium and potassium. As was previously noted, calcium and sodium compete for internal binding sites on the cell membrane. It also appears that there is an exchange mechanism by which (in a manner reminiscent of the sodium-potassium exchange pump) sodium is exchanged on a 2:1 equal-charge basis for calcium, sodium leaving the cell and calcium entering. The details of this exchange are unsettled and it is difficult to measure electrically because equal charge is swapped. But it does represent an interactive flow in which the extracellular level of calcium directly affects a flow of sodium out of the cell.

Calcium also affects the flow of sodium into the cell. In a poorly understood manner (that is to say, experimentally observed but theoretically obscure), high levels of extracellular calcium make the sodium conductance less sluggish when G_{Na} turns on. Calcium seems to sharpen the distinction between G_{Na} being shut off and being full on. The effect is to make the turn-on of G_{Na} a more sensitive function of membrane voltage. Thus cells having a hard time firing because, for example, their resting potentials are high and G_{Na} is consequently sluggish can typically be made to fire more easily by the administration of calcium, which improves the briskness of the action potential upstroke.

On the other hand, it is *intracellular* calcium that affects potassium flows. In recent years, it has been shown that increasing intracellular calcium levels increase the repolarizing potassium conductance and consequently raise both the magnitude and rate at which potassium flows out to end the action potential. The net effect is to shorten the duration of the action potential. This is unexpected; increase extracellular calcium increases the magnitude of the slow inward current and thereby the height of the plateau. One would expect that keeping the plateau up would, if anything, prolong the action potential. Thus for years it has seemed a paradox that administration of calcium substantially *shortened* the action potential. Clinically this is recognized as a shorter QT interval on the ECG when serum calcium is elevated. But the reason is now clear: increased extracellular calcium increases the calcium influx, which increases the intracellular calcium level, which increases G_K, which increases the repolarizing potassium efflux, which increases the speed with which the membrane voltage returns to resting potential, which shortens the action potential. Note the synergism here

with β-catecholamines, which independently increase G_K and shorten the action potential and which also increase G_{Ca} and calcium influx. This calcium influx raises the intracellular calcium level, which in turn shortens the action potential even further by the aforementioned effect on G_K. Clinically this is quite apparent. Administration of calcium and β-catecholamine together produces a very short systole and QT interval.

CALCIUM EFFLUX

A substantial beat-by-beat flow of calcium into the cell has been described. How, in turn, does calcium leave the cell? The truth is that much of it doesn't, but in fact is stored within the cell, either on internal membranes, in the sarcoplasmic reticulum (SR), or in the mitochondria.

The mitochondria have a huge *passive* calcium storage capacity. Mitochondria load or unload calcium stores very slowly. Thus, while they play a role in the long-term internal cellular level, they play no role on a beat-by-beat time scale.

The SR is at the other extreme. This system also has a substantial calcium storage capacity (probably less than mitochondria, however) where the calcium is stored at very high concentrations (about 10^{-1} M) until it is needed on the next beat. There are pumps in the wall of the SR that are voracious in their ability to gather up calcium from the cytoplasm and pump it up an extreme gradient to the internal storage. These pumps will bring the intracellular calcium concentration down from approximately 10^{-5} M (the peak level during contraction) to the resting neighborhood of 10^{-7} M. These are the most powerful ionic pumps in the human body, in terms of the high concentration gradient against which they pump effectively. They consume enormous energy; well over half the energy consumption of the heart goes to fuel these pumps. In other words, the majority of the heart's energy supply is consumed in *relaxing* the heart, bringing the internal calcium concentration down from 10^{-5} to 10^{-7} M. This explains why a heart which is short of

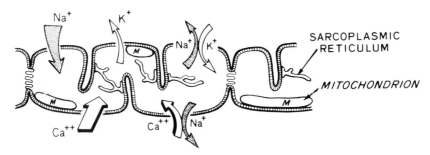

Fig. 3-13. Calcium movement and storage within the cell.

energy stores and is thus unable to adequately power this SR calcium pump, dies in hard contraction (stone heart) with extremely high intracellular calcium levels.

Finally there is cell membrane storage. This is a relatively small amount, certainly insufficient to raise the cytoplasmic calcium level to the 10^{-5} M full contraction levels. Nevertheless there is growing evidence that calcium released from the surface membrane or coming through the membrane, or both, during the action potential is a trigger (mechanism unclear) that causes the full amount needed for contraction to be released somehow by the SR (mechanism also unclear). This is an active area of research that hopefully will provide answers in the next few years. There is a consensus, though, that (1) contraction cannot take place unless some calcium comes in through the membrane, (2) this surface-originating calcium is insufficient for full contraction, and (3) the SR is the most likely source for the remainder required. These mechanisms are summarized in Figure 3-13.

Equally unclear is where, when, and how calcium actually leaves the cell—perhaps by ion exchange at the membrane or perhaps diffusing down the transverse tubules delivered there by the connecting SR. It is obviously not important on a beat-by-beat basis but it is intriguing; it must go out somewhere.

Parenthetically, xanthines (*e.g.,* caffeine, aminophyllin, theophyllin) partially poison the SR calcium pump and thereby cause the intracellular calcium to rise. This leads to increased contractility and increased cardiac output. This is why the heart beats more strongly after that second cup of coffee. (See references 7–13 for further reading.)

CONTRACTION

Pause for a moment to look back over the discussion so far. It began with drift and diffusion and is now at the point where the intracellular calcium concentration is cycling up and down. Crudely speaking, the role of the cell membrane is to generate a steady train of action potentials; the role of the action potential is to turn on and off the channel through which calcium enters the cell as a pulse. The role of the sodium pump in the cell membrane and the calcium pump in the SR is to mop up the mess and restore things to order. Finally, the way in which an increased level of intracellular calcium makes the cell contract must be determined.

Consider the part of the cell that performs the contraction, namely, the myofibrils. These are organized into sarcomeres, small motor units, each of which contract, connected end to end like links in a chain. Many such chains (of varying length) may be in one cell, running from one end to the other. As the sarcomere "links" contract, the chains contract and the cell contracts.

Each sarcomere is constructed of numerous thin, longitudinal strands (actin proteins) interdigitating with thicker strands (myosin proteins). Actin and myosin have great mutual attraction, and, left together, they form crossbridges that fuse the two strands together into a conglomerate actomyosin.

In heart muscle, there is some overlap of

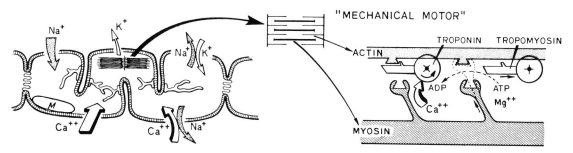

Fig. 3-14. The mechanisms of contraction.

the actin and myosin strands. The overlap region understandably appears more dense when viewed in the microscope. This dense region has been termed the *A-band*. The non-overlapped region is called the *I-band*. The partition between sarcomeres to which the actin strands attach is called the *Z-line* (see Fig. 3-3).

When actin and myosin form crossbridges they slide together to maximize their overlap, virtually eliminating the I-band. This sliding together is what shortens the sarcomere length (distance between Z-lines) and thus collectively, if all sarcomeres shorten together, contracts the cell.

There are two additional proteins, however, intermingled with the actin and myosin strands: tropomyosin and a complex called troponin. Tropomyosin inhibits the crossbridge formation between actin and myosin. Troponin, which is attached to tropomyosin, can prevent this inhibition if, and only if, calcium ions are bound to a certain part of the troponin complex. Thus, if calcium ions are freely available to the myofibrils, they bind to troponin, which in turn releases the inhibition that tropomyosin has been imposing an actin to prevent crossbridge formation with myosin. With this inhibition gone, crossbridges are formed and contraction occurs. In brief, applying calcium ions to the myofibrils causes contraction; removing calcium causes relaxation (Fig. 3-14). The process is entirely reversible: more calcium, more contraction; less calcium, less contraction. Nothing can go wrong.

Well, almost nothing. The crossbridge for-

mation is the active part of the process, where energy is required. On the end of the myosin crossbridge is an ATPase that splits ATP to provide the energy. This enzyme critically requires magnesium. Thus both ATP and magnesium must be present for contraction. For reasons not understood, halothane (and undoubtedly other halogenated anesthetics) seems to partially interfere with this crossbridge formation process, in addition to its membrane effects reducing G_{Ca}. Both actions depress contractility, explaining the substantial negative inotropic effect of halothane on the heart. Conversely, both actions can be counteracted by administering intravenous calcium.

Administration of magnesium is rational therapy when all else fails to establish satisfactory contraction (*e.g.*, normothermia, adequate coronary perfusion, catecholamine, normocalcemia), especially if there has been massive blood/fluid replacement that has depleted serum magnesium (see Chap. 14).

Because sarcomeres are like links in a chain, all must contract in order for the chain to contract. If only some contract, they will pull out to full extension those others in the chain that are still relaxed and, as a result, little or no overall chain contraction will occur. A similar argument holds for cells. All the cells must contract *together* in order for the heart muscle as a whole to contract. This is why cell-to-cell action potential conduction through the entire heart is critical; all cells must beat synchronously.

A serious nonsynchrony is ventricular fibrillation. Here most, if not all, cells are firing and contracting, but they are doing so quite asynchronously. Consumption of ATP continues in crossbridge formation, but without synchrony there is no effective pumping of blood and no perfusion of the heart. High consumption with no energy supply is lethal unless terminated quickly by countershock. Note that countershock essentially causes all cells to first depolarize and then contract simultaneously, stimulated by the large current passing through each cell. All cells then repolarize to resting potential at their own characteristic rate. The first cell that spontaneously develops an action potential triggers the cell-to-cell network and the heart contracts synchronously once again. Generally, and hopefully, that first spontaneous cell is from the sinus node and normal sinus rhythm will ensue. But there are no guarantees. Several attempts at countershock may be necessary as well as treatment (*e.g.,* xylocaine) to suppress spontaneous action potentials from other parts of the heart.

A final observation: anything that increases intracellular calcium level increases contraction; anything that decreases intracellular calcium causes relaxation. There are two ways to raise intracellular calcium: increase the influx (*e.g.,* catecholamines) or decrease the intracellular binding (*e.g.,* digitalis). Conversely, there are two ways to lower intracellular calcium: decrease the influx (*e.g.,* verapamil) or increase intracellular capture (*e.g.,* optimize metabolic conditions for SR pumping). The maximum pulse pressure occurs when there is the widest swing in intracellular calcium level during a single beat. This requires that influx be maximized for maximum contraction at the same time that mop-up is maximized for maximum relaxation. In practical terms, influx is maximized when both catecholamine and calcium are administered simultaneously (*e.g.,* combination epinephrine + calcium drip) and relaxation is maximized when the SR pumps are optimally tuned (*e.g.,* normothermia, excellent coronary perfusion, and with ample oxygen and metabolic substrates).

One last maneuver to maximize cardiac output is to maximize the efficiency of mechanical coupling from sarcomeres (contrac-

tile source) to ejected blood (final output). This is done by optimizing the length of the muscle fibers during contraction, which is accomplished by adjusting the intraventricular blood volume at end diastole. Such adjustment can be made by transfusion, to increase volume, or venodilation, to reduce volume. The optimal point is where all sarcomeres in all cells and all cells in all muscles are stretched out at end diastole so they can develop full contraction force.

If heart muscle is examined microscopically under contraction with a light load, one sees that the cells are not all aligned perfectly longitudinally, but rather have a wavy serpentine appearance. Contraction in this wavy condition causes some straightening out, but until all cells are aligned there are nonlongitudinal (transverse) forces developed which are not transmitted to the ends of the muscle and thus contribute to inefficiency. Increasing the load on the muscle stretches out the waviness. The optimal point is the minimum load where all waviness just disappears. Overstretching the muscle cells beyond this point causes progressively more sarcomeres to become overextended to the point where there becomes inadequate overlap of actin and myosin strands to develop maximum crossbridge force. Any stretch beyond this point is accompanied by progressively less peak force capability.

In clinical practice, this phenomenon is evidenced by progressively higher peak contraction forces as intraventricular filling volume is increased until a maximum is reached beyond which force decreases with increased volume. This proportional relationship between peak developed force and filling volume is called the Frank-Starling Law in honor of two independent observers of this behavior. The peak of the Frank-Starling curve is the end diastolic filling volume that just stretches the cells and sarcomeres to optimal length. This is *the most efficient operating point for the heart.* Thus to the list of ways to effectively maximize cardiac output, both transfusion and vasodilators can be added. They are used to adjust end diastolic filling volume and thereby optimize mechanical coupling efficiency (see Chap. 2).

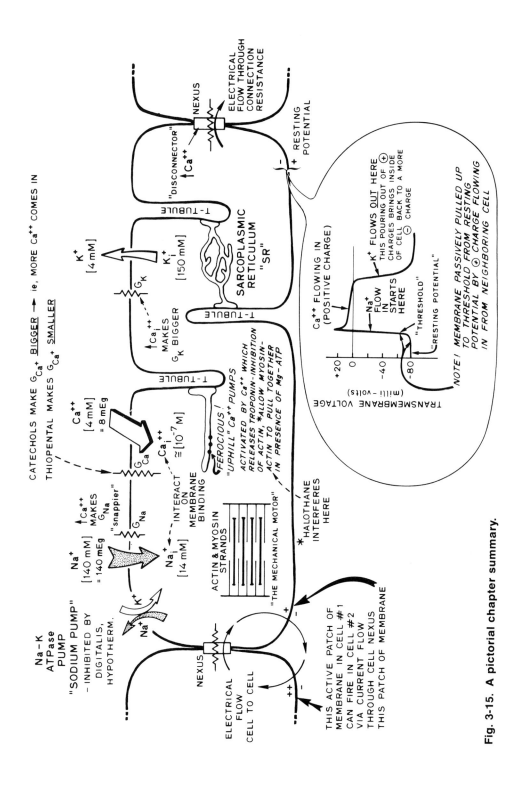

Fig. 3-15. A pictorial chapter summary.

SUMMARY

The discussion has ranged from ion forces to mechanical contraction while examining some interesting electrical behavior along the way. At each step of the way, another piece of the puzzle was explored. They are all assembled in Figure 3-15. It is appropriate to look back now at the conclusions stated at the beginning:

1. All electrical and mechanical activity of the heart (and other muscles, for that matter) is determined at the cellular level by the concentration, flow, and interactions of ions.
2. Calcium is a ubiquitous ion of central importance.
3. Electromechanical behavior of the heart can be modified (for better or for worse) by physiochemical influences on ions.
4. Cardiac anesthesia and intensive care can be usefully conceptualized as the beneficial control of ionic behavior, especially that of calcium.

It is hoped that the reader will agree with the last conclusion. Think about it, then reread this chapter after reading the rest of this book.

" 'Begin at the beginning,' the King said, gravely, 'and go on till you come to the end: then stop.' "[14]

REFERENCES

GENERAL REFERENCES

1. Katz B: Nerve, Muscle and Synapse. New York, McGraw–Hill, 1966, paper. A classic primer on cellular electrophysiology.
2. Aidley DJ: The Physiology of Excitable Cells. Cambridge, England, Cambridge University Press, 1971, paper. An intermediate, more difficult but complete electrophysiology text.
3. Berne RM, Levy MN: Cardiovascular Physiology, 3rd ed. St. Louis, C.V. Mosby, 1977, paper. The best available primer on clinical cardiac physiology.
4. Katz AM: Physiology of the Heart. New York, Raven Press, 1977. The best all-round reference on basic science of cardiac cellular physiology tied to clinical need. Biased toward basic science.
5. Braunwald E (ed): The Myocardium: Failure and Infarction. New York, HP Publishing Co, 1974. An excellent reference on basic science and clinical physiology. Biased toward clinical application.
6. Langer GA, Brady AJ: The Mammalian Myocardium. New York, John Wiley & Sons, 1974. A summation of major concepts for a clinician wishing to do research at the cellular level.

CALCIUM INFLUX

7. New W, Trautwein W: The ionic nature of slow inward current and its relation to contraction. Pflugers Arch 334:24–38, 1972. Status of basic science, 1972. First actual quantitive calcium flow measurements.
8. Kohlhardt M, Mnich Z: Studies on the inhibitory effect of verapamil on the slow inward current in mammalian ventricular myocardium. J Mol Cell Cardiol 10:1037–1052, 1978. A recent calcium current reference in the basic science literature.
9. Opie LH: Calcium antagonists. Lancet 1:806–809, 1980. Most recent review, showing clinical application.
10. Ikemoto Y: Reduction by thiopental of the slow channel-mediated action potential of canine papillary muscle. Pflugers Arch 372:285–286, 1977. Example of testing for clinical relevance.
11. Vogel S, Sperelakis N: Blockade of myocardial slow inward current at low pH. Am J Physiol 2:C99–103, 1977. Example of testing for clinical relevance.
12. Price HL: Calcium reverses myocardial depression caused by halothane. Anesthesiology 41:576–579, 1974. Best anesthetic study to date.
13. Kass RS, Tsien RW: Control of action potential duration by calcium ions in cardiac Purkinje fibers. J Gen Physiol 67:599–617, 1976. Why calcium and catecholamines share certain properties.

SUMMARY

14. Carroll L: Alice's Adventures in Wonderland. London, Macmillan, 1865

4

Interpretation of Cardiac Catheterization

ROBERT E. FOWLES

INTRODUCTION

HISTORICAL PERSPECTIVE

Our current understanding of heart disease is based extensively on knowledge gained through cardiac catherization studies. The first cardiac catheterization of a living person was performed in 1929 by a German surgical resident, Werner Forssman.[1, 2] Using himself as a subject he directed a ureteral catheter from an antecubital vein into his own right atrium while observing the fluoroscopic image in a mirror held by his nurse. The practical value of cardiac catheterization was proved in the early 1940s by Cournand and Richards,[3] who, with Forssmann, later shared the 1956 Nobel Prize in Medicine or Physiology for their invasive studies of right heart physiology.[4, 5] Subsequent developments included measurement of oxygen saturations to detect congenital shunting disorders (1947),[6] indirect determination of left-sided filling pressures by ''wedging'' the right-sided catheter in the distal pulmonary artery (1949),[7, 8] retrograde left-heart catheterization (1950),[9] percutaneous (Seldinger) vessel catheterization (1953),[10] transseptal left-heart catheterization (1959),[11, 12] and selective coronary arteriography (1959).[13]

Modern cardiac catheterization techniques have evolved as indispensible, safe tools for the diagnosis and treatment of patients with cardiovascular disease. New diagnostic uses include sensitive electrophysiologic intracardiac mapping, endomyocardial biopsy, and extended hemodynamic monitoring during acute myocardial infarction or perioperative period. Therapeutic applications include permanent placement of intracardiac pacing catheters for treatment of heart block or dysrhythmias, catheter retrieval of foreign bodies, intravascular placement of filters in venous thromboembolic disease, enlargement of atrial septal defects in cases of large shunts, and percutaneous balloon angioplasty in the treatment of obstructive atherosclerotic cardiovascular disease.

OPTIMAL USE OF CARDIAC CATHETERIZATION STUDIES

The proper use of cardiac catheterization requires careful planning with specific diagnostic questions in mind. All members of the cardiovascular care team should understand and be able to interpret and apply the information gained from an invasive study.

There are several general indications for performing cardiac catheterization. Hemodynamic or angiographic data is used to (1) reach a diagnosis (such as in atypical chest pain); (2) define anatomy (such as in congenital heart disease); (3) assess the severity of a lesion (such as in the consideration of bypass surgery for coronary atherosclerosis or of valve replacement for valvular heart disease); (4) evaluate an intervention (such as in the administration of ''afterload reducing'' agents); and (5) determine prognosis (such as in congestive cardiomyopathy).

Just as risks must be considered before a diagnostic procedure, potential complications of cardiac catheterization should be recognized by any physicians evaluating the patient after invasive study.[14] Certain patients are vulnerable to complications. Elderly persons and young children are especially fragile. Patients in congestive heart failure, renal failure, or those who have poor myocardial reserve may not tolerate the injection of large amounts of angiographic contrast material. Patients with critical aortic stenosis or idiopathic hypertrophic subaortic stenosis may develop profound shock, low output states, or dangerous arrhythmias. Pulmonary angiography is similarly hazardous in patients with extreme pulmonary hypertension. The nature of the procedure also determines the risks. Right-heart catheterization is generally safer than left heart procedures. Angiography introduces additional hazards and special procedures such as transatrial puncture require still more vigilance.

GENERAL CONSIDERATIONS IN INTERPRETING CATHETERIZATION DATA

Cardiac catheterization data must be reviewed critically because there are several sources of possible error. Mechanical factors such as wave-form distortion from fluid-filled catheters,[15, 16] or electronic factors, such as faulty calibration or inherent drift, may yield erroneous data. Technical considerations must also be kept in mind. Catheter location is important because damping of pressures may occur with the tip against a vessel wall or within ventricular trabeculae. Radiographic exposure technique may be inadequate, as may be the amount or rate of contrast injected. Oxygen saturation sampling may be incomplete and thereby lead to misdiagnosis of shunting. Simultaneous pressure measurements must be obtained in certain cases of valvular heart disease and idiopathic hypertrophic subaortic stenosis, or gradient estimates may be inaccurate. Finally, if exercise studies are performed to assess the severity of a valvular lesion, the load must be sufficient to stress cardiovascular reserve or to duplicate clinical symptoms.

It is important to appreciate any change in the patient's condition which may have occurred since cardiac catheterization. Alterations in fluid balance may greatly affect cardiac output. The cardiac patient with relatively normal hemodynamics at catheterization may, if fluid depleted, become unstable under physiologic stress. Patients undergo catheterization under minimal sedation: oral benzodiazepines (diazepam, 10 mg) or barbiturates (secobarbital, 100 mg) are most common. The patient's cardiovascular system may respond quite differently during induction of anesthesia. Varying myocardial ischemia or interposed arrhythmias, or both, can significantly alter cardiac performance.

Even if catheterization data are accurate, faulty interpretations can result unless care and judgement are used. To conclude that valve replacement is necessary solely on the basis of calculated orifice area, or that coronary artery bypass grafting is required merely because of an abnormal arteriogram may be erroneous without full consideration of the clinical circumstances. Detailed discussion of catheterization results, possible errors in their interpretation, and patient risks should always be carried out with the proposed surgical team.

BASIC CATHETERIZATION METHODS

RIGHT-HEART CATHETERIZATION

The techniques of right-heart catheterization are relatively standard. Venous access points include the antecubital-basilic, internal jugular, and femoral veins. The method of entry, percutaneous or cutdown, will vary according to vein accessibility and site. The site of catheterization chosen will depend upon operator experience and preference and upon the nature of the study to be performed, including any concomitant arterial procedures. For example, if coronary arteriography using brachial arteriotomy is planned, then an antecubital vein is usually chosen for venous access. If atrial septal defect is suspected, then the femoral approach is favorable because of the greater ease of crossing the defect from below. Approaching the right heart from the superior vena cava allows easier placement into the pulmonary artery, especially in cases of right ventricular outflow tract narrowing or hypertrophy. The Cournand (end-hole) and Goodale–Lubin (end-hole and side-hole) catheters are most uniformly used in right-heart catheterization (Fig. 4-1); they have a slight distal bend which allows directional guidance under fluoroscopic observation. Presssure tracings and blood samples are taken from various sites, depending on diagnostic needs.

Once the catheter is in the pulmonary artery it can usually be advanced until it becomes "impacted" or "wedged" in a tapering distal branch. At that point, an end-hole catheter communicates directly with the capillary-venous compartment of the lung, measuring what is known as the *pulmonary wedge (PW) pressure, pulmonary artery wedge (PAW) pressure, pulmonary capillary wedge (PCW) pressure,* or *pulmonary artery occlusive pressure (PAOP)* (Fig. 4-2). This wedge pressure reflects left atrial pressure in most cases.[17, 18] However, recent studies have raised some questions as

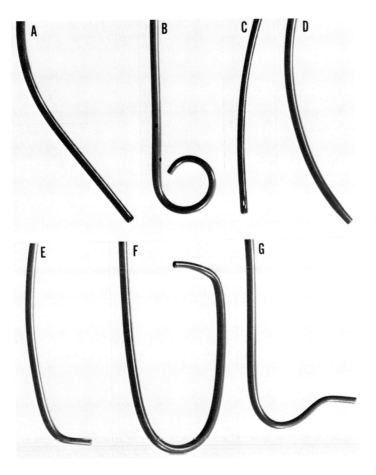

Fig. 4-1. Various cardiovascular catheters. The distal ends are shown for A. Cournand (single end hole, right heart catheterization); B. Pigtail (end and side holes, left sided cinéangiography); C. Sones (end and side holes, selective left, right coronary arteriography and left ventriculography); D. graft catheter (end hole, aortocoronary bypass graft angiography); E. Judkins right (end hole, selective right coronary arteriography); F. Judkins left (end holes, selective left coronary arteriography; and G. Amplatz (end hole, coronary and graft angiography).

Fig. 4-2. Comparison between right atrial (RA), pulmonary artery wedge (PA Wedge) and left atrial (LA) pressure waveforms. Note the A and V waves. The scale is the same for each tracing and the left-sided filling pressures (Wedge, LA) are elevated in this case of mitral regurgitation and congestive heart failure. The ECG is at the top and the time scale at lower right. Pressures in torr.

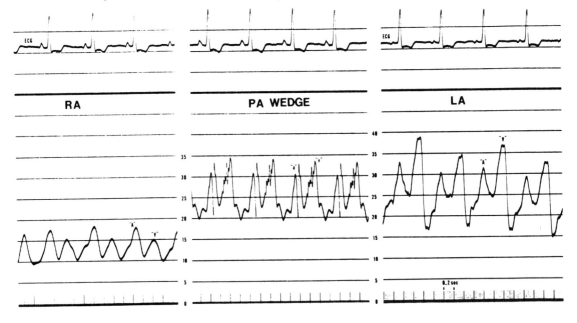

to the uniform validity of PAW pressure as an index of left-sided filling pressure.[19-21] Technical causes of an inadequate or inaccurate wedge pressure include incomplete wedging (resulting in a mixed pulmonary artery and wedge tracing) or wedging of the catheter tip against the wall of a sharply angulated pulmonary artery branching vessel. In certain conditions, such as those producing large *a* waves (atrial hypertrophy, mitral stenosis) or *v* waves (mitral regurgitation), the mean wedge pressure will be falsely elevated, and not reflect true left ventricular end diastolic pressures. In some cases the pul-

monary artery diastolic (PAD) pressure may be a good estimator of left-sided filling pressure, unless pulmonary vascular resistance is elevated or the patient is undergoing mechanical ventilation with positive end expiratory pressure (PEEP).

The flow-directed, balloon-tipped, right-heart catheter is now common, having been clinically introduced by Swan, Ganz and coworkers in 1970[22] (Fig. 4-3). It should be noted that a self-guiding, balloon-tipped catheter was described in 1953 by Lategola and Rahn in animal experiments.[23] Although this catheter is familiar in the operating room,

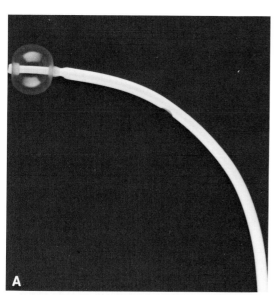

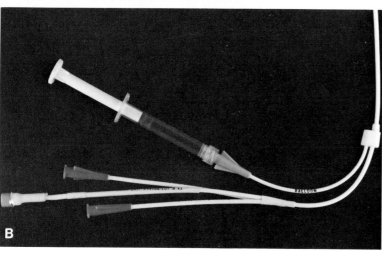

Fig. 4-3. Balloon flotation (Swan–Ganz) catheter. *A.* The distal catheter with inflated balloon and thermistor (indentation on catheter). *B.* The syringe for balloon inflation, the distal and proximal ports, and the electronic connector from the thermistor.

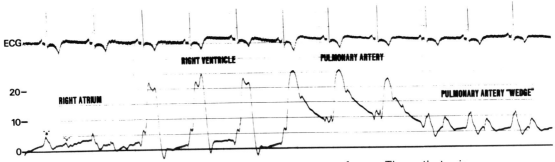

ECG

20—

RIGHT ATRIUM

10—

0—

RIGHT VENTRICLE

PULMONARY ARTERY

PULMONARY ARTERY "WEDGE"

Fig. 4-4. Right heart catheterization—normal pressure waveforms. The catheter is advanced (left to right) through the right atrium (*RA*, note *a* and *v* waves), the right ventricle (*RV*), the pulmonary artery (*PA*), and into the pulmonary artery wedge (*PAW*) position, reflecting left atrial pressure. The pressure scale is given in torr; ECG at *top*.

Fig. 4-5. Diagram of left and right heart catheterization values in the normal adult. Systolic and diastolic pressures are shown for each chamber and the great vessels. Mean pressures are given for the atria. The blood oxygen saturation percentages are expressed in italics. These are typical (median) normal values.

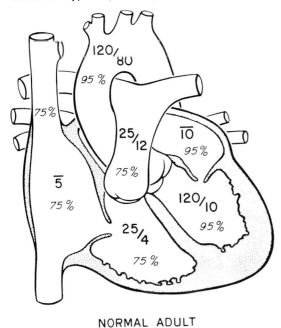

NORMAL ADULT

intensive care unit, and coronary care unit, it is also used in the cardiac catheterization laboratory. For example, in some laboratories, multiple-lumen, thermistor-tipped flotation catheters are used for determination of cardiac output by the thermodilution technique.[24] The use of the flow-directed right-heart catheter has been reviewed elsewhere.[25]

Normal pressure waveforms obtained during right-heart catheterization are illustrated in Figure 4-4. The accompanying normal ranges of pressure are shown in Table 4-1 and Figure 4-5. Pressures are measured with strain-gauge transducers in most laboratories, but in many centers (especially for research purposes) micromanometers are used.[26, 27] These miniaturized pressure transducers are small enough to fit within the end of standard catheters, thus reducing the distortion and artifacts associated with fluid filled systems.

Most cardiac catheterization laboratories use some form of computerized data analysis.[28] Several commercial systems are available. Advantages of computers include the automatic measurement of pressures, more accurate integration of the area under a curve (for valve gradient and dye dilution determination), rapid output of results allowing instant modification of the diagnostic procedure, quantitative analysis of left ventricular volumes and function, and hard-copy printout suitable for insertion into the patient's medical record (Figs. 4-6, 4-7).

STANFORD UNIVERSITY HOSPITAL
CARDIAC CATHETERIZATION: HEMODYNAMIC AND ANGIOGRAPHIC EVALUATION   PAGE 5A
   3/11/80 11:24 AM   VENTRICULOGRAPHY
MOOSE, BULLWINKLE   SEX: M   ANGIO #:   12
MEDICAL RECORD #: 12   HEIGHT: 180.0 cm   WEIGHT: 80.0 kg
BIRTHDATE: 1/ 1/1911   AGE: 69 yrs   BODY SURFACE AREA: 2.01 sq M

        LEFT VENTRICULAR ANGIOGRAPHY

Left Ventricle
        moderate enlargement
        mural thrombus

Left Ventricular Volumes:
        End diastolic volume   150 cc
        End systolic volume   90 cc
        Ejection fraction (post normal beat)   40%

Left Ventricular Contractility:

                    WALL SEGMENT   WALL MOTION
                1   Anterobasal   normal
                2   Anterolateral   moderately hypokinetic
                3   Apical   moderately hypokinetic
                4   Diaphragmatic   dyskinetic
                5   Posterobasal   normal
                6   Basal Septal   normal
                7   Apical Septal   moderately hypokinetic
                8   Posterolateral   akinetic
                9   Inferior Lateral   severely hypokinetic
               10   Superior Lateral   normal

Mitral Valve
        prolapse
        2+ regurgitation

Aortic Valve
        normal

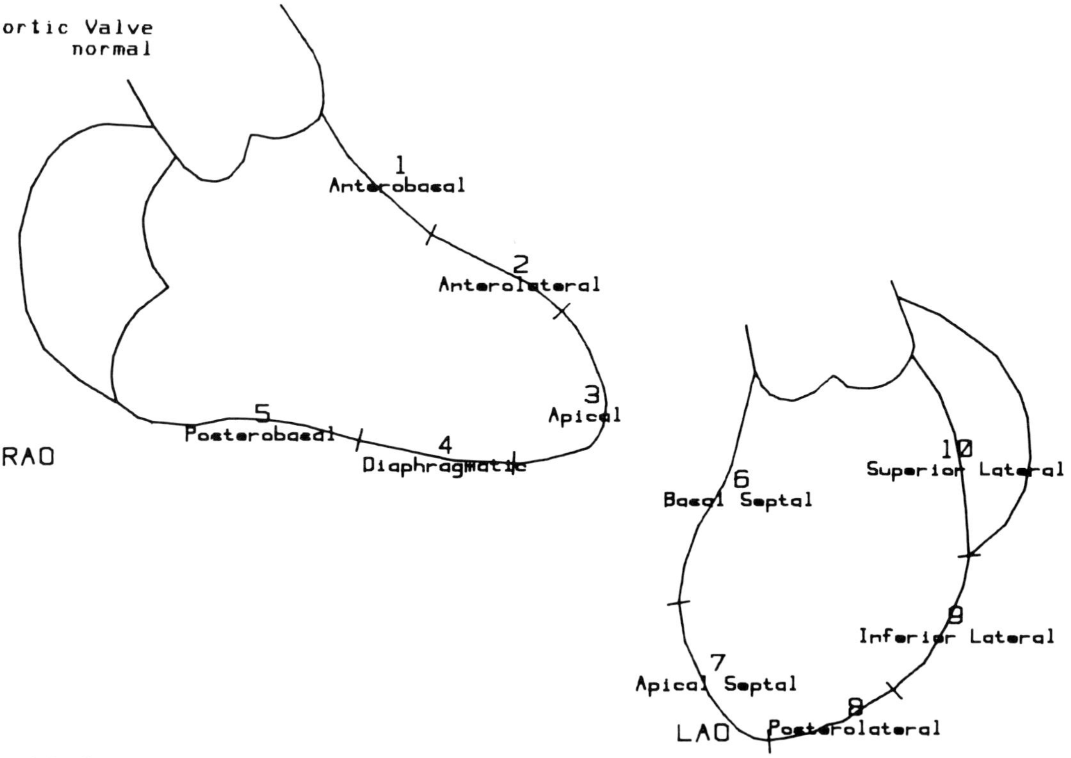

Fig. 4-6. Computerized cardiac catheterization/angiography report used at Stanford University Medical Center. The wall segments of the left ventriculogram are shown for *RAO* and *LAO* projections.

CARDIAC CATHETERIZATION: HEMODYNAMIC AND ANGIOGRAPHIC EVALUATION   PAGE 4A
    3/11/80 11:24 AM   CORONARY ARTERIOGRAPHY
  MOOSE, BULLWINKLE   SEX: M   ANGIO #:   12
  MEDICAL RECORD #: 12   HEIGHT: 180.0 cm   WEIGHT: 80.0 kg
  BIRTHDATE: 1/ 1/1911   AGE: 69 yrs   BODY SURFACE AREA: 2.01 sq M

        CORONARY ARTERIOGRAPHY
Anatomy of native coronary arteries:
    Dominance: Right
    LAD branches: Diag 1....medium   Diag 2....medium   Diag 3....small
                       Dist LAD..large
    Cx branches: Intermed..absent
                       ObMarg 1..medium   ObMarg 2..medium   ObMarg 3..small
                       Dist Cx...small
Right Coronary Artery:
    Prox RCA...90% discrete stenosis
                    discrete aneurysm
    Mid RCA ...is normal
    Dist RCA...is normal
Left Main Coronary Artery:
    LMCA   ....90% discrete stenosis
Left Anterior Descending:
    Prox LAD....75% tubular stenosis
    Mid LAD ...is normal
    Dist LAD...is normal
Left Circumflex Artery:
    Prox Cx.....60% tubular stenosis
    Mid Cx ...is normal
    Dist Cx ...is normal
Assessment of Bypassability of vessels with lesions > 50%
    (based on the angiographic size and morphology of the distal vessel)
                RCA....... is bypassable
                LAD....... is bypassable
                Cx........ is bypassable

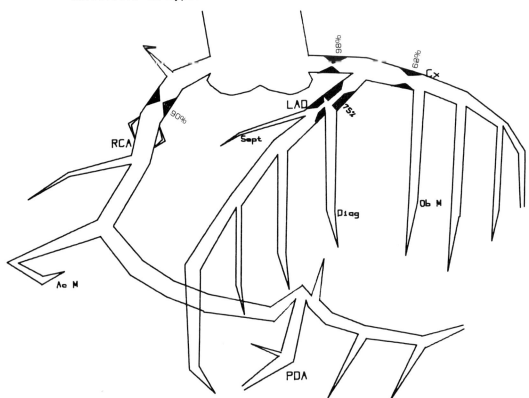

Fig. 4-7. Computerized graphic coronary arteriography report used at Stanford University Medical Center. Individual coronary lesions are entered and edited by the angiographer, who interprets the arteriogram.

LEFT-HEART CATHETERIZATION

There are several equally feasible approaches to catheterization of the left ventricle. It is routine to catheterize a peripheral artery and then enter the left ventricle by retrograde passage across the aortic valve. The easiest and least complicated approach is percutaneous femoral artery catheterization; brachial arteriotomy is also simple in experienced hands. In cases of tortuous, stenotic, or occluded aortic or iliofemoral vessels, percutaneous axillary artery catheterization is common. A normal aortic valve will allow retrograde catheter passage in practically all cases. In severe aortic stenosis, aortic valve prostheses, or idiopathic hypertrophic subaortic stenosis (IHSS), it is often necessary or desirable to enter the left ventricle by transatrial puncture. Transseptal left-heart catheterization is performed from the right femoral vein with a long, relatively rigid Brockenbrough needle-catheter assembly[29] (Fig. 4-8).

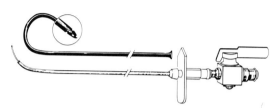

Fig. 4-8. Brockenbrough-type (Ross needle) catheter assembly. The flexible rubber catheter is placed high in the right atrium, and then the needle is introduced into the catheter, but not out of the catheter tip, until the catheter is drawn down over the aortic arch and up into the fossa ovalis. The needle is then gently advanced into the left atrium, the catheter follows, and the needle is withdrawn.

Table 4-1. Normal Cardiac Catheterization Values (Adults)

	NORMAL VALUE	RANGE
Pressure (Torr):	*a/v/mean*	
Right atrium (RA)	6/6/5	2–10/2–10/1–8
Left atrium (LA) or		
	12/12/10	4–16/4–18/2–12
Pulmonary artery wedge (PAW)		
	systolic/diastolic/mean	
Pulmonary artery (PA)	25/12/16	15–30/4–12/9–19
Systemic artery	120/80/93	100–140/60–90/70–105
	systolic/diastolic/end diastolic	
Right ventricle (RV)	25/ 0/ 4	15–30/0–8/0–8
Left ventricle (LV)	120/ 0/10	100–140/0–8/2–12
Oxygen Saturation, Consumption:		
RA, RV, PA oxygen saturation	70%	65–75
LA, LV, arterial saturation	95%	94–100
arteriovenous oxygen difference [$\Delta(A–V)O_2$]	4.0 ml/dl	3–5
oxygen consumption (VO_2)	130 l/min/m²	110–150
Flows		
Cardiac output (CO)	(varies with patient size)	3–8 l/min
Cardiac index (CI)	3.0 l/min/m²	2.8–4.2
Stroke volume index (SVI)	40 ml/beat/m²	30–60
Resistances (dyne·sec·cm⁻⁵)		
Total systemic vascular resistance (SVR)	1000	800–1200
Pulmonary vascular resistance (PVR) (or pulmonary arteriolar resistance)	80	50–150

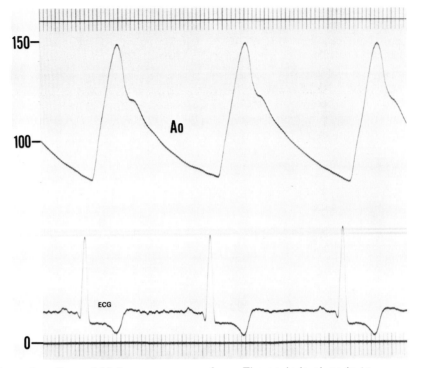

Fig. 4-9. Normal aortic root (Ao) pressure waveform. The scale is given in torr.

Fig. 4-10. Normal left ventricular (LV) pressure waveform, scale in torr. Note the *A* wave produced by atrial contraction. The *LV* end diastolic pressure is at the nadir of the post *A* wave curve.

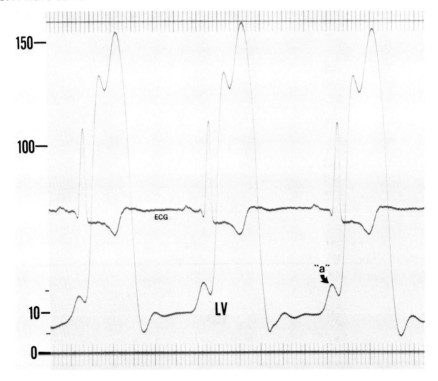

The technique is common and relatively safe in experienced hands. The procedure and its possible complications are reviewed elsewhere.[30-32] In rare instances, percutaneous puncture of the left ventricle through its apex is performed.[33, 34] Normal left-sided pressures and wave forms are depicted in Table 4-1 and Figures 4-9 and 4-10, respectively.

MEASUREMENT OF BLOOD FLOW

Accurate determination of cardiac output is essential to any cardiac catheterization procedure. Two methods are commonly used: (1) The Fick principle; and (2) indicator dilution.

In 1870 Adolph Fick theorized that "the total uptake or release of a substance by an organ is the product of the blood flow to the organ and of the arteriovenous concentration of the substance."[35] This principle may be applied to the lungs and stated as follows:

$$O_2 \text{ uptake} = \text{(ml/min)}$$
$$\text{pulmonary blood flow} \times \text{(l/min)}$$
$$\text{arteriovenous } O_2 \text{ difference} \text{ (ml/l)}^2$$

In practice, pulmonary blood flow equals cardiac output in the absence of shunts. Also, systemic arterial O_2 content may be used rather than the pulmonary venous value. Mixed venous blood is obtained from the pulmonary artery and oxygen consumption is measured by collecting a 3-minute expired air sample (stable, resting condition). The above equation can then be reexpressed:

$$\frac{\text{Cardiac output}}{\text{(l/min)}} = \frac{O_2 \text{ uptake (ml/min)}}{\text{(A-V) } O_2 \text{ difference (ml/l)}}$$

Potential errors in determining cardiac output by this method include faulty collection of expired air, collection of blood or air samples in a nonsteady state, and contamination of blood samples with air bubbles or flush solution. The cumulative error in Fick oxygen determination of cardiac output has been found to be approximately 10 percent.[36] Additionally, it is clear from the equation above

that small (A-V)O_2 differences will introduce more error; therefore, the Fick method is most accurate in patients with high (A-V)O_2 differences (i.e., low cardiac output).

The other major method of cardiac output determination is indicator dilution, based on the principle that an unknown volume of fluid can be calculated by adding a known quantity of an indicator to that volume and measuring the indicator concentration.

$$\text{volume (l)} = \frac{\text{Amount of indicator added (mg)}}{\text{Final indicator concentration (mg/l)}}$$

This principle is valid for fluids in motion[37] and in particular for cardiac output.[38] To calculate flow, this equation becomes

$$\frac{\dot{V}}{\text{(l/min)}} = \frac{A \text{ (mg)}}{\bar{c} \times t}$$
$$\text{(mg/l) (min)}$$

where $\dot{V}$ is flow, A is total amount of indicator, $\bar{c}$ is the average indicator concentration during its appearance, and t is the time over which the indicator's appearance is observed. In practice, an indicator is injected in the pulmonary artery and its appearance is observed in a peripheral artery, producing a concentration curve such as that diagrammed in Figure 4-11. This procedure is simplified by microprocessors which automatically compute the cardiac output. There are several substances that are sufficiently nontoxic, soluble, and physiologically inert to serve as indicators. These include indocyanine green dye and the gases nitrous oxide, krypton-85, and hydrogen. A recent and very popular development is the use of cold fluid as an indicator in the thermodilution technique of cardiac output determination.[39, 40] Cooled saline or 5% dextrose solution is injected through the proximal port of a balloon flotation catheter placed in the pulmonary artery, and the temperature drop of the mixed blood is detected by a thermistor in the catheter tip.[41] The indicator dilution method is least accurate in low-output states or in valvular regurgitation, in which nonexponential decay of indicator concentration may be observed or in which the onset of recirculation may be unclear (see Fig. 4-11).

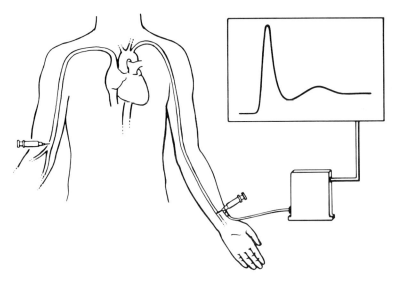

Fig. 4-11. Indicator dilution technique for cardiac output determination. The indicator is injected into a vein and arterial blood is sampled continuously, producing a concentration curve as shown to the right. The concentration reaches a peak during its first pass through the circulation, with a smaller, secondary rise caused by recirculation of indicator.

It is clear from the above paragraphs that several techniques for cardiac output determination are advantageous in the cardiac catheterization laboratory. Blood gas analysis remains the primary method, with indicator dilution serving as a supplementary technique.

FLOW PROBES

In several situations it is desirable to measure local, pulsatile blood flow. The development of electromagnetic catheter-tip, velocity-sensitive flow probes has allowed determination of instantaneous phasic flow at chosen sites in the cardiovascular tree.[42, 43] These miniature probes generate a small magnetic field within the electrically conductive surrounding blood. This creates a local voltage difference proportional to the velocity of the blood stream that is measured by tiny electrodes in the catheter. Because the magnetic field is induced by a small electrical current, although insulated from the catheter surface, a current leak detector automatically turns off power to the probe if even a minute short occurs, thus preventing accidental cardiac fibrillation. These velocity probes are mainly used for research protocols, but may in the future aid in the quantification of tricuspid insufficiency, intracardiac shunts,[44] and in diagnosis of constrictive pericardial disease.[45]

PULSATILE BLOOD FLOW

The concept of resistance to flow has become increasingly important in cardiology. Pulmonary vascular resistance is a major determinant of the feasibility of surgical repair of cardiac lesions involving left-to-right shunts.[16, 17] Pulmonary vascular resistance may decrease significantly after valve repair or replacement for mitral stenosis.[48] Pulmonary vascular resistance (PVR) or pulmonary arteriolar resistance (PAR) is given by the equation

$$PVR = \frac{PA_m - LA_m}{Q_p}, \left(\frac{torr}{l/min}\right) \text{ or } \left(\frac{dynes/cm^2}{cm^3/sec}\right)$$

where PA_m is mean pulmonary artery pressure, LA_m is mean left atrial pressure (estimated by mean PW pressure), and Q_p is pulmonary blood flow (cardiac output in absence of shunts). PVR is usually expressed as above in arbitrary "Wood units" but may be converted to absolute physical resistance, expressed as dynes-seconds-cm^{-5}, by multiplying by 80.

$$Resistance = \frac{mean\ pressure\ (dynes/cm^2)}{mean\ flow\ (cm^3/sec)}$$

To describe resistance by the above equation is somewhat simplified, for blood flow is pulsatile and occurs within an elastic, nonlinear, frequency-dependent vascular bed.

The concept of *vascular impedance* (the ratio of pulsatile pressure to pulsatile flow) takes into account both vascular resistance and compliance in characterizing blood flow.[49]

Systemic vascular resistance (SVR) is expressed as

$$SVR = \frac{MAP - CVP_m}{Q_s}$$

where MAP is mean systemic arterial pressure, CVP_m is mean central venous (or right atrial) pressure, and Q_s is systemic blood flow (or cardiac output). SVR has recently become a very important parameter in light of afterload reduction therapy for low output states.[50, 51]

DETECTION AND QUANTIFICATION OF SHUNTS

Intracardiac shunting commonly occurs in congenital malformations such as atrial or ventricular septal defects, patent ductus arteriosus, and anomalous pulmonary venous drainage. Shunting of blood may also result from certain acquired abnormalities such as trauma, ruptured interventricular septum, or ruptured sinus of Valsalva aneurysm. It is usually important not only to detect shunting, but also to determine its amount.

Left-to-right shunts are most commonly detected by oximetry. Oxygen saturation is measured in a diagnostic run with samples being withdrawn at multiple sequential sites, from pulmonary artery to vena cava. A significant *step up* in oxygen saturation indicates shunting of blood from the left-heart circulation. The criteria for significance of a step up in saturation depends upon the chamber from which the sample is taken, for the degree of mixing of venous blood increases from right atrium to right ventricle to pulmonary artery. Formulas for calculating the amount of left to right shunt are given below. Oximetry is only consistently able to detect shunts of greater than 25 percent of the systemic blood flow.

During left-heart catheterization, angiocardiography may be useful in defining the anatomy of a shunting defect but it cannot quantitate the shunt. It is currently popular to combine oximetry and angiocardiography in shunt detection because of their simplicity and ease.

Where greater sensitivity is required, the indicator dilution method can detect some shunts too small to discover by oximetry.[52] For example, tricarbocyanine green dye, when injected into a distal pulmonary artery branch, can be accurately detected by another catheter more proximal in the right-heart circulation. This allows discovery and localization of left-to-right shunts as small as 5 percent of systemic flow. Similarly, inhaled gases (such as nitrous oxide, krypton-85, or hydrogen) will appear prematurely in the right-heart circulation with a left-to-right shunt. Most commonly, inhaled hydrogen gas is detected by a sensitive platinum electrode placed near the site of a shunt or distal to it.[53]

Right-to-left intracardiac shunting produces arterial hypoxemia, but so may pulmonary disease. It is therefore important to locate and quantify any shunt as accurately as possible in order to differentiate an anatomic cardiac defect from intrinsic lung disease.

Right-to-left shunts as small as 5 percent of systemic flow can be detected by injection of an indicator in the right side of the heart. Indicators such as indocyanine green dye or ascorbic acid will appear prematurely in the left circulation. Dye is detected by a densitometer receiving blood from the catheter; ascorbic acid (a strong reducing agent) is sensed by a platinum electrode at the tip of the catheter. The ascorbate method is safe and avoids withdrawal of blood (which can be difficult in infants and small children). Substances normally cleared by the lungs after venous injection can also serve as indicators. Saline-dissolved hydrogen gas or krypton-85, when introduced into the right-heart circulation, will reveal a right to left shunt if they appear in the systemic circuit.

Although angiography does not allow quantification, it is a valuable technique for demonstrating right-to-left shunting. It is especially helpful in pulmonary arteriovenous fistulas, where the shunt is distal and close enough to the capillary bed that early appearance of indicator cannot be detected. Indicator methods cannot distinguish between shunting and valve incompetence. Newly developed nuclear medicine techniques can identify and quantitate shunts noninvasively and will be discussed below.

ASSESSMENT OF VENTRICULAR FUNCTION

The continuing development of new therapeutic techniques for heart disease has intensified the need to accurately assess ventricular performance. Cardiac output is only the end result of a complex network of cardiovascular phenomena and cannot be equated with the contractile state of the heart. Even in the presence of advancing heart disease, cardiac output is maintained by adaptive, compensatory mechanisms. It is important to know the degree of myocardial dysfunction in treating the cardiac patient. One should ask (1) to what extent are symptoms related to a mechanical problem (such as valvular stenosis) and therefore potentially reversible? (2) what are the patient's risks as reflected by intrinsic ventricular dysfunction? (3) how much myocardial reserve does the patient have while undergoing smooth anesthetic induction and withstanding the stress of cardiac surgery? (4) in reevaluating a patient, has a particular drug or operation improved cardiac function?

These questions are often critically important in the clinical management of heart disease because intrinsic myocardial function can determine the outcome of cardiac surgery.

The conventional hemodynamic parameters of instantaneous pressure and mean blood flow are indirect and rather insensitive indicators of myocardial function. Therefore, any values derived from these parameters will also be limited. In searching for sensitive methods for detecting abnormal myocardial function, cardiac physiologists view the heart as an elastic muscle responsive to various extrinsic factors. Theoretical considerations in myocardial mechanics have been discussed in Chapter 2.

The output of the heart beat, stroke volume, is determined by three factors: (1) pre-load, analogous to the stretching force upon the muscle in the relaxed state, determined in practice by end diastolic pressure; (2) afterload, the force distributed in the ventricular wall during ejection, related to outflow impedance and instantaneous cardiac output, as well as to ventricular volume and wall thickness according to the LaPlace relationship; and (3) contractility, analogous to shortening velocity of a muscle segment, the intensity of contraction. Preload and afterload are extrinsic influences which affect the developed performance of the heart. For example, in the operating room or intensive care unit, the cardiac output of the ailing heart can be augmented by adjusting preload with volume infusion or diuretics as is commonly practiced by monitoring left-sided filling pressures, or by reducing afterload with vasodilators. However, none of these maneuvers improves the heart's intrinsic contractility, the limiting factor. Ideally, contractility should be separately determined without influence from whatever preload or afterload conditions exist at the time of evaluation. Practically, there is no perfect index of absolute myocardial contractility independent of pre- and afterload that is able to clearly and sensitively detect the abnormal myocardium in early stages of disease.

Many indices of cardiac performance have been developed in an attempt to accurately characterize basal myocardial contractility. These methods have recently been reviewed, and the parameters are detailed in Table 4-2.[54, 55] Measurements derived from the rate of change of left ventricular pressure during the preejection phase of systole are termed isovolumic phase indices (see Table 4-2), but correlate poorly with clinical status.* Values obtained during ventricular emptying are termed ejection phase indices, and they include ejection fraction (EF), velocity of circumferential shortening (V_{CF}), mean normalized systolic ejection rate (MNSER), and left ventricular stroke work index (LVSWI). The left ventricular end diastolic pressure (LVEDP) is often a useful diastolic-phase index of cardiac performance.

---

*See discussion in Chapter 2.

Table 4-2. Indices of Cardiac Performance

PARAMETER	HOW OBTAINED	NORMAL VALUES	ADVANTAGES	DISADVANTAGES
peak dP/dt (maximum rate of rise of ventricular pressure)	Electronic differentiation of pressure signal or construction of steepest tangent to ventricular pressure curve	900–2400 $\frac{torr[56, 57]}{sec}$	Independent of afterload[58–60] (peak occurs before aortic valve opens.) Sensitive to known inotropic interventions such as digitalis,[61] isoproterenol,[62] and calcium,[63] or to diminished contractility,[64, 65] therefore probably most useful in detecting acute changes in a single patient[66]	Slightly sensitive to preload[67–69] and to heart rate[70, 71] The normal range is too wide to allow meaningful interpatient evaluation Better for assessing acute changes than basal state
$\dfrac{\text{peak dP/dt}}{\text{DP}}$ (DP = *developed* isovolumic pressure)	Measure DP as difference between isovolumic pressure (at point of peak *dP/dt*) and end diastolic pressure	$54 \pm 6\ sec^{-1}$	Virtually independent of preload[72, 73]	Difficult to measure DP accurately because of steep pressure waveform
$\dfrac{dP/dt}{DP_{40}}$	Values measured at a developed pressure of 40 torr	$32.5 \pm 2.1\ sec^{-1}$[74]	Virtually independent of preload[75] Preferable in low aortic diastolic pressure because of earlier measuring point than peak *dP/dt*	Variable with time; useful in acute studies of same patient
peak $\left(\dfrac{dP/dt}{kP}\right) = V_{pm}$ or peak V_{CE}	This value is theoretically equivalent to the peak velocity of the myocardial contractile element, V_{CE}, the sum of the velocities of muscle fiber shortening and of elongation of the series elastic element. *k* is the series elastic constant determined empirically to be between 24 and 32[77]	>1.6 circ/sec[76] (k = 28)	Peak value relatively easy to derive	Perhaps too sensitive to acute changes in preload.[78]

Table 4-2. Continued

PARAMETER	HOW OBTAINED	NORMAL VALUES	ADVANTAGES	DISADVANTAGES
V_{max}	$\left(\frac{dP/dt}{kP}\right)$ is plotted against pressure, P, and V_{max} is obtained by extrapolating the resulting force velocity curve back to $P = O$, or "no load."	2.37 ± 0.12 sec^{-1}	No significant afterload dependence[79] Independent of preload when calculated from developed pressure.[80, 81] Most sensitive to contractility changes[82, 83] Narrowest range of normal values Theoretically founded on basic muscle fiber physiology[84]	Felt by some to be less sensitive than LVEDP or ejection fraction[85] but more studies needed[86] Need hi-fidelity measurements, extrapolation
Ejection fraction (EF)	Angiocardiography with calculation of volume from RAO left ventriculogram $EF = \frac{SV}{EDV} = \frac{EDV-ESV}{EDV}$ where SV = stroke volume; EDV = end diastolic volume; ESV = end-systolic Noninvasive methods (echocardiography,[88] radionuclide scintigraphy[89])	0.67 ± 0.08[87]	Valid for interpatient comparisons Helps detect myocardial dysfunction in presence of a mechanical lesion (valvular stenosis/regurgitation)[90–92] Prognostic indicator of cardiac surgical outcome[93] May be measured noninvasively	Highly affected by preload, afterload, and heart rate[94] (↑ in hypovolemia, tachycardia, and ↑ afterload; ↓ in hypervolemia) Relatively insensitive to known contractility depression by propranolol[95] May be less sensitive than V_{CF}[96]
V_{CF} velocity of circumferential fiber shortening	Left ventriculogram; equatorial mid-LV circumference calculated from single plane diameter $mean\ V_{CF} = \frac{C_{ED} - C_{ES}}{C_{ED} \times ET} = \frac{D_{ED} - D_{ES}}{D_{ED} \times ET}$ where C_{ED} and D_{ED} are diastolic circumference and diameter; C_{ES} and D_{ES} are systolic circumference and diameter; ET is ejection time	>1.2 circ/sec[97]	Relatively preload independent[98, 99] Sensitive to known changes in contractility[100, 101] Added time dimension makes V_{CF} more sensitive to contractility changes than EF.[102] More sensitive assessment of basal contractility than isovolumic indices[103, 104]	Very sensitive to afterload[105] and to heart rate; therefore values obtained should be accompanied by concomitant BP and heart rate.
peak V_{CF}	$peak\ V_{CF} = peak\ \left(\frac{dC/dt}{C}\right)$ where C = instantaneous circumference, calculated for each cineangiographic frame	>2.4 circ/sec[106]	Peak V_{CF} better than mean V_{CF} in separating normal from abnormal LV function[108] May be measured noninvasively	Peak V_{CF} more difficult to measure than mean V_{CF}

Abbreviation and name	Method	Normal value	Advantages	Disadvantages
	Echocardiogram; mid-LV diameter used in above equation for mean V_{CF}[107]		More sensitive than EF in detecting abnormal LV function in setting of mitral regurgitation[109]	Highly preload and afterload dependent and therefore insensitive to isolated ventricular performance per se
MSER mean systolic ejection rate	$MSER = \dfrac{SI}{sep}\left(\dfrac{ml/sec \text{ of ejection}}{m^2\,BSA}\right)$ where SI = stroke index $\left(\dfrac{ml/beat}{m^2\,BSA}\right)$ sep = systolic ejection period per beat h_2 = (sec/beat)	159 ± 39[110] $\left(\dfrac{ml/sec}{m^2}\right)$	Easily calculated More sensitive for detecting abnormal LV performance than isovolumic indices[104]	
MNSER mean normalized systolic ejection rate	$MNSER = \dfrac{MSER \text{ (ejection/sec.)}}{EDV}$ where EDV = end diastolic volume	$2.29 \pm .05$[111] (sec^{-1})	Normalization (division by EDV) corrects for preload dependence[112]	
LVSWI left ventricular stroke work index	$LVSWI = SI \times \overline{LV}_s \times 0.0136$ $\left(\dfrac{g \cdot m/m^2\,BSA}{beat}\right)$ where SI = stroke index $\left(\dfrac{ml/beat}{m^2\,BSA}\right)$ $\overline{LV}_s$ = mean LV pressure during ejection (torr) 0.0136 = factor for conversion of torr from cm^3 to g·m	65 ± 17[113] $\left(\dfrac{g \cdot m/m^2}{beat}\right)$	Probably superior to V_{max} in coronary heart disease[114] as an indicator of pump performance	Depends on all the nonmyocardial factors affecting stroke volume and LV pressure, such as heart rate Not very sensitive Neglects ventricular size and therefore wall tension; myocardial mechanical efficiency may vary greatly. To correct for this, *contractility index* $\left(\dfrac{LVSW}{EDV}\right)$ may be used (normal value >0.5 $\dfrac{g \cdot m/cm^3}{beat}$)
LVEDP left ventricular end-diastolic pressure	Measure post-a wave LV pressure	<12 torr[115]	*As sensitive or more sensitive than contractile indices (such as V_{max}, V_{pm})[116]* *Simple technique* *Useful in unmasking LV dysfunction during stress such as dynamic exercise,[117] isometric exercise,[118] or pressure administration[119]*	*Wide normal range* *Affected by preload and afterload* *Exercise or post-pacing LVEDP is more sensitive in detecting abnormal LV function.* *May be elevated by pericardial or restrictive myocardial disease independent of contractility*

Indices derived from preejection pressure measurements (isovolumic phase) are limited in their ability to define basal contractility, and are better applied in studying acute changes in myocardial performance.* Wide divergence in these values causes significant overlap between normal and abnormal LV function, and therefore *isovolumic phase* indices are more applicable in studies on the same patient over a short period of time. As a result of chronic adaptations (hypertrophy stabilizes wall stress in chronic increasing afterload; dilatation stabilizes sarcomere length in chronic increased preload), it may not be necessary to evaluate basal contractility with indices that are independent of preload and afterload.[120]

Ejection-phase indices appear to be useful in measuring basal myocardial contractility. They are more sensitive than *isovolumic indices* in separating abnormal from normal left ventricular function. Their dependence on afterload may explain their sensitivity, inasmuch as inclusion of extrinsic stress helps unmask the failing myocardium.[121] A further advantage to EF and V_{CF} is their measurability by noninvasive methods.[122, 123]

The value of cardiac performance indices can be enhanced by measuring them during various stresses upon the heart. By introducing dynamic exercise, isometric exercise or pressor administration, LVEDP becomes a better detector of LV dysfunction (see Table 4-2). Atrial pacing also improves the diagnostic sensitivity of LVEDP[124] and preejection isovolumic contractile indices.[125] The contractile response of cardiac muscle to a perturbation in the rate and pattern of stimulation (such as in a programmed premature beat) is termed the *force-interval relationship* and appears to be a contractile index with improved diagnostic sensitivity.[126]

New techniques are appearing which will undoubtedly improve our ability to account for segmental wall motion abnormalities in evaluating left ventricular performance. These include noninvasive tools such as ra-

dionuclide angiography[127] and two-dimensional echocardiography.[128]

ANGIOGRAPHIC METHODS

VENTRICULOGRAPHY

Left ventriculography is currently the standard technique for evaluating left ventricular performance. Providing reliable, precise information about changes in anatomy and function occurring with disease, the left ventriculogram is a valuable complement to conventional pressure and flow measurements.

The methods employed in left ventriculography are relatively simple and uniform. Usually a pigtail or Sones catheter (See Fig. 4-1) is placed in the mid-left ventricle by retrograde passage across the aortic valve or by transseptal puncture, and then across the mitral valve. The catheter has side holes to reduce recoil or myocardial injection, and is 7F or 8F in diameter to permit delivery of a large bolus (30 to 60 ml in adults) of contrast fluid by flow-controlled mechanical injection over a relatively short time (3–4 sec). The angiocardiographic image is simultaneously recorded on video tape and on 35-mm film (at a frame rate of 30–60 frames/sec). Extra systoles during injection are usually avoided or minimized by removing the catheter from irritable areas (such as outflow tract or apex), by performing a preliminary manual test injection to assure proper position and by modifying injection rate. Ciné recording permits frequent measurements during the cardiac cycle, relatively accurate visualization of end diastole and end systole, and greater ease of viewing than large cut roentgenograms.

Angiographic determination of ventricular volumes has been extensively developed and empirically confirmed by forming casts of postmortem hearts.[129, 130] Dodge's original area-length approximation of left ventricular volume is preferred,[131] the left ventricle is assumed to be *ellipsoid* in shape and its volume is calculated according to the formula

---

*See discussion in chapter 2.

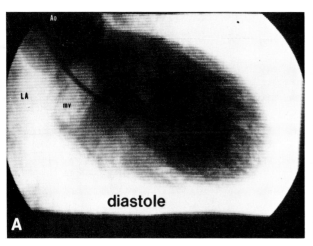 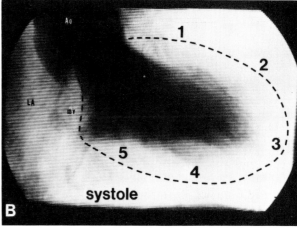

Fig. 4-12 A, B. Normal left ventriculogram, 30° right anterior oblique (RAO) projection. The diastolic ventricular outline is shown (*dashed line*) with the wall segments labelled as follows: (1) anterobasal, (2) anteroapical, (3) apical, (4) posteroapical, and (5) posterobasal. (*AO:* aortic root; *LA:* left atrium; *MV:* mitral valve)

$$V = \left(\frac{4}{3}\pi\right) \times \frac{D_a}{2} \times \frac{D_l}{2} \times \frac{L_m}{2}$$

where L_m is the longest measured length of the ventricle (major axis) and D_a and D_l are the anteroposterior and lateral view diameters of the minor axes, derived from the planimetered areas (A) of these views according to the formula $\dfrac{D}{2} = \dfrac{2A}{\pi L_m}$. (Measurements are corrected by regression equations for distortion-magnification caused by the point source of x-ray beams and short filming distance.) In this biplane method, simultaneous views 90° apart are recorded by separate cameras. Several studies have more recently shown that single plane filming (usually anteroposterior or 30° RAO [right anterior oblique]) yields results comparable in most patients to those of biplane studies.[132–134] In patients with coronary artery disease displaying segmental wall motion abnormalities, single plane ventriculography may be inaccurate.[135]

Interpretation of the left ventriculogram is both descriptive and quantitative. The pattern of contraction is described according to standard nomenclature in which the left ventricular walls are divided into standard segments[136] in both RAO and LAO views (Fig.

4-12). Wall motion may be *normal* (concentric inward movement during systole), *reduced* or *hypokinetic* (velocity or amplitude or both diminished), *absent* or *akinetic* (without appropriate motion), or *dyskinetic* (moving outward or paradoxically during systole). Detailed analysis of wall motion abnormalities and interventions are described below in the section on coronary artery disease. The left ventriculogram is also described according to presence and degree of mitral regurgitation (best seen in the 30° RAO view), ventricular septal defect with left-to-right shunting (best seen in the 60° LAO view), and filling defects, obstruction, or aneurysmal dilation (either or both views). Ejection fraction is calculated from the end diastolic and end systolic volumes. It is easily and reliably determined except in the presence of atrial fibrillation or a series of premature beats, *and must be measured after adequate hydration and with a heart rate between 60 and 100.* It correlates with the prognosis of patients with coronary heart disease, valvular heart disease, or myocardial disease, and gauges the risk of cardiac surgery.[137] An abnormal ejection fraction is less than 0.55. Between 0.55 and 0.40 corresponds with mild left ventricular impairment, compensated function, and no symptoms of heart failure; between 0.40 and 0.25 corresponds with moderate symptoms of heart failure (New York Heart Association class III); and less than 0.25 with severe ventricular impairment or destruction with profound symptoms (New York Heart Association class IV).

Right ventriculography is most often performed for investigation of congenital heart disease. Biplane full-size films may be desirable for demonstration of anatomy, but ciné filming is better for detecting a small shunt. Again, a side-hole catheter (usually NIH, Eppendorf, or Gensini) is used; the duration of filming varies according to the nature of the investigation, with approximately 12 seconds being required to opacify the left heart. The lateral view displays the right ventricular outflow tract and pulmonic valve well; biplane or RAO are used for suspected tetralogy of Fallot and Ebstein's anomaly.

Modern contrast media are various salts of tri-iodinated benzoic acids, the iodine content conferring radiopacity upon the solution, which has a very high osmolarity. Sodium salts are less viscous but more toxic to myocardium and brain than methylglucamine salts, so contrast media usually contain a mixture of both.

The complications of ventriculography are summarized in Table 4-3, and include mechanically-related problems such as extrasystoles, intramyocardial injection and embolism, as well as pharmacologic, allergic and toxic effects.[212, 213]

SELECTIVE CORONARY ARTERIOGRAPHY

Coronary arteriography is a highly developed technique which has become the definitive method for diagnosing and describing coronary artery abnormalities. Original attempts at visualizing the coronary arteries involved flooding the aortic root with contrast material, injecting during diastole with an electronically-triggered device,[214] injecting during transient acetylcholine-induced cardiac arrest,[215, 216] and elevating intrabronchial pressure to cause decreased thoracic blood flow and improve coronary artery opacification.[217] None of these methods was as effective as selective catheterization of the coronary artery itself, first reported by Sones in 1959.[218]

Selective coronary arteriography may be performed by either of two main methods. In the *Sones* technique, a gently curved, thin-walled, woven catheter with tapering tip (see Fig. 4-1) is introduced through a surgical cutdown and brachial arteriotomy; it may then be manipulated into the left and right coronary ostia and also into the left ventricle).[219, 220] Several injections of from 2 to 5 ml of contrast fluid are made in multiple projections and recorded on 35-mm ciné-angiographic film, affording detailed visualization of the entire coronary arterial tree. In the *Judkins* technique, preformed, "coronary seeking" catheters[221] (see Fig. 4-1) are introduced percutaneously into the femoral artery and manipulated into the respective coronary ostia, with separate catheters (Judkins or Amplatz) being required for the left and right coronary arteries.[222, 223] A recently developed technique using the Schoonmaker–King catheter [221] combines the advantageous percutaneous femoral artery approach of Judkins and the single catheter feature of Sones.

The basic procedure of coronary arteriography is relatively standard. Premedication usually includes an orally administered sedative such as diazepam or a barbiturate. Maintenance medications are often discontinued; nitrates are not withheld unless provocative maneuvers to elicit coronary spasm are planned, and propranolol is continued if needed to control angina. The patient is brought to the catheterization laboratory in the fasting state or after light oral intake of liquids only. Central venous access is usually obtained before arterial cannulation, although some laboratories rely on a peripheral intravenous line. Atropine (0.6 mg) is often administered routinely as prophylaxis against the bradycardia resulting from intracoronary contrast injections. Systemic heparinization[225, 226] is carried out at the beginning of the procedure and later reversed with protamine. The patient with a prior history of hypersensitivity to contrast media is usually successfully studied if premedicated with antihistamines and corticosteroids, but epinephrine and resuscitative equipment are available in the event of anaphylaxis. If congestive heart failure is aggravated, the patient may be positioned head-up and given oxygen, nitrates, and furosemide. Blood pressure decreases with each coronary injection but usually recovers after voluntary coughing (which raises aortic pressure, enhancing clearance of contrast material). Continuing hypotension is hazardous and may warrant administration of a vasopressor. Hypertension, angina, or both are usually relieved by sublingual nitroglycerin; in persistent episodes accompanied by tachycardia, IV propranolol is helpful.

The adequate coronary arteriography report should include a complete account of the patient's status throughout the procedure (including ECG appearance and rhythm), any significant events or problems encountered, and all drugs administered. This will aid the anesthesiologist in planning for anesthesia induction and management, and in avoiding or coping with deleterious stresses in the operating room and intensive care unit.

Although complete description of the interpretation of coronary arteriograms is beyond the scope of this chapter, there are several points with which the cardiovascular anesthesiologist should be familiar:

1. *The grading of coronary artery stenosis is subjective*, therefore interobserver variability is wide.[227, 228] Stenosis is usually described in terms of percent reduction in lumen diameter. Therefore a 50 percent reduction in diameter represents a 70 percent reduction in cross-sectional area; above this range a gradient begins to appear across a constriction,[229] and symptoms may occur.[230] At 85 to 90 percent diameter reduction, coronary blood flow begins to decrease steeply.[231]

2. *The area of the heart supplied by coronary ar-*

tery branches may be important. The sinoatrial node (and much of the atrium) is supplied by the sinoatrial mode artery, arising from the right coronary artery in 55 percent of patients and from the left circumflex in 45 percent. Severe stenosis of this artery may cause atrial dysrhythmias, especially at surgery. The atrioventricular (AV) node and posterior myocardium are fed by the right coronary artery in 90 percent of cases and by the distal circumflex in 10 percent, hence the occasional observation of various degrees of AV block (usually mitigated by collateral supply) in patients with posterior wall infarction or ischemia. The left bundle branch is supplied by septal branches of the left anterior descending artery (LAD), as well as proximally by the AV nodal artery. Ischemia or infarction in this area may be accompanied by more severe AV conduction disturbances, often requiring a pacemaker. The anterolateral or free wall of the left ventricle is supplied by diagonal branches of the LAD and obtuse marginal branches of the left circumflex artery. Extensive disease in these vessels may cause profound left ventricular dysfunction or aneurysm formation.

3. *Some patterns of coronary artery stenosis render the patient particularly fragile*. Foremost is left main coronary artery stenosis[232] (of 70% or greater) because of the large area of left ventricle supplied by this vessel (Fig. 4-13). Episodes of myocardial ischemia or hypotension may be disastrous in this condition, and may be compounded by significant stenosis of the right coronary artery. Significant proximal obstruction of the LAD and left circumflex coronary arteries has been termed *left main equivalent disease* and deserves special attention, as does high-grade *three vessel disease*, stenosis of right coronary, LAD, and left circumflex arteries. The degree of left ventricular dysfunction, as determined by ejection fraction and LVEDP, further jeopardizes the coronary artery disease patient undergoing surgery.

Table 4-3. Complications Associated With Cardiac Catheterization and Angiography

PROCEDURE	HIGH-RISK SUBJECTS	POTENTIAL COMPLICATIONS	AVOIDANCE OR TREATMENT OF COMPLICATIONS
1. *Arterial puncture or arteriotomy* with cannulation and retrograde catheterization	Young patients; less than 10 years old have three times the complication rate[138] Anticoagulated patients; four times the complication rate Atherosclerotic patients; irregular intimal surfaces, tortuous, stiff vessels; four times the complication rate Hypertensive patients; three times the complication rate Aortic insufficiency; increased pulse pressure; seven times the complication rate Higher risk of vascular complications in coronary arteriography with brachial arteriotomy (0.93%) than with percutaneous femoral approach (0.13%)[139]	*Major* (2.6% incidence)[140] Obstruction (thrombosis)[141] Embolization[142] Hemorrhage (0.12%)[143] Massive ecchymosis Creation of false aneurysm (0.06%)[144] Spasm (especially in small patients)	→ Heparinization Thrombectomy if required Do not totally obliterate flow when compressing artery at conclusion of procedure.[146] → Correct abnormal coagulation Surgically repair lacerations and the like → May require surgical drainage → Closely observe patient to rule out vessel occlusion, expanding mass, and so on
		Minor (10% incidence)[145] Pain Ecchymosis Mass (hematoma) Arteriospasm (especially in children)	→ Avoid lengthy procedures.
2. *Catheter and guide wire manipulations; equipment failure* (less than 0.01% incidence)[147]	Patients with abnormal anatomy or tortuous non-compliant or obstructed vessels or chambers	Kinking and knotting of catheters Fractured guide wire (occurs with difficult passages or turns) Guide wire exiting *side* hole of angiocatheter rather than end hole; wire becomes lodged	→ Avoid rigorous manipulations. Inspect equipment carefully before insertion. → Withdrawal through insertion site may avulse vessel; withdraw as distally as possible, incise vessel, and remove catheter and guide.
3. *Right- and left-heart catheterization*	Infants and other patients with small hearts	*Arrhythmias* (overall incidence 1.2%)[150] Ventricular fibrillation; 0.2% overall during manipulation of catheter in *right* ventricle;[151] current conduction through catheter may be a factor in rare cases[152]	→ Continuous ECG monitoring, prompt DC cardioversion

Possible increased risk in patients on digitalis

Hypovolemia, especially in children[148]

Critical valvular stenosis

Cyanotic infants

Other patients with congenital heart disease, rheumatic heart disease, or WPW syndrome[149]

Marked bradycardia or asystole (0.3% incidence);[153] multiple causes include vasovagal reactions, catheter manipulation, vessel damage, cardiac perforation, and hemopericardium

→ Oxygen, atropine, sympathomimetics, closed chest massage.

→ Consider possible hemopericardium.

Supraventricular tachyarrhythmias (0.28% incidence);[154] mostly caused by catheter manipulation, especially in right atrium or right ventricle

→ Often disappears spontaneously
IV digoxin, propranolol, and the like
DC cardioversion
Overdrive pacing

Bundle branch block (<1% incidence); occurs mostly during right ventricular catheterization, probably due to mechanical irritation of conduction system.

→ Consider prophylactic pacing in patients with prior intermittent block.

Patients with severe valvular disease (especially calcific aortic stenosis) or prosthetic valves

Systemic arterial embolism (0.1[155] to 0.4%[156] incidence)

→ In Judkins technique, exchange catheters over guide wire distal to brachiocephalic vessels, flush before advancing.[160]

Embolism to coronary artery during manipulation of catheter in aortic root may cause MI or be fatal.

Air embolism may occur without careful attention to connections, catheter exchanges, and so on.

→ Heparin may be helpful.

Patients with small ventricles and/or valvular stenosis

Infants

Patients with aortic atheromata

Perforation of heart or great vessels (0.8% incidence)[157]

Right atrial perforation usually occurs during transseptal catheterization. Right ventricular perforation may occur during contrast injection or pacemaker placement.

Left atrial perforation, usually occurs during catheter or guide manipulation.

Left ventricular perforation may occur during contrast injection (see below).

Aortic root perforation may occur during transseptal puncture.

→ Cautious manipulations
Monitor hemodynamic status carefully.
Pericardiocentesis as required
Thoracotomy in extreme cases

Table 4-3. Continued

PROCEDURE	HIGH-RISK SUBJECTS	POTENTIAL COMPLICATIONS	AVOIDANCE OR TREATMENT OF COMPLICATIONS
	Patients with rheumatic heart disease or cardiomyopathy	*Pulmonary complications* Pulmonary embolism and/or infarction (<0.01% incidence)[158] may be caused by femoral vein thrombosis or prolonged wedge position of pulmonary artery catheter; symptoms usually occur by 6 days. Pulmonary edema; may occur without angiography; caused by prolonged recumbency	→ Careful post-procedure monitoring
	Valvular heart disease, congenital heart disease patients.	*Infections* (0.1% incidence)[159] Bacterial endocarditis Localized infections (usually at site of catheter insertion) Fever without infection may occur frequently as result of pyrogen reaction to contrast media or other unknown factors.	→ Consider antibiotic prophylaxis in high-risk patients. → Strict aseptic technique
4. *Contrast ventriculography and aortography*	Infants or other patients with small hearts Severely ill patients	*Arrhythmias* (0.1% incidence)[164] Ventricular fibrillation; usually associated with contrast injection or manipulation of catheter; may or may not be preceded by premature beats Bradycardia and the like (see below)	→ Prompt DC cardioversion May consider antiarrhythmic prophylaxis in patients with ventricular irritability
	Patients with small or hypertrophic hearts	*Intramural injections* (1–2% incidence) Usually results in ventricular irritability Cardiac perforation occurs rarely (0.2%),[165] mostly in right ventricular injections (0.46% incidence).[166]	→ Assure free-moving catheter tip on fluoroscopy with undamped pressure tracing. Use flexible catheter with multiple side holes. Preliminary, manual test injection Avoid high-pressure machine injections.

Atopic individuals; previous allergic reactions to various medications, contrast fluids, and so on; asthmatic patients[161]	*Contrast effects* Cerebral reactions:[167] toxic encephalopathy: convulsions, altered mental status, probably caused by cerebral edema. Vomiting (5% incidence):[168] not usually a major problem; transient Hypotension: probably a combination of decreased myocardial contractility and peripheral vasodilation; severe reactions occur in 0.03% of cases[169]	→ Low-sodium salts; avoid high-volume injections.
Patients with previous reactions to contrast material experience a repeat in only 25% of cases.[162] Patients in congestive heart failure with high filling pressures.	*Allergic Reactions to Contrast* (very rare: 0.04%[170]–0.1%[171] incidence) Pruritus, erythema, urticaria, edema, hypotension, or wheezing Usually good recovery after prompt treatment	→ Careful history taking Pretest "challenge" not helpful[174] Consider premedication with antihistamine and possibly corticosteroids. Treat with IV epinephrine, corticosteroids, and antihistamines.
	Acute pulmonary edema (rare) Probably result of volume effect of hyperosmolar contrast and its myocardial depressant effect May also occur during coronary arteriography	→ Minimize volume of contrast material. Monitor patient condition and ventricular/pulmonary artery pressures. Prompt treatment with oxygen, diuretics, and the like
Patients with renal disease.[163] Dehydration or laxative use	*Renal complications* Incidence in abdominal aortography was once as high as 0.2%, but introduction of less-toxic diatrizoate contrast media has substantially lowered complication rate. Apparent renal damage with current angiography is extremely rare.[171, 173]	→ Avoid administering more than 0.5 g/kg of contrast material.[175] Ensure adequate hydration; protect against hypotension.

Table 4-3. Continued

PROCEDURE	HIGH-RISK SUBJECTS	POTENTIAL COMPLICATIONS	AVOIDANCE OR TREATMENT OF COMPLICATIONS
5. *Coronary arteriography*	Left main coronary artery stenosis (≥50% narrowing), mortality rate up to 6%[176] Extensive (combined multiple lesions) coronary disease Severe symptoms[177] (*e.g.*, angina at rest or longstanding angina) Left ventricular dysfunction (eject on fraction <0.30)[178] Multiple PVCs on resting ECG[179] Congestive heart failure[180] Hypertension (past or present) Extensive coronary disease Unstable angina[181]	*Death* 0.76%[182]–3.8%[183] in high-risk patients 0.05%–0.12%[184] in low-risk patients Usually caused by shock and/or ventricular tachyarrhythmias unresponsive to treatment.	→ Consider risk versus benefit; many deaths may occur *before* catheterization in high-risk patients.[201, 202] Possible addition of circulatory assist devices (such as intraaortic balloon pump) with OR standby Possible limitation of examination to extraostial or sinus of Valsalva injections
		Myocardial infarction Overall rate is approximately 0.25%[185–188] with 3.4-fold greater risk in patients with unstable angina[189] May rarely occur because of acute dissection of coronary artery during injection.	→ Some studies suggest systemic heparinization helpful,[203] others find no effect.[204] → Recognized coronary artery dissection may be favorably treated by prompt bypass surgery.
	Age >50 years Carotid or cerebrovascular disease	*CNS disturbances* Occur in 0–1% of cases;[190, 191] more recent surveys indicate 0.1[192]–0.03%[193] Presumably caused by embolization; other causes include *in situ* thrombosis (especially with preexisting disease, hypovolemia, hypotension) and diffuse toxic reaction to contrast (such as in occipital cortical blindness). Air emboli to CNS may cause focal deficits, agitation, confusion, or coma. Most patients eventually recover.[194]	→ Avoid hypotension and hypovolemia. Limit duration of study. Heparinization may be helpful.[205–208] Catheter exchanges and other manipulations should be performed distal to brachiocephalic arteries.[209]

Patients with known sinoatrial disease Patients with high-grade proximal right coronary stenosis	*Arrhythmias* Sinus bradycardia; probably caused by contrast effect and/or sinoatrial node ischemia; more frequent with right coronary injections;[195] in extreme cases, may progress to asystole Conduction defects.[196, 197]	→ Atropine (0.5–1.0 mg IV) Prophylactic atrial pacing as standby in vulnerable patients Minimize volume and rate of dye injection Use non-ionic contrast. → Prophylactic right ventricular temporary pacemaker.
Patients with preexisting conduction defects (AV block, bundle branch block) Severe coronary disease, recent myocardial infarction, preexisting ventricular ectopy	Ventricular fibrillation (<1% incidence);[198–200] ventricular ectopy may precede fibrillation.	→ Immediate defibrillation (DC cardioversion) Avoid large bolus coronary injections. Avoid high- or low-sodium salt contrast. Lidocaine prophylaxis
6. *Pulmonary angiography*		
Patients with bronchial asthma Ill patients with massive pulmonary embolism and low cardiac output Primary pulmonary hypertension patients; already compromised pulmonary vascular bed	*Contrast reactions* Includes bronchospasm (0.6% incidence); also angioneurotic edema and anaphylaxis (both <0.2% incidence)[210] *Death* (0.4% incidence),[211] usually caused by cardiogenic shock in a patient with already low cardiac output and pulmonary hypertension	→ IV administration of dilute epinephrine if necessary → Perform selective, segmental injections rather than mainstream.

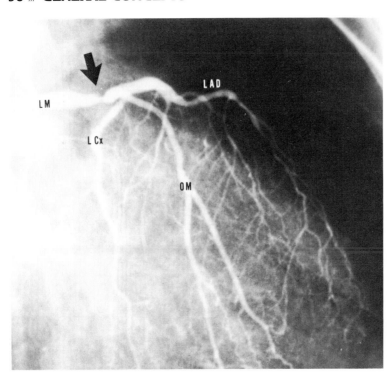

Fig. 4-13. Selective left coronary arteriogram, RAO projection. The left main coronary artery (LMCA) has a high-grade stenosis (*arrow*). (*LAD:* left anterior descending; *LCx:* left circumflex; and *OM:* obtuse marginal)

4. *Collateral supply to proximally stenosed vessels probably correlates* with severity (or chronicity or both) of ischemia, and appears to predict in some cases the success of revascularization procedures.[233]

5. *There are several sources of potential error in the interpretation of coronary arteriograms.* The coronary catheter may induce proximal vessel spasm, distinguishable from fixed obstruction by its reversibility after nitroglycerin administration. Nonpathologic coronary arterial impingement may appear in focal areas as a result of perivascular myocardial bands, constricting the vessel only during systole, but allowing full relaxation during diastole—the predominant period of coronary blood flow. Layering of contrast material, crossing or overlapping of vessels in the two-dimensional roentgenographic image, foreshortening of vessel segments and eccentricity of lesions all may give erroneous impressions of vessel caliber, which can be overcome by observing arteriograms from multiple projections.[234, 235]

Anatomic anomalies of the coronary arteries may occur in normal patients or in those with congenital heart disease. Some coronary artery anomalies are inconsequential and others may have pathologic significance.[236] The most common variations occurring without associated congenital heart disease or pathologic consequences are the following: coronary ostia located in the ascending aorta, independent ostial origin of the right coronary conus branch, origin of left circumflex from right coronary sinus or from right coronary artery, absent left main coronary artery (branches originate independently from sinus of Valsalva), variable distribution of branches feeding ventricular segments, and duplication of a coronary artery or its main branches. Pathologic coronary artery anomalies in otherwise normal individuals may include anomalous origin of the left coronary artery from right coronary sinus with passage between the aorta and pulmonary artery (possible left main coronary artery compression, leading to myocardial infarction or sudden death),[237] congenital absence of the left circumflex coronary artery without compensatory development of the distal right coronary artery (localized myocardial dysfunction and posterior papillary muscle prolapse), and primary fistulas (usually right coronary artery to right ventricle, right atrium, or pulmonary artery, with variable consequences depending on magnitude of shunt).

Further details on the performance and interpretation of coronary arteriograms are available in several recent reviews.[238-240] The potential complications of coronary arteriography are presented in Table 4-3.

AORTOGRAPHY

Aortic angiography is useful in the diagnosis of a wide variety of conditions. It is therefore important that aortography be performed and interpreted by experienced physicians.

Adequate opacification of the aortic root or lumen requires a high rate of injection, usually 30 ml/sec. In adults, 30 to 50 ml is injected; in children, 0.5 ml/lb of body weight is injected.

In the patient with *aortic regurgitation,* the best view of the aortic valve is the LAO (left anterior oblique) projection, usually at 45°. This allows visualization of the left ventricle clear of the bony spine shadows. Aortic regurgitation is graded 1+ to 4+ in severity by the following criteria: *1+* is a small amount of dye entering the left ventricle but clearing with each systole; *2+* is faint, incomplete opacification of the left ventricle, not clearing with each systole; *3+* represents progressive opacification of the entire left ventricle; and *4+* is complete opacification of the left ventricle with the first diastole, remaining so during the succeeding cardiac cycles.[241] This grading scale usually approximates true severity of aortic valvular insufficiency in terms of mild, moderate, or severe,[242, 243] it may be inaccurate especially in cases of mild disease[244] (Fig. 4-14).

Other projections may be required for investigation of various conditions. If mitral insufficiency is suspected as well as aortic, the 45° right anterior oblique (RAO) projection is used (Fig. 4-15). For visualization of the brachiocephalic vessels, a steeper LAO (45°–60°) view is employed to unfold the aorta. Shunting in patent ductus arteriosus (PDA) is best observed in 45° LAO. Aortic coarctation is often studied in two planes, one being LAO 20° to 45°.

Dissecting aortic aneurysm is a dangerous condition which, despite risks, requires aortography for diagnosis and definition of extent. Site of intimal tear, aortic valve and coronary artery status, size of dissecting hematoma, integrity of branching vessels, and reentry site should be determined.[245-247] (Fig. 4-16).

In abdominal aortic aneurysm, abdominal ultrasound is the primary diagnostic method, with confirmation by angiography.[248] Abdominal aortography may however be misleading because the dilated lumen may be filled with laminated thrombus.

PULMONARY ANGIOGRAPHY

The chief indications for pulmonary angiography are (1) suspicion of pulmonary thromboembolism; (2) elucidation of congenital malformations; and (3) anatomic visualization of the pulmonary artery or left atrium.

Certain patients, such as those with primary pulmonary hypertension, are at high risk in pulmonary arteriography. The risks and complications of this procedure are listed in Table 4-3.

The pulmonary angiogram is performed through venous access, usually from the median antecubital vein; the femoral vein may be the site of thrombi in patients with suspected pulmonary emboli and the antecubital vein is more hemostatically controllable in heparinized patients. A flexible side-hole catheter is used. Positioning the catheter tip correctly is important for an adequate study. Main pulmonary artery injections require 30 to 40 ml/second of 20 to 40 ml of contrast fluid; visualization of a left-to-right shunt or of the left heart requires 40 to 60 ml. Selective

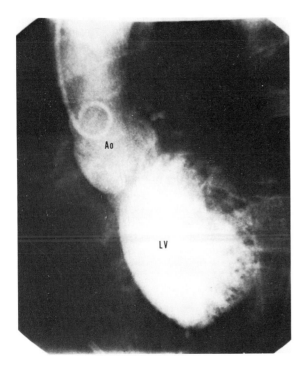

Fig. 4-14. Supravalvular aortogram, 60° LAO projection, in severe aortic regurgitation. The left ventricular (*LV*) cavity becomes more densely opacified than the aortic root (*Ao*) because of a large amount of regurgitant flow.

Fig. 4-15. Left ventriculogram, 30° RAO projection, in severe mitral regurgitation. The left atrium (*LA*) is enlarged and is well opacified by contrast material injected into the left ventricle (*LV*, diastolic outline shown; Ao: aortic root).

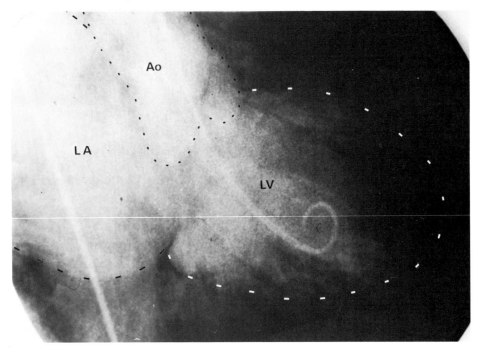

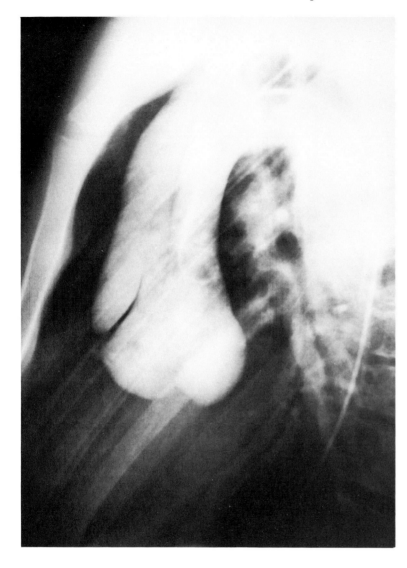

Fig. 4-16. Supravalvular aortogram in aortic dissection. Note the intimal flap (curvilinear nonopacified form) within the aortic root.

right or left pulmonary artery injections are safer, requiring less contrast media (15–25 ml) at slower rates (15–20 ml/sec). The study is recorded in the AP projection on large, separate roentgenographs for optimal resolution.

Interpretation of the pulmonary angiogram in suspected pulmonary embolism involves inspection for *intraluminal filling defects* or *abrupt cut offs* and also for areas of asymmetric delayed filling or relative oligemia (Fig. 4-17). These latter findings may occur in chronic lung disease and are not in themselves diagnostic of pulmonary thromboembolism. Problem areas can be better delineated by specific local injection.

Pulmonary angiography for shunting (as in arteriovenous malformation or anomalous pulmonary venous return) or for left-heart visualization requires that films be taken throughout the course of dye travel into the left heart, or *levo* phase. There are several good reviews and studies of pulmonary angiography in the literature.[249]

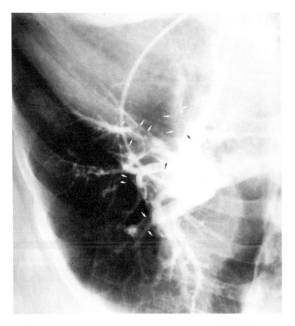

Fig. 4-17. Pulmonary arteriogram. Multiple pulmonary emboli are present in several branches of the left pulmonary artery in this left posterior oblique view. The black arrows indicate the filling defects caused by thrombus and the white arrows outline the walls of vessels containing emboli. The curvilinear shadow is the pulmonary artery catheter.

COMPLICATIONS ASSOCIATED WITH CARDIAC CATHETERIZATION

The complications of cardiac catheterization include death, cardiac injury (such as myocardial infarction), arrhythmias, cerebral disturbances (such as stroke), and local vascular damage. Potential hazards as well as their setting and treatment are detailed in Table 4-3.

The overall mortality rate associated with cardiac catheterization has been quoted in the past as 0.45 percent.[250] It is important to note that over two-thirds of these deaths occurred in infants (typically, cyanotic patients with congenital malformations and congestive failure); the risk of dying for patients studied in the first month of life is 6.2 percent, but only 0.15 percent for all patients over two years of age. The vast majority of patients dying at catheterization are critically ill at the time of study. Thus, the risk of catheterization must be carefully weighed against the potential benefits expected from the planned investigation. Cardiac catheterization may merely precipitate death which would occur in the course of severe illness anway; if the patient would probably benefit from crucial information gained by invasive study, such a procedure should be considered as a guide for needed therapy such as surgery. Some reports indicate that in precariously ill adult patients with coronary artery disease, there may be more deaths in the 24 hours preceding angiography than in the 24 hours following the procedure.[251, 252]

In addition to the severity and nature of the patient's illness, there are other factors which influence the likelihood of complications, such as the duration and complexity of the procedure. Certain techniques are associated with greater hazard: transseptal catheterization, for example, is somewhat riskier than other procedures.[253] Some studies of coronary arteriography have reported a higher mortality rate (0.78%) with the femoral percutaneous (Judkins) technique than with the brachial arteriotomy (Sones) method (0.13%).[254] A more recent multicenter cooperative trial has observed a higher mortality rate (0.51% versus 0.14%) with the brachial technique. In experienced hands, the brachial method was proven just as safe as the femoral;[255] however, the safety of both techniques has improved in recent years.[256, 257] Experienced centers achieve a mortality rate near 0.1 percent for coronary arteriography. The most recent survey of complications of this procedure is from 7553 consecutive patients in a multicenter study, reporting an overall mortality rate of 0.2 percent; myocardial infarction, 0.25 percent; and of CNS embolic complications, 0.03 percent.[250]

SPECIAL INVASIVE METHODS

ELECTROPHYSIOLOGIC STUDIES

Many rhythm and conduction disorders can now be effectively diagnosed by intracardiac electrocardiography, a technique first introduced in humans in 1969.[257] Information from these studies allows better understanding of cardiac electrophysiology and affords a rational approach to pharmacologic, pacemaker, or surgical therapy.

By appropriately positioning an electrode-tipped catheter (Fig. 4-18) within various cardiac chambers, impulses can be recorded which are not detected on the usual 12-lead surface ECG. For example, with the electrodes along the right ventricular surface of the interventricular septum, depolarization of the right atrium, the Bundle of His, and the ventricles can be recorded, revealing the site of atrioventricular conduction delay. The morbidity of such a procedure is similar to that of routine right-heart catheterization.

More recently, intracardiac recordings have been used to localize the site of anomalous atrioventricular pathways or bypass tracts in preexcitation conditions, such as the Wolff–Parkinson–White syndrome.[258] This may guide pharmacologic therapy or surgical ablation of the abnormal conducting tissue.

Electrode-catheter techniques may be used to initiate certain tachyarrhythmias. A programmable impulse generator allows stimulation of various intracardiac sites in a predetermined sequence. Induction of supraventricular or ventricular tachycardia in patients with these arrhythmias allows reliable selection and evaluation of pharmacotherapy.[259] This is important in patients with life-threatening arrhythmias, in whom clinical trial and error can be costly and perhaps risky.

The most recent application of electrophysiologic techniques has been in the treatment of recurrent, sustained ventricular tachycardia (see Chap. 8). This dangerous arrhythmia may occur in survivors of myocardial infarction, often in association with a ventricular scar or aneurysm. If antiarrhythmic drugs are not effective, the abnormal tissue causing the tachycardia may be surgically removed. Routine or "blind" ventricular aneurysmectomy appears less successful than specific endocardial resection guided by electrophysiologic mapping to locate and re-

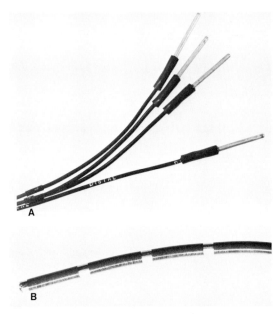

Fig. 4-18. Intracardiac electrode catheter.
Multiple leads (*A*) at proximal end of catheter are connected to the distal electrodes (*B*).

move the origin of the tachycardia.[260] Before surgery, the inducibility of the tachycardia and the approximate location of its origin are established by electrode-catheter studies in the catheterization laboratory. In the operating room, the heart is exposed and bipolar electrograms are recorded from multiple epicardial sites using an electrode-probe mounted on the fingertip of the surgeon. This is then repeated after initiating ventricular tachycardia with epicardial pacing electrodes. Cardiopulmonary bypass is begun and aneurysmectomy or ventriculotomy is performed. Endocardial mapping is then repeated with the probe-electrode. The site of earliest electrical activation is considered the origin of the tachycardia (Fig. 4-19). This area is nearly always on the endocardial surface. The site is resected to a depth of 1 to 2 mm in as wide an excision as is practical. An encircling ventriculotomy is performed around any scar in order to electrically isolate the site. After ventricular repair, induction of tachycardia is reattempted to assess the result. Although new, this technique is prom-

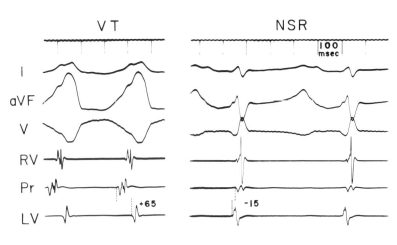

Fig. 4-19. Intracardiac electrogram. At left, during ventricular tachycardia (*VT*), abnormal early electrical activation occurs at the probe site (*Pr*), preceding left ventricular reference electrode (*LV*) depolarization by 65 msec. During normal sinus rhythm (*NSR*) the usual sequence is observed. (*I, aVF,* and *V* are standard surface ECG leads; *RV:* right ventricular reference electrode).

Fig. 4-20. Catheter bioptome. The handle (*A*) can be engaged, closing the distal jaws (*B*) for endomyocardial biopsy. The catheter is introduced through a 9-French sheath.

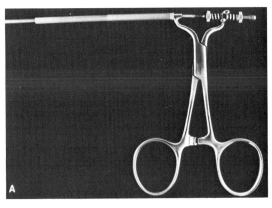

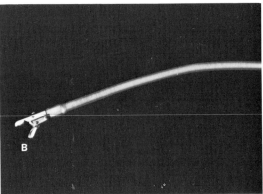

ising and offers potential therapy in an increasingly frequent and frustrating clinical setting.

CARDIAC BIOPSY

Diagnostic myocardial biopsy in humans began in 1956, requiring limited thoracotomy.[261] This was followed by variations of needle biopsy techniques with a relatively high complication rate. In the 1960s, the transvascular endomyocardial biopsy technique was developed, allowing the procedure to be performed much more safely and easily during routine cardiac catheterization without surgical assistance.

The techniques of endomyocardial biopsy have been reviewed extensively.[262–264] The Stanford method has been used substantially and is representative of the general technique. In it, a catheter-mounted bioptome (Fig. 4-20) is introduced percutaneously into the right internal jugular vein and advanced under fluoroscopic control (Fig. 4-21) into the right ventricular apex, pointing toward the interventricular septum. The jaws of the bioptome are opened, gently advanced against the septal wall, closed, and a 2 to 3 mm diameter specimen removed. This procedure has been performed in over 3000 cases without any deaths and with a complication rate of less than 1 percent.[265] It can be performed repeatedly (one transplant patient

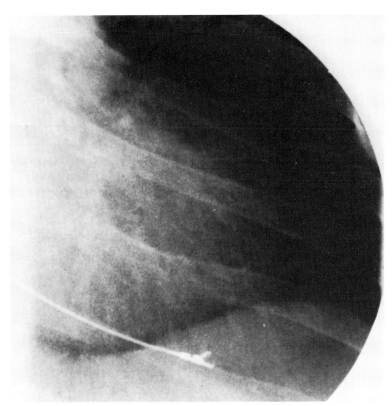

Fig. 4-21. Fluoroscopic image of catheter bioptome within the right ventricle, posteroanterior projection. The catheter has been advanced from the right internal jugular vein, across the tricuspid valve, and into the right ventricular apex (below the left diaphragm shadow in this view). The catheter is then withdrawn slightly, opened, and gently readvanced, whereupon the jaws are closed to perform the biopsy.

has had over 30 biopsies) and yields enough tissue for adequate histologic examination. Left ventricular percutaneous endomyocardial biopsy can also be performed with a catheter bioptome and is as safe as the right-sided procedure.

Catheter biopsy of the heart has been used for specific diagnosis in several diseases: cardiac allograft rejection, myocarditis, adriamycin cardiac toxicity, cardiac amyloidosis, sarcoidosis and hemochromatosis, endocardial fibrosis and fibroelastosis, carcinoid disease, Fabry's disease of the heart, glycogen storage disease, and others. Nonpathognomonic myocardial changes have been observed in idiopathic congestive cardiomyopathy, IHSS, thyroid heart disease, myotonic dystrophy, and mitral valve prolapse. *General* clinical use of endomyocardial biopsy is probably not justified, however, because of the low diagnostic yield. When employed for specific clinical questions or for research purposes, this technique appears quite useful.

Further development will undoubtedly make it a more valuable clinical tool.

PERCUTANEOUS TRANSLUMINAL CORONARY ANGIOPLASTY

A nonsurgical treatment for obstructive coronary atherosclerosis would have obvious advantages over the sometimes hazardous and clearly expensive operative procedures currently so extensively used. In 1977, Dr. Andreas Grüntzig in Zürich performed the first transluminal coronary angioplasty in humans, using a special balloon catheter.[266] This procedure enjoyed early notoriety among the public as well as the medical profession because of its innovative approach to a widespread disease.

The technique involves the percutaneous insertion of a preshaped guiding catheter into the region of the coronary ostium. A second catheter is then advanced through the guiding channel into the coronary artery. This

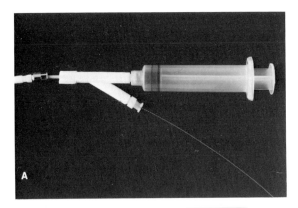

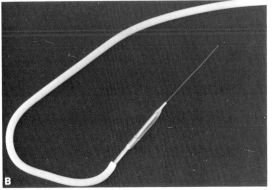

Fig. 4-22. Percutaneous transluminal angioplasty catheter assembly. The guide wire is shown entering the catheter (*A*) and exiting via the distal end (*B*). The syringe fills the distal balloon (*B*) with contrast under manually controlled pressure. The dilating catheter is placed into the vessel with a preformed guiding sheath, in this case for the left coronary artery.

dilation catheter contains a thin guide wire which facilitates its advance across proximal coronary obstructions (Fig. 4-22). A slender balloon is then inflated with contrast fluid to a pressure of 4 to 6 atmospheres for a few seconds, dilating the putty-like atheromatous narrowing, as verified by pressure gradient measurements and subsequent angiography.

Percutaneous angioplasty is currently applicable to less than 10 percent of all coronary artery disease patients: those with proximal noncalcified lesions, usually in a single vessel, and patent enough to allow passage of the balloon catheter. Initial experience[267] indicates that this is a very specialized technique best performed by highly experienced physicians. Symptomatic and hemodynamic improvement occurs, but is offset by an immediate mortality rate of 1 percent, a need for early bypass surgery in nearly 10 percent of patients, and restenosis in another 10 percent.

Further development of transluminal angioplasty may include refinement of equipment, improvement of technique, extension to a larger fraction of coronary patients, and use in the operating room as an adjunct to bypass surgery.

NONINVASIVE DIAGNOSTIC METHODS COMPLEMENTING INVASIVE STUDIES

Modern cardiology is largely founded on advances in cardiac catheterization and open-heart surgery. However, a small revolution has been taking place over the past two decades involving new noninvasive diagnostic methods. Noninvasive techniques have the virtues of safety, simplicity, and economy, and are now approaching the diagnostic accuracy of invasive methods, the "gold standard" with which they have long been compared. Rather than replacing cardiac catheterization, noninvasive methods currently enhance invasive techniques; the noninvasive test is useful in screening patients and determining the appropriate time for catheterization and surgery. Noninvasive methods are particularly helpful in multiple serial studies and in the evaluation of critically ill, high-risk patients. This section will highlight the noninvasive methods which currently complement cardiac catheterization.

PHONOCARDIOGRAPHY AND SYSTOLIC TIME INTERVALS

The recording of heart sounds and external pulses may help determine the presence and severity of certain cardiac lesions. For example, tricuspid insufficiency causes ventricularization of the jugular venous pulse (loss of x-descent and appearance of a regurgitant wave in systole whose amplitude often correlates with severity of regurgitation); the severity of pulmonic stenosis may be estimated by measuring the time interval between the aortic and pulmonic components of the second heart sound.[268]

The noninvasive determination of systolic time intervals (STIs) was developed quite early and still remains very useful in evaluating left ventricular performance in many diseases.[269, 270] There are three fundamental systolic time intervals: (1) $Q - S_2$ (electromechanical systole, QRS onset to second heart sound); (2) *LVET* (left ventricular ejection time, carotid pulse upstroke to dicrotic notch); (3) *PEP* (preejection period; PEP = $(Q - S_2)$ − LVET (Fig. 4-23). Because these intervals vary inversely with heart rate and sex, they may be corrected and expressed as indices (Table 4-4).

Several conditions influence STIs.[271] LVET may be prolonged in left ventricular outflow tract obstruction as a result of aortic stenosis or shortened in conditions with reduced effective stroke volume, such as cardiomyopathy. PEP is prolonged in delayed left ventricular electrical conduction, such as left bundle branch block. In normal conduction, prolongation of the PEP suggests a reduced rate of left ventricular early systolic pressure rise *(dP/dt)*, which may be caused by left ventricular failure or diminished filling pressure. Conversely, a shortened PEP occurs with increased inotropy (Table 4-5).

The PEP consists of the electromechanical interval (EMI; time between ECG Q wave onset and beginning of left ventricular pressure rise) and the pressure rise time (PRT; time between beginning of left ventricular pressure rise and opening of aortic valve). In the absence of conduction delay, the PEP depends chiefly on the PRT. It can be shown that the PRT (in msec) is approximately equal to

$$(Ao_{dp} - LVEDP)/(\Delta P/\Delta T)$$

where Ao_{dp} is diastolic aortic pressure (afterload), LVEDP is left ventricular end diastolic pressure (preload), and $\Delta P/\Delta T$ is mean rate of left ventricular pressure rise (contractility). Expressed differently,

$$\frac{\Delta P}{\Delta T} \cong \frac{Ao_{dp} - PAWP}{PEP} \left(\frac{torr}{milliseconds} \right)$$

Thus, $\Delta P/\Delta T$ (mean electromechanical $\Delta P/\Delta T$) is an index of left ventricular performance, which can be obtained from combined findings of right-heart catheterization and noninvasive STIs. In a small series of patients, $\Delta P/\Delta T$ correlated well with left ventricular dp/dt obtained by left ventricular catheterization.[272]

The ratio PEP/LVET is essentially independent of heart rate variation below 110 beats/min and is the most useful and sensitive measurement of left ventricular performance derived from STIs. PEP/LVET correlates well (r = −0.90) with angiographic ejection fraction in various cardiac diseases:[273] a PEP/LVET of greater than 0.5 predicts an ejection fraction of less than 40 percent, with 95 percent confidence. PEP/LVET is almost always abnormal when the cardiac index is reduced because cardiac index is less sensitive than other left ventricular performance indices. However, there may be patients with abnormal PEP/LVET yet normal cardiac index. Normal PEP/LVET at rest is 0.345 ± 0.036.[274]

ECHOCARDIOGRAPHY

During the 1960s and 1970s, echocardiography advanced from a new, relatively crude technique to its current position as a highly useful and reliable clinical tool, involving in-

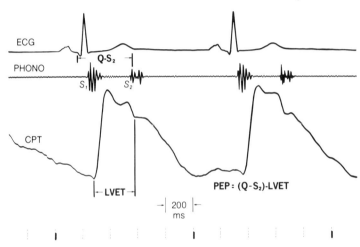

Fig. 4-23. Systolic time intervals. From the ECG and phonocardiogram (Phono), total electromechanical systole ($Q - S_2$) is measured. The left ventricular ejection time (*LVET*) is obtained from the carotid pulse tracing (*CPT*). Preejection period (*PEP*) is the difference between $Q - S_2$ and *LVET*.

Table 4-4. Systolic Time Intervals: Regression Equation for Predicted Values of STIs

	MALE	FEMALE
$Q-S_2$	$[546 - (2.1) \text{ HR}] \pm 14$	$[549 - (2.0) \text{ HR}] \pm 14$
PEP	$[131 - (0.4) \text{ HR}] \pm 13$	$[133 - (0.4) \text{ HR}] \pm 11$
LVET	$[413 - (1.7) \text{ HR}] \pm 10$	$[418 - (1.6) \text{ HR}] \pm 10$

Values are given as msec $\pm$ SD
Normal PEP/LVET is 0.345 ± 0.036.[274]
(Weissler AM, Harris WS, Schoenfeld C: Systolic time intervals in heart failure in man. Circulation 37:149, 1968)

Table 4-5. Systolic Time Intervals: Changes With Disease and Drugs

	Q-S₂	PEP	LVET	PEP/LVET
Coronary artery disease				
Chronic ischemic left ventricular dysfunction		— or ↑	— or ↓	↑ In angina, CHF; may improve after surgical revascularization
Acute myocardial infarction	↓ In-creased adrener-gic tone	Variable	↓	— or ↑
Valvular heart disease				
Aortic stenosis without CHF	↑	↓	↑	↓
(values tend to normalize in AS with CHF)				
Aortic regurgitation		↓	↑	↓
(LVET decreases with CHF)				
Mitral stenosis with CHF		↑	↓	↑ Usually with de-creased ejection fraction
Mitral regurgitation		↑	↓	↑ Accentuated with left ventricular dysfunction
Myocardial disease		↑	↓	↑
Rhythm disturbances				
Left bundle branch block	↑	↑	— or ↓	↑
Atrial fibrillation, rate >75/min		↑	↓	↑
Atrial pacing	↓		↓	
Drugs				
Digitalis	↓	↓	↓	↓
Isoproterenol	↓	↓	↓	↓
Propranolol		↑	↑	↑
Methoxamine (increased afterload)	↑	↑	↑	
Phenotolamine		↓	↑	↓
Atropine	↓		↓	

creasingly sophisticated electronic equipment. Although definitely limited in its ability to diagnose cardiac disorders, echocardiography already provides accurate, free-standing diagnoses of many conditions. This section will outline some of the clinical conditions in which echocardiography is most useful. For more complete information, the reader is referred to several good review articles and books.[275-277]

Clinical ultrasound depends upon three acoustical principles: (1) the transmission speed of ultrasound through soft tissues is relatively constant (approximately 1540 m/sec for the frequency range 2–5 million cps or megaHz); (2) any interface between two materials with different densities will reflect a portion of the incident sound (producing an echo); and (3) the location of sonoreflective objects or interfaces along an ultrasound beam may be displayed accurately by an electronic instrument. *M-mode* (or motion mode) echocardiography is the one-dimensional array of various tissue interfaces swept in time across an oscilloscope or inscribed by a strip-chart recorder, producing characteristic motion patterns (Fig. 4-24). The echo transducer contains a piezoelectric crystal which emits a sound impulse lasting approximately one millionth of a second and then acts as a sound receiver until the next pulse. This cycle occurs rapidly enough to allow approximately 1000 depth readings per second and thus echocardiography can be very precise.

The echocardiographic abnormalities of some cardiac conditions are specific enough to allow a positive diagnosis solely by ultrasound. These include pericardial effusion and rheumatic mitral stenosis: two conditions in which echocardiography found early application. The echocardiographic findings in other heart disorders may not provide an absolute diagnosis but can confirm a clinical suspicion, localize an abnormality, or indicate further diagnostic tests. Table 4-6 lists current clinical applications of M-mode echocardiography in the diagnosis of acquired and congenital heart disease.

Conventional M-mode echocardiography has limited diagnostic value in some cases, such as mitral regurgitation. With the new technique of Doppler echocardiography, the severity of mitral regurgitation may be estimated.[278] Commercially available instruments employ circuitry using the ultrasound transducer as a receiver of reflected sound waves for graphic presentation (echo) as well as for electronic analysis of frequency shift (Doppler).

Two-dimensional, cross-sectional echocardiography is a recent development which has greatly extended the diagnostic power of ultrasound. This technique, which is still undergoing rapid development, allows two-dimensional imaging of the heart in multiple planes from multiple angles (Fig. 4-25). This spatial orientation proves valuable in estimating the severity of mitral and aortic stenosis, detecting intracardiac tumors and valvular vegetations, revealing anatomy in congenital disease, assessing wall motion abnormalities, and detecting ventricular aneurysms. Two-dimensional echocardiography has proven more sensitive than the M-mode technique in certain cases, but is not necessarily wholly superior and is still a subject of active research.

NUCLEAR CARDIOLOGY

Nuclear cardiology is a rapidly developing field which has already become extremely popular in several clinical settings. Radioactive isotopes, or radionuclides, are injected intravenously and their activity recorded by complex scanners or cameras positioned over the heart. There are currently three main types of radionuclide scans: (1) *perfusion imaging*, for evaluating myocardial blood flow; (2) *infarction scintigraphy*, for detecting necrotic or injured myocardium; and (3) *blood-pool scanning*, for determining ventricular performance.

Myocardial perfusion imaging relies on uptake by normal cardiac cells of the potassium analogue, [201]thallous chloride. Thallium accumulates rapidly and uniformly within normal myocardium within minutes after intravenous injection, but unevenly or not at all

Table 4-6. Clinical Applications of M-Mode Echocardiography

CONDITION	ECHO FINDINGS DIAGNOSTIC	ECHO FINDINGS SUGGESTIVE

Acquired	Rheumatic mitral stenosis
	Mitral valve prolapse
	Calcified mitral annulus
	Aortic regurgitation
	Atrial masses
	Asymmetric septal hyper-
	  trophy
	Dilated (congestive)
	  cardiomyopathy
	Pericardial effusion
		Aortic stenosis
		Aortic root dissecting
		  aneurysm
		Valvular vegetations
		Ruptured chordae tendi-
		  neae
		Pericardial thickening
		Left ventricular dysfunc-
		  tion

Congenital	*Cyanotic*
	Ebstein's anomaly
	Hypoplastic left heart
	D-transposition of great ar-
	  teries
	Tetralogy of Fallot
	
	Shunts
	Primum ASD
	Malalignment VSD
	Complete AV canal
		Tricuspid atresia
		Pulmonary atresia with in-
		  tact septum
		Double outlet right ventri-
		  cle
		
		Secundum ASD, anoma-
		lous pulmonary venous
		  return
		Patent ductus arteriosus
		  with L → R shunt
		
		Other
		Bicuspid aortic valve
		Congenital mitral stenosis
		  (parachute mitral valve)
		Cor triatriatum
		Subaortic stenosis
		L-transposition of great ar-
		  teries

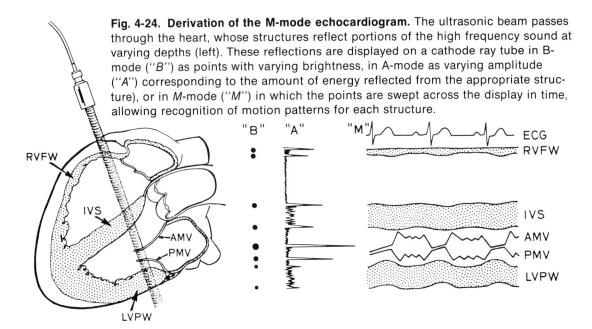

Fig. 4-24. Derivation of the M-mode echocardiogram. The ultrasonic beam passes through the heart, whose structures reflect portions of the high frequency sound at varying depths (left). These reflections are displayed on a cathode ray tube in B-mode ("*B*") as points with varying brightness, in A-mode as varying amplitude ("*A*") corresponding to the amount of energy reflected from the appropriate structure), or in M-mode ("*M*") in which the points are swept across the display in time, allowing recognition of motion patterns for each structure.

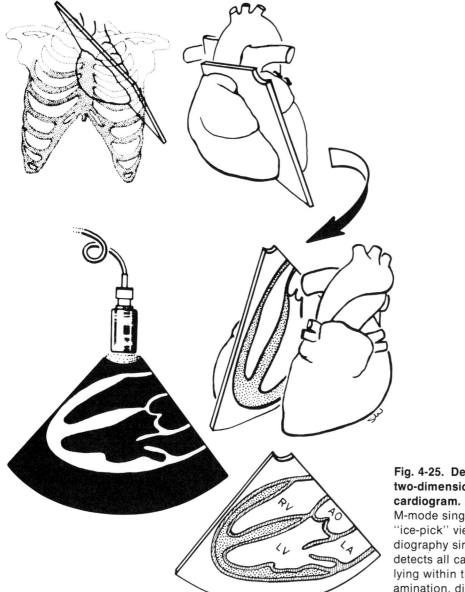

Fig. 4-25. Derivation of the two-dimensional (2-D) echocardiogram. Rather than the M-mode single dimensional, "ice-pick" view, 2-D echocardiography simultaneously detects all cardiac structures lying within the plane of examination, displaying the image on a video screen.

in hypoperfused or infarcted tissue.[279] The abnormal areas without thallium uptake produce "cold spots" on the image; the size and severity of these defects depends on the ratio of blood flow in the abnormal area to that in the surrounding areas. Blood flow during exercise increases more in normal coronary arteries than in stenosed vessels and may therefore intensify a resting thallium defect

or produce a new one not observed as rest. For this reason, [201]thallium perfusion imaging is most useful in conjunction with exercise electrocardiography; the combination of both techniques can detect coronary artery disease with greater sensitivity than either method alone. Thallium scanning is less likely to result in a false-positive diagnosis of coronary artery disease than is exercise electrocardiography, especially in the setting of an abnormal ECG or digitalis effects. Other advantages of thallium imaging include its value in screening patients with atypical chest pain and an equivocal exercise ECG, assessing the physiologic significance of a known coronary arterial lesion, and in determining coronary graft patency. The disadvantages of thallium imaging include its decreased sensitivity to the diffuse hypoperfusion abnormalities of multi-vessel coronary disease and its inability to always distinguish infarcted tissue from ischemic myocardium.

Infarction scintigraphy involves the increased uptake of ^{99m}technetium pyrophosphate by acutely damaged myocardium.[280] Thus areas of acute myocardial infarction will register a "hot spot" on the image in contrast to unlabelled normal tissue. Technetium pyrophosphate scintigrams become positive from 12 to 72 hours after infarction and usually revert to normal in about ten days. This technique can be particularly useful in diagnosing myocardial infarction in several clinical settings, such as immediately after coronary artery bypass grafting. However, because it is a sensitive detector of all types of myocardial necrosis, technetium pyrophosphate scanning may also be positive in myocardial contusion, high-energy cardioversion, ventricular aneurysms, or even old myocardial infarctions.

Blood pool scanning is the display and analysis of radioactivity remaining in the bloodstream after an intravenous injection. ^{99m}Technetium human serum albumin is the most common intravascular marker used. There are currently two blood pool scanning methods: *first-pass* radionuclide angiocardiography and *equilibrium-gated* blood pool imaging. The first-pass technique follows the marker as it moves through the cardiac chambers, allowing detection of shunts or valvular regurgitation. The equilibrium technique measures the marker after it has equilibrated within the vasculature, permitting repeated scans over several hours and during acute interventions. By "triggering" or "gating" the camera to the ECG, the left ventricular image or representative counts can be recorded in end diastole and end systole, giving ejection fraction. The main problem with radionuclide scanning as an angiocardiographic method is resolution. However, ejection fraction derived from gated imaging correlates well with that from contrast ventriculography.

CARDIAC CATHETERIZATION IN SPECIFIC CARDIAC DISORDERS (Table 4-7)

CORONARY ARTERY DISEASE

The definitive diagnostic method for coronary artery disease is *selective* coronary cinéarteriography (see p. 88). Rapid developments in recent years have liberalized the indications for coronary arteriography. Indications will also differ somewhat between various centers, but in general the following guidelines apply:

1. *Angina pectoris unresponsive to medical therapy.* Such patients will probably benefit from coronary artery bypass surgery,[281, 282] and coronary arteriography is performed to assess the feasibility of bypass in any given patient.
2. *Patients undergoing planned open-heart surgery.* The patient with surgically treatable valvular disease may have significant coronary atherosclerosis (for example, patients with aortic stenosis[283]) and should in many cases have coronary arteriography as part of the preoperative evaluation, especially if angina pectoris is present.
3. *Patients suspected of having left main coronary artery stenosis.* Although clinical characteristics cannot fully identify this group, increased severity of angina and markedly abnormal exercise electrocardiography may raise the suspicion of left main or extensive three-vessel coronary disease. Because of the ominous natural prognosis and improved survival with surgical treatment in these patients,[284] they should un-

dergo coronary arteriography (see Fig. 4-12).

4. *Patients with uncertain diagnosis.* This includes patients with significant chest pain syndromes in whom noninvasive tests are unclear and in whom it is important to determine the cause of chest pain and the extent of coronary disease if present.

5. *Unstable angina pectoris.* These patients, especially those in whom medical therapy is not fully effective, should probably receive coronary arteriography because there is the possibility of severe and extensive coronary atherosclerosis, often with poor intrinsic collateralization.[285-287]

6. *Angina pectoris with life-threatening, recurrent ventricular arrhythmias.* Investigation of the coronary circulation may reveal significant and surgically approachable disease, which in some cases is responsive to myocardial revascularization.

7. *Other indications.* Varying according to medical center and individual cases, include
   a. *possible coronary artery spasm,* whose treatment differs from atherosclerotic disease and warrants specialized investigation;[288, 289]
   b. *need for evaluation of graft patency after bypass surgery;*
   c. *myocardial infarction, angina, or abnormal ECG in youthful patients or in persons with crucial occupations* (pilots, drivers);
   d. *patients undergoing ventriculotomy for congenital heart disease*—since anomalous coronary circulation may be harmed if not known preoperatively; and
   e. *research applications.*

Coronary arteriography is highly useful when performed appropriately. With an estimated 300,000 to 400,000 of these procedures per year, there may be many instances of inappropriate use;[290] this means all members of the medical care team must be aware of correct indications and contraindications.

Contraindications to coronary arteriography include severe or uncontrolled conges-

tive heart failure or arrhythmias, febrile illnesses, hypokalemia, and acute myocardial infarction.[291] These are somewhat relative and depend on the patient, center, and urgency of study. Perhaps the most absolute contraindication has been acute myocardial infarction, but some have reported no increased mortality or clinical worsening if coronary arteriography is performed selectively and properly.[292, 293]

Several special techniques have emerged which are useful for evaluating the patient with coronary artery disease. Angiographic visualization of bypass grafts is an important method for assessing the results of surgical revascularization and has recently been extensively reviewed.[294] Coronary artery spasm has become better recognized in recent years; in appropriate patients, coronary arteriography is performed with ergonovine maleate challenge in order to disclose focal coronary spasm.[295] Measurement of coronary blood flow is currently a research procedure. Radioisotope and krypton perfusion techniques have been disappointing, but newly developed thermodilution methods are promising. Determination of flow, combined with measurement of arteriovenous oxygen differences, should yield valuable data regarding uptake and discharge of myocardial metabolites. Intracoronary infusion of streptokinase during the first few hours of myocardial infarction is a novel therapeutic catheter technique. This is designed to lyse thrombi which have acutely precipitated nearly reversible or reversible ischemia.

Left ventriculography remains the standard for detecting and measuring the segmental contraction abnormalities associated with infarcted or ischemic zones in the hearts of coronary artery disease patients (see p. 86). Mitral regurgitation caused by papillary muscle dysfunction is assessed most reliably by the ventriculogram (see Fig. 4-15), which can yield stroke volume, regurgitant fraction (when combined with forward cardiac output), and approximations of contractility, such as V_{CF} (velocity of circumferential shortening), and ejection fraction.

Table 4-7. Diagnostic Approaches to Various Diseases

DISEASE CATEGORY	DEFINITIVE DIAGNOSTIC METHODS	SCREENING OR SUPPORTIVE DIAGNOSTIC METHODS
Coronary artery disease (CAD)	*Selective coronary arteriography* Presence, severity, distribution of coronary athero-sclerosis; extent of intercoronary collateralization; success of revascularization surgery; progression of intrinsic atherosclerosis; addition of *ergonovine challenge* unmasks focal coronary spasm. *Left ventriculography* Degree and distribution of segmental contraction abnormalities; presence and location of ventricular aneurysms or focal dyskinetic sites; presence of mitral regurgitation caused by papillary muscle dysfunction or infarction; intervention ventriculography (e.g., ventriculography after administration of nitroglycerin) may reveal left ventricular segments with reversible contraction abnormalities.	*Right heart catheterization* Exercise or pacing may cause elevation in pulmonary artery wedge pressure or pulmonary artery diastolic pressure; such stress-induced hemodynamic changes may help assess extent of left ventricular ischemic disease or improvement after surgery. *Exercise electrocardiography* Can help diagnose ischemic heart disease, especially in a population with increased risk of coronary atherosclerosis; although limited in its reliability for detecting ischemia or severity of disease, may be most useful in postoperative or post MI rehabilitation and prognosis assessment. *Radionuclide studies* Perfusion scanning (cold spot) for detection of relative or absolute ischemia at rest or during exercise; blood pool scanning for measurement of ejection fraction and for noninvasive left ventriculography; infarct scintigraphy (hot spot) for detection of acute myocardial infarction *Myocardial metabolic studies* Coronary sinus sampling of lactate and so on; measurement of coronary blood flow, assessment of significance of coronary lesions by observing lactate production (anaerobiosis) during stress (such as atrial pacing)
Valvular heart disease *Aortic stenosis (AS)*	*Hemodynamics* Direct determination of aortic valve gradient and area by left-heart catheterization; left ventricular compliance estimated by LVEDP; most stenotic valves allow retrograde catheter passage into left ventricle but occasionally transseptal catheterization is required. *Angiography* Left ventriculogram evaluates left ventricle size, performance, and wall thickness (hypertrophy); supravalvular aortogram can usually identify bicuspid aortic valves; both techniques can localize congenital sub- or supravalvular stenosis.	*Cardiac fluoroscopy* Detects calcification of aortic valve *Phonocardiography and external pulse recording* Slow carotid pulse rise, diminished aortic component of second heart sound, late-peaking ejection murmur, and increased apexcardiogram A wave usually indicate severity of stenosis. *Two-dimensional echocardiography* Can stratify stenosis severity according to maximum systolic cusp separation; can also detect sub- or supravalvular stenosis.

Aortic regurgitation (AR)	*Angiography* Supravalvular aortography qualitatively estimates severity according to amount of dye entering left ventricle; left ventriculography reveals left ventricle size, contractility, and, combined with forward cardiac output, regurgitant fraction and volume. *Indicator Dilution Technique* May be more accurate in assessing regurgitant volume in severe AR with enlarged left ventricle.	*Hemodynamics* Difference between central aortic and femoral arterial pulse pressures correlates with regurgitant fraction; LVEDP elevation reveals left ventricular failure. *External pulse recording* May show diminished dicrotic notch *Phonocardiography* Shows diastolic murmur; S_3 in left ventricular dysfunction *Echocardiography* Shows anterior mitral leaflet diastolic flutter or "buzz."
Mitral stenosis (MS)	*Hemodynamics* Elevated LA pressure; persistent diastolic LA-LV pressure gradient, reflecting valve orifice area; decreased y descent in LA pressure curve because of slow LA emptying; when transseptal catheterization is not performed, LA pressure curve may be approximated by PA wedge tracing; pulmonary hypertension and increased pulmonary vascular resistance are present in severe, chronic MS.	*Phonocardiography* Loud S_1; opening snap (OS) recorded, and S_2-OS interval decreases with more severe MS *Echocardiography* Typical rheumatic pattern for mitral valve motion (posterior leaflet moves anteriorly); posterior aortic root motion indicates slow LA emptying.
Mitral regurgitation (MR)	*Left ventriculography* Qualitative assessment of MR according to amount of dye entering LA; reveals left ventricular size, performance *Indicator dilution* Technique allows more quantitative results, but requires transseptal catheterization (indicator injected in LV, sampled from LA). *Hemodynamics* Large v wave in LA (or PA wedge) pressure curve, reflecting flow; elevated LVEDP reflects LV failure.	*Phonocardiography* Shows holosystolic murmur; S_3 present in left ventricle dysfunction.
Tricuspid regurgitation (TR)	Difficult to quantitate by any method. *Hemodynamics* Large right atrial v wave; in extreme cases ventricularization of RA pressure with rapid y descent (caused by rapid RA emptying through a nonobstructed tricuspid valve) and diminished x descent (regurgitant v wave begins earlier) in severe cases.	

Table 4-7. Continued

DISEASE CATEGORY	DEFINITIVE DIAGNOSTIC METHODS	SCREENING OR SUPPORTIVE DIAGNOSTIC METHODS
Congenital heart disease *Valvular and vascular lesions* Patent ductus arteriosus (PDA)	*Saturation studies* The venous catheter is manipulable into the descending aorta; at the main PA level, a L → R shunt (O_2 step-up) is seen.	*Angiography* Usually not necessary; this shows prompt opacification of the pulmonary artery through the PDA upon injection of contrast media into the aorta.
Coarctation of the aorta	*Hemodynamics* Pre- and postcoarctation pressures may be obtained through upper and lower extremity retrograde arterial catheterization.	*Angiography* May be helpful in ruling out associated abnormalities (such as bicuspid aortic valve).
Vascular rings	*Angiography* Anatomy defined by angiogram	
Pulmonic stenosis	*Hemodynamics* RV-PA gradient on pull-back (catheter withdrawn from PA into RV). RV pressure is greater than 30–35 torr with PS gradients of 10 torr or more. RV pressures in extreme cases may reach 250 torr.	*Angiography* Lateral view right ventriculogram shows domed pulmonic leaflets with jet of contrast through orifice. Narrowed, hypertrophied infundibulum may be seen. *Saturation studies* Occasional R → L shunting across foramen ovale if RA pressures rise
Aortic stenosis	*Hemodynamics* Transobstruction gradient across subvalvular, valvular, or supravalvular stenoses. Gradients of greater than 75 torr usually signify severe stenosis.	*LV angiogram* May show a ring-like obstruction in subvalvular, a thickened, domed valve in valvular, or an "hourglass"-like aortic root narrowing in supravalvular aortic stenosis.
Ebstein's anomaly of the tricuspid valve	*Hemodynamic* Electrocardiographic combined study shows RV ECG with RA pressure curves as catheter is withdrawn from RV across the displaced tricuspid valve into the atrialized portion of the RV.	*Angiography* Of RV shows tricuspid valve displaced towards apex, with tricuspid regurgitation.
Intracardiac lesions with L → R shunt Secundum atrial septal defect (ASD) and patent foramen ovale	*Saturation studies* Increased O_2 content in RA quantification of shunt may be difficult if right pulmonary veins drain anomalously into superior vena cava.	*Angiography* Main PA injection will demonstrate L → R (LA → RA) shunt.

Hemodynamics
Right-sided pressures are usually normal; because of high *flow*, there may be a systolic gradient of up to 20 torr across the normal pulmonic valve.

Indicator dilution curves
Are best estimators of shunt in case of anomalous pulmonary venous connection.

Endocardial cushion defect (ECD)

Hemodynamics
In complete ECD, RV pressure may rise to systemic (LV) level, with increased pulmonary blood flow. Eventually, right-sided pressures may rise sufficiently to reverse the shunting slightly, yielding a net R → L shunt.

Catheter manipulation
On fluoroscopy reveals passage of the catheter across a partial ECD (ostium primum defect) at a lower level than the secundum ASD; in complete ECD, the venous catheter is usually easily manipulated into all 4 cardiac chambers.
Saturation studies
Large L → R shunt at RA (and RV in complete ECD)
Angiography
In partial or full ECD, LV angiogram shows "gooseneck" deformity of outflow tract; abnormal anterior mitral leaflet insertion onto crest of muscular septum; also cleft mitral valve

---

Ventricular septal defect (VSD)

Hemodynamics
LV end-diastolic pressure may be elevated, especially in large shunt, with CHF.

Saturation studies
Large O$_2$ step up in RV caused by L → R shunt.
Angiography
LV angiogram in LAO view shows size and location of defect(s).

Intracardiac lesions with R → L shunt
Tetralogy of fallot

Coronary arteriography
Is performed to rule out associated anatomic abnormalities and to indicate coronary artery distribution over the infundibulum, where ventriculotomy may be contemplated in attempting total correction.

Saturation studies
Aortic saturation shows mixed input from both ventricles.
Hemodynamics
RV-PA gradient by catheter pullback
Angiography
Right ventriculogram shows size, location of R → L shunt, size of pulmonic annulus, presence of infundibular chamber, and size and anatomy of the pulmonary trunk and its branches

---

Tricuspid atresia

Catheter manipulation
Catheter cannot pass from RA to RV

Saturation studies
R → L shunt at atrial level
Angiocardiography
Injection into RA sequentially opacifies the LA, LV, RV (through VSD) and PA.

Pulmonary atresia with intact ventricular septum

Hemodynamics
High RV pressures; left-sided pressures normal
Saturation studies
Reduced O$_2$ content in LA, LV, aorta

Angiography
Upon RV injection, PA does not opacify. RV may be hypoplastic. Aortic injection demonstrates PA through PDA.

Table 4-7. Continued

DISEASE CATEGORY	DEFINITIVE DIAGNOSTIC METHODS	SCREENING OR SUPPORTIVE DIAGNOSTIC METHODS

Intracardiac lesions with bidirectional shunts
Total anomalous pulmonary venous return (TAPVR)
	Saturation studies
	  O_2 content in systemic artery (aorta) similar to that in RA and PA; in most cases, sole communication to systemic circuit is through a patent foramen ovale.
	Angiography
	  Injection in PA reveals anomalous pulmonary venous return into persistent left SVC (supracardiac drainage), into coronary sinus or RA (cardiac drainage) or into portal, hepatic veins, ductus venous, or IVC (infracardiac).
		Hemodynamics
		  Obstruction to return through pulmonary veins may be noted, causing increased pulmonary venous pressure and pulmonary edema; if obstruction is caused by insufficient interatrial communication, *balloon* septostomy may be life-saving. In cases without obstruction, pulmonary blood flow increases after birth with lessening cyanosis, but eventual RV volume overload and pulmonary hypertension may ensue.

Truncus arteriosus	*Angiography*
	  Injection into proximal truncus reveals abnormal origin of the pulmonary arteries (important for surgical planning).
	Saturation studies
	  Admixture within truncus causes aortic and PA saturations to be similar; L → R shunting may be noted in RV outflow tract.
		Hemodynamics
		  Equal systolic pressures in truncus and both ventricles; pulmonary blood flow is determined by size of pulmonary arteries and pulmonary arteriolar resistance.

Transposition of the great vessels	*Saturation studies*
	  Low O_2 content in systemic artery, RV, RA. Occasionally, a small L → R shunt at the atrial level may occur. Pulmonary venous, LV, and LA (through patent foramen ovale) saturations are normal.
	Angiography
	  Injections in both ventricles reveal relationship between chambers and great vessels. Lateral view shows A-P relationship of great vessels to each other, and the presence of any VSD. Frontal view shows opacification of pulmonary branches if ductus is patent, and shows relationship between ventricles and great vessels.
		Hemodynamics
		  Reveals whether PS is present; if so, or if VSD has placed volume load on LV, increased end diastolic pressures and CHF may be found.

Myocardial disease

Hypertrophic cardiomyopathy

Hemodynamics
1. Arterial pressure rapid upstroke, midsystolic fall, and second late systolic rise
2. Elevated left ventricular end diastolic pressure, increased left atrial a wave
3. Cardiac output usually normal; may decrease in late stages of disease with congestive failure
4. Intracavitary left ventricular outflow systolic pressure gradient, often latent or intermittent, elicitable by maneuvers

Angiography
1. Small left ventricular cavity with systolic near obliteration
2. LAO left ventriculogram may show disproportionately thickened interventricular septum.

Congestive cardiomyopathy

Angiography (left ventriculogram)
1. Grossly enlarged LV
2. Diffuse hypokinesis, reduced ejection fraction
3. Possible secondary mitral regurgitation, usually mild and probably related to globular ventricular dilation
4. Occasional mural filling defects caused by thrombus.

Hemodynamics
1. Reduced cardiac index, rate of pressure rise (*dp/dt*)
2. Frequently elevated LV end diastolic pressure
3. Pulmonary hypertension in severe disease or late stages

Restrictive cardiomyopathy

Hemodynamics
1. Increased pulmonary and systemic venous pressures (RA, LA) with large a and v waves
2. Ventricular diastolic dip and plateau pressure pattern greater than right
3. Left-sided filling pressures greater than right
4. Decreased cardiac index (reduced ventricular filling)

Pericardial disease

Constrictive pericarditis

Hemodynamics
1. Elevated venous pressure with prominent diastolic y descent and inspiratory rise in RA mean pressure (Küssmaul's sign)
2. Ventricular diastolic dip and plateau pressure pattern
3. Equalization of diastolic filling pressures, right-left.

Cardiac tamponade

Hemodynamics
1. *Pulsus paradoxus*, inspiratory fall in arterial systolic pressure, usually greater than 10 torr, with inspiratory decrease in pulse pressure
2. Elevated venous pressure, prominent systolic x descent, Küssmaul's sign less frequent than in constrictive pericarditis (above)
3. Elevated intrapericardial pressure, relieved by pericardiocentesis, with accompanying reversal of above signs and improved cardiac output.

Left ventricular aneurysm is frequently found in patients with coronary artery disease, usually following myocardial infarction. The term *aneurysm* has been adopted by most angiographers to describe any localized area of akinesis (no systolic motion) or dyskinesis (paradoxically outward systolic motion). A strict pathologic definition requires that the outpouching aneurysm consist of all layers, including muscle, of the ventricular wall. In many cases an aneurysm consists solely of smoothly lined, thick scar tissue replacing the muscular wall. This lesion may produce ventricular arrhythmias or congestive heart failure, and can be surgically approached. Resection (or plication, in some cases) of left ventricular aneurysm has been reported effective for selected patients in relieving congestive heart failure. Functional improvement is not always accompanied by an increase in cardiac output, however, and the full effects of this operation remain a subject of ongoing clinical research. Some patients may benefit from the revascularization procedure often accompanying aneurysm resection. By subtracting or ignoring the noncontractile segment on the ventricular angiogram, an estimated ejection fraction for the contractile portion can be obtained. Such a corrected ejection fraction of less than 40 percent implies a lower probability of functional improvement from the operation.

Recent developments in nuclear cardiology have been very rewarding in studying coronary artery disease. Perfusion imaging, infarct scintigraphy, and blood pool scanning are described above. Echocardiography, especially two-dimensional, cross-sectional *sector scanning*, can estimate ejection fraction and identify abnormal wall motion, may easily be performed in the coronary care unit in patients with acute myocardial infarction, and allows serial study.

VALVULAR HEART DISEASE

Although many clinical and noninvasive signs may estimate the severity of valvular lesions, cardiac catheterization is required to fully evaluate valve stenosis or regurgitation

or both. Additionally, accurate assessment of ventricular function is important in determining the patient's ability to survive or benefit from cardiac surgery.

The grading of valvular stenosis requires measurement of both flow and pressure gradient across the valve in question. Normal flow across an unobstructed valve orifice requires a small (< 5 torr) pressure gradient. Gorlin established the following basic formula for valve orifice area:[296]

$$\text{area (cm}^2) = \frac{\text{flow (cm}^3/\text{sec})}{\text{velocity (cm/sec)}} = \frac{\text{flow}}{k\sqrt{\Delta P}}$$

where ΔP is the mean pressure gradient across the orifice and k is a constant for the valve in question (k = 31 for the mitral valve, 44.5 for the aortic valve; (Figs. 4-26, 4-27). Of course, valve flow occurs only during the portion of the cardiac cycle in which the valve is open: the diastolic filling period (sec/min) for the mitral valve and the systolic ejection period (sec/min) for the aortic valve. Valve flow for the equation above is then calculated from cardiac output as follows:

mitral flow (cm³/sec) =
$$\frac{\text{cardiac output (cm}^3/\text{min})}{\text{diastolic filling period (sec/min)}}$$
aortic flow (cm³/sec) =
$$\frac{\text{cardiac output (cm}^3/\text{min})}{\text{systolic ejection period (sec/min)}}$$

From the equation giving valve orifice *area*, the pressure gradient is inversely related to the square of the orifice area (Fig. 4-28). Thus, for a significant (*i.e.*, 20 torr or 4× normal) detectable gradient, valve area must be diminished by one-half. As valve area is reduced further, the gradient must increase as the square of that reduction to maintain the same flow. If increased flow is required (as in exercise) the gradient must increase. Eventually the necessary gradient cannot be maintained even at rest, and cardiac output falls. For these reasons, flow and gradient must be accurately measured in order to assess the severity of valve stenosis. The increased transvalvular flow in *mixed* lesions of stenosis and regurgitation requires particular caution in interpreting the degree of stenosis; the se-

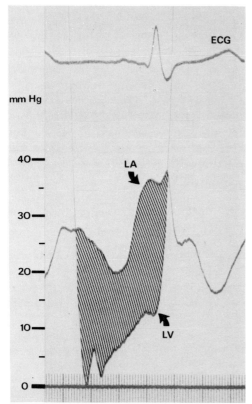

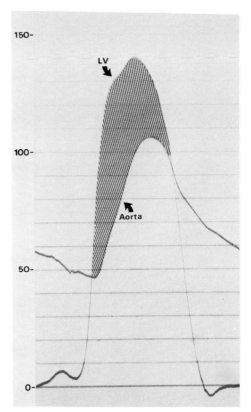

Fig. 4-26. Mitral stenosis. Simultaneous pressures in the left atrium (*LA*) and left ventricle (*LV*) reveal a gradient throughout diastole (*hatched area*). The mean gradient, ΔP, can be determined by measuring the total area between the pressure curves and dividing by the base—the diastolic filling period (dfp)—for that beat.

Fig. 4-27. Aortic stenosis. Simultaneous pressures in the left ventricular (*LV*) and aortic pressures, with a gradient throughout systole. The mean pressure gradient calculation is analogous to that described for Fig. 4-25.

Fig. 4-28. Aortic valve variation between pressure and flow. A family of curves is generated for each aortic valve orifice area (indicated in cm²). Note that for a given pressure gradient, the flow across the valve varies according to orifice area. For augmented flow across an orifice of fixed maximal area, the measured pressure gradient must increase accordingly.

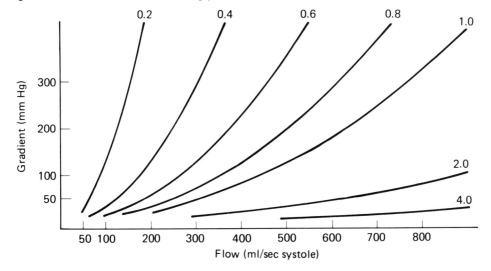

verity of stenosis may be greatly exaggerated if regurgitation is not taken into account. The amount of regurgitant flow (F_{reg}) may be calculated by comparing the cardiac outputs derived from the Fick or indicator methods (forward flow only, CO_{Fick}) with that derived from ventriculography (total flow, CO_{Angio}) thus

$$F_{reg} = CO_{Angio} - CO_{Fick}$$

and for consideration of valve stenosis, the total flow across the valve should be used. From the equation above and that for area and Figure 4-28, if the *angiographically determined* aortic valve systolic flow is 400 ml/sec of systole and the *Fick-determined* flow is 200 ml/sec of systole (50% regurgitant fraction), for a given mean gradient of approximately 50 torr, the *estimated* valve area could be 0.6 cm^2—critical stenosis—whereas the *true* area would be closer to 1.3 cm^2!

Quantification of valvular regurgitation is more difficult than that of stenosis. It is common practice with both aortic and mitral valves to qualitatively estimate the severity of regurgitation by judging during angiography the amount of contrast material entering the upstream chamber from the downstream chamber. Thus, for aortic regurgitation, supravalvular aortography is performed and severity is graded as follows (see Fig. 4-14):

1+ = small amount of contrast material entering left ventricle during diastole but clearing completely with each systole;
2+ = left ventricle faintly and incompletely opacified during diastole, contrast material not clearing with each systole;
3+ = left ventricle becoming progressively opacified during diastole, eventually completely opacified; and
4+ = left ventricle completely opacified after first diastole, remaining so for several cardiac cycles.

The scale for mitral regurgitation is analogous (see Fig. 4-14). Large *v* waves in the left atrial or pulmonary artery wedge tracing may indicate the presence of mitral regurgitation (Fig. 4-29).

A more quantitative approach to the estimation of valvular regurgitation is use of indicator dilution curves. This requires an injecting catheter in the downstream chamber and a sampling catheter in the upstream chamber, so it is less popular in common clinical practice. With either the indicator method or cinéangiography, the regurgitant fraction can be calculated and is the best indicator of severity. For the indicator method in aortic regurgitation

regurgitant fraction =

$$\frac{\text{dye sampled in left ventricle (regurgitant volume)}}{\text{dye sampled in aorta (total volume, forward plus regurgitant)}}$$

For the cinéangiographic method

regurgitant volume = total stroke volume (from left ventriculogram) − forward stroke volume (*cardiac output heart rate*)

$$\text{regurgitant fraction} = \frac{\text{regurgitant volume}}{\text{total stroke volume}}$$

Radionuclide angiography is a promising technique for the noninvasive estimation of regurgitant fractions in these lesions, but does not stand alone as the definitive diagnostic approach.

It is important to assess left ventricular function in both aortic and mitral regurgitation, for severe, chronic valvular insufficiency is accompanied by progressive myocardial deterioration. Ejection fraction and forward net cardiac output currently seem the most often used parameters to estimate the state of left ventricular function.

Tricuspid regurgitation occurs most commonly as a result of right ventricular failure. Other causes include endocarditis, chest trauma, and Ebstein's anomaly. It is not possible to accurately measure the amount of regurgitation; a catheter in the right ventricle for either contrast or indicator injection induces a variable amount of regurgitation itself. Generally, ventricularization (extremely large *v* wave) of the right atrial pressure curve is accepted as suggestive of severe tricuspid regurgitation, but any condition with venous hypertension and cardiomegaly can mimic this condition. Electromagnetic flow probes

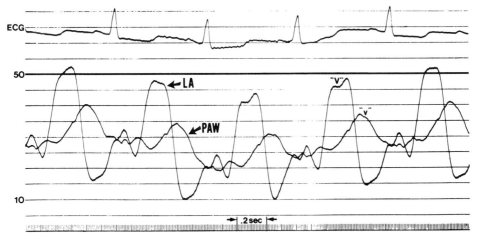

Fig. 4-29. Mitral regurgitation. Simultaneous left atrial (*LA*) and pulmonary artery wedge (*PAW*) pressure. Note the predominant *v* wave in the *PAW* tracing, which is even more marked (*V*) in the *LA*. Pressure scale is given in torr.

CONGENITAL HEART DISEASE

Indications for cardiac catheterization in children vary according to age and nature of presentation. For example, the neonate or infant presenting with cardiac symptoms or signs (cyanosis, congestive heart failure, respiratory problems) should undergo cardiac catheterization. This may be emergent in certain cases of transposition of the great vessels, total anomalous pulmonary venous return, or tricuspid atresia, in which balloon septostomy may be life-saving. In this procedure, a balloon-tipped catheter, 4 to 6.5 French in diameter is placed from the right atrium through the fossa ovalis into the left atrium; the balloon is inflated with contrast material to a diameter of from 12 to 15 mm and the catheter is abruptly drawn across the interatrial septum, rupturing the septum primum of the fossa ovalis. In children, any significant change in the course of their congenital heart disorder should prompt consideration of invasive study. Cardiac catheterization is used preoperatively in all cases, and often postoperatively to assess results and provide a postoperative baseline for future comparison.

The techniques of cardiac catheterization in children differ from those in adults in several ways. During the first week of life, right-heart catheterization may be performed through the umbilical vein, for example. Left-heart catheterization in many infants and children can be carried out through a patent foramen ovale.

Potential complications of cardiac catheterization in children are particularly threatening because of their relatively increased frequency in this age group. Neonates undergoing invasive studies are at increased risk because they are usually severely ill at the time; they are less tolerant of changes such as hypoxemia or acidosis; they are subject to hypothermia, catheter perforation of heart chambers, and vascular complications (because of vessel size); and they may not tolerate angiography or the removal of blood samples very well because of their small blood volume. Aside from the special problems of neonates, most children with congenital heart disease are vulnerable in three areas: (1) their small hearts are more likely to manifest ventricular ectopy; (2) cardiac output may be severely decreased by contrast injections (such as one into a reactive or resistive pulmonary vascular bed); and (3) arterial hypoxemia can readily occur. This may be caused by sedation, and may appear also in cases of right-to-left shunting, such as tetralogy of Fallot, if systemic vascular resistance fails and pulmonary blood flow then decreases. Catheterization is performed under local anesthesia with judicious sedation, usually employing combinations of meperidine and hydroxyzine, droperidol, or chlorpromazine. Chlorpromazine, because of its systemic vasodilatory properties, is avoided in cases such as tetralogy of Fallot, where a fall in systemic resistance could significantly reduce pulmonary blood flow.

Table 4-7 indicates the applications of cardiac catheterization to particular congenital heart disorders. As in adult cardiovascular disorders, hemodynamic findings and angiographic visualization of anatomy are important. Because of the preponderance of abnormal venous-arterial intracardiac communications, the calculation of shunts is essential in the evaluation of congenital heart disease. Most commonly this relies upon the measurement of oxygen saturation at various cardiovascular locations (Table 4-1). The list below gives the equations for calculation of left-to-right, right-to-left, and bidirectional shunts.

Shunt Calculation

1. *Systemic blood flow* (cardiac output; l/min)

$$= Q_S = \frac{\dot{V}O_2 \text{ (ml/min)}}{(SAO_2 - MVO_2) \times 10 \text{ (vol \%)}}$$

where $\dot{V}O_2$ = oxygen consumption, measured from expired air

SAO_2 = oxygen content, systemic arterial blood

MVO_2 = oxygen content, mixed venous blood; equivalent to pulmonary artery valve except in L → R shunt where a weighted mean of inferior and superior vena cava values is used in a ratio of 2:1

and oxygen content = O_2 capacity × O_2 saturation (vol %)

O_2 capacity = blood hemoglobin content (mg/dl) × 1.36 (ml/g) + 0.00326 (vol %/torr) × PO_2 (torr)

2. *Pulmonary blood flow* (l/min)

$$= Q_P = \frac{\dot{V}O_2 \text{ (ml/min)}}{(PVO_2 - PAO_2) \times 10 \text{ (vol \%)}}$$

where PVO_2 = oxygen content, pulmonary venous blood (equivalent to systemic arterial sample if there is no R → L shunt, or calculated assuming 95% saturation)

PAO_2 = oxygen content, pulmonary arterial blood

3. Effective pulmonary blood flow (the portion of mixed venous return that flows through the pulmonary vascular bed to be oxygenated)

$$= Q_P \text{ eff} = \frac{\dot{V}O_2 \text{ (ml/min)}}{(PVO_2 - MVO_2) \times 10 \text{ (vol \%)}}$$

4. *Shunt Calculation*

   a. *L → R shunt* = $Q_P - Q_P$ eff (= $Q_P - Q_S$, no R → L shunt)

   b. *R → L shunt* = $Q_S - Q_P$ eff (= $Q_S - Q_P$, no L → R shunt)

   c. *Bidirectional shunt* = calculate each shunt according to a and b above; the *net* shunt is the difference.

5. *Pulmonary to systemic flow ratio* = Q_P/Q_S = from 1 and 2 above,

$$\frac{\dfrac{\dot{V}O_2}{(PVO_2 - PAO_2) \times 10}}{\dfrac{\dot{V}O_2}{(SAO_2 - MVO_2) \times 10}} = \frac{SAO_2 - MVO_2}{PVO_2 - PAO_2}$$

MYOCARDIAL DISEASE

Cardiac catheterization is valuable in answering many clinical questions regarding myocardial diseases. Thus, a functional classification of these disorders is most helpful in describing their diagnostic approaches. In the temperate climates, three main types of heart muscle disorders exist: hypertrophic, congestive, and restrictive. The term *cardiomyopathy* has been applied to many heart muscle disorders, but may be more appropriately reserved for those entities of unknown cause, the balance being named according to the underlying disease affecting the myocardium.

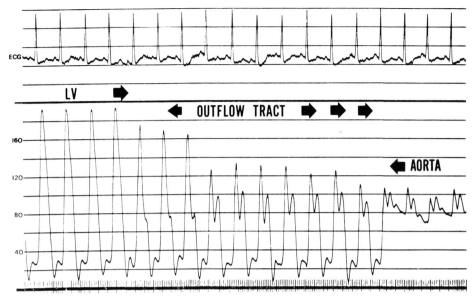

Fig. 4-30. Pullback pressure tracing in idiopathic hypertrophic subaortic stenosis (IHSS). There is nearly a 100-mm gradient between left ventricular cavity (*LV*) and *aorta* because of an obstruction within the *LV*. This is demonstrated by slowly withdrawing the catheter across the outflow tract.

Hypertrophic cardiomyopathy, because of the thick, inelastic ventricular wall, is characterized by resistance to ventricular filling, usually reflected by elevated end diastolic pressures. Systolic "pump" function is preserved. In the obstructive form known as idiopathic hypertrophic subaortic stenosis (IHSS) the outflow of blood is impeded by the disproportionately thickened interventricular septum, producing an intracavitary gradient (Fig. 4-30). This systolic pressure gradient can be extremely variable and during catheterization may be provoked by several maneuvers, including infusion of an inotrope (isoproterenol) or induction of extrasystoles by catheter manipulation (the Brockenbrough maneuver, in which the heightened contractility of the postextrasystolic beat produces a gradient across the left ventricular outflow tract). Cardiac catheterization is useful not only in diagnosing obstructive cardiomyopathy but may guide therapy; if the gradient is severe enough and not satisfactorily ameliorated with medical therapy, surgical treatment (septal myectomy) may be indicated.[297]

Congestive cardiomyopathy is often diagnosed by noninvasive means; the clinical history, physical exam, chest film, and echocardiogram are usually characteristic. Cardiac catheterization is used to confirm the diagnosis, reveal the severity of the disorder, estimate myocardial reserve (after exercise or angiography), guide medical therapy (such as afterload reduction), and exclude certain conditions (such as coronary artery disease or myocarditis). Left ventricular angiography reveals a diffusely enlarged chamber with overall hypokinesis and reduced ejection fraction, occasional secondary mitral regurgitation and left ventricular filling defects caused by mural thrombi. The hemodynamics include low cardiac index, although in mild or early forms of the condition, ventricular dilation may compensate for the myocardial insufficiency, which may be disclosed by resting or exercise-provoked increases in left ventricular end diastolic pressure. The coronary arteries are usually patent despite occasional segmental wall motion abnormalities in congestive cardiomyopathy. In rare instances (approximately 10% of cases), a treatable condition such as myocarditis may be found, and thus endomyocardial biopsy by catheter bioptome (Fig. 4-21) has recently found limited usefulness when indicated by appropriate clinical circumstances.[298]

Restrictive cardiomyopathy is typified by reduced ventricular filling due to diminished compliance. Restrictive features may be present in hypertrophic myocardial disease, idiopathic or caused by arterial hypertension or aortic stenosis. In its isolated form, restrictive myocardial disease is usually caused by infiltrative disorders or extensive fibrosis. The main hemodynamic characteristics are (1) elevated left- and right-sided venous pressures with large *a* and *v* waves; (2) ventricular diastolic dip and plateau (square root sign) pattern caused by late diastolic limitation of filling; (3) left-filling pressures usually greater than right; and (4) reduced cardiac output caused by limited diastolic filling rather than an intrinsic contraction defect. Restrictive myocardial disease notoriously mimics constrictive pericarditis and must therefore be carefully ruled out, for example, before proceeding to thoracotomy for pericardiectomy. This may be difficult; the most reliable distinguishing feature is probably the fact that in restrictive disease, left-sided filling pressures (left atrial or pulmonary artery wedge mean and left ventricular end diastolic) usually exceed right sided filling pressures by at least 10 torr. This differential may be latent until provoked by maneuvers which preferentially stress the left side of the heart, such as exercise or afterload augmentation by isometric exertion (handgrip) or pharmacologic means. Because cardiac amyloidosis usually presents with restrictive features, endomyocardial biopsy may be helpful in achieving a diagnsis (Fig. 4-21).

PERICARDIAL DISEASE

Constrictive pericarditis as noted above may be imitated by restrictive myocardial disease. Cardiac catheterization may distinguish the two entities, usually by the differential left- and right-sided filling pressures in restriction, as opposed to the uniform equalization

of these pressures in constrictive disease. Venous pressure is elevated, but because the limit of ventricular filling is not reached until the latter portion of diastole, a prominent right atrial *y* descent is usually recorded. If venous return is acutely augmented, the limitation in flow through the *encased* ventricles will be exceeded, and the venous pressure will rise. This is manifested in Küssmaul's sign (inspiratory rise in mean right atrial pressure) or with rapid infusion of crystalloid as a provocative maneuver.

Cardiac tamponade is compression of the heart by pericardial fluid, usually sufficient to cause circulatory compromise.[299] Hemodynamically it may be detected by the presence of paradoxical pulse or pulsus paradoxus, an exaggeration of the physiologic inspiratory fall in peak systolic arterial pressure. This sign may, however, be absent in several important cases such as localized cardiac compression (often postoperative), aortic regurgitation, left ventricular hypertrophy, or preexisting elevated pulmonary artery wedge pressure. Küssmaul's sign is more suggestive of constrictive disease than of tamponade. Echocardiography can detect pericardial effusion, but cannot reliably diagnose tamponade. Pericardiocentesis is often performed in the cardiac catheterization laboratory for therapeutic and diagnostic purposes[300] as well as for optimal gathering of hemodynamic information in cases of mixed effusive (tamponade) and constrictive disease.[301]

SUMMARY

Beginning as a bold, innovative technique with initially limited applicability, cardiac catheterization has become a relatively safe and indispensible tool in the diagnosis and treatment of cardiovascular disorders. It has also revealed most of our current understanding of cardiovascular physiology and continues to play an important role in modern research. For example, the genesis of certain heart sounds can now be studied with intracardiac microphones, pressure transducers, and flow probes only recently developed. Fundamental research areas such as myocardial metabolism and platelet activity are studied by catheterization of the coronary arteries, the coronary sinus and cardiac veins.

This chapter has underscored the need for an integrated, rational approach to invasive techniques in the investigation of heart disease. The cardiovascular team—cardiologist, radiologist, surgeon, anesthesiologist, intensive care specialist, and others—must carefully select diagnostic procedures with specific questions in mind, using the most appropriate technique for a given query. For example, the best way to detect pericardial effusion is by echocardiography, but the way to accurately diagnose constrictive pericarditis is by invasive, hemodynamic study.

The basics of each catheterization technique used in modern cardiology have been outlined as have heart disease categories, indicating the manner in which various studies can be used for a given type of disorder. Possible complications, their likelihood in certain high-risk patients, and their avoidance or treatment have also been listed.

Newly developed and highly specialized invasive procedures have also been reviewed. Of current interest are intracardiac electrophysiologic studies for the detection and treatment, medically or surgically, of life-threatening arrhythmias. Catheter biopsy of the endomyocardium, pharmacologic induction of coronary spasm, and percutaneous coronary arterial angioplasty by balloon catheter are also discussed.

It is important to emphasize that many new, *noninvasive* techniques promise to complement substantially, or perhaps partially replace, invasive methods. Cardiovascular care specialists should become increasingly familiar with these modern techniques, which include echocardiography and radionuclide studies.

The improved safety of cardiac catheterization combined with rapidly advancing supportive technology has revolutionized the investigation and care of the cardiovascular patient. In this age of superspecialization,

prudent use and correct interpretation of diagnostic procedures is challenging but potentially very rewarding.

GLOSSARY

afterload. The pressure seen by the left ventricle on opening the aortic valve. In the study of isolated cardiac muscle, *afterload* is the *force* opposing muscular contraction.

cardiac output (CO). The net forward or effective blood flow reaching the systemic circulation, expressed usually in liters/minute.

compliance. The ratio of change in volume (dV) to change in pressure (dP) expressed in $\frac{ml}{torr}$. Stiffness is the reciprocal of compliance. Note that because compliance changes with pressure, $dV/dP \neq V/P$.

contractility. The intensity or forcefulness of cardiac contraction.

diastolic filling period (DFP). The time during the cardiac cycle during which ventricular filling occurs. DFP (sec/min) is the total number of diastolic filling seconds in each minute as opposed to *dfp*, the number of diastolic filling seconds per beat.

$$DFP\ (sec/min) = \frac{dfp\ (seconds\ of\ diastole/beat)}{duration\ of\ 1\ cardiac\ cycle\ (seconds/beat)} \times 60\ (sec/min)$$

ejection fraction (EF). The portion of ventricular diastolic volume ejected with systole. EF is the ratio of the difference between end diastolic volume (EDV) and end systolic volume (ESV) to end diastolic volume. EF = (EDV − ESV)/EDV

impedance. The opposition to *pulsatile* flow through a given segment of the circulation. Impedance depends upon vascular caliber and elasticity and varies with frequency. Impedance is determined by the resistance and compliance of the vascular system. The *impedance modulus* is the ratio of pressure to flow for all possible driving frequencies in the system. An elevated impedance modulus at all frequencies implies decreased distensibility of the large vessels. A change in the frequency at which maxima and minima appear implies altered wave velocity or reflection. Increased frequency dependence of impedance oscillations implies increased reflection in the microcirculation. In the pulmonary vascular bed, autonomic control of *resistance* and *impedance* are unassociated; increased sympathetic tone elevates impedance without an accompanying degree of change in resistance.[302]

preload. The end diastolic pressure in the ventricle. The stretching force applied to a muscle before contraction.

regurgitant flow (F_{reg}). The amount of flow that does not effectively reach the systemic circulation because of valvular insufficiency. $F_{reg} = F_{tot} - F_{eff}$, where F_{tot} is total forward flow and F_{eff} is effective flow or cardiac output.

regurgitant fraction (RF). The proportion of regurgitant flow, F_{reg}, to total forward flow, F_{tot} (*see* total forward flow).

$$RF = \frac{F_{reg}}{F_{tot}} = \frac{F_{reg}}{F_{reg} + F_{eff}}$$

resistance. The opposition to flow through a given segment of the circulation, according to the hemodynamic analog of Ohm's Law

$$\left(R = \frac{\Delta P \text{ (dyne/cm}^2)}{F \text{ (cm}^3/\text{sec)}}\right) \quad \text{where } R \text{ is resistance,}$$

ΔP is *mean* pressure gradient across the segment, and F is *mean* flow through the segment; R is expressed in dyne·cm^{-5} or as $\frac{torr}{l/min}$).

shunt. Abnormal communication between right and left sides of the circulation. A *right-to-left* shunt bypasses the pulmonary vascular bed, causing blood of low oxygen content to enter the systemic circulation (cyanosis). A left-to-right shunt causes already-oxygenated blood to reenter the pulmonary vascular bed (pulmonary overcirculation).

shunt ratio ($Q_P:Q_s$). The ratio of pulmonary flow Q_P to systemic flow Q_s. A shunt ratio of 2:1 means that twice as much blood flows through the pulmonary vascular bed as thru the systemic.

systolic ejection period (SEP). The time during the cardiac cycle during which ventricular ejection occurs. SEP (sec/min) is the total number of systolic ejection seconds in each minute as opposed to *sep*, the number of systolic ejection seconds in each beat.

$$SEP \text{ (sec/min)} = \frac{sep \text{ (sec of systole/beat)}}{duration \text{ of cardiac cycle (sec/beat)}} \times 60 \text{ (sec/min)}$$

total forward flow (F_{tot}). The entire flow across a valve, including (1) the amount regurgitated backward across an insufficient valve (*regurgi-tant flow,* F_{reg}) and (2) the amount which effectively enters the systemic circulation (*effective flow,* F_{eff}). Total forward flow can be derived from the left ventricular angiogram by measuring the stroke volume (end diastolic volume minus end systolic volume). Effective flow can be measured as cardiac output by the Fick or indicator dilution methods.

valvular orifice area. The mathematically calculated area used to estimate the severity of valvular stenosis. The equation of Gorlin and Gorlin is derived by combining the following formulas:[303]

1. $v^2 = 2 \, gh \, C_c^2$ (conservation of energy) and
2. $F = vA \, C_v$ (flow), where v is velocity (cm/sec), g is gravity acceleration (980 cm/sec^2), h is mean pressure gradient (cm H$_2$O), F is flow (ml per diastolic filling sec or systolic ejection sec), A is valve orifice area (cm^2), C_c is the coefficient to compensate for orifice contraction during flow and C_v is velocity conversion coefficient. The resulting Gorlin equation is obtained by substituting ΔP, the mean transvalvular gradient for h. The equation is

$$A = \frac{F}{C \, (44.5) \, \sqrt{\Delta P}} \text{ (ml/sec)}$$

where C = 1 for aortic and pulmonic valves
C = 0.85 for mitral valve (if the diastolic filling period is derived from simultaneous left atrial/PA wedge and LV pressures).

REFERENCES

GENERAL REFERENCES

Historical Perspective

1. Forssmann W: Die Sondierung des rechten Herzens. Klin Wochenschr 8:2085–2087, 1929
2. Steckelberg JM, Vlietstra RE, Lundwig J, Mann RJ: Werner Forssmann (1904–1979) and his unusual success story. Mayo Clin Proc 54:746–748, 1979
3. Cournand A, Ranges HA: Catheterization of the right auricle in man. Proc Soc Exp Biol Med 46:462–466, 1941
4. Richards DW: Cardiac output by the catheterization technique in various clinical conditions. Fed Proc 4:215–220, 1945

. Cournand AF, Riley RL, Breed ES et al: Measurement of cardiac output in man using the technique of catheterization of the right auricle or ventricle. J Clin Invest 24:106–116, 1945

6. Dexter L, Haynes FW, Burwell CS et al: Studies of congenital heart disease. II. The pressure and oxygen content of blood in the right auricle, right ventricle, and pulmonary artery in control patients, with observations on the oxygen saturation and source of pulmonary "capillary" blood. J Clin Invest 26:554–576, 1947

7. Hellems HK, Haynes FW, Dexter L: Pulmonary "capillary" pressure in man. J Appl Physiol 2:24–29, 1949

8. Lagerlöf H, Werkö L: Studies on circulation of blood in man. Scand J Clin Lab Invest 1:147–161, 1949

9. Zimmerman HA, Scott RW, Becker NO: Catheterization of the left side of the heart in man. Circulation 1:356–359, 1950

10. Seldinger SI: Catheter placement of the needle in percutaneous arteriography: a new technique. Acta Radiol 39:368–376, 1953

11. Ross J Jr: Transseptal left heart catheterization: a new method of left atrial puncture. Ann Surg 149:395–401, 1959

12. Cope C: Technique for transseptal catheterization of the left atrium: preliminary report. J Thoracic Surg 37:482–486, 1959

13. Sones FM Jr, Shirey EK, Proudfit WL, Westcott RN: Cine-coronary arteriography (abstr). Circulation 20:773–774, 1959

14. Thomas MM, Longo MR Jr: Care of patients after cardiac catheterization. Aviat Space Environ Med 47:192–198, 1976

15. Scroggs V, Pietras RJ, Rosen KM: Frequency response of fluid filled catheter-micromanometer systems used for measurement of ventricular pressure. Am Heart J 89:619–62, 1975

16. Falsetti HL, Mates RE, Carroll RJ et al: Analysis and correction of pressure wave distortion in fluid-filled catheter systems. Circulation 49:165–172, 1974

Basic Catheterization Methods

17. Humphrey CB, Oury JH, Virgilio RW et al: An analysis of direct and indirect measurements of left atrial filling pressure. J Thorac Cardiovasc Surg 71:643–647, 1976

18. Batson G, Chandrasekhar KP, Payas Y, Rickards DF: Comparison of wedge pressure measured by the flow directed Swan–Ganz catheter with direct left atrial measurement. Cardiovasc Res 6:748–752, 1972

19. Pace NL: A critique of flow-directed pulmonary arterial catheterization. Anesthesiology 47:455–465, 1977

20. Walston AH, Kendall ME: Comparison of pulmonary wedge and left atrial pressure in man. Am Heart J 86:159–164, 1973

21. Smith HC, Butler J: Pulmonary venous waterfall and perivenous pressure in the living dog. J Appl Physiol 38:304–308, 1975

22. Swan HJC, Ganz W, Forrester J et al: Catheterization of the heart in man with the use of a flow-directed balloon-tipped catheter. N Engl J Med 283:447–451, 1970

23. Lategola M, Rahn H: A self-guiding catheter for cardiac and pulmonary arterial catheterization and occlusion. Proc Soc Exp Biol Med 84:667–668, 1953

24. Forrester JS, Ganz W, Diamond G et al: Thermodilution cardiac output determination with a single flow-directed catheter. Am Heart J 83:306–311, 1972

25. Editorial: Swan-Ganz catheters. Lancet 2:357–358, 1978

26. Gould KL, Trenholme S, Kennedy JW: In vivo comparison of catheter manometer systems with the cather-tip micromanometer. J Appl Physiol 34:263–267, 1973

27. Jacobs R, Killam H, Barefoot C, Millar H: Human application of a catheter with tip-mounted pressure and flow transducers. Review of Surgery 149–152, 1972

28. Alderman EA, Spitz AL, Sanders WJ, Harrison DC: Use and value of the computer in the cardiac catheterization laboratory. Chest 71:526–530, 1977

29. Brockenbrough EC, Braunwald E: A new technique for left ventricular angiocardiography and transseptal left heart catheterization. Am J Cardiol 6:1062–1064, 1960

30. Brockenbrough ED, Braunwald E, Ross J Jr: Transseptal left heart catheterization, review of 450 studies and description of improved technique. Circulation 25:15–21, 1962

31. Cope C: Transseptal left heart catheterization: details of technique. Circulation 27:758–761, 1963

32. Ross J Jr: Considerations regarding the technique for left heart catheterization. Circulation 34:391–399, 1966

33. Davies H: Left ventricular puncture. In Mendel, D (ed): A Practice of Cardiac Catheterisation, 2nd ed. Oxford, Blackwell Scientific Publications, 1974
34. Semple T, McGuinness JB, Gardner H: Left heart catheterization by direct ventricular puncture. Br Heart J 30:402–406, 1968

Measurement of Blood Flow

35. Fick A: Ueber die Messung des Blutquantums in den Herzventrikeln. Verhandl. d. phys-med. Ges. zu Würzburg 2:16, 1870. In Hoff HE, Scott HJ (trans): N Engl J Med 239:120–126, 1948
36. Visscher MB, Johnson JA: The Fick Principle: analysis of potential errors in its conventional application. J Appl Physiol 5:635–636, 1953
37. Stewart GN: The output of the heart in dogs. Am J Physiol 57:27–50, 1921
38. Moore JW, Kinsman JM, Hamilton, WF, Spurling RG: Studies on the circulation. II. Cardiac output determinations: comparison of the injection method with the direct Fick procedures. Am J Physiol 89:331–339, 1929
39. Branthwaite MA, Bradley RD: Measurement of cardiac output by thermodilution in man. J Appl Physiol 24:434–438, 1968
40. Swan HJC: Balloon flotation catheters: their use in hemodynamic monitoring in clinical practice. JAMA 233:865–867, 1975
41. Forrester JS, Ganz W, Diamond G et al: Thermodilution cardiac output determination with a single flow-directed catheter. Am Heart J 83:306–311, 1972

Flow Probes

42. Warbasse JR, Hellman BH, Gillilan RE et al: Physiologic evaluation of a catheter tip electromagnetic velocity probe: a new instrument. Am J Cardiol 23:424–433, 1969
43. Bond RF, Barefoot CA: Evaluation of an electromagnetic catheter tip velocity-sensitive blood flow probe. J Appl Physiol 23:403–409, 1967
44. Frøysaker T: Intraoperative measurement of the superior vena caval flow pattern in patients with intracardiac shunts. Scand J Thor Cardiovasc Surg 6:218–226, 1972
45. Frøysaker T: The influence of constrictive pericarditis on the superior vena caval flow pattern. Scand J Thor Cardiovasc Surg 6:227–233, 1972

Pulsatile Blood Flow

46. Wood P: The Eisenmenger syndrome or pulmonary hypertension with reversal of central shunt. Br Med J 2:701–709, 755–762, 1958
47. Kimball KG, McIlroy MB: Pulmonary hypertension in patients with congenital heart disease. Am J Med 41:883–897, 1966
48. Braunwald E, Braunwald NS, Ross J Jr, Morrow AG: Effects of mitral valve replacement on the pulmonary vascular dynamics of patients with pulmonary hypertension. N Engl J Med 273:509–514, 1965
49. Milnor WR: Pulsatile blood flow. N Engl J Med 287:27–34, 1972
50. Cohn JN, Franciosa JA: Vasodilator therapy of heart failure. N Engl J Med 297:27–31, 1977
51. Parmley WW, Chatterjee K: Vasodilator Therapy. In Harvey WP (ed): Current Problems in Cardiology, pp 57–62. Chicago, Year Book Medical Publishers, 1978

Detection and Quantification of Shunts

52. Hyman AL, Myers W, Hyatt K et al: A comparative study of the detection of cardiovascular shunts by oxygen analysis and indicator dilution methods. Ann Intern Med 56:535–544, 1962
53. Wilson MR, Gontana ME, Wooley CF: Routine use of the hydrogen platinum electrode system in shunt detection. Cathet Cardiovasc Diagn 1:207–221, 1975

Assessment of Left Ventricular Function

54. Braunwald E, Ross J Jr, Sonnenblick EH: Methods for assessing cardiac contractility. In Braunwald E, Ross J Jr Sonnenblick EH (eds): Mechanisms of contraction of the normal and failing heart, 2nd ed, pp 131–165. Boston, Little Brown and Co, 1976
55. Sonnenblick EH, Strobeck JE: Derived indexes of ventricular and myocardial function. N Engl J Med 296:978–982, 1977
56. Quinones MA, Gaasch WH, Alexander JK: Influence of acute changes in preload, afterload, contractile state, and heart rate on ejection and isovolumic indices of myocardial contractility in man. Circulation 53:293–302, 1976

57. Mahler R, Ross J Jr, O'Rourke RA et al: Effects of changes in preload, afterload and inotropic state on ejection and isovolumic phase measures of contractility in the conscious dog. Am J Cardiol 35:626–634, 1972

58. Quinones MA, Gaasch WH, Alexander JK: Influence of acute changes in preload, afterload, contractile state, and heart rate on ejection and isovolumic indices of myocardial contractility in man. Circulation 53:293–302, 1976

59. Mahler R, Ross J Jr, O'Rourke RA et al: Effects of changes in preload, afterload and inotropic state on ejection and isovolumic phase measures of contractility in the conscious dog. Am J Cardiol 35:626–634, 1972

60. Grossman W, Haynes F, Paraskos JA et al: Alterations in preload and myocardial mechanics in the dog and in man. Circ Res 31:83–94, 1972

61. Mason DT, Braunwald E, Covell JW et al: Assessment of cardiac contractility. The relation between the rate of pressure rise and ventricular pressure during iso-volumic systole. Circulation 44:47–58, 1971

62. Quinones MA, Gaasch WH, Alexander JK: Influence of acute changes in preload, afterload, contractile state, and heart rate on ejection and isovolumic indices of myocardial contractility in man. Circulation 53:293–302, 1976

63. Cohn PF, Liedtke AJ, Serur J et al: Maximal rate of pressure fall (peak negative dP/dt) during ventricular relaxation. Cardiovasc Res 6:263–267, 1972

64. Mahler R, Ross J Jr, O'Rourke RA et al: Effects of changes in preload, afterload and inotropic state on ejection and isovolumic phase measures of contractility in the conscious dog. Am J Cardiol 35:626–634, 1972

65. Wiggers CJ: Dynamics of ventricular contraction under abnormal conditions. Circulation 5:321–348, 1952

66. Davidson DM, Covell JW, Malloch CI et al: Factors influencing indices of left ventricular contractility in the conscious dog. Cardiovasc Res 8:299–312, 1974

67. Quinones MA, Gaasch WH, Alexander JK: Influence of acute changes in preload, afterload, contractile state, and heart rate on ejection and isovolumic indices of myocardial contractility in man. Circulation 53:293–302, 1976

68. Mahler R, Ross J Jr, O'Rourke RA et al: Effects of changes in preload, afterload and inotropic state on ejection and isovolumic phase measures of contractility in the conscious dog. Am J Cardiol 35:626–634, 1972

69. Grossman W, Haynes F, Paraskos JA et al: Alterations in preload and myocardial mechanics in the dog and in man. Circ Res 31:83–94, 1972

70. Quinones MA, Gaasch WH, Alexander JK: Influence of acute changes in preload, afterload, contractile state, and heart rate on ejection and isovolumic indices of myocardial contractility in man. Circulation 53:293–302, 1976

71. Wallace AG, Skinner NS Jr, Mitchell JH: Hemodynamic determinants of the maximal rate of rise of left ventricular pressure. Am J Physiol 205:30–36, 1963

72. Mason DT, Braunwald E, Covell JW et al: Assessment of cardiac contractility. The relation between the rate of pressure rise and ventricular pressure during iso-volumic systole. Circulation 44:47–58, 1971

73. Veragut UP, Krayenbühl HP: Estimation and quantification of myocardial contractility in the closed-chest dog. Cardiologia 47:96–112, 1965

74. Quinones MA, Gaasch WH, Alexander JK: Influence of acute changes in preload, afterload, contractile state, and heart rate on ejection and isovolumic indices of myocardial contractility in man. Circulation 53:293–302, 1976

75. Mahler R, Ross J Jr, O'Rourke RA et al: Effects of changes in preload, afterload and inotropic state on ejection and isovolumic phase measures of contractility in the conscious dog. Am J Cardiol 35:626–634, 1972

76. Mehmel H, Krayenbühl HP, Rutishauser W: Peak measured velocity of shortening in the canine left ventricle. J Appl Physiol 29:637–645, 1970

77. Mirsky I, Pasternac A, Ellison RC: General index for the assessment of cardiac function. Am J Cardiol 30:483–491, 1972

78. Stein PD, McBride GG, Sabbah HN: Ventricular performance and energy of compression, power and rate of change of power during isovolumic contraction. Cardiovasc Res 9:29–37, 1975

79. Quinones MA, Gaasch WH, Alexander JK: Influence of acute changes in preload, afterload, contractile state, and heart rate on ejection and isovolumic indices of myocardial contractility in man. Circulation 53:293–302, 1976

80. Grossman W, Haynes F, Paraskos JA et al: Alterations in preload and myocardial mechanics in the dog and in man. Circ Res 31:83–94, 1972

81. Davidson DM, Covell JW, Malloch CI et al: Factors influencing indices of left ventricular contractility in the conscious dog. Cardiovasc Res 8:299–312, 1974

82. Quinones MA, Gaasch WH, Alexander JK: Influence of acute changes in preload, afterload, contractile state, and heart rate on ejection and isovolumic indices of myocardial contractility in man. Circulation 53:293–302, 1976

83. Dodge HT, Baxley WA: Left ventricular volume and mass and their significance in heart disease. Am J Cardiol 23:528–537, 1969

84. Pollack GH: Maximum velocity as an index of contractility in cardiac muscle: a critical evaluation. Circ Res 26:111–127, 1970

85. Mirsky I, Pasternac A, Ellison RC: General index for the assessment of cardiac function. Am J Cardiol 30:483–491, 1972

86. Pollack GH: Maximum velocity as an index of contractility in cardiac muscle: a critical evaluation. Circ Res 26:111–127, 1970

87. Jones JW, Rackley CE, Bruce RA et al: Left ventricular volumes in valvular heart disease. Circulation 29:887–891, 1964

88. Ross J Jr, Peterson KL: Editorial: On the assessment of cardiac inotropic state. Circulation 47:435–438, 1973

89. Ross J Jr, Covell JW, Mahler F: Contractile responses of the left ventricle to acute and chronic stress. Eur J Cardiol 1:325–322, 1974

90. Jones JW, Rackley CE, Bruce RA et al: Left ventricular volumes in valvular heart disease. Circulation 29:887–891, 1964

91. Braunwald E: On the difference between the heart's output and its contractile state. Circulation 43:171–174, 1971

92. Dodge HT: Hemodynamic aspects of cardiac failure. In Braunwald E (ed): The myocardium: Failure and Infarction, pp 70–78. New York, Hospital Practice Publishing Co, 1974

93. Cohn FP, Gorlin R, Cohn LH et al: Left ventricular ejection fraction as a prognostic guide in the surgical treatment of coronary and valvular heart disease. Am J Cardiol 34–136–141, 1974

94. MacGregor DC, Covell JW, Mahler F et al: Relations between afterload, stroke volume, and the descending limit of Starling's curve. Am J Physiol 227:884–890, 1974

95. MacGregor DC, Covell JW, Mahler F et al: Relations between afterload, stroke volume, and the descending limit of Starling's curve. Am J Physiol 227:884–890, 1974

96. Eckberg DL, Gault JH, Buchard RL et al: Mechanics of left ventricular contraction in chronic severe mitral regurgitation. Circulation 47:1252–1259, 1973

97. Hernandez-Lattuf PR, Quinones MA, Gaasch WH: Usefulness and limitations of circumferential fibre shortening velocity in evaluating segmental disorders of left ventricular contraction. Br Heart J 36:11667–1174, 1974

98. Quinones MA, Gaasch WH, Alexander JK: Influence of acute changes in preload, afterload, contractile state, and heart rate on ejection and isovolumic indices of myocardial contractility in man. Circulation 53:293–302, 1976

99. Quinones MA, Gaasch WH, Cole JS et al: Echocardiographic determinations of left ventricular stress-velocity relations in man: with reference to the effects of loading and contractility. Circulation 51:689–700, 1975

100. Quinones MA, Gaasch WH, Alexander JK: Influence of acute changes in preload, afterload, contractile state, and heart rate on ejection and isovolumic indices of myocardial contractility in man. Circulation 53:293–302, 1976

101. Quinones MA, Gaasch WH, Cole JS et al: Echocardiographic determinations of left ventricular stress-velocity relations in man: with reference to the effects of loading, and contractility. Circulation 51:689–700, 1975

102. Karliner JS, Gault HG, Eckberg D et al: Mean velocity of fiber shortening: a simplified measure of left ventricular myocardial contractility. Circulation 44:323–333, 1971

103. Mirsky I, Pasternac A, Ellison RC: General index for the assessment of cardiac function. Am J Cardiol 30:483–491, 1972

104. Peterson KL, Skloven D, Ludbrook P et al: Comparison of isovolumic and ejection phase indices of myocardial performance in man. Circulation 46:1088–1101, 1974

105. Quinones MA, Gaasch WH, Cole JS et al: Echocardiographic determinations of left ventricular stress-velocity relations in man: with reference to the effects of loading and contractility. Circulation 51:689–700, 1975

106. Hernandez-Lattuf PR, Quinones MA, Gaasch WH: Usefulness and limitations of

circumferential fibre shortening velocity in evaluating segmental disorders of left ventricular contraction. Br Heart J 36:1167–1174, 1974

107. Quinones MA, Gaasch WH, Cole JS et al: Echocardiographic determinations of left ventricular stress-velocity relations in man: with reference to the effects of loading and contractility. Circulation 51:689–700, 1975

108. Karliner JS, Gault HG, Eckberg D et al: Mean velocity of fiber shortening: a simplified measure of left ventricular myocardial contractility. Circulation 44:323–333, 1971

109. Hernandez-Latuff PR, Quinones MA et al: Usefulness and limitations of circumferential fibre shortening velocity in evaluating segmental disorders of left ventricular contraction. Br Heart J 36:1167–1174, 1974

110. Levine HJ, Neill WA, Wagman RJ et al: The effect of exercise on mean left ventricular ejection rate in man. J Clin Invest 41:1050–1058, 1962

111. Johnson LL, Ellis K, Schmidt S et al: Volume ejected in early systole: a sensitive index of left ventricular performance in coronary artery disease. Circulation 52:378–389, 1975

112. Johnson LL, Ellis K, Schmidt S et al: Volume ejected in early systole: a sensitive index of left ventricular performace in coronary artery disease. Circulation 52:378–389, 1975

113. Parmley WW, Tomoda H, Diamond G et al: Dissociation between indices of pump performance and contractility in patients with coronary artery disease and acute myocardial infarction. Chest 67:141–146, 1975

114. Parmley WW, Tomoda H, Diamond G et al: Dissociation between indices of pump performance and contractility in patients with coronary artery disease and acute myocardial infarction. Chest 67:141–146, 1975

115. Braunwald E, Brockenbrough EC, Frahm CJ et al: Left atrial and left ventricular pressures in subjects without cardiovascular disease: observations in eighteen patients studied by transseptal left heart catheterization. Circulation 24:267–269, 1961

116. Mirsky I, Pasternac A, Ellison RC: General index for the assessment of cardiac function. Am J Cardiol 30:483–491, 1972

117. Ross J Jr, Gault JH, Mason DT et al: Left ventricular performance during muscular exercise in patients with and without cardiac dysfunction. Circulation 34–597–608, 1966

118. Kivowitz C, Parmley WW, Donoso R et al: Effects of isometric exercise on cardiac performance: the grip test. Circulation 45:994–1002, 1971

119. Ross J Jr, Braunwald E: The study of left ventricular function in man by increasing resistance to ventricular ejection with angiotensin. Circulation 29:739–749, 1964

120. Ross J Jr, Peterson KL: Editorial: On the assessment of cardiac inotropic state. Circulation 47:435–438, 1973

121. Ross J Jr, Covell JW, Mahler F: Contractile responses of the left ventricle to acute and chronic stress. Eur J Cardiol 1:325–332, 1974

122. Pombo JF, Troy BL, Russell RO Jr: Left ventricular volumes and ejection fraction by echocardiography. Circulation 43:480–490, 1971

123. Strauss HW, Zaret BL, Hurley PJ et al: A scintigraphic method for measuring left ventricular ejection fraction in man without cardiac catheterization. Am J Cardiol 28:575–580, 1971

124. Arbogast R, Baurassa MG: Myocardial function during atrial pacing in patients with angina pectoris and normal coronary arteriograms: comparison with patients having significant coronary artery disease. Am J Cardiol 32:257–263, 1973

125. Graber JD, Conti CR, Lappe KL, Ross RS: Effect of pacing-induced tachycardia and myocardial ischemia on ventricular pressure-velocity relationships in man. Circulation 46:74–83, 1972

126. Anderson PW, Manring A, Serwer GA et al: The force-interval relationship of the left ventricle. Circulation 60:334–348, 1979

127. Pitt B, Strauss HW: Current concepts: Evaluation of ventricular function by radioisotopic technics. N Engl J Med 296:1097–1099, 1977

128. Kisslo JA, Robertson D, Gilbert BW et al: A comparison of real-time, two-dimensional echocardiography in detecting left ventricular asynergy. Circulation 55:134–141, 1977

ANGIOGRAPHIC METHODS

Ventriculography

129. Bentivoglio LG, Griffith LD, Cuesta AJ et al: Radiographic evaluation of formulas for left ventricular volume using canine casts. J Appl Physiol 33:365–374, 1972

130. Dodge HT, Sandler H, Ballew DW et al: The

use of biplane angiocardiography for the measurement of left ventricular volume in man. Am Heart J 60:762–776, 1960

131. Dodge HT, Sander H, Ballew DW et al: The use of biplane angiocardiography for the measurement of left ventricular volume in man. Am Heart J 60:762–776, 1960

132. Sandler H, Hawley RR, Dodge HT et al: Calculation of left ventricular volume from single plane (A-P) angio-cardiograms. J Clin Invest 44:1094–1095, 1965

133. Sandler H, Dodge HT: The use of single plane angiocardiograms for the calculation of left ventricular volume in man. Am Heart J 75:325–334, 1968

134. Greene DG, Carlisle R et al: Estimation of left ventricular volume by one-plane cineangiography. Circulation 35:61–69, 1967

Complications

135. Vogel JHK, Cornish D, McFadden RB: Underestimation of ejection fraction with single plane angiography in coronary artery disease: role of biplane angiography. Chest 64:217–221, 1973

136. Austin WG, Edwards JE, Frye RL et al: A reporting system on patients evaluated for coronary artery disease. Report of the ad hoc Committee for Grading of Coronary Artery Disease, Council on Cardiovascular Surgery, American Heart Association. Circulation (Suppl IV) 51:5–40, 1975

137. Cohn FP, Gorlin R et al: Left ventricular ejection fraction as a prognostic guide in the surgical treatment of coronary and valvular heart disease. Am J Cardiol 34:136–141, 1974

138. Mortensen JD: Clinical sequelae from arterial needle puncture, cannulation, and incision. Circulation 35:1118–1123, 1967

139. Davis K, Kennedy JW, Kemp HG Jr et al: Complications of coronary arteriography from the Collaborative Study of Coronary Artery Surgery (CASS). Circulation 59:1105–1112, 1979

140. Mortensen JD: Clinical sequelae from arterial needle puncture, cannulation, and incision. Circulation 35:1118–1123, 1967

141. Amplatz K, Haut G: Complication rates of transfemoral and transaortic catheterization. Surgery 63:594–596, 1968

142. Formanek G, Frech RS, Amplatz K: Arterial thrombus formation during clinical percutaneous catheterization. Circulation 41:833–839, 1970

143. Adams DF, Fraser DB, Abrams HL: The complications of coronary arteriography. Circulation 48:609–618, 1973

144. Adams DF, Fraser DB, Abrams HL: The complications of coronary arteriography. Circulation 48:609–618, 1973

145. Mortensen JD: Clinical sequelae from arterial needle puncture, cannulation, and incision. Circulation 35:1118–1123, 1967

146. Silverman JF, Wexler L: Complications of percutaneous transfemoral coronary arteriography. Clin Radiol 27:317–321, 1976

147. Braunwald E, Swan HJC (eds): Cooperative study on cardiac catheterization. Circulation (Suppl III) 37, 1968 (Also available as American Heart Association Monograph #20)

148. Braunwald E, Swan HJC (eds): Cooperative study on cardiac catheterization. Circulation (Suppl III) 37, 1968 (Also available as American Heart Association Monograph #20)

149. Braunwald E, Swan HJC (eds): Cooperative study on cardiac catheterization. Circulation (Suppl III) 37, 1968 (Also available as American Heart Association Monograph #20)

150. Braunwald E, Swan HJC (eds): Cooperative study on cardiac catheterization. Circulation (Suppl III) 37, 1968 (Also available as American Heart Association Monograph #20)

151. Braunwald E, Swan HJC (eds): Cooperative study on cardiac catheterization. Circulation (Suppl III) 37, 1968 (Also available as American Heart Association Monograph #20)

152. Ream AK, Lipton MJ, Hyndman BH: Reduced risk of cardiac fibrillation with use of a conductive catheter. Ann Biomed Eng 5:287–301, 1977

153. Braunwald E, Swan HJC (eds): Cooperative study on cardiac catheterization. Circulation (Suppl III) 37, 1968 (Also available as American Heart Association Monograph #20)

154. Braunwald E, Swan HJC (eds): Cooperative study on cardiac catheterization. Circulation (Suppl III) 37, 1968 (Also available as American Heart Association Monograph #20)

155. Braunwald E, Swan HJC (eds): Cooperative study on cardiac catheterization. Circulation (Suppl III) 37, 1968 (Also available as American Heart Association Monograph #20)

156. Karnegis JN, Heinz J: The risk of diagnostic cardiovascular catheterization. Am Heart J 97:291–297, 1979

157. Braunwald E, Swan HJC (eds): Cooperative study on cardiac catheterization. Circulation (Suppl III) 37, 1968 (Also available as American Heart Association Monograph #20)

158. Braunwald E, Swan HJC (eds): Cooperative study on cardiac catheterization. Circulation (Suppl III) 37, 1968 (Also available as American Heart Association Monograph #20)

159. Braunwald E, Swan HJC (eds): Cooperative study on cardiac catheterization. Circulation (Suppl III) 37, 1968 (Also available as American Heart Association Monograph #20)

160. Silverman JF, Wexler L: Complications of percutaneous transfemoral coronary arteriography. Clin Radiol 27:317–321, 1976

161. Witten DM: Reactions to urographic contrast media. JAMA 231:974–977, 1975

162. Witten DM: Reactions to urographic contrast media. JAMA 231:974–977, 1975

163. Maher JF: Toxic and irradiation nephropathies, chap 43. In Early LE, Gottschalk CW (eds): Strauss and Welt's Diseases of the Kidney, 3rd ed. Boston, Little, Brown & Co, 1979

164. Braunwald E, Swan HJC (eds): Cooperative study on cardiac catheterization. Circulation (Suppl III) 37, 1968 (Also available as American Heart Association Monograph #20)

165. Braunwald E, Swan HJC (eds): Cooperative study on cardiac catheterization. Circulation (Suppl III) 37, 1968 (Also available as American Heart Association Monograph #20)

166. Braunwald E, Swan HJC (eds): Cooperative study on cardiac catheterization. Circulation (Suppl III) 37, 1968 (Also available as American Heart Association Monograph #20)

167. Braunwald E, Swan HJC (eds): Cooperative study on cardiac catheterization. Circulation (Suppl III) 37, 1968 (Also available as American Heart Association Monograph #20)

168. Witten DM: Reactions to urographic contrast media. JAMA 231:974–977, 1975

169. Braunwald E, Swan HJC (eds): Cooperative study on cardiac catheterization. Circulation (Suppl III) 37, 1968 (Also available as American Heart Association Monograph #20)

170. Braunwald E, Swan HJC (eds): Cooperative study on cardiac catheterization. Circulation (Suppl III) 37, 1968 (Also available as American Heart Association Monograph #20)

171. Witten DM: Reactions to urographic contrast media. JAMA 231:974–977, 1975

172. Braunwald E, Swan HJC (eds): Cooperative study on cardiac catheterization. Circulation (Suppl III) 37, 1968 (Also available as American Heart Association Monograph #20)

173. Grainger RG: Complications of cardiovascular radiologic investigations. Br J Radiol 38:201–215, 1965

174. Witten DM: Reactions to urographic contrast media. JAMA 231:974–977, 1975

175. Maher JF: Toxic and irradiation nephropathies, chap 43. In Early LE, Gottschalk CW (eds): Strauss and Welt's Diseases of the Kidney, 3rd ed. Boston, Little, Brown & Co, 1979

176. Bourassa MG, Noble J: Complication rate of coronary arteriography: a review of 5250 cases studied by a percutaneous femoral technique. Circulation 53:106–114, 1976

177. Wolfson S, Grant D, Ross AM, Cohen LS: Risk of death related to coronary arteriography: role of left coronary arterial lesions. Am J Cardiol 37:210–216, 1976

178. Davis K, Kennedy JW, Kemp HG Jr et al: Complications of coronary arteriography from the Collaborative Study of Coronary Artery Surgery (CASS). Circulation 59:1105–1112, 1979

179. Davis K, Kennedy JW, Kemp HG Jr et al: Complications of coronary arteriography from the Collaborative Study of Coronary Artery Surgery (CASS). Circulation 59:1105–1112, 1979

180. Davis K, Kennedy JW, Kemp HG Jr et al: Complications of coronary arteriography from the Collaborative Study of Coronary Artery Surgery (CASS). Circulation 59:1105–1112, 1979

181. Davis K, Kennedy JW, Kemp HG Jr et al: Complications of coronary arteriography from the Collaborative Study of Coronary Artery Surgery (CASS). Circulation 59:1105–1112, 1979

182. Davis K, Kennedy JW, Kemp HG Jr et al: Complications of coronary arteriography from the Collaborative Study of Coronary Artery Surgery (CASS). Circulation 59:1105–1112, 1979

183. Wolfson S, Grant D, Ross AM, Cohen LS: Risk of death related to coronary arteriography: role of left coronary arterial lesions. Am J Cardiol 37:210–216, 1976

184. Davis K, Kennedy JW, Kemp HG Jr et al: Complications of coronary arteriography from the Collaborative Study of Coronary Artery Surgery (CASS). Circulation 59:1105–1112, 1979

185. Silverman JF, Wexler L: Complications of percutaneous transfemoral coronary arteriography. Clin Radiol 27:317–321, 1976

186. Adams DF, Fraser DB, Abrams HL: The complications of coronary arteriography. Circulation 48:609–618, 1973

187. Davis K, Kennedy JW, Kemp HG Jr et al:

Complications of coronary arteriography from the Collaborative Study of Coronary Artery Surgery (CASS). Circulation 59:1105–1112, 1979

188. Sones FM Jr: Complications of coronary arteriography and left heart catheterization. Cleve Clin Q 45:21–23, 1978

189. Davis K, Kennedy JW, Kemp HG Jr et al: Complications of coronary arteriography from the Collaborative Study of Coronary Artery Surgery (CASS). Circulation 59:1105–1112, 1979

190. Wolfson S, Grant D, Ross AM, Cohen LS: Risk of death related to coronary arteriography: role of left coronary arterial lesions. Am J Cardiol 37:210–216, 1976

191. Dawson DM, Fischer EG: Neurologic complications of cardiac catheterization. Neurology 27:496–497, 1977

192. Abrams HL, Douglass FA: The complications of coronary arteriography (abstr). Circulation (Suppl II)51, 52:II-27, 1975

193. Davis K, Kennedy JW, Kemp HG Jr et al: Complications of coronary arteriography from the Collaborative Study of Coronary Artery Surgery (CASS). Circulation 59:1105–1112, 1979

194. Dawson DM, Fischer EG: Neurologic complications of cardiac catheterization. Neurology 27:496–497, 1977

195. Higgins CB, Feld GK: Direct chronotropic and dromotropic actions of contrast material: ineffectiveness of atropine in the prevention of bradyarrhythmias and conduction disturbances. Radiology 121:205–209, 1976

196. Higgins CB: Effect of contrast material on the conducting system of the heart. Radiology 124:599–606, 1977

197. Langou RA, Sheps DS, Wolfson S et al: Intraventricular conduction during coronary arteriography in patients with pre-existing conduction abnormalities. Invest Radiol 12:505–509, 1977

198. Davis K, Kennedy JW, Kemp HG Jr et al: Complications of coronary arteriography from the Collaborative Study of Coronary Artery Surgery (CASS). Circulation 59:1105–1112, 1979

199. Braunwald E, Swan HJC (eds): Cooperative study on cardiac catheterization. Circulation (Suppl III) 37, 1968 (Also available as American Heart Association Monograph #20)

200. Sones FM Jr: Complications of coronary arteriography and left heart catheterization. Cleve Clin Q 45:21–23, 1978

201. Hildner FJ, Javier RP, Ramaswamy K et al: Pseudo complications of cardiac catheterization. Chest 63:15–17, 1973

202. Gensini GG: The coronary circulation. In Zimmerman HA (ed): Intravascular Catheterization. Springfield, (Ill), Charles C Thomas, 1966

203. Walker WJ, Mundall SJ, Broderick HG et al: Systemic heparinization for femoral percutaneous coronary arteriography. N Engl J Med 288:826–828, 1973

204. Davis K, Kennedy JW, Kemp HG Jr et al: Complications of coronary arteriography from the Collaborative Study of Coronary Artery Surgery (CASS). Circulation 59:1105–1112, 1979

205. Silverman JF, Wexler L: Complications of percutaneous trransfemoral coronary arteriography. Clin Radiol 27:317–321, 1976

206. Walker WJ, Mundall SJ, Broderick HG et al: Systemic heparinization for femoral percutaneous coronary arteriography. N Engl J Med 288:826–828, 1973

207. Wallace S, Medellin H, DeJongh D, Gianturco C: Systemic heparinization for angiography. AJR 116:204–209, 1972

208. Nelson RM, Osborne AG: Systemic heparinization for percutaneous catheter arteriography (abstr). Circulation (Suppl II) 44:II-205, 1971

209. Silverman JF, Wexler L: Complications of percutaneous transfemoral coronary arteriography. Clin Radiol 27:317–321, 1976

210. Alpert JS, Dalen JE: Pulmonary angiography in the diagnosis of pulmonary embolism. International Medical Digest 9:17–22, 1974

211. Alpert JS, Dalen JE: Pulmonary angiography in the diagnosis of pulmonary embolism. International Medical Digest 9:17–22, 1974

212. Lipton MJ, Higgins C, Winkle R: Drug hazards in coronary arteriography. In Prezer L (ed): Diagnosis and Management of Industrial Drug and Radiation Hazards: Selected Topics, vol I, pp 77–92. New York, Grune and Stratton, 1980

213. Gensini GG, DiGiorgi S: Myocardial toxicity of contrast agents used in angiography. Radiology 82:24–34, 1964

Selective Coronary Arteriography

214. Richards LS, Thal AP: Phasic dye injection control system for coronary arteriography in

the human. Surg Gynecol Obstet 107:739–741, 1958

215. Lehman, JS, Boyer RA, Winter FS: Coronary arteriography. American Journal of Roentgenology, Radium Therapy and Nuclear Medicine 81:749–763, 1959
216. Bilgutay AM, Lillihei CW: New method for coronary arteriography: acetylcholine asystole with controlled return of heart rate using a cardiac pacemaker. JAMA 180:1095–1099, 1962
217. Nordenström B, Ovenfors C, Törnell G: Coronary angiography in 100 cases of ischemic heart disease. Radiology 78:714–724, 1962
218. Sones FM Jr, Shirey EK, Proudfit WL, Westcott RN: Cine-coronary arteriography (abstr). Circulation 20:773–774, 1959
219. Sones FM Jr, Shirey EK: Coronary arteriography. Mod Concepts Cardiovasc Dis 31:735–738, 1962
220. Sewell WH: Coronary arteriography by the Sones technique: tecnical considerations. American Journal of Roentgenology, Radium Therapy and Nuclear Medicine 95:673–683, 1965
221. Ricketts HJ, Abrams HL: Percutaneous selective coronary cine arteriography. JAMA 181:620–624, 1962
222. Judkins MP: Percutaneous transfemoral selective coronary arteriography. Radiol Clin North Am 6:467–492, 1968
223. Amplatz K, Formanck G, Stranger P, Wilson W: Mechanics of selective coronary artery catheterization via femoral approach. Radiology 89:1040–1047, 1967
224. Schoonmaker FW, King SB III: Coronary arteriography by the single catheter percutaneous femoral technique: experience with 6,800 cases. Circulation 50:735–740, 1974
225. Walker WJ, Mundall SJ, Broderick HG et al: Systemic heparinization of femoral percutaneous coronary arteriography. N Engl J Med 288:826–828, 1973
226. Eyer KM: Complications of transfemoral coronary arteriography and their prevention using heparin. Am Heart J 86:428, 1973
227. Zir LM, Miller SW, Dinsmore RE et al: Interobserver variability in coronary angiography. Circulation 53:627–632, 1976
228. Grondin CM, Dyrda I, Pasternac A et al: Discrepancies between cineangiographic and postmortem findings in patients with coronary artery disease and recent myocardial revascularization. Circulation 49:703–708, 1974
229. Gould KL, Lipscomb K, Calvert C: Compen-

satory changes of the distal coronary vascular bed during progressive coronary constriction. Circulation 51:1085–1094, 1975
230. Abrams HL, Adams DF: The coronary arteriogram. N Engl J Med 281:1276–1285, 1336–1342, 1969
231. Gould KL, Lipscomb K, Calvert C: Compensatory changes of the distal coronary vascular bed during progressive coronary constriction. Circulation 541:1085–1094, 1975
232. Wolfson S, Grand D, Ross AM, Cohen LS: Risk of death related to coronary arteriography: role of left coronary arterial lesions. Am J Cardiol 37:210–216, 1976
233. Glassman E, Spencer FC, Krauss KR et al: Changes in the underlying coronary circulation secondary to bypass grafting. Circulation (Suppl II) 49, 50:II-80–II-83, 1974
234. Conti CR: Coronary arteriography. Circulation 55:227–237, 1977
235. Helfant RH, Banka VA: A Clinical and Angiographic Approach to Coronary Heart Disease. Philadelphia, F.A. Davis, 1978
236. Morettin LB: Coronary Arteriography (Chapter 14, pp 443–509). In Radiology of the Heart and Great Vessels, 3rd ed., Cooley RN, Schreiber MH (eds), William and Wilkins, Baltimore, 1978
237. Cheitlin MD, deCastro CM, McAllister HA: Sudden death as a complication of anomalous left coronary origin from the anterior sinus of Valsalva, a not-so-minor congenital anomaly. Circulation 50:780–787, 1974
238. Conti CR: Coronary arteriography. Circulation 55:227–237, 1977
239. Helfant RH, Banka VA: A Clinical and Angiographic Approach to Coronary Heart Disease. Philadelphia, F.A. Davis, 1978
240. Morettin LB: Coronary Arteriography (Chapter 14, pp 443–509). In Radiology of the Heart and Great Vessels, 3rd ed., Cooley RN, Schreiber MH (eds), William and Wilkins, Baltimore, 1978

Aortic and Pulmonary Angiography

241. Cohn LH, Mason DT, Ross J Jr et al: Preoperative assessment of aortic regurgitation in patients with mitral valve disease. Am J Cardiol 19:177–182, 1967
242. Cohn LH, Mason DT, Ross J Jr et al: Preoperative assessment of aortic regurgitation in patients with mitral valve disease. Am J Cardiol 19:177–182, 1967

243. Lehman JS, Boyle JJ, Debbas JN: Quantitation of aortic valvular insufficiency by catheter thoracic aortography. Radiology 79:361–370, 1962

244. Marrel RG, Joyner CR, Thompson PD et al: The preoperative and operative assessment of aortic regurgitation. Am J Cardiol 29:360–364, 1972

245. Beachley MC, Ranniger K, Roth FJ: Roentgenographic evaluation of dissecting aneurysm of the aorta. American Journal of Roentgenology, Radium Therapy and Nuclear Medicine 121:617–625, 1974

246. Dinsmore RE, Willerson JT, Buckley MJ: Dissecting aneurysm of the aorta: aortographic features affecting prognosis. Radiology 105:567–572, 1972

247. Eisen S, Elliott LP: The roentgenology of cystic medial necrosis of the ascending aorta. Radiol Clin North Am 6:437–449, 1968

248. Gore I, Hirst AE Jr: Arteriosclerotic aneurysms of the abdominal aorta: a review. Prog Cardiovasc Dis 16:113–150, 1973

Pulmonary Angiography

249. Dotter CT, Steiner RE, Milne ENC et al: Pulmonary and bronchial arteriography: section III. In Abrams HL (ed): Angiography, 2nd Edition. Boston, Little, Brown & Co, 1971

COMPLICATIONS ASSOCIATED WITH CARDIAC CATHETERIZATION

250. Braunwald E, Swan HJC (eds): Cooperative study on cardiac catheterization. Circulation (Suppl III) 37, 1968 (Also available as American Heart Association Monograph #20)

251. Hildner FJ, Javier RP, Ramaswamy K et al: Pseudo complications of cardiac catheterization. Chest 63:15–17, 1973

252. Schlant RC, Abrams HL, Gensini GG, Mullins CB:Indications for and hazards of coronary arteriography. Am J Cardiol 29:139, 1973

253. Braunwald E, Swan HJC (eds): Cooperative study on cardiac catheterization. Circulation (Suppl III) 37, 1968 (Also available as American Heart Association Monograph #20)

254. Silverman JF, Wexler L: Complications of percutaneous transfemoral coronary arteriography. Clin Radiol 27:317–321, 1976

255. Sones FM Jr: Complications of coronary arteriography and left heart catheterization. Cleve Clin Q 45:21–23, 1978

256. Braunwald E, Swan HJC (eds): Cooperative study on cardiac catheterization. Circulation (Suppl III) 37, 1968 (Also available as American Heart Association Monograph #20)

SPECIAL INVASIVE METHODS

Electrophysiologic Studies

257. Scherlag BJ, Lan SH, Helfant RH et al: Catheter technique for recording His bundle activity in man. Circulation 39:13–18, 1969

258. Josephson ME, Seides SF: Preexcitation syndromes, chap 11. In Josephson ME, Seides SF (eds): Clinical Cardiac Electrophysiology: Techniques and Interpretations. Philadelphia, Lea & Febiger, 1979

259. Mason JW, Winkle RA: Electrode-catheter arrhythmia induction in the selection and assessment of antiarrhythmic drug therapy for recurrent ventricular tachycardia. Circulation 58:971–985, 1978

260. Horowitz LN, Harken AH, Kaston JA, Josephson ME: Ventricular resection guided by epicardial and endocardial mapping for treatment of recurrent ventricular tachycardia. N Engl J Med 302:589–593, 1980

Cardiac Biopsy

261. Sutton DC, Sutton GC, Kent G: Needle biopsy of the human ventricular myocardium. Quarterly Bulletin of the Northwestern University Medical School 30:213, 1956

262. Mason JW: Techniques for right and left ventricular endomyocardial biopsy. Am J Cardiol 41:887–892, 1978

263. Konno S, Sekiguchi M, Sakakibara S: Catheter biopsy of the heart. Radiol Clin North Am 4:491, 1971

264. Richardson PJ: King's endomyocardial bioptome. Lancet 1:660–661, 1974

265. Mason JW: Techniques for right and left ventricular endomyocardial biopsy. Am J Cardiol 41:887–892, 1978

Percutaneous Transluminal Coronary Angioplasty

266. Grüntzig AR: Transluminal dilatation of coronary artery stenosis. Lancet 1:263, 1978
267. Grüntzig AR, Senning A, Siegenthaler WE: Nonoperative dilation of coronary-artery stenosis. N Engl J Med 301:61–68, 1979

NONINVASIVE DIAGNOSTIC METHODS COMPLEMENTING INVASIVE STUDIES

Phonocardiography and Systolic Time Intervals

268. Leatham A, Weitzman D: Auscultatory and phonocardiographic signs of pulmonary stenosis. Br Heart J 19:303–317, 1957
269. Weissler AM, Garrard CL Jr: Systolic time intervals in cardiac disease (I). Mod Concepts Cardiovasc Dis 40:1–4, 1971
270. Weissler AM, Garrard CL Jr: Systolic time intervals in cardiac disease (II). Mod Concepts Cardiovasc Dis 40:5–8, 1971
271. Lewis RP, Rittgers SE, Forester WF, Boudoulas H: A critical review of systolic time intervals. Circulation 56:146–158, 1977
272. Diamond G, Forrester JS, Chatterjee K: Mean electro-mechanical $\Delta P/\Delta t$. Am J Cardiol 30:338–341, 1972
273. Garrard CL Jr, Weissler AM, Dodge HT: The relationship of alterations in systolic time intervals to ejection fraction in patients with cardiac disease. Circulation 42:445–462, 1970
274. Garrard CL Jr, Weissler AM, Dodge HT: The relationship of alterations in systolic time intervals to ejection fraction in patients with cardiac disease. Circulation 42:445–462, 1970

Echocardiography

275. Feigenbaum H: Echocardiography, 2nd ed. Philadelphia, Lea & Febiger, 1976
276. Williams RG, Tucker CR: Echocardiographic Diagnosis of Congenital Heart Disease. Boston, Little, Brown & Co, 1977
277. Popp RL: Echocardiographic assessment of cardiac disease. Circulation 54:538–552, 1976
278. Abbasi AS, Allen MW, DeCristofaro D, Ungar I: Detection and estimation of the degree of mitral regurgitation by range-gated pulsed Doppler echocardiography. Circulation 61:143–155, 1980

Nuclear Cardiology

279. Strauss HW, Harrison K, Langan JK et al: Thallium[201] for myocardial imaging: relation of thallium[201] to regional myocardial perfusion. Circulation 51:641–645, 1975
280. Willerson JT, Parkey RW, Bonte FJ et al: Technetium stannous pyrophosphate myocardial scintigrams in patients with chest pain of varying etiology. Circulation 51:1046–1052, 1975

CARDIAC CATHERIZATION IN SPECIFIC CARDIAC DISORDERS

Coronary Artery Disease

281. Dunkman WB, Perloff JK, Kastor JA, Shelburne JC: Medical perspectives in coronary artery surgery: a caveat. Ann Intern Med 81:817–837, 1974
282. Mathur VS, Guinn GA: Prospective randomized study of coronary bypass surgery in stable angina. Circulation (Suppl I) 51, 52:I-133, 1975
283. Hancock EW: Aortic stenosis, angina pectoris, and coronary artery disease. Am Heart J 93:382–393, 1977
284. Takaro T, Hultgren HN, Lipton MJ et al: The VA cooperative randomized study of surgery for coronary arterial occlusive disease. II. Subgroup with significant left main lesions. Circulation (Suppl III) 54:III-107–III-117, 1976
285. Fischl SJ, Herman MV, Gorlin R: The intermediate coronary syndrome: clinical, angiographic and therapeutic aspects. N Engl J Med 288:1193–1198, 1973
286. Scanlon PJ, Nemickas R, Moran JF et al: Accelerated angina pectoris: clinical, hemodynamic, arteriographic and therapeutic experience in 85 patients. Circulation 47:19–26, 1973
287. National cooperative study group to compare medical and surgical therapy in unstable angina pectoris: I. Report of protocol and patient population. Am J Cardiol 37:896–902, 1976

288. Maseri A, Severi S, DeNes M et al: ''Variant'' angina: one aspect of a continuous spectrum of vasospastic myocardial ischemia. Am J Cardiol 42:1019–1035, 1978
289. Waters DD, Chaitman BR, Dupras G et al: Coronary artery spasm during exercise in patients with variant angina. Circulation 59:580–585, 1979
290. Phibbs B: The abuse of coronary arteriography. N Engl J Med 301:1394–1396, 1979
291. Bristow JD et al: Report of the ad hoc committee on the indications for coronary arteriography. Circulation 55:969–974, 1977
292. Kasparian H et al: Coronary arteriography in patients with impending and evolving myocardial infarction. Cardiovasc Clin 7:143–148, 1975
293. Levine FH et al: Management of acute myocardial ischemia with intraaortic balloon pumping and coronary artery bypass surgery. Circulation (Suppl I) 58:I-69–I-72, 1978
294. Guthaner D, Wexler L: The radiologic evaluation of patients with coronary bypass. Curr Probl Diagn Radiol 6:1–32, 1976
295. Maseri A, Severi S, DeNes M et al: ''Variant'' angina: one aspect of a continuous spectrum of vasospastic myocardial ischemia. Am J Cardiol 42:1019–1035, 1978

Valvular Disease

296. Gorlin R, Gorlin SG: Hydraulic formula for calculation of the area of the stenotic mitral valve, other cardiac valves, and central circulating shunts. Am Heart J 41:1–29, 1951
297. Morrow AG, Rietz BA, Epstein SE et al: Operative treatment in hypertrophic subaortic stenosis: techniques and the results of pre- and postoperative assessments in 83 patients. Circulation 52:88–102, 1975
298. Mason JW: Techniques for right and left ventricular endomyocardial biopsy. Am J Cardiol 41:887–892, 1978

Pericardial Disease

299. Reddy PS, Curtiss EI, O'Toole JD, Shaver JA: Cardiac tamponade: hemodynamic observations in man. Circulation 58:265–271, 1978
300. Krikorian JG, Hancock EW: Pericardiocentesis. Am J Cardiol 65:808–814, 1978
301. Hancock EW: Subacute effusive-constrictive pericarditis. Circulation 43:183–192, 1971

GLOSSARY

302. Milnor WR: Pulsatile blood flow. N Engl J Med 287:27–34, 1972
303. Gorlin R, Gorlin SG: Hydraulic formula for calculation of the area of the stenotic mitral valve, other cardiac valves, and central circulating shunts. Am Heart J 41:1–29, 1951

5

Monitoring Concepts and Techniques

ALLEN K. REAM

INTRODUCTION

Although the word *monitoring* is often thought to refer to the act of obtaining a measurement, the proper use of the term in anesthesia is to observe *and* control. That is, monitoring is both the obtaining and the use of information. Because conditions in the cardiovascular system change rapidly and physiologic control loops are relatively fast-acting, control becomes at least as difficult as measurement. Thus, we discuss both the measurement and its use. We examine use first because it determines the necessary measurements, then measurement, and conclude with selected clinical examples.

In the space available, we cannot discuss all specific measurement applications and techniques, which are covered thoroughly in the cited references.[1-3] Renal monitoring is discussed in Chapter 25. Respiratory monitoring is discussed in Chapter 16 and the provided references.[4,5] Further clinical examples are provided in Chapter 2 and all of the clinical chapters. Here, we examine the most essential measurements and use them to illustrate the central concepts.

THEORY

LOOP BEHAVIOR

We may think of the anesthesiologist and patient as components of a control loop, as illustrated in Figure 5–1d. *Input* and *response* are

INPUT

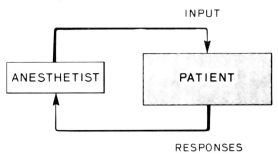

RESPONSES

Fig. 5-1. The monitoring loop of patient and anesthesiologist. Inputs are activities which influence the patient. Patient responses are activities of the patient which can usually be measured by the anesthesiologist.

defined with respect to the patient. An input might be halothane concentration in the airway and the response might be mean blood pressure. This example shows a response which is not a direct result of the input, the most common situation. We presume the existence of the intervening body mechanisms but do not need to consider them in using the concept, unless more detail is clinically useful.

In some situations, we may require more than one measurement to fully control a response. An example is measurement of the mixed venous partial pressure of oxygen to estimate tissue oxygenation. But a concomitant measure, arterial partial pressure of oxygen, helps determine whether a deficiency is cardiovascular or pulmonary in origin. When more than one variable must be measured, *simultaneous* measurement enhances control accuracy.

The behavior of the *control loop* defined in Figure 5-1 is complex because effects may pass all the way around, often more than once. The phenomenon of an input influencing itself through the system response is called *feedback.* Because of feedback, a change in any element of a control loop affects all the others, making it very difficult to separate cause and effect.

Gain, response time and *delay time* are quantitative measures of the way in which the entire loop responds. They are essential to predict loop behavior. And, they are the factors, together with inputs, which the anesthesiologist can use to maintain control.

GAIN

In order to improve our understanding of loop behavior, it is useful to consider an abnormal situation. Consider the previous example: control of blood pressure by administration of halothane. Cut the loop, as shown in Figure 5-2, so that simulated patient responses can be provided to the anesthesiologist, who will then change the halothane concentration, resulting in changed patient blood pressure. The numerical ratio of the change in patient response to the change in simulated patient response provided the anesthesiologist is the *gain* of the system.

If the value of loop gain is less than minus one or greater than one, then, when the loop is closed, each change in input to the anesthesiologist (patient response) will result in a change of greater magnitude next time around the loop. The change in patient response will increase until the patient is unable to respond further. This is an *unstable* loop because disturbances grow with each passage around the loop. Instability occurs when the loop gain is less than −1 or greater than +1, but the results are not the same.

If the loop gain is positive, the resulting change, each time around the loop, will be in the same direction as the original change (*positive feedback*). An unstable monitoring loop with positive feedback usually signifies an inappropriate response by the anesthesiologist. An example would be the attempt to control blood pressure using a methoxamine drip, believing (in error) that the drug was nitroprusside.

Negative loop gain is called *negative feedback.* In this case, each change in patient response with a transit around the loop is in the opposite direction. If the magnitude of the gain is greater than one, it will grow, as illustrated in Figure 5-3. A clinical example

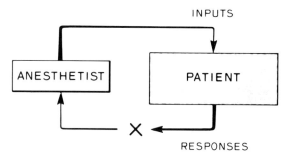

INPUTS

ANESTHETIST   PATIENT

X ←

RESPONSES

Fig. 5-2. The monitoring loop of Fig. 5-1 has been interrupted so that patient responses can be measured, but they are not communicated to the anesthesiologist. Simulated patient responses can be provided to the anesthesiologist to determine how he will change input to the patient and what patient response will result. The numerical ratio of the magnitude of the patient response to the simulated response given the anesthesiologist is called the *loop gain.* This information can be used to predict the response of the system when the loop is *closed.*

Fig. 5-3. The undesirable patient response to a positive perturbation in an unstable monitoring loop (gain greater than unity) with negative feedback. A negative perturbation would start the response in the opposite direction, but would also produce growing oscillations.

of instability with negative feedback is the infusion of sodium nitroprusside for blood pressure control, but with excessive change in dosage each time the blood pressure changes. If the correction is too large, each correction brings a progressively larger change in blood pressure.

When the magnitude of gain is less than one, each succeeding loop response to a perturbation is smaller, finally dying out. The loop is *stable.* Stable negative feedback ($-1 <$ gain < 0) is the desired state for a monitoring loop because it is most effective in maintaining a stable value of the monitored patient response. This is illustrated in Figure 5-4.

RESPONSE AND DELAY TIME

These attributes are difficult to mentally separate but are of immense practical value. *Response time* is the time required for the patient response to be *complete* after an input is provided. *Delay time* is the time from the beginning of the input to the beginning of the response. In these definitions, the input is that of the anesthesiologist, and the response is that of the patient.

The mathematics defining response and delay time can be tedious and are very sen-

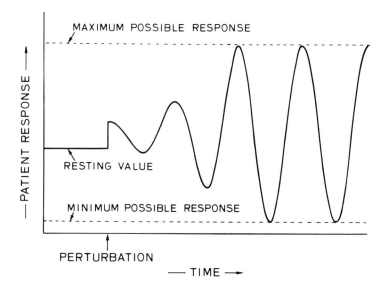

MAXIMUM POSSIBLE RESPONSE

PATIENT RESPONSE →

RESTING VALUE

MINIMUM POSSIBLE RESPONSE

PERTURBATION

— TIME →

sitive to the precise nature of the control loop. But in general, allowing the *response time* of a system with negative feedback *to increase reduces oscillation.* Allowing *delay to increase* usually *increases* the probability of *oscillation.*

In the practical world of the anesthesiologist, the most common approach is to exercise control by altering loop gain; that is, the magnitude of the management response to a change in patient state. However, controlling response and delay time, when possible, is a superior approach because it permits a faster system response.

For example, in cooling a patient, one can minimize the possibility of overcooling by reducing the rate of cooling (loop gain). But one can reduce delay time by administration of vasodilators, using nasal temperature in preference to rectal temperature. This approach permits more rapid cooling without increasing the risk of overcooling. In this ex-

ample, vasodilators decrease both response and delay time. The further reduction in delay time by improving the temperature measurement is sufficient to reduce the likelihood of overcooling.

DITHERING

The first step in determining a desired patient response, such as mean blood pressure, is to identify the patient subgroup, and presume the desirable norm for that subgroup is the desirable value for the patient. The response to previous insults, current debilities, and laboratory data help to identify the patient's subgroup, and reduce the uncertainty about his most desirable physiologic state.

However, this estimate can be refined by observing the patient response to management. With this technique, the input is continuously varied by a small amount, and the

Fig. 5-4. The patient response to a perturbation in a stable monitoring loop (gain less than unity) with negative feedback. This control loop forces the patient response to return close to the resting value. Three curves are presented, showing the effect of varying damping. The *underdamped* case shows the response of a stable system with negative feedback when loop response time is short enough to permit overcorrection before the system comes to rest. The system is *stable* because the response to changed input finally settles near the resting value. When damping is added, the system response is slowed; sufficient damping prevents overshooting the final value during the response. *Critical damping* is defined as the amount of damping that is just sufficient to prevent overshoot. *Overdamping* results in a longer response time.

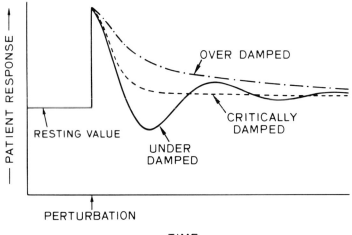

response is observed. With experience, the response to a large input can be predicted using the response to a small input.

For example, with a nitrous oxide-sodium thiopental anesthetic, the anesthesiologist may watch for signs of lightness before giving each dose of thiopental. The ideal state is when the patient is just sleepy enough not to move or recall the operation. Because signs of deeper anesthesia are clinically difficult to detect reliably, the small oscillations into a lighter plane clearly define the desired state. This technique is well-known in control theory, and is referred to as *dithering!*

In other instances, perturbation may determine whether the patient requires a change in therapy. For example, it is common practice to administer rapidly a small bolus of intravenous fluid to a patient with low blood pressure. It is presumed that if the blood pressure increases and the central venous pressure does not become undesirably high, there is evidence of the need for further infusion. In practice, dithering is the only effective approach to assuring that a compromised patient is operating on the most effective portion of his own Starling curve (see Chap. 2).

MAINTAINING HOMEOSTASIS

In control loops, the concept of an *error signal* has proven quite useful. This is the difference between the actual status of the patient and that which is desired.

Two control responses to an error signal are common. One, *proportional control,* changes the input to the patient in proportion to the error signal. When the error signal diminishes, so does the corrective input. This kind of response is illustrated by the acute ventilatory response to a change in pH. Ventilation is altered to bring the pH toward normal. The change in error signal reduces the response until an equilibrium is reached. For this reason, proportional control never provides complete correction. But it can be quite rapid.

The second, *integral control,* is illustrated by the renal response to a change in pH. Cor-

rective action continues so long as any imbalance exists. This control response is very effective, but must act more slowly to assure loop stability.

As a general rule in monitoring, proportional control is a safer technique. It preserves functioning of normal physiologic mechanisms, permits smoother control with changing state, and is less likely to produce dangerous overcorrection. It is always acutely preferable when rapidly changing variables, such as blood pressure, are controlled. When integral control is used, complete correction must be obtained very slowly. For example, too rapid correction of serum hyperosmolarity can produce lethal cerebral edema.

APPROPRIATE MEASUREMENTS

The obvious approach is to select those measurements which permit adequate control of homeostasis in the short run. With more sophistication, however, investigators have begun to search quantitatively for correlation of ultimate outcome with monitored (presumably measured and controlled) variables. Three studies provide insight into the techniques for evaluating the value of possible measurements that are more likely to be used in the future.

Cullen employed straightforward statistical techniques to assess the relative merit of systolic, diastolic, pulse, and mean pressure in correlation with each other, heart rate, stroke volume, and peripheral vascular resistance.[6] He concluded that systolic pressure alone was adequate. Although the conclusions appear correct as reported, the difficulty in using the results of this analysis clinically is that it presumed that only one measure could be used, and did not address the question of whether a combination of measurements provided more information or improved prediction of long-term outcome. In fact, as discussed with reference to arterial pressure measurements they do provide more information.

Schneider examined the relevance of monitored variables in 66 patients undergoing general surgical procedures.[7] The factors most highly correlated with risk, as measured by outcome, are presented in the list below.

The 6 most significant risk factors of 254 were evaluated. High absolute value of skewness means that more high or low values were seen than normally expected. The negative CUSUM means an abnormal decrease in value as the surgery progressed. Thus the risk factors fell into three categories: (1) increased preoperative risk (elevated preoperative systolic blood pressure and anesthesia within the previous year); (2) abnormal variability intraoperatively (in pulse pressure and systolic blood pressure); and (3) an abnormal decrease in value as surgery progressed (systolic blood pressure and cardiac work index).

We interpret these data to suggest that underlying disease and hemodynamic instability during surgery increase the risk of postoperative morbidity and mortality.

Similarly, Shoemaker examined the correlation of 35 monitored variables used in postoperatively monitoring 113 critically ill patients. He noted that the accuracy of single variables in predicting outcome varied from 91 to 60 percent, but varied markedly during each successive stage of postoperative shock. He found that the commonly monitored variables, such as heart rate, temperature, central venous pressure, and hemoglobin, were less successful in predicting outcome than per-

fusion-related variables, such as efficiency of tissue oxygen extraction, red cell mass, and oxygen transport.[8] In this case the correlation was with actual values, rather than with variability.

The lesson of these studies seems straightforward. The adequacy of short-term monitoring must first be assured because, even after a period of stability, a short-term instability can be catastrophic. Thus, the examples at the end of this chapter dwell on the problems of achieving control adequate to assure patient stability. Given the ability to assure stability, correlations with long-term favorable outcome may be expected to be highest where the variables relate to preservation of biologic function, particularly energy supply and waste removal. By analogy, one must first learn to stay on the road; then one can do more sophisticated studies to learn the acceptable speed limit. And while the more sophisticated approaches may be expected to ultimately be of great value, progress is likely to be slow, because of the effort necessary to phrase and answer the proper questions.

INSTRUMENTS

MAN-MACHINE INTERFACE

The effective use of instruments requires that one be sensitive to human and machine limitations. In particular, the largest rate of information transfer is through the eyes, with the ears a distant second. Thus detailed monitoring information should be presented visually. *True* alarms should be auditory, so the observer need not be looking at the instrument to receive the message.

Also, human observers cannot maintain uninterrupted periods of observation without unusual self-discipline. This suggests that the regular measurement of baseline variables, such as blood pressure and heart rate, is best performed by an instrument. This option is likely to become a requirement as prices decline and instrument reliability continues to improve. The anesthesiologist must support

---

Monitored Variables Associated With Increased Operative Risk

1. Systolic blood pressure, maintenance, negative cumulative sum of the differences (CUSUM)
2. Pulse pressure, maintenance data*, absolute value of skewness
3. Systolic blood pressure, all data, absolute value of skewness
4. Cardiac work index, all negative CUSUM
5. Preoperative systolic blood pressure
6. Anesthesia within the previous year

*Beginning 8 minutes after induction.

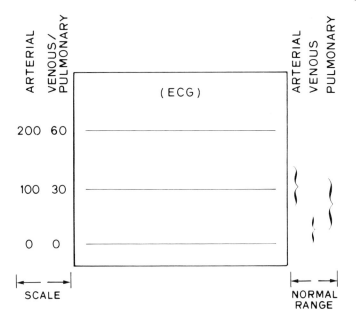

Fig. 5-5. An illustration of the recommended method of setting up a calibrated graphic display showing several values simultaneously. The pertinent points are (1) a common zero position for all of the variables (except ECG in which the DC value is ignored), (2) the use of the entire screen for the range of each variable, and (3) a selection of scales for the pressures involved which leads, under usual circumstances, to visual separation and is of sufficient range to encompass nearly all eventualities.

this requirement by establishing a routine, rhythmic pattern for reviewing his monitored variables. Another benefit of this approach is the early detection of conditions requiring correction. Early detection usually averts major difficulties.

Particularly in cardiovascular monitoring, a regular pattern of displays helps the observer assimilate more information more rapidly. Nonfade video displays are preferable, and should always be in the *moving black bar* mode, rather than the *moving strip chart* mode, to make detail easier to appreciate. We strongly recommend using the full screen when several signals are presented simultaneously; detail is easier to observe, a calibrated screen is more useful, and quantitative comparison is easier. It is best to use a single *y*-axis point for calibration of all pressures because it provides the eye a single reference level, reducing the amount of information that must be remembered. Gains may be different, however, to help separate signals on the screen, such as a 200 torr full scale for arterial pressure, 60 torr for pulmonary artery pressure, and 30 torr for central venous pressure (Fig. 5-5). Some new concepts, such as differential sweep rates for the different signals or the use of color are quite

effective, but must be seen to be fully appreciated.

When multiple pressures are numerically displayed, they should be in the same sequence as shown on the screen. The most common sequence for complete monitoring is ECG, arterial, venous, and pulmonary pressures. Both position and labelling then reinforce correct interpretation.

Equipment should be placed where it will be used. One is less likely to follow urine output if the collector is at the other end of the table. Much information is missed when the monitor is behind the anesthesiologist. It should be placed so that the visual angle from patient to monitor is as small as possible. The practice common in early cardiovascular surgery of placing the monitor so that it is most conveniently viewed by the surgeon is inappropriate but self-reinforcing: when the anesthesiologist is not able to note changes promptly, the surgeon is more anxious to perform his own monitoring. In the complex activities associated with open-heart surgery, dividing attention in this way is counterproductive for both anesthesiologist and surgeon.

When a measurement is easier, it will be performed more consistently. If comfortable, one is more likely to concentrate on the task at hand. If fatigued by standing, one should sit, unless sitting prevents adequate observation or communication. Extraneous noise should be discouraged and lighting should be adequate.

Modern cardiovascular management is impossible without quantitative monitoring devices. Yet the anesthesiologist should never discount information from any source, for at least two reasons. Available quantitative monitors (such as ECG and pressure) do not consider all variables of interest. As documented in Chapters 2 and 14 for example, both the assessment of inotropic state and end diastolic volume are considerably improved by visual observation during the time the chest is open. Similarly, attention to conversation and observation of the field will invariably detect rapid blood loss before it is revealed by a changing mean pressure. Second, effective monitoring demands that each conclusion be supported by independent measurements. The alternative is the possibility of serious error. The reliability of modern pressure measurement, for example, leads to a tendency to miss occasional but serious errors in instrument-obtained values. Corroboration can be obtained both between instruments, as with comparison of the waveform on the screen with the digital readout, and between instruments and direct observation, as in observing the rapidity of bleeding when the aorta is vented during air maneuvers before terminating bypass.

EQUIPMENT MAINTENANCE

Because aggressive therapeutic decisions are made during cardiovascular surgery, accurate pressure calibration is essential. And presently available instruments are not well enough designed to permit the physician to ignore their design characteristics.

Calibrating part of the pressure measurement system is not an adequate substitute for complete calibration. For example, pressure is measured by obtaining an electrical signal from a pressure transducer, which is amplified, and presented to a screen or meter (Fig. 5-6). The electrical calibration signal provided with most pressure measurement systems checks only the part of this sequence after the pressure transducer, which is the part most likely to fail. In order to calibrate the complete system, a known pressure must be applied to the transducer, and the output

Fig. 5-6. The sequence of information flow in pressure measurement. When the system is calibrated, a signal of known value is provided as input, and the output is adjusted to read the proper value. Only the portion between input and output is calibrated. Electrical calibration does not include the most common source of error, the pressure transducer. One must apply a known pressure at the transducer to include it in system calibration.

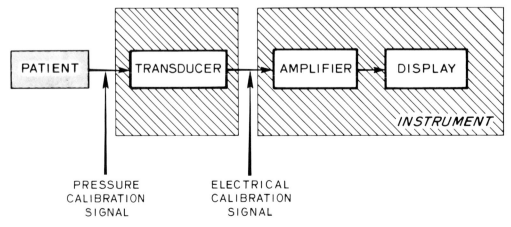

set to display the correct value. This technique is illustrated in Figure 5–7.

The physician should also review the equipment maintenance system to assure that it is adequate. Routine preventive maintenance, technician-performed full calibration, and regular checks are essential to optimal performance. Similarly, the physician should be involved in equipment selection and purchase, to assure that the equipment is adequate for professional needs.[9]

SPECIFIC MEASUREMENTS

ECG

This discussion concerns practical application; interpretation is fully discussed in Chapter 6. The ECG provides three kinds of information: rate, rhythm, and waveform. The first two are best measured from a signal which may contain distortion, but which is consistently present. Waveform analysis requires a signal with minimal distortion.

The operating room is a particularly noisy electrical environment, largely because of the electrocautery (which is essential to modern cardiovascular surgery). Early monitor designs inadequately reject electrical noise, and are not acceptable. Some recent monitors have excellent rejection, but at the expense of waveform distortion, apparently occasioned by the failure of manufacturers to appreciate the need for fidelity and by the technical difficulty of achieving it. The Association for the Advancement of Medical Instrumentation has developed draft standards which define two levels of accuracy for ECG measurement; the stricter standard is preferable for cardiac monitoring.*

In the operating room, the principal source of instrument failure is the connection to the patient. The leads should always be checked if the instrument exhibits erratic behavior. Dry electrodes or a different resistance be-

*Available from Association for the Advancement of Instrumentation, 1901 North Fort Myer Drive, Suite 602, Arlington, VA 22209.

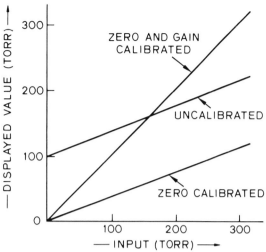

Fig. 5-7. The proper sequence of calibration of a pressure measuring system. Normally a transducer is calibrated over a range of values (*e.g.*, 0–300 torr) rather than for a single value. If the measurement system is linear (output proportional to input), the output plotted against the input is a straight line. Most clinical instruments use a hybrid calibration system, implemented in the following fashion. One pressure value—zero, gauge, or atmospheric—does not require an instrument. The pressure transducer is vented to atmosphere, and the instrument adjusted with a knob (usually marked "zero") until the display output is zero. The zero must always be set BEFORE the gain. To set gain, a calibration button is pushed to supply a known electrical signal, as shown in Fig. 5-5. The "gain" knob is adjusted to give the expected output. (In some instruments the steps following venting the transducer to air are automated, but the sequence is the same.) If the transducer gain is calibrated, this completes the system calibration. Also, transducer gain drift is significantly greater than electronic gain drift in modern instruments. Thus, frequent calibration for drift in instrument gain should be unnecessary, but scheduled calibration for drift in transducer gain is essential.

tween different electrodes and the skin substantially increase sensitivity to noise.

It is not generally recognized that it is not necessary to grossly abrade the skin to minimize resistance. The source of resistance is the level of maturation of intercellular bridges in the epidermis. Removal of superficial layers of epithelium, until the skin is shiny, is sufficient. Abrasion to the point of punctate bleeding means that the capillary loops of the dermis have been injured, well below the layer of interest. Normally, rubbing with an alcohol sponge is sufficient; in extreme cases repeated application of a fresh surface of adhesive tape to a one centimeter square area before affixing the electrode will suffice. Dry skin has very high resistance and the measurement will not be stable until the superficial squamous cells under the electrode are moistened all the way down to the underlying living tissue.

All monitors draw minute currents through the electrode that can polarize the electrode and reduce current carrying capacity. A silver-silver chloride amalgam electrode provides charge carriers which alleviate this problem, but is not ordinarily required.

Place the electrocautery return electrode as close to the site of surgery as possible to reduce interference. When significant electrocautery interference is noted, a poor electrocautery return path should be suspected.

The ECG can be monitored through the esophagus; this has the advantage of enhancing the size of the P wave.[10] In an emergency, it is possible to pace a patient through this electrode.[11]

Shock hazard is much greater with the use of an internally placed catheter because the fibrillation threshold is specified by the current density at the heart.[12, 13] Monitoring in this way requires that the instrument be tested to assure a leakage current of less than 100 microamp. Some suggest 10 microamp, but this appears unduly strict.

ARTERIAL PRESSURE

The single most valuable measurement still appears, by consensus, to be arterial pressure.[14] Ideally, pressure is measured in the aortic root, but this is not yet clinically reliable and is quite expensive. Thus most direct arterial measurements are made through a fluid-filled catheter, connected to an external pressure transducer. In most cases, the arterial catheter ends in the radial artery, so that the fluid column connecting aortic root and transducer passes through the brachial artery.

The pathway between the aortic root and external transducer alters the shape of the pressure waveform. A common form of distortion is *ringing* or oscillation of the arterial waveform after the upstroke. Many clinicians insert a small air bubble in the catheter to damp this oscillation, but the bubble reduces the frequency response of the catheter, introducing distortion by slowing the rapidly changing components of the waveform, and rounding sharp corners. Also, damping reduces the measured pulse pressure.

The characteristics of the artery between the aortic root and the radial artery can also increase or decrease the pulse pressure. It can be shown, however, that the mean pressure is not sensitive to these influences, and is therefore more reliable with a system that is accurately calibrated, but has poor damping or frequency response. Both pulse pressure and mean pressure yield useful information.[15]

Direct measurement of arterial pressure is essential for any situation where the pressure must be continuously monitored. The risk of placing the catheter is small if appropriate criteria are observed,[16, 17] principally removal of the catheter as soon as blood cannot be withdrawn through it.[18] Disposable continuous flushing devices are available to keep the catheter patent.

The most common site for placement of an arterial catheter is the radial artery. The clinician first assures that Allen's test is normal by digitally occluding the ulnar and radial arteries, having the patient open and close his hand until the palm is blanched, then releasing the ulnar artery and ensuring that the palm turns pink within three seconds. The skin is prepped under sterile conditions, and a small full-thickness incision made with a needle or blade after instillation of local anesthetic. An 18- or 20-gauge, over-needle catheter is then advanced until blood returns, the catheter is advanced into the artery (do not first withdraw the needle!), air is withdrawn, and the system is then filled with heparinized saline. The catheter and connecting tubing are taped to the wrist (not hand) of the patient (Figs. 5–8 through 5–12).

Calibration of the transducer has already been discussed and is summarized in Figure 5–7. However, one additional concept requires discussion. Many clinicians have great practical difficulty with the concept of the reference level. In brief, the pressure transducer measures pressure at the transducer diaphragm. This pressure is the same as that in the aortic root, except for the vertical offset between transducer and aortic root. The correction can be made during calibration by opening a port in the fluid filled catheter at heart level, and setting the indicated pressure to zero. This approach works by introducing an electrical offset to the measured pressure at the transducer. However, it requires that the vertical distance between transducer and heart be kept constant because the calibration is correct only for the vertical distance at the time of calibration. Most experienced clinicians recommend using a port on the transducer, keeping it at heart level, because visual inspection will then more easily reveal if the port is in the calibrated position.

Indirect systolic and diastolic blood pressures are less satisfactory because of diminished accuracy and the inability to obtain continuous measurements. Nonetheless, convenience and speed sometimes make it the preferred mode. Most accept the following recommendations of the American Heart Association: (1) the cuff should be 20 percent wider than the diameter of the limb, (2) "Korotkoff" sounds are detected by listening over the brachial artery distal to the cuff, (3) systolic pressure is the cuff pressure at which sounds first appear on two consecutive beats as the cuff is deflated, and (4) diastolic pressure is the cuff pressure at which sounds abruptly become muffled with further deflation.[19]

Many anesthesiologists employ the oscillometric technique. Systolic and diastolic pressures are obtained by observing the vibration of the mercury column or aneroid needle of the sphygmomanometer. Analogous criteria are observed; the point of appearance of an unequivocal upward bounce is taken as systolic pressure, the point of muffling of the bounce is taken as diastolic pressure. The rate of fall of pressure must be kept *slow* and *constant*. The best available study shows that the oscillometric technique is more accurate, even when variations in hearing acuity are eliminated.[20]

Recently, noninvasive, microprocessor-controlled devices have become available which accurately measure mean blood pressure.[21] It appears likely that these instruments will achieve widespread use because of the accuracy, which is greater than possible with noninvasive systolic/diastolic measurements[22] and the intrinsic value of mean blood pressure.[15] The most important single value is *mean blood pressure*. This value is required to calculate peripheral vascular resistance, and with resistance, to recognize changes in cardiac output between flow measurements. Pulse pressure is influenced by peripheral resistance, central arterial compliance, and stroke volume. With other information, the pulse, systolic, and diastolic pressures are also of value to the clinician.

VENOUS CATHETERS: MANAGEMENT CONCEPTS

While the management of peripheral venous lines appears obvious, some major points are worthy of discussion. The number of lines must be sufficient to assure an adequate transfusion rate. With blood warming, under normal circumstances, one line, using a blood pump and catheter no smaller than 16 gauge (14 gauge is preferable) is sufficient. Many clinicians prefer two lines if the patient has had a prior cardiotomy, chest irradiation, or currently has a coagulopathy. However, a significant risk with two large lines is overtransfusion; this must be anticipated and avoided.

Ringer's lactate should not be infused with blood; the calcium content is sufficient to cause coagulation and emboli.

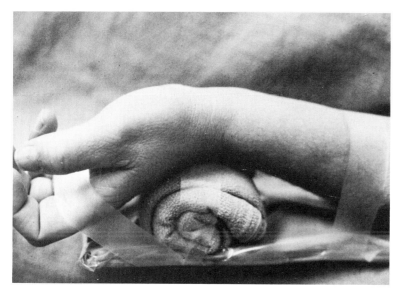

Fig. 5-8. Positioning of the hand for radial artery cannulation. The hand must be extended over a roll, but not sufficiently to compromise arterial flow or pulsation. (Courtesy of Dr. J. Kent Garman)

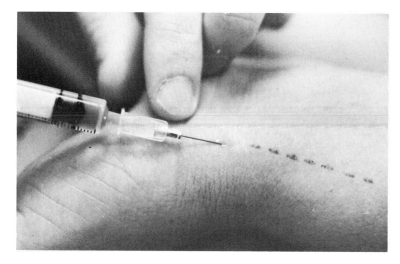

Fig. 5-9. Local anesthetic should be injected before radial artery cannulation, intradermally and on both sides of the artery. Two percent lidocaine is preferred to assure a longer lasting block. (Courtesy of Dr. J. Kent Garman)

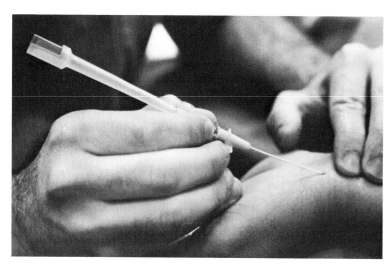

Fig. 5-10. Inserting the cannula. The artery should be located by palpation, continued gently while advancing. First, make a relieving small incision with the needle so that the catheter tip is not damaged while passing through the skin and "feel" is preserved. The artery should be entered bevel up. Some fill the reservoir with clear fluid to protect against clot. The reservoir should be used to show return and avoid spilling blood. (Courtesy of Dr. J. Kent Garman)

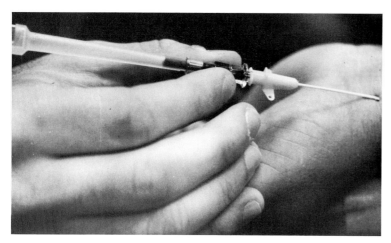

Fig. 5-11. Cannulating the artery. When blood enters the reservoir, one should attempt to thread the needle into the artery. The return should "flash" back quickly. A very slow return may be caused by venous blood, or inadequate entry. Then, advance the catheter off the needle, without withdrawing the needle. Return should be visible during advance. Advancing without return usually makes subsequent cannulation at that site impossible. If there is no return and the needle is within the artery, advance the needle further (through-and-through technique), and withdraw the needle only about 2 mm, leaving the catheter in place. Slowly withdraw the catheter-needle combination. (Courtesy of Dr. J. Kent Garman)

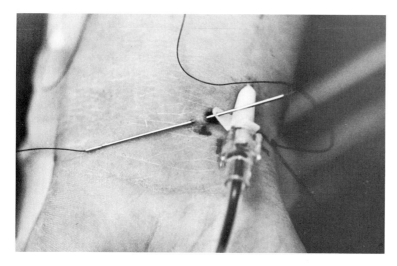

Fig. 5-12. The catheter must be firmly fixed in place. It should not be taped or sewn to both the hand and wrist; wrist flexion will destroy the catheter. It is advisable to attach an automatic flushing unit to the catheter immediately; even if failure to do so does not immediately compromise sampling or pressure measurement, it appears to shorten the duration of acceptable measurements. (Courtesy of Dr. J. Kent Garman)

The purposes of placing a central venous line are to measure pressure, to sample blood, and to permit drug infusions with immediate mixing (such as sclerosing agents) and minimal delay (such as rapid- and short-acting drugs).

These considerations lead to specific requirements for drug infusions. It is preferable to give only nonirritating drugs through the peripheral line. Bolus injections have a slower onset when given peripherally, often a desirable consequence during induction. When speeding up the drip rate to pass in a bolus injection, the volume of the line should be noted. It is common to give excessive fluid during this maneuver.

Concentrated drip infusions should always be administered in parallel with a crystalloid carrier infusion ("piggyback"). The length of common line should always be as short as possible because it represents both infusion delay and an obligatory bolus if the rate of carrier flow is increased. A sample calculation may help the reader's intuition. If a drip chamber giving 60 drops/ml is running at 5 drops/minute, and the priming volume is 2 ml, typical for the shortest small-volume extension lines, then if no carrier is running, 24 minutes are required for the drug to reach the patient! If the carrier is running at 60 drops/minute, it still requires more than 2 minutes for a change in drug rate to affect the patient. Conversely, infusion through a peripheral line (such as during induction) is acceptable if pharmacologically dilute, and may be preferable to avoid interfering with central pressure measurement.

Despite custom, it is better not to add heparin to the central venous infusion. Heparin coats the inside of the line, and is partially eluted when blood samples are withdrawn. On occasion this can significantly distort the ACT measurement.

We prefer gravity-controlled infusion units (Sorenson: Dial-a-Flow), which are precisely calibrated, to pumps. Reproducibility is more important than accuracy because all of the active drugs are titrated to patient response. Pumps require more precious space and are more expensive, less reliable, and do not appear to offer improved reproducibility.

At Stanford, four stopcocks are attached to the central venous line, as close to the point of entering the patient as is physically possible. The closest port is reserved for blood sampling (smallest cleansing volume and the drips can be temporarily interrupted with a single stopcock). Drug infusions are connected to the most distal ports, with the most rapid acting drug closest to the patient. A carrier drip is always used; otherwise dangerous quantities of drug can be given with sampling and flushing.

CENTRAL VENOUS PRESSURE

The central venous pressure is of value in assessing the filling pressure (preload) of the right heart. If the right heart and pulmonary vascular resistance are normal, it provides an estimate of the left ventricular preload as well. Measurement convenience, reliability, and accuracy are enhanced by using a direct catheter measurement. The catheter also provides a convenient pathway for withdrawing venous blood samples, administering drugs where infusion delays must be minimized, and administering drugs with undesirable side effects in high concentration (*e.g.*, the sclerosing effects of many antibiotics).

In the past, venous pressure was often measured peripherally or via a line passed centrally through a brachial vein. Because peripheral lines permit measurement error because of intervening venous valves, and a central line through a brachial entry is both more difficult to pass and requires fluoroscopy for adequate assurance of proper tip placement, the majority of centers are changing to central placement.

Subclavian lines work well, but are discouraged because this approach has no inherent advantage over a higher approach, carries an obligatory risk of pneumothorax, and, if bleeding occurs (as from accidental arterial puncture), there is risk of cardiac tamponade or obligatory thoracotomy.

The external jugular vein is satisfactory, but more difficult to enter than the internal jugular vein. Occasionally the catheter cannot be advanced, passage into an inadequate sidebranch occurs, or measurement is compromised because of a venous valve.

The most acceptable site, on the average, is the internal jugular vein. The catheter is usually placed on the right side because of the more direct course of the vascular sheath. The patient is placed supine, with no pillow, and the head is fully rotated to the left while the skin is prepped under sterile conditions. After tilting the patient 20° head down (Trendelenberg's position), or until external jugular distention is noted, a 20-gauge needle is passed to verify the location of the vessel. Typically the site of insertion is about 5 mm medial to the center of a triangle formed by three soft tissue landmarks: the lateral margin of the medial head of the sternocleido-

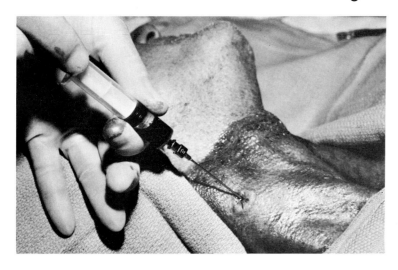

Fig. 5-13. Placing an internal jugular catheter. The needle is aimed at the ipsilateral nipple. (Courtesy of Dr. J. Kent Garman).

mastoid, the course of the external jugular vein, and a transverse plane passing through the cricothyroid membrane (see Fig. 5–13). The needle is advanced at an angle of 30° to the skin, toward the ipsilateral nipple. A flexible guidewire is then placed through an 18-gauge thinwall needle, and the catheter passed over it (Seldinger technique). Rarely, a *J* wire (a guidewire with the tip forming a flexible *J*) is helpful to pass an obstruction. The *J* wire is more often necessary to catheterize the left internal jugular vein.

The possibility of arterial puncture is minimized by rotation of the patient's head and initial passage of the probing needle slightly lateral to the most probable location of the vein. Entry is high to avoid pneumothorax and to assure that, should arterial puncture occur, locally applied pressure will occlude the hole and bleeding will not result in cardiac tamponade. Under ordinary circumstances, this procedure should not be performed in a fully anticoagulated patient. The small exploring needle reduces the risks of brachial plexus laceration and significant arterial bleeding. Palpation of the carotid sheath before entering is strongly recommended for the novice, but is of little additional value with greater experience. The internal jugular is often visible by pulsation or, by refilling after compression in the head-down position. The patient should always be

kept head down, until the port is closed, to avoid aspiration of air. If the open port is large, the patient should maintain a gentle Valsalva maneuver until it is occluded. With proper technique, the risk of any complication is small. Comparison of data with other centers suggests that the incidence of all complications is less than 3 percent in experienced hands; permanent sequelae are much less likely.

Other complications have been reported, such as tearing the thoracic duct and entry into the trachea. With normal anatomy and skilled supervision or adequate experience, these events are extremely rare.

PULMONARY ARTERY MONITORING

The advent of the balloon flotation (Swan–Ganz) catheter, has made possible direct measurement of pulmonary artery pressure and sampling of pulmonary artery (mixed venous) blood. With a tip thermistor and a second lumen ending in the vena cava, thermal dilution cardiac output measurement is also possible.

The primary attraction of pulmonary artery pressure measurement is the opportunity to estimate left atrial pressure. This was first accomplished by placing the catheter tip in the *wedge* position, so that inflation of the balloon occluded the vessel, permitting the tip catheter to measure the runoff pressure. This is presumed equal to (or, in more precise studies, to correlate with) left atrial pressure, unless intrathoracic pressure is abnormal,[23] such as with PEEP.[24] More recently, it has been shown that an excellent estimate of left atrial pressure can be obtained from pulmonary artery diastolic pressure, though accuracy requires either simple automated calculation or an unusually compulsive clinician.[25, 26] This approach permits avoidance of the risks associated with the wedge position.

Left atrial pressure determines left ventricular preload. As noted in Chapters 2, 4, and 16, this measure is extremely helpful in assessing and modifying left ventricular function, and is less accurately estimated from central venous pressure under many circumstances, including abnormal pulmonary vascular resistance, alveolar capillary dysfunction, and right-heart failure. It is not correct, however, to say that central venous pressure is of no help in estimating left-heart filling pressure and function. The central venous pressure correlates well with the pulmonary capillary wedge pressure in normal patients.[27] It is less likely to correlate well in the presence of pulmonary hypertension, edema, or elevated pulmonary vascular resistance. It may correlate, but is likely to be offset, in patients with left-heart dysfunction.

As with central venous pressure, the most acceptable site for percutaneous placement is the right internal jugular vein. The guide wire is placed as previously described, and the sheath passed after a minimal, relieving, full-thickness skin incision with a number eleven (tapered, straight-edged) blade. The previously balloon-tested, flushed, instrumented, and calibrated catheter is passed after removing the inner sheath. The balloon is inflated when beyond the tip of the sheath (approximately 15 cm), and slowly advanced while the tip pressure waveform is observed on the monitor screen.

A typical sequence of pressures, illustrated in Figure 5–14, is seen as the tip passes from vena cava to right atrium, right ventricle, and pulmonary artery. Placement should always be by slow advance, observing the waveform on the screen, and the length of catheter passed to assure that unacceptable coiling has not occurred. Typical adult values are from 25 to 40 cm to enter the right ventricle and from 35 to 60 cm to enter the pulmonary artery. Once in the artery, the catheter is advanced until wedged, as measured by loss of arterial pulsation and a stable pressure after flushing (to rule out tip occlusion). On occasion it can be difficult to assure a wedge (*e.g.*, with severe mitral regurgitation) because the waveforms are similar, but the difference is clear-cut in the normal patient. The catheter should then be slowly withdrawn, with the balloon deflated, but verifying the wedge every 1 to 2 cm, until the wedge is lost. The sheath is then withdrawn, the patient returned to a level (or comfortable) position, and the catheter gently sewn in place.

The catheter is associated with many complications and the possibility of injury should always be considered before proceeding. A defibrillator and lidocaine should always be present to treat any arrhythmias. They are most commonly caused by unnecessary pressure of the catheter tip against the wall of the heart.[28] The catheter should never be withdrawn with the balloon inflated; serious injury could result if it were withdrawn

Fig. 5-14. An illustration of pressures observed with passage of a Swan–Ganz catheter.

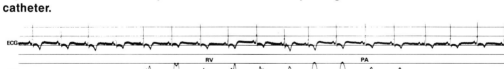

through a valve. One should never forget that significant amounts of air can be aspirated despite slow return bleeding and should ensure that patient position or Valsalva maneuvers, or both, assure positive pressure while aspiration can occur. Aseptic technique is essential because in many instances the catheter will remain for days. The catheter must be withdrawn after obtaining a wedge (if required) because some coiling occurs during placement. If not straightened by withdrawal, subsequent straightening is likely to produce vessel occlusion, thrombus formation, and local infarction. Excessive pressure on the vessel wall can also erode the vessel wall and produce hemorrhage, particularly if the catheter is left in place more than 48 hours. It is possible to tie a knot in the catheter by withdrawal after coiling in the right ventricle, but this risk is minimized by keeping track of the length advanced (to avoid unnecessary advancement with failure to pass the pulmonary valve), and slow withdrawal with the balloon deflated if another try is necessary. Head movement can move the catheter tip, causing injury or incorrect measurements.[29] Finally, in some instances, such as post-pneumonectomy, a wedge pressure measurement may decrease pulmonary blood flow. This may cause pulmonary hypertension and right-heart failure.[30]

TEMPERATURE

Temperature is monitored by two common techniques: the thermocouple and the thermistor. The thermocouple (discovered by a physician, Thomas Johann Seebeck, 1780–1831) is a series of two junctions between two dissimilar metals which generate an electrical potential proportional to the temperature difference between the two junctions. Typically, one junction is placed at the desired site of measurement and the other in a location at room temperature. The advantage is that the potential is solely a function of the temperature difference and the materials used. The disadvantage is that the voltage generated is quite small.

The thermistor is a semiconductor device which varies in resistance with changing temperature. Its behavior is sensitive to the technique of manufacture, so that no two devices are ever exactly alike. But the range of resistance can be selected so that an inexpensive electronic circuit provides adequate performance, and no reference temperature is required. Most clinical temperature monitors are of this type.

The primary clinical concern is the site of temperature monitoring. Suggested sites include the rectum, mouth, nose, esophagus, and tympanic membrane. The rectum is preferred by some because it is acceptable in the awake patient (though not attractive), and it appears to give trunk temperature. Measurements within the head are close to rapid blood flow, and therefore give a more accurate estimate of central blood temperature. Air flow over moist tissues near a sensor can provide misleading results, however, and this situation should be avoided. (Use a nasal probe with oral intubation.) The nasal probe appears particularly attractive because it is also close to the high blood flow through the turbinates. The argument for tympanic membrane temperature measurement is based on the observation that a branch of the internal carotid artery supplies the tympanic membrane. However, observations of the author suggest that the temperature measured is really the equilibrium temperature of the auditory canal, and that if the auditory meatus is occluded, the sensor gives equivalent results when withdrawn slightly. Avoiding tympanic membrane contact should reduce the risk of injury to the membrane.

Differences in measured temperature between these sites is usually caused by a significant source of heat loss or gain which is not uniformly applied. Under such circumstances, monitoring at several sites provides information of practical value. As shown in Figure 26–7, both measurements are required in clinical hypothermia for adequate control and patient protection. The nasal temperature reveals the true core temperature and the rectal temperature permits an estimate of the thermal lag, or time required for equilibration. With mild hypothermia, two measurements are desirable but not mandatory. A nasal measurement is more precise, but the rectal measurement is more convenient.

DIRECT OBSERVATION

Information that is difficult to quantify must not be ignored. An example is heart size. For example, the concept of maximizing the efficiency of cardiac function under Starling's Law presumes that one can relate preload to end diastolic ventricular volume. During open-heart surgery, ventricular compliance is often abnormal, and visual correlation of heart size with measured pressures can noticeably improve patient management. Similarly, heart size, through the Law of Laplace, directly influences myocardial oxygen demand. The clinician who prefers to watch only his electronic monitors is often not aware of their limitations. See Chapter 2 for further discussion.

APPLICATION

Although the concepts of biological control loops and feedback are generally known, it is difficult to apply them in a specific way, because the details of the loop behavior are usually not known. Yet, these lessons can be applied in ways which permit increased insight and management control before obtaining complete understanding.

Most people have difficulty in following the description of control loop behavior presented below by simply reading the text. The reader is urged to draw the control loop under discussion, and follow each event on the copied diagram as it is presented in the text. Generally, this approach makes the discussion clear the first time through.

An example is the relationship between the carotid baroreceptors and central arterial blood pressure. In casual discussion of this mechanism, the usual concept is that the baroreceptors change their neural output with changes in mean arterial blood pressure, and that this neural output alters heart rate through the vagus nerve. In fact, the baro-

receptors respond to both mean pressure and pulse pressure,[31] and the response is expressed by a change in heart rate and peripheral vascular resistance. By taking the full relationship into account, as shown in Figure 5-15, one can add considerably to the precision of patient management. Even here, we have ignored inotropic changes, but with lesser effect. Also the system uses proportional, rather than integral control. Thus, an error signal must persist to sustain the response. (It is interesting to note that there is evidence of long-term integral control, demonstrated in patients who have their baroreceptors surgically removed. After surgery the blood pressure moves toward the presurgical value over a period of days.)

Consider the patient response to hemorrhage. The immediate response is a decrease in arterial mean blood pressure, secondary to a decreased cardiac output. Now, the baroreceptor response increases systemic vascular resistance, increasing mean blood pressure. The baroreceptor response also increases heart rate, further reducing stroke volume and pulse pressure.

This compensatory decrease in pulse pressure further stimulates the baroreceptor-mediated response, increasing both heart rate and peripheral vascular resistance. In the awake patient who is frightened or in pain, the result is often a return of mean blood pressure to a normal or even slightly elevated value, despite the previous statement that an error signal must persist to stimulate a continued response. The remaining error signal is the decreased pulse pressure supplemented by general stimulation of sympathetic tone.

This understanding of the control loop behavior makes the classic observations reported in hemorrhagic shock understandable. The pulse is thready because the pulse pressure is so small. The patient is pale and diaphoretic because of the significantly elevated peripheral vascular resistance and the consequent diminution in peripheral blood flow.

These findings also explain the commonly believed but false presumption that the mean blood pressure is significantly reduced. In reality, the high peripheral vascular resistance makes a peripherally measured blood pressure difficult to obtain, leading to the presumption that it is depressed. In the author's experience, in those patients coming to the emergency room in shock in which a peripheral blood pressure, measured by cuff, was unobtainable, the majority were found to have a slightly elevated mean pressure when a direct arterial line was placed by cutdown in the next few minutes. In fact, a significant decrease in mean blood pressure, associated solely with hemorrhage, represents a failure of the physiologic mechanisms to adequately compensate. If not immediately treated, it is usually quickly followed by circulatory collapse and death.

These data make clear that in hemorrhagic shock it is necessary to monitor heart rate, mean blood pressure, and pulse pressure. Cardiac output, when obtainable, increases monitoring (management) precision.

In this example, another consideration also affects the desirable approach to monitoring. With the increase in peripheral vascular resistance, the vascular volume is decreased (see Chap. 2) and blood flow to the medium and slow compartments is decreased, leaving flow to the fast compartment (the vital organs) relatively less affected. This has an immediate effect on any drugs administered. For agents administered through a centrally placed catheter, the response time is normal or slightly decreased. The drug effect is also enhanced, not because of an unusual susceptibility associated wth cellular injury in shock, but because the reduced circulation blood volume, further reduced in the fast compartment by obligatory trapping of blood in the now under-perfused slow compartments, results in a much higher blood concentration for the same drug dose.

Two serious errors can result from a failure to appreciate this result: (1) anesthetic overdose, with subsequent paralysis of homeostatic mechanisms which are compensating for the blood loss, resulting in circulatory collapse; and (2) subsequent anesthetic underdose, as the drug is ultimately distributed

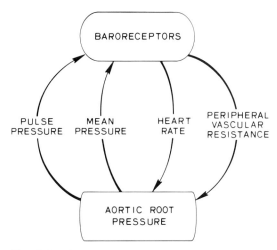

Fig. 5-15. An illustration of the control loop involving the aortic baroreceptors and aortic root pressure. Note that the usual discussion of this control loop considers only *mean pressure* and *heart rate*. It is necessary to consider the two additional factors: *pulse pressure* (or derivative of arterial pressure) and *peripheral vascular resistance* to adequately explain physiologic behavior under clinical conditions.

throughout the body, and cumulative drug requirements return toward normal.

Then, in order to assure adequate management, monitoring must be enhanced to reduce the risk of overshoot. A number of the previously discussed techniques are helpful. Dithering, with a very small excursion, can yield valuable information about the degree of patient stability, avoiding the possibility of a large swing in blood pressure because a drug dose proved to be too large. Reducing loop delay is a very effective way to improve response accuracy, either by better measurements (*e.g.,* a direct arterial line) or by more rapid anesthetist response (*e.g.,* more frequent blood pressure measurements).

It is evident that loop behavior makes it impossible to construct a manageable series of open-loop therapeutic recipes which together will address all of the commonly encountered clinical situations. A much better way to develop monitoring (and hence management) skill, is first to understand the basic behavior of the control loops that must be affected. Secondly, a list of priorities should be drawn up for the situations that must be corrected (*e.g.,* deciding whether to first treat hypovolemia, low blood pressure, low cardiac output, or edema). Thirdly, monitoring should be done in a way which provides the management information required. Fourthly, therapy should be provided according to the previously determined priorities. Fifth, through monitoring, it should be determined whether the response is that desired, and therapy should be adjusted accordingly.

Many corollaries to this approach can be elaborated, but most are obvious, such as the need to select, when possible, modes of therapy that address more than one problem, and to avoid approaches that solve one problem while exacerbating others. Not so obvious is the way in which this approach avoids other pitfalls. A commonly verbalized frustration is the feeling that inadequate understanding of physiologic mechanisms impairs the use of the concept in clinical practice, and the associated feeling that, in such situations, the use of a recipe is better. Rather, it is simpler, and therefore less stressful for the practitioner with incomplete understanding. But the hallmark of a control loop is that negative feedback works surprisingly well when one does not understand the precise nature of the loop but observes certain general rules.

What is needed is an understanding of limitations. Some kinds of control loops are less stable. If one understands how to measure and increase stability, one can still achieve control without fully understanding the characteristics of a particular control loop. But one must understand a few of the basic concepts; the untutored instinctive response is often incorrect. An example from the earlier discussion: increasing the size of your response when the patient overshoots often makes matters worse. And note the paradoxical behavior of two closely related concepts: *increasing response time* increases stability, but *decreasing delay time* does also! With these basic concepts, control can usually be obtained, even when understanding of the loop is grossly incomplete.

The closed-loop approach is much safer when two major effects are finely balanced.

For example, there exist directly conflicting recipes for treating myocardial ischemia under anesthesia: either increasing or decreasing mean arterial blood pressure (in addition to other therapy). The use of feedback means that the anesthesiologist is able to detect an inappropriate patient response and select the appropriate therapy. Other examples are the choice of an inotropic or vasopressor agent in treating the patient with aortic stenosis, and selection of the appropriate preload for optimizing cardiac performance using Starling's Law.

The recipe approach has its place, in starting treatment and in selecting therapy when loop behavior is completely uncertain. But once the anesthetist-patient interaction is well under way, the recipe approach is (by itself) a grossly inadequate means of managing the cardiovascular patient. Stability requires feedback, and the anesthetist is part of the loop. Adequate management of the many interacting cardiovascular mechanisms requires attention to the patient response. This approach provides needed protection against the possibility that the recipe is inappropriate to the patient's most urgent needs.

Thus, the traditional approach in the anesthetic literature to monitoring (the techniques required for specific measurements) is incomplete. The selection of appropriate measurements is influenced by the equipment and skills available. But the major determinant of what is measured and how often, is the information needed for adequate patient management. The concept of monitoring includes the concept of management.

GLOSSARY

monitoring system. The anesthetist, patient, surgeon, and instruments which interact during monitoring activities; an interconnected group of system components
event. An interaction between system components
input. An event which acts on the patient
response. An event which originates at the patient

loop. A group of interconnections between monitoring system components forming a path which an event can traverse more than once in the same direction; a closed path

gain. A term which defines how an event grows or shrinks with each transit around a loop

stability. A stytem of the type discussed in this chapter is stable when the magnitude of the gain is less than one—that is, when the change in an event shrinks in magnitude with each transit around the loop. Thus, the response to a stimulus of short duration dies away, leaving the patient in equilibrium.

negative feedback. A loop has negative feedback if, when an event is transmitted around the loop, the result is subtracted from the original perturbation—that is, the loop gain is negative.

delay. The time required for an event to travel around a loop. Longer delays yield a system which responds more slowly, and is less likely to be stable. The user is usually interested in minimizing delay.

response time. The time required for the system to complete a response to an event. A slower response usually increases the likelihood of a stable system. The user usually wants the fastest response time which permits acceptable stability.

dithering. A control technique which assures that the loop is maintained in the best state by constantly slightly changing imput to the patient, to know the change in patient state which results from a change in input.

error signal. The difference between the actual patient response and the desired patient response.

integral control. A control loop which continues correction so long as any error signal is present. This form of loop control provides complete correction.

proportional control. A control loop in which the correction is proportional to the error signal. This form of loop control never provides complete correction.

REFERENCES

GENERAL REFERENCES

1. Ream AK: Monitoring Principles. Monitoring Techniques. Both in Wollman H and Larsen CP: Anesthesiology. Philadelphia, JB Lippincott, in press

2. Saidman L, and Smith NT (eds): Monitoring and Anesthesia. New York, John Wiley & Sons, 1978
3. Hill DW: Intensive Care Instrumentation. New York, Academic Press, 1976
4. Bryan–Brown CW, Shapiro BM, Miller CM et al: A less invasive approach to monitoring acute respiratory failure. Med Instrum 13:327–329, 1979
5. Osborn JJ, Fagan LM, Fallat RJ et al: Managing the data from respiratory measurements. Med Instrum 13:330–336, 1979

THEORY

Appropriate measurements

6. Cullen DJ: Interpretation of blood pressure measurements in anesthesia. Anesthesiology 40:6–12, 1974
7. Schneider AJL, Knoke JD, Zollinger RM et al: Morbidity prediction using pre- and intra-operative data. Anesthesiology 51:4–10, 1979
8. Shoemaker WC, Czer LS: Evaluation of the biologic importance of various hemodynamic and oxygen transport variables: which variables should be monitored in post operative shock? Crit Care Med 7:424–429, 1979

Equipment Maintenance

9. Ream AK: Future trends in monitoring and biomedical instrumentation. In Saidman L, Smith NT (eds): Monitoring and Anesthesia. New York, John Wiley & Sons, 1978

SPECIFIC MEASUREMENTS

ECG

10. Severinghaus JW: The telecor, an esophageal monitoring probe. Anesthesiology 18:145–149, 1957
11. Rose GE, Terry W, Neblett I: Cardiac pacing with an esophageal electrode. Am J Cardiol 24:548–550, 1969
12. Lipton MJ, Ream AK, Hyndman BH: A conductive catheter to improve patient safety during cardiac catheterization. Circulation 58:1190–1195, 1978

13. Ream AK, Lipton MJ, Hyndman BH: Reduced risk of cardiac fibrillation with use of a conductive catheter. Ann Biomed Eng 5:287–301, 1977

Arterial Pressure

14. Gravenstein JS, Newbower RS, Ream AK, Smith NT (eds): Patient Monitoring. Springfield (Ill), Charles C Thomas, 1978
15. Ream AK: Systolic, diastolic, mean or pulse pressure: which is the best measurement of arterial pressure? In Gravenstein JS, Newbower RS, Ream AK, Smith NT (eds): Essential Noninvasive Monitoring, pp 53–74. New York, Grune and Stratton, 1980
16. Lowenstein E, Little JW, Lo HH: Prevention of cerebral embolization from flushing radial artery cannulas. New Engl J Med 285:1414–1415, 1971
17. Weinstein RA, Stamm WE, Kramer L et al: Pressure monitoring devices: an overlooked source of nosocomial infection. JAMA 236:936–938, 1976
18. Bedford RF, Wollman H: Complications of percutaneous radial artery cannulation: an objective prospective study in man. Anesthesiology 38:228–236, 1973
19. Kirkendall WM, Burton AC, Epstein FH: Recommendations for Human Blood Pressure Determination by Sphygmomanometers. New York: American Heart Association, 1967
20. Van Bergen FH, Weatherhead DS, Treloar AE et al: Comparison of indirect and direct methods of measuring arterial blood pressure. Circulation 10:481–490, 1954
21. Yelderman M, Ream AK: A microprocessor-based automated noninvasive blood pressure device for the anesthetized patient. Proceedings of the San Diego Biomedical Symposium 17:57–64, 1978
22. Yelderman M, Ream AK: Indirect measurement of mean blood pressure. Anesthesiology 51:253–256, 1979

Pulmonary Artery Monitoring

23. Buda AJ, Pinsky MR, Ingels NB Jr et al: Effect of intrathoracic pressure on left ventricular performance. New Engl J Med 301:453–459, 1979
24. Geer RT: Interpretation of pulmonary artery wedge pressure when PEEP is used. Anesthesiology 46:383–384, 1977
25. Yelderman ML, New W: Estimation of left atrial mean pressure from right heart measurements. Anesthesiology 51:S210, 1979
26. Yelderman M, New WJ Jr, Rosenthal M et al: Improved clinical measurement of pulmonary vascular resistance. Anesthesiology 52:365–369, 1980
27. Risk C, Rudo N, Falltrick R et al: Comparison of right atrial and pulmonary capillary wedge pressures. Crit Care Med 6:172–175, 1978
28. Thomson IR, Dalton BC, Lappas DG et al: Right bundle-branch block and complete heart block caused by the Swan–Ganz catheter. Anesthesiology 51:359–362, 1979
29. Lingenfelter AL, Guskiewicz RA, Munson ES: Displacement of right atrial and endotracheal catheters with neck flexion. Anesth Analg 57:371–373, 1978
30. Berry AJ, Geer RT, Marshall BE: Alteration of pulmonary blood flow by pulmonary-artery occluded pressure measurement. Anesthesiology 51:164–166, 1979

APPLICATION

31. Ead HW, Green JH, Neil E: A comparison of the effects of pulsatile and nonpulsatile blood flow through the carotid sinus on the reflexogenic activity of the sinus baroreceptors in the cat. J Physiol (Lond) 118:509–519, 1952

Part II

ELECTRICAL ACTIVITY OF THE HEART

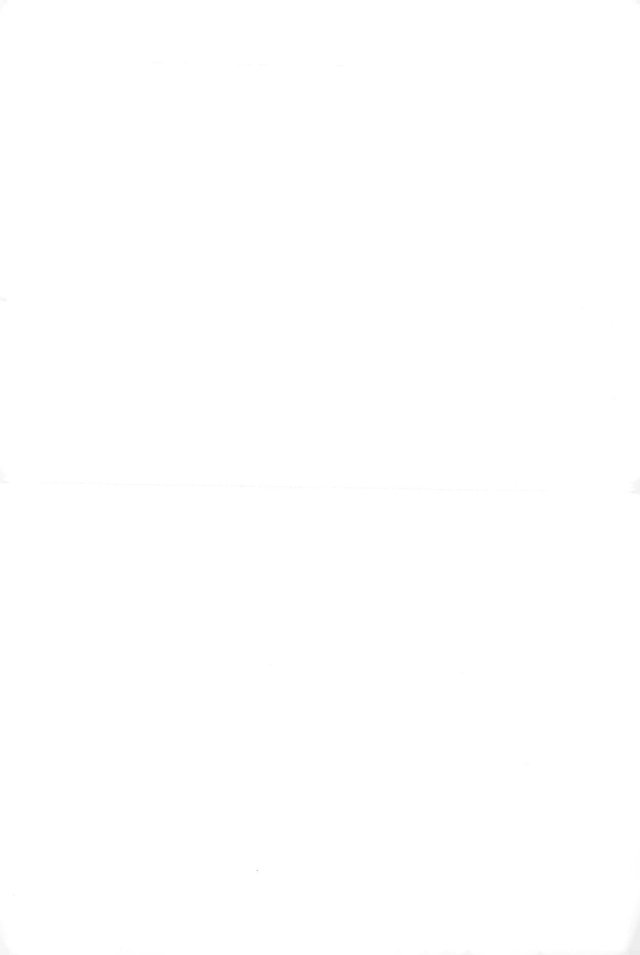

6

Electrocardiographic Monitoring

JOEL A. KAPLAN
PHILIP H. WELLS

INTRODUCTION

The electrocardiogram (ECG) is a graphic representation of the electrical potential produced by the heart and its conduction system. Since the clinical introduction of the ECG in 1903 by Einthoven, increasing importance has been placed on its interpretation and use throughout all areas of medicine, to the extent that it now comprises one of the most useful clinical aids to the practicing physician. Through close scrutiny of its patterns, acute rhythm changes, muscular enlargement, and areas of infarction may be discerned. To the anesthesiologist, the ECG should serve as a close ally, enlightening him during his preoperative evaluation, providing safety and reassurance throughout the intraoperative period, and reassuring him into the recovery or intensive care periods. Because of its widespread use, a thorough comprehensive understanding of the ECG is necessary. The purposes of this chapter, therefore, are to review the basic principles underlying cardiac electrophysiology, electrocardiography, and vectorcardiography; discuss the various means of monitoring the electrocardiogram; evaluate antiarrhythmic therapy; and evaluate the various patterns found on the standard ECG.

ELECTROCARDIOGRAPHIC MONITORING IN THE OPERATING ROOM

The ECG monitor is almost routine in today's operating room and is certainly routine in all patients with cardiac disease.[1] It is useful for monitoring arrhythmias, ischemia, heart block, and drug and electrolyte effects. However, it does not give any useful information about myocardial function or cardiac output. Arrhythmia detection has been the main function of the ECG in the operating room, with lead II being used most commonly. Lead II has frequently been selected because a good P wave is seen, and junctional or ventricular rhythms are easy to identify. The reported incidence of arrhythmias during surgery ranges from 10 percent to more than 60 percent of cases.[2] At the present time, many patients with coronary artery disease are coming to surgery, and the ECG is equally useful to diagnose ischemic changes. A precordial lead (V_5) has been very useful in diagnosing ischemia during surgery. The simultaneous display of leads II and V_5 in all patients with coronary artery disease allows monitoring of both the left (V_5) and right (II) sides of the coronary circulation.[3]

During surgery, the ECG is viewed from an oscilloscope and may be recorded if indicated. All operating rooms where cardiac surgery is performed should have ECG recording capabilities, and portable recorders should be available to all other operating rooms for interesting diagnostic problems. The recorder is needed to make accurate measurements of the S-T segment changes and accurate diagnoses of complex arrhythmias. In addition, the recorder is frequently needed to be certain artifacts are not being incorrectly interpreted from the oscilloscope. A recorder should make the tracing directly from the patient without first going through the oscilloscope's filter circuits.

Artifacts on the oscilloscope can be a major problem and lead to incorrect diagnoses.[4] Unfortunately, most physicians do not know enough about the electronics of the monitors to be able to distinguish these artifacts from real changes. The low-frequency filters of the ECG circuitry are the main source of the problem because these can be selected by the physician or nurse using the equipment. The *diagnostic* mode filters frequencies below 0.14 Hz. A second mode frequently available is called the *monitor* mode and this filters all frequencies below 4 Hz. The diagnostic mode should be used (especially for recording S-T segment changes), but, unfortunately, it is susceptible to baseline wandering caused by respiration, movement, or poor electrode contact. As more filtration is added (monitor mode), the baseline becomes more stable, but the ECG complex becomes more distorted. The P and T waves may be decreased in amplitude, but the main problem is change in the S-T segment. An isoelectric S-T segment may be elevated or depressed, resembling ischemic changes, or elevated or depressed S-T segments may be shifted toward the iso-electric line. High-frequency filters are less of a problem. They are usually set at about 50 Hz to eliminate 60-cycle interference. Arrhythmias have also been inappropriately diagnosed due to ECG artifacts. Broken electrode wires have been reported to produce an ECG pattern mistaken for atrial flutter. Also, hypothermia with shivering has been reported to be misdiagnosed as atrial flutter. Artifacts produced by the roller pumps on cardiopulmonary bypass can also create an ECG pattern that looks like atrial flutter. Another electrical problem with ECG monitoring in the operating room is the electrocautery. When the cautery is used, the standard ECG is totally lost because of electrical interference. The interference is a combination of radiofrequency current (800–2,000 kHz), AC line frequency (60 Hz), and low frequency (0.1–10 Hz). Doss has shown that it is possible to modify the ECG preamplifiers so they will function well in the presence of the electrocautery.[5] It is surprising that this has not been done to more monitoring units designed for use in the operating room.

In addition to the usual causes of ECG changes that may occur during surgery, there are mechanical factors that can also affect the ECG. Respiratory variation can alter the height of the QRS complex, most marked in leads III and AVF. This is caused either by a shift of the mediastinum with respiration or by a change in volume of the heart due to respiratory effects on venous return. Studies have shown that increases in the ventricular end-diastolic volume lead to an increased height of the QRS complex; and hemorrhage leads to a decreased height of the QRS.[6] Catheters or wires in the heart frequently lead to arrhythmias. Premature ventricular contractions are very common (58% as reported by Zaidan) with placement of the Swan–Ganz catheter. There are also ECG changes related to age alone. There is a decreasing amplitude of the QRS complex and T wave with increasing age, and PVCs occur more frequently over the age of 40 years.

BASIC ELECTROPHYSIOLOGY AND CARDIAC LEAD SYSTEMS

The electrical conduction system of the heart and its anatomic relationships are described below. The initiation of the cardiac impulse begins at the sinoatrial (SA) node. This consists of a bundle of specialized neural tissue which lies on the endocardial surface of the right atrium at the junction of the superior vena cava and right atrial appendage. The SA node is the pacemaker of the heart because it has the most rapid spontaneous *phase* 4 depolarization of any normal cardiac tissue. If the SA node fails to function, a secondary slower pacemaker will take over. The SA node normally fires from 60 to 100 times per minute, while the atrioventricular junctional tissue (AV node) will fire from 45 to 50 times per minute, and the ventricular Purkinje system will fire from 30 to 40 times per minute. Thus, the rate will become slower as the pacemaker moves away from the SA node.[7]

The SA node impulse spreads through the internodal pathways and atrial muscle, providing the P wave of the ECG, and arrives at the AV junction. This area, composed of specialized muscular tissue, is located on the endocardial surface on the right atrial side of the interatrial septum near the tricuspid valve, just inferior to the opening of the coronary sinus. In the recent past, the term *AV node* was used to define a single functioning area. However, as more is understood about the conduction system, it has become clearer that this is a more complex region than formerly thought. Presently, this area is divided anatomically by the bundle of His. Those areas above the bundle of His (supra-Hissian) and those areas below the bundle of His (infra-Hissian) constitute the two major areas of the AV junction.

The rapidly moving impulse from the SA node is abruptly delayed in the AV junctional area because of its complex conducting system. This delay is normally from 70 to 100 milliseconds. After passage through the bundle of His located on the right side of the atrial septum immediately above the intraventricular septum, the conduction system divides into the right bundle, the anterior-superior division, and the much broader posterior-inferior division of the left bundle. There is very little scientific evidence anatomically confirming that such a trifurcation exists. Nevertheless, the concept of such a trifurcation aids in the understanding of certain electrographic patterns and conduction abnormalities which occur. Thus, the conduction system distant to the bundle of His is divided into the right bundle branch and the left bundle branch, and the latter is subdivided into its two divisions: the anterior-superior division and posterior-inferior division. These arise from the lower portion of the bundle of His in the membranous portion of the interventricular septum and are located on either side of the interventricular septum. These are the most rapidly conducting tissues of the heart, and the passage of the impulse through them does not even appear on the standard surface ECG. After passing through the bundles, the impulse arrives in the Purkinje system which covers the subendocardial surfaces of both ventricles. The electrical impulse passes initially from the endocardial to the epicardial surface of the ventricular muscle, producing the QRS complex of the ECG.

The normal ECG tracing and definition of wave forms and intervals are shown in Figure 6–1. The P wave represents atrial depolarization. The Ta wave of atrial repolarization is not routinely seen because it is usually buried in the QRS complex. Ventricular depolarization is represented by the QRS complex and ventricular repolarization by the T wave. One may see a U wave following the T wave; it should have the same polarity as the T wave. Its precise significance is uncertain, but it most likely represents *phase 3* repolarization of the Purkinje system. The PR interval should be less than 0.20 seconds, the QRS interval less than 0.10 seconds, and the Q-T interval less than one half the R-R interval.

The ECG is the recording of the electrical forces produced by the heart.[8] The myocardium is composed of a variety of excitable cells with a potential to create or conduct electrical current. These excitable cells are further subdivided into two specific types: those with the ability to spontaneously depolarize, and those that require a stimulus for depolarization. For a cell to be excitable, a potential energy difference must be present between the inside and outside of its cell membrane produced by a difference in concentrations of the extracellular ions (Na^+ and Cl^-) and intracellular ions (K^+ and PO_4^{-2}). Because the cellular membrane is more permeable to K^+ at rest, the resting membrane potential remains at -90 mv secondary to this K^+ gradient. With stimulation, a rapid change in the cellular membrane permeability to ions occurs with the production of an action potential (*phase 0*). Upon reaching the threshold of excitation (-70 mv), a rapid influx of Na^+ ions (Na^+ gate opens) occurs with a rapid reversal of the electrical charge to $+30$ mv. This creates cellular depolarization of the myocardium. In addition to the rapid influx of Na^+, recent voltage clamp studies have demonstrated a slower influx of

Fig. 6-1. A normal ECG is demonstrated with the P, QRS, and T waves. PR and QT intervals are also shown.

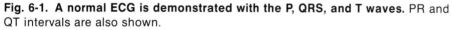
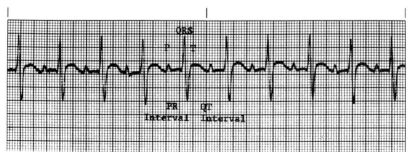

Ca^{+2} ions in the latter part of depolarization. These studies demonstrate the separation of the "fast-channel response" to sodium and the "slow-channel response" carried largely by Ca^{+2} but also by Na^+.

Following this depolarization (*phase 0*), a sudden decrease in membrane permeability to Na^+ occurs with an increased permeability to K^+ ions. *Phase 1,* or rapid depolarization, is considered secondary to decreased Na^+ influx as well as increased Cl^- permeability into the cell. *Phase 2,* or the plateau phase, results from a lack of ion flow, except possibly for the slow channel flow whose inactivation has a long time constant. *Phase 3* begins repolarization, which is primarily the function of an outward current carried largely by potassium ions.

In those excitable cells showing spontaneous depolarization (pacemaker cells), there is a continuous, slow leakage of sodium into the cells and potassium out of the cells until threshold potential is reached with spontaneous depolarization. This slow leakage of ions, termed *phase 4 depolarization*, determines the automatic firing of certain myocardial cells (cellular automaticity). Various factors can affect *phase 4* depolarization. Calcium ions are felt to regulate the sodium influx channels and, thus, changing calcium levels can alter the threshold potential. Hypocalcemia will lower the threshold potential to approximately -80 mv, resulting in an earlier depolarization; increased calcium has the opposite effect. With a decreased sodium concentration, less sodium influx is generated and the maximum action potential is lower than normal ($+15$ mv rather than $+30$ mv). A decrease in intracellular potassium raises the resting membrane potential (*e.g.,* -90–-80 mv) with an unchanged threshold potential; thus, depolarization requires less change and the cell is more excitable. Other factors which alter *phase 4* depolarization and increase excitability are ischemia and catecholamines. Vagal stimulation inhibits *phase 4* depolarization with a reduction in cellular excitability. An increase in the extracellular fluid potassium makes the resting membrane potential less negative (-90–-80 mv);

whereas a decrease in extracellular fluid potassium increases the resting membrane potential (-90–-100 mv). An increase in the extracellular calcium or sodium concentration can antagonize the increased excitability secondary to hyperkalemia.

During *phase 3*, the excitable cell membrane is being repolarized, and the cell is completely refractory before it reaches the threshold potential. After it reaches threshold potential, but before it again begins *phase 4* depolarization, the cell is considered relatively refractory, requiring an increased stimulus to depolarize.

With myocardial cell depolarization, an electrical impulse is generated which can be recorded from the epicardium or precordium. Each cell that depolarizes creates a miniature dipole consisting of a positive and negative charge. The entire myocardium, therefore, consists of a multitude of these dipoles varying in their polarity and spatial orientation; and which, at any instant, can be represented by an integrated single dipole. This is graphically recorded as an arrow, the length representing the magnitude of the recorded current, the position of the arrow representing the spatial orientation, and the tip of the arrow oriented toward the more positive portion of the dipole. With the construction of many of these instantaneous vectors, a composite of the electrical forces throughout depolarization can be depicted. The tips of these vectors, if connected, form a continuous (vectoral) loop, which can be used to graphically describe the entire QRS cycle. Figure 6–2 demonstrates a typical, two-dimensional vector loop. In a similar fashion, vectoral representation can be made of all portions of the cardiac cycle including the P, T, and U waves and ST segments (Fig. 6–3).

The classic approach to electrocardiography depends on the memorization of patterns from the scalar ECG, which reflects normal events and certain abnormalities. Because the vectoral approach allows a more graphic, three-dimensional view of the cardiac electrical cycle, using the vectorcardiogram (VCG) one can better appreciate the standard ECG. When dealing with the scalar

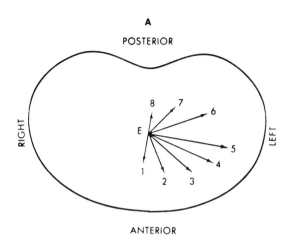

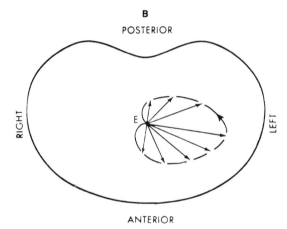

Fig. 6-2. A typical two-dimensional vectoral loop is demonstrated.

Fig. 6-3. Vectoral loops for P wave, QRS complex, and T wave are demonstrated.

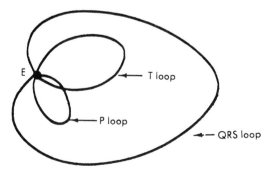

ECG, an isolated area of the precordial surface is selected and the entire electrical sequence is viewed from that one area. Using the standard ECG leads defined by Einthoven (I, II, III), the electrical cycle is observed in a two-dimensional, frontal plane. Einthoven's leads divide this plane into six equal 60° sections.[9] Each of the leads measures the electrical potential between the two electrodes. Lead I compares the electrical potential between the right and left arms; lead II, the right arm and left leg; and lead III, the left arm and left leg. The electrodes can be attached anywhere on the extremities or on the trunk at the root of an extremity (*e.g.,* shoulder). Figure 6–4 demonstrates the polarity and orientation of the standard limb leads. The three standard limb leads are the most frequently used leads in the operating room.[10] They allow accurate evaluation of the cardiac rhythm since the P and QRS waves most often show the largest amplitude in these leads. Conduction disturbances, inferior ischemia and infarction, and axis changes can best be determined by these leads.

A further refinement in viewing the frontal ECG can be made by utilizing the unipolar limb leads (aVR, aVL, aVF). In these, the electrodes from two extremities (*e.g.,* right arm and left arm) are made the central, inactive terminal and the other extremity (left leg) is made the active electrode (in this ex-

Fig. 6-4. Einthoven's triangle is demonstrated. Leads I, II, and III are shown with their electrical polarity.

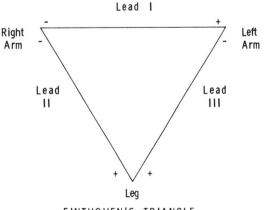

ample the aVF lead). Thus, three additional axes are determined, further dividing the frontal plane into twelve 30° sections. By using the six leads, a precise placement of the frontal QRS vector can be made demonstrating the augmented limb leads in addition to the standard limb leads and their relationship to the frontal plane.

The standard limb leads have the following disadvantages:

1. Each is derived from two points (bipolar) distant from the heart.
2. All three leads are in the same frontal body plane.

The precordial *V* leads are unipolar; the four extremity electrodes form a central indifferent terminal, and an active exploring electrode is placed at one of the six usual chest lead positions. The exploring electrode is thus able to view the electrical sequence in a horizontal plane, perpendicular to the frontal plane. The V_1 lead has the active electrode to the right of the sternum in the fourth interspace. It is thus best able to visualize the anterior (right ventricular or septal) myocardial surface. Leads V_5 and V_6 are in the fifth interspace in the anterior axillary and midaxillary lines, respectively. These leads best visualize the lateral myocardial (left ventricular) surface. Leads V_2 to V_5 are placed in intermediate positions and view progressively more of the left ventricle as they proceed from V_2 to V_5. The precordial leads are most helpful in diagnosing rotational changes of the heart, ventricular hypertrophy, bundle branch patterns, and ischemia of the anteroseptal, anterior, or lateral areas of the left ventricle.

The electrical pattern of the heart is three-dimensional, and the VCG is able to visualize these three dimensions.[11] The VCG is recorded in three planes: frontal, right sagittal, and horizontal. The frontal plane corresponds to the six frontal ECG leads, the horizontal plane to the precordial leads, and the sagittal surface is a composite of these two planes. The ability to transpose the VCG to its corresponding ECG leads is critical in interrelating these two systems. For example, frontal plane leads I and aVF, and horizontal plane leads V_1 and V_6 can be transcribed. For each lead, a perpendicular line is constructed through the origin of the VCG. All forces lying on the positive side of this perpendicular line show an upward deflection on the ECG, and all forces directed away from the perpendicular line are negative and show a downward deflection on the ECG. In a reverse fashion, a VCG tracing can be constructed from a known ECG tracing.

By comparing the vector loop in all three planes, a better appreciation of the magnitude and direction of the vector loop is obtained. The QRS loop is visualized initially as being spatially oriented to the right, anterior and superior. This represents the initial septal QRS forces and may occasionally be to the left and anterior, but normally the initial forces are not posterior. The forces then progress to the left, posterior and inferior, with the predominance of left ventricular forces. The loop's terminal forces are to the right, posterior and inferior.

In addition to the standard frontal, augmented, and precordial electrocardiographic leads, other lead systems are frequently utilized in specific situations. During exercise stress testing, other lead systems have been used to identify ischemia. Many of these have used a bipolar lead system with a positive electrode in the V_5 position. The CM_5 lead has the positive electrode at V_5 and the negative electrode on the upper sternum (manubrium); the CS_5 lead has the negative electrode just below the right clavicle. The CM_5 is the most popular lead for stress testing because of its simplicity (two electrodes) and high incidence of positive findings. Unipolar esophageal leads have been used to record atrial complexes and diagnose arrhythmias. The active electrode is placed in the esophagus and thus the posterior surface of the left ventricle and the atrioventricular junction can be explored. The MCL_1 lead is popular for cardiac monitoring, arrhythmia detection, and conduction disturbance monitoring in coronary care units. The MCL_1 lead is a modified lead V_1, the best single lead to detect arrhythmias. This is a bipolar lead with the positive electrode to the right of the sternum in the fourth interspace (V_1 position);

the negative electrode is placed near the left shoulder under the left clavicle. Another lead that can be looked at when trying to record clear atrial complexes (P waves) takes advantage of the atrial vector forces oriented anteriorly, inferiorly, and leftward. The right-arm electrode is placed just to the right of the manubrium of the sternum, and the left-arm electrode on the zyphoid sternum.

Intracardiac ECG also has been used for diagnostic purposes because it is relatively easy to obtain. A long central venous pressure catheter with a metal hub filled with saline is attached to the V lead of the ECG with an alligator clip, and is advanced into the upper superior vena cava. When the catheter reaches the superior vena cava, the ECG tracing appears similar to a normal lead aVR with inverted P, QRS, and T waves. On reaching the high right atrium, the P wave is large and deeply inverted; in the midatrium, the P is biphasic; and in the low atrium it becomes upright. When the right ventricle is entered, the QRS complex becomes very large. By utilizing this ECG method, a CVP catheter tip can be accurately placed in the low right atrium. Recently, a multipurpose pulmonary artery catheter with atrial and ventricular ECG or pacing electrodes has become available. In the patient requiring this monitoring device, the catheter permits recording of a bipolar atrial electrogram and diagnosis of complex arrhythmias.[12]

An additional method of ECG diagnosis involves the recording of the bundle of His electrogram using an intracardiac catheter.[13] Conduction through this part of the heart is so rapid that it does not appear on the standard ECG. In patients with intact atrioventricular conduction, the PR interval can be divided into two subintervals:

1. P-H interval: from the atrial complex to the His bundle electrogram, which reflects AV nodal conduction time.
2. H-R interval: from the His bundle to ventricular complex, which reflects conduction time in the His bundle and bundle branches

This His-bundle electrogram may be used to localize heart blocks to certain areas of the conduction system or diagnose the mechanism of complex arrhythmias.

HEART RATE

ECG paper usually has markers in the margin at 3-second intervals. One method of rapidly obtaining the heart rate is to count the number of cycles in 6 seconds and multiply by 10. In addition, the thick lines on the ECG paper are 0.2 seconds (1/5 of a second) apart, and the thin lines are 0.04 seconds apart with a usual paper speed of 25 mm/sec. Marriott has described a rapid system to estimate the heart rate based on the thick (1/5 of a second) lines (Fig. 6–5).[14] By Marriott's method, if a heart beat occurs on every thick line, 0.2 seconds, the overall heart rate is 300 beats per minute. Additionally, if a QRS falls on every other thick line, the rate is 150 beats per minute; every third line, 100 beats per minute; every fourth line, 75 beats per minute; and so on. This system is useful only if the rhythm is regular. It is best, in this method, to find two beats which fall precisely on the heavy lines. However, heart rate can be estimated if the second beat falls between two lines (*e.g.*, if

---

A Systematic Approach to the ECG

In examining an ECG the following features should always be checked:

1. Heart rate
2. Rhythm
3. Cardiac axis
4. P wave
5. P-R interval
6. QRS complex and interval
7. S-T segment
8. T wave
9. U wave
10. Q-T interval

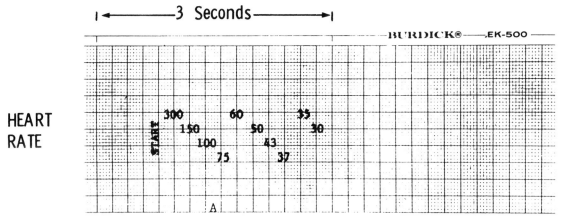

Fig. 6-5. A strip of electrocardiographic paper is shown with a 3-sec interval used to determine the heart rate. This is an adaptation of Marriott's system for determining heart rates.

the second beat occurred at point A on Fig. 6–5, the heart rate would be approximately 87 beats per minute).

RHYTHM

To define the cardiac rhythm, it must be first ascertained whether each QRS complex is preceded by a P wave. This generally reflects the presence of a sinus mechanism initiating the cardiac beat (SA node). The PR interval should then be measured to determine whether any degree of AV block is present (PR > 0.20 sec = 1° AV block; a changing PR interval = 2° or 3° AV block). The regularity or irregularity of the QRS should then be defined. If the QRS rhythm is irregular, any pattern to the irregularity should be noted (*e.g.,* bigeminy). This will be discussed in more detail in the section below on arrhythmias.

CARDIAC AXIS

The axis of the heart is the heart's electrical vector described in the frontal plane. To quickly calculate this vector, it is necessary only to use leads I and aVF from the frontal plane. If the QRS complex in leads I and aVF are both positive, the vector must fall in the left lower quadrant (between 0 and 90°) and constitutes a normal axis. Similarly, if lead I is positive and aVF is negative, the patient's

vector falls in the left upper quadrant tending toward left-axis deviation. If lead I is negative and aVF is positive, the patient's vector falls in the right lower quadrant tending toward right-axis deviation. Thus, by quickly scanning two of the frontal limb leads, a quick appraisal of a normal axis versus an axis deviation can be gained. Additionally, if a lead is isoelectric, having equal positive and negative deflections, the vector generally runs parallel to that lead (*e.g.,* if isoelectric to lead I, the axis is approximately 0°, and, if isoelectric to aVF, the axis is approximately +90°). P and T wave axes (vectors) can be derived in the same manner. Abnormal right-axis deviation may be caused by a right bundle branch block, left posterior hemiblock, right ventricular hypertrophy or pulmonary pathology. Abnormal left-axis deviation may be caused by left bundle branch block, left anterior hemiblock, inferior myocardial infarction, or ectopic beats.

P WAVE

This wave is normally upright, except in aVR and sometimes in lead III. The P wave is inverted when an abnormal conduction pathway exists or an atrial site other than the SA node is the pacemaker. A classic example of an inverted P wave in lead II is that of the *coronary sinus rhythm,* which originates near the coronary sinus. The P wave's amplitude should not exceed 2.5 mm, and its duration should not exceed 0.11 seconds. Increased amplitude or width indicates atrial hypertrophy. There are a few specific configurations seen in the P wave that are diagnostic:

1. P-pulmonale: Tall pointed P waves are seen with the P in lead III being taller than in I (right-atrial hypertrophy).
2. P-mitrale: Wide and notched P waves are seen with the P being taller in I than in III (left-atrial hypertrophy).

P-R INTERVAL

This interval occurs from the beginning of the P wave to the beginning of the QRS complex, and is normally from 0.12 to 0.20 seconds at normal heart rates. It is prolonged in first-degree heart block and in patients taking digitalis. It is shortened in junctional rhythms, Wolff–Parkinson–White syndrome, and Lown–Ganong–Levine syndrome.

QRS COMPLEX AND INTERVAL

The normal duration is from 0.05 to 0.10 seconds; above 0.12 seconds is indicative of ab-normal intraventricular conduction. Low voltage in all three standard leads (I, II, III: less than 5 mm) may be seen in myxedema, heart failure, pericardial effusions, diffuse coronary artery disease, or emphysema. Voltage criteria can be used to diagnose left- and right-ventricular hypertrophy (LVH and RVH). LVH is diagnosed by any one of these criteria (Fig. 6–6):[14]

1. S_{V_1} and $R_{V_5} \geq 35$ mm
2. $R_{AVL} \geq 12$ mm
3. Any precordial lead deflections ≥ 30 mm

LVH may occur with strain, which is probably caused by associated ischemia or conduction abnormalities. In leads V_5 and V_6, the S-T segments are depressed and the T waves deeply depressed. This is most often produced by hypertension or aortic stenosis. RVH is diagnosed by a reversal of the normal precordial pattern. The R waves are large in the right precordial leads and the S waves are deep in the left precordial leads. Thus, V_1 on the anterior chest wall "sees" the increased muscular electrical forces in the right (anterior) ventricle. If the R:S ratio exceeds 1 in V_1, RVH is present (Fig. 6–7). This is frequently associated with a right axis deviation

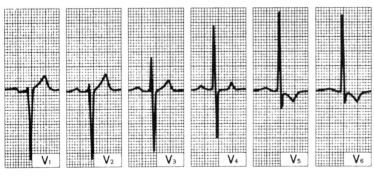

Fig. 6-6. An ECG of left ventricular hypertrophy is demonstrated. The S wave in V_1 plus the R wave in V_5 equals more than 35 mm. (The Electrocardio Guide, Merck, Sharp, & Dohme)

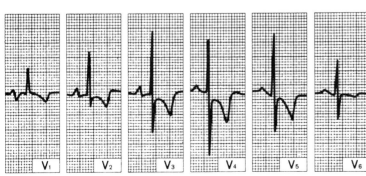

Fig. 6-7. Right ventricular hypertrophy is demonstrated. The R:S ratio exceeds one in lead V_1. (The Electrocardio Guide, Merck, Sharp, & Dohme)

and a right bundle branch block, especially in patients with mitral stenosis. Other causes of RVH are congential heart disease and cor pulmonale.

The Q wave is the first wave of the QRS complex, and is negative in direction. Pathologic Q waves should be over 0.04 seconds in width, and should be bunched in a pattern. For example, inferior infarctions show Q waves in II, III, and aVF; anteroseptal infarctions have Q waves in V_1 to V_3; and anterolateral infarcts have Q waves in V_4 to V_6.

S-T SEGMENT

The point at which the S-T segment takes off from the QRS complex is called the J (*junction*) *point.* Normally it is isoelectric with the T-P segment. However, it may normally be elevated less than 1 mm in standard and precordial leads. It is not normally depressed. The level of the S-T segment relative to the T-P segment should be observed, as well as its shape and slope. Upsloping, downsloping, or horizontal S-T segment depression, and J-junction depression may have different meanings (see the section on ischemia). Occasionally, the Ta (atrial repolarization) wave may be seen to alter the S-T segment.

T WAVE

The T wave is normally upright in leads I, II and $V_3 - V_6$, inverted in aVR, and variable in the other leads. It normally does not exceed 5 mm in height in standard leads, or 10 mm in precordial leads. Larger T waves may be indicative of myocardial ischemia or hyperkalemia.

U WAVE

The U wave is best seen in lead V_3, and has the same polarity as the T wave. It is enlarged in hypokalemia, and inverted in ischemia.

QT INTERVAL

The QT interval is measured from the beginning of the Q wave to the end of the T wave. It should be less than one half of the preceding R-R interval, and is affected by heart rate. It is called the QT_c when corrected for heart rate. It is prolonged by hypocalcemia, quinidine, procainamide, disopyramide, and myocarditis. It is shortened by digitalis, hypercalcemia, and hyperkalemia.

ISCHEMIA AND INFARCTION

Electrocardiographic monitoring of myocardial ischemia is a relatively new technique in the operating room. Studies of intraoperative ECG monitoring by Cannard in 1960, and Russell in 1969, did not even mention the use of the ECG to diagnose ischemia; they only discussed the use of the ECG to diagnose arrhythmias.[15, 16] In recent years, coronary artery disease has become the number one health problem in the United States. Patients coming for all types of surgical procedures have significant coronary artery disease, and many have histories of acute myocardial infarctions or angina pectoris. In these patients, the ECG should be used to identify myocardial ischemia during the stresses of anesthesia and surgery, as well as to recognize arrhythmias. It is important to realize that a substantial number of patients with severe coronary artery disease may have a normal resting ECG. Benchimol found that 17 of 106 patients with documented triple vessel coronary artery disease had normal resting ECGs.[17] Therefore, it is important to monitor the ECG for ischemic changes in all patients with potential coronary artery disease (*e.g.,* obese or hypertensive patients); probable coronary artery disease (*e.g.,* patients with atherosclerosis undergoing vascular surgery, such as a carotid endarterectomy); or known coronary artery disease (*e.g.,* documented myocardial infarction, positive coronary arteriogram)

The cardiologist frequently states in his consultations for all patients with coronary artery disease that the ECG should be monitored. However, he or she has never told the anesthesiologist or surgeon the specific techniques learned during exercise stress testing (*e.g.*, lead placement, criteria for the diagnosis of ischemia). Therefore, until recently, the older ECG lead systems designed primarily for arrhythmia detection have been used during surgery when monitoring of ischemic changes was desired.

LEAD SYSTEMS

As early as 1931, it was noted that the precordial leads gave a greater sensitivity in detecting S-T segment depression of ischemic origin than did the standard leads. Since then, a number of lead systems have been developed to monitor myocardial ischemia, and they have been studied extensively during stress testing. Blackburn has done many studies of the lead systems and found that the most sensitive exploring electrode was at the V_5 chest position.[18] He showed that 89 percent of the S-T segment information contained in a conventional 12-lead ECG is found in lead V_5. Mason studied 174 patients using a multiple lead ECG during exercise, and he found that leads V_4, V_5, and V_6 were the most valuable, and that lead I was the least informative.[19] Of the 56 patients with a positive test, 30 had left ventricular ischemia (V_3–V_6), 8 had inferior ischemia (II, III, aVF), and 18 had a combined pattern. As can be seen from this study, isolated anterior wall (V_1–V_2) or inferior wall ischemia can still be missed by single V_5 lead monitoring. Because of this, most authors have recommended the observation of multiple leads when monitoring for myocardial ischemia.

It was not until 1976 that any information on the use of precordial leads for monitoring of ischemia during anesthesia first appeared. Dalton recommended placing a sterile spinal needle in the V_4 position after the skin was "prepped" for cardiac surgery.[20] Kaplan recommended that a multiple lead ECG system be used in all patients with coronary artery disease.[21] Using this system, four disposable electrocardiographic pads are placed on the extremities and a fifth is placed in the V_5 position covered with a small piece of steri-drape. The V_5 lead and steri-drape are placed

before the induction of anesthesia and can be "prepped over" by the surgical team. This V_5 lead does not interfere with the performance of cardiac surgery through a median sternotomy. Many instances of severe ischemic changes have been observed before and after the skin prep, when little was seen in the other leads.

Using the five electrodes, seven different ECG leads may be selected for observation (I, II, III, aVR, aVL, aVF, or V_5). All seven leads are observed before the start of anesthesia and *recorded* for later reference. In patients undergoing coronary revascularization, all seven leads are recorded and then two leads (V_5 and II) are viewed simultaneously using two different ECG channels on the oscilloscope. Thus, the left ventricular (V_5) and inferior (II) walls of the heart can be observed continuously throughout the operative procedure. Robertson has shown that there is some degree of correlation between the site of coronary artery obstruction and the lead in which ischemia is detected.[22] S-T segment changes in leads II, III and aVF correspond to disease of the right coronary artery; and ischemic changes in V_4–V_6 indicate disease of the left anterior descending or circumflex coronary artery. However, the correlation between ECG zonal ischemia and coronary anatomy is not always this precise.

The five-electrode system discussed above, including the true V_5 lead, is preferable for precise intraoperative monitoring. However, most operating room ECG systems have only three or four electrode wires. A modification of the V_5 lead can be readily used in those cases, as is frequently done during exercise stress testing. The most popular modified leads during stress testing have been the CM_5 and CS_5 bipolar leads. These leads are good for the detection of ischemia, but recently Froelicher has shown that they are not as good as V_5.[23] In the operating room, the right-arm electrode can be placed just under the clavicle or on the right shoulder, and the left-arm electrode placed in the V_5 position. Lead I can then be selected to observe the anterior heart wall (a modified CS_5) and lead II for the inferior wall. Another alternative in a four-electrode system is to place the left-arm lead in the V_5 position and observe lead aVL, a modified V_5 lead.

S-T SEGMENT CHANGES

The criteria for ischemic changes on the ECG are still not entirely agreed upon. However, there is more agreement than there has been in the past as a result of extensive studies during exercise stress testing. Surgery and anesthesia are certainly a good stress test for the patient with coronary artery disease, and therefore, exercise testing information is transferable to the operating room. When patients with coronary artery disease are exercised, the first abnormality seen is depression of the J-point. This J-point depression evolves into a progressively more depressed horizontal S-T segment and then anginal pain frequently occurs. The pain always, however, *follows* the S-T segment depression. At the end of the test, the S-T segment may either return to the up-sloping J-point depression, or convert to a down-sloping S-T segment with a deeply inverted T wave. Significant subendocardial myocardial ischemia is defined as greater than 1 mm of horizontal or down-sloping S-T segment depression measured from a point 0.06 seconds from the J-point.[24] Downsloping S-T segment depression greater than 1 mm and beginning at the J-point is the most specific sign of myocardial ischemia. There is general agreement that an increased magnitude of S-T segment depression denotes an increased degree of ischemia. J-point depression with up-sloping S-T segments may reflect ischemia (especially if over 2 mm), but is not a specific sign. Also, T wave changes may reflect ischemia, but again are not specific. All S-T segment elevations of greater than 1.0 mm are considered significant. This is a manifestation of more severe myocardial ischemia reflecting transmural, rather than subendocardial, ischemia. In patients with Prinzmetal angina (coronary spasm), the S-T segments are also elevated with pain (Fig. 6-8).

The S-T segments and T waves can be affected by many factors other than myocardial ischemia. These other factors produce the "nonspecific ST-T wave changes." Drugs that can affect the S-T segments include digitalis, diuretics which deplete potassium, and reserpine. Hypokalemia or glucose infusion can affect the S-T segment by altering the membrane-potassium relationships. The S-T segments may appear to be depressed by the Ta wave of atrial repolarization, and altered by conduction disturbances such as LBBB or WPW. S-T segment depression and T wave inversion have been reported with changes in respiration alone.[25]

MYOCARDIAL INFARCTION

The classic ECG pattern of ischemia progresses to infarction as follows:

1. S-T segment depression and T wave inversion; possible ischemia
2. S-T segment elevation; pattern of injury
3. Q wave appearance; pattern of necrosis; only the Q waves are diagnostic of definite infarction.

The Q waves are diagnostic if they are more than 0.04 seconds in width; the S-T segment elevation shows an upward convexity; and the T waves are symmetrical and pointed. These *indicative* changes of an infarction are seen in the leads of the ECG facing the necrotic area. The opposite surface of the heart shows *reciprocal* changes consisting of an increased height of the R wave, depressed S-T segments, and tall upright T waves.

The location of a myocardial infarction is described by the wall of the heart affected. However, this is only an approximation because there are no clear-cut boundaries between areas of the heart. The four walls usually referred to are anterior, lateral, inferior, and posterior (Table 6-1).

Acute myocardial infarctions tend to evolve electrocardiographically through various stages. Soon after the onset of pain the S-T segments are elevated and the T waves are taller and upright (hyperacute changes). Then the T waves become symmetrically in-

Table 6-1. ECG Changes With Different Anatomic Locations of Myocardial Infarction

LOCATION OF INFARCTION	INDICATIVE CHANGES	RECIPROCAL CHANGES
Anterior	V_1–V_4, I, AVL	II, III, AVF
Lateral	V_5–V_6, I, AVL	V_1, AVR
Inferior	II, III, AVF	V_1–V_4, I, AVL
Posterior	None	V_1–V_2

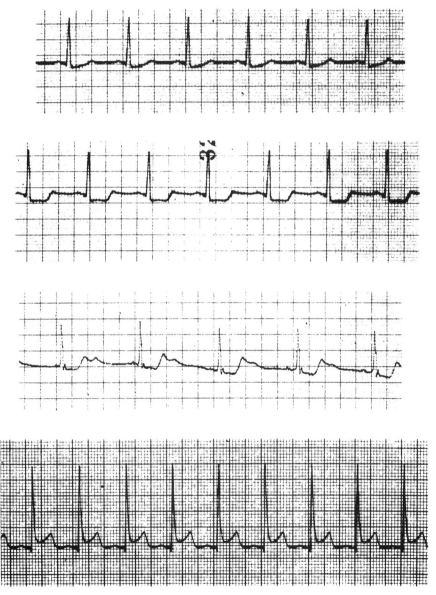

Fig. 6-8. Various types of *ST*-segment changes associated with myocardial ischemia are demonstrated.

verted (coving) as the S-T segments return to baseline. Finally, the T waves return to their baseline position. The Q waves usually appear within 12 to 24 hours of the infarction, but may be delayed to a much later time. Persistent S-T elevation is usually caused by either pericarditis or ventricular aneurysm.

Not all infarctions are as easy to diagnose as it would appear from the above discussion. In some cases, the diagnosis is made from the history and enzyme studies, not from the ECG. Some of these difficult situations occur in patients with left bundle branch block, previous infarctions, lack of development of Q waves (loss of R waves only), or subendocardial infarctions. The diagnosis of an acute subendocardial infarction depends on the following (Fig. 6-9):

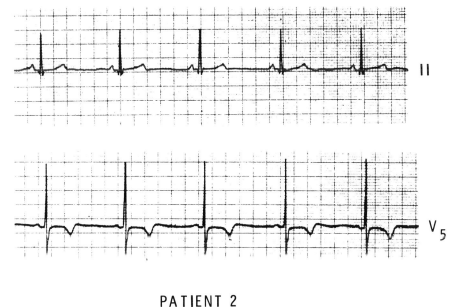

PATIENT 2

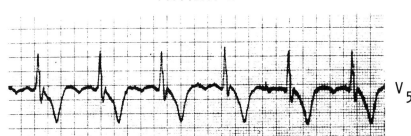

Fig. 6-9. Two patients with subendocardial myocardial infarctions are demonstrated. Symmetrical T-wave inversion is demonstrated in both patients in the V₅ lead.

1. The clinical history of chest pain
2. S-T segment depression and symmetrical T wave inversion in the precordial leads
3. No Q wave development
4. Elevation of the CPK enzyme and the CPK-MB isoenzyme

Myocardial infarctions after coronary artery revascularization have been extremely difficult to define and diagnose. This partially accounts for the great variability of the infarction rates, ranging from 5 to 40 percent, reported from different institutions. The two primary techniques for detecting perioperative infarctions have been (1) development of new Q waves on the ECG and (2) elevation of serum enzymes. In the past, less specific enzymes, such as LDH and SGOT, were reported. In one study in patients with acute myocardial infarctions, elevations of at least two enzymes were noted to levels of SGOT greater than 200, LDH greater than 400, or CPK greater than 800.[26]

Recently, the myocardial isoenzymes of creatine phosphokinase (CPK-MB) and of lactic dehydrogenase (LDH₁) have been used with much greater specificity. The LDH₁ isoenzyme is predominantly myocardial but is also present in red blood cells, kidney, brain, stomach, and pancreas. Therefore, it has not correlated with acute infarctions as well as the CPK-MB isoenzyme, which is only found in the heart muscle. The normal total CPK is less than 40 mIU/ml and CPK-MB is 2 ± 1 mIU/ml. During an acute infarction, the total CPK frequently exceeds 800 and the peak CPK-MB has been found to range from 25 to 400 mIU/ml. The initial CPK-MB is detectable within three hours after the onset of chest pain, and peak values usually occur within 12 hours. Dixon studied a series of 100 patients undergoing coronary revascularization and divided them into groups according to the presence or absence of postoperative CPK-MB.[27] Group I (49 patients) had no CPK-MB postoperatively and had a peak total CPK of about 900 and peak LDH of 500; group II (4 patients) had CPK-MB in a low concentration (less than 40 mIU/ml) for only one day and peak total CPK of about 650 and LDH of 400; group III (17 patients) had CPK-MB activity ranging from 40 to 400 mIU/ml lasting 31 hours, and peak total CPK of 1100 and LDH of 500. These groups correlated with the ECG findings as well. Groups I and II had no ECG changes; Group III had changes characteristic of acute infarctions.

The other standard method of diagnosing an infarction after coronary artery surgery is by the appearance of new Q waves on the ECG. Steinberg found that new Q waves correlated well with the appearance of localized abnormalities of left ventricular wall motion on repeat cardiac catheterization.[28] However, Basson reported that all new Q waves may not be a new infarction, but rather an un-

masking of a preexisting inferior infarction by anterior wall ischemia.[29] To complicate things even further, Kennedy reported the disappearance of Q waves after coronary revascularization caused by either reperfusion of an ischemic area or a "cancelling effect" of new perioperative myocardial damage upon the old ECG evidence of a myocardial infarction.[30] Righetti compared the ECG changes with CPK-MB measurements and concluded that (1) new Q waves on the ECG *underestimate* the incidence of myocardial damage after coronary artery surgery; (2) CPK-MB alone *overestimates* the incidence of infarction; and (3) the two techniques should possibly be combined along with a Tcm⁹⁹ pyrophosphate myocardial scan to best detect perioperative infarction.[31]

OTHER CONDITIONS THAT AFFECT THE ECG

EFFECTS OF DRUGS ON THE ECG[32]

Digitalis

Digitalis preparations have many effects on the ECG. The usual effects include prolongation of the PR interval to a first-degree heart block, but no change in the QRS complex. Marked ventricular repolarization effects include (1) depression of the S-T segment; (2) decreased amplitude of the T wave and sometimes inversion of the T wave; (3) shortening of the QT_c interval; and (4) increase of the U wave amplitude.

Because of increased automaticity of ectopic pacemaker fibers, digitalis intoxication can produce almost any arrhythmia. The most common arrhythmias seen with toxicity are PVCs of multifocal origin which proceed to ventricular bigeminy. The most characteristic supraventricular arrhythmia is paroxysmal atrial tachycardia. This is frequently associated with atrioventricular block because digitalis prolongs AV conduction. All forms of heart block have been produced by digitalis toxicity; the most common being a Mobitz type 1 block.

Quinidine

Therapeutic doses of quinidine decrease the "upslope" of the action potential and decrease automaticity. They may prolong the P wave and PR interval, but increasing doses always prolong the QRS complex. At high plasma levels, the QRS complex can be widened by 50 percent. The S-T segments may be depressed, the T wave depressed or inverted, and the U waves increased, as with digitalis. However, with quinidine, the QT_c interval *lengthens,* while it *shortens* with digitalis. Two types of toxic reactions may occur: (1) dose-dependent widening of the QRS, heart block, and severe bradycardia; and (2) dose-independent ventricular ectopy resulting from reentry promoted by slow conduction.

Procainamide and Other Cardiac Drugs

Procainamide has effects very similar to quinidine, but because it is frequently given intravenously and is a shorter-acting drug, its effects on the ECG appear sooner and last for a shorter period of time. Therapeutic doses of lidocaine, diphenylhydantoin, and propranolol have no definite effects on the ECG. Diuretics have no direct effect on the ECG, but can affect it profoundly by altering electrolytes. The antihypertensive drugs do not affect the ECG directly, but only through changes in electrolytes and the autonomic nervous system.

Psychotropic Drugs

Several phenothiazines produce dose-dependent abnormalities of ventricular repolarization. These are most commonly seen with thioridazine (Mellaril), but are also seen with chlorpromazine and other major tranquilizers. Widening of the QT_c interval and T wave, and increased U wave amplitude are seen, but no changes occur in the P, QRS, or S-T segment. Ectopic rhythms have also been reported, probably secondary to reentry. Imipramine hydrochloride, the non-MAO inhibitor antidepressant drug, has been associated with marked ECG changes. It prolongs the QT_c interval, depresses the S-T segment and T waves, widens the QRS complex, and produces supraventricular and ventricular arrhythmias.

EFFECTS OF ELECTROLYTES ON THE ECG[33]

Because depolarization and repolarization of myocardial cells depend on potassium, calcium, and magnesium ions, it would be expected that abnormalities of these electrolytes would markedly alter the ECG.

Potassium

The ECG is the best measurement of the relationship between intracellular and extracellular potassium. Hypokalemia produces characteristic changes on the ECG. When the serum potassium is reduced to 3 to 3.5 meq/L, the T wave is lowered and a tall U wave is seen. This appears to prolong the QT interval but in fact does not; it is the fused QTU interval that is observed. When the serum potassium is under 3 meq/L, the S-T segment is also depressed.

Hyperkalemia can produce profound changes on the ECG. Narrowing and peaking of the T wave, along with shortening of the QT interval, are seen when the serum potassium reaches 6.0 meq/L. This is caused by an increased velocity of repolarization. When the serum potassium exceeds 6.5 meq/L, the QRS complex begins to widen and simulates a left bundle branch block. The PR interval increases when the potassium exceeds 7 meq/L, and by a potassium of 8.8 meq/L, the P wave is lost. Potassium levels greater than 10 to 12 meq/L produce ventricular asystole or fibrillation.

High levels of potassium also block AV conduction and this is now being seen with increasing frequency because hyperkalemic solutions are being used to arrest the heart on cardiopulmonary bypass. In this situation, the potassium frequently has to be driven into the cells to reestablish the membrane potential and allow repolarization and conduction. This is done by administering either calcium chloride, sodium bicarbonate, or glucose and insulin.

Calcium and Magnesium

Hypocalcemia prolongs the QT interval by elongating the S-T segment. This must be differentiated from the prolonged QU interval of hypokalemia. In patients with a low ionized calcium, the U wave is usually absent. In hypercalcemia, the QT interval is shortened and the proximal limb of the T wave abruptly rises to its peak. In animal experiments, the pattern of hypocalcemia is exaggerated by hypomagnesemia and corrected by hypermagnesemia. Early magnesium deficiency is characterized by tall, peaked T waves (not narrow as in hyperkalemia) and a normal QT interval. Later changes include a prolonged PR interval, widened QRS, S-T segment depression, and low T waves.

EFFECTS OF HYPOTHERMIA ON THE ECG[34]

The ECG findings of hypothermia can be quite marked. As the temperature decreases, there is a progressive slowing of the sinus rate, inversion of the T waves, and prolongation of the PR, QRS, and QT intervals. Atrial fibrillation or flutter is frequently encountered, and ventricular arrhythmias appear below 30°C. Further decreases below 28°C produce ventricular fibrillation. In addition, a secondary deflection at the end of the QRS complex called the *J wave, Osborn wave,* or *"camel hump"* is frequently seen. Figure 6-10 demonstrates progressive hypothermic changes on the ECG. The top panel is at 37°C; the second panel at 29°C demonstrates the camel hump; and the third and fourth panels show course and fine ventric-

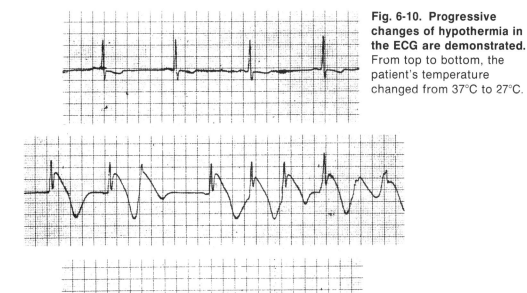

Fig. 6-10. Progressive changes of hypothermia in the ECG are demonstrated. From top to bottom, the patient's temperature changed from 37°C to 27°C.

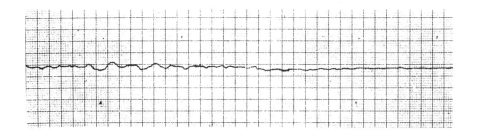

ular fibrillation, which occurred at 27°C. The J wave is seen in hypothermia below 28°C, but is not diagnostic because it has also been reported with central nervous system disease.

CARDIAC ARRHYTHMIAS

Arrhythmia detection has been the most important use of the ECG during and after surgery. Intraoperative arrhythmias were reported in the early 1900s, but the first large series of ECG studies during anesthesia was reported in 1936 by Kurtz.[35] In 109 patients, he found that sinus arrhythmia, extra systoles, and downward displacement of the pacemaker site predominated, and that 79 percent of the patients developed some rhythm disturbance during surgery. More recent studies, as summarized by Katz, have found the incidence of intraoperative arrhythmias to vary from 16.3 to 61.7 percent.[36] Bertrand studied 100 patients, using continuous electromagnetic taperecording during surgery, and reported an 84 percent incidence of supraventricular and ventricular arrhythmias.[37] Arrhythmias were most common at the times of intubation and extubation of the trachea. Patients with preexisting cardiac disease had a higher incidence of ventricular arrhythmias (60% versus 37%) than patients without known heart disease. Twenty-four of twenty-five patients with heart disease had a rhythm disturbance during surgery. In a study of patients undergoing cardiac surgery, Angelini reported that 29 of 50 patients (58%) having valve surgery, and 35 of 78 patients (45%) having coronary revascularization developed significant postoperative arrhythmias.[38] These arrhythmias tended to correlate with the severity of the heart disease, prolonged the hospital stay, and were responsible for up to 80 percent of surgical mortality.

Hypercarbia, hypocarbia, and hypoxia have all been shown to precipitate the development of arrhythmias, especially with the use of halothane or cyclopropane anesthesia. Edwards showed that hyperventilation to a $PaCO_2$ of 30 or 20 torr (pH 7.51 and 7.61) lowered a normal serum potassium level

(4.03 meq/L) to 3.64 and 3.12 meq/L, respectively.[39] If serum and total body potassium start at lower levels, it is possible to decrease the serum potassium into the 2 meq/L range by hyperventilation and precipitate severe cardiac dysrhythmias. Kochstrop recently showed that drugs such as cocaine and ketamine that block the uptake of norepinephrine can facilitate the development of epinephrine-induced arrhythmias.[40] Endotracheal intubation is probably the most common cause for arrhythmias during surgery, and Fox recently reported on the severe hypertension and arrhythmias that can occur during this procedure.[41] Many ECG abnormalities have been reported with intracranial pathology, especially subarachnoid hemorrhages, including changes in QT intervals, development of Q waves, S-T segment changes, U waves, and all types of arrhythmias. The mechanism of the arrhythmias appears to be changes in the autonomic nervous system. Dental surgery has been one of the types of surgery most often associated with arrhythmia formation. Junctional rhythms are very common and may be caused by stimulation of the autonomic nervous system through the fifth cranial nerve.

However, arrhythmias also may be *corrected* by general anesthesia. Borg and others have reported the disappearance of chronic arrhythmias following the induction of general anesthesia.[42] This could be caused by the relief of anxiety and loss of sympathetic stimulation, an antiarrhythmic property of the anesthetic agent itself, or the correction of abnormalities of respiration, blood gases, and electrolytes.

PHYSIOLOGICAL BASIS OF CARDIAC ARRHYTHMIAS

Arrhythmias may result from abnormalities of impulse formation (automaticity), impulse conduction (block, reentry), or both.[43] The cells of the SA node undergo a rapid spontaneous *phase 4* depolarization and are thus the pacemakers of the normal heart; ventricular cells normally do not undergo spontaneous *phase 4* depolarization. If, however, the higher pacemaker cells do not fire, the lower cells will undergo slow spontaneous *phase 4* depolarization, taking over as pacemakers. Factors that selectively decrease the rate of *phase 4* depolarization of the higher pacemaker sites, leaving the lower cells unaffected, favor the movement of the pacemaker to a lower area in the heart. In addition, factors that increase the spontaneous *phase 4* depolarization of a lower pacing site favor the take-over of these lower areas as the cardiac pacemaker. Factors tending to slow pacemaker sites above the AV node are primarily vagal influences, such as digitalis, parasympathomimetic drugs, and halothane. Factors tending to enhance automatic pacemaker activity below the AV node are catecholamines, hypercarbia, hypoxia, and digitalis overdose. Therefore, the combination of halothane to depress the atrial pacemaker, and hypercarbia to increase ventricular automaticity may lead to ventricular arrhythmias. Increased automaticity is usually caused by an increase in the slope of *phase 4* depolarization, but it may also be caused by an increase in the resting membrane potential or a decrease in the threshold potential (Figure 6-11*A*).

Abnormal impulse conduction is the second major mechanism of arrhythmia formation. With a localized depression of the normal conduction system, a reduction in impulse transmission may occur leading to a form of blocked conduction (*e.g.*, Wenckebach's phenomenon). In addition, increased impulse transmission may occur when abnormal conduction circuits are formed. These abnormal circuits may be present anatomically (Bundle of Kent) or may develop transiently, secondary to various drugs (digitalis) or secondary to local tissue abnormalities (ischemia, hypoxia, acidosis) leading to the most common form of abnormal conduction called *reentry excitation*.[44] A reentrant pathway is potentially formed when a difference in the rate of impulse transmission is present in adjacent conductive tissues. In the tissue with abnormal impulse transmission, an antegrade block develops, slowing impulse conduction in a forward direction but allowing normal retrograde conduction. In the adjacent tissue with normal conduction, the im-

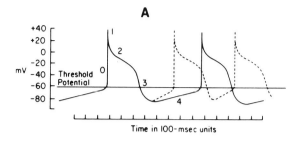

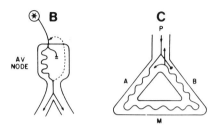

Fig. 6-11. Panel A demonstrates an increase in slope of phase 4 depolarization, while panels B and C demonstrate reentry mechanisms for supraventricular and ventricular tachycardias. (Lurie AJ: Rapid overdrive pacing for refractory tachyrhythmias in patients with open heart surgery. J Thorac Cardiovasc Surg 72:458, 1976)

pulse passes the conduction block and proceeds along the normal distal pathways. In addition, an impulse is passed retrograde through the abnormal tissue. This impulse returns to the area that conducted normally, finding it repolarized and capable of rapidly reinitiating impulse formation. Thus, a reentrant or circus loop is created.

For an impulse to complete a reentrant circuit, it must be unidirectionally blocked, travel slowly over another pathway, and reexcite in retrograde manner the tissue proximal to the block, after its refractory period. This results in a coupled premature contraction. The two key features are slow conduction and unidirectional block of the AV node or Purkinje network. This may be the mechanism of most arrhythmias. Reentry can occur throughout the conduction system both above and below the AV junction. The reentry mechanism for supraventricular tachyarrhythmias (*e.g.*, PAT) is shown in Figure 6-11*B*. The impulse comes from the SA node and is partially blocked in the AV node. The retrograde reentry is shown with the *dashed line*. The mechanism of reentrant ventricular tachyarrhythmias (*e.g.,* bigeminy) is similarly shown in Figure 6-11C.

The mechanism of action of the antiarrhythmic drugs can be integrated with the above discussion. Many of the commonly used antiarrhythmic drugs suppress automaticity in pacemaker fibers by decreasing the slope of *phase 4* spontaneous depolarization. For example, propranolol, by reducing beta-adrenergic stimulation, reduces the spontaneous depolarization. In addition, reentry mechanisms that produce arrhyth-

mias can be treated by slowing conduction in the abnormal tissue, by converting the unidirectional block to a bidirectional block (propranolol, quinidine, procainamide), or by reducing or eliminating the unidirectional block by increasing impulse transmission (lidocaine, diphenylhydantoin).

TREATMENT OF ARRHYTHMIAS

Antiarrhythmic Drugs: Categories

In order to understand more clearly the effects of the antiarrhythmic drugs, their mode

Table 6-2. Antiarrhythmic Drugs

DRUG	CLASS	IV DOSE	BLOOD LEVEL DESIRED	TOXICITY
Procainamide (Pronestyl)	I	100 mg q5 min up to 1000 mg; may infuse at 1–4 mg/min	4–6 µg/ml	Myocardial depression, hypotension, widened QRS; lupus (chronic)
Quinidine (Quinaglute)	I	200 mg PO not IV	4–8 µg/ml	Fever, chills, nausea, diarrhea, hypotension
Disopyramide (Norpace)	I	150 mg PO q6h 1–2 mg/kg IV over 5–10 min, max 150 mg	2–4 µg/ml	Parasympatholytic symptoms: dry mouth, constipation, nausea, urinary retention, blurred vision; contraindicated in CHF, sick sinus node syndrome, A-V block; may widen QRS
Mexiletine	I	10–14 mg/kg/day average 12 mg/kg/day	0.75–2.0 µg/ml	Fine tremor of hands; CNS stimulation → dizziness, blurred vision, dysarthria, generalized confusional state; hypotension, sinus bradycardia, widened QRS
Tocainide	I	PO 400–600 mg q8h	6–12 µg/ml	Anorexia, nausea, vomiting, constipation, abdominal pain; CNS stimulation
Aprindine	I	PO loading 200–300 mg then 100–150 mg/day	1–2 µg/ml	Ataxia, tremors, cholestatic jaundice, serious agranulocytosis
Lidocaine (Xylocaine)	I	1.0–1.5 mg/kg bolus followed by constant infusion 1–4 mg/min	2–5 µg/ml	> 5 µg/ml→ CNS excitation, muscle twitching and fasciculations, dizziness, tinnitus, convulsions and respiratory arrest; dosage must be reduced in CHF and liver dysfunction; with A-V block may increase conduction with marked increase in ventricular response

of action must be understood in relation to their effects on the various phases of the cardiac action potential, particularly with regard to the inward and outward membrane currents. In the normal heart, cardiac rhythm is determined by a single dominant pacemaker, a rapid uniform conduction system, and an action potential and refractory period of long duration. Changes in any of these variables will enhance the likelihood of an abnormal cardiac rhythm. Thus, shortening of the action potential, increasing conduction veloc-

ity, or diminishing the refractory period may potentiate the development of an arrhythmia. To better understand the various drugs classified as antiarrhythmic agents, it is best to divide them into four electrophysiologic categories.[45, 46] All of the agents have one dominant action on the myocardial cell justifying their categorization. There is some overlap among groups and controversy continues as to the classifications of lidocaine, diphenylhydantoin, and propranolol (Table 6-2).

Table 6.2 (Continued)

DRUG	CLASS	IV DOSE	BLOOD LEVEL DESIRED	TOXICITY
Diphenylhydantoin (Dilantin)	I	100 mg q5 min up to 500 mg	8–16 μg/ml	Hypotension and myocardial depression, rapid IV injection → ventricular fibrillation, asystole, respiratory arrest, death
Propranolol (Inderal)	II	0.5 mg q2 min up to total dose 5 mg	25–50 ng/ml	Myocardial depression, hypotension, bronchospasm; contraindicated in CHF, bradycardia, and AV block
Bretylium (Bretylol)	III	5 mg/kg diluted in 50–100 ml over 10–20 min; PO 600 mg q6h		Orthostatic hypotension, myocardial depression, hypotension especially if used subsequent to other antifibrillatory agents
Amiodarone (Cordarone)	III	IV 5–10 mg slowly PO 200–800 mg/day		Nausea, vomiting, diarrhea; slate-grey skin discoloration; thyroid dysfunction; yellowish-brown granular corneal pigments
Verapamil (Isoptin, Cordilox)	IV	IV 10 mg over 15–60 sec (0.145 mg/kg) Repeat q30 min or infuse 5 μg/kg/min; PO 40–80 mg q8h		Contraindicated in CHF, SA node disease, unstable AV block, hypotension; synergistic depression with beta-adrenergic blockers
Digoxin (Lanoxin)	Glycoside	0.25–0.50 mg → 1.5 mg	2 ng/ml	Bradycardia, CHB; toxicity potentiated by $K^+ < 3.5$
Ouabain	Glycoside	0.1–0.2 mg → 1.0 mg		Bradycardia, CHB; toxicity potentiated by $K^+ < 3.5$
Edrophonium (Tensilon)	Cholinergic	5–10 mg IV, may use test dose 2 mg esp. in presence of digitalis or heart block		Sinus bradycardia, AV block, dizziness, abdominal cramps, cardiac arrest
Neosynephrine	α-adrenergic receptor stimulator	50–100 μ IV		Hypertension, ↑ MVO_2 → ischemia
Atropine	Parasympatholytic	0.3–2 mg		Tachycardia, ↑ MVO_2 → ischemia; fever, mouth dryness

Class I. These agents are potent local anesthetics for nerve cells as well as myocardial membranes. They are divided into class IA and IB drugs. The former have the ability to reduce the maximal rate of depolarization in cardiac muscle (block the fast inward sodium channel), and therefore, increase the threshold of excitability, depress the conduction velocity, produce a marked prolongation in the effective refractory period, and inhibit spontaneous depolarization in automatic cells. These changes occur without any alteration in the action potential duration or resting membrane potential. These drugs include quinidine, procainamide, disopyramide, mexiletine, aprindine, and tocainide. Some authors also include propranolol and some other beta-blockers in class IA because of their local anesthetic properties in high doses. Lidocaine and diphenylhydantoin differ from the class IA drugs in two ways: (1) they shorten the action potential duration and (2) they increase conduction velocity; they are called class IB drugs by Singh.

Class II. These drugs are the beta-adrenergic receptor blocking agents. Overactivity of the sympathetic nervous system is considered significant in the development of certain cardiac arrhythmias, and this can be inhibited with class II agents. They work by way of depression of *phase 4* depolarization with a resultant decrease in cellular automaticity. This group includes propranolol, practolol, metoprolol, oxyprenolol, alprenolol, pindolol, and nadolol.

Class III. Bretylium and the antianginal agent amiodarone produce pure prolongation of the action potential with prolongation of repolarization of both atrial and ventricular muscle. These agents are not local anesthetics nor beta blockers. Their lengthening of the effective refractory period reduces the ability for reentry and constitutes their major antiarrhythmic mechanism.

Class IV. Calcium blockers, which inhibit the slow inward calcium response (selective calcium antagonists), include verapamil, nife-dipine, perhexiline, and diltiazem. Class IV antiarrhythmics, which also serve as antianginal agents through coronary artery vasodilation, affect phase 0 polarization with slowing of the cardiac action potential throughout the conduction system.

This classification of antiarrhythmic drugs allows a clearer understanding of the cellular mechanism of action of the various antiarrhythmic agents. Table 6-2 lists the various current and investigational antiarrhythmic agents, their intravenous or oral doses, therapeutic plasma levels (when known), and toxicities or contraindications. Table 6-3 serves as a rapid reference for the treatment of the important cardiac arrhythmias. Treatment is divided into the first, second, third, and occasionally fourth choice for each arrhythmia.

Additional information concerning the currently available antiarrhythmic drugs is readily available in most standard reference texts and will not be presented in greater detail at this time. Many exciting new antiarrhythmic agents are increasingly available. These drugs extend the physician's ability to treat previously untreatable and recalcitrant arrhythmias. Because of their increasing importance and their relative newness, a short section dealing with each of the most promising agents is presented.[46]

Antiarrhythmic Drugs: Newer Agents

Disopyramide. Disopyramide (Norpace) is currently available in oral form to control recurrent premature ventricular contractions and other ventricular arrhythmias. It appears to be effective in reducing life-threatening arrhythmias resistant to other treatments, especially those associated with acute myocardial infarction. In addition, antegrade and retrograde accessory pathway slowing in Wolff–Parkinson–White syndrome (WPW) has been found valuable in the control of the ventricular response in atrial fibrillation and atrial flutter associated with WPW. This class I drug resembles quinidine but is associated with a reduced frequency of side effects.

Mexiletine. This class I agent resembles lidocaine and is a primary experimental agent for the chronic oral prophylaxis of ventricular arrhythmias. By depressing fast depolarization of the cardiac action potential, it reduces the maximal rate of depolarization, decreases the conduction velocity, and prolongs the effective refractory period. It has been shown to be beneficial in digitalis and ouabain toxicity and to be particularly effective in ventricular arrhythmias associated with a recent myocardial infarction. Mexiletine is recommended as the oral treatment of ventricular arrhythmias when lidocaine was the primary intravenous treatment. Some depression of myocardial contractility may occur, but can be lessened with a reduction in the dosage of medication.

Table 6-3. Arrhythmia Treatment Summary

RHYTHM	FIRST TREATMENT CHOICE	SECOND TREATMENT CHOICE	THIRD TREATMENT CHOICE
Ventricular fibrillation Ventricular tachycardia	Electrical defibrillation; 200 watt/sec (3 watt/sec/kg) increase energy as required	Lidocaine (Xylocaine) 1.0–1.5 mg/kg initial IV bolus Infusion 1–4 mg/min (2 g/ 500 ml D_5W)	Propranolol (Inderal) 0.5 mg q2 min up to 5 mg Fourth choice: Refractory ventricular fibrillation Bretylium 5 mg/kg qs 50–100 ml D_5W up to 30 mg/kg total dose
Premature ventricular contractions	Lidocaine (Xylocaine) 1.0–1.5 mg/kg initial bolus; followed by infusion 1–4 mg/min	Propranolol (Inderal) 0.5 mg q2 min up to 5 mg	Procainamide (Pronestyl) 100 mg q5 min up to 1000 mg; may infuse 1–4 mg/ min
Atrial fibrillation Atrial flutter	Digitalis (Lanoxin) 0.25–0.5 mg IV Ouabain 0.1–0.2 mg IV	Propranolol (Inderal) 0.5 mg q2 min to 5 mg	Cardioversion—*external*— synchronized-flutter: 50 watt/sec, fibrillation: 200 watt/sec. *Internal*: 5–30 watt/sec-synchronized
Paroxysmal atrial tachycardia	Edrophonium 2 mg→10 mg; can be used to improve response by increasing parasympathetic tone Carotid sinus massage: Care must be exercised with carotid vascular disease.	Neosynephrine 50–100 μg/ dose: ↑ BP and convert through carotid sinus reflex	Propranolol (Inderal) *0.5 mg q2 min up to 5 mg* Fourth treatment choice cardioversion as in atrial flutter above Fifth: verapamil 5–10 mg IV
Sinus tachycardia	Usually no treatment required. If ↑ HR → ischemia, go to second treatment	Propranolol (Inderal) 0.5 mg q2 min up to 5 mg	
Sinus bradycardia	Usually no treatment required. If hypotension or ventricular escape beats present go to →	Atropine 0.3–2.0 mg	Ephedrine 5–10 mg Fourth treatment choice: atrial pacing if heart exposed
1° AV block 2° AV block Mobitz I Mobitz II	No treatment required No treatment required More ominous; requires transvenous or epicardial pacemaker		
3° AV block Complete heart block	Atropine 0.3–2.0 mg may be helpful if suprahissian block	Isuprel 1–4 μg/min (1 mg/250 ml D_5W)	Transvenous or epicardial pacemaker

Tocainide. Tocainide is orally active with a spectrum identical to lidocaine and mexiletine. It is a potent antiarrhythmic for the elective long-term control of ventricular arrhythmias.

Aprindine. Aprindine is a class I agent effective against both supraventricular and ventricular arrhythmias. It decreases *phase 0* depolarization with a resultant decrease in ventricular, atrial, and Purkinje fiber diastolic depolarization without an effect on the slow-channel calcium activity. Orally, aprindine may be effective when other antiarrhythmic agents are ineffective. One particularly useful area involves control of ventricular tachyarrhythmias in the mitral valve prolapse syndrome. It also slows both AV node and accessory pathway conduction in atrial fibrillation or flutter caused by WPW. Marked side effects, including cholestatic jaundice and agranulocytosis, have been reported. A narrow toxic-to-therapeutic ratio must be balanced against its remarkable effectiveness in recalcitrant ventricular arrhythmias.

Verapamil. Verapamil is a synthetic papaverine derivative which selectively inhibits calcium flux across the cell membrane. By blocking the slow inward current of calcium (and possibly sodium), *phase 4* diastolic depolarization is prolonged. Its antiarrhythmic effect is produced by slowing atrial depolarization, delaying AV conduction secondary to prolonging the AV refractory period, and impeding the conduction proximal to the His bundle without affecting SA or ventricular conduction. Intravenous verapamil is rapidly effective in correcting both atrial and ventricular arrhythmias. However, by inhibiting intranodal reentry or circus-type preexcitation, it is most effective with supraventricular tachycardias. Verapamil is not effective in the treatment of ventricular arrhythmias. Because of its effect on excitation-contraction coupling, it should be used with caution in patients with significant myocardial dysfunction. Verapamil is available both in oral and intravenous formulations. Nifedipine and diltiazem, two other selective calcium blockers, although also effective as antiarrhythmics, are now primarily utilized as antianginal medications and coronary vasodilators.

Amiodarone. Amiodarone (Cordarone) is a benzofuran derivative combining antianginal and antiarrhythmic properties without appreciable negative inotropism in the failing heart. It produces a decrease in the slope of diastolic depolarization, isolated prolongation of the atrial and ventricular action potentials, and depression of the AV node. It is useful in the chronic prophylaxis of recalcitrant arrhythmias associated with preexcitation. It is effective in both supraventricular and ventricular tachyarrhythmias. The production of corneal pigments, a gray skin discoloration, and thyroid dysfunction must be weighed against its benefits.

Bretylium. Bretylium is capable of markedly reducing the vunerability to recurrent ventricular tachycardia and fibrillation associated with an acute myocardial infarction. This agent has a biphasic response. First, there is a release of norepinephrine with increased conduction velocity, increased spontaneous heart rate, and a decreased refractory period. This is followed by a depletion of norepinephrine stores, which tends to lengthen action potential duration and the effective refractory period. It is not effective in the treatment of supraventricular arrhythmias, but can be dramatic in the control of resistant ventricular tachycardia or ventricular fibrillation unresponsive to other antiarrhythmic agents.

The majority of the newer drugs presented are still investigational. These agents, in addition to many other drugs, will add to the armamentarium of the physician dealing with chronic and refractory arrhythmias.

Chest Thump

This was recommended to treat ventricular tachycardia by Pennington in 1970.[47] He reported its use in terminating twelve episodes of ventricular tachycardia in five patients with coronary heart disease. The chest thump is performed by hitting the mid-sternum with a fist raised 12 inches (30 cm) off the chest. This moderate thump should be delivered only one time. This will deliver from 4 to 5 watt/sec of energy which may convert ventricular tachycardia to sinus rhythm. This small energy discharge works by interrupting a reentry mechanism similar to a pacemaker spike converting an arrhythmia. The present American Heart Association recommendation is to use the chest thump *only* in two situations: (1) a witnessed cardiac arrest and (2) a monitored cardiac arrest. In both of these situations, the heart is oxygenated and the thump can be applied within 15 seconds of the arrest. If it fails to convert the arrhythmia to regular sinus rhythm, cardiopulmonary resuscitation should be instituted immediately.

Cardioversion

Since its introduction by Lown in 1962, direct current cardioversion has been widely utilized in the treatment of cardiac arrhythmias.[48] It is used to treat ventricular tachycardia and acute or chronic atrial fibrillation or flutter, and is performed by using a *synchronized DC shock* applied either directly to the heart or through the chest wall. Pulse discharge is synchronized to occur within 20 msec of the peak of the R wave on the ECG, thereby avoiding the period of ventricular vulnerability at the peak of the T wave. The shock depolarizes all the fibers that are excitable at that instant and allows the SA node to reinitiate the normal cardiac rhythm. Synchronization is important to avoid inadvertant ventricular fibrillation, which will occur about 2 percent of the time in nonsynchronized cardioversion.[49] All recent cardioverter/defibrillator machines have a synchronizer switch which must be turned on to achieve synchronization.

For *external* cardioversion, the paddles are placed in the same position as for defibrillation: one paddle over the apex of the heart and the other to the right of the sternum. Atrial flutter is the easiest rhythm to convert

and usually requires about 50 watt/sec externally. For atrial fibrillation or ventricular tachycardia, 200 watt/sec externally frequently is effective, but 300 to 400 watt/sec may be required. For *internal* cardioversion, the paddles are placed across the atria for treatment of supraventricular arrhythmias and on the ventricles for treatment of ventricular tachycardia. Much lower energy levels are needed for internal cardioversion than for external cardioversion. All supraventricular tachycardias are treated with 5 to 10 watt/sec; ventricular arrhythmias are also initially treated with 10 watt/sec, but may require an increase to 30 watt/sec to be effective.

Internal cardioversion may be very useful during cardiac surgery. Atrial arrhythmias are frequently produced by cannulation of the right atrium for cardiopulmonary bypass. These arrhythmias are often very rapid, and poorly tolerated by these cardiac patients. Their occurrence appears to be more frequent in patients with right coronary artery disease, hypovolemia, hypokalemia, or with rough surgeons. If cannulation is almost complete, it is preferable to go directly on bypass to support the circulation. However, if cannulation is not completed, the heart should be cardioverted immediately back into sinus rhythm rather than beginning with pharmacologic therapy.

Elective external cardioversion is indicated for patients with recent onset (less than one year) of atrial fibrillation or flutter. Elective cardioversion in postoperative open-heart patients should be deferred for at least 3 weeks after surgery. Contraindications include long-term atrial fibrillation, underlying heart block, recent systemic embolization, a giant left atrium, or digitalis toxicity. Digitalis intoxication is especially important because cardioversion of these patients can produce serious arrhythmias or even resistant ventricular fibrillation. Therefore, digitalis is discontinued 24 to 48 hours before elective cardioversion. Quinidine is frequently begun at this time in an effort to maintain sinus rhythm after the cardioversion. Anticoagulants are not routinely used but may be utilized for patients with a prior history of embolization.

Defibrillation

In 1899, Prevost and Batelli, in France, observed that an electric shock could cause ventricular fibrillation and a second shock could stop it. In 1933, Kouwenhoven confirmed that a dog with a fibrillating heart could be converted to regular sinus rhythm by an electric countershock. In 1940, Wiggers studied ventricular fibrillation and showed that an alternating current (AC) shock (termed a *countershock*) could normalize the heart rhythm. The first successful human defibrillation was performed by Beck in 1947 with an AC defibrillator.[49] Because of their long discharge time, tendency to produce tissue damage, and the inability to be synchronized, AC defibrillators have been replaced by DC defibrillators.

In 1966, Nachlas demonstrated the superiority of DC over AC defibrillators. DC defibrillators have the following advantages:

1. Small size and portability
2. Ability to synchronize
3. More powerful and shorter discharge time (3–5 msec)
4. More effective than AC defibrillators

Considerable controversy exists regarding the proper amount of delivered energy that should be utilized for external defibrillation.[50] Recent reports suggesting megadose defibrillation (500–1000 watt/sec) have been proposed but appear excessive and unwarranted. Animal studies have demonstrated increased myocardial cellular injury and increased cardiac arrhythmias when large dose defibrillation was undertaken. Human studies have demonstrated cellular damage with ECG changes, increased myocardial isoenzyme concentrations, and abnormal radioactive imaging with increased delivered energy. High-dose defibrillation may produce irreversible myocardial cell damage and reduce the possibility of subsequent successful defibrillation.

Adgey and coworkers cite the effectiveness of a 200 watt/sec dose to patients up to 100 kg with a success rate of 95 percent.[51] If unsuccessful, a second or third dose at the same 200 watt/sec level increases the success rate even further. Various factors exclusive of delivered energy may be important to determine success of defibrillation: (1) quality of CPR (acidosis, hypoxia), (2) length of delay before the first defibrillatory attempt, (3) underlying disease state, (4) length of fibrillation, and (5) transthoracic resistance (paddle position and size, pressure, pads, or gels). The presence of antiarrhythmic drugs (quinidine, lidocaine, procainamide) increases the threshold to defibrillation and may alter the effectiveness of defibrillation. Certain causes of ventricular fibrillation (*e.g.*, digitalis toxicity) may preclude effective defibrillation regardless of energy delivered.

The current American Heart Association guidelines for ventricular defibrillation suggest from 3.5 to 6.0 watt/sec/kg should be delivered in patients under 50 kg; in patients over 50 kg, 400 watt/sec should be used initially. However, because of the present trend toward studying delivered energy, many physicians would agree with Adgey and Taylor's suggestion of an initial 200 watt/second dose of delivered energy, or 4 watt/sec/kg, which may be repeated as needed. If unsuccessful, then the energy should be increased to higher levels.

With internal defibrillation, significant epicardial damage has occurred with delivered energy greater than 30 watt/sec and with short time intervals between successive shocks. Therefore, attempts at energy levels less than 30 watt/sec are recommended for initial internal defibrillation.

To terminate ventricular defibrillation, a DC shock is the recommended treatment. When performing external cardiac defibrillation, proper electrode position should always be used: one electrode just to the right of the upper sternum below the clavicle, the other electrode adjacent to the cardiac apex or left nipple. An effective conductive medium must be applied to the electrode surface to minimize skin resistance and allow optimum energy delivery. Improper electrode positioning over the sternum or other large boney structures reduces delivered energy because of the poor conductivity of bone. Standard electrode gel reduces skin resistance, but often its slipperiness impairs effective cardiac compression with simultaneous CPR. Saline-soaked gauze sponges are excellent conductors and effectively reduce the skin resistance. Firm pressure to the electrode paddles also increases the energy delivered.

1. What is the heart rate?
2. Is the rhythm regular?
3. Is there one P wave for each QRS? (Is there block?)
4. Is the QRS complex normal?
5. Is the rhythm dangerous?
6. Does the rhythm requires treatment?

APPROACH TO ARRHYTHMIAS[52, 53]

The best leads, in order of preference, to diagnose arrhythmias are the following:

1. V_1: Use four limb electrodes and the V electrode placed in the fourth intercostal space to the right of the sternum. However, this requires a five-electrode system. It shows a good atrial deflection and QRS complex.
2. MCL_1 (Modified chest lead one): A three-electrode system most easily set up by placing the left-arm electrode under the left clavicle (negative electrode); the left-leg electrode in the V_1 position in the fourth intercostal space to the right of the sternum (positive electrode); and the right-arm electrode in the usual position (ground). The lead selector switch is placed on lead III.
3. II: Standard lead II is the third choice. It reflects a good atrial deflection, but not necessarily a good QRS complex.

The six key diagnostic questions to ask are:

Supraventricular arrhythmias

Sinus Arrhythmia. The sinus node irregularly forms impulses. There are two types of sinus arrhythmias: (1) varies with respiration, heart rate accelerates with inspiration; and (2) no relationship to respiration (rare type) (Fig. 6-12).

1. Heart rate: 60–100
2. Rhythm: Irregular
3. P:QRS: 1:1; all P waves the same
4. QRS complex: Normal
5. Significance: Normal finding; do not confuse with more serious problems
6. Treatment: None

Premature Atrial Contractions (PAC). These arise from an atrial focus other than the SA node and, therefore, are ectopic. They discharge the atria before the next SA nodal impulse and are, therefore, premature. They are recognized by a premature, abnormally shaped P wave, and usually a normal QRS

Fig. 6-12. Sinus arrhythmia.

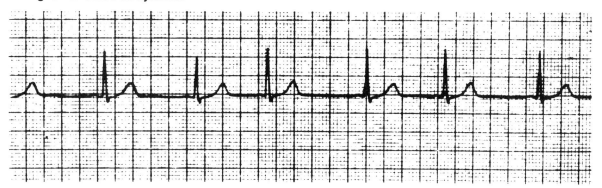

complex. They tend to reset the SA node and cause a slight pause, but not a full compensatory pause (Fig. 6-13).

1. Heart rate: variable, depending on frequency of PACs
2. Rhythm: Irregular
3. P:QRS: Usually 1:1; the P waves have various shapes and may even be lost in the QRS or T waves. Occasionally, the P wave will be so early as to find the ventricle refractory. Then it will not be conducted, and will have no QRS complex.
4. QRS complex: usually normal; occasionally, the PAC may find part of the ventricular conduction system refractory. Then it will travel down an aberrant pathway, and create an abnormal QRS complex. This is called a premature atrial contraction with *ventricular aberration*, and can be very easily confused with a premature ventricular contraction.

Helpful points in telling a PAC with aberration from a PVC are (1) there is a pre-ceding P wave that is usually abnormally shaped; (2) the complex is frequently of a right bundle branch configuration; (3) there is a rSR' in V_1; and (4) the initial vector force is *identical* with the preceding beat, but is usually the opposite with a PVC.

5. Significance: Usually not dangerous, but very frequent PACs can lead to other supraventricular tachyarrhythmias.
6. Treatment: Usually none; rarely, digitalis or propranolol, if the arrhythmia is causing poor hemodynamic function

Sinus Bradycardia. Discharge site is the SA node but at a slower than normal rate. Occasionally, other pacemaker sites will try to take over and cause premature beats (*e.g.,* PVCs)(Fig. 6-14).

1. Heart rate: 40 to 60 beats/min; in patients taking chronic propranolol therapy, this arrhythmia has been redefined as a heart rate less than 50 beats/min.

Fig. 6-13. Premature atrial contractions are demonstrated at the arrows.

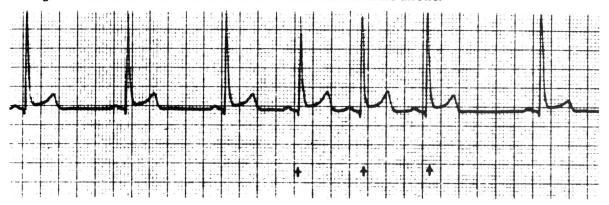

Fig. 6-14. Sinus bradycardia.

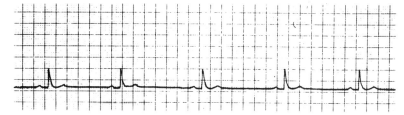

2. Rhythm: Regular, except for premature "escape" beats which occasionally occur
3. P:QRS: 1:1
4. QRS complex: Normal
5. Significance: This is the goal for patients treated with propranolol for ischemic heart disease. It may be seen with acute inferior myocardial infarction, and many drugs (*e.g.*, morphine and neostigmine). It is of little significance unless it is affecting peripheral or cardiac perfusion (such as in aortic insufficiency) or is associated with hypotension or PVCs. Heart rates below 40 beats/min are rarely tolerated very long and require treatment. This may be part of the *sick sinus syndrome* in which sinus node dysfunction can precipitate bradycardia, heart block, various tachyarrhythmias, or alternating bradytachyarrhythmias.
6. Treatment: Usually none; atropine (0.3–2.0 mg IV) if associated with hypotension or PVCs; rarely, isoproterenol infusion (4 μg/ml) or a pacemaker will be required.

Sinus Tachycardia. Discharge site is the SA node, but at a faster than normal rate. This is a very common arrhythmia during and after surgery. Determining its cause is frequently the main problem. Included among the possible etiologies are pain, hypovolemia, fever, emotion, heart failure, and hyperthyroidism (Fig. 6-15).

1. Heart rate: Above 100 beats/min; the top rate is 150 to 170 beats/min, which is usually seen with a high fever.

2. Rhythm: Regular
3. P:QRS: 1:1
4. QRS complex: Normal
5. Significance: Prolonged rapid heart rates in patients with underlying heart disease can precipitate congestive heart failure. The fast heart rate decreases coronary perfusion time, which can cause secondary ST-T wave changes and can precipitate angina in patients with coronary artery disease. The usual problem is finding the underlying cause of the problem; light anesthesia and hypovolemia are the most common intraoperative causes.

If the heart rate is *150 beats/min*, it can be a major diagnostic problem. This is a common heart rate for three arrhythmias: (1) sinus tachycardia; (2) paroxysmal atrial tachycardia (PAT); and (3) atrial flutter with 2:1 block.

There are three diagnostic maneuvers to try to separate these three arrhythmias.

a. Carotid sinus massage: A sinus tachycardia will gradually slow and then speed up again or it will be unaffected; a PAT will usually break and revert to sinus rhythm or it will be unaffected; and atrial flutter with 2:1 block will usually increase the heart block and make the atrial flutter waves more obvious.
b. Edrophonium (Tensilon): A dosage of 1–10 mg IV will accentuate the carotid massage effects.
c. Atrial or esophageal ECG leads to better observe the P waves.

Fig. 6-15. Sinus tachycardia.

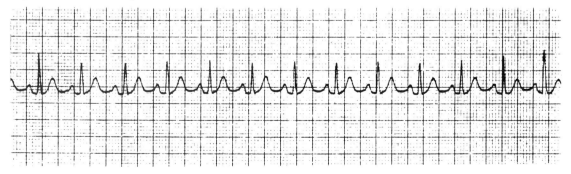

6. Treatment: Treat the underlying cause. While determining the cause, propranolol may be used in patients with ischemic heart disease or in those who develop ST-T wave changes, in an effort to prevent further myocardial ischemia.

Paroxysmal Atrial Tachycardia (PAT). This is a run of rapidly repeated supraventricular premature beats from a site other than the SA node (Fig. 6-16). This rhythm is frequently very rapid and can lead to severe ST-T wave changes that may persist even after the rate slows (the post-tachycardia syndrome). This arrhythmia is frequently seen in patients with the Wolff–Parkinson–White syndrome in which an abnormal conduction pathway is present.

Wolff–Parkinson–White is characterized by normal P wave contour, a PR interval less than 0.12 m, and an abnormal ventricular complex which includes the inscription of an abnormal delta wave. A normal impulse begins in the SA node and proceeds down interatrial pathway tissue to the AV node area where a transient delay occurs before activation through the His bundle to the ventricular Purkinje system. In the preexcitation syndrome, the delay at the AV node is bypassed by way of various anomalous pathways (Kent fibers in Wolff–Parkinson–White, James fibers in Lown–Ganong–Levine; and Mahaim fibers in Mahaim pathway) with activation of the His bundle by the more rapid anomalous conduction. Ventricular excitation is a composite of the normal as well as the anomalous stimulus resulting in an abnormal QRS inscription (*e.g.*, delta wave in Wolff–Parkinson–White). In the Lown–Ganong–Levine syndrome, an anomalous pathway is present with a shortened PR interval, but no ventricular abnormality is noted.

Because of the anomalous pathways, the tendency to frequent supraventricular arrhythmias, especially PAT and atrial fibrillation with rapid conduction over the anomalous pathway, is present. Atrial flutter is rarer in the preexcitation syndrome. These syndromes are frequently associated with the following cardiac disorders: balloon mitral valve, Ebstein's anomaly of the tricuspid valve, and coronary artery disease. Frequent tachyarrhythmias develop through a reentry mechanism whereby antegrade conduction occurs down the abnormal AV pathway with retrograde conduction through the anomalous path.

1. Heart rate: 150 to 250 beats/min
2. Rhythm: Usually regular except if a multifocal atrial tachycardia (MAT) exists
3. P:QRS: 1:1; P waves frequently abnormal
4. QRS complex: Normal; ST-T depression common
5. Significance: This may occur under anesthesia and produce severe hemodynamic deterioration. It can be precipitated by changes in the autonomic nervous system, drug effects, or volume shifts. It may be seen in 5 percent of normal young adults and many patients with Wolff–Parkinson–White. It may be associated with atrioventricular block caused by the fast atrial rate and slow AV conduction. PAT with 2:1 block represents digitalis intoxication in 50 percent of the cases. PAT is seen often in elderly patients with advanced heart disease.
6. Treatment: This arrhythmia frequently has to be treated because of its rapid rate and associated poor hemodynamic function.

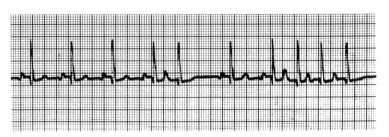

Fig. 6-16. Paroxysmal atrial tachycardia.

a. Carotid sinus massage is frequently effective, but should only be applied to one side, and used carefully in elderly patients with cerebrovascular disease. Eyeball pressure to achieve vagal stimulation should not be used.

b. Edrophonium (Tensilon) in 1 to 10 mg doses slowly given intravenously frequently increases vagal tone enough to make carotid massage effective.

c. If the patient is hypotensive, an alpha-adrenergic stimulator such as neo-synephrine can be used in 100 μg doses to increase the blood pressure and achieve a reflex vagal slowing.

d. Propranolol in 0.5 mg doses will frequently slow the PAT and may be used in combination with digitalis (propranolol 0.5 mg and digoxin 0.25 mg).

e. Lidocaine (50–100 mg) may be tried, and may work if the mechanism of the arrhythmia and conduction are over an anomalous pathway.

f. Rapid overdrive pacing may be used to capture the ectopic focus and then the rate progressively slowed.

g. Cardioversion with appropriate synchronization may occasionally be required. This is used less now than in the past because propranolol is so effective.

h. Quinidine and procainamide have also frequently been used in the past, especially for prevention of these episodes in patients with Wolff–Parkinson–White.

i. Surgery is now occasionally used to excise the aberrant conduction pathway of the bundle of Kent in patients with Wolff–Parkinson–White who have frequent attacks of PAT even when receiving maximal medical therapy (see Chap. 8).

Atrial Flutter. This represents a *faster discharge* from an irritable focus in the atria than does a rapid atrial tachycardia. It is usually associated with AV block because the atrial rate is so fast. Classical saw-toothed flutter waves (F waves) are usually present (Fig. 6-17).

1. Heart rate: Atrial rate is 250 to 350 beats/min and the ventricular rate around 150 beats/min.
2. Rhythm: Atrial rhythm is regular, but ventricular may be regular if a fixed block or irregular if a variable block exists.
3. P:QRS: Usually 2:1 block with atrial rate of 300 and a ventricular rate of 150, but may vary between 2:1 and 8:1. F waves best seen in leads V_1 and II.
4. QRS complex: Normal; T waves lost in F waves
5. Significance: Usually associated with severe heart disease
6. Treatment: Two main forms of treatment are used. If the rhythm is being tolerated, it can be treated pharmacologically with digitalis and propranolol which will slow it and possibly convert it to atrial fibrillation. If there is acute hemodynamic deterioration, cardioversion, using very low voltage (10–40 watt/sec), is effective in more than 90 percent of cases.

Atrial Fibrillation. This is an excessively rapid and irregular atrial focus. There are no P waves on the ECG, but, instead, a fine fibrillatory activity called *f* waves. This is the most irregular rhythm and is thus called irregularly irregular. It is frequently associated with a pulse deficit (Fig. 6-18).

1. Heart rate: Atrial rate is 350 to 500 beats/min and ventricular rate, depending on treatment, is 60 to 170 beats/min.
2. Rhythm: Irregularly irregular

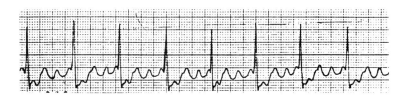

Fig. 6-17. Atrial flutter.

3. P:QRS: P waves are absent and replaced with f waves or there is no obvious atrial activity at all.
4. QRS complex: Normal; may have some aberrancy.
5. Significance: Usually associated with severe heart disease; loss of atrial contraction tends to decrease cardiac output. This rhythm must be differentiated from (1) atrial flutter with varying block (atrial fib-flutter); (2) frequent premature beats; (3) sinus rhythm with varying block; (4) gross sinus arrhythmia; and (5) wandering atrial pacemaker. Atrial fibrillation or flutter commonly occur during cannulation of the right atrium for cardiopulmonary bypass.
6. Treatment: Digitalis is usually used to slow the ventricular response. Propranolol may also be added. In atrial fibrillation of recent onset, especially after cardiac surgery, cardioversion may be used to reestablish sinus rhythm. Lidocaine should be avoided or used cautiously in patients with atrial fibrillation because it can markedly increase atrioventricular conduction and lead to an accelerated ventricular response. Internal cardioversion should be used if this rhythm occurs during cannulation for bypass.

Junctional Rhythm (Nodal). The impulse arises in the AV juctional tissue. It travels down into the ventricles in the normal fashion and travels retrograde into the atrium (the P wave may be distorted). There are three varieties of this rhythm:

High-nodal rhythm: The impulse reaches the atrium before the ventricle and, therefore, the P wave precedes the QRS but has a shortened PR interval (less than 0.1 second).
Mid-nodal rhythm: The impulse arrives in the atrium and the ventricle at the same time and the P wave is lost in the QRS (Fig. 6-19).
Low-nodal rhythm: The impulse reaches the ventricle first and then the atrium, so that the P wave follows the QRS complex.

1. Heart rate: Variable (40–180 beats/min); nodal bradycardia to nodal tachycardia
2. Rhythm: Regular
3. P:QRS: 1:1, but appears variable depending on the location of the P wave

Fig. 6-18. Atrial fibrillation.

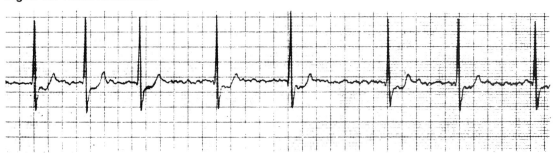

Fig. 6-19. Nodal (Junctional) rhythm.

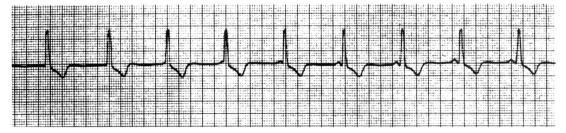

4. QRS complex: Normal, unless altered by the P wave
5. Significance: Junctional rhythms are common under anesthesia (about 20% of cases), especially with halogenated anesthetic agents or the ether drugs. The nodal rhythm frequently decreases blood pressure and cardiac output by about 15 percent, but it can decrease it by up to 30 percent in patients with heart disease.
6. Treatment: Usually no treatment is required and the rhythm reverts spontaneously. If hypotension and poor perfusion are associated with the rhythm, treatment is indicated. Atropine, ephedrine, or isoproterenol can be used in an effort to increase the activity of the SA node so it will take over as the pacemaker. A small dose of succinylcholine (10 mg intravenously) may revert a nodal rhythm to a sinus rhythm during anesthesia with halothane and enflurane. This probably works because of succinylcholine's effect as a sympathetic ganglionic stimulator.

Ventricular Arrhythmias

Premature Ventricular Contractions (PVCs). These are premature ectopics arising from a focus below the AV junction, and are one of the most common arrhythmias seen in anesthesia and in patients with cardiac disease. They are usually identified as premature, having a wide QRS complex, an ST-segment that slopes in the opposite direction from the QRS, and a compensatory pause associated with these premature beats. There is no P wave visible with these beats in most situations. Interpolated PVCs occur between two normal beats and there is no compensatory pause. Usually, PVCs are coupled to regular beats (fixed coupling); however, occasionally they are not coupled and thus fire off at their own rate. This latter pattern is called *parasystole* (variable coupling), and is identified by an irregular interval between the normal beat and the PVCs (Fig. 6-20).

1. Heart rate: Depends on the frequency of the PVCs
2. Rhythm: Irregular
3. P:QRS: No P waves are seen.
4. QRS complex: Wide and bizarre with a width of over 0.12 sec. The T wave is directed in the opposite manner.
5. Significance: Potentially a very dangerous arrhythmia that can proceed to ventricular tachycardia or fibrillation. The most dangerous forms are multiple PVCs (> 5 per minute), multifocal PVCs (several ectopic ventricular foci), coupled PVCs (bigeminy), short runs of PVCs (more than three in a row is frequently considered ventricular tachycardia), or the R-on-T phenomenon (PVCs near the vulnerable period which can precipitate ventricular fibrillation). The PVCs also decrease coronary blood flow and saphenous vein bypass-graft blood flow.
6. Treatment: The first step is to correct any underlying abnormalities, such as a low potassium, reduced arterial oxygen tension, increased arterial carbon dioxide tension, or acid-base disturbance. Lidocaine is the treatment of choice with an initial dose of 1.0 to 1.5 mg/kg intravenously as a bolus. If PVCs persist or recur, another lidocaine bolus (1.0 mg/kg) followed im-

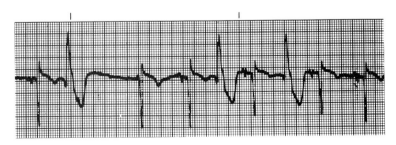

Fig. 6-20. Premature ventricular contractions.

mediately with a lidocaine infusion (1–4 mg/min) is generally effective in suppressing the ventricular ectopy. Propranolol, procainamide, and quinidine are excellent second-line drugs for control of premature ventricular ectopic beats. These must be used with caution when administered intravenously because of their marked myocardial depressant properties. A relatively recent addition, bretylium, is effective in controlling resistant ventricular arrhythmias, especially those complicating an acute myocardial infarction. Bretylium has also been helpful in the correction of ventricular fibrillation resistant to defibrillation. Caution should be used, particularly in the patient who still has a recordable blood pressure, because bretylium can produce severe hypotension.

Ventricular Tachycardia. This arrhythmia consists of rapidly repeated ectopic beats which can be life-threatening. Three coupled PVCs constitute ventricular tachycardia. Diagnostic criteria include the presence of (1) fusion beats (the ventricle is activated partially by the atrial impulse and partially by the ventricular impulse), (2) capture beats (these are conducted SA nodal beats), and (3) AV dissociation in which unrelated P waves can be identified (Fig. 6-21).

1. Heart rate: 100 to 250 beats/min
2. Rhythm: Usually regular but may be irregular if the ventricular tachycardia is paroxysmal

3. P:QRS: No fixed relationship; ventricular tachycardia is a form of atrioventricular dissociation. The P waves can be seen marching through the QRS complex.
4. QRS complex: Wide, over 0.12 sec in width with P waves marching through
5. Significance: Acute onset, life-threatening, and requires immediate treatment; however, many patients have chronic ventricular tachycardia and tolerate it quite well.
6. Treatment: A lidocaine bolus will frequently convert this to sinus rhythm. Cardioversion is needed in some patients.

Ventricular Fibrillation. The ventricles discharge in a completely chaotic, asynchronous fashion without effective output. There is no clear-cut ventricular complex seen on the ECG. The most important conditions precipitating this arrhythmia are myocardial ischemia, electrolyte imbalance, hypoxia, hypothermia, slow conduction, and drugs increasing automaticity (Fig. 6-22).

1. Heart rate: Rapid and grossly disorganized
2. Rhythm: Totally irregular
3. P:QRS: None are seen
4. QRS complex: Not present
5. Significance: There is no effective cardiac output and life must be sustained by artificial means (external massage or extracorporeal circulation). Ventricular fibrillation has been of great concern to anesthesiologists since first reported by Guedel in 1936.

Fig. 6-21. A short run of ventricular tachycardia.

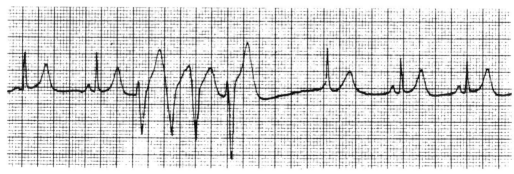

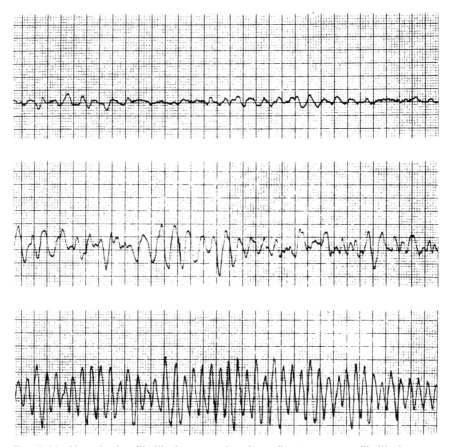

Fig. 6-22. Ventricular fibrillation, ranging from fine to course fibrillation.

6. Treatment: Cardiopulmonary resuscitation must be initiated immediately. Defibrillation is the standard definitive treatment, the external dosage being 200 to 400 watt/sec, the internal dosage 10 to 60 watt/sec. This is frequently unsuccessful if electrolyte or acid-base status is out of balance. Pharmacologic therapy has occasionally been successful with bretylium, lidocaine, or propranolol, even when defibrillation has not been successful.

Ventricular Asystole. No ventricular activity is present. In association with a cardiac arrest this suggests an extremely grave prognosis. Occasionally, patients have had transient atrioventricular standstill lasting up to 20 seconds as a result of vagal stimuli or drugs, producing cerebral ischemia and requiring resuscitation. During cardiac surgery, asystole is frequently produced by injecting a hypothermic, hyperkalemic cardioplegic solution into the coronary circulation to reduce oxygen requirements (Fig. 6-23).

1. Heart rate: None present
2. Rhythm: Straight line on the ECG (Must be sure ECG is not disconnected from the patient)
3. P:QRS: None present
4. QRS complex: Absent
5. Significance: Second most common rhythm associated with a cardiac arrest (ventricular fibrillation is first). It is difficult to treat, and an attempt should be made to convert it to ventricular fibrillation.

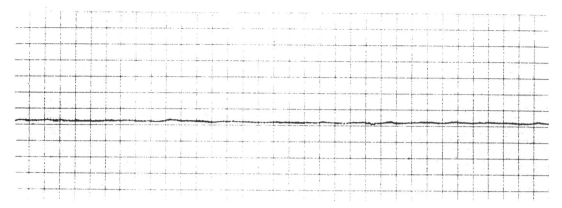

Fig. 6-23. Ventricular asystole.

6. Treatment: Maintain cardiopulmonary resuscitation while administering calcium chloride, isoproterenol, epinephrine, $NaHCO_2$, and inserting a transvenous pacemaker.

HEART BLOCKS:
DIAGNOSIS AND TREATMENT

Two types of blocks will be discussed in this section: intraventricular conduction disturbances and atrioventricular heart block.[54] Bundle of His electrograms have greatly improved understanding of AV conduction. A normal ECG and His bundle electrogram (HBE) are shown in Figure 6-24 along with their recording locations.

The normal intervals are as follows:

1. The P-H Interval: From the onset of P wave to the His complex (normal = 119 ± 38 msec). This complex is made up of
   a. A-H interval: From the atrial electrogram to the His complex (normal = 92 ± 38 msec)
   b. P-A interval: From the onset of the P wave to the atrial electrogram (normal = 27 ± 18 msec)

2. H-R or H-V interval: From the His complex to the R wave or ventricular electrogram (normal = 43 ± 12 msec).

Intraventricular Conduction Disturbances

Left Bundle Branch Block (LBBB). The impulse reaches the ventricles exclusively through the right bundle branch and there is a wide QRS complex of more than 0.12 sec and a wide, notched R wave seen in leads I, AVL, and V_6. Also, there is no Q wave in V_6. The most important leads to study in bundle branch blocks are I, V_1 and V_6.

The pattern of LBBB in V_6 is similar to LVH but exaggerated. The QRS complex interval is longer and the ST-T changes are more pronounced because of the slow conduction in LBBB. A similar pattern with a QRS duration of less than 0.12 sec (0.10–0.11) occurs when there is an incomplete LBBB. The H-V interval is almost always prolonged in LBBB.

Right Bundle Branch Block (RBBB). The QRS complex exceeds 0.11 seconds, leads V_1 to V_3 have broad RSR' complexes, and leads I and V_6 have wide S waves. An incomplete RBBB is diagnosed if the QRS duration is from 0.09 to 0.10 seconds with the RBBB configuration. Unlike LBBB, which is always associated with heart disease, RBBB may be of no clinical consequence. Its overall incidence is about 1 percent in hospitalized patients. Incomplete RBBB is frequently present in patients with elevated right ventricular pressures (*e.g.*, chronic lung disease or atrial septal defects).

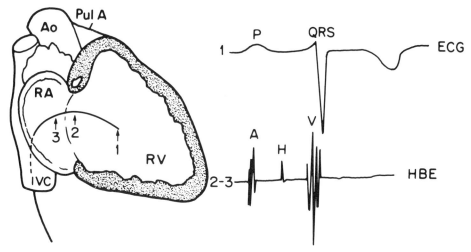

Fig. 6-24. An intracardiac electrocardiographic lead is shown coming up thorough the inferior vena cava, the right atrium, and across the tricuspid valve, with the tip in the right ventricle. A normal ECG is shown as well as the intracavitary HIS bundle electrograph. (Akhtar M, Damato AN: Clinical use of HIS bundle electrocardiography. Am Heart J 91:520, 1976)

Hemiblocks. This is the term for blockage of one of the two main divisions of the *left* bundle branch. If both divisions are blocked, then LBBB exists. Even though hemiblocks are a form of intraventricular block, the QRS complex is not prolonged. The order and direction of ventricular activation is altered, but the time required for depolarization is not markedly prolonged. Marriott's criteria for a left anterior hemiblock (LAH) are:

1. Left axis deviation greater than $-60°$
2. Small Q in lead I, small R in III
3. Normal QRS duration

The criteria for left posterior hemiblock (LPH) are:

1. Right axis deviation greater than $+120°$
2. Small R in lead I, small Q in III
3. Normal QRS duration
4. No RVH

The hemiblocks can occur by themselves, but LAH and LPH are frequently associated with RBBB to form a bilateral bundle branch block. Hearts with RBBB and LAH progress to complete heart block (trifascicular block) in

only 10 percent of patients; while hearts with RBBB and LPH usually proceed to complete heart block.

The anesthesiologist must be concerned with these conduction defects because of the possibility of complete heart block developing during or after anesthesia, and the need to decide if a pacemaker is indicated in the perioperative period. Rooney studied 27 patients undergoing surgery who had RBBB and LAH. None of these patients developed further conduction problems, and routine use of a pacemaker was found not to be needed.[55] Patients with RBBB and LPH are more controversial. If they are symptomatic, the author feels that they *possibly* should have a temporary pacemaker placed before major surgical procedures.

Intermittent Block. Rate-related bundle branch blocks are not uncommon and have been reported during general anesthesia. When a critical heart rate is exceeded, conduction through a diseased bundle branch can become blocked. Heart rates above 120 beats/min can produce either RBBB or LBBB and can be mistaken for a ventricular tachycardia because both have wide QRS complexes and abnormal ST-T changes.

Atrioventricular Heart Block (A-V Block)

AV block may be incomplete or complete. First and second degree A-V blocks are incomplete, while third-degree A-V block is complete heart block.

First-Degree Heart Block. This is a delay in passage of the impulse through the A-V node with the PR interval greater than 0.21 sec. The A-H interval is prolonged on the HBE (Fig. 6-25).

1. Heart rate: Normal
2. Rhythm: Regular
3. P:QRS: 1:1 with no dropped beats
4. QRS complex: Normal
5. Significance: May be normal; also seen in patients taking digitalis or those with rheumatic fever
6. Treatment: Usually none; the PR interval may be shortened with atropine or catecholamines.

Second-Degree Heart Block. There are two types of second degree block:

1. Mobitz type I block: Reflects disease of the AV node
2. Mobitz type II block: Reflects disease of the His bundle-Purkinje tissues. In both of these blocks, some P waves are not followed by QRS complexes.

Mobitz I Block (Wenckebach). There is a progressive lengthening of the PR interval until a QRS complex is dropped. This form of block is *relatively benign,* frequently reversible (*e.g.,* digitalis intoxication), and does not require a pacemaker (Fig. 6-26).

1. Heart rate: Atrial rate is normal and the ventricular rate depends on the degree of AV block
2. Rhythm: Irregular ventricular response caused by the varying PR interval
3. P:QRS: More P waves than QRS complexes
4. QRS complex: Normal
5. Significance: Generally caused by digitalis toxicity or myocardial infarction; it is transient and does not require pacing.
6. Treatment: Discontinue digitalis; if the rate is very slow, atropine, isoproterenol, or pacing can be used.

Mobitz II Block. This is the less common and *more serious* form of second-degree heart block. P waves occur without subsequent QRS complexes. These are just "dropped beats" without any lengthening of the PR interval (Fig. 6-27).

1. Heart rate: Atrial rate is normal, and the ventricular rate depends on the number of dropped beats.
2. Rhythm: Irregular ventricular response caused by the irregularly dropped beats.
3. P:QRS: More P waves than QRS complex. The PR intervals are normal when present.
4. QRS complex: Normal, but a bundle branch block is frequently present
5. Significance: This is seen only when the block occurs in the His–Purkinje system, and has a *serious prognosis* because it frequently progresses to complete heart block.
6. Treatment: Atropine or isoproterenol can usually restore 1:1 conduction. Pacemaker insertion should be considered for major surgery.

Third-Degree Heart Block (Complete Heart Block). In this situation, no impulses from the atrium can reach the ventricle, and the

Fig. 6-25. First-degree (1°) heart block.

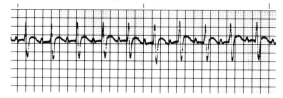

Fig. 6-26. Second-degree (2°) Mobitz I block.

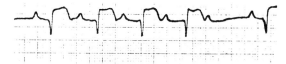

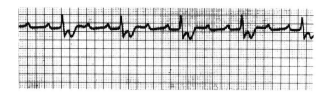

Fig. 6-27. Second-degree (2°) Mobitz II block.

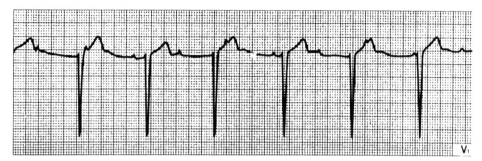

Fig. 6-28. Third-degree (3°) heart block.

ventricles act as the pacemaker of the heart. There is no relationship between the P waves and QRS complexes (Fig. 6-28).

1. Heart rate: 30 to 40 beats/min
2. Rhythm: Regular
3. P:QRS: No relationship; more P waves than QRS complexes
4. QRS complex: May be normal if the pacer site is in the AV node, but usually is widened to longer than 0.12 seconds with the pacer site in the ventricle.
5. Significance: The heart rate is too slow to maintain adequate cardiac output, and syncope (Stokes–Adams syndrome) and heart failure will occur.
6. Treatment: Pacemaker. Atropine or isoproterenol may temporarily increase the heart rate.

SUMMARY

Although the ECG does not provide direct information about pump performance, it is helpful in detecting arrhythmias that affect pump performance, and ischemia, which can result in muscle death. In order to use the ECG properly, however, lead placement must be modified from that customary for acquiring a written record to supplement a cardiologist's evaluation during nonacute care. The anesthesiologist must master the rules of interpretation most useful in monitoring situations. And, the effects of physiologic disruption, due to illness or the techniques of care (as electrolyte abnormalities, hypothermia, etc.) must be taken into consideration in evaluating the ECG.

Though this approach may seem complex, the careful practitioner soon realizes that an orderly approach makes therapy quite manageable. One must first decide how significant the findings are (immediate and life threatening, an indicator of undesirable trends, or academically interesting, or unchangeable); select the appropriate therapy (usually a change in life support, drugs or electrolytes, or electric shock); and titrate the response, with an appropriate understanding of the nature of the time course that can be expected. And one must be particularly careful not to overlook the simpler but accessible modalities available during intensive care (as oxygenation, electrolyte adjustment, and control of pH) in using the newer, more esoteric and aggressive alternatives.

Finally, one must avoid ascribing too much meaning to a measurement that has become classic in application because of its convenience and reliability. An adequate ECG does not guarantee adequate pump performance, and other measurements also must be used. It does provide, however, an early warning system, and is extraordinarily valuable, because of the reliability and simplicity of present ECG monitoring instruments.

REFERENCES

ECG Monitoring in the Operating Room
1. Kaplan JA: Electrocardiographic monitoring. In Kaplan JA (ed): Cardiac Anesthesia, pp 117–166. New York, Grune & Stratton, 1979
2. Katz RL, Bigger JT: Cardiac arrhythmias during anesthesia and operation. Anesthesiology 33:193–213, 1970
3. Kaplan JA, King, SB: The precordial electrocardiographic lead (V$_5$) in patients who have coronary artery disease. Anesthesiology 45:570–574, 1976
4. Arbeit SR, Rubin IL, Gross H: Dangers in interpreting the ECG from the oscilloscope monitor. JAMA 211:453–456, 1970
5. Doss JD, McCabe CW, Weiss GK: Noise free ECG data during electrosurgical procedures. Anesth Analg (Cleve) 52:156–160, 1973
6. Voukydis PC: Effect of intracardiac blood on the ECG. Am Heart J 82:55–61, 1971

Basic Electrophysiology and Cardiac Lead Systems
7. Titus JL: Normal anatomy of the human conduction system. Anesth Analg (Cleve) 52:508–514, 1973
8. Cranefield PF, Wit AL, Hoffman BF: Genesis of cardiac arrhythmias. Circulation 47:190–204, 1973
9. Marriott JHL: Practical Electrocardiology, 5th ed. Baltimore, Williams & Wilkins, 1972
10. Kaplan JA: Electrocardiographic monitoring. In Kaplan JA (ed): Cardiac Anesthesia, pp 117–166. New York, Grune & Stratton, 1979
11. Pozzi L: Basic Principles in Vector Electrocardiology. Springfield (Ill), Charles C Thomas, 1961
12. Mantel JA, Massing GK, James TN et al: A multipurpose catheter for electrocardiographic and hemodynamic monitoring plus atrial pacing. Chest 72:285–290, 1977
13. Akhtar M, Damato AN: Clinical uses of HIS bundle electrocardiography, part I. Am Heart J 91:520–526, 1976

A Systematic Approach to the ECG
14. Marriott JHL: Practical Electrocardiology, 5th ed. Baltimore, Williams & Wilkins, 1972

Ischemia and Infarction
15. Cannard TH, Dripps RD, Helwig J et al: The ECG during anesthesia and surgery. Anesthesiology 21:194–202, 1960
16. Russell PH, Coakley CS: Electrocardiographic observation in the operating room. Anesth Analg (Cleve) 48:784–788, 1969
17. Benchimol A, Harris CL, Desser KB et al: Resting ECG in major coronary artery disease. JAMA 224:1489–1492, 1973
18. Blackburn H: The exercise electrocardiogram: technological procedural, and conceptual development. In Henry Blackburn (ed): Measurements in Exercise Electrocardiography. Springfield (Ill) Charles C Thomas, 1967
19. Mason RE, Likar I, Biern RO et al: Multiple lead exercise electrocardiography. Circulation 36:517–525, 1967
20. Dalton B: A precordial ECG lead for chest operations. Anesth Analg (Cleve) 55:740–741, 1976
21. Kaplan JA, King SB: The precordial electrocardiographic lead (V$_5$) in patients who have coronary artery disease. Anesthesiology 45:570–574, 1976
22. Robertson D, Kostuk WJ, Ahuja SP: The localization of coronary artery stenosis by 12 lead ECG response to graded exercise test. Am Heart J 91:437–444, 1976
23. Froelicher VF, Wolthius R, Keiser N et al: A comparison of two bipolar exercise ECG leads to lead V$_5$. Chest 70:611–616, 1976
24. Ellestad MH: Stress-testing: Principles and Practice, pp 25–46. Philadelphia, FA Davis, 1975
25. Adams CW: T wave changes with inspiration. JAMA 216:1019–1022, 1971
26. Ghani MF, Parker BM, Smith JR: Recognition of myocardial infarction after cardiac surgery and its relation to cardiopulmonary bypass. Am Heart J 88:18–22, 1974
27. Dixon SA, Limbird LE, Roe CR et al: Recognition of postoperative acute myocardial infarction: application of isoenzyme techniques. Circulation (Suppl III) 47, 48:III-137–140, 1973
28. Steinberg L, Wisneski JA, Ullyot DJ et al: Significance of new Q waves after aortocoronary bypass surgery: correlation with changes in ventricular wall motion. Circulation 52:1037–1044, 1975

29. Bassan MM, Oatfield R, Hoffman I et al: New Q waves after aortocoronary bypass surgery: unmasking of an old infarction. N Engl J Med 290:349–353, 1974
30. Kennedy FB, Ticzon AR, Duffy FC et al: Disappearance of ECG pattern of inferior wall myocardial infarction after aortocoronary bypass surgery. J Thorac Cardiovasc Surg 74:585–593, 1977
31. Righetti A, Crawford MH, O'Rourke RA et al: Detection of perioperative myocardial damage after coronary artery bypass graft surgery. Circulation 55:173–178, 1977

Other Conditions Affecting the ECG
32. Surawicz B, Lasseter KC: Effect of drugs on the ECG. Prog Cardiovasc Dis 13:26–50, 1970
33. Surawicz B: Relationship between ECG and electrolytes. Am Heart J 73:814–834, 1967
34. Trevino A, Razi B, Beller BM: The characteristic ECG of accidental hypothermia. Arch Intern Med 127:470–473, 1971

Cardiac Arrhythmias
35. Kurtz CM, Bennett JH, Shapiro HH: ECG studies during surgical anesthesia. JAMA 106:434–440, 1936
36. Katz RL, Bigger JT: Cardiac arrhythmias during anesthesia and operation. Anesthesiology 33:193–213, 1970
37. Bertrand CA, Steiner NV, Jameson AG et al: Disturbances of cardiac rhythm during anesthesia and surgery. JAMA 216:1615–1617, 1971
38. Angelini L, Feldman MI, Lufschonowski R et al: Cardiac arrhythmias during and after heart surgery: diagnosis and management. Prog Cardiovasc Dis 16:469–495, 1974
39. Edwards R, Winnie AL, Ramamurthy S: Acute hypocapnic hypokalemia: an iatrogenic anesthetic complication. Anesth Analg (Cleve) 56:786–792, 1977
40. Koehntop DE, Liao JC, Van Bergen FH: Effects of pharmacologic alterations of adrenergic mechanisms by cocaine, tropolone, aminophylline, and ketamine on epinephrine-induced arrhythmias during halothane-nitrous oxide anesthesia. Anesthesiology 46:83–93, 1977
41. Fox EJ, Sklar GS, Hill CH et al: Complications related to the pressor response to endotracheal intubation. Anesthesiology 47:524–525, 1977
42. Borg DE: Paradox of cardiac arrhythmias in anaesthesia. Br J Anaesth 41:709–710, 1969

Physiologic Basis of Arrhythmias
43. Cranefield PF, Wit AL, Hoffman BF: Genesis of cardiac arrhythmias. Circulation 47:190–204, 1973
44. Moe GK, Mendez C: Physiologic basis of premature beats and sustained tachycardia. N Engl J Med 288:250–253, 1973

Treatment of Arrhythmias
45. Carson IW, Lyons SM, Shanks RG: Antiarrhythmic drugs. Br J Anaesth 51:659–670, 1979
46. Singh BN, Collett JT, Chew CY: New prospectives in the pharmacologic therapy of cardiac arrhythmia. Prog Cardiovasc Dis 22:243–301, 1980
47. Pennington JE, Taylor J, Lown B: Chest thump for reverting ventricular tachycardia. N Engl J Med 283:1192–1195, 1970
48. Glassman E: Direct current cardioversion. Am Heart J 82:128–130, 1971
49. Resnekov L: Present status of electroversion in the management of cardiac dysrhythmias. Circulation 47:1356–1363, 1973
50. Tacker WA, Ewy GA: Energy defibrillation dose: recommendations and rationale. Circulation 60:223, 1979
51. Adgey AA: Ventricular defibrillation: appropriate energy levels. Circulation 60:219, 1979

Approach to Arrhythmias
52. Schamroth L: How to approach an arrhythmia. Circulation 47:420–425, 1973
53. Kaplan JA: Electrocardiographic Monitoring. In Kaplan JA (ed): Cardiac Anesthesia, pp 117–166. New York, Grune & Stratton, 1979
54. Hecht HH, Kossman EC, Childers RW et al: Atrioventricular and intraventricular conduction: Revised nomenclature and concepts. Am J Cardiol 31:232–242, 1973
55. Rooney S–M, Goldiner PL, Muss E: Relationship of right bundle-branch block and marked left axis deviation to complete heart block during general anesthesia. Anesthesiology 44:64–66, 1976

7

Cardiac Pacing

JERRY C. GRIFFIN

INTRODUCTION

In the two decades since the first success, the use and quality of cardiac pacemakers have greatly increased. The number of indications has steadily increased and the efficacy of pacing for the management of these indications has been documented. Tremendous strides have been made in the reliability and complexity of pacing systems. [1-5] Approximately 1300 physicians, operating in 2515 hospitals, implanted pacemakers in the United States in 1978. In that year, these physicians implanted pacemakers in 66,000 new patients and replaced pacemakers in an additional 30,000. There are presently over 300,000 patients in the United States with cardiac pacemakers, or 1 for each 800 population.[6] Therefore, the perioperative management of patients with pacemakers and pacemaker implantation has become a significant and legitimate concern of the anesthesiologist, surgeon, and cardiologist.

ELECTROPHYSIOLOGY OF ARTIFICIAL CARDIAC PACING

ELECTRICAL STIMULATION

Cardiac contraction may be initiated by the passage of current through the myocardium between two electrodes. The electric field created between the two electrodes causes hyperpolarization of the membrane nearest the anodal electrode and reduction of membrane potential in that portion nearest the cathode.[7] If sufficient energy is applied, threshold voltage will be reached and a propagating depolarization will be initiated. The amount of electrical energy necessary to result in a spontaneous propagated depolarization is defined

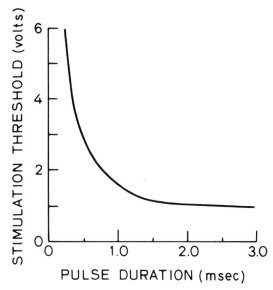

Fig. 7-1. Stimulus strength versus duration at threshold. The relationship between the voltage and duration of the stimulating pulse required for myocardial depolarization is not linear. However, above 1 msec, further increases in pulse duration have limited effect and, above 3–5 msec, no effect at all (rheobase).

as the *threshold of excitability* or *pacing threshold*. This is an intrinsic property of the myocardium and may be altered by certain drugs and physiologic states as described below. In addition, certain properties of the pacing system also play a major role in the determination of the measured threshold in any given instance.[8] Threshold may be described using several measures of electrical activity, most commonly the voltage or current necessary to induce reliable depolarization. However, threshold may also be defined as the charge (current times pulse duration) or energy (pulse duration times current times voltage) delivered.

There are three basic determinants of threshold. The first is the intrinsic excitability of the myocardium. A minimum current is necessary to induce depolarization. The second is the current density at the electrode-myocardial cell interface. Current density is defined as the current flow per square milli-

meter of effective electrode surface area. Electrodes of larger surface area will have correspondingly greater thresholds because current density is less for a fixed value of current. Likewise, because of the growth of a layer of fibrous tissue over the electride tip (effectively increasing the electrode surface area) thresholds on a given electrode tend to be higher after months or years than at the time of placement. The third important but nonlinear determinant of measured threshold is pulse duration. As pulse duration is increased, threshold decreases until a pulse duration of approximately 2 to 3 msec is reached. Varying pulse duration beyond this point has little effect (Fig. 7-1). In general, pulse durations in the range from 0.5 to 1.5 msec represent the best balance between low threshold and charge conservation.[9]

EXCITABILITY

In general, the intrinsic myocardial threshold for excitation remains relatively stable in a given patient with a well-placed electrode. However, small changes, usually within 50 percent of the resting threshold, do occur in certain physiologic situations as listed below.

Westerhom has shown that conditions of moderate hypoxia, or hypercarbia with or without hypoxia, result in a significant increase in stimulation threshold.[10] However, Doenecke observed a decrease in threshold

---

Determinants of Pacing Threshold

1. Myocardial factors
   a. Increased: Moderate hypoxia, hypercarbia, increased intracellular potassium, hypernatremia, sleep, post-parandial state.
   b. Decreased: Extreme hypoxia, hyperkalemia, exercise

2. Electrode factors
   a. Current Density (milliamperes/area of electrode surface)
   b. Impulse Duration

with extreme hypoxia and acidosis.[11] Increased oxygen tension, hypocarbia, and alkalosis seem to have little effect on threshold.

Altered electrolyte levels, particularly rapid changes in serum, sodium, and potassium also have a significant effect on excitability threshold. Potassium infusion with resulting increased serum potassium concentration tends to reduce threshold, while potassium administered in combination with insulin (thereby raising intracellular potassium) tends to increase threshold. Elevation of extracellular sodium by sodium infusion increases threshold. Infusion of calcium intravenously has little effect on excitability threshold (see Chap. 3).

The physiologic state of the patient may significantly alter threshold values. Simple orthostatic changes may result in small increases in threshold. Sleep results in a 30 to 40 percent increase in threshold. The postparandial state also results in an increase in threshold. However, exercise may result in an 30 to 40 percent decrease in threshold from the resting state.

Several drugs have an effect on excitability thresholds, but in general these effects are quite small, usually resulting in changes of less than 50 percent. Antiarrhythmic drugs are particularly striking in their lack of effect on stimulation threshold. Propranolol, procainamide, verapamil, and quinidine tend to increase threshold slightly. Diphenylhydantoin and lidocaine have been found to have essentially no effect while epinephrine and most catecholamines tend to decrease threshold. Digitalis seems to have little effect.

Although a wide variety of agents and physiologic conditions are capable of making alterations in excitability threshold, these changes are usually small and individually clinically insignificant. But in patients who have marginal thresholds under basal conditions, the effects of several of these conditions occurring simultaneously may result in clinically significant threshold changes and inadequate pacing. Therefore, any patient with inconsistent pacemaker capture should be screened for blood gas, electrolyte, and acid base abnormalities, and the drug history should be reviewed.

ELECTROCARDIOGRAPHY

The electrocardiographic rhythm strip and 12-lead ECG contain significant information about a pacemaker system and its function.[12] Each pacemaker impulse can usually be seen and distinguished from the resulting myocardial depolarization. The 12-lead ECG is helpful in determining the location of the pacing electrode. Patients with left-ventricular pacing electrodes have a right bundle branch block (RBBB) pattern with rightward terminal vectors in lead I and terminal anterior vectors in lead V_1. In patients with right ventricular endocardial electrodes, the proper placement of the electrode in the right ventricular apex can also be established. The resultant QRS vector with proper electrode placement is directed leftward, superior, and posterior, a left bundle branch block (LBBB) pattern. With the electrode tip displaced into the right ventricular outflow tract, a QRS complex is produced with a vector directed leftward inferior and posterior. Frequent observation of the 12-lead ECG is therefore a useful technique for assessing the stability of placement of a transvenous electrode (Fig. 7-2).

The appearance of an RBBB pattern in a patient with a right ventricular endocardial electrode is almost always abnormal. The differential diagnosis of this is reviewed in detail by Barold and includes 1) right ventricular perforation with epicardial stimulation, 2) inadvertent catheterization of the coronary sinus with left ventricular stimulation, 3) inadvertent cannulation of the subclavian artery with left ventricular endocardial stimulation, and 4) fusion of paced beats with spontaneous beats having right bundle branch pattern.[13]

The pacemaker stimulus artifact of unipolar and bipolar pacemakers will appear slightly different. The unipolar pacing spike is characterized by a large amplitude and prominent voltage decay curve. The bipolar pacemaker impulse is characterized by small

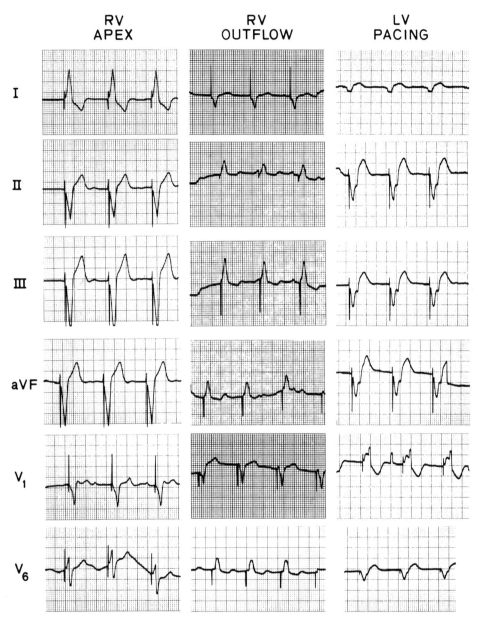

Fig. 7-2. The QRS vector during ventricular pacing at different sites. Left ventricular pacing produces a QRS complex directed anterior, superior, and rightward, resembling the complex seen with right bundle branch block. Pacing from the right ventricular apex produces an ARS complex directed left, superior, and posterior (*left bundle branch pattern*). If the pacing catheter should displace toward the outflow tract of the right ventricle, the complex will shift to a horizontal or inferior orientation.

amplitude and the absence of a voltage decay curve. This is because of the much larger dipole of a unipolar pacemaker system because the anode (usually the pulse generator case) is widely separated from the cathode (the electrode tip) located in the heart. In contrast, the bipolar dipole is small with the electrodes usually only 1.5 to 2 cm apart.

BASIC CONCEPTS OF PACEMAKER DESIGN AND FUNCTION

COMPONENTS

The basic functional components of a cardiac pacemaker are essentially the same for both temporary and permanently implantable devices (Fig. 7-3). The pacemaker is connected to the heart by the electrode, which serves both to carry pacing stimuli to the heart and to transmit the cardiac electrogram retrograde to the pacemaker amplifier circuits. The power source for a pacemaker is a bat-

tery, one of several varieties for implantable units and an ordinary mercury transistor battery for temporary pacemakers. This source of current is connected to the heart by an output circuit which stores and regulates the energy for the pulse. The output stage is in turn controlled by a timer which determines the pulse duration and interpulse interval. These functional units constitute an asynchronous pacemaker.

The more complex, noncompetitive demand pacemaker also has electrical circuits for detecting spontaneous cardiac activity and regulating the timer circuit. The electrode is connected to an amplifier which greatly augments the low voltage cardiac electrogram. This signal is then passed through a filter circuit which tends to attenuate signals of a higher (muscle artifact, electromagnetic interference) and lower (P waves, T waves) frequency. The filtered signal, essentially the QRS complex, is then passed through a level detector to determine whether the signal is sufficiently large to be considered a QRS complex (*i.e.*, whether it

Fig. 7-3. Functional block diagram of an artificial demand cardiac pacemaker.
(EMI: electromagnetic interference)

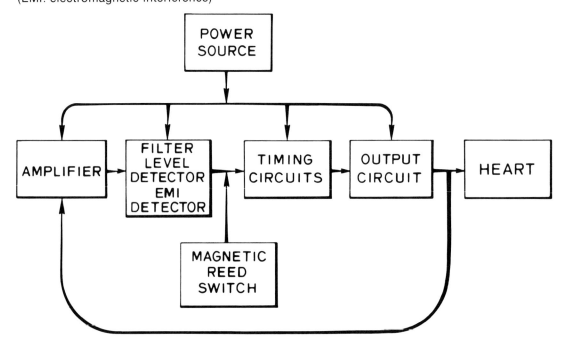

Table 7-1. Comparison of Bipolar and Unipolar Electrodes

	BIPOLAR	UNIPOLAR
Thresholds		
Voltage	Higher	
Current	Same	
Sensing	Variable	
EMI		Susceptible
VF hazard	more susceptible	Rare
Size		Smaller
Perforation	More common	
Redundancy	Feasible	None

should be sensed or ignored). If spontaneous cardiac activity is sensed at the level detector, the timing circuit is reset to begin a new cycle.

Implantable cardiac pacemakers also have a magnetic switch which, when closed, disables the sensing circuit, converting the pacemaker to a fixed rate of asynchronous operation. The function of the various circuit elements of newer implantable pacemakers may be altered by an additional circuit designed to receive instructions in the form of external electromagnetic or radio frequency signals. This capability, termed *programmability*, allows for the noninvasive alteration of pacemaker functions by the physician.[14,15]

ELECTRODE DESIGN AND FUNCTION

Cardiac electrodes may be described in three ways. They are bipolar or unipolar, endocardial or epicardial, and actively or passively fixed to the myocardium.

"Unipolar" means that the anode (positive electrode) is not in contact with myocardium, but is remote. In implantable pacemakers, it is usually the generator case. With temporary pacemakers, it may be a plaque electrode attached to the skin by a conductive medium. A bipolar electrode, on the other hand, has both the anode and cathode in contact with active myocardium. Differences in pacing between the two methods are slight (Table 7-1). Bipolar pacemakers require slightly greater voltage at threshold, but current thresholds are equal. This is because in unipolar pacemakers the remote anode has a large surface area and low resistance, thereby decreasing

the impedance of the lead system and allowing more current to flow per unit of applied voltage. Because of the larger dipole between cathode and anode, the unipolar pacemaker makes a larger more easily identifiable stimulus artifact in the ECG.[16,17]

The most significant difference in the two methods is the mode of sensing myocardial depolarization. Pacemaker sensing circuits detect differences in potential between anode and cathode. In bipolar systems this is caused by passage of the activation wavefront, resulting in a change in potential at one pole before the other. Unipolar systems detect the potential difference between the myocardial electrode and some remote nonelectrically changing location. The bipolar format is therefore subject to the effects of orientation of the electrode dipole on the activation wavefront (Fig. 7-4). Bipolar electrodes, because of their short interelectrode distance, are much more resistant to far-field signals, such as electromagnetic interference and skeletal muscle potentials. The bipolar electrogram permits better discrimination of P wave and QRS complex on the atrial electrogram. In terms of sensing the ventricular electrogram, the two methods appear to be equally efficient. However, in situations where bipolar sensing is impaired because of the orientation of the electrodes to the activation wavefront, a unipolar arrangement may allow excellent sensing.[18,19]

The heart is more susceptible to ventricular arrhythmias and fibrillation from anodal than cathodal stimuli. For this reason, bipolar systems in which the anode is in contact with myocardium have been thought to be more

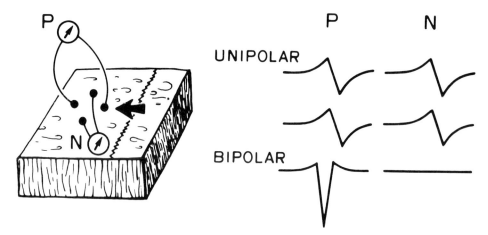

Fig. 7-4. Sensing myocardial depolarization. Two pairs of electrodes are shown: one set perpendicular (*P*) and one set normal (*N*) to an advancing wavefront (*arrow*). The electrograms recorded during passage of the wavefront are shown on the *right*. Unipolar recordings from each of the four electrodes are identical. In contrast, bipolar recordings from the two pairs of electrodes are markedly different. A large amplitude, symmetrical complex is recorded from the electrode pair oriented perpendicular to the wavefront because a large voltage difference between the two occurs when the wavefront has reached only one of the electrodes. No voltage difference ever exists in the pair oriented normal to the wavefront; therefore no complex is seen.

hazardous. The available data supports this view; all but one of the documented cases of ventricular fibrillation secondary to pacemaker R on T phenomenon have occurred in bipolar systems. This problem has been largely eliminated in permanent pacing systems by increasing anodal surface area to more then four times cathodal area, decreasing the likelihood of stimulation occurring at the anode. This design change has not been incorporated in temporary electrodes. Consequently, the hazard of ventricular fibrillation caused by pacemaker stimulation during the relative refractory period is noteworthy, particularly in patients with a lowered threshold for ventricular fibrillation.[20]

Since the demonstration of transvenous pacing in 1958 by Furman, this approach has become dominant.[21] Epicardial pacing presently is used in less than 10 percent of the implants in this country. It is customarily reserved for cases known to require cardiac pacing at the time of thoractomy for other procedures such as aortic valve replacement.

Epicardial pacing is generally favored in small children. Epicardial pacing is also indicated in that very small fraction of patients in whom repeated attempts at transvenous electrode placement have been unsuccessful.

Recently, new endocardial electrodes have allowed fixation of the tip to myocardium. A variety of designs exist, including tines, small screws, and pop-out pins (Fig. 7-5). These designs are in contrast to those described as *passive fixation leads,* which simply wedge beneath the trabeculae of the right ventricle. In general, active fixation leads have a lower incidence of early displacement and may be particularly helpful in patients with a high likelihood of electrode placement problems, such as right ventricular dilatation and tricuspid regurgitation.[22]

PROGRAMMABILITY

Programmability may be defined as the noninvasive, persistent alteration of pacemaker characteristics within a preset range. Programmable pacemakers have been available since the early 1970s, but programmability has enjoyed a recent resurgence of interest and an increase in complexity. Currently, pacemakers are available offering programmability of some or all of the following variables: *stimulus rate, energy output* (variation of pulse width, amplitude, or both), *refractory period, input sensitivity threshold, mode* (inhibited versus triggered versus asynchronous), and *hysteresis.* Hysteresis is the capacity of a pacemaker to have separate escape and pacing intervals. This enables the device to remain inhibited at slow heart rates, but once pacing commences, it occurs at a faster rate. In addition, information may now be retrieved from the pacemaker by telemetry, such as battery voltage and impedance, electrode impedance, current drain, and hermaticity (Table 7-2).

Programmability allows the physician much greater flexibility in patient management. Initially the pacemaker may be tailored to suit each patient's exact requirements. Following implantation, programmability allows the physician to adjust pacemaker function to meet any departure from those initial requirements, thus helping to preserve the functional life of the pacemaker and reduce the likelihood of operative intervention before battery depletion.

Programmability allows the physician to minimize current drain from the pacemaker by reducing rate and output to the minimal safe levels, significantly improving pacemaker longevity. Increasing pacemaker output may allow maintenance of adequate pacing during temporary or permanent periods of increased threshold which otherwise might result in unreliable pacing. Stimulation of noncardiac tissue, such as the pectoral

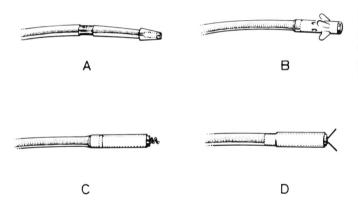

Fig. 7-5. Permanent pacemaker electrodes. *A.* Standard flange or wedge tip. *B.* Tined tip. *C.* Endocardial screw fixation electrode. *D.* Pronged fixation electrode.

Table 7-2. Currently Available Programmable Variables

Programmability	
Rate	30–130 ppm
Output	
Amplitude	1.3–7.5 volts
Impulse duration	0.08–2.3 msec
Sensitivity	0.6–8 mv
Refractory period	180–450 msec
Hysteresis	0–60 bpm
Mode	Asynchronous, inhibited, triggered
Telemetry	
Battery voltage and impedance	
Electrode impedance	
Programmed settings	
Current drain	
Hermaticity	

muscles and the diaphragm, may be lessened or eliminated by decreasing pacemaker output.

The quality of the electrogram may vary widely during the life of a pacing system. Sensitivity programmability helps to prevent both under- and oversensing. In circumstances in which sensitivity adjustment is inadequate to meet these objectives, mode programmability from the standard demand-inhibited to either asynchronous or ventricular-triggered modes is frequently useful. Conversion to the asynchronous mode may also significantly decrease energy consumption and improve pacemaker longevity. A programmed increase in the refractory period allows exclusion of T-wave potentials which may cause oversensing, and shortening the refractory period may allow the perception of otherwise unsensed early premature beats.

MODES OF PACING

Cardiac pacing may be carried out in a variety of modes tailored to the patient's specific physiologic needs (Fig. 7-6).[23] The inhibited mode of function refers to a pacemaker which resets its timer upon detection of spontaneous cardiac activity *without* producing any impulse. The triggered-mode pacemaker on the other hand *releases* its stored charge each time spontaneous cardiac activity is detected and the timing oscillator is reset. Each system will provide an impulse if no spontaneous cardiac activity is sensed within the specified time interval. The pulse released by triggered-mode pacing simply falls within the period of depolarization when the ventricle is totally refractory, therefore there is no possibility for the genesis of arrhythmias. The advantage of triggered-mode pacing is that it

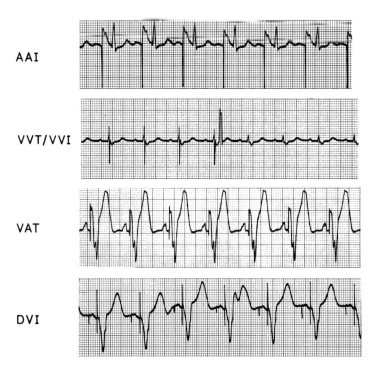

AAI

VVT/VVI

VAT

DVI

Fig. 7-6. The ECG during various modes of cardiac pacing. The upper ECG strip shows atrial-inhibited pacing (*AAI*). R-wave synchronous or triggered pacing (*VVT*), seen in the left portion of the second strip, is converted by programming (large deflection in center) to R-wave inhibited pacing (*VVI*). Atrial synchronous ventricular pacing (*VAT*) is illustrated in the third strip and AV sequential pacing (*DVI*) in the final one. The letters accompanying each ECG trace form the three-letter code which has been adopted for the description of pacing systems. The first letter represents the chamber(s) *paced*, the second the chamber(s) *sensed*, and the third the *mode of response* to sensing. (*A:* atrial; *V:* ventricular; *I:* inhibited; *T:* triggered; and *D:* dual.

cannot be falsely inhibited by electromagnetic interference or skeletal muscle potentials. The obvious disadvantage is that it wastes considerable amounts of energy in patients with only an intermittent need for pacing.

Atrial, inhibited, or triggered pacing may be used in patients requiring only rate support who have intact A-V conduction. This would include patients with sinus bradycardia and sinus pauses or arrest. For patients with normal atrial function and A-V conduction abnormalities, two forms of pacing are available. Simple ventricular pacing has been the predominant method used in these patients and provides adequate function, particularly in patients with good cardiac reserve. However, in patients with limited reserve or in younger patients, desirous of the capacity for vigorous physical activity, a pacing mode that preserves the proper A-V sequence is preferable. The best available at present for this setting is atrial/synchronous-ventricular pacing. In this mode of pacing, sensing of atrial depolarization triggers a stimulus to the ventricle after an appropriate delay. Several pacemakers with this mode of operation are available and significant differences exist between these units: the capacity for inhibition by spontaneous ventricular activity, the mode of limitation of atrial tracing at rapid atrial rates, and the range of upper and lower rates available. The advantage of this system is that it restores essentially normal A-V conduction, allowing the patient's natural atrial rhythm to control heart rate in a proper A-V sequence. The disadvantages are the increased complexity of the system and the need for both atrial and ventricular electrodes. Finally, in those patients with atrial bradyarrhythmias and A-V conduction abnormalities, the A-V sequential pacemaker is the mode of choice. Present versions of this pacemaker allows only asynchronous pacing in the atrium with triggered pacing in the ventricle after an appropriate delay. The ventricular or both impulses may be inhibited by spontaneous ventricular activity. No atrial sensing function is present. Initial designs of more complex dual-chambered pacing and sensing pacemakers, which provide for A-V

sequential pacing during atrial bradycardia and atrial synchronous pacing at more rapid spontaneous atrial rates, have been implanted and offer significant advantages over present systems.

INDICATIONS FOR ARTIFICIAL PACING

HEMODYNAMIC CONSEQUENCES OF A-V BLOCK AND TACHYARRHYTHMIAS

Complete A-V block results in several alterations in cardiac function. The most important is probably the loss of control of heart rate by the sinoatrial (SA) node. Lower centers, such as A-V junctional tissue and idioventricular foci, are slower and less responsive to the usual controlling factors of heart rate, such as autonomic tone. Junctional rhythms at a rate of 40 to 60 beats/min may provide normal cardiac output at rest. In patients with normal ventricles and the capacity to augment output by increases in stroke volume, some increase in cardiac output with exercise may also be seen. Because heart rate is generally more important than stroke volume in increasing cardiac output in sinus rhythm, a decreased capacity to alter heart rate has significantly deleterious effects on cardiac output, particularly in those patients with ventricular dysfunction and an impaired ability to alter stroke output.[24, 25]

Idioventricular rhythms usually have a rate of 20 to 40 beats/min and are rarely adequate to sustain a normal resting output for significant periods of time. Bradycardia of this severity coupled with abnormal ventricular function may be devastating.

The effects of atrioventricular dys-synchrony have also received considerable attention in recent years. During period of A-V dissociation, cyclic variations in left ventricular function occur as the relationship between atrial and ventricular systole change. Benchimol found that these differences were compensated in normal hearts, but were significant in patients with myocardial disease, particularly those with decreased ventricular compliance.[26]

Cardiac pacing offers significant improvement in patients with marked bradycardia. With ventricular pacing, the abnormal sequence of ventricular activation does not result in hemodynamic problems. In most patients, the choice of the specific site of atrial or ventricular pacing is primarily influenced by other factors. However, the contribution of properly timed atrial contraction may be highly significant in two groups: (1) those patients with diminished ventricular compliance who are largely dependent upon atrial contribution for adequate ventricular filling, and (2) patients who have retrograde conduction of ventricular depolarization, resulting in atrial systole occurring during closure of the A-V valves.[27] These patients may benefit from some form of A-V sequential pacing.

Proper timing of atrial and ventrical systole can be provided with several new pacing systems. In patients with normal SA node function and A-V block, atrial synchronous ventricular pacing provides not only a proper A-V sequence, but also allows for natural control of ventricular rate by the SA node. If SA node disease exists in the absence of A-V conduction abnormalities, atrial pacing from either the right atrial appendage or coronary sinus may provide a stable atrial rate without competition with normal atrial function. In patients with both atrial bradyarrhythmias and A-V conduction abnormalities, A-V sequential pacing provides a single atrial paced rate with properly related ventricular noncompetitive pacing. Soon to be available are dual-chambered pacing systems providing for noncompetitive pacing in both atrial and ventricular chambers and atrial synchronous ventricular pacing throughout the range of normal sinus rhythm and sinus tachycardia. It is this form of pacing that will most efficiently solve the hemodynamic consequences of atrial bradycardia and A-V block.[28, 29]

CONSEQUENCES OF SUDDEN A-V BLOCK

The intermittent development of complete A-V block may place the patient at considerable risk. The risk is greater with lower sites of block because lower pacemakers are slower and less reliable. Prolonged periods of ventricular asystole may result, producing severe cerebrovascular and myocardial ischemia, which may result in ventricular tachycardia, fibrillation, or both. Prolonged bradycardia, such as with an idioventricular rhythm, may also predispose the patient to the development of ventricular tachyarrhythmias. The sudden conversion from sinus rhythm to a bradyarrhythmia with A-V dissociation is likely to have significannt hemodynamic consequences, resulting in at least transient dizziness or syncope. These unexpected lapses in consciousness are a significant additional risk.

SPECIFIC ABNORMALITIES

Indications for Pacing in Bradyarrhythmias Including A-V Block

A-V conduction disturbances constitute a significant indication for cardiac pacing.[30, 31] These blocks may be intermittent or permanent and located in either the A-V node or more distally in the Purkinje system. In general, patients with A-V conduction abnormalities are symptomatic, manifesting either the symptoms or prolonged bradycardia or of sudden periodic cessation of cardiac output. Because lower pacemakers are usually less reliable and of inadequate rate, permanent pacing is usually indicated in patients with sustained complete A-V block.

Less pronounced forms as A-V block are also frequently observed in the symptomatic patient. In these patients, every effort must be made to demonstrate intermittent higher grade of complete A-V block using techniques such as continuous or intermittent patient-activated ambulatory monitoring and invasive endocardial electrophysiologic study with measurement of atrioventricular conduction times. Patients with partial block below the His bundle (usually Mobitz type II) are at greater risk of complications of catastrophic A-V block, such as sustained asystole, ventricular fibrillation, or tachycardia, than are patients with higher block in the A-V node (usually Wenckebach or Mobitz I block). These can be differentiated on the surface ECG except for cases of 2:1 A-V block in which progressive lengthening of A-V conduction time before block, characteristic of Mobitz type I block, cannot be observed. The ECG pattern of 2:1 block is most often the result of infrahisian block. This may be confirmed by electrophysiologic study. Permanent pacing is the therapy of choice.

Evidence of bilateral bundle branch block, RBBB with alternating left-anterior fascicular and left-posterior fascicular block, and the unusual case of infrahisian Wenckebach phenomenon are all indications for permanent pacing in the presence of symptoms of high grade A-V block. The risk of complete block in asymptomatic patients with bifascicular block is an area of significant controversy.[32–35] It is usually unnecessary to pace these patients, unless additional abnormalities of A-V conduction, such as a split His potential or a long H-V interval, are demonstrated. Likewise, pacing in the presence of an isolated prolonged H-V interval is also controversial, but a recent report favors pacing if symptoms are present.[36] In these patients, A-V conduction abnormalities do not preclude other causes of syncope and associated symptoms. A careful search should be made for neurologic abnormalities, carotid sinus hypersensitivity, and evidence of sinus node dysfunction.

Indications for permanent pacing in patients without symptoms of transient A-V conduction block are more stringent, but valid in certain circumstances. The asymptomatic patient with documented intermittent Mobitz II block should probably be paced while those with Wenckebach or intranodal block should not. Pacing in asymptomatic patients with long H-V intervals or split His potentials is not supported by current evidence.

The appearance of A-V block in the presence of atrial fibrillation is a frequent clinical problem. In general, these patients may be divided into groups having regular and irregular ventricular responses. In the first group, the emergence of regular, wide QRS complexes or narrow complexes with a rate less than 40 per minute is evidence of complete A-V block and pacing should be instituted. If the rhythm remains irregular, Fontaine has recommended observing the distribution of RR intervals over a period of half an hour.[37] A shift to the right of this curve associated with the presence of intervals exceeding 1.2 seconds in the absence of drugs affecting A-V nodal conduction is evidence of advanced A-V conduction block and an indication for pacing.

Drugs such as digitalis and β-blocking drugs may significantly affect A-V conduction, particularly in the A-V node. The presence of such drugs or the need for future use of such drugs must be considered when permanent pacing is considered. Other drugs such as Ajmaline may produce His-Purkinje block.

A-V block also results from cardiovascular surgical procedures, such as aortic valve replacement, tetrology of Fallot repair, and VSD closure. Placement of epicardial electrodes at the time of surgery facilitates subsequent pacemaker placement if required.

In children with congenital complete A-V block, the indications for pacing are usually symptoms of syncope or inadequate cardiac output caused by bradycardia. In asymptomatic patients, evidence of an unreliable pacemaker focus (*i.e.*, widened QRS complex with a rate less than 40 beats/min) is also an adequate indication.

Syncope without demonstrable A-V conduction abnormalities is a significant diagnostic problem. Persistent study of neurologic and cerebrovascular function is frequently rewarding. If A-V conduction and cardiac electrical activity are normal during symptoms, pacemaker therapy should be resisted.

A common indication for cardiac pacing is the sinus node dysfunction syndrome. Many arrhythmias may be observed, including sinus arrest, sinus bradycardia, paroxysmal supraventricular tachycardia, and atrial fibrillation. In a significant fraction, abnormalities of A-V conduction are also present. The present therapeutic strategem in these cases is to treat the bradyarrhythmias and A-V conduction disturbances with ventricular or A-V sequential pacing. This prevents the exaggerated bradycardia sometimes seen in response to antiarrhythmic drugs used in the treatment of the tachyarrhythmias. Syncope resulting from hyperactivity of the carotid sinus is also an indication for permanent pacing.

A-V block following cardiac surgery or myocardial infarction may not be permanent. If the block persists longer than one to two weeks, permanent pacing is indicated. In patients in whom the block resolves, therapy is more controversial. Some authors recommend electrophysiologic study in postoperative patients having complete A-V block with regression. After acute myocardial infarction, patients developing conduction defects (such as bifascicular block) without progression to higher degrees of A-V block also present a therapeutic dilemma. Some suggest that these patients, particularly those demonstrating abnormalities of H-V conduction, are at high risk of early death. The role of permanent pacing in this circumstance is controversial.[38, 39]

Tachyarrhythmias

Since the first report of the termination of atrial flutter by Haft in 1967, pacing has assumed a steadily widening role in the management of tachyarrhythmias.[40] At least three approaches to the management of tachyarrhythmias are currently used. These are

1. the suppression of abnormal rhythms;
2. the conversion of one type of abnormal rhythm to a more easily managed arrhythmia; and
3. termination of the abnormal rhythms.

Patients with bradycardia are frequently noted to have ectopic beats which initiate runs of tachyarrhythmia. Pacing these patients at a normal heart rate frequently will suppress these ectopic rhythms. If normal rate pacing fails, pacing the chamber at more

rapid rates may also be effective. In general, overdrive pacing requires rates in excess of 90 beats/min and often as rapid as 120 to 130 beats/min.[41] In particular, the ventricular tachycardia "Torsades de Pointes" associated with Q-T interval prolongation may be effectively suppressed by rapid pacing.[42]

Patients with supraventricular arrhythmias may be converted to atrial fibrillation by pacing. Atrial fibrillation can then be more easily managed with pharmacologic A-V nodal blockade or may spontaneously revert to sinus rhythm. Patients with a persistent paroxysmal supraventricular arrhythmia may be managed by continuous pacing at a rapid rate with pharmacologically induced 2:1 or 3:1 A-V block. This approach prevents the symptoms of paroxysmal tachycardia.

The preferable pacing technique for the management of other arrhythmias is arrhythmia termination. These techniques are based on the recognition that reentrant arrhythmias may be interrupted by an appropriately timed stimulus which depolarizes a portion of the circuit at a time inappropriate to sustain the reentrant process. This may be carried out by the use of single stimuli applied throughout the cardiac cycle in a random fashion, such as with asynchronous pacing, or by a single programmed extra stimulus progressively delayed from the preceding beat until the entire refractory period and diastole is scanned. Perhaps the most useful pacing technique in the managment of tachyarrhythmias is the application of bursts of rapid stimuli. This technique involves the use of short trains of stimuli at rates usually greater than 130 percent of the tachycardia rate[43]

These methods are effective in hospitalized patients using temporary pacing electrodes, and are also effective in selected patients using permanently implanted automatic or patient-activated systems. Used acutely, pacing termination causes less trauma than DC cardioversion, and is safer, less unpleasant, and quicker than pharmacologic methods. Pacing termination may also be effective when initial pharmacologic attempts have been unsuccessful. A disadvantage of acute pacing termination is the placement of a temporary electrode catheter in those patients not already having one. However, these arrhythmias are often recurrent and repeated pacing termination is much better tolerated than frequent cardioversion. Even in well-selected patients, pacing termination techniques are occasionally ineffective and cardioversion is necessary. There is a small incidence of both atrial and ventricular fibrillation which may also require subsequent cardioversion. For this reason, pacing termination techniques should not be applied unless facilities and personnel for immediate DC cardioversion are available.[44, 45]

Atrial flutter with or without some degree of A-V block usually responds to pacing termination techniques. The most effective is rapid atrial stimulation delivered at a rate of approximately 130 to 140 percent of the tachycardia rate. Paroxysmal atrial tachycardial is also usually responsive to pacing termination techniques, either rapid atrial stimulation or single stimuli. Accessory pathway tachycardias such as those complicating Wolf–Parkinson–White syndrome are usually responsive to single stimuli in either the atrium or ventricle or to rapid atrial stimulation. However, rapid atrial stimulation in patients with intact anterograde conduction in the accessory pathway presents a special hazard. The induction of atrial fibrillation in these patients may result in rapid conduction through the accessory pathway producing ventricular rates in excess of 200 beats/minute. Similarly, rapid pacing in the atrium may be conducted 1:1 to the ventricles. Either may result in ventricular fibrillation. Ectopic supraventricular tachycardias, such as those complicating digitalis excess, are unresponsive to pacing termination techniques. Atrial fibrillation cannot be managed using pacing techniques.

Ventricular tachycardia may be suppressed by pacing techniques for the prevention of tachyarrhythmias described above. It may be terminated with single or paired stimuli, but is more reliably terminated by bursts of rapid ventricular stimulation. Like atrial stimulation, this occasionally results in ventricular fibrillation requiring cardioversion.

TECHNIQUES FOR CARDIAC PACING

GENERAL ANESTHETIC MANAGEMENT

More than 90 percent of cardiac pacemakers are implanted by a transvenous route. A major advantage of this technique is that the procedure can be performed without general anesthesia.[46] Preoperative evaluation of the patient should address the nature and status of the rhythm disturbance and associated underlying heart disease. Particular attention should be given to conditions predisposing to altered cardiac excitability such as hypokalemia, hyperkalemia, digitalis intoxication, and other cardiac drugs. Local anesthesia is usually best. Rarely, some patients require significant sedation with short duration agents. General anesthesia is not appropriate for the typical patient, and it is not necessary to manage the anxious patient or surgeon. Accurate monitoring of the ECG is essential for assessment of the patient, the adequacy of electrode placement, and pacemaker function. A pulse monitor and blood pressure cuff should also be used.

Occasionally, patients with incomplete heart block will progress to complete block with asystole during the procedure. The anesthesiologist should be familiar with the pharmacologic agents useful in the management of this situation. Block at the A-V node, induced by parasympathetic stimulation may be alleviated with intravenous atropine. Failing this, the emergence and rate of lower cardiac pacemakers, such as junctional and idioventricular, may be enhanced by the administration of chronotropic catecholamines, such as isoproterenol. Likewise, the anesthesiologist should be familiar with techniques for temporary electrode placement.

A variety of complications may rarely occur during pacemaker implantation and these are listed below. Most of these involve the cardiopulmonary system and may be life-threatening. They include hemorrhage, particularly if the surgery involves the internal jugular venous system. For this reason, adequate venous access is an important facet of prepa-

Complications

1. Rhythm: Asystole, atrial tachycardia/fibrillation, ventricular tachycardia/fibrillation
2. Hemorrhage
3. Pneumothorax, hemothorax
4. Perforation with or without hemopericardium and tamponade

ration of the patient for pacemaker implantation. A variety of cardiac arrhythmias may occur, particularly during passage of the electrode through the right atrium and ventricle. These rarely require therapy, but the operating suite should be fully equipped for cardiopulmonary resuscitation and a defibrillator should be readily available. Cardiac perforation with hemopericardium and acute cardiac tamponade can occur and is characterized by a rapidly declining blood pressure in the face of tachycardia and decreased cardiac motion on fluoroscopic examination of the heart. Dissection in the area of the subclavian vein or percutaneous puncture of the subclavian vein may result in pneumothorax and even tension pneumothorax.

Pacemaker implantation generally does not require extensive post-procedure monitoring in the recovery area. In general these patients may be returned directly to their hospital room with the provision that continuous electrocardiographic monitoring be carried out and a chest film performed upon arrival. The choice of anesthetic agents should take this into consideration. Long-acting sedatives and narcotics should be used sparingly, if at all, and scopalomine has no rational purpose in this situation. Patients may be up within hours after the procedure and thereafter may move about as they desire. Monitoring should be continued for three to four days after the implantation of a new transvenous electrode. If the electrode is undisturbed and only the generator is changed, patients may be discharged within 6 to 24 hours after the procedure. Pacemaker function should be checked before discharge and again within the first two to three weeks postimplantation.

TECHNIQUES FOR ELECTRODE PLACEMENT

In order to fully use newer pacing techniques, it is important to be able to pace from a variety of sites within the heart. Pacing has been carried out by stimulating the ventricles, either by placing an electrode catheter into the right ventricular apex through the venous system or by placing an electrode directly on the epicardial surface of the right or left ventricle. The former technique is generally used because it obviates the need for thoracotomy to place a pacing electrode. However, epicardial electrodes still play a very useful role in pacing in special situations (see p. 212).

The most important test of electrode function is that of pacing threshold. If the patient has a spontaneous rate adequate to maintain normal cardiac function, the analyzer is adjusted to the minimum output, the pulse duration of the pacemaker to be implanted, and a rate of 10 to 20 beats/min faster than the spontaneous rate. The voltage output is gradually increased until reliable capture occurs. The amount of current passed at threshold voltage should also be recorded. The threshold in volts divided by the current in amperes gives the resistance in ohms of the electrode system. In general, for modern small-tipped electrodes, the resistance should range from 500 to 1000 ohms and the threshold should be less than one volt. In those patients not having an adequate spontaneous rhythm, the pacing analyzer should be set to approximately 5 to 6 volts, which will allow immediate pacing. The output may then be gradually decreased until capture is transiently lost. In general, the pacing threshold is slightly higher when determined by increasing voltage to initial capture than when determined by decreasing voltage until capture is lost. For programmable pacemakers, threshold voltage and current should be determined at several pulse durations spread over the range of settings available. The strength-duration curve can thus be accu-

Table 7-3. Tests for Adequate Placement of Electrode

Threshold	< 1 volt @ 1 msec
Sensing	> 6 mv consistently
Fluoroscopic appearance	
PA	RV apex
Lateral	Anterior
ECG pattern	Appropriate bundle branch block pattern

rately characterized. This is particularly important when using a chronic lead with increased threshold values at shorter pulse durations.[47]

Reliable atrial pacing is less easily accomplished. Atrial pacing is required in many newer strategies. A number of catheters are available for pacing the right atrium, including atrial appendage J-shaped electrodes with tines, corkscrew-tipped electrodes, septal-penetrating electrodes, wire loops that expand within the atrium, and ordinary electrode catheters lodged in a stable position within the atrium. In addition, the atrium may be stimulated both acutely and chronically by an electrode catheter placed in the proximal portion of the coronary sinus.[48, 49]

When a catheter or electrode has been placed in a location which appears appropriate, tests may be done to ensure the adequacy of electrode function (Table 7-3). These tests are made easier and more accurate by using a pacing systems analyzer, available from several manufacturers. Perhaps the simplest and most commonly used unit is the Medronic 5300 (Fig. 7-7). This unit is essentially a voltage-source pacemaker, allowing continuous adjustment of voltage output, pulse duration, and stimulus rate. In addition, it has measurement functions allowing the determination of the amount of current being passed at any given voltage setting, the magnitude of the endocardial electrogram, and the voltage output, pulse duration, and stimulus rate of a pacemaker.[50, 51]

Demand cardiac pacing requires not only low pacing thresholds but also an adequate electrogram for proper sensing. This quality of the electrogram may be determined by the pacing system analyzer by turning to the R wave threshold position. The button marked

R test is depressed, allowing the analyzer to temporarily stop pacing. Any spontaneous activity is then filtered as it would be in a permanent pacemaker and the amplitude measured. Slight variations in how this is accomplished are found among the various analyzers that are available. In general, it is most accurate to use an analyzer and pacemaker from the same manufacturer; filtering and measuring techniques then tend to be consistent between the analyzer and pacemaker. A more reliable technique is to record the electrogram on a physiologic recorder with a high-frequency response. From this recording, the amplitude of various portions of the signal can be measured as well as the slew rate, or $\Delta v/\Delta t$, of the intrinsic deflection (Fig. 7-8) and the magnitude of ST displacement. The measured amplitude should be

Fig. 7-7. The pacing system analyzer.

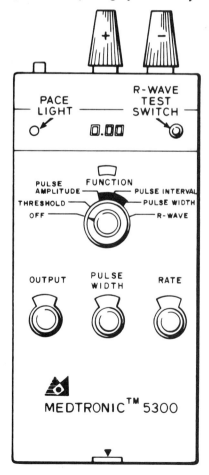

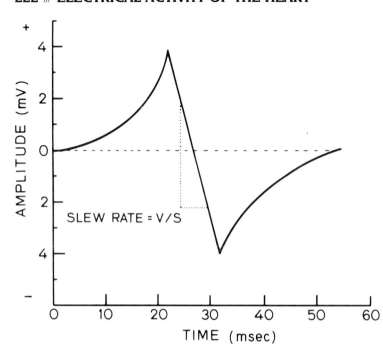

Fig. 7-8. Analysis of the cardiac electrogram. A unipolar intracardiac electrogram is shown greatly expanded in time. The slew rate is the rate of change in voltage with time of the intrinsic deflection of the signal; it can be calculated directly from the tracings and is an index of the frequency content of the signal. In general, electrograms of higher slew rate are more easily sensed, while those of a lower slew rate (<0.5 V/S) may be less easily sensed because they are more highly attenuated by the filter circuit of the pacemaker.

greater than 6 mv and the slew rate greater than 1 to 1.5 v-/sec for an acute lead. Because amplitude, slew rate, and ST segment displacement all decrease or disappear with time, less stringent requirements are held for chronic leads. An amplitude of 4 mv with a slew rate of 0.6 to 0.8 v/sec is generally adequate.[52]

The pacing system analyzer may also be used to test pacemaker function. In connecting both the analyzer and pacemaker to the electrode, the following precautions should be observed. The cathode or negative pole of the pacemaker or analyzer should always be attached to the distal electrode in a bipolar system or to the intracardiac electrode in a unipolar system. The anode or positive pole should be connected to the ring electrode of a bipolar system and is the generator case in a unipolar system. In an epicardial electrode system, the cathode should be connected to the electrode having the lowest pacing threshold. When using the pacing systems analyzer for testing a unipolar electrode, the anodal lead should be placed in contact with subcutaneous tissue in the pacemaker pocket. The contact should have a large surface area similar to that of the generator case. Small area contact, such as clipping the alligator connector to subcutaneous tissue, will significantly alter the recorded electrogram and may alter pacing threshold and lead resistance.

Finally, radiographic confirmation of adequate position must be obtained, including the lateral view. The proper placement of an electrode in the right ventricle or atrium cannot be completely ascertained in the PA projection because no perception of anterior versus posterior location can be gained. For proper right ventricular placement, the catheter in the lateral projection should pass anteriorly toward the sternum. A posterior orientation of the catheter suggests its location in the coronary sinus or one of the descending coronary veins. Catheter placement in the right atrial appendage will show an anterior orientation of the J-shaped electrode in the lateral projection.[53]

As described above, the 12-lead ECG is also useful in gauging the location of a right ventricular electrode.

CONSIDERATIONS IN TEMPORARY PACING

The nature of cardiac conduction disturbances frequently dictates that some rapid temporary means of sustaining cardiac rhythm be used. External pulse generators connected to temporary pacing electrodes are designed to accomplish these objectives. Although a wide variety of electrodes are available, most temporary pacing is accomplished using the bipolar configuration with a small, flexible, semi-floating catheter. This has the advantage of a decreased likelihood of perforation and can frequently be implanted under electrocardiographic guidance only. The electrode is connected to a standard electrocardiograph by the method described above and the waveform monitored as the catheter is passed through the superior vena cava and right atrium into the apex of the right ventricle. Adequate pacing is confirmed by threshold measurement, the appearance of the cardiac electrogram, and the appearance of the 12-lead ECG. The best entry site is usually at the subclavian or internal jugular vein. With fluoroscopic guidance, catheters may also be inserted into the brachial and femoral veins as well. In general, these entry sites require more immobility of the patient and are less desirable for long-term therapy. Larger, less flexible catheters can also be used for temporary pacing, particularly if multipolar catheters for the recording of simultaneous electrograms is required.

The bipolar format for pacing provides protection from leakage currents and electromagnetic interference. It also eliminates the possibility of poor indifferent electrode contact causing pacing failure, as may be seen with a unipolar indifferent electrode placed on the skin surface. Disadvantages, however, include more variable electrograms, which may create difficulty in sensing and a lower ventricular fibrillation threshold in the acute setting. Recently, an electrode has been described which attempts to combine the best features of both unipolar and bipolar pacing by having an internal anode remote from the heart and providing the redundancy of two electrodes (both cathodes) at the catheter tip.[54]

Atrial pacing can be accomplished by the use of an electrode having a wire loop at its distal end which expands to contact the right atrial endocardium.[55] An alternative method is the use of a catheter placed in the proximal portion of the coronary sinus. The preferred catheter is the quadrapolar, which allows better anchoring in the coronary sinus and multiple electrode combinations for better pacing.

A variety of temporary pulse generators are available providing for single-chambered demand pacing or multichambered A-V sequential pacing. The Medtronic 5375 is a typical external single chambered demand pacemaker (Fig. 7-9). It has an output of approximately 8 to 10 v providing up to 20 milliamperes of current through a normal resistance. The device is current-limited and the current output is adjustable by the operator. The pacing rate is adjustable from 50 to

Fig. 7-9. The temporary cardiac pacemaker.

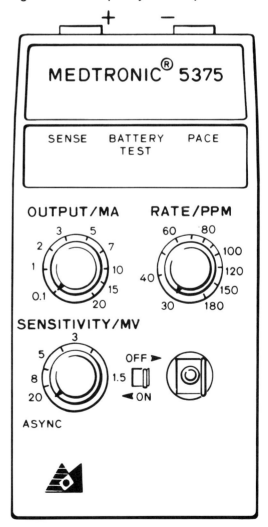

150 beats/min. The input sensitivity level is adjustable from asynchronous to a maximally sensitive level in a continuous, but noncalibrated scale. At the time of implantation, the current threshold in milliamperes should be determined and the pacemaker adjusted to an output level approximately two to two and a half times greater. The sensitivity threshold for sensing both the R wave and any additional signals or noise, such as the P and T wave, should both be determined and the sensitivity adjusted midway between these levels.

After an acceptable electrode position is found the electrode should be anchored to the skin securely and the entry site covered with a dry sterile dressing. Great care should be taken that this area remain clean and dry. It should be examined daily for any evidence of bleeding, inflammation, or infection. Continuous electrocardiographic monitoring is optimal and the 12-lead ECG should be inspected daily for evidence of changes in the electrode position or improper function. Chest films, preferably posteroanterior and lateral views, should be obtained immediately following implantation. Pacing and sensitivity thresholds should be evaluated at least daily and appropriate adjustments made to provide adequate safety margins for sensing and pacing. At the termination of temporary pacing, the sutures anchoring the catheter are severed and the catheter is simply withdrawn. Pressure over the vein entry site for 3 to 5 minutes is usually sufficient to control bleeding at that point.

Complications of temporary pacing include infection plebitis or both at the site of vein entry. The most effective treatment is removal of the old catheter and replacement at a remote site. The incidence of this complication can be decreased by meticulous care of the entry site area. The presence of a catheter within the heart may induce ectopic activity, which is usually transient. Irritability may be enhanced by drugs or circumstances promoting increased cardiac excitability. Perforation of the heart occasionally occurs during temporary pacing. Perforation of the right ventricle rarely results in significant hemo-

pericardium. Occasionally hemodynamic symptoms do result and pericardiocentesis or open drainage is necessary. Perforation may result in inadequate pacing or pacing of the hemidiaphragm. This is generally corrected simply be withdrawing and repositioning the electrode catheter.

CONSIDERATIONS IN PERMANENT PACING

Unless special circumstances require, permanent cardiac pacing is accomplished through transvenous electrodes.[56] The preferred route is through the subclavian vein, either directly by Seldinger technique using an introducer-sheath system[57, 58] or indirectly by dissection and cannulation of the cephalic vein. Alternate routes would include the external and internal jugular and femoral veins. The electrode is passed into the apex of the right ventricle under fluoroscopic guidance. When the tip location is appropriate, the adequacy of placement is tested by the techniques described above. The choice of electrode is in part dependent upon the presumed anatomy of the right ventricle. The standard flange-tip or tined electrode is adequate for patients with small or normal-sized right ventricular cavities, while an electrode offering some method of active fixation is preferable in those patients with enlarged right ventricles, tricuspid regurgitation, hypertrophic right ventricles, or congenital variations of the pulmonic ventricle, such as corrected transposition of the great vessels. A variety of electrodes are available for permanent atrial pacing from either the coronary sinus or the atrial appendage. Following satisfactory electrode placement, the pulse generator is connected and implanted in a subcutaneous subclavicular pocket.

Cardiac pacing in children presents special problems with regard to the maintenance of cardiac pacing systems. The general reliability and life span of electrode systems is decreased. Special techniques in their management have been recently reviewed by Furman and Young[59] and Williams and coworkers.[60]

Pulse generator replacement presents a

slightly different problem in that an electrode already present and presumably firmly anchored must be evaluated for adequacy of continued use. Structural continuity of the electrode can be assessed by measuring its impedance. A low impedance suggests a short circuit or current leakage path such as would result from an insulation break. A high resistance indicates discontinuity of the conductor such as would occur with a fracture of the wire. The expected range of resistance is dependent on a variety of factors such as material, length, and electrode surface area. In general, electrodes of typical construction and of larger surface area (15–25 mm²) have a resistance of approximately 300 to 500 ohms, while those with smaller electrode areas (5–15 mm²) have a higher electrode impedance, 500 to 900 ohms. Because the physiologic changes in excitation threshold have long since occurred and the electrode thresholds are presumed to be stable, higher values can be accepted than can be for a new lead implant. In general, at least a 100 percent safety margin in voltage or current threshold should be present. For most permanent pacemakers, this dictates that the upper limits of acceptability of a chronic threshold is from 2.5 to 2.8 v. If a pulse duration programmable pacemaker is to be implanted, the strength-duration curve should be determined throughout the limits of programmability of the device. This is the only way in which the full capabilities of the generator can be determined with respect to the electrode to be used. If a nonprogrammable pacemaker is to be implanted, the threshold should be determined at the fixed-pulse duration of the generator to be implanted.[61]

The approach to the malfunctioning pacing system is similar to that of the evaluation of chronic electrodes. Pacing failure may be characterized by either a lack of the appearance of a stimulus artifact on the surface ECG in the asynchronous mode or the appearance of such an artifact without producing cardiac excitation. The former implies a defect in the transmission of current to the myocardium caused by either discontinuity of the electrode system or failure of output from the pulse generator itself. The latter suggests insufficient energy delivered to the electrode tip to cause myocardial excitation. This in turn may result from dislocation of the electrode tip from viable myocardium, fibrosis around the electrode tip sufficient to reduce current density to levels below the excitation threshold, or to leakage of current through a defect in the insulation of the electrode. As previously described, both the pulse generator and integrity and function of the electrode may be tested with the pacing system analyzer. Insulation defects are characterized by having normal voltage and a high current threshold with a low electrode resistance. Conductor fractures are characterized by normal current, high voltage threshold, and high resistance. Pulse generator malfunction is usually readily apparent. Care must be taken to check all attachments and connections between the pacemaker or electrode and the analyzer so that misleading data are not obtained.[62]

PRECAUTIONS FOR PACEMAKER PATIENTS UNDERGOING OTHER SURGICAL PROCEDURES

Certain precautions are necessary in dealing with patients who have cardiac pacemakers and who are undergoing surgical procedures.[63] In general, no particular operation or technique of anesthesia is contraindicated, but certain general hazards common to the operating room should be identified. Before the induction of anesthesia, the adequacy of pacemaker function should be determined by the methods described above. Because pacing may frequently be life-sustaining, it is mandatory that pacemaker support be available during stress, such as anesthesia and surgery.

The most common hazard encountered in the perioperative management of pacemaker patients is that of electromagnetic interference. The operating room may contain several sources, including electrocautery, diathermy, and occasionally radio frequency and microwave radiation. Electrocardiographic monitoring is frequently inadequate to assess pacemaker function because of interference. Electrocautery may so completely disrupt the ECG signal that it is not possible to follow cardiac function. During these periods the anesthesiologist must rely on other techniques, such as the esophageal or precordial stethoscope, blood pressure, or a finger pulse monitor. In general, electrocautery should be kept to a minimum, administered for only brief periods, and never used within 15 cm of the pacemaker or electrode. Application of electrocautery too near the pacemaker or electrode may result in permanent damage to it or to the electrode tissue interface. During unavoidable periods of interference, the grounding plate of the electrocautery system should be located near the area of cautery and far away from the generator case. A magnet may also be placed over the pacemaker to convert it to the asynchronous mode of operation during cautery.

Manipulation of the patient or the intrathoracic structures may result in dislodging a transvenous electrode system.

Large amounts of electrical energy are passed through the thorax during external defibrillation. Cardiac pacemakers are designed to resist such insults but occasionally may be permanently damaged in this way. The likelihood of this can be minimized by appropriate spacing of the defibrillating electrodes. The defibrillating electrodes preferably should be placed in an anteroposterior orientation. If this is not possible, an attempt should be made to place them equidistant from the pulse generator. Following defibrillation, pacemaker function should be carefully checked to ensure that no permanent damage has been sustained by the pacemaker.

A wide variety of pharmacologic agents and physiologic events may significantly alter threshold. These may become clinically important in patients with marginal electrodes and a failure of pacing may result. Counter

measures, such as administration of potassium to the hypokalemic patient, may be lifesaving. The anesthesiologist must be aware of these factors, their prevention, and means for correction.

REFERENCES

GENERAL REFERENCES

1. Chung EK (ed): Artificial Cardiac Pacing: Practical Approach. Baltimore, Williams & Wilkins Company, 1978
2. Varriale P, Naclerio EA (eds): Cardiac Pacing: A Concise Guide to Clinical Practice. Philadelphia, Lea & Febiger, 1979
3. Thalen HJ, Meere C (eds): Fundamentals of Cardiac Pacing. The Hague, Martinez Nijoff, 1979
4. Samet P, El Sherif N (eds): Cardiac Pacing. New York, Grune & Stratton, 1980
5. Josephson ME: Key references: pacemakers. Circulation 63:230–234, 1981
6. Meere C: Cardiac pacing: State of the Art 1979. Proceeding of the Sixth World Symposium on Cardiac Pacing. Montreal, PACESYMP, 1979

ELECTROPHYSIOLOGY OF ARTIFICAL PACING

Electrical Stimulation

7. Parker B: Electrode design and longevity. In Chung EK (ed): Artificial Cardiac Pacing: Practical Approach, pp 270–282. Baltimore, Williams & Wilkins, 1978
8. Mansfield PB: Myocardial stimulation: the electrochemistry of electrode-tissue coupling. Am J Physiol 212:1475–1488, 1967
9. Furman S, Harzeler P, Mira R: Cardiac pacing and pacemakers. IV. Threshold of cardiac stimulation. Am Heart J 94:115–124, 1977

Excitability

10. Westerholm JC: Threshold studies in transvenous cardiac pacemaker treatment. Scand J Thorac Cardiovasc Surg [Suppl] 8:1–35, 1971

11. Donacke P, Flothner R, Rettig G, Bette L: Studies of short and long term threshold changes. In Shaldag M, Furman S (eds): Advances in Pacemaker Technology, pp 283–296. New York, Springer–Verlag, 1979

Electrocardiography

12. Pupillo JA: ECG of artificial pacemakers. Parma, Vismar Publishing, 1979
13. Barold SS: Clinical problems with temporary ventricular pacing. In Furman S, Escher D (eds): Modern Cardiac Pacing: A Clinical Overview, pp 115–134. Maryland, JW Charles Press, 1975

BASIC CONCEPTS OF PACEMAKER DESIGN AND FUNCTION

Components

14. Chardack W, Greatbach W: The implantable pacing system. In Thalen HJ, Meere C (eds): Fundamentals of Cardiac Pacing, pp 3:29–58. The Hague, Martinez Nijoff, 1979
15. Hauser RG, Giuffre VW: Clinical assessment of cardiac pacemaker performance. Journal of Continuing Education in Cardiology 14:19–55, 1979

Electrode Design and Function

16. Furman S, Harzeler P, Mira R: Cardiac pacing and pacemakers. IV. Threshold of cardiac stimulation. Am Heart J 94:115–124, 1977
17. Parker B: Electrode design and longevity. In Chung EK (ed): Artificial Cardiac Pacing: Practical Approach, pp 270–277. Baltimore, Williams & Wilkins, 1978
18. Furman S, Herzeler P, De Caprio V: Cardiac pacing and pacemakers. III. Sensing the cardiac electrogram. Am Heart J 93:794–801, 1977
19. Herzeler P, Caprio V, Furman S: Endocardial electrograms and pacemakers sensing. Med Instrum 10:178–183, 1976
20. Mehra, R, Furman S, Crump J: Vulnerability of the mildly ischemic ventrical to cathodal anodal and bipolar stimulation. Circ Res 41:159–166, 1977
21. Furman S, Robinson G: The use of an intra-cardiac pacemaker in the correction of total heart block. Surg Forum 9:245–248, 1958
22. Furman S, Pannizzo F, Campo I: Comparison of passive and active adhering leads for endocardial pacing. PACE 2:417–427, 1979

Modes of Pacing

23. Hawthorn JW: Different modes of artificial cardiac pacing. In Chung EK: Artificial Cardiac Pacing: Practical Approach, pp 252–260. Baltimore, Williams & Wilkins, 1978

INDICATIONS FOR ARTIFICIAL PACING

Hemodynamic Consequences of A-V Block and Tachyarrhythmias

24. Segel N, Samet P: Physiologic aspects of cardiac pacing. In Samet P, El Sherif N (eds): Cardiac Pacing, pp 111–148. New York, Grune & Stratton, 1980
25. Walsh RA, O'Rourke RA: Hemodynamic effects of pacing. In Varriale P, Naclerio EA: Cardiac Pacing, pp 123–131
26. Benchimol A, Ellis JG, Diamond EG: Hemodynamic consequences of atrial and ventricular pacing in patients with normal and abnormal hearts. Am J Med 39:911–922, 1965
27. Ogawa S, Dreifus LS, Shenoy PN et al: Hemodynamic consequences of atrioventricular and ventriculoatrial pacing. PACE 1:8–15, 1978
28. Leinbach RC, Chamberlain DA, Kastor JA et al: A comparison of the hemodynamic effects of ventricular and sequential AV pacing in patients with heart block. Am Heart J 78:502–508, 1978
29. Herzeler P, Heffery O, Maloney JD et al: Hemodynamic benefits of atrioventricular sequential pacing after cardiac surgery. Am J Cardiol 40:232–236, 1977

Specific Abnormalities

30. Fontaine G: Current indication of pacemaker therapy. In Thalen HJ, Meere C (eds): Fundamentals of Cardiac Pacing, pp 57–58. The Hague, Martinez Nijoff, 1979
31. Furman S: Cardiac pacing and pacemakers. I.

Indications for pacing bradyarrhythmias. Am Heart J 93:658–668, 1977

32. Ventakaraman K, Madias JE, Hood WB: Indications for prophylactic preoperative insertions of pacemakers in patients within right bundle branch block and left anterior hemiblock. Chest 68:501–506, 1975

33. McAnaulty JH, Rahimtoola SH, Murphy ES et al: A prospective study of sudden death "high risk" bundle branch block. N Engl J Med 299:209–215, 1979

34. Dhiugra RC, Denes P, Dclou W et al: Syncope in patients with chronic bifascicular block. Ann Intern Med 81:302–306, 1974

35. Peters RW, Scheinman MM, Modin G et al: Prophylactic permanent pacemakers for patients with chronic bundle branch block. Am J Med 66:978–985, 1979

36. Altschuler H, Fischer JD, Furman S: Significance of isolated H-V interval prolongation in symptomatic patients without documented heart block. Am Heart J 97:19–26, 1979

37. Fontaine G: Current indication of pacemaker therapy. In Thalen HJ, Meere C (eds): Fundamentals of Cardiac Pacing, pp 57–58. The Hague, Martinez Nijoff, 1979

38. Mullins CB: Indications for pacing after acute myocardial infarction in patients with fascicular blocks. J Electrocardiol 8:297–298, 1978

39. Hindman MC, Wagner GS, Jaro M et al: The clinical significance of bundle branch block complicating acute myocardial infarction (I, II). Circulation 58:679–688, 689–699, 1978

40. Haft JI, Kosowsky BD, Lau SH et al: Termination of atrial flutter by rapid electrical pacing of the atrium. Am J Cardiol 20:239–244, 1967

41. Sowton E, Leathman A, Carson P: The suppression of arrhythmias by artificial pacing. Lancet 2:1098–1100, 1964

42. Smith WM, Gallagher JJ: "Les Torsades de Pointes": An unusual ventricular arrhythmia. Ann Intern Med 93:578–584, 1980

43. Fisher JD, Cohen HL, Mehra R et al: Cardiac pacing and pacemakers. II. Serial electrophysiologic-pharmacologic testing for control of recurrent tachyarrhythmias. Am Heart J 93:658–668, 1977

44. Waldo AL, MacLean WAH: Diagnosis and Treatment of Cardiac Arrhythmias Following Open Heart Surgery. New York, Futura Publishers, 1980

45. Preston TA: The use of pacemaking for the treatment of acute arrhythmias. Heart Lung 6:249–255, 1977

TECHNIQUES FOR CARDIAC PACING

General Anesthetic Management

46. Wynands JE: Anesthesia for patients with heart block and artificial pacemakers. Anesth Analg (Cleve) 55:626–632, 1976

Techniques for Electrode Placement

47. Furman S, Harzeler P, Mira R: Cardiac pacing and pacemakers. IV. Threshold of cardiac stimulation. Am Heart J 94:115–124, 1977

48. Smyth NPD: Atrial programmed pacing. PACE 1:104–113, 1978

49. Moss AJ: Therapeutic uses of permanent pervenous atrial pacemakers: a review. J Electrocardiol 8:373–380, 1975

50. Calvin JW: Intraoperative pacemaker electrical testing. Ann Thorac Surg 26:165–176, 1978

51. Varriale P, Kwa RP, Niznik J, Naclerio EA: Electrical testing in cardiac pacing. In Varriale P, Naclerio EA (eds): Cardiac Pacing, pp 247–264. Philadelphia, Lea & Febiger, 1979

52. Furman S, Herzeler P, De Caprio V: Cardiac pacing and pacemakers. III. Sensing the cardiac electrogram. Am Heart J 93:794–801, 1977

53. Kaul TK, Bain WH: Radiographic appearances of implanted transvenous endocardial pacing electrodes. Chest 72:323–326, 1977

Consideration in Temporary Pacing

54. Preston TA: Temporary unipolar pacing using a dual cathode. J Electrocardiol 9:193–197, 1976

55. Berens S, Kolin A, MacAlpin R: A new stable temporary atrial pacing loop. Am J Cardiol 34:325–332, 1974

Considerations in Permanent Pacing

56. Furman S, Fischer JD: Cardiac pacing and pacemaker. V. Technical aspects of implantation and equipment. Am Heart J 94:250–259, 1977

57. Littleford PO, Darsonnet V, Spector SD: Method for the rapid and atraumatic insertion of permanent endocardial pacemaker elec-

trodes through the subclavian vein. Am J Cardiol 43:980–982, 1979

58. Miller FA, Holmes DR, Gerch BJ, Maloney JD: Permanent transvenous pacemaker implantation via the subclavian vein. Mayo Clin Proc 55:309–314, 1980

59. Furman S, Young D: Cardiac pacing in children and adolescents. Am J Cardiol 39:550–558, 1977

60. Williams WG, Izukawa PM, Olley GA et al: Permanent cardiac pacing in infants and children. PACE 1:439–447, 1978

61. Barold SS, Winner JA: Techniques and signif-icance of threshold measurement for cardiac pacing. Chest 70:760–766, 1976

62. Furman S: Cardiac pacing and pacemaker. VI. Analysis of pacemaker malfunction. Am Heart J 94:378, 1977

Precautions for Pacemaker Patients Undergoing Other Surgical Procedures

63. Simon AB: Preoperative management of the pacemaker patient. Anesthesiology 46:127–131, 1977

8

Cardiac Mapping: A New Anesthetic Challenge

RICHARD P. FOGDALL

INTRODUCTION

Surgical intervention to correct *mechanical* cardiac disorders (valvular, shunting, obstructive, and so on) is commonplace. Surgical intervention to correct electrophysiologic disorders is presently uncommon, but undergoing active investigation in several centers.[1-7] Surgical therapy is instituted upon the failure of both traditional and experimental antiarrhythmic drug therapy.

There are two basic patient populations requiring such intervention: those with preexcitation syndromes (such as the Wolff–Parkinson–White [WPW] syndrome), and those with intractable ventricular tachyarrhythmias, usually of ischemic origin. Sophisticated electrophysiologic studies are necessary for patient selection and intraoperative success. Some considerations of importance to the cardiovascular anesthesiologist have been summarized briefly for the Wolff–Parkinson–White syndrome,[8] but there is little available information describing the patient group afflicted with intractable ventricular tachyarrhythmias undergoing corrective cardiac surgery.

Some background information is necessary to understand the physiologic status of these patients, their selection, and perioperative events and concerns. In other areas of this text, background data has been provided on myocardial cellular function (Chap. 3), electrocardiography and antiarrhythmic drug therapy (Chap. 6), cardiac catheterization and electrophysiologic investigations (Chap. 4), and understanding of artificial pacemaker physiology and function (Chap. 7). Because an understanding of all of these areas is required to provide optimal care for patients undergoing cardiac mapping, the reader is referred to them for review. In addition, an excellent recent electrophysiology review article is available.[9]

All electrical events germane to the clinical events discussed in this chapter are the result of normal or abnormal cellular function. Abnormal cellular function is the result of derangements in cellular membrane ion flow and concentrations, especially the calcium ion. Drug and surgical therapies will alter such membrane ion flow, and produce good or bad effects in the myocardium.

The recent introduction of intracardiac recording and programmed cardiac electrical stimulation has enhanced greatly our understanding of ventricular and supraventricular tachyarrhythmias. The ability to activate certain cardiac areas assists in delineating the origin or sequence of electrical depolarization. His-bundle electrocardiography and cardiac pacing techniques, coupled with evaluations of QRS morphology, assist in differentiating ventricular from supraventricular arrhythmias.

The initiation and termination of ventricular tachycardia (VT) by electrical pacing, coupled with cardiac mapping techniques, has permitted a more accurate assessment of the origin of ventricular tachyarrhythmias in a given patient. The induction of VT is enhanced by catecholamines, alcohol, myocardial ischemia, and occassionally antiarrhythmic drugs.[9] However, most antiarrhythmic drugs, administered in sufficient doses, suppress the induction of VT by pacing.[9] Thus the plasma concentration of an antiarrhythmic drug may be important to know during the perioperative period.

A review of the effects of cardiac dysrhythmias on cerebral perfusion may be helpful in understanding the severity of some of the rhythm alterations seen in these patients.[10] This brief chapter will not be an exhaustive review of the surgical or medical literature. Other authors have done so.[1-7, 11] Very re-

cent investigational therapies with implantable automatic defibrillators will not be covered.[12] The focus here will be upon those specific details and concerns of direct interest to the cardiovascular anesthesiologist and intensivist confronted with a patient requiring intraoperative mapping, and surgical ablation or excision of abnormal electrical pathways or foci.

EPICARDIAL MAPPING IN THE PATIENT WITH VENTRICULAR PREEXCITATION SYNDROMES

PHYSIOLOGY AND PHARMACOLOGY

Preexcitation of ventricular muscle occurs when electrical pathways other than the normal conduction system are used, thus producing ventricular depolarization earlier than normally expected. These pathways have various anatomic configurations and names (Fig. 8-1): Kent bundle, atrio–Hisian fiber (fiber of Brechenmacher), Mahaim fiber,[13] and Lown–Ganong–Levine pathway (James fiber).[14] Nomenclature and consolidation of terminology is presently in a state of flux. The most common example of preexcitation through an abnormal pathway is seen in the patient with WPW.

The basic physiologic problem in WPW syndrome is the sudden production of reentry tachyarrhythmias (Fig. 8-2). Atrial fibrillation or ventricular fibrillation or both then also may occur,[13, 15] associated with a profound decrease in cardiac output. Detailed discussions of this syndrome complex are presented by Gallagher,[13] Farshidi,[16] and Wu.[17] Various therapies for chronic use, such as lidocaine, procainamide, quinidine, propranolol, verapamil, disopyramide phosphate, and pacemakers, have been partially successful (Tables 8-1, 8-2).[13] Digitalis preparations are controversial because the incidence of ventricular fibrillation appears higher in the patient receiving digitalis.[13, 15] The syndrome is seen in infants and may be associated with congenital cardiac defects or sudden death.[18]

Table 8-1. Electrophysiologic Effect of Drugs Used in Patients with Wolff–Parkinson–White Syndrome

DRUG	DURATION OF EFFECTIVE REFRACTORY PERIOD					SHORTEST R-R INTERVAL BETWEEN TWO PREEXCITED BEATS DURING AF
	Atrium	A-V Node	His–Purkinge	Ventricle	Accessory Pathway	
Digitalis	±	+	0	±	−	−
Quinidine*	+	−	+	+	+	+
Procainamide*	+	−	+	+	+	+
Lidocaine*	±	±	−	+	+	+
Disopyramide*	+	−	±	+	+	?
Aprindine†	+	+	?	+	+	+
Amiodarone†	+	+	+	+	+	+
Ajmaline (IV)†	+	0	+	+	+	+
Propranolol	0	+	0	0	0	0
Diphenylhydantoin	±	−	−	±	±	?
Verapamil	±	+	0	±	±	?

* Best combination may be a drug which *prolongs* the effective refractory period of the *accessory* pathway and *shortens* the effective refractory period of the *A-V node*. This is a controversial concept presently.

† Presently investigational

+ Prolonged

− Shortened

0 No change

± Variable

? Unknown

Modified from Gallagher JJ, Pritchett ELC, Sealy WC et al: The Pre-excitation syndromes. Prog Cardiovasc Dis 20:285–327, 1978

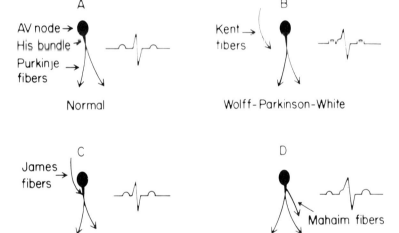

Fig. 8-1. Preexcitation syndromes—types of accessory pathways. Conduction in the (*A*) normal, (*B*) WPW, (*C*) Lown–Ganong–Levine, and (*D*) Mahaim pathways. (Sadowski AR, Moyers JR: Anesthetic management of the Wolff–Parkinson–White syndrome. Anesthesiology 51:553–556, 1979)

SURGICAL PROCEDURE

The surgical ablation of abnormal electrical pathways in WPW syndrome using epicardial mapping techniques is described in detail by Gallagher (Figs. 8-3, 8-4).[19] Intraoperative technical problems must be minimized, including electrical interference from monitoring, heating, and cautery equipment. Additional surgical problems include the identification of multiple accessory pathways and septal accessory pathways. In addition, severe alterations may occur in hemodynamic or electrical cardiac function caused by cardiac manipulation or injury to normal cardiac tissue (especially conductive tissue). Performance of the procedure while the patient receives *normothermic* hemodynamic support on cardiopulmonary bypass (CPB) appears to be the most effective, and least disruptive, to patient homeostasis. Because the intact, warm (normothermic), beating heart is being perfused by the aortic root pressure provided during CPB, mean arterial pressure (MAP) may require manipulation to assure adequate coronary perfusion. A MAP of 70 to 90 torr often is provided.

ANESTHETIC MANAGEMENT

Anesthetic management of the patient with WPW syndrome requires the minimizing or avoidance of tachyarrhythmias. Various anesthetic plans are summarized by Sadowski and range over virtually all of the available anesthetic armamentarium.[20] Thiopental appears to be innocuous with respect to alter-

Table 8-2. Drug Therapy in Wolff–Parkinson–White Syndrome

Goal ↓ Conduction in accessory pathway(s)
↑ Conduction in normal pathway
↓ Premature beats
↑ Refractory period: accessory pathway(s)
↓ Refractory period: normal pathway
Useful
Lidocaine
Procainamide
Quinidine
Propranolol
Disopyramide phosphate
Diphenylhydantoin
Controversial
Digitalis, especially if irregular VT
Verapamil
Contraindicated:
Ketamine
Pancuronium
Atropine/scopolamine?
"Alternatives"
Pacemakers
Cardioversion

Fig. 8-2. Reentry and reciprocating tachycardia. Mechanisms of tachycardia in Wolff–Parkinson–White syndrome. *A.* NSR fusion. *B.* Premature beat dissociates normal and accessory pathways. *C.* Reentry established antegrade conduction over AV node. *D.* Reentry confined to AV junction with reciprocation. (Gallagher JJ, Pritchett ELC, Sealy WC et al: The preexcitation syndromes. Prog Cardiovasc Dis 20:285–327, 1978)

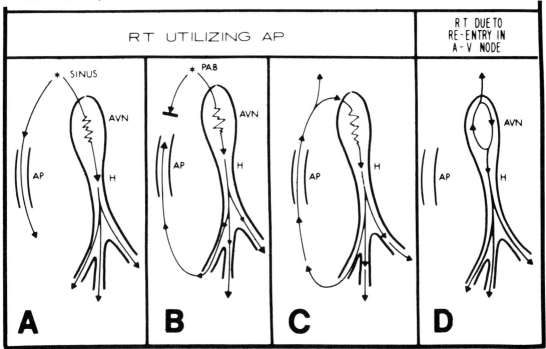

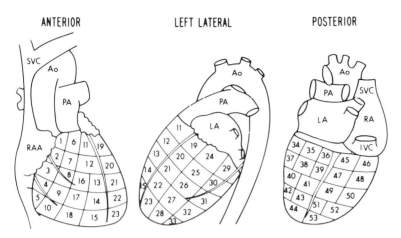

ANTERIOR   LEFT LATERAL   POSTERIOR

Fig. 8-3. Epicardial mapping grid. There are 53 areas from which activation data are recorded. Surface landmarks serve as references. (Gallagher JJ, Kasell J, Sealy WC et al: Epicardial mapping in the Wolff–Parkinson–White syndrome. Circulation 57:854–866, 1978. By permission of the American Heart Association, Inc.)

ations in cardiac conduction, based upon clinical reports of success.[20] There are no satisfactory prospective data on which to base solid conclusions regarding the use or avoidance of other intravenous anesthetic agents.

Any drug which produces an increase in circulating catecholamines, cardiac catecholamine release, vagolytic effects, or direct cardiac stimulating effects would best be avoided, pending outcome of any prospective investigations to the contrary. Thus it would seem appropriate to avoid atropine or scopolamine, except for specific treatment of sinus bradycardia with atropine. Following similar logic, pancuronium should be avoided in favor of metocurine, unless there is a contraindication for metocurine use. And, it would seem *reasonable,* but not proven, that "deep" anesthesia with an inhalation agent such as enflurane, to supplement any narcotic analgesia, should provide more complete sympathetic blockade. Theoretically, enflurane (Ethrane) is preferable to halothane in order to minimize ventricular irritability; its advantage in WPW syndrome is unproven. Isoflurane (Forane) carries the same advantages as enflurane without the degree of myocardial depression seen with either enflurane or halothane. Ketamine is best avoided, also on theoretical grounds, because of its sympathomimetic effects. Again, there are no clinical data which clearly document the advantage of one drug over another. A definitive study would be wel-

comed. Table 8-2 summarizes drug therapy in the patient with WPW. Additional concerns in this patient population are highlighted further during discussions of endocardial mapping.

ENDOCARDIAL MAPPING IN THE PATIENT WITH INTRACTABLE VENTRICULAR TACHYARRHYTHMIAS

An increasing number of patients is receiving intraoperative endocardial electrophysiologic mapping to locate, and to guide excision of, abnormal arrhythmogenic ventricular tissue.[21–26] These patients are refractory to both accepted and experimental antiarrhythmic drug therapy. This surgical procedure is an alternative to multiple daily defibrillation episodes, chronic low cardiac output syndrome, multiple drug infusions with toxic side effects, or perhaps death. It is undertaken in most cases after all other avenues have failed. Early results indicate surgical success rates approximating 80 to 90 percent.[21, 25]

PATIENT POPULATION AND PROBLEMS

With the application of recent advances in pharmacologic and pacemaker therapy, many of these patients have survived ventricular dysrhythmias to reach preoperative electrophysiologic study and endocardial/epicardial operative mapping. These patients usually have abnormal ventricular electrical foci resulting from distortions of anatomy and physiology. Various associated conditions include ventricular aneurysm, previous ventricular surgery, previous ventriculotomy, and LV or RV cardiomyopathy. Occassionally, patients have normal ventricular structure.

Almost all have ischemic myocardial disease. They often have associated coronary heart disease producing left ventricular compliance abnormalities and papillary muscle dysfunction. The presence of a left ventricular aneurysm of substantial size may severely compromise effective stroke volume. Performance of a standard aneurysmectomy (without mapping) may fail to resect the electrical focus.[27, 28] This focus is often in or near the endocardial surface of the aneurysm border,

and may extend several centimeters from the margin of the aneurysm or infarction.[29] Thus, it is hoped that mapping will offer a clearer delineation of the focus or foci intraoperatively and a subsequently greater degree of surgical success.

A discussion of ventricular arrhythmias in ischemic heart disease is beyond the scope of this chapter. In addition to Chapter 6, several reviews are offered for the reader's further enlightenment.[30–33] The anesthesiologist may be presented with a critically ill patient with multiple problems, including ongoing myocardial ischemia, low cardiac output, altered systemic and pulmonary vascular resistances, multiple arrhythmias refractory to all drugs, varying drug regimens, electrolyte imbalance, toxic drug responses, and investigative drugs being administered. The anesthesiologist then is requested to provide a

Fig. 8-4. Epicardial mapping "sock" electrode system. The nylon mech sock is shown with button electrodes placed in the mesh. Colored beads identify electrode sequence. This system is not used at Stanford. A hand-directed probe is preferred. (Gallagher JJ: Surgical treatment of arrhythmias: current status and future directions. Am J Cardiol 41:1035–1044, 1978)

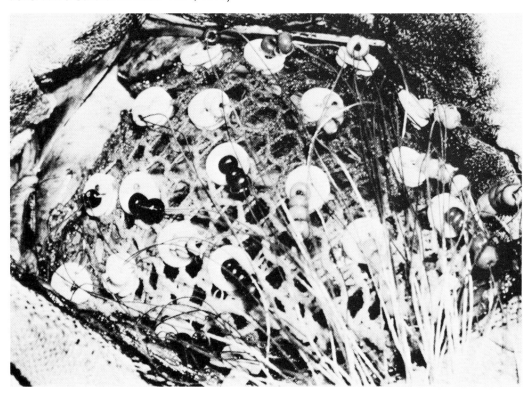

safe, smooth, and trouble-free anesthetic course, often on an emergency basis. Such an anesthetic course must be planned and performed carefully.

PREOPERATIVE ANESTHETIC CONSIDERATIONS

In addition to the usual considerations in a patient about to undergo cardiopulmonary bypass (see also Chap. 13), there are numerous questions which need to be addressed.

When all of these questions have been answered to the satisfaction of the patient, family, and all physicians caring for the patient, mapping may proceed. Premedication with drugs such as dizaepam and narcotics (morphine, hydromorphone) should be provided for optimal patient comfort. Atropine or scopolamine should not be administered. Continuously administered infusion drugs should be adjusted for optimal infusion rate and effect. A *working* nonmetal intravenous cannula should be in place before patient transport. All routine precardiac surgical procedures should be completed (blood type/crossmatch, laboratory results available, and so on). The patient should not have had food or drink for at least six hours. The expected roles of anesthesiologist, surgeon, and electrophysiologist should all be discussed preoperatively to avoid intraoperative conflicts.

Rhythm

Exactly what rhythm disturbances are present, and which therapies appear to work best?

What problems might occur, if any, or all, antiarrhythmic agents are discontinued? Has this been attempted?

Has the patient displayed signs of antiarrhythmic drug toxicity?

At which plasma level of each drug has toxicity occurred?

What plasma level of each drug (or total of drugs) is acceptable in order to perform a successful intraoperative mapping study inducing ventricular tachycardia (VT)?

Does this patient's VT respond to DC countershock? What current is needed?

Will this patient's VT spontaneously disappear? In what time period?

Does the patient lose consciousness with VT?

Can a pacemaker be used to stop VT?

Is a pacemaker in place and operationally effective?

Surgical Plans

Exactly what are the surgical plans?

Is coronary artery bypass grafting probable?

Will the preinduction placement of a pulmonary artery catheter likely trigger VT during placement?

Is anxiety or stress in this patient known to increase the incidence of arrhythmias?[34, 35] If so, how should premedication be planned?

Does the patient or family or both comprehend the seriousness of the anticipated procedure?

Is the planned ventricular excision too large for survival?

Are the complications of prolonged CPB understood and anticipated (Table 8-3)?

Are the non-CPB complications of endocardial mapping understood and anticipated (Table 8-3)?

Are all required personnel ready, and is all equipment working?

PREOPERATIVE PATIENT TRANSPORT

The patient should be transported to the operating suite accompanied by one or more anesthesiologists. The family should not accompany the patient. There should be sufficient assistance so that monitoring and treatment is the anesthesiologist's only job. If myocardial ischemia is present, supplemental inspired oxygen should be provided continuously. Sufficient IV sedation and analgesia should be provided before and during transport, and nitroglycerin infusion or tablets should be available. A working portable ECG monitor should be connected to the patient, and there should be a tested defibrillator on or near the transport bed. Resuscitation drugs and equipment should be available readily throughout the transport. Halls and elevators should be clear of obstructions. At any stage of transport, the team should be prepared fully to perform complete cardiopulmonary resuscitation. The trip should be quick, and efficiently performed.

PREBYPASS MANAGEMENT

Upon arrival in the operative area, ECG monitoring should continue, including now a modified V_5 lead system. Intravascular cannulas should be placed in the operative suite or similarly equipped area (see chapter 13 on routine prebypass management). If a pulmonary artery catheter is not placed because of an "irritable" ventricular response to intrachamber catheters, the surgeons should be agreeable to the surgical placement of a PA or LA pressure monitoring catheter intraoperatively if needed. A *minimum* amount of 0.5 percent lidocaine should be used for local anesthesia during vascular cannulation, the less the better. A separate, extra set of ECG leads capable of triggering an intraaortic counterpulsation balloon (IACPB) should be placed *preinduction* in dry skin areas and protected from the surgical "prep." Induction should begin only when perfusionist and surgeons are available, and *all* equipment to be used is fully operational.

Induction of anesthesia should be a controlled transition to unconsciousness. Drugs used should be compatible with the institution's protocols and standards, and consistent with the patient's anticipated physiologic reactions to known pharmacologic effects (see chapter 9 on anesthetic agents for further detail.) This may contraindicate agents such as halothane,[36] pancuronium, or ketamine, so that the likelihood of an increase in ventricular irritability or an increase in myocardial oxygen demand or both does not occur. Intravenous lidocaine anesthesia is not used, in order to avoid excessive plasma lidocaine levels which could interfere with the mapping procedure. There are no data in this patient population to specifically indicate or contraindicate other anesthetic agents. Hydromorphone (Dilaudid), diazepam, fentanyl, barbiturates, enflurane, isoflurane, and nitrous oxide all appear to be acceptable anesthetic agents if tailored to the patient's requirements for analgesia, sympathetic blockade, and optimal cardiovascular function.

The trachea must *not* be sprayed with li-

Table 8-3. Possible Complications During Endocardial Mapping

Rhythm	Unsuccessful procedure
	Ventricular tachycardia, irritability
	Supraventricular arrhythmias
	Catecholamine-induced arrhythmias
	Electrolyte abnormalities (K^+, Ca^{++}, Mg^{++}, etc.)
	Need for pacing
Hemodynamic	Low cardiac output
	Small stroke volume
	Ischemia
	Myocardial depression from antiarrhythmic drugs
	Myocardial injury from multiple DC countershocks or surgical manipulations
	Myocardial ischemia
	Problems secondary to use of an intraaortic counterpulsation balloon (IACPB)
	Hypovolemia secondary to blood loss
	Mitral insufficiency
	Ventricular septal defect
	Technical errors or problems

Emboli (air, intraventricular clot or debris)
Complications related to prolonged CPB
   Coagulopathies
   Prolonged myocardial ischemia
   Hemolysis
   Other organ injuries?
   Hypothermia
   Protein denaturation?
CNS injury secondary to decreased cerebral perfusion during dysrhythmias
CNS toxicity secondary to antiarrhythmic drug therapy
Infection or vascular injury from indwelling vascular devices

docaine in any patient for cardiac mapping, nor should lidocaine be used to lubricate the endotracheal tube or artificial airway. While the topical anesthetic effects would attenuate the circulatory effects of tracheal intubation,[37] the levels of lidocaine produced in the plasma may impair the ventricle's response to inducing VT during mapping. A lidocaine whole blood level greater than 2.5 μg base/ml is obtained easily with lubricant and spray combination,[38] even higher if the patient is small or if lidocaine has been used for local anesthesia at multiple cannulation sites.[39] The lidocaine level which can impair electrophysiologic studies is in the range of from 1 to 1.2 μg base/ml.[39] It is easy to overlook the accu-

Sources of Lidocaine Leading to Accumulation of Drug Which May Impair Cardiac Mapping Procedures

1. Cannulation sites: IV, arterial, CVP, PA, cutdowns, angiography, electrophysiologic studies, and so on
2. IV infusions used for arrhythmia control
3. Endotracheal tube lubricants
4. Oral/nasal airway lubricants
5. Laryngotracheal spray devices

mulated effects of lidocaine used in multiple areas for multiple effects.

Prebypass management should be concerned with hemodynamic and rhythm stability, provision of appropriate anesthesia, and avoidance of any complications which will interfere with the mapping procedure. All other standard prebypass concerns, discussed in other chapters, are operational in these patients as well. Approximately 30 minutes before CPB, a plasma specimen should be drawn to assess the plasma level of lidocaine (or other recently-used antiarrhythmic drug). This will assist in sorting out technical problems from drug problems if there is difficulty inducing VT during mapping.

BYPASS MANAGEMENT

The actual surgical mapping and excision procedures performed during or before bypass will vary somewhat with the patient and institution. Basically, these will involve the induction of VT by electrical means while examining either the exterior surface of the heart (epicardial) or interior surface within the ventricle(s) (endocardial) for ECG recordings, delineating the abnormal electrical focus or foci. Predetermined probe location sites are used (Fig. 8-3). Epicardial-activation and endocardial-activation maps are constructed during mapping, in an effort to establish the site of earliest depolarization. Comparisons between movable surface, reference, and stimulating electrodes assist in delineating the site. The interior of the heart will be exposed during endocardial mapping.

During most of bypass, the body and heart will be maintained at normothermia, and

thus bypass pressure and flow must be adequate to sustain total body perfusion. The heart remains perfused during mapping, to ensure myocardial oxygenation and well-being. Therefore, MAP needs to be maintained at a level sufficient to provide for adequate coronary blood flow, usually at 70 to 90 torr. As soon as mapping is completed and surgical correction instituted, cardiac and body hypothermia and cardioplegic solutions may be employed. The ascending aorta will be cross-clamped, and MAP may be decreased to levels routinely used during CPB at that institution.

Once the site of earliest electrical activity (focus) has been established, this area of endocardium is resected along with any aneurysmal area which requires resection for hemodynamic reasons. If there is not an associated aneurysm, or if involved tissue cannot be resected, the area of focus instead

Fig. 8-5. Encircling endocardial ventriculotomy. Cross section of left ventricle, with an area of extensive subendocardial infarction (*stippling*). *Dashed line* is ventriculotomy incision at border of infarction. Ao: aorta; MV: mitral valve; and PPM: posterior papillary muscle) (Gallagher JJ: Surgical treatment of arrhythmias: current status and future directions. Am J Cardiol 41:1035–1044, 1978)

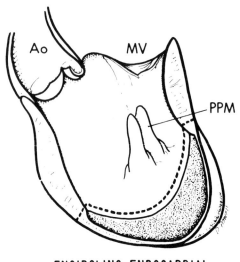

ENCIRCLING ENDOCARDIAL
VENTRICULOTOMY OF GUIRAUDON

may be surrounded by an encircling endo-cardial ventriculotomy (Fig. 8-5). Intraven-tricular clot may be dislodged from the en-docardial surface of an aneurysm during this procedure. Care is required to see that all intraventricular debris is removed before closing the ventriculotomy.

If substantial left ventricular mass is ex-cised, the post-bypass stroke volume (SV) may be very small, necessitating a higher post-CPB heart rate (HR) to provide an ade-quate cardiac output (CO) that will be life-sustaining [CO = SV × HR]. Further details of the actual surgical procedure are beyond the scope of this chapter and are presented by Horowitz,[40] Gallagher,[41] and Harken.[42]

CPB time may be extensive, depending upon technical details, inducibility of VT, sur-gical expertise, and the time required for analyzing mapping data. If endocardial map-ping, ventricular aneurysmectomy, and cor-onary artery bypass grafting are all per-formed, bypass time can exceed several hours. Some of the complications of pro-longed CPB are listed in Table 8-3. Additional complications referable to the procedure(s), not specifically caused by CPB itself, are listed also in Table 8-3. These possibilities must be anticipated because successful post-bypass management will involve the avoid-ance of many of these complications or ma-nipulations to improve them. The length of CPB will provide ample time for the anesthe-siologist to prepare IV drug infusions neces-sary for post-CPB management (lidocaine, dopamine, isoproterenol, dobutamine, nitro-prusside, nitroglycerin, and the like), prepa-rations for the treatment of post-CPB coagu-lopathies (platelets, fresh frozen plasma, and occasionally factor concentrates), correction of electrolyte abnormalities (K^+, Ca^{++}, acid-base, and so on), and to assure availability and proper function of an intraortic counter-pulsation balloon (IACPB) if indicated.

POSTBYPASS MANAGEMENT

All of the principles which I have outlined and discussed in Chapter 15 on routine post-bypass management should be followed. The reader is referred to that chapter for a thor-ough discussion of all aspects of routine post-bypass management; highlights of specific in-terest in the care of the patient post-mapping are presented here.

The guiding principles of post-mapping management and the general sequence of events in the cardiovascular aspects of man-agement are outlined below. Rhythm man-agement is preeminent and is summarized in Figure 8-6. Sinus rhythm is preferred with vigorous treatment of ventricular irritability. A pacemaker may be required, but a backup tested ventricular pacing system is manda-tory. IACPB therapy may provide relief for left ventricular work demand during systole, while allowing an increase in diastolic coro-nary perfusion. Often, IACPB use will solve rhythm disturbances thought intractable when using other therapies.

Inotropic and chronotropic drug support may be necessary. However, sympathomi-metic (and thus arrhythmogenic) drugs should be avoided if possible, or used in min-imum concentrations. Heart rate should be maintained in the 90 to 150 bpm range, the

Guiding Principles and Goals for Post-Mapping Management*

Maintain, through effective monitoring, all variables to where benefit exceeds risk.
Maintain myocardial oxygen supply > demand.
Maintain cardiac output sufficient for total body needs.
Maintain heart rate at 90–130 bpm: sinus rhythm.
Optimize preload for best cardiovascular function.
Maintain cardiac output by adjusting vascular volume, vascular resistance, and then contractility.
Maintain renal function by adequate CO and volume status; diuretics only as a secondary concern.
Maintain coagulation status within normal limits: prot-amine, platelets, fresh frozen plasma, factor IX con-centrate.
Plan to have PCV in early postop period above 30%.
Return rectal temperature, if possible, to normal, at least ≥35°C.
Maintain serum K^+ at 5.0 – 5.5 meq/L.
Maintain serum ionized calcium in normal range.
Anticipate the conceivable, and plan!
Transport with ECG monitoring, defibrillation equip-ment, and CPR drugs.

* See Chapter 15 for more details.

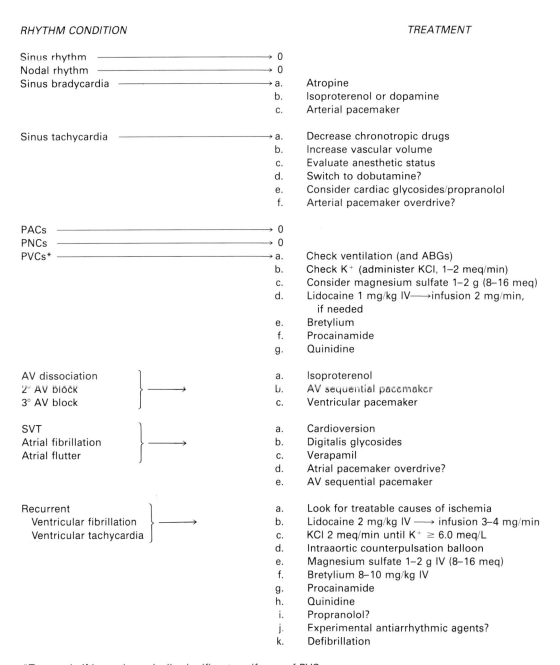

*Treat only if hemodynamically significant, or if runs of PVCs.

Fig. 8-6. Arrhythmia management postmapping.

General Sequence of Events: Cardiovascular Management Postmapping*

1. Cardiac rhythm
   Sinus rhythm preferred
   Pacemaker if necessary
   Vigorously control myocardial irritability (*e.g.*, lidocaine)
2. Cardiac rate (beats/minute)
   90–130 (higher range if small stroke volume postaneurysmectomy)
   < 90: Chronotropic support (dopamine, at lowest possible dose)
   > 130: Volume corrections or decrease chronotropic support or both
3. Adequate MAP and CO
   MAP < 60 torr: Volume, inotropic support, IACPB
   MAP 60 – 80 torr
   a. If CO OK, vasodilation and volume infusion until volume OK
   b. If CO low, also add inotropic support
   MAP > 80 torr:
   Reduce peripheral vascular resistance.
4. Readjust each of the above as needed, one variable at a time.

* See Chapters 8 and 15 for more detail.

higher limits required postaneurysmectomy if stroke volume is small. Lidocaine is infused intravenously to provide a whole-blood concentration satisfactory to suppress ventricular irritability (at least 2–3 μg/ml). This often requires a continuous infusion of from 2 to 4 mg/min. If pacing is required, ventricular or A-V sequential pacing is used (see Chap. 7 on pacemakers).

Control of coagulation mechanisms is provided by a three-part sequence. Initially, heparin effect is reversed with protamine, until the ACT returns to control value or to its lowest obtainable value. A normal thrombin time signifies sufficient protamine therapy. Platelets then are infused to provide a platelet count of greater than 100,000/mm^3 (and a bleeding time of less than 6 to 7 minutes). This often requires the administration of 3 to 6 platelet pack units, depending upon the initial platelet count, the length of CPB, aspirin use by the patient, and so on. Fresh frozen plasma and, rarely, factor IX concentrate (Proplex, Konyne) are administered as

needed to produce a normal prothrombin time or normal prothrombin/proconvertin time. (For a further discussion of coagulation therapy, see chapter 24, and a separate new coagulation textbook.[43])

SUMMARY

Endocardial and epicardial mapping are performed intraoperatively in critically ill patients. Patient selection provides patient populations refractory to nonsurgical forms of treatment. Especially in patients for endocardial mapping, the procedure may be a last hope for life. The anesthesiologist must be familiar with the disease entities under treatment and the physiologic and pharmacologic aspects of care. Absolute attention to detail is critical, as well as a well-coordinated team approach involving a skilled, experienced cardiovascular anesthesiologist, cardiac surgeon, electrophysiologist, perfusionist, and surgical nurses. Future improvements in electrophysiologic equipment, antiarrhythmic drugs, computerization and miniaturization of equipment for intraoperative data analysis should provide an even higher success rate for these procedures than presently seen.

REFERENCES

INTRODUCTION

1. Horowitz LN, Harken AH, Kastor JA et al: Ventricular resection guided by epicardial and endocardial mapping for treatment of recurrent ventricular tachycardia. N Engl J Med 302:589–593, 1980
2. Collins JJ: Editorial: Surgery for intractable ventricular arrhythmias. N Engl J Med 302:627–628, 1980
3. Gallagher JJ, Cox JL: Editorial: Status of surgery for ventricular arrhythmias. Circulation 60:1440–1442, 1979

4. Gallagher JJ: Surgical treatment of arrhythmias: Current status and future directions. Am J Cardiol 41:1035–1044, 1978
5. Josephson ME, Harken, AH, Horowitz LN: Endocardial excision: A new surgical technique for the treatment of recurrent ventricular tachycardia. Circulation 60:1430–1439, 1979
6. Zipes DP: Editorial: New approaches to antiarrhythmic therapy. N Engl J Med 304:475–476, 1981
7. Harken AH, Horowitz LN, Josephson ME: Comparison of standard aneurysmectomy and aneurysmectomy with directed endocardial resection for the treatment of recurrent sustained ventricular tachycardia. J Thorac Cardiovasc Surg 80:527–534, 1980
8. Sadowski AR, Moyers JR: Anesthetic management of the Wolff–Parkinson–White syndrome. Anesthesiology 51:553–556, 1979
9. Kastor JA, Horowitz LN, Harken AH et al: Clinical electrophysiology of ventricular tachycardia. New Eng J Med 304:1004–1020, 1981
10. Sand BJ, Rose HB, Barker WF: Effect of cardiac dysrhythmia on cerebral perfusion. Arch Surg 111:787–791, 1976
11. Willerson JT: Editorial: Prevention and control of ventricular arrhythmias. N Engl J Med 303:332–334, 1980
12. Mirowski M, Reid PR, Mower MM et al: Termination of malignant ventricular arrhythmias with an implanted automatic defibrillator in human beings. N Engl J Med 303:322–324, 1980

EPICARDIAL MAPPING

13. Gallagher JJ, Pritchett ELC, Sealy WC et al: The preexcitation syndromes, Prog Cardiovasc Dis 20:285–327, 1978
14. Sadowski AR, Moyers JR: Anesthetic management of the Wolff–Parkinson–White syndrome. Anesthesiology 51:553–556, 1979
15. Klein, GJ, Bashore TM, Sellers TD et al: Ventricular fibrillation in the Wolff–Parkinson–White syndrome. N Engl J Med 301:1080–1085, 1979
16. Farshidi A, Josephson ME, Horowitz LN: Electrophysiologic characteristics of concealed bypass tracts: Clinical and electrocardiographic correlates. Am J Cardiol 41:1052–1060, 1978
17. Wu D, Denes P, Amat-Y-Leon F et al: Clinical, electrocardiographic and electrophysiologic observations in patients with paroxysmal supraventricular tachycardia. Am J Cardiol 41:1045–1051, 1978
18. Mantakas ME, McCue CM, Miller WW: Natural history of Wolff–Parkinson–White syndrome discovered in infancy. Am J Cardiol 41:1097–1103, 1978

Surgical Procedure

19. Gallagher JJ, Kasell J, Sealy WC et al: Epicardial mapping in the Wolff–Parkinson–White syndrome. Circulation 57:854–866, 1978

Anesthetic Management

20. Sadowski AR, Moyers JR: Anesthetic management of the Wolff–Parkinson–White syndrome. Anesthesiology 51:553–556, 1979

ENDOCARDIAL MAPPING

21. Horowitz LN, Harken AH, Kastor JA et al: Ventricular resection guided by epicardial and endocardial mapping for treatment of recurrent ventricular tachycardia. N Engl J Med 302:589–593, 1980
22. Collins JJ: Editorial Surgery for intractable ventricular arrhythmias. N Engl J Med 302:627–628, 1980
23. Gallagher JJ, Cox JL: Editorial Status of surgery for ventricular arrhythmias: Circulation 60:1440–1442, 1979
24. Gallagher JJ: Surgical treatment of arrhythmias: Current status and future directions. Am J Cardiol 41:1035–1044, 1978
25. Josephson ME, Harken AH, Horowitz LN: Endocardial excision: A new surgical technique for the treatment of recurrent ventricular tachycardia. Circulation 60:1430–1439, 1979
26. Harken AH, Horowitz LN, Josephson ME: Comparison of standard aneurysmectomy and aneurysmectomy with directed endocardial resection for the treatment of recurrent sustained ventricular tachycardia. J Thorac Cardiovasc Surg 80:527–534, 1980

Patient Population and Problems

27. Horowitz LN, Harken AH, Kastor JA et al: Ventricular resection guided by epicardial and endocardial mapping for treatment of recur-

rent ventricular tachycardia. N Engl J Med 302:589–593, 1980

28. Gallagher JJ: Surgical treatment of arrhythmias: Current status and future directions. Am J Cardiol 41:1035–1044, 1978

29. Harken AH, Horowitz LN, Josephson ME: Comparison of standard aneurysmectomy and aneurysmectomy with directed endocardial resection for the treatment of recurrent sustained ventricular tachycardia. J Thorac Cardiovasc Surg 80:527–534, 1980

30. Hillis LD, Braunwald E: Myocardial ischemia, Part 1. N Engl J Med 296:971–978, 1977

31. Hillis LD, Braunwald E: Myocardial ischemia, Part 2. N Engl J Med 296:1034–1041, 1977

32. Hillis LD, Braunwald E: Myocardial ischemia, Part 3. N Engl J Med 296:1093–1096, 1977

33. Bigger JT Jr, Dresdale RJ, Heissenbuttel RH et al: Ventricular arrhythmias in ischemic heart disease: Mechanism, prevalence, significance, and management. Prog Cardiovasc Dis 19:255–300, 1977

Preanesthetic Considerations

34. Lown B, DeSilva RA, Lenson R: Roles of psychologic stress and autonomic nervous system changes in provocation of ventricular premature complexes. Am J Cardiol 41:979–985, 1978

35. Rosenfeld J, Rosen MR, Hoffman BF: Pharmacologic and behavioral effects on arrhythmias that immediately follow abrupt coronary occlusion: A canine model of sudden coronary death. Am J Cardiol 41:1075–1081, 1978

Prebypass Management

36. Johnston RR, Eger EI, Wilson C: A comparative interaction of epinephrine with enflurane, isoflurane, and halothane in man. Anesth Analg 55:709–712, 1976

37. Denlinger JK, Ellison N, Ominsky AJ: Effects of intratracheal lidocaine on circulatory responses to tracheal intubation. Anesthesiology 41:409–412, 1974

38. Viegas O, Stoelting RK: Lidocaine in arterial blood after laryngotracheal administration. Anesthesiology 43:491–493, 1975

39. Nattel S, Rinkenberger RL, Lehrman LL et al: Therapeutic blood lidocaine concentrations after local anesthesia for cardiac electrophysiologic studies. New Engl J Med 301:418–420, 1979

Bypass Management

40. Horowitz LN, Harken AH, Kastor JA et al: Ventricular resection guided by epicardial and endocardial mapping for treatment of recurrent ventricular tachycardia. N Engl J Med 302:589–593, 1980

41. Gallagher JJ: Surgical treatment of arrhythmias: Current status and future directions. Am J Cardiol 41:1035–1044, 1978

42. Harken AH, Horowitz LN, Josephson ME: Comparison of standard aneurysmectomy and aneurysmectomy with directed endocardial resection for the treatment of recurrent sustained ventricular tachycardia. J Thorac Cardiovasc Surg 80:527–534, 1980

Postbypass Management

43. Fischbach DP, Fogdall RP: COAGULATION: The Essentials. Baltimore, Williams & Wilkins, 1981

ADDITIONAL REFERENCES

[The following references may be useful for the reader. Several were in press at time of page proofing]

Boineau J: Mapping: Cardiac activation and repolarization (key references). Circulation 64:208–213, 1981. [A list of 223 references, grouped in sections of interest to the reader.]

Mason et al: Comparison of mapping to aneurysm resection. Circulation (In press)

Mason et al: Relative efficacy of conventional surgery for VT. Am J Cardiol (In press)

Mason et al: Editorial: Uncertainty of mechanism for VT. Am Heart J (In press)

Part III PHARMACOLOGIC AGENTS

9

Anesthetic Agents and the Patient with Cardiovascular Disease

CARL C. HUG, JR.

INTRODUCTION

This chapter is *not* intended as a review of the general pharmacology of anesthetic drugs; this has been done elsewhere.[1] Rather it discusses those features of anesthetic drugs that suggest their use or avoidance in patients with cardiovascular disease. In devising an anesthetic plan, the anesthesiologist chooses a particular anesthetic technique and specific drugs on the basis of the demands of surgery, the pathophysiologic status of the patient, and the potential of individual drugs to produce certain desired effects while avoiding or minimizing side-effects and toxicity. In the case of the patient with cardiovascular disease, the focus of the anesthesiologist's attention is on the hemodynamic effects of anesthetic drugs, and these are emphasized below. However, it is obviously necessary for the anesthesiologist to be fully aware of the whole patient and to take the functional status of all organ systems into account when choosing among anesthetic drugs.

CARDIOVASCULAR DISEASE

Cardiovascular disease includes a broad spectrum of functional abnormalities of the heart and vasculature. Certainly the anesthesiologist should be well-informed about the intricate details of the specific disease(s) he encounters in an individual patient. A thorough understanding of the hemodynamic conditions in each patient is essential if the anesthesiologist is to achieve the lowest possible incidence and degree of anesthetic morbidity and mortality. The hemodynamic problems

---

Primary Determinants of Cardiac Output That May Be Affected By Anesthetic Drugs

Heart rate
Heart rhythm
Ventricular contractility
Ventricular filling (venous return of blood)
Vascular resistance

---

of specific cardiovascular diseases have been reviewed in detail by others.[2,3]

In more general terms, the choice of anesthetic agents from among those currently available involves recognition of their effects on the hemodynamic factors listed above and discussed elsewhere in this text. None of the drugs curently available is ideal; some have minimal effects on cardiovascular function but fail to control the hemodynamic responses to surgical stress. The key to using any of the drugs effectively and safely is monitoring.

In the case of the surgical patient with cardiovascular disease, monitoring includes both the adequacy of anesthesia and the hemodynamic alterations associated with anesthesia and surgery. Moreover, monitoring should extend into the postoperative period when residual effects of anesthesia and surgery may have adverse consequences for the patient with cardiovascular disease.

Another aspect of cardiovascular disease of importance to the anesthesiologist is the influence of altered hemodynamics on the pharmacokinetics of the drugs he administers. The influence of perfusion abnormalities on the uptake and distribution of inhalational anesthetics has been reviewed by Eger.[4] Alterations of distribution, biotransformation, and excretion of intravenous drugs have been described in the presence of abnormal hemodynamics.[5] A great deal remains to be learned about the pharmacokinetics of anesthetic drugs in patients with cardiovascular disease, but important clues are already available from the studies of other drugs, especially lidocaine.[6]

Anesthesia has traditionally had three objectives:

1. *Analgesia* or the insensibility to pain; often extrapolated to include the suppression of responses to noxious stimulation
2. *Unconsciousness* or the lack of awareness of the surgical environment and *amnesia* for perioperative events
3. *Muscular relaxation* to facilitate the operation and to reduce somatic reflex responses to noxious stimuli

As the anesthesiologist has assumed greater responsibility for life support of the critically ill patient in the perioperative period, other objectives have been added. Often these additional objectives have to do with the maintenance of hemodynamic stability. This may be particularly difficult in the patient who will not tolerate the cardiovascular depression of potent general anesthetics and in whom autonomic reflex activity and the associated hemodynamic changes are elicited by surgical stimulation under light levels of anesthesia. The solution to this quandray often involves the use of nonanesthetic drugs that act directly on the autonomic and cardiovascular systems.

Another problem related to light levels of anesthesia has to do with the use (and abuse) of skeletal muscle relaxants. Muscular tone is maintained under light levels of anesthesia and this may impede certain types of operations. The patient may move in a dangerous manner in response to surgical stimulation. Continued muscular activity in response to hypothermia may increase oxygen demand beyond the limits of tissue perfusion under surgical conditions. For any of these reasons, the use of a neuromuscular blocking drug may be indicated (see Chapter 10). It is most important to remember, however, that the most reliable signs of anesthetic depth (*e.g.,* movement, ventilatory pattern) are suppressed in the paralyzed patient who appears to be anesthetizd even when he is conscious and experiencing pain.[7] The anesthesiologist must remain congnizant of this possibility and keenly alert to subtle signs of awareness by the patient (Table 9-1). This job is made easier by avoiding the use of muscle relaxants except when they are specifically indicated and by producing only the minimally required degree of paralysis. Total paralysis is seldom, if ever, necessary. Adequate muscular relaxation can be achieved and maintained precisely by the application of dose-response principles and the use of peripheral nerve stimulator.[8] It should be noted that there is a less than satisfactory correlation between autonomic sympathetic signs of light anesthesia and awareness.[9]

Table 9-1. Signs of Light Anesthesia

Skeletal muscular activity*
    Withdrawal or non-purposeful movement
    Grimacing, wincing
    Opening eyes
    Tensing abdomen and diaphragm (decreased ventilatory compliance)
    Coughing, vocalization
    Increased rate and depth of spontaneous ventilation
Sympathetic activity†
    Hyptertension and tachycardia
    Mydriasis and tearing
    Sweating
    Cold, clamy skin

*Reduced or eliminated by neuromuscular blocking drugs
†Awareness and recall have been reported in the absence of sympathetic signs.

DOSE-RESPONSE RELATIONSHIP

The dose-response relationship is essential to the anesthesiologist who seeks to provide adequate anesthesia and hemodynamic stability in the patient with cardiovascular disease. Almost all of the drugs currently used to alter cardiovascular and central nervous system function follow the general rule that the degree of the response is proportional to the logarithm of the dose. The anesthesiologist administers most drugs intravenously or by inhalation, and therefore, has the opportunity to determine the dose-response relationship in each and every patient, providing he monitors the patient's responses appropriately. In other words, because there is relatively little delay in the onset of drug action after inhalational or intravenous administration, the anesthesiologist can titrate drug dosages against the patient's needs. This is performed beginning with a small dose and increasing the dose in logarithmic (1,3,10,30 . . . units) or geometric fashion (1,2,4,8,16 . . . units) until a response is detected. This approach is especially important in the care of critically ill patients whose responsiveness to anesthetic and cardiovascular drugs is highly variable.

This variability usually can be demonstrated by noting the smaller doses of anesthetic drugs required for the induction of anesthesia in a patient with chronic mitral insufficiency and progressive heart failure compared to the doses required for a physically fit patient with coronary artery disease recently manifest by angina pectoris.

Another important source of variability is drug interaction. Such interactions may be of a pharmacodynamic nature (*i.e.*, change in the sensitivity of the responding organ) or of a pharmacokinetic type (*i.e.*, one drug alters the disposition of another). Propranolol provides good examples of the complexity of drug interactions in that it (1) slows the elimination of lidocaine,[10] (2) may prolong paralysis caused by d-tubocurarine,[11] (3) exaggerates the vasoconstrictor responses to epinephrine, (4) adds to the cardiovascular depression of halothane, (5) appears to potentiate the cardiovascular depression of methoxyflurane, and (6) limits the hemodynamic responses to sympathetic activation by noxious stimulation thereby reducing the dosage requirements for anesthetic drugs.[12, 13]

The dose-response and concentration-response relationships must be recognized in any meaningful discussion of drugs, including those used for anesthesia. A small dose is expected to produce a small effect. Thus, halothane is a cardiac depressant at anesthetic concentrations ($> 0.7\%$), but may have minimal effects on cardiac performance in subanesthetic concentrations ($\leq 0.25\%$) that are useful for supplementing the anesthetic effects of other drugs. On the other hand, investigators report that fentanyl is able to block alpha-adrenergic receptors *in vitro* at concentrations of 10^{-6} M (336 ng/ml) and greater.[14] However, these data have little or no relevance to the clinical situation where plasma concentrations of fentanyl are unlikely to exceed 50 ng/ml even after doses of 60 to 70 µg/kg.[15–17] These concentrations represent both free and protein-bound fentanyl. Only free fentanyl is pharmacologically active and in equilibrium across capillary and cellular membranes. More than 80 percent of fentanyl in plasma is protein-bound in normal subjects.[18]

Thus, it is necessary for the anesthesiologist to think and to communicate about drugs in quantitative terms. More often than not, blanket statements, such as, "It's contraindicated and should never be used in this situation," are incomplete and misleading. The important point is to recognize that while a large dose may be contraindicated, a small dose of the same drug may be used safely, and perhaps more effectively than any other available alternative for achieving a particular objective.

In relation to anesthetic drugs and their hemodynamic effects, it is important to note that almost every healthy volunteer and surgical patient is apprehensive before the induction of anesthesia (unless he has received adequate preanesthetic medication, which is often omitted in research subjects). The apprehension is associated with increased activity of the sympathetic nervous system and often produces hemodynamic effects. Thus, it is important to report data in absolute as well as relative (*e.g.*, percent of control) terms and to demonstrate that increasing increments of dose produce corresponding increases in response.

It is especially important to recognize that the depth of anesthesia represents a balance between the degree of depression induced by drugs and the intensity of stimulation produced by operative procedures. As the stimulus intensity increases so do anesthetic requirements. These relationships are readily demonstrated during cardiac surgery before and after cardiopulmonary bypass. Anesthetic dose requirements increase progressively for the patient to tolerate catheterization of the urinary bladder, an oral airway, endotracheal intubation, skin incision, electrocautery, sternal sawing and retraction in the prebypass period.

Anesthetic requirements are minimal under hypothermic conditions but increase progressively as body temperature returns to normal, pulsatile blood flow is reestablished, and, particularly, as electrocautery is used in the postbypass period. It is not uncommon for patients to become responsive to commands at one of these stages. It is likely that their recovery reflects the elimination of anesthetic drugs during bypass, although few studies are yet available to document this widely held belief. [19-21] Again it is to be emphasized that excessive doses of muscle relaxants will mask signs of the patient's return to consciousness.

THE PHASES OF ANESTHESIA

The phases of anesthesia include preanesthetic medication, induction and maintenance of anesthesia, and postoperative care. Tradi-

tionally, the emphasis of *preanesthetic medication* has been on allaying the patient's anxiety (*i.e.,* sedation). This is an important objective, but it should be remembered that communication between the anesthesiologist and patient is every bit as important as antianxiety drug therapy.[22] There are other objectives of preanesthetic medication for the patient with cardiovascular disease (Table 9-2). These medications are appropriately ordered by the anesthesiologist to be administered the night before and morning of surgery. It

Table 9-2. Objectives That Can Be Realized With Drugs Used for Preanesthetic Medication of the Patient with Cardiac Disease

DRUG CLASS	OBJECTIVES
Barbiturates and benzodiazepines	Sedation and sleep Reduction of anesthetic requirements Amnesia (benzodiazepines only)
Narcotic analgesics	Prevention of pain caused by percutaneous needle puncture Relief of existing pain Sedation and sleep Reduction of anesthetic requirements Postoperative pain relief (short operation)
Major tranquilizers	Reduction of nausea and vomiting Increased sedative and analgesic effects of narcotic analgesics
Anticholinergics	Drying of mucous membranes (rarely indicated, always uncomfortable) Prevention of bradycardia (rarely effective) Decreased gastric secretions (partially effective) Amnesia (scopolamine only)
Antihistamines	Sedation Drying of mucous membranes (atropine-like)
H₂ blockers	Decreased gastric secretions and acidity Minimization of the responses to histamine (*e.g.,* released by d-tubocurarine, morphine)
Antacids	Neutralization of gastric acidity
Antihypertensives	Maintenance of blood pressure control in the perioperative period Reduction of hypertensive responses to noxious stimulation under light anesthesia
Antianginal drugs	Less myocardial ischemia in the perioperative period
Pilocarpine (for patients with glaucoma)	Eyedrops to maintain miosis and prevent mydriasis in response to systemic anticholinergics
Insulin (for patients with diabetes mellitus)	Preservation of glucose uptake into tissues during the perioperative period

is noteworthy that many of the drugs are useful both before and during anesthesia. For example, beta-adrenergic receptor blocking drugs (*e.g.,* propranolol [Inderal]) are indicated not only for the preanesthetic control of angina pectoris and hypertension, but also because they limit intraoperative tachycardia resulting from noxious stimulation or from the use of vasodilators to produce deliberate hypotension.[23] There is a growing trend to continue *essential* chronic drug therapy up to the time of surgery in order to prevent the consequences of its withdrawal (*e.g.,* rebound hypertension, angina pectoris, psychological depression and anxiety) and to provide a smoother intraoperative course.

The induction of general anesthesia is an event abounding in risks for the patient with cardiovascular disease. Hemodynamic changes can be anticipated in response to anesthetic drugs, especially when they are administered rapidly in large doses. Hence, the risks attendant with a rapid sequence of anesthetic induction and endotracheal intubation are to be avoided whenever possible in favor of a gradual induction of anesthesia with careful titration of drug dosage in accordance with anesthetic requirements and hemodynamic changes. An adequate depth of anesthesia should be achieved before laryngoscopy and other procedures likely to stimulate autonomic reflexes.

The choice of drugs for rapid induction of anesthesia is usually dictated by hemodynamic considerations. Chief among these is the dependence of cardiovascular performance on sympathetic tone. For example, the hypovolemic patient (*e.g.,* dehydration, hemorrhage) will not tolerate anesthetics that interfere with sympathetic function; ketamine may be the drug of choice under such circumstances (see below).

Maintenance of general anesthesia in the patient with cardiovascular disease should be based on considerations of the demands of the surgical procedure and on the cardiovascular status of the patient (Table 9-3). Remember that minor surgery may demand a major effort on the part of the anesthesiologist in order to achieve a satisfactory anes-

Table 9-3. Considerations in the Choice of Technique for Maintenance of Anesthesia in the Patient With Cardiovascular Disease

Surgical procedure
    Intensity of noxious stimulation
    Requirements for muscular relaxation
    Use of drugs by the surgeon (*e.g.,* epinephrine, neomycin)
    Procedures compromising cardiovascular function (*e.g.,* position of patient,
        surgical manipulation, high risk of sudden or excessive blood loss)
    Requirements for postoperative care (*e.g.,* ventilatory support, intensive
        care)
Cardiovascular status of the patient
    Sympathetic nervous system activity
        Compensation of cardiac failure
        Maintenance of venous return with a low circulating blood volume (*e.g.,*
            hemorrhage, dehydration)
    Chronic hypertension
        Reduced circulating blood volume
        Left ventricular hypertrophy ($\uparrow$ risk myocardial ischemia)
    Cerebrovascular-carotid artery disease
        Maintenance of cerebral perfusion pressure
    Coronary artery disease
        Factors influencing myocardial oxygen balance
    Ventricular function (see list below)
        Determinants of cardiac output (see list above)
    Valvular heart disease
        Specific pathophysiologic features for each type of lesion

thetic state while supporting vital functions at optimal levels.

The choice of monitoring techniques can influence the selection of anesthetic drugs especially for the hemodynamically unstable patient for whom the earliest detection of adverse trends is indicated. It may be necessary for the anesthesiologist to maintain a delicate balance between adequate anesthetic depth and excessive hemodynamic depression. Without careful monitoring of both hemodynamics and anesthetic depth, errors are likely. In terms of hemodynamics, the selection of drugs for the maintenance of anesthesia is made with regard to their effects on cardiac performance, specifically their effects on ventricular function, which can be classified as good or poor for practical purposes (see list below). Drugs depressing myocardial contractility and sympathetic tone in anesthetic concentrations (*e.g.*, halothane) may be useful in the patient with good ventricular function to limit sympathetic and hemodynamic responses to noxious stimulation and to minimize myocardial oxygen demand, especially in the patient with coronary artery disease. Myocardial depression and suppression of autonomic sympathetic activity is poorly tolerated by patients with impaired ventricular function for any reason (*i.e.*, infarction, valvular disease, dysrhythmias, hypovolemia). In such cases, light anesthetic levels produced by narcotic analgesics (in combination with muscle relaxants and perhaps hypnotic drugs) may be indicated along with cardiovascular drugs to control specific problems as they develop (*e.g.*, nitroglycerin infusion for myocardial ischemia).

Postoperative care is obviously influenced by intraoperative anesthetic management, and in some cases, plans for postoperative care dictate the selection (or avoidance) of specific drugs. Long-acting narcotic analgesics (*e.g.*, morphine or fentanyl in large doses) are usually inappropriate if provisions for postoperative ventilatory support are not made. When ventilatory assistance is planned for the postanesthetic period, these narcotic analgesics may be ideal because they promote the pa-

Characteristics of Poor Ventricular Function

Signs and symptoms of congestive heart failure
History of multiple myocardial infarctions
Cardiac catheterization reveals the following:
　Left ventricular end-diastolic pressure > 18 torr
　Ejection fraction < 0.5
　Cardiac index < 2.5 l/min/M²
　Abnormal ventriculogram (dysfunction, aneurysm)

tient's tolerance of the endotracheal tube and they provide sedation and analgesia.

REGIONAL ANESTHESIA

Regional anesthesia has a very limited role in the management of patients undergoing cardiac surgery for obvious reasons. Local anesthesia may be appropriate in some circumstances (*e.g.*, transvenous pacemaker insertion, opening a pericardial window). Intercostal nerve blocks may be useful for short-term control of post-thoracotomy pain. Some have employed local anesthetics for cervical sympathetic ganglionic blockade in an attempt to control postoperative hypertension.[24] The hemodynamic consequences of such procedures are discussed elsewhere.[25–27] The indications for regional anesthesia in peripheral vascular surgery are presented in Part 6 of this text.

BASIS OF THIS REVIEW

The cardiovascular pharmacology of anesthetic drugs and their applications in anesthesia for cardiac surgery was reviewed early in 1978 by the author of this chapter.* A large amount of additional information has accumulated in the intervening time, especially for the narcotic analgesic, fentanyl. In addition, the "new" inhalational anesthetic, isoflurane (Forane), is now available for general use. These agents and the newer references

---

* Hug CC Jr: Pharmacology: anesthetic drugs. In Kaplan (ed): Cardiac Anesthesia. New York, Grune & Stratton, 1979

are included in this chapter; most of the 92 references published before 1970 and cited in the earlier review have been omitted. In fact, only 21 of the bibliographic citations cited in this chapter were published before 1970; 40% of the citations have appeared since the beginning of 1978. The hemodynamic effects of muscle relaxants are considered in Chapter 10.

NITROUS OXIDE

Nitrous oxide (N_2O) is the most widely used anesthetic, but its limited potency makes supplementation with other CNS depressants and muscle relaxants necessary in order to achieve the classic triad of anesthetic objectives. Conversely, nitrous oxide is used to supplement other anesthetic agents: (1) to produce unconsciousness and amnesia in combination with narcotic analgesics; (2) to provide analgesia and reduce responses to noxious stimulation in combination with barbiturates, benzodiazepines, and other hypnotics; and (3) to reduce the dosage requirements of potent inhalational anesthetics.[28]

Besides some of the cardiovascular effects discussed below, there are a number of other features about this anesthetic gas that restrict its use. The requirement for oxygen supplementation of the inspired gases may limit the concentration of nitrous oxide that can be administered. (Incidentally, nitrous oxide is often administered intraoperatively when it is desirable to reduce the partial pressure of oxygen in the inspired mixture; it would be more logical to use nitrogen or air for such purposes, especially if the other side-effects of nitrous oxide are to avoided.)

Nitrous oxide readily diffuses into air-filled cavities inside the body and expands those that are distensible and increases the pressure in those that are rigid.[29] Thus, it will enlarge air emboli in blood, exacerbate a pneumothorax, and expand the air-filled cuff on an endotracheal tube or increase the pressure it exerts on the tracheal mucosa.[30] These are of particular concern in the patient undergoing cardiac surgery because air emboli are frequent after open-heart surgery and may occur in the aorta and vein grafts during coronary bypass procedures. Also, cardiac surgery is frequently complicated by pneumothorax, and it is common to leave the endotracheal tube in place for prolonged periods.

Nitrous oxide exacerbates the truncal rigidity induced by narcotic analgesics (discussed below) and this can impair both spontaneous and mechanical ventilation of the lungs.

The *cardiovascular effects* of nitrous oxide appear to be the result of two actions: (1) a direct depression of myocardial contractility[31] and (2) a stimulation of autonomic sympathetic centers with the CNS.[32] In normal subjects, these actions are manifested by small and somewhat inconsistent changes in cardiovascular variables and by modest increases in circulating catecholamines.[33, 34]

Hemodynamic changes may be more marked in the patient with cardiac disease, especially in those with impaired ventricular function. The depression of cardiac output is relatively greater and is further exacerbated by the rise in systemic and pulmonary vascular resistances.[35-37] Significant degrees of hypotension may occur, wherein a reduction of the inspired concentration of nitrous oxide or discontinuation of its use is necessary.

These same actions of nitrous oxide are evident when it is combined with other drugs, especially the narcotic analgesics or benzodiazepines or both, which have little or no effect on myocardial contractility.[38-42] The degree of hypotension may be somewhat greater than with nitrous oxide alone to the extent that the intravenous drugs interfere with activation of the sympathetic nervous system by nitrous oxide.

Combinations of nitrous oxide with potent inhalational anesthetics produce complex hemodynamic effects that are not always predictable but are usually understandable in light of the following facts.[28, 43-46]

1. Nitrous oxide deepens the level of anesthesia when it is added to a potent inhalational anesthetic.

2. Nitrous oxide reduces the dose of an inhalational anesthetic required for a given anesthetic depth. To the extent that less of the potent agent is required, it is anticipated that the cardiovascular depression by that potent agent will be less.

3. Potent volatile anesthetics tend to depress autonomic function and would be expected to block the sympathetic stimulating actions of nitrous oxide. Hence, vascular resistance may not increase and blood pressure may fall because of the myocardial depressant effects of nitrous oxide and the volatile agent.

4. Myocardial depression by the potent anesthetics may be sufficient to overshadow the weaker actions of nitrous oxide.

5. In most circumstances the hemodynamic consequences of nitrous oxide are small, especially in relation to the numerous other factors that influence cardiovascular function. Under some conditions, the hemodynamic changes associated with the administration of nitrous oxide are transient (10–20 min).[46]

In summary, it is important to recognize that nitrous oxide can affect the cardiovascular system and the changes it elicits may dictate its discontinuation. Usually the hemodynamic changes revert toward the pre-nitrous oxide state within a few minutes because this gaseous anesthetic is eliminated rapidly through the lungs.[47] Should the situation demand immediate correction, nitrous oxide will not interfere with the actions of drugs acting on the autonomic and cardiovascular systems. (*e.g.*, ephedrine, calcium).

VOLATILE ANESTHETIC AGENTS

The number of potent inhalational anesthetics commonly used for surgical anesthesia has dwindled to three: halothane (Fluothane), enflurane (Ēthrane), and isoflurane (Forane). Each of these is sufficiently potent to produce all of the objectives of anesthesia when used in sufficiently high concentrations. A standard index of anesthetic potency is the Minimum Alveolar Concentration (MAC) of anesthetic at 1 atmosphere that produces immobility in 50 percent of subjects exposed to a noxious stimulus (*e.g.*, skin incision).[48, 49] MAC is the same as a median effective dose or ED50.[50] The standard deviation of an average MAC value equals 10 to 20 percent of that value; thus, MAC plus 2 standard deviations will prevent movement of 95 percent of subjects in response to stimulation. (*i.e.*, ED$_{95}$). The MAC values for the three anesthetics to be discussed below are:

	ED50 (MAC)	APPROXIMATE ED95
Halothane	0.75%	1.0%
Isoflurane	1.15%	1.5%
Enflurane	1.68%	2.0%

It is important to keep these end-tidal (alveolar) concentrations in mind when discussing and comparing the effects of these anesthetics. One should also be aware of the factors that influence MAC (*i.e.*, increase or decrease anesthetic requirements; Table 9-4).

Nitrous oxide interacts additively with the potent volatile anesthetics.[51] The MAC of nitrous oxide is approximately 100 percent. Thus, the use of 50 percent nitrous oxide (at sea level) will reduce the anesthetic requirements of the potent volatile anesthetics by one-half. In other words, 1 percent halothane alone or 0.5 percent halothane combined with 50 percent nitrous oxide will produce about the same anesthetic depth.

It is apparent that the requirement for oxygen in the inspired anesthetic mixture precludes the use of nitrous oxide alone for general anesthesia. The potent volatile agents can produce any depth of anesthesia with oxygen concentrations approaching 98 percent in the inspired mixture.

Each of the volatile anesthetics produces skeletal muscle relaxation, but the concentrations required for the desired degree of relaxation often exceed those that will be tolerated because of the cardiovascular side-effects of the anesthetics, especially in ill patients. Thus, muscle relaxants are frequently used in conjunction with the volatile anesthetics. It is important to note that the combination

Table 9-4. Factors Influencing or Not Influencing Anesthetic Requirements (MAC)[49]

MAC DECREASED	MAC UNCHANGED	MAC INCREASED
Increasing Age	Duration of anesthesia	Alcoholism (chronic abuse)
CNS depressants	Circadian rhythm	Drugs increasing CNS catecholamines
Alcohol (acute intake)	Gender	Cocaine
Barbiturates	Species	Dextroamphetamine
Benzodiazepines	Hypertension	Ephedrine
Bromide ion	Propranolol	Hypernatremia and other factors
Lidocaine (systematically)	Hyperkalemia	increasing brain sodium
Narcotic analgesics	Hypocarbia	Hyperthermia $> 42°C$
Nitrous oxide and other	Metabolic acidosis or	Hypercarbia (PaCO$_2$ > 95 torr,
anesthetics	alkalosis	CSF pH < 7.1)
Phenothiazines (with		Hypoxemia (PaO$_2$ < 38 torr)
sedative actions)		Anemia (Arterial O$_2$ content < 4.3
Δ-9-tetrahydrocannabinol		ml/dl)
Drugs decreasing CNS catecholamines		
(*e.g.*, reserpine, alphamethyldopa)		
Pancuronium		
Cholinesterase inhibitors		
Pregnancy		
Hypercalcemia		
Hypotension		
Hypothermia		

of one of these potent anesthetics with a skeletal muscle relaxant reduces the dosage requirements of *both* drugs.[52]

Unconsciousness can be induced with the inhalational anesthetics at concentrations well below MAC, especially in the presence of other drugs (*e.g.*, preanesthetic medication) and factors that reduce anesthetic requirements.[49] Recognition of this fact allows the potent agents to be used as anesthetic supplements in small concentrations that may not adversely affect hemodynamics in the patient with impaired cardiovascular function. Similarly low concentrations of one of the volatile anesthetics are also useful to blunt the hemodynamic and autonomic sympathetic responses to noxious stimulation in patients already lightly anesthetized with intravenous drugs.

The choice of one or the other of the volatile anesthetics for a particular patient and operation is usually based on a consideration of its side-effects, especially those related to the cardiovascular system. Side-effects related to the CNS (*e.g.*, seizure-like activity), lung (*e.g.*, bronchodilation for asthmatics), liver (*e.g.*, hepatitis), and kidney (*e.g.*, release of fluoride ion) are widely discussed and debated in the anesthesia literature and will not be considered here. The actions of these

agents on the cardiovascular system are detailed below.

Cardiovascular changes occur with the inhalation of halothane, enflurane, or isoflurane. Each produces a concentration-dependent depression of contractility in the isolated heart and hypotension in proportion to dose in the intact animal and man.[53] Nevertheless, significant differences exist in the hemodynamic effects of these anesthetics, and some of these are important in the management of patients, especially those with cardiovascular disease. It is noteworthy that there is no exact relationship between their anesthetic potency and their ability to depress cardiac contractility either *in vitro* or *in vivo*. And in the intact subject, neurogenic and hormonal mechanisms may be more or less effective in compensating for the cardiovascular actions depending on the particular anesthetic and the depth of anesthesia (*i.e.*, the balance of CNS depression and noxious stimulation).

In comparing the cardiovascular changes induced by these anesthetics, it is important to recognize that a number of factors influence the responses that are observed. Obviously, the dose of anesthetic is important and it is essential that measurements be reported at a defined, stable level of anesthetic partial pressure in arterial blood and end-tidal gas; the latter is usually more convenient to measure. The depression of spontaneous ventilation leads to accumulation of carbon dioxide (and perhaps hypoxia) which stimulates the autonomic nervous system and relaxes vascular smooth muscle. The interactions of each of these potent volatile anesthetics with other drugs (*e.g.*, nitrous oxide, propranolol) may differ in terms of hemodynamic effects.

The cardiovascular effects of halothane, enflurane and isoflurane are summarized in Table 9–5 for healthy volunteers whose respiration was controlled.[54–56] Details about the individual agents are discussed below.

Halothane (Fluothane) produces dose-dependent hypotension, which persists for the duration of its administration. Moderate anesthetic concentrations (1–1.5 MAC) initially reduce cardiac output with little or no change in systemic vascular resistance. As the duration of anesthesia is prolonged (up to 5 hours), heart rate and cardiac output tend to increase while vascular resistance and central venous pressure decrease. The reason for these time-dependent changes is unknown; they are also seen with diethyl ether and to a much lesser degree with other volatile anesthetics.[57] The mechanisms underlying the

cardiovascular depression by halothane include (1) direct depression of contractile mechanisms in myocardial and vascular smooth muscle and (2) reduction of sympathetic nervous system activity (multiple sites of action).[57, 58]

The practical implications of these actions of halothane can be summarized as follows.

1. Halothane can produce cardiovascular collapse even in fit individuals when unusually high concentrations are administered. Severe hypotension may occur at moderate anesthetic concentrations in those with limited cardiovascular reserve. The usual compensatory mechanisms for cardiac failure, namely tachycardia and peripheral vasoconstriction, are also depressed by halothane.
2. Patients dependent on sympathetic nervous system activity for maintenance of circulatory function are unusually susceptible to halothane, and its use in anesthetic doses is contraindicated in those with hypovolemia or congestive heart failure.
3. Propranolol and other beta-adrenergic receptor blocking drugs add to the cardiovascular depression of halothane.[59, 60] This additive interaction is predictable and

Table 9-5. Cardiovascular Effects of Volatile Inhalational Anesthetics at 1–1.5 MAC in Healthy Volunteers With Normal PaCO$_2$

VARIABLE	HALOTHANE[54]	ENFLURANE[55]	ISOFLURANE[56]
Blood pressure	↓↓	↓↓	↓↓
Vascular resistance	0	↓	↓↓
Cardiac output	↓↓	↓↓	0
Cardiac contraction*	↓	↓↓	0
Central venous pressure	↑	↑	0
Heart rate	0	↑↑	↑
Sensitization of the heart to epinephrine	↑↑↑	± ↑	0?

*Estimated from change in amplitude of the IJ wave of the ballistocardiogram.

  0 = no change (< 10%)
  ± = variable change
  ↓ = 10 − 20% decrease
  ↓↓ = 20 − 40% decrease
  ↑ = increase

reversible by reducing the concentration of halothane. The administration of beta-adrenergic receptor blocking drugs up to the time of surgery does not contraindicate the use of halothane,[61] but the maximum safe concentration of halothane may be lower and it may be necessary to discontinue halothane administration because of excessive circulatory depression.[62]

4. Halothane is useful in patients with labile hypertension because it limits their sympathetic and circulatory responses to noxious stimulation during surgery.[63] Patients with chronic severe hypertension (diastolic blood pressure greater than 120 torr) tend to have a reduced blood volume and may show an exaggerated decrease in arterial pressure during halothane anesthesia.

5. Halothane is effective in controlling elevated perfusion pressures by lowering peripheral vascular resistance during cardiopulmonary bypass.

6. By virtue of its cardiovascular and sympathetic nervous system depressant actions, halothane can be used to limit myocardial work and oxygen demand.[64] The limiting factor in this application of halothane is the development of arterial hypotension which reduces coronary perfusion. Experiments in dogs suggest that in the absence of ventricular failure, the oxygen supply/demand relationship is shifted in a beneficial direction and the severity of myocardial ischemia caused by temporary occlusion of a coronary artery reduced.[65] The benefit of halothane anesthesia in limiting myocardial ischemia results primarily from its ability to reduce tachycardia, thereby reducing oxygen demand, and to increase diastolic coronary perfusion time, thereby increasing oxygen supply. These benefits may be offset by the development of systemic hypotension, and thus reduced coronary perfusion pressure.[66]

7. Should hypotension become excessive during halothane anesthesia it can be reversed by (1) eliminating halothane from the inspired gas (at least temporarily until some recovery is evident), (2) maintaining adequate cardiac filling pressures by elevating the legs, infusing fluids, and administering a noncatecholamine vasopressor with both alpha- and beta-adrenergic receptor stimulating properties (*e.g.*, ephedrine); and (3) counteracting the depression of cardiac contractility by the injection of calcium or a noncatecholamine sympathomimetic, such as ephedrine. The avoidance of catecholamines is dictated by halothane-induced sensitization of the heart to their arrythmogenic actions. Thus, calcium is the preferred inotropic drug to counteract the depressant actions of halothane.[67]

In addition to its negative inotropic effects, halothane can reduce cardiac output by altering cardiac rhythm. All types of dysrhythmias have been observed during halothane anesthesia.[68] Nodal rhythms are common and can result in marked hypotension because cardiac output is reduced by lower ventricular filling in the absence of an appropriately timed atrial contraction. Cardiac output is similarly reduced by premature nodal and ventricular beats. These rhythm disturbances may revert to normal spontaneously but require treatment if they persist or recur frequently and are occasioned by significant hypotension. The specific therapy depends on the circumstances because the same dysrhythmias may be seen under light or moderately deep anesthesia. Thus it may be appropriate to increase or to decrease the inspired concentration of halothane; if uncertain about the cause, decrease it! Equally important steps include (1) increasing the inspired oxygen concentration and alveolar ventilation to correct any hypoxia or hypercarbia, the two most frequent causes of dysrhythmias under anesthesia; (2) correcting sinus bradycardia which allows latent AV nodal and ectopic pacemakers to become dominant, either atropine (0.2–0.4 mg increments IV) or ephedrine (5–10 mg increments IV) are effective, but the latter may be preferred when the level of halothane anesthesia is deep; (3) administering antiarrhythmic drugs as indicated, lidocaine (1 mg/kg bolus IV doses) for nodal and ventricular premature beats, propranolol (0.25–1 mg increments IV) for sinus or atrial tachycardia, ouabain (0.3–0.5 mg IV; 0.125–0.25 mg IV in the digitalized patient) to control supraventricular tachycardia and the associated rapid ventricular responses; (4) cardioversion of atrial fibrillation with DC current synchronized to the QRS wave on the ECG;* and (5) sternal compression or direct cardiac massage until ventricular fibrillation or tachycardia with severe hypotension can be treated with DC countershock.†

One action of halothane predisposing to the development of ventricular premature beats and fibrillation is its sensitization of the myocardium to the actions of epinephrine and other catecholamines.[69] Sensitization occurs to a lesser degree to noncatecholamine sympathomimetics which may be used to treat cardiovascular depression induced by halothane, although calcium is a more logical choice.[67, 70] Administration of catecholamines is essentially contraindicated during halothane anesthesia except for local hemostasis in very restricted doses (i.e., 1–1.5 µg/kg subcutaneously or submucosally every 10 min not to exceed 4 µg/kg/hr). This recommendation is based on those put forth by Johnston and coworkers[69] and Katz and coworkers.[71] A relationship between the degree of sensitization and halothane concentration has not been established, but it is important to note that the supplementation of anesthesia with halothane earlier in the surgical procedure (e.g., before or during cardiopulmonary bypass) does not preclude the use of sympathomimetic catecholamines (e.g., for inotropic support) after bypass when halothane administration has been discontinued for 20 to 30 minutes (i.e., to allow halothane concentrations to decline to low levels).

Hypoxemia contributes to the development of cardiac arryhthmias. Two actions of halothane on the lung are important in this regard. First, halothane reduces pulmonary vascular resistance in a dose-dependent manner but appears to be less inhibitory of hypoxic pulmonary vasoconstriction than other inhalational anesthetics.[72] Thus, the degree of hypoxemia resulting from venous admixture (shunt) may not be increased by modest anesthetic concentrations of halothane. Secondly, halothane relaxes bronchial smooth muscle and for that reason is often chosen as an anesthetic for patients with asthma.[73] Several facts should be remembered when using halothane for this purpose. Light levels of anesthesia, regardless of the anesthetic, predisposes to asthmatic attacks; once in progress, it is foolhardy to attempt to break it with halothane because its uptake will be slowed and it predisposes to arrythmias that are likely in the presence of hypoxia, hypercarbia, and the associated sympathoadrenal stimulation. Also, the use of isoproterenol, epinephrine, and other sympathomimetic bronchodilators in the presence of halothane anesthesia is risky, even if they are administered as aerosols. Terbutaline (Brethine, Bricanyl) may be an exception because its arrhythmogenic dose is much higher (at least in dogs) than that required for bronchodilation.[74] Lastly, enflurane is an effective bronchodilator and sensitizes the heart to a much lesser degree than halothane; it should be considered as an alternative to halothane before beginning the induction of anesthesia in an asthmatic patient.[69, 73]

Interestingly, halothane anesthesia counteracts the arrythmogenic actions of digitalis glycosides and may be considered the anesthetic of choice for emergency surgery in a patient with digitalis intoxication.[75] (Elective surgery should be postponed.)

Enflurane (Ēthrane) produces a pattern of circulatory changes very similar to those described for halothane (Table 9–5).[76, 77] In volunteers, it tended to produce slightly greater depression of cardiac contractility and vascular resistance than did halothane. Compared to halothane, it was associated with an

---

*External application of the paddles to the chest wall: 50 watts/sec (or joules)–400 watts/sec; internal application of the paddles to the heart: 5–10 watts/sec.

†External defibrillation: 400 watts/sec; internal 10–50 watts/sec depending on the size of the heart, paddle contact, and response

increase in heart rate but much less sensitization of the heart to catecholamines. The ED50 of epinephrine for premature beats was over 10 μg/kg at 1.25 MAC enflurane compared to 2 μg/kg at 1.25 MAC halothane.[78]

The following experimental observations seem to be important although their clinical significance has not yet been determined. First, a stable degree of circulatory depression was maintained in volunteers at 1 to 1.5 MAC enflurane for more than 5 hours, but progressive cardiovascular depression was evident when an attempt was made to sustain 2 MAC levels of enflurane. The circulatory effects were reversed when enflurane was eliminated.[77] Secondly, the addition of propranolol to enflurane produced greater circulatory depression than when it was added to an anesthetically equivalent concentration of halothane. Moreover, the superimposition of blood loss was more poorly tolerated in dogs anesthetized with enflurane than in halothane-anesthetized animals.[79] Thirdly, the addition of nitrous oxide to enflurane produced minimal changes in hemodynamics in contrast to the transient sympathomimetic effects produced by nitrous oxide addition to halothane.[80-82] On the other hand, the substitution of nitrous oxide for a portion of the volatile anesthetic dose resulted in less cardiovascular depression by either enflurane or halothane. All of these observations suggest the possibility that enflurane may be somewhat more depressant of the sympathetic nervous system than is halothane, especially at higher concentrations. This speculation must be tempered by the observations of similar effects of halothane and enflurane on autonomic and circulatory functions in cats.[83, 84]

Regardless of the above-mentioned differences between halothane and enflurane, they are used interchangeably in terms of their cardiovascular effects except in patients for whom epinephrine injection is anticipated for local hemostasis; enflurane is preferable to halothane in that case.[78] Potential effects of the two anesthetics on other organ systems more frequently form the basis for choosing between them. Certainly, enflurane is an appropriate general anesthetic for patients with normal ventricular function whose hemodynamic stability is not dependent on higher than normal sympathetic activity. Like halothane it can be used as an anesthetic supplement to control labile hypertension, to obtund sympathetic and circulatory responses to noxious stimulation, to limit myocardial work and oxygen demand, and to reduce elevated perfusion pressures during cardiopulmonary bypass. When excessive circulatory depression is induced by enflurane, the same sequence of therapy is used as in the case of halothane overdosage (see above).

Isoflurane (Forane) was released for general clinical use just before the submission of this manuscript. Relatively little is known about its hemodynamic effects under clinical conditions of cardiac surgery. Observations in healthy volunteers (Table 9–5) suggest that it is less of a cardiac depressant than either halothane or enflurane, which may offer an advantage in anesthetizing patients with impaired cardiac function.[85, 86] On the other hand, it is the most potent of the three volatile anesthetics in reducing peripheral vascular resistance, and this is a definite disadvantage when the maintenance of blood pressure and coronary perfusion are essential for meeting the oxygen demands of the heart (*e.g.,* aortic valvular stenosis, coronary artery disease). Also, the decrease in resistance is attributed largely to vascular beds in skeletal muscle. Increased perfusion of skeletal muscle in the anesthetized patient represents wasted cardiac work. The decrease in vascular resistance appears to be reversed by sympathetic responses to surgical stimulation. The addition of nitrous oxide to isoflurane increased peripheral vascular resistance and lessened the degree of hypotension, but did not reduce blood flow in skeletal muscle, especially when the subject's ventilation was controlled.[87]

Just what place isoflurane will take in anesthesia for cardiovascular surgery remains to be seen. In one study of patients undergoing coronary artery surgery, the hemodynamic changes under halothane and isoflurane anesthesia were similar.[88]

Other considerations that may enter into the decision to use or to avoid isoflurane are as follows: (1) isoflurane is a potent inhibitor of hypoxic pulmonary vasoconstriction in the dog and may increase venous admixture in patients with abnormal distribution of pulmonary ventilation;[89] (2) in its sensitization of the heart to the actions of catecholamines, isoflurane is intermediate (epinephrine ED50 = 6.7 μg/kg) between halothane (2.1 μg/kg) and enflurane (10.9 μg/kg);[90] and (3) isoflurane appears to produce less depression through more variable changes in the conduction of impulses through the atrioventricular node, and it has been suggested that nodal rhythms based on impulse reentry are less likely to develop.[91]

There appears to be little difference between isoflurane and halothane in the degree of their depression of isolated cardiac muscle; the depression of both is exacerbated to the same degree by the presence of congestive heart failure.[92] The interactions of propranolol and isoflurane are similar to those of propranolol and halothane in the dog.[93, 94] Like halothane, isoflurane depresses sympathetic nervous system function probably in a dose-dependent fashion. Although its significance for man is unknown, isoflurane has a greater margin of safety between anesthetic concentrations and those producing either respiratory or cardiac arrest in the rat than either enflurane or halothane.[95]

INTRAVENOUS ANESTHETIC AGENTS

Despite the heading, none of the drugs discussed in this section is truly an anesthetic in terms of achieving fully the major objectives of anesthesia (discussed previously) in a practical range of doses. It is a common practice to combine drugs in order to meet the anesthetic requirements for a specific patient and type of surgery. This is usually most appropriately done by selecting a specific drug for a specific effect (Table 9-6). This combined use of individual drugs for specific effects has a number of misnomers, including "balanced anesthesia." Ideally, all types of anesthesia, whether inhalational or intravenous drugs are used, should be balanced in every conceivable manner. In fact, it is appropriate to supplement intravenous agents with low, subanesthetic concentrations of

Table 9-6. Anesthetic Objectives and the Selection of Drugs to Meet Them

OBJECTIVE	DRUGS*
Sleep → unconsciousness	N_2O†, barbiturates, benzodiazepines, etomidate
Amnesia	N_2O, benzodiazepines, scopolamine
Analgesia: suppression of responses to noxious stimulation	N_2O, narcotic analgesics
Muscular relaxation	Neuromuscular blocking drugs (see Chapter 10)
Autonomic reflex control	
Parasympathetic blockers	Atropine, glycopyrrolate (Robinul)
Sympathetic blockers	
α (hypertension)	Phentolamine (Regitine), prazosin (Minipress)‡
β (tachycardia)	Propranolol (Inderal)
Ganglionic blockers	Trimethaphan (Arfonad), pentolinium (Ansolysen)
CNS-autonomic depression	Volatile anesthetics,* major tranquilizers

*Volatile anesthetics such as halothane and enflurane can be used in low, subanesthetic concentrations to supplement other drugs in achieving any one of the anesthetic objectives.
†N_2O is the chemical formula for nitrous oxide.
‡Prazosin is not yet available for intravenous use; it has the advantage over phentolamine of blocking both α_1- and α_2-adrenergic receptors.

volatile anesthetics in order to achieve any one of the objectives. Note that the techniques of intravenous anesthesia developed in part as a means of supplementing the deficiencies of nitrous oxide. The latter is used almost always as part of an "intravenous anesthetic" unless its effects are not tolerated or its use is contraindicated (see section on nitrous oxide).

One concern frequently registered in regard to intravenous anesthetics is that they are not "controllable and retrievable" as are the inhalational anesthetics. It is true that greater knowledge and skill are required to achieve anesthetic objectives satisfactorily and precisely with the intravenous drugs than with the inhalational drugs, the elimination of which can be facilitated by adjusting the ventilation of the patient and the anesthetic concentration in the inspired gas mixture. The key to precision with intravenous anesthetics is titration of dose size and frequency of administration to the response of the patient. Knowledge of the pharmacokinetics of each intravenous anesthetic is essential to perform this titration efficiently.[96, 97] In general, a drug that traverses biologic membranes rapidly (i.e., most intravenous anesthetics) will have a rapid onset after intravenous injection and will undergo rapid redistribution (short-lasting effect) until its storage sites equilibrate with plasma; thereafter the decline of its effects will parallel its elimination from the body. Slow elimination results in long-lasting effects. Because of the nature of drug disposition, it is necessary initially to give larger doses more frequently to achieve and to maintain an effect, and then as storage sites (e.g., muscle, fat) come into equilibrium with other body tissues, smaller doses are required less frequently to maintain the effect. These patterns of intravenous drug administration and disposition are analogous to those of the inhalational anesthetics.[97, 98] The use of intravenous priming and maintenance infusions offers the potential of as much control and precision as is possible with inhalational anesthetic.[99] As is the case with inhalational anesthetics, it is necessary for the anesthe-

siologist to anticipate the end of surgery and to discontinue the administration of intravenous drugs appropriately. And it is noteworthy that cardiovascular function is a major determinant of the elimination of both inhalational and intravenous drugs.[98, 100] In the face of cardiovascular collapse, the anesthesiologist cannot retrieve an inhalational anesthetic any better than the body can metabolize and excrete an intravenous drug. Again, titration of dosage to response is the key to precision in anesthesia and the avoidance of complications with both inhalational and intravenous drugs.

The maintenance of a stable tissue level of an anesthetic (or other drug) is essential to the measurement of its cardiovascular actions. Failure to do so in the case of intravenous anesthetic drugs presents a major problem in the interpretation of hemodynamic changes that have been reported to date. For a given effect to be ascribed to a drug, definition of the dose-response relationship, previously discussed, is essential. Actually, it is the drug concentration-response relationship that is fundamental, and in the case of drugs administered as bolus doses intravenously, the drug concentration at its site of action may fluctuate widely. Moreover, a large number of factors influence the relationship between drug dosage and the concentration achieved at its site of action so that considerable variation may be observed when different subjects receive the same mg/kg dose. One solution to this problem is to maintain a stable drug concentration by continuous infusion and to measure its plasma concentration, which is proportional to and closely reflects changes in the concentration at the sites of action to lipid-soluble drugs which are able to equilibrate rapidly across biologic membranes (i.e., most intravenous anesthetic drugs).[97] Thus far, this approach has been applied to a very limited extent.[99, 101–106]

BARBITURATES

This class of CNS depressants includes a large number of drugs used to produce sedation, sleep, and unconsciousness. The pharmacology of these drugs is thoroughly reviewed elsewhere.[107–109] The longer lasting ones (*e.g.*, pentobarbital—Nembutal) are used for anesthesia in experimental animals, but rarely in humans. The ultrashort-acting barbiturates (*e.g.*, thiopental—Pentothal; methohexital—Brevital) are used primarily for the induction of anesthesia and occasionally for its maintenance in patients undergoing surgery, electroconvulsive therapy, cardioversion, diagnostic, and other types of procedures, especially brief ones. Only thiopental and methohexital will be considered here because they are widely used and the hemodynamic effects of anesthetic doses have been studied in humans. Except as specifically noted below, methohexital is qualitatively identical to thiopental. Quantitatively, it is two to four times more potent than thiopental and is eliminated more rapidly ($t\frac{1}{2}\beta$ for methohexital = 1.5 hr; $t\frac{1}{2}\beta$ for thiopental = 7 hr)[110, 111]

Thiopental (Pentothal) is still the drug most widely used for induction of anesthesia because the onset of unconsciousness is almost instantaneous and it is well-accepted by patients. It is seldom used alone for maintenance of anesthesia because it does not efficiently suppress responses to noxious stimulation or relax skeletal muscle. Moreover, the effects of an induction dose (1–4 mg/kg) are short lasting (7–15 min) and larger or repeated doses result in accumulation of thiopental which is only slowly eliminated from the body.[111]

The hemodynamic effects of anesthetic doses of thiopental (or methohexital) consist of a mild, transient hypotension reflecting decreased cardiac output that is of little significance in healthy subjects.[112, 113] The decrease in cardiac output results from a reduction in stroke volume that is partially compensated for by an increase in heart rate.[114] Thiopental acts directly on the heart to depress contractility.[115] It also reduces sympathetic activity emanating from the CNS.[116] The consequences of these actions may be evident as severe hypotension in patients with heart failure and those dependent on sympathetic tone for maintenance of

blood pressure (*e.g.*, hypovolemia, sitting position). Accompanying these actions is an increase in the capacitance of veins with variable changes in central venous pressure (*i.e.*, decreased venous return versus raised end-diastolic pressure caused by depressed ventricular ejection).[117, 118] Although the barbiturates act directly on vascular smooth muscle to relax it,[119] changes in arterial resistance after anesthetizing doses in healthy subjects are small and variable, perhaps reflecting a compensatory increase in sympathetic activity to maintain blood pressure through an increase in systemic vascular resistance. It may be that baroreceptor-sympathetic reflex mechanisms are only partially inhibited by the usual doses of thiopental, and that the inhibition is evident only when the system is stressed by hypovolemia or an upright body position. Excessive doses are likely to obtund reflex mechanisms and to produce a decrease in systemic vascular resistance.

The increased heart rate is probably responsible for the increased myocardial oxygen consumption that is satisfied by a proportionally increased coronary blood flow in subjects with normal coronary arteries and minimal hypotension.[114] However, the actions of thiopental offer the potential for disaster in the patient with coronary artery disease. Hypotension caused by depressed cardiac contractility may be exaggerated in the patient with impaired left ventricular function caused by ischemia or infarction. Coronary perfusion pressure will decrease because of systemic hypotension, and myocardial oxygen demand will increase because of tachycardia and left ventricular distension (less emptying). An imbalance in oxygen supply and demand will develop or worsen and lead to further ischemic impairment of ventricular function and thereby create a vicious cycle. Although not contraindicated, thiopental should be used cautiously in patients with coronary artery disease, especially in the face of impaired ventricular function.

Thiopental may be used in anesthesia for cardiac surgery for the following:

1. Produce sleep (0.5–1.5 mg/kg IV bolus)
2. Induce unconsciousness (*i.e.*, anesthesia) in incremental IV doses of 1–2 mg/kg up to a total of 5 mg/kg in fit subjects
3. Accomplish a rapid sequence induction of anesthesia and endotracheal intubation; thiopental 4 mg/kg IV bolus followed immediately by succinylcholine (1 mg/kg IV bolus without, or 1.5 mg/kg 3–5 min after a 3–mg dose of d-tubocurarine to reduce fasciculations)
4. Control an acute episode of hypertension and tachycardia caused by surgical or other noxious stimulation under light anesthesia (0.5–1 mg/kg IV bolus)
5. Reduce arterial perfusion pressure during cardiopulmonary bypass (0.5–1 mg/kg as a bolus into the oxygenator reservoir).

Because of the risks noted above, the use of a rapid sequence induction and intubation ("crash") is to be avoided if at all possible. In the event that surgery cannot be delayed, the anesthesiologist must determine the best way to protect the airway in a patient presumed to have a full stomach, and at the same time prevent additional stress on the cardiovascular system. Besides thiopental-succinylcholine the anesthesiologist can consider other combinations to be discussed later, such as ketamine-succinylcholine, or perhaps fentanyl-pancuronium, for a rapid induction-in-tubation sequence.[120] Alternatively, topical anesthesia of the airway in an awake-sedated patient may be appropriate for tracheal intubation, in the author's opinion. Strong contraindications to thiopental include history of an allergic-anaphylactic response, history of prophyria, hypovolemia, and congestive heart failure.

As suggested above, large or repeated doses can lead to prolonged effects, primarily sedation and somnolence in the postanesthetic period. The ventilatory depressant effects are proportional to dose. In the somnolent, arousable patient the degree of ventilatory depression approximates that of natural sleep.[108] Of course, residual effects of thiopental add to or potentiate the depressant actions of other drugs.

In the absence of analgesic drugs, the patient's response to pain may be exaggerated by the barbiturates.[121] (Antanalgesia may be a form of disinhibition.) Under such conditions, the patient may be unmanageable and exhibit sympathomimetic signs including hypertension and tachycardia. The situation should be avoided, and may be remedied by an appropriate dose of a narcotic analgesic.

BENZODIAZEPINES

Only diazepam (Valium) and lorazepam (Ativan) are currently available in the United States for intravenous injection, and there are specific recommendations offered to reduce the incidence and severity of phlebitis caused by irritating characteristics of the injectable solutions. (Each milliliter contains 5 mg diazepam, 40% propylene glycol, 10% ethyl alcohol, 5% sodium benzoate, and 1.5% benzyl alcohol; or each milliliter contains 2 or 4 mg lorazepam, 0.18 ml polyethylene glycol 400 in propylene glycol, and 2% benzyl alcohol.[122]) A water-soluble benzodiazepine, midazolam, is undergoing clinical trials and offers the following advantages over diazepam and lorazepam: (1) less irritation of veins with lower incidences of painful injection and phlebitis; (2) shorter duration of action; (3) more rapid elimination from the body ($t_{\frac{1}{2}}\beta$ = 2 hr versus 21 to 37 hr for diazepam and 16 hr for lorazepam) without accumulation of pharmacologically active metabolites; and (4) avoidance of potential pharmacologic activity of the injection solution vehicle. Preliminary reports indicate that midazolam is approximately twice as potent as diazepam and that equipotent doses produce the same spectrum and intensity of effects.[123, 124]

Other nonparenteral benzodiazepines (*e.g.*, oxazepam—Serax) are used by anesthesiologists for preanesthetic medication (sedation, sleep, amnesia). They differ from orally administered diazepam and lorazepam primarily in their rate of elimination and the nature of their metabolites.[125] The pharmacology of benzodiazepines has been reviewed by many authors.[126, 127]

Diazepam or lorazepam may be administered orally as a preanesthetic medication to allay anxiety. Diazepam is more reliably absorbed from the gastrointestinal tract than from sites of intramuscular injection, which causes considerable pain. Both are administered intravenously to produce sedation, sleep, or unconsciousness and have anticonvulsant effects including the elevation of the seizure threshold dose of local anesthetics.[128] As with other CNS depressants, the net effect is dependent on the balance between dose and the intensity of stimulation. It is common for a patient with atrial fibrillation to become unarousable to command (0.5–0.7 mg/kg IV) and then awaken to the jolt of direct current cardioversion. Some of these patients remember the experience, especially the pain associated with the DC shock; diazepam and lorazepam have no analgesic actions.[129] Amnesia occurs in some patients, but it is more reliably produced when diazepam is combined with other amnestic drugs (*e.g.*, scopolamine or nitrous oxide).[126, 130, 131]

The *cardiovascular effects* of intravenous diazepam are benign and unrelated to the dose in the vast majority of people; there is a slight lowering of blood pressure equivalent to that which is expected when the subject goes to sleep.[132–137] A small decrease in stroke volume ($<20\%$) is compensated for by slight increases in heart rate and systemic vascular resistance, so that cardiac output and blood pressure tend to be maintained. The decrease in stroke volume is associated with a decline in central venous pressure, indicating that decreased venous return rather than depressed myocardial contractility is responsible.[138] Studies in rats suggest that the injectable form of diazepam as well as the vehicle alone can dilate vena caval smooth muscle and obtund its response to norepinephrine.[139] However, no sympatholytic effect has been demonstrated in man and he does not exhibit orthostatic hypotension after diazepam.[140] Considering the widespread and frequent use of diazepam, the reports of serious degrees of hypotension are indeed rare and the mechanism is unknown.[141]

Myocardial oxygen balance may be shifted in a favorable direction by diazepam even in patients with coronary artery disease.[142, 143] Total coronary blood flow increases, but it is not known if subendocardial and ischemic areas get their share of the increase. Myocardial oxygen demand may be lowered to the extent that left ventricular end diastolic volume decreases. During cardiac catheterization studies, the usual rise in left ventricular end diastolic pressure following injection of the contrast medium appeared to be blunted in patients receiving diazepam.[144]

Because diazepam lacks analgesic properties, it is frequently combined with a narcotic analgesic for anesthetic purposes and for postoperative comfort. Diazepam and narcotic analgesics complement one another in achieving a pain-free, unconscious state using much lower doses of both drugs than would be required if both objectives were to be sought using one or the other drug alone.[145] The hemodynamic consequences of such combinations have not been explored fully. The degree of change in cardiovascular dynamics when 10 mg of diazepam was added to morphine (2 mg/kg) or fentanyl (50 μg/kg) was about the same as that reported for diazepam alone (*i.e.*, $<20\%$), but it was suggested that the changes reflect a mild degree of depression of myocardial contractility by the combination because central venous pressures tended to rise rather than remain unchanged or fall as reported for diazepam alone.[146, 147] In most cases, the hemodynamic changes are likely to be clinically insignificant and represent a small cost for the benefits of greater assurance of unconsciousness and amnesia than can be provided by using much larger doses of a narcotic analgesic alone.

Thus, diazepam provides obtundation of consciousness with minimal hemodynamic alterations. Its major limitations as an anesthetic are its limited potency, lack of analgesic effects, and prolonged duration of action.

OTHER HYPNOTICS

There are a number of hypnotic drugs being used for the induction and maintenance of anesthesia in countries outside the United States. Some of these are unlikely to be approved by the Food and Drug Administration. For example, propanidid and althesin (a mixture alphaxalone and alphadalone) are poorly soluble in water and are dissolved in Cremophor EL for injection; a very high incidence of thrombophlebitis is attributed to the vehicle and makes these agents unacceptable for general use.

Etomidate, a water-soluble imidazole derivative, is a potent, short-acting hypnotic developed by Janssen Pharmaceutica. Clinical trials in the United States confirm the findings in other countries that etomidate produces a rapid induction of anesthesia, equivalent in onset and duration to that produced by thiopental. It is associated occasionally with pain when injected into peripheral veins (local irritation) and with involuntary, myoclonic-type movements (*not* associated with abnormal EEG patterns).[148, 149] Except for these effects the incidence of adverse responses is very low, and the effects of etomidate on the cardiovascular system appear to be minimal.[150, 151] A relatively large dose (0.45 mg/kg) produced slight reductions in cardiac index, stroke volume, left ventricular work, and arterial blood pressure that averaged less than a 10 percent change from the preanesthetic values in unpremedicated surgical patients. Minimal changes were seen in other hemodynamic variables including heart rate, which tended to increase by less than 10 percent from the control state.[151] Etomidate, like thiopental, failed to block the hemodynamic responses to endotracheal intubation.[149] Just what place etomidate will take among intravenous drugs for the induction of anesthesia remains to be seen. With its minimal effects on the cardiovascular system, etomidate may prove useful in the anesthetic management of patients with unstable hemodynamics.

NARCOTIC ANALGESICS

By far, the drugs most frequently used today along with muscle relaxants for the anesthetic management of critically ill patients and for those with cardiovascular disease are the narcotic analgesics. In sufficient doses, these drugs produce freedom from pain and sleep with minimal cardiac depression and clinically insignificant hemodynamic alterations, providing certain precautions are taken (see below). They certainly are not without side-effects; but with the exception of their depression of brain stem respiratory centers (easily managed in the setting of general anesthesia), most of the narcotic analgesics have no direct, unreversible, or detrimental effects on the function of vital organs including the brain, lung, heart, liver, and kidney. Of course, the function of these vital organs can be grossly impaired if ventilation is not supported and precautions are not taken to prevent or to treat circulatory side-effects largely caused by vascular dilation. Some of the indications for using a narcotic analgesic as a primary drug for general anesthesia are summarized in the list below.

The narcotic analgesics comprise a large number of compounds, more than 20 of which are used clinically. They differ in chemical structure, physical properties, analgesic potency, intensity of side-effects, onset and duration of action, and in a number of other ways as well.[152] But in terms of their pharmacologic actions, they closely resemble morphine except for a few effects of the narcotic antagonist analgesics such as pentazocine (Talwin), butorphanol (Stadol) and nalbuphine (Nubain). These are discussed briefly below.

The narcotic analgesics most widely used for anesthetic purposes are morphine, meperidine (Demerol), hydromorphone (Dilaudid),* and fentanyl (Sublimaze). For purposes here, it is appropriate to consider the actions of morphine in detail and then to compare the other narcotic analgesics to it.

Morphine as a Prototype

Morphine has been used in conjunction with general anesthesia since 1850 when Lorenzo Bruno described its combination with chlo-

---

* Hydromorphone is used commonly at Stanford University by University cardiac anesthesiologists. There are no data reported on its use; it will not be disccused further in this chapter.

roform. In 1869, Claude Bernard reported that morphine reduced the dosage requirements of chloroform, and in the early 1900s a number of reports described the use of morphine in doses approximating 1 mg/kg in conjunction with 1 to 3 mg of scopolamine for surgical anesthesia.[153] The latter use was short-lived because of the demanding requirements for restraining the patient during surgery (though none of the patients recalled the events) and because there was a high incidence of death, probably caused by respiratory depression (artificial respiration was not known). The use of narcotic analgesics as anesthetic agents languished until Neff and coworkers reported the supplementation of nitrous oxide with meperidine in 1947.[154] Bailey and colleagues described in 1958 the use of meperidine and 100 percent oxygen for heart surgery after the induction of sleep with thiopental.[155] But it was in the mid-1960s at the Massachusetts General Hospital where Lowenstein and his colleagues rediscovered the use of morphine as a primary anesthetic agent in combination with muscle relaxants.[156] (Ether anesthesia was *rediscovered* at the same hospital!) Since the 1969 report of Lowenstein and coworkers, the use of morphine and other narcotic analgesics in anesthesia for cardiac surgery has increased dramatically. And the application of anesthetic techniques based on narcotic analgesics has spread to all types of surgery in critically ill patients, especially those with cardiovascular instability.

It is important to recognize that the narcotic analgesics act selectively on certain areas of the CNS in contrast to general anesthetics which are capable of depressing all CNS functions. The effects of morphine and the other narcotic analgesics will be considered in relation to the objectives of general anesthesia previously discussed.

Analgesia is a dose-dependent effect of morphine and its surrogates. In the setting of anesthesia, the dosage requirement depends primarily on the intensity of noxious stimulation and it is presumed that even the most intense pain can be obtunded if the dose is increased sufficiently. At least patients who

---

Advantages of a Narcotic Analgesic as a Primary Anesthetic Agent

Minimal cardiac depression
No myocardial sensitization to catecholamines
Circulatory autoregulation maintained in CNS and kidney
Can awaken patient intraoperatively
Postoperative analgesia
Decreased cough reflexes (↑ toleration of endotracheal tube)
Ventilatory depression (facilitates mechanical ventilation)
Antagonist available
No hepatic or renal toxicity
No environmental pollution (but high abuse potential)
Not teratogenic
Not a trigger of malignant hyperthermia

---

awaken enough to respond appropriately to commands often indicate that they are not experiencing pain even though the operation is proceeding. Others have reported after surgery that they were pain-free even though they can recall (and were frightened by) intraoperative events.[157, 158] The particular type of pain (*i.e.*, somatic versus visceral), personality of the patient, and other factors that modify the effectiveness of analgesic doses (morphine 0.1–0.3 mg/kg) seem to be of little practical importance in the face of anesthetic doses of morphine (1–3 mg/kg) or its congeners.

Analgesic actions of morphine and most other narcotic analgesics are still evident when the patient awakens postoperatively. This is an obvious benefit of anesthetic techniques based on morphine, but the cost may be mechanical support of ventilation and continued intubation of the trachea well into the postanesthetic period. The narcotic antagonists (*e.g.*, naloxone) will reverse both analgesia and respiratory depression in a parallel fashion.[152, 153] It may be necessary to accept some degree of ventilatory depression in order to preserve some degree of analgesia. If the decision is made to use naloxone (Narcan), it is essential that the dose be titrated carefully according to the patient's response for the sake of both comfort and safety (see below).

Unconsciousness can be induced by large, anesthetic doses (1–3 mg/kg) of morphine, especially in debilitated and elderly patients. It is not reliably produced in physically fit subjects even by doses of 3 to 4 mg/kg.[158] Some have claimed that unconsciousness will occur in every subject when the dose of morphine reaches 8 to 11 mg/kg, but this dose is associated with generalized edema and such prolonged respiratory depression and coma that it is impractical.[159] Equivalently large doses of fentanyl (70–150 µg/kg) result in ventilatory depression lasting as long as 18 to 36 hours after surgery but do not cause edema and prolonged coma; it remains to be seen whether fentanyl alone can produce unconsciousness reliably for the duration of surgery in physically fit patients.[160–165]

The problem is that the patient may go to sleep in the absence of stimulation but remain arousable, especially by noxious surgical maneuvers. If he is completely paralyzed with neuromuscular blocking drugs, his awakening may go undetected and his recall of this predicament is likely because morphine and the other narcotic analgesics have no amnestic effects. These circumstances can be prevented by (1) combining morphine with general CNS depressants (*e.g.*, diazepam, barbiturates, nitrous oxide; see cardiovascular effects below), (2) limiting the degree of paralysis so that awakening can be detected (*e.g.*, facial movement in response to noxious stimulation or to command), (3) administering a drug producing amnesia as a part of preanesthetic medication or intraoperatively (*e.g.*, scopolamine, diazepam, nitrous oxide), and (4) most importantly, the anesthetist and others remaining alert to signs of lightening anesthesia and awareness. The appearance of sympathetic responses to surgical stimulation (*e.g.*, mydriasis, tearing, sweating, tachycardia, hypertension) may indicate lightening of anesthesia. However, awareness without any signs of sympathetic activity has been reported.[166]

Skeletal muscular relaxation is not produced by anesthetic doses of morphine or any other narcotic analgesic. Quite the opposite may occur in the form of truncal rigidity which appears as a board-like abdomen and chest.[167–169] Occasionally the rigidity extends into the limb muscles. Besides the fact that rigidity may impede surgery, it reduces chest wall compliance and restricts inflation of the lungs by positive pressure ventilation in a patient whose spontaneous ventilatory effort has been reduced or eliminated by narcotic analgesic depression of the respiratory centers in the brain stem.[170] The high intra-thoracic pressure produced by attempts at ventilation is transmitted to the venous circulation and heart so that cardiac output is reduced and signs suggesting the occurrence of pericardial tamponade may appear. The rigidity-inducing actions of morphine and fentanyl are greatly potentiated in a reversible manner by nitrous oxide.[167] Rigidity can be prevented or controlled by the administration of general anesthesia (*e.g.*, thiopental,[167] halothane[171]), or neuromuscular blocking drugs (*e.g.*, succinylcholine,[171] pancuronium[172]). Premedication with centrally acting "muscle relaxants" (*e.g.*, diazepam) will not prevent the rigidity.[171] It can be relieved by narcotic analgesic antagonists.[173]

Rigidity is usually noted during the induction and maintenance of anesthesia with any of the narcotic analgesics,[174–176] and it has been observed in the postoperative period.[171] Its occurrence and intensity have not been clearly related to the size of the dose or to the rapidity of its administration. It has been observed after as little as 250 µg of fentanyl,[177] and it has occurred during a very slow infusion of fentanyl (35 µg/min to a total dose of only 10 µg/kg) in adult patients with valvular heart disease.[178] Rigidity and apnea often occur before the patient is unconscious.[163, 169, 176, 179] Administration of a muscle relaxant to facilitate ventilation may leave the patient paralyzed and conscious. Furthermore, the following points should be remembered: (1) rigidity will recur when the muscle relaxant effects are eliminated;[171] (2) if unconsciousness is achieved by the rapid administration of fentanyl, the concentrations of fentanyl decline rapidly to levels below those producing unconsciousness;[160, 180,]

[181] (3) it is difficult to detect the return of consciousness in a paralyzed patient;[157] and (4) the problem of awareness can be largely avoided by combining the narcotic analgesic with a hypnotic such as diazepam.

Suppression of reflex activity by morphine and the other narcotic analgesics is quite selective. On one hand, doses that produce apnea profoundly obtund the cough reflex to the point that airway manipulation and the presence of an endotracheal tube are tolerated without coughing, gagging or choking (somatic responses).[182] On the other hand, the autonomic sympathetic responses to noxious stimulation (*e.g.*, tracheal intubation, skin incision, sternotomy) are not reliably suppressed by anesthetic doses; consequently tachycardia and hypertension may occur.[158, 163, 183, 184] (The effects of narcotic analgesics on autonomic and endocrine reflexes are discussed below in conjunction with their actions on the cardiovascular system.)

Small doses of morphine stimulate the chemoreceptor trigger zone (CTZ) and large doses depress the vomiting center.[185] Thus, nausea and vomiting are often associated with analgesic doses, especially when stimulation of the CTZ by the semicircular canals in response to movement is superimposed on that by morphine. Anesthetic doses of morphine and its surrogates are rarely associated with nausea or vomiting except perhaps in the recovery period when their concentrations have declined. Nausea and vomiting can be prevented and treated by antiemetic drugs (*e.g.*, scopolamine, droperidol, or one of the phenothiazines).

Other narcotic analgesic actions of importance to the anesthesiologist include those affecting respiration, histamine release, the gastrointestinal tract and other smooth muscle, and the psyche.[153, 185, 186] These have been reviewed elsewhere in detail. However, a few statements about these actions in patients with cardiovascular disease follow.

Respiratory depression is a dose-dependent effect that leads to the accumulation of carbon dioxide, which produces hemodynamic changes as a result of central stimulation of the sympathetic nervous system and the local vasodilatory effects of carbon dioxide.[186, 187] The well-known consequences of hypoxia also include sympathetic stimulation initially. These consequences are routinely prevented in the operating room by mechanical support of ventilation, which is also the safest and most benign therapy for postoperative respiratory depression in the patient with cardiovascular instability. The use of naloxone (Narcan) or other narcotic analgesic antagonists in the postoperative period on a *routine* basis is to be condemned for the reasons listed below. Certainly there are indications for these valuable drugs, and the following should be remembered in using them properly. First, they are competitive antagonists;[185] the dose of the antagonist should be titrated in small increments (*e.g.*, naloxone 0.5–1 μg/kg) to the *desirable* endpoint.[188] Secondly, *complete* antagonism of ventilatory depression may be accompanied by elimination of the analgesic actions and is seldom necessary. A moderate elevation of carbon dioxide ($Pa_{CO_2} < 50$ torr) is well tolerated by most patients who should be observed for an unfavorable progression rather than treated with naloxone unless they are at risk from increased levels of carbon dioxide. Even patients with elevated intracranial pressure or cardiac dysrhythmias present a therapeutic dilemma; increased Pa_{CO2} may exacerbate their condition and so may the sudden antagonism of narcotic analgesic actions by naloxone. In most of these cases, mechanical assistance of ventilation is preferable to the use of a narcotic analgesic antagonist which may unmask pain and exacerbate the same risks.[188–194] Thirdly, the kinetics of elimination of the antagonist usually differ from those of the analgesic.[195–197] Ventilatory depression may recur. Intramuscular doses of naloxone have been suggested as a means of prolonging the antagonism,[194] but these may be undependable because of erratic rates of absorption, especially in the hemodynamically unstable patient.[198] A constant infusion of naloxone has also been used to antagonize the effects of large doses of morphine.[195, 196]

Hazards of Improper Use of Narcotic Analgesic Antagonists in Surgical Patients

Unmask pain
Increase sympathetic responses
    Hypertension
    Tachycardia
    Dysrhythmias
Restoration of airway reflexes (*e.g.*, coughing on endotracheal tube)
Increase incidence of nausea and vomiting
Precipitate acute abstinence syndrome in physically dependent (addicted) patient
Recurrence of CNS and ventilatory depression

Histamine release occurs as a result of morphine and certain other narcotic analgesics displacing histamine from its binding sites in mast cells.[186] This is a competitive interaction and the amount of histamine liberated can be minimized by keeping the circulating levels of morphine as low as possible. One means of doing so is to administer intravenous morphine slowly (5 mg/min in a full-size adult). Even so, cutaneous signs (*e.g.*, erythema in flush areas, hives, pruritis), hypotension (see below) and, very rarely, bronchospasm may occur. Antihistamines (H_1-receptor blockers) do not prevent the release of histamine and only partially reduce the vascular responses to it.[186, 199] Cimetidine (Tagamet) is an H_2-histamine receptor blocker that in combination with one of the standard antihistamines (*e.g.*, diphenhydramine Benadryl) antagonizes the vasodilatory responses to histamine more completely.[200] Very potent narcotic analgesics are administered in small doses (fewer molecules) that are likely to release proportionally less histamine. In fact, fentanyl in doses as high as 50 μg/kg does not increase the circulating levels of histamine,[201] although all 17 of the author's volunteers noted transient pruritis after a 10 μg/kg bolus dose.[171, 202]

The *gastrointestinal tract and other smooth muscle* are directly affected by all narcotic analgesics.[185] Besides the longer term problems of postoperative ileus, constipation, and urinary retention, the anesthesiologist should be aware of narcotic analgesic-induced smooth muscle spasm as a cause of pain. Of particular importance to the patient with cardiovascular disease is the occurrence of substernal discomfort and pain after an analgesic or premedicant dose of a narcotic analgesic. It results from spasm of the sphincter of Oddi and the build-up of pressure in the biliary tract. The important differential diagnosis is angina pectoris. In the case of sphincter spasm, naloxone will provide prompt relief, but it will only intensify cardiac pain to the extent it was suppressed by the narcotic analgesic. (The administration of a narcotic antagonist to the patient exibiting angina pectoris is not recommended.) Nitroglycerin may relieve both.[203] In most cases, a combination of history and the ECG will point to the correct diagnosis. Incidentally, the narcotic analgesics are about equally potent as analgesics and as spasmodics, with the possible exception of the narcotic antagonist analgesic, pentazocine (Talwin).[204, 205]

The *psychological effects* of morphine-like drugs include dysphoria, euphoria, and psychic dependence. These effects are excerbated by the development of physical dependence. These phenomena are well-described elsewhere and they are important to the anesthesiologist.[185, 206] Dysphoria is more likely to occur in the patient who is not experiencing pain when a narcotic analgesic is administered. Euphoria and the development of psychic dependence are rare in patients receiving these drugs for acute pain or anesthesia, but they pose a substantial hazard to the anesthesiologist *per se* if self-administered for whatever reason. The acute development of tolerance to, and physical dependence on, the narcotic analgesics are possible consequences of the use of anesthetic doses, but their occurrence has not yet been documented in man.[207, 208]

Cardiovascular Effects of Narcotic Analgesics

Morphine. As initially demonstrated by Lowenstein and coworkers, and subsequently confirmed by others, the intravenous administration of morphine at a rate of 5 mg/

min (adult) to a total dose of 1 to 2 mg/kg produces relatively small changes in the hemodynamics of normal subjects and patients with cardiac disease.[209–211] On the average, systemic vascular resistance decreased and cardiac index increased; changes in mean arterial blood pressure were variable but the tendency was toward a slight decrease. More rapid administration of morphine was associated with significant degrees of hypotension in some patients.[210] On the other hand, the introduction of surgical stimulation was accompanied by marked degrees of hypertension in a large proportion of patients.[211, 212] The mechanisms underlying the deviations from generally stable hemodynamics are still not completely known but the following have been considered.

1. Morphine depresses contractility of the isolated heart only in concentrations around 10^{-3}M which is equivalent to 285 μg/ml.[213] Plasma concentrations of less than 0.1 μg/ml are associated with a satisfactory anesthetic state in combination with 70 percent nitrous oxide in physically fit children and the peak plasma concentrations of morphine only momentarily exceed 1 μg/ml immediately after an intravenous dose of 2 mg/kg.[214, 215] Thus, it is highly unlikely that direct myocardial depression occurs as the result of morphine administration to surgical patients.

2. Morphine tends to slow the heart rate in experimental animals by an activation of the vagal nerves.[216] Bradycardia is occasionally seen in surgical patients, and it is readily reversed or prevented by atropine-like drugs.[216, 217] The vagomimetic actions of morphine may explain the mild or absent reflex tachycardia that is expected when hypotension occurs.

3. Morphine reduces arteriolar resistance and increases venous capacitance (i.e., venodilation) in experimental animals and man.[216, 218–220] A number of mechanisms may contribute to these effects. Histamine release is probably the predominant one in the case of anesthetic doses of morphine and it is discussed above. A selec-

tive reduction in sympathetic nervous system activity is postulated, but blockade of alpha adrenergic receptors has been ruled out.[220–223] The possibility of a direct action of morphine on vascular smooth muscle remains uncertain.[220, 222–224] Carbon dioxide accumulation caused by ventilatory depression can produce vasodilation by its local action, especially if sympathetic reflex mechanisms are attenuated by morphine or other drugs.[218]

Regardless of the mechanism, the following points should be remembered by the anesthesiologist in preventing and treating hypotension caused by the vascular effects of morphine.

a. Maintain the patient in a supine position to prevent orthostatic hypotension and elevate the legs as necessary to restore or to increase the venous return of blood to the heart.

b. Correct hypovolemia before the administration of morphine and infuse fluids as needed to restore ventricular filling pressures to normal.

c. Support pulmonary ventilation to prevent the accumulation of carbon dioxide.

d. Administer morphine slowly to minimize the release of histamine. (See the above discussion of histamine release.)

e. Administer vasopressors if the above measures fail to correct clinically significant hypotension. An alpha-adrenergic receptor stimulant (e.g., phenylephrine) will correct the vasodilation; a mixed alpha- and beta-receptor stimulant (e.g., ephedrine) will also correct any morphine-induced bradycardia. (The initiation of surgery may substitute for the injection of exogenous sympathomimetics.)

4. Morphine alone fails to block the hemodynamic responses to noxious stimulation reliably. Hypertension and tachycardia may develop to a severe degree within a minute or two after endotracheal intubation or surgical stimulation in a substantial number of patients given 1 to 3 mg/kg doses of morphine.[209, 211, 212, 225] Only

rarely is the cardiovascular stimulation reversed by the administration of additional doses of morphine. The mechanisms responsible for the hyperdynamic responses have not been clearly defined. Morphine has been shown to block the adrenergic and cardiovascular responses to skin incision in a dose-related fashion when combined with 60 percent nitrous oxide.[226] Nitrous oxide's depression of myocardial contractility may predominate in the presence of anesthetic doses of morphine, which may attenuate sympathetic stimulation by the anesthetic gas. (See earlier discussion of nitrous oxide.) On the other hand, morphine's blockade of sympathetic mechanisms appears to be quite selective and its effects on other systems mediating hypertension are not fully understood. While anesthetic doses of morphine depress the surgically-induced release of antidiuretic hormone (vasopressin),[227] they fail to prevent the increases in plasma renin and aldosterone that occur in response to surgical stimulation.[228] In any event, the anesthesiologist usually has to resort to other drugs to prevent or to correct the hypertension and tachycardia elicited by noxious stimulation of patients receiving morphine anesthesia. These include the following:

a. Administration of thiopental, nitrous oxide, halothane or similar drugs to deepen the anesthetic level and to depress sympathetic and cardiovascular functions

b. Injection of adrenergic receptor blocking drugs to reduce the responsiveness of the heart (*e.g.,* propranolol) and vasculature (*e.g.,* phentolamine) to sympathetic nervous system activity

c. Infusion of vasodilators

Rapid control of these responses is indicated in hemodynamically unstable patients, especially those with coronary artery disease, because of the increased cardiac work and oxygen demand in the face of a relatively fixed oxygen supply.

5. The mechanisms underlying the increased requirements for fluids and blood by patients receiving anesthetic doses of morphine (1–3 mg/kg) and the development of edema after huge doses (8–11 mg/kg) are unknown.[229] Similarly, the beneficial effects of morphine in the treatment of pulmonary edema are not yet explained. The reader should refer to the writings of Zelis and coworkers and Green and coworkers for summaries of available information.[220, 223, 230, 231]

Fentanyl (Sublimaze). Hemodynamic changes following large doses of fentanyl (25–75 µg/kg) administered over a 15-min period are slight.[232–235] Mild degrees of hypotension may be seen in association with bradycardia or decreases in systemic vascular resistance. Usually the changes are clinically insignificant even when large doses are administered rapidly. Nevertheless, caution is advised because the author and others have observed unexpected and profound hypotension closely following the injection of fentanyl in a very few patients with coronary artery and valvular heart disease.

The following facts about the cardiovascular effects of fentanyl are noteworthy.

1. Fentanyl, like morphine, exerts no direct depressant effect on the cardiac or vascular smooth muscle in the concentrations that result from anesthetic doses. That is, fentanyl concentrations of 10^{-6}M (equivalent to 0.34 µg/ml) produced only minimal depression of vascular smooth muscle *in vitro*,[236] and even greater concentrations (approximately 10–30 µg/ml) were required to depress contractility of the isolated heart.[237–239] The peak plasma levels of fentanyl in patients given intravenous doses of 75 µg/kg averaged 0.05 µg/ml.[232, 240, 241] The lack of myocardial depression by high doses of fentanyl was also evident in the dog heart-lung preparation[242, 243] and in intact dogs receiving other drugs for anesthesia.[244–248]

2. Histamine levels in the blood do not rise after intravenous injection of fentanyl and this is probably the primary reason for the lower incidence and lesser degree of hypotension after fentanyl than after morphine.[249]

3. The requirement for intravenous fluid infusion seems to be less in patients anesthetized with fentanyl for cardiac surgery than in those receiving large doses of morphine. Edema is not evident after fentanyl doses of 120 µg/kg which are equivalent to morphine doses of 9 mg/kg, assuming a potency ration of 75:1.[250, 251]

4. Fentanyl, like morphine, can produce bradycardia.[233–235, 243–246, 248, 252, 253] It occurs perhaps more frequently under clinical conditions after fentanyl than after morphine, but it is usually limited in degree and easily reversed by anticholinergic drugs, including pancuronium. Several points should be noted however. Occasionally the bradycardia is marked and associated with hypotension that requires treatment with *either* an anticholinergic *or* sympathomimetic drug. One or the other type drug should be used, but not both; the combination can lead to undesirable degrees of tachycardia. Tachycardia and hypertension associated electrocardiographic signs of myocardial ischemia have resulted when paralyzing doses of pancuronium have been administered intravenously as a bolus in order to facilitate ventilation impaired by truncal rigidity.[251] In such cases it is likely that the effects of pancuronium were enhanced by sympathetic stimulation caused by accumulation of carbon dioxide, endotracheal intubation, or other noxious stimulation. If the bradycardia is moderate in degree and not associated with significant degrees of hypotension, it need not be treated and may even be beneficial in terms of myocardial oxygen balance. For example, fentanyl-induced bradycardia is credited with a reduction of myocardial ischemia induced experimentally by an acute occlusion of a coronary artery.[248] The benefit may not be realized, however, if coronary perfusion decreases as a result of hypotension.[243, 246] In dogs studied 2 to 3 hours after an acute myocardial infarction, fentanyl (50 µg/kg) produced decreases in heart rate, left ventricular contractility, and cardiac output; all of these were reversed by atropine.[254]

5. The causes of the very rare occurrence of profound hypotension (in the absence of or out of proportion to the degree of bradycardia) associated with the administration of fentanyl are unknown. Certainly most patients tolerate intravenous bolus doses of 10–25 µg/kg without hypotension providing bradycardia is prevented. Experiments in animals indicate that high doses of fentanyl can reduce the outflow of sympathetic activity from the central nervous system.[252, 255] Interference with sympathetic nerve activity at peripheral sites is an unlikely mechanism of fentanyl-induced cardiovascular changes because the concentrations required to reduce catecholamine output from nerve endings and to block adrenergic receptors are much larger than those likely to be achieved even after very large doses of fentanyl (see previous discussion of dose-response).[236, 256] The direct effects of fentanyl on the systemic and pulmonary vasculature have not been investigated adequately.[257, 258] In most studies of patients, there has been a small decrease or no change in vascular resistance following the administration of fentanyl.[233–235, 259] Of course, the local vascular effect of carbon dioxide accumulation resulting from fentanyl-induced ventilatory depression can lead to hypotension as it does in the case of morphine.[244, 259, 260] On the other hand, factors activating the sympathetic nervous system (*e.g.,* hypercarbia, surgical and other types of noxious stimulation) can lead to an increase in vascular resistance.[235] The author has found an increasing pulmonary artery pressure to be a sensitive clue to carbon dioxide accumulation during the induction of anesthesia with fentanyl.[235]

6. As in the case of patients anesthetized with morphine, the introduction of noxious stimulation (*e.g.,* endotracheal intubation, skin incision, sternotomy) results in hypertension and tachycardia in some patients even after the administration of very large doses of fentanyl (over 100 µg/kg).[235, 261] It is not yet clear why these episodes of cardiovascular stimulation occur only in certain patients, and it is not

yet proven that larger doses of fentanyl will prevent them. Additional fentanyl definitely will *not* control the hypertension and tachycardia once they are in progress, and the anesthesiologist will find it necessary to employ other drugs to treat these signs of cardiovascular stimulation.[250, 251]

Even though they may provide better hemodynamic stability, these enormous doses of fentanyl do not solve all the problems associated with the use of narcotic analgesics as anesthetics. Intraoperative awareness and postoperative recall have been observed after large doses of fentanyl.[251, 262] Muscular rigidity of the body trunk is more common and much more intense after fentanyl than after morphine, and it has been observed in the postanesthetic recovery phase even after the patient has demonstrated satisfactory spontaneous ventilation and been extubated.[251] Fentanyl is no longer a short-acting narcotic analgesic after anesthetic doses;[263] in fact, the half-time of elimination of fentanyl is longer than that of morphine in man (*i.e.*, 4 versus 2 hr).[264-266] Finally, fentanyl is more expensive than morphine. The dosage requirements for fentanyl can be reduced considerably by its combination with other depressant drugs (*e.g.*, nitrous oxide, diazepam) but at the cost of incurring the hemodynamic side-effects of these drugs.[232, 233]

Newer analogues of fentanyl are in various stages of development for clinical use. None are available yet commercially in the United States. Sufentanyl is a more potent analgesic than fentanyl and it also has a larger difference than fentanyl between the dose producing analgesia and that causing convulsions in animals.*[267, 268] Except for these potency differences, sufentanyl appears to be similar to fentanyl in terms of duration of action, side-

effects, and hemodynamic changes observed under conditions of anesthesia and surgery.[261, 268-270] It remains to be determined whether or not it is a superior narcotic analgesic for anesthetic purposes.

Alfentanil is a less potent analogue of fentanyl that has a very short duration of action.[271] Because of the latter property, it is less useful for maintenance of anesthesia during cardiac surgery. It appears to be similar to fentanyl in terms of the hemodynamic changes and side-effects noted during the induction of anesthesia.[272]

Other Narcotic Analgesics. Morphine and fentanyl are the two narcotic analgesics most widely used in anesthesia for cardiac surgery. Morphine has been the most intensely studied drug in its class, and in general, the other narcotic analgesics produce the same spectrum of actions and side-effects. The published experience with the other narcotic analgesics is very limited, especially with regard to their use in anesthesia.

Meperidine (Demerol) has been used widely as an anesthetic supplement for the past 30 years.[273, 274] It is approximately one-tenth as potent as morphine as an analgesic. Doses of 1 to 3 mg/kg have been used during the induction of anesthesia and supplemented as needed with 0.3 mg/kg intravenous doses during the maintenance of anesthesia with nitrous oxide or other general anesthetics. It shares the same spectrum of actions as morphine,[275-277] but its use in large quantities equivalent to anesthetic doses of morphine is limited by cardiovascular depression and the potential for neurotoxicity.

Cardiovascular depression is attributable to all the mechanisms described for morphine (*i.e.*, histamine release, interference with certain sympathetic reflexes, bradycardia under certain conditions) plus a negative inotropic effect that is evident at concentrations of meperidine close to those achieved after its intravenous administration to intact animals and man.[278-280] In terms of equivalent analgesic doses, meperidine is estimated to be 100 to 200 times more potent a myocardial depressant than either fentanyl or mor-

*Providing that ventilation is supported mechanically, the maximum dose of morphine and the other narcotic analgesics that can be tolerated is that producing convulsions. The maximum or convulsant dose becomes a practical consideration when an attempt is made to produce complete anesthesia with the narcotic analgesics. The ratios for analgesic to lethal, convulsant doses in dogs are approximately 67 for morphine, 400 for fentanyl, and 800 for sufentanyl.

phine.[278] Severe hypotension has limited the use of meperidine in anesthesia.[281, 282]

In addition, meperidine is metabolized to normeperidine which is a weak analgesic but potent CNS stimulant.[275] Seizures have been observed in association with accumulation of this metabolite in animals and man.[283] This potential for CNS toxicity further limits the use of meperidine as a primary anesthetic drug.

Alphaprodine (Nisentil) is an analogue of meperidine with a very similar spectrum of pharmacologic actions. The similarities appear to include marked depression of the cardiovascular system.[284]

NARCOTIC ANTAGONIST ANALGESICS

The discovery of an analgesic potency equivalent to that of morphine in the narcotic antagonist, nalorphine, led to the study of other compounds that combined agonistic (*e.g.*, analgesia) and antagonistic actions (*e.g.*, reversal of morphine-induced apnea). Nalorphine and many of the other agonist-antagonist compounds were not acceptable as analgesics because they also had psychotomimetic effects.[285] Three drugs with a lesser incidence of mental aberrations associated with their analgesic actions are currently available for clinical use: pentazocine (Talwin), butorphanol (Stadol), and nalbuphine (Nubain). Studies to date suggest that (1) their antagonistic actions are relatively weak; (2) their ability to produce respiratory depression is limited; (3) their cardiovascular effects in analgesic doses are relatively benign; (4) their incidence of psychotomimetic reactions is low but not absent; (5) their potential for abuse is low but not nil.[286–289]

The major question about the cardiovascular effects of these drugs focuses on the changes in vascular resistance, especially in the pulmonary circulation. Both pentazocine and butorphanol in analgesic doses have been reported to increase pulmonary vascular resistance.[287, 288, 290] In the case of pentazocine, systemic vascular resistance increased and left ventricular ejection decreased in patients with acute myocardial

infarctions; morphine and meperidine did not produce these potentially detrimental effects in the same patients.[291] The mechanisms underlying these hemodynamic changes are unknown. Nalbuphine (like morphine) in analgesic doses (10 mg) produced no hemodynamic changes in patients with or without coronary artery disease.[292, 293]

The cardiovascular effects of larger doses have not been reported for humans, but a preliminary report of a study in dogs indicates that butorphanol in doses up to 0.2 mg/kg produced myocardial depression manifested by elevated right atrial pressures, hypotension, and bradycardia (not reversed by atropine); there was no change in vascular resistance. The myocardial depression was exacerbated and the systemic vascular resistance was increased by the addition of 60 percent nitrous oxide to the inspired mixture.[294]

These narcotic antagonist analgesics are being used in analgesic doses to supplement general and regional anesthesia. But they are unlikely to be useful as primary anesthetic agents because their analgesic and CNS depressant effects are limited in the same manner as their respiratory depressant actions.[295] In fact, patients receiving doses of butorphanol (20–30 mg) or nalbuphine (60–100 mg) equivalent to anesthetic doses of morphine (1–2 mg/kg) under clinical conditions do not go to sleep, and their hemodynamic responses to noxious stimulation are not satisfactorily obtunded even after the administration of thiopental, nitrous oxide or other drugs to induce unconsciousness.[296, 297] With the information currently available, their potential usefulness in anesthesia for cardiac surgery seems very limited.

KETAMINE

Ketamine (Ketalar, Ketaject) is unique among the drugs used for anesthesia because of its effects on the cardiovascular and central nervous systems.[298, 299] It has important but limited applications in anesthesia for cardiac surgery as indicated below.

The effects of ketamine on the central nervous system include analgesia, amnesia, un-consciousness, increased muscular tone and occasionally involuntary movements, emer-gence delirium, minimal depression of res-piration and airway reflexes, and activation of the sympathetic nervous system.[298, 299] The fact that ketamine can produce uncon-sciousness within seconds after an intrave-nous injection while maintaining or increas-ing sympathetic activity makes it a useful agent (replacing cyclopropane) for the rapid induction of anesthesia in patients depen-dent on sympathetic activity for maintenance of cardiovascular function (e.g., in hypovo-lemia, congestive heart failure, pericardial tamponade; see below) and for bronchodila-tion (e.g., asthmatic bronchitis).[300–302] Anes-thetic uses in other situations is limited by the tendency of ketamine to produce hyper-tension and tachycardia intraoperatively and to cause emergence delirium (prolonged re-covery with recurring dreams, hallucina-tions, disorientation, agitation, restlessness excitement and visual disturbances).[298] New interest and clinical applications have arisen in recognition of its potent analgesic actions and the selectivity of action of its isomers.[303] Its analgesic effects are evident at subanesth-etic doses,[304] and they may be mediated by opiate receptors, although the latter point is controversial.[305–307] In one study, the (+) ke-tamine isomer was 3.5 times more potent than the (−) isomer as an analgesic and an-esthetic, produced less cardiovascular stim-ulation, and had a lower incidence of unde-sirable post anesthetic emergence reactions although dreaming was still prevalent.[303] The possibility of reducing postoperative compli-cations by the use of the (+) isomer, or the combination of ketamine with other drugs (e.g., diazepam) offers the prospect of some-what broader applications of ketamine in the future.[299, 308–312]

The cardiovascular effects of ketamine are the result of two basic actions: (1) a central activation of the sympathetic nervous sys-tem[313] and (2) direct depression of the heart.[314] The former predominates when ketamine is administered alone in moderate doses or in combination with other drugs that enhance sympathetic activity (e.g., pancuro-

nium).[315] The latter is evident when very high doses of ketamine are administered alone,[316] when ketamine is combined with drugs that depress the sympathetic nervous system (e.g., halothane, adrenergic receptor antagonists),[317] or in patients with interrup-tion of sympathetic outflow from the CNS (e.g., spinal cord transection, epidural anes-thesia).[318, 319]

Thus, the cardiovascular changes induced by ketamine are greatly dependent on the conditions under which it is administered. In the normal individual, tachycardia and hy-pertension predominate, reflecting an in-crease in cardiac output and a variable, usu-ally transient elevation of systemic vascular resistance.[320] Pulmonary artery pressure also increases. In patients with normal hearts, right atrial and left ventricular end diastolic pressures did not increase; nevertheless, it is likely that ventricular wall tension rose be-cause of the increased afterload. Cardiac work increases along with all of the deter-minants of myocardial oxygen demand: heart rate, contractility, and wall tension. Thus, myocardial oxygen utilization increases while the opportunity for supply decreases as a re-sult of tachycardia (i.e., reduced diastolic per-fusion time). This represents an unfavorable change in the myocardial oxygen demand-supply relationships for the patient with cor-onary arterial obstructive disease; the poten-tial risks of these changes to such patients has limited the use of ketamine for coronary artery surgery even though the one pub-lished prospective study demonstrated no more unfavorable hemodynamic conse-quences with ketamine-N_2O than with mor-phine-N_2O anesthesia.[321] Of course, mor-phine has its own limitations as an anesthetic as discussed above. The combination of ke-tamine (2 mg/kg initially, then an infusion of 1 mg/kg/hr) with diazepam (0.4 mg/kg) and nitrous oxide (50%) proved to be a satisfac-tory alternative to morphine (3 mg/kg) as an anesthetic regimen for valvular heart sur-gery;[311] the suitability of this technique for coronary artery surgery remains to be deter-mined. A note of caution has been sounded by investigators who observed significant in-creases in ventricular preloading without increased contractility in some subjects given ketamine. These effects could be detrimental to the patient with severely impaired ventricular function who already is dependent on maximal preloading (the Frank–Starling mechanism) to maintain cardiac output.[322]

Some incidental findings that may be important in certain situations include the following. Ketamine has a cocaine-like action on sympathetic nerve endings and potentiates the actions of catecholamines.[323, 324] Ketamine has an antiarrhythmic action but it may be offset by its potentiation of catecholamine actions.[314, 324] Adrenergic beta-receptor blocking drugs limit the chronotropic but not the hypertensive responses to ketamine.[325]

Thus, the use of ketamine anesthesia for cardiac surgery remains controversial, except perhaps for the patient dependent on sympathetic nervous system activity to maintain hemodynamic function. It is usually contraindicated in the patient with hypertension, and probably should only be used in combination with other drugs (to control sympathomimetic responses) in patients with coronary artery disease.

MAJOR TRANQUILIZERS (NEUROLEPTICS)*

This classification includes the phenothiazines (*e.g.*, chlorpromazine-Thorazine) and butyrophenones (*e.g.*, droperidol—Inapsine).[326] These drugs are unsuitable in their own right for anesthetic purposes because they do not produce sleep, amnesia, analgesia, or muscular relaxation, or even relieve the situational anxiety associated with surgery. Moreover, they may cause anxiety, confusion, dysphoria, extrapyramidal reactions, and hypotension.[326, 327–337] They are sometimes useful as supplements to the narcotic analgesics, and perhaps ketamine, because

they enhance their analgesic actions and reduce the emetic and other side-effects.[328, 338, 339] However, it should be noted that the combination of a major tranquilizer and a narcotic analgesic (*i.e.*, neuroleptanalgesia) does not reliably induce either sleep or amnesia.[340] Also noteworthy is the observation that the unpleasant effects of the long-acting neuroleptics may appear as the effects of a short-acting narcotic analgesic wear off.[341]

Several other actions of the major tranquilizers may be useful to the anesthesiologist. In some cases, they can control systemic hypertension through their actions on the CNS and blockade of adrenergic alpha-receptors on vascular smooth muscle.[336, 337] Droperidol has the potential to block the vasodilating effect of dopamine on the renal vasculature.[342, 343] The neuroleptic agents interfere with body temperature regulation and may facilitate the production of deliberate hypothermia and reduce shivering. (The latter is more certainly prevented by neuromuscular blocking drugs.) The phenothiazines and butyrophenones are potent antiemetics.[326] Droperidol has antidysrhythmic actions and may reduce the sensitization of the myocardium to catecholamines by anesthetics such as halothane.[344] (Lidocaine is more reliable for this purpose.[345])

OTHER DRUGS[346]

The anesthesiologist may find certain actions of non-CNS drugs useful in an anesthetic regimen. *Scopolamine* has sedative, amnesic, and antiemetic effects. The *antihistamines* (*e.g.*, diphenhydramine—Benadryl) have sedative properties and, in combination with cimetidine (Tagamet), can reduce the hypotensive responses caused by histamine release by d-tubocurarine and some of the narcotic analgesics (see previous discussion). *Hydroxyzine* (Vistaril) combines antihistaminic, sedative, and weak analgesic properties, but is not approved for intravenous administration. And of course, there are a variety of *drugs acting on the cardiovascular system* that are useful in controlling the adverse hemodynamic consequences of disease, surgery, and anesthetic drugs.

---

*Minor tranquilizers are similar to sedatives and hypnotics in that they relieve anxiety and can induce sleep after adequate doses. They include the benzodiazepines (*e.g.*, diazepam) and hydroxyzine (Vistaril). The latter drugs have virtually none of the actions of the major tranquilizers.

SUMMARY

In the choice of anesthetic drugs for the patient with cardiovascular disease, the anesthesiologist must recognize anesthetic, hemodynamic, and surgical objectives. Combinations of drugs usually are required to fulfill the objectives. Each drug has desirable effects as well as unwanted or detrimental side-effects. It is important that the cardiovascular anesthesiologist or intensivist understand the pharmacologic effects of each drug, or combinations of drugs, and understand the pathophysiologic state of the patient. Only then can the choice of drugs be optimal and side-effects minimized. There is no ideal anesthetic or "cookbook" protocol for all patients. Drug use must be individualized and the dosage titrated to the desired degree of effect. In the patient with cardiovascular disease, hemodynamic monitoring is an essential guide to therapy.

REFERENCES

INTRODUCTION

1. Gilman LS, Goodman LS, Gilman AG: The Pharmacological Basis of Therapeutics, 6th ed. New York, Macmillan, 1980. The standard textbook of pharmacology with chapters on anesthetic drugs written by anesthesiologists.

Cardiovascular Disease

2. Hurst JW, Logue RB, Schlant RC, Wenger NK: The Heart, 5th ed. New York, McGraw–Hill, 1981. The standard encyclopedic reference on cardiovascular disease.
3. Braunwald E: Heart Disease, Philadelphia, WB Saunders, 1980
4. Eger EI II: Anesthetic Uptake and Action. Baltimore, Williams & Wilkins, 1974. Chapters 7 and 8 are particularly pertinent to the uptake and elimination of inhaled anesthetics by patients with cardiovascular disease.
5. Benowitz NL, Meister W: Pharmacokinetics in patients with cardiac failure. Clin Pharmacokinet 1:389–405, 1976
6. Benowitz NL, Meister W: Clinical Pharmaco-

kinetics of Lignocaine. Clin Pharmacokinet 3:177–201, 1978
7. Mainzer J Jr: Awareness, Muscle Relaxants and Balanced Anaesthesia. Can Anaesth Soc J 26:386–393, 1979
8. Ali HH, Savarese JJ: Monitoring of Neuromuscular Function. Anesthesiology 45.216–249, 1976
9. Abouleish E, Taylor FH: Effect of morphine-diazepam on signs of anesthesia, awareness, and dreams of patients under N_2O for Cesarean section. Anesth Analg (Cleve) 55:702–705, 1976

Dose-Response Relationship

10. Ochs HR, Carstens G, Greenblatt DJ: Reduction in lidocaine clearance during continuous infusion and by coadministration of propranolol. N Engl J Med 303:373–377, 1980
11. Rozen MS, Whan FMcK: Prolonged durarization associated with propranolol. Med J Aust 1:467–468, 1972
12. Prys–Roberts C: The Circulation in Anaesthesia, pp 394–428. Oxford, Blackwell Scientific Publications, 1980
13. Gilman LS, Goodman LS, Gilman AG: The Pharmacological Basis of Therapeutics, 6th ed. New York, Macmillan, 1980. The standard textbook of pharmacology with chapters on anesthetic drugs written by anesthesiologists.
14. Toda N, Hatano Y: Alpha-adrenergic blocking action of fentanyl on the isolated aorta of the rabbit. Anesthesiology 46:411–416, 1977
15. Lunn JK, Stanley TH, Eisele J et al: High dose fentanyl anesthesia for coronary artery surgery: plasma fentanyl concentrations and influence of nitrous oxide on cardiovascular responses. Anesth Analg (Cleve) 58:390–395, 1979
16. Murphy MR, Olson WA, Hug CC Jr.: Pharmacokinetics of ^{3}H-fentanyl in the dog anesthetized with enflurane. Anesthesiology 50:13–19, 1979
17. Bovill JG, Sebel PS: Pharmacokenitics of high-dose fentanyl. Br J Anaesth 52:795–801, 1980
18. McClain DA, Hug CC Jr: Intravenous fentanyl kinetics. Clin Pharmacol Ther 28:106–114, 1980
19. Hug CC Jr: Pharmacokinetics of morphine during cardiac surgery, pp 305–306 (abstr). Chicago, American Society of Anesthesiologists Annual Meeting, 1978
20. Hug CC Jr., Kaplan JA, Rigel EP: The effect of cardiopulmonary bypass on plasma propranolol concentrations and the response to iso-

proterenol, pp 501–502 (abstr). New Orleans, Society of Anesthesiologists Annual Meeting, 1977

21. Moldenhauer CC, Hug CC Jr.: Continuous infusion of fentanyl for cardiac surgery. Anesth Analg (Cleve) 61: (In press), 1982

The Phases of Anesthesia

22. Egbert LD, Battit GE, Turndorf H et al: The value of the preoperative visit by an anesthetist. JAMA 185:553–555, 1963
23. Prys–Roberts C: The Circulation in Anaesthesia. Blackwell, Oxford, 1980, pp. 394–428.

Regional Anesthesia

24. Bidwai AV, Rogers CR, Pearce M, Stanley TH: Preoperative stellate-ganglion blockade to prevent hypertension following coronary artery-operations. Anesthesiology 51:345–347, 1979
25. Covino BG, Vassallo HG: Local Anesthetics: Mechanisms of Action and Clinical Use. New York, Grune & Stratton, 1976
26. Greene NM: Physiology of Spinal Anesthesia, 2nd ed, Huntington (NY), RE Krieger, 1976
27. de Jong RH: Local Anesthetics, 2nd ed. Charles C Thomas, Springfield (Ill), 1977

NITROUS OXIDE

28. Torri G, Damia G, Fabiani ML: Effect of nitrous oxide on the anaesthetic requirements of enflurane. Br J Anaesth 46:468–472, 1974
29. Munson ES: Transfer of nitrous oxide into body air cavities. Br J Anaesth 46:202–209, 1974
30. Stanley TH: Nitrous oxide and pressures and volumes of high- and low-pressure endotracheal-tube cuffs in intubated patients. Anesthesiology 42:637–640, 1975
31. Price HL: Myocardial depression by nitrous oxide and its reversal by Ca^{++}. Anesthesiology 44:211–215, 1976
32. Fukunaga AF, Epstein RM: Sympathetic excitation during nitrous oxide-halothane anesthesia in the cat. Anesthesiology 39:23–36, 1973
33. Kawamura R, Stanley TH, English JB, Hill GE, Liu W-S, Webster LR: Cardiovascular responses to nitrous oxide exposure for two hours in man. Anesth Analg (Cleve) 59:93–99, 1980

34. Eisele JH, Smith NT: Cardiovascular effects of nitrous oxide in man. Anesth Analg (Cleve) 51:956–963, 1972
35. Eisele JH, Reitan JA, Massumi RA et al: Myocardial performance and N_2O analgesia in coronary artery disease. Anesthesiology 44:16–20, 1976
36. Lappas DA, Buckley MJ, Laver MB et al: Left ventricular performance and pulmonary circulation following addition of nitrous oxide to morphine during coronary-artery surgery. Anesthesiology 43:61–69, 1975
37. Hilgenberg JC, McCammon RL, Stoelting RK: Pulmonary and systemic vascular responses to nitrous oxide in patients with mitral stenosis and pulmonary hypertension. Anesth Analg (Cleve) 59:323–326, 1980
38. Lunn JK, Stanley TH, Eisele J et al: High dose fentanyl anesthesia for coronary artery surgery: Plasma fentanyl concentrations and influence of nitrous oxide on cardiovascular responses. Anesth Analg 58:390–395, 1979
39. Wong KC, Martin WE, Hornbein TF et al: The cardiovascular effects of morphine sulfate with oxygen and with nitrous oxide in man. Anesthesiology 38:542–549, 1973
40. Stoelting RK, Gibbs PS: Hemodynamic effects of morphine and morphine-nitrous oxide in valvular heart disease and coronary-artery disease. Anesthesiology 38:45–52, 1973
41. Stoelting RK, Gibbs PS, Creasser CW, Peterson C: Hemodynamic and ventilatory responses to fentanyl, fentanyl-droperidol, and nitrous oxide in patients with acquired valvular heart disease. Anesthesiology 42:319–324, 1975
42. McCammon RL, Hilgenberg JC, Stoelting RK: Hemodynamic effects of diazepam and diazepam-nitrous oxide in patients with coronary artery disease. Anesth Analg (Cleve) 59:438–441, 1980
43. Smith NT, Eger EI II, Stoelting RK et al: The cardiovascular and sympathomimetic responses to the addition of nitrous oxide to halothane in man. Anesthesiology 32:410–421, 1970
44. Bahlman SH, Eger EI II, Smith NT et al: The cardiovascular effects of nitrous oxide-halothane anesthesia in man. Anesthesiology 35:274–285, 1971
45. Dolan WM, Stevens WC, Eger EI II et al: The cardiovascular respiratory effects of isoflurane-nitrous oxide anesthesia. Can Anaesth Soc J 21:557–568, 1974
46. Smith NT, Calverley RK, Prys–Roberts C et al:

Impact of nitrous oxide on the circulation during enflurane anesthesia in man. Anesthesiology 48:345–349, 1978

47. Eger EI II: Anesthetic Uptake and Action. Baltimore, Williams & Wilkins, 1974 Chapters 7 and 8 are particularly pertinent to the uptake and elimination of inhaled anesthetics by patients with cardiovascular disease.

VOLATILE ANESTHETIC AGENTS

48. Eger EI II: Anesthetic Uptake Action, Baltimore, Williams & Wilkins, 1974
49. Quasha AL, Eger EI II, Tinker JH: Determination and applications of MAC. Anesthesiology 53:315–334, 1980
50. Gilman LS, Goodman LS, Gilman AG: The Pharmacological Basis of Therapeutics, 6th ed. New York, Macmillan, 1980.
51. Torri G, Damia G, Fabiani ML: Effect of nitrous oxide on the anaesthetic requirements of enflurane. Br J Anaesth 46:468–472, 1974
52. Miller RD, Way WL, Dolan WM, et al: The dependence of pancuronium- and d-Tubocurarine-induced neuromuscular blockades on alveolar concentrations of halothane and forane. Anesthesiology 37:573–581, 1972

Cardiovascular Effects

53. Hickey RF, Eger EI II: Circulatory effects of inhaled anaesthetics, In Prys-Roberts C (ed): The Circulation in Anaesthesia. Oxford, Blackwell Scientific Publications, 1980
54. Eger EI II, Smith NT, Stoelting RK et al: Cardiovascular effects of halothane in man. Anesthesiology 32:396–409, 1970
55. Calverley RK, Smith NT, Prys–Roberts C et al: Cardiovascular effects of enflurane anesthesia during controlled ventilation in man. Anesth Analg (Cleve) 57:619–628, 1978
56. Stevens WC, Cromwell TH, Halsey MJ et al: The cardiovascular effects of a new inhalation anesthetic, Forane, in human volunteers at constant arterial carbon dioxide tension. Anesthesiology 35:8–16, 1971

Halothane

57. Hickey RF, Eger EI II: Circulatory effects of inhaled anaesthetics. In Prys–Roberts C (ed): The Circulation in Anaesthesia. Oxford, Blackwell Scientific Publication, 1980

58. Eger EI II, Smith NT, Stoelting RK, Cullen DJ, Kadis LB, Whitcher CE: Cardiovascular effects of halothane in man. Anesthesiology 32:396–409, 1970
59. Roberts JG, Foex P, Clarke TNS, Bennett MJ: Haemodynamic interactions of high-dose propranolol pretreatment and anaesthesia in the dog. I. Halothane dose-response studies. Br J Anaesth 48:315–325, 1976
60. Slogoff S, Keats AS, Hibbs CW et al: Failure of general anesthesia to potentiate propranolol activity. Anesthesiology 47:504–508, 1977
61. Kopriva CJ, Brown ACD, Pappas G: Hemodynamics during general anesthesia in patients receiving propranolol. Anesthesiology 48:28–33, 1978
62. Lowenstein E, Foex P, Francis CM et al: Narrowed coronary arteries, halothane, and paradox. Anesthesiology 51:s62, 1979
63. Prys–Roberts C, Foex P et al: Studies of anaesthesia in relation to hypertension. V. Adrenergic beta-receptor blockade. Br J Anaesth 45:671–680, 1973
64. Kistner JR, Miller ED, Lake CL, Ross WT Jr: Indices of myocardial oxygenation during coronary-artery revascularization in man with morphine versus halothane anesthesia. Anesthesiology 50:324–330, 1979
65. Verrier ED, Edelist G, Consigny PM: Greater coronary vascular reserve with halothane. Anesthesiology 51:63, 1979
66. Kissin I, Stanbridge R, Bishop SP et al: Effect of halothane on myocardial infarct size in rats. Canad Anaesth Soc J 28:239–247, 1981
67. Price HL: Calcium reverses myocardial depression caused by halothane: site of action. Anesthesiology 41:576–579, 1974
68. Marshall BE, Wollman H: General anesthetics. In Gilman, Goodman, Gilman (eds): The Pharmacological Basis of Therapeutics, 6th ed. New York, Macmillan, 1980
69. Johnston RR, Eger EI II, Wilson C: A comparative interaction of epinephrine with enflurane, isoflurane, and halothane in man. Anesth Analg (Cleve) 55:709–712, 1976
70. Tucker WK, Rackstein AD, Munson ES: Comparison of arrhythmic doses of adrenaline metaraminol, ephedrine and phenylephrine during isoflurane and halothane anaesthesia in dogs. Br J Anaesth 46:392–396, 1974
71. Katz RL, Matteo RS, Papper EM: The injection of epinephrine during general anesthesia with halogenated hydrocarbons and cyclopropane in man. Anesthesiology 23:597–600, 1962

72. Mathers J. Benumof JL, Wahrenbrock EA: General anesthetics and regional hypoxic pulmonary vasoconstriction. Anesthesiology 46:111–114, 1977

73. Coon RL, Kampine JP: Hypocapnic bronchoconstriction and inhalation anesthetics. Anesthesiology 43:635–641, 1975

74. Little RR, Hug CC Jr, Frederickson EL: Arrhythmogenicity of terbutaline in anesthetized dogs. Anesthesiology 53:55, 1980

75. Morrow DH, Haley JV, Logic JR: Anesthesia and digitalis. VII. The effect of pentobarbital, halothane and methoxyflurane on the AV conduction and inotropic responses to ouabain. Anesth Analg (Cleve) 51:430–438, 1972

Enflurane

76. Hickey RF, Eger EI II: Circulatory effects of inhaled anaesthetics, In Prys–Roberts C (ed): The Circulation in Anesthesia. Oxford, Blackwell Scientific Publications, 1980

77. Calverley RK, Smith NT, Prys-Roberts C et al: Cardiovascular effects of enflurane anesthesia during controlled ventilation in man. Anesth Analg 57:619–628, 1978

78. Johnston RR, Eger EI II, Wilson C: A comparative interaction of epinephrine with enflurane, isoflurane, and halothane in man. Anesth Analg 55:709–712, 1976

79. Horan BF, Prys–Roberts C, Hamilton WK, Roberts JG: Haemodynamic responses to enflurane anaesthesia and hypovolaemia in the dog, and their modification by propranolol. Br J Anaesth 49:1189–1197, 1977

80. Smith NT, Eger EI II, Stoelting RK et al: The cardiovascular and sympathomimetic responses to the addition of nitrous oxide to halothane in man. Anesthesiology 32:410–421, 1970

81. Bahlman SH, Eger EI II, Smith NT et al: The cardiovascular effects of nitrous oxide-halothane anesthesia in man. Anesthesiology 35:274–285, 1971

82. Smith, NT, Calverley RK, Prys–Roberts C et al: Impact of nitrous oxide on the circulation during enflurane anesthesia in man. Anesthesiology 48:345–349, 1978

83. Skovsted P, Price ML, Price HL: The effects of halothane on arterial pressure, preganglionic sympathetic activity and barostatic reflexes. Anesthesiology 31:507–514, 1969

84. Skovsted P, Price HL: The effects of ethrane on arterial pressure, preganglionic sympathetic activity, and barostatic reflexes. Anesthesiology 36:257–262, 1972

Isoflurane

85. Stevens WC, Cromwell TH, Halsey MJ et al: The cardiovascular effects of a new inhalation anesthetic, Forane, in human volunteers at constant arterial carbon dioxide tension. Anesthesiology 35:8–16, 1971

86. Cromwell TH, Stevens WC, Eger EI II et al: The cardiovascular effects of compound 469 (Forane) during spontaneous ventilation and CO2 challenge in man. Anesthesiology 35:17–25, 1971

87. Dolan WM, Stevens WC, Eger EI II et al: The cardiovascular and respiratory effects of isoflurane-nitrous oxide anaesthesia. Can Anaesth Soc J 21:557–568, 1974

88. Mallow JE, White RD, Cucchiara RF, Tarhan S: Hemodynamic effects of isoflurane and halothane in patients with coronary artery disease. Anesth Analg (Cleve) 55:135–138, 1976

89. Mathers J, Benumof JL, Wahrenbrock EA: General anesthetics and regional hypoxic pulmonary vasoconstriction. Anesthesiology 46:111–114, 1977

90. Johnston RR, Eger EI II, Wilson C: A comparative interaction of epinephrine with enflurane, isoflurane, and halothane in man. Anesth Analg 55:709–712, 1976

91. Blitt CD, Raessler KL, Wightman MA et al: Atrioventricular conduction in dogs during anesthesia with isoflurane. Anesthesiology 50:210–212, 1979

92. Kemmotsu O, Hashimoto Y, Shimosato S: Inotropic effects of isoflurane on mechanics of contraction in isolated cat papillary muscles from normal and failing hearts. Anesthesiology 39:470–477, 1973

93. Horan BF, Prys–Roberts C, Roberts JG et al: Haemodynamic responses to isoflurane anaesthesia and hypovolaemia in the dog, and their modification by propranolol. Br J Anesth 49:1179–1187, 1977

94. Philbin DM, Lowenstein E: Lack of beta-adrenergic activity of isoflurane in the dog: a comparison of circulatory effects of halothane and isoflurane after propranolol administration. Br J Anaesth 48:1165–1170, 1976

95. Wolfson B, Hetrick WD, Lake CL, Siker ES: Anesthetic indices: further data. Anesthesiology 48:187–190, 1978

INTRAVENOUS ANESTHETIC AGENTS

96. Ghoneim MM, Korttila K: Pharmacokinetics of intravenous anaesthetics: implications for clinical use. Clin Pharmacokinet 2:344–372, 1977
97. Hug CC Jr: Pharmacokinetics of drugs administered intravenously. Anesth Analg (Cleve) 57:704–723, 1978
98. Eger EI II: Anesthetic Uptake and Action. Baltimore, Williams & Wilkins, 1974
99. Hug CC Jr: Improving analgesic therapy. Anesthesiology 53:441–443, 1980
100. Hug CC Jr: Drug disposition in abnormal flow states. (In preparation), 1982
101. Becker KE Jr: Plasma levels of thiopental necessary for anesthesia. Anesthesiology 49:192–196, 1978
102. Becker KE Jr, Tonnesen AS: Cardiovascular effects of plasma levels of thiopental necessary for anesthesia. Anesthesiology 49:197–200, 1978
103. Hengstmann JH, Stoeckel H, Schuttler J: Infusion model for fentanyl based on pharmacokinetic analysis. Br J Anaesth 52:1021–1025, 1980
104. Stapleton JV, Austin KL, Mather LE: A pharmacokinetic approach to postoperative pain: Continuous infusion of pethidine. Anaesth Intensive Care 7:25–32, 1979
105. Stanski DR, Ham J, Miller RD, Sheiner LB: Pharmacokinetics and pharmacodynamics of D-tubocurarine during nitrous oxide-narcotic and halothane anesthesia in man. Anesthesiology 51:235–241, 1979
106. Ramzan MI, Shanks CA, Triggs EJ: Pharmacokinetics of tubocurarine administration by combined I.V. bolus and infusion. Br J Anaesth 52:893–899, 1980

Barbiturates

107. Gilman LS, Goodman LS, Gilman AF: The Pharmacological Basis of Therapeutics, 6th ed. New York, Macmillan, 1980.
108. Marshall BE, Wollman H: General anesthetics. In Gilman, Goodman, Gilman: The Pharmacological Basis of Therapeutics, 6th ed. New York, Macmillan, 1980
109. Dundee JW, Wyant GM: Intravenous Anaesthesia. London, Churchill Livingstone, 1974
110. Breimer DD: Pharmacokinetics of metho-

hexitone following intravenous infusion in humans. Br J Anaesth 48:643–649, 1976
111. Christensen JH, Andreasen F, Jansen JA: Pharmacokinetics of thiopentone in a group of young women and a group of young men. Br J Anaesth 52:913–918, 1980
112. Becker KE Jr, Tonnesen AS: Cardiovascular effects of plasma levels of thiopental necessary for anesthesia. Anesthesiology 49:197–200, 1978
113. Conway CM, Ellis DB: The haemodynamic effects of short-acting barbiturates. Br J Anaesth 41:534–542, 1969
114. Sonntag H, Hellberg K, Schenk H-D et al: Effects of thiopental (Trapanal) on coronary blood flow and myocardial metabolism in man. Acta Anaesthesiol Scand 19:69–78, 1975
115. Price HL, Helrich M: The effect of cyclopropane, diethyl ether, nitrous oxide, thiopental, and hydrogen ion concentration on the myocardial function of the dog heart-lung preparation. J Pharmacol Exp Ther 115:206–216, 1955
116. Skovsted P, Price ML, Price HL: The effects of short-acting barbiturates on arterial pressure, preganglionic sympathetic activity and barostatic reflexes. Anesthesiology 33:10–18, 1970
117. Eckstein JW, Hamilton WK, McCammond JM: The effect of thiopental on peripheral venous tone. Anesthesiology 22:525–528, 1961
118. Watson WE, Seelye E, Smith AC: The action of thiopentone on the vascular distensibility of the hand. Br J Anaesth 34:19–23, 1962
119. Altura BT, Altura BM: Barbiturates and aortic and venous smooth-muscle function. Anesthesiology 43:432–444, 1975
120. Kentor ML, Schwalb AJ, Lieberman RW: Rapid high dose fentanyl induction for CABG. Anesthesiology 53:s95, 1980
121. Dundee JW: Alterations in response to somatic pain associated with anaesthesia. II. The effect of thiopentone and pentobarbitone. Br J Anaesth 32:407–414, 1960

Benzodiazepines

122. Physicians' Desk Reference, 35th ed. Oradell (NJ), Medical Economics, 1981
123. Brown CR, Sarnquist FH, Canup CA, Pedley TA: Clinical, electroencephalographic and pharmacokinetic studies of a water-soluble

benzodiazepine, midazolam maleate. Anesthesiology 50:467–470, 1979

124. Reves JG, Samuelson PN, Lewis S: Midazolam maleate induction in patients with ischaemic heart disease: haemodynamic observations. Can Anaesth Soc J 26:402–409, 1979
125. Greenblatt DJ, Shader RI: Pharmacokinetic understanding of antianxiety drug therapy. South Med J 71:2–9, 1978
126. Dundee JW, Haslett WHK: The benzodiazepines: a review of their actions and uses relative to anesthetic practice. Br J Anaesth 42:217–234, 1970
127. Greenblatt DJ, Shader RI: Benzodiazepines. N Engl J Med 291:1011–1015, 1239–1243, 1974
128. de Jong RH: Local Anesthetics, 2nd ed. Springfield (Ill), Charles C Thomas, 1977, p 97
129. Kahler RL, Burrow GN, Felig P: Diazepam: induced amnesia for cardioversion. JAMA 200:997–998, 1967
130. Pandit SK, Dundee JW, Keilty SR: Amnesia studies with intravenous premedication. Anaesthesia 26:421–428, 1971
131. Frumin MJ, Herekar VR, Jarvik ME: Amnesic actions of diazepam and scopolamine in man. Anesthesiology 45:406–412, 1976
132. McCammon RL, Hilgenberg JC, Stoelting RK: Hemodynamic effects of diazepam and diazepam-nitrous oxide in patients with coronary artery disease. Anesth Analg 59:438–441, 1980
133. Rao S, Sherbaniuk RW, Prasad K et al: Cardiopulmonary effects of diazepam. Clin Pharmacol Ther 14:182–189, 1973
134. Clarke RSJ, Lyons SM: Diazepam and flunitrazepam as induction agents for cardiac surgical operations. Acta Anaesthesiol Scand 21:282–292, 1977
135. D'Amelio G, Volta DS, Stritoni P et al: Acute cardiovascular effects of diazepam in patients with mitral valve disease. Eur J Clin Pharmacol 6:61–63, 1973
136. Cote P, Campeau L, Bourassa MG: Therapeutic implications of diazepam in patients with elevated left ventricular filling pressure. Am Heart J 91:747–751, 1976
137. Landis C: Changes in blood pressure during sleep as determined by the Erlanger method. Am J Physiol 73:551–555, 1925
138. Zsoter TT, Gospodarowicz M: The effect of diazepam and pentazocine on the venomotor reflexes in man. J Clin Pharmacol 12:89–94, 1972

139. Bradshaw EG: The vasodilator effects of diazepam in vitro. Br J Anaesth 48:817–818, 1976
140. Katz J, Finestone SC, Pappas MT: Circulatory response to tilting after intravenous diazepam in volunteers. Anesth Analg (Cleve) 46:243–246, 1967
141. Falk RB, Denlinger JK, Nahrwold ML, Todd RA: Acute vasodilation following induction of anesthesia with intravenous diazepam and nitrous oxide. Anesthesiology 49:149–150, 1978
142. Ikram H, Rubin AP, Jewkes RF: Effect of diazepam on myocardial blood flow of patients with and without coronary artery disease. Br Heart J 35:626–630, 1973
143. Cote P, Noble J, Bourassa MG: Systemic vasodilation following diazepam after combined sympathetic and parasympathetic blockade in patients with coronary artery disease. Cathet Cardiovasc Diag 2:369–380, 1976
144. Cote P, Campeau L, Bourassa MG: Therapeutic implications of diazepam in patients with elevated left ventricular filling pressure. Amer Heart J 91:747–751, 1976
145. Rosen M: Recent advances in pain relief in childbirth. I. Inhalation and systemic analgesia. Br J Anaesth 43:837–848, 1971
146. Stanley TH, Bennett GM, Loeser EA et al: Cardiovascular effects of diazepam and droperidol during morphine anesthesia. Anesthesiology 44:255–258, 1976
147. Stanley TH, Webster LR: Anesthetic requirements and cardiovascular effects of fentanyl-oxygen and fentanyl-diazepam-oxygen anesthesia in man. Anesth Analg (Cleve) 57:411–416, 1978

Other Hypnotics (Etomidate)

148. Horrigan RW, Moyers JR, Johnson BH et al: Etomidate vs. thiopental with and without fentanyl: a comparative study of awakening in man. Anesthesiology 52:362–364, 1980
149. Korttila K, Tammisto T, Aromaa U: Comparison of etomidate in combination with fentanyl or diazepam, with thiopentone as an induction agent for general anesthesia. Br J Anaesth 51:1151–1156, 1979
150. Gooding JM, Corssen G: Effect of etomidate on the cardiovascular system. Anesth Analg (Cleve) 56:717–719, 1977
151. Criado A, Maseda J, Navarro E et al: Induction of anaesthesia with etomidate: haemo-

dynamic study of 36 patients. Br J Anaesth 52:803–806, 1980

Narcotic Analgesics

152. Jaffe JH, Martin WR: Opioid analgesics and antagonists. In Gilman, Goodman, Gilman (eds): The Pharmacological Basis of Therapeutics, 6th ed. New York, Macmillan, 1980
153. Foldes FF, Swerdlow M, Siker ES: Narcotics and Narcotic Antagonists, Springfield (Ill), Charles C Thomas, 1964
154. Neff W, Mayer EC, Perales M de la Luz: Nitrous oxide and oxygen anesthesia with curare relaxation. California Medicine 66:67–69, 1947
155. Bailey P, Gerbode F, Garlington L: An anesthetic technique for cardiac surgery which utilizes 100% oxygen as the only inhalant. AMA Arch Surg 76:437–440, 1958
156. Lowenstein E, Hallowell P, Levine FH et al: Cardiovascular response to large doses of intravenous morphine in man. N Engl J Med 281:1389–1393, 1969
157. Mainzer J Jr: Awareness, Muscle Relaxants, and Balanced Anaesthesia. Canad Anaesth Soc J 26:386–393, 1979
158. Lowenstein E: Morphine "anesthesia": a perspective. Anesthesiology 35:563–565, 1971
159. Stanley TH, Gray NH, Stanford W, Armstrong R: The effects of high-dose morphine on fluid and blood requirements in open heart operations. Anesthesiology 38:536–541, 1973
160. Lunn JK, Stanley TH, Eisele J et al: High dose fentanyl anesthesia for coronary artery surgery: Plasma fentanyl concentrations and influence of nitrous oxide on cardiovascular responses. Anesth Analg 58:390–395, 1979
161. Stanley TH, Webster LR: Anesthetic requirements and cardiovascular effects of fentanyl-oxygen and fentanyl-diazepam-oxygen anesthesia in man. Anesth Analg 57:411–416, 1978
162. Stanley TH, Philbin DM, Coggins CH: Fentanyl-oxygen anesthesia for coronary artery surgery: Cardiovascular and antidiuretic hormone responses. Can Anaesth Soc J 26:168–172, 1979
163. Waller JL, Hug CC Jr, Nagle DM, Craver JM: Hemodynamic changes during fentanyl–oxygen anesthesia for aortocoronary bypass operation. Anesthesiology 55:212–217, 1981
164. Mummaneni N, Rao TLK: Awareness and

165. recall with high dose fentanyl-oxygen anesthesia. Anesthesiology (in press)
165. Editorial: High-dose fentanyl. Lancet 1:81–82, 1979 (Replies: Feb. 3, 1979)
166. Abouleish E, Taylor FH: Effect of morphine-diazepam on signs of anesthesia, awareness, and dreams of patients under N_2O for cesarean section. Anesth Analg 55:702–705, 1976
167. Freund FG, Martin WE, Wong KC, Hornbein TF: Abdominal-muscle rigidity induced by morphine and nitrous oxide. Anesthesiology 38:358–362, 1973
168. Sokoll MD, Hoyt JL, Gergis SD: Studies in muscle rigidity, nitrous oxide, and narcotic analgesic agents. Anesth Analg (Cleve) 51:16–20, 1972
169. Comstock MK, Scamman FL, Carter JG et al: Rigidity and hypercarbia on fentanyl-oxygen induction. Anesthesiology 51:s28, 1979
170. Kallos T, Wyche MZ, Garmen JK: The effects of Innovar on functional residual capacity and total chest compliance in man. Anesthesiology 39:558–561, 1973
171. Hug CC Jr: Unpublished observations
172. Hill AB, Nahrwold ML, De Rosayro AM et al: Prevention of rigidity during fentanyl-oxygen induction. Anesthesiology 53:68, 1980
173. Gergis SD, Hoyt JL, Sokoll MD: Effects of Innovar and Innovar plus nitrous oxide on muscle tone and "H" reflex. Anesth Analg (Cleve) 50:743–747, 1971
174. Hamilton WK, Cullen SC: Supplementation of nitrous oxide anesthesia with opiates and a new opiate antagonist. Anesthesiology 16:22–28, 1955
175. Spierdijk J, van Kleef J, Nauta J, Stanley TH, de Lange S: Alfentanyl: A new narcotic anesthetic induction agent. Anesthesiology 53:s32, 1980
176. deLange S, Stanley TH, Boscoe MJ: Comparison of sulfentanyl-O_2 and fentanyl-O_2 anesthesia for coronary artery surgery. Anesthesiology 53:s64, 1980
177. Grell FL, Koons RA, Denson JS: Fentanyl in anesthesia: a report of 500 cases. Anesth Analg 49:523–532, 1970
178. Stoelting RK, Gibbs PS, Creasser CW, Peterson C: Hemodynamic and ventilatory responses to fentanyl, fentanyl-droperidol, and nitrous oxide in patients with acquired valvular heart disease. Anesthesiology 42:319–324, 1975
179. Spierdijk J, van Kleef J, Nauta J et al: Alfen-

tanyl: A new narcotic anesthetic induction agent. Anesthesiology 53:32, 1980

180. Bovill JG, Sebel PS: Pharmacokenitics of high-dose fentanyl. Br J Anaesth 52:795–801, 1980

181. Moldenhauer CC, Hug CC Jr.: Continuous infusion of fentanyl for cardiac surgery. Anesth Analg (Cleve) 61: (In press), 1982

182. Calvert JR, Steinhaus JE, Martin GA, McFarland JC: Interrelation of cough suppression and respiratory depression. Anesthesiology 24:127, 1963

183. Arens JF, Benbow BP, Ochsner JL, Theard R: Morphine anesthesia for aortocoronary bypass procedures. Anesth Analg (Cleve) 51:901–909, 1972

184. Conahan TJ, Ominsky AJ, Wollman H, Stroth RA: A prospective random comparison of halothane and morphine for open-heart anesthesia: one year's experience. Anesthesiology 38:528–535, 1973

185. Jaffe JH, Martin WR: Opioid analgesics and antagonists. In Gilman, Goodman, Gilman: The Pharmacological Basis of Therapeutics, 6th ed. New York, Macmillan, 1980

186. Eckenhoff JE, Oech SR: The effects of narcotics and antagonists upon respiration and circulation in man. Clin Pharmacol Ther 1:483–524, 1960

187. Zelis R, Flaim SF, Eisele JH: Effects of morphine on reflex arteriolar constriction induced in man by hypercapnia. Clin Pharmacol Ther 22:172–178, 1977

188. Heisterkamp DV, Cohen PJ: The use of naloxone to antagonize large doses of opiates administered during nitrous oxide anesthesia. Anesth Analg 53:12–18, 1974

189. Michaelis LL, Hickey PR, Clark TA, Dixon WM: Ventricular irritability associated with the use of naloxone hydrochloride. Ann Thor Surg 18:608–614, 1974

190. Patschke D, Eberlein HJ, Hess W et al: Antagonism of morphine with naloxone in dogs: cardiovascular effects with special reference to the coronary circulation. Br J Anaesth 49:525–533, 1977

191. Flacke JW, Flacke WE, Williams GD: Acute pulmonary edema following naloxone reversal of high-dose morphine anesthesia. Anesthesiology 47:376–378, 1977

192. Desmonts JM, Bohm G, Couderc E: Hemodynamic responses to low doses of naloxone after narcotic-nitrous oxide anesthesia. Anesthesiology 49:12–16, 1978

193. Azar I, Turndorf H: Severe hypertension and multiple atrial premature contractions following naloxone administration. Anesth Analg (Cleve) 58:524–525, 1979

194. Longnecker DE, Grazis PA, Eggers GWN: Naloxone antagonism of morphine-induced respiratory depression. Anesth Analg (Cleve) 52:447–453, 1973

195. Evans JM, Hogg MIJ, Lunn JN, Rosen M: Degree and duration of reversal by naloxone of effects of morphine in conscious subjects. Br Med J 2:589–591, 1974

196. Johnstone RE, Jobes DR, Kennell EM et al: Reversal of morphine anesthesia with naloxone. Anesthesiology 41:361–367, 1974

197. Ngai SH, Berkowitz BA, Yang JC et al: Pharmacokinetics of naloxone in rats and in man: basis for its potency and short duration of action. Anesthesiology 44:398–401, 1976

198. Hug CC Jr: Drug disposition in abnormal flow states. (In preparation), 1982

199. Hsu HO, Hickey RF, Forbes AR: Morphine decreases peripheral vascular resistance and increases capacitance in man. Anesthesiology 50:98–102, 1979

200. Philbin DM, Moss J, Rosow CE et al: The use of H_1 and H_2 histamine blockers with morphine: a double blind study. Anesthesiology 53:67, 1980

201. Rosow CE, Moss J, Philbin DM, Saverese JJ: Histamine in human plasma following administration of morphine or fentanyl (abstr), p 285. Hamburg, 7th World Congress of Anesthesiologists, September 14–21, 1980

202. McClain DA, Hug CC Jr: Intravenous fentanyl kinetics. Clin Pharmacol Ther 28:106–114, 1980

203. Jones RM, Fiddian–Green R, Knight PR: Narotic-induced choledochoduodenal sphincter spasm reversed by glucagon. Anesth Analg (Cleve) 59:946–947, 1980

204. Economou G, Ward–McQuaid JN: A crossover comparison of the effect of morphine, pethidine, pentazocine, and phenazocine on bilary pressure. Gut 12:218–221, 1971

205. Radnay PA, Brodman E, Mankikar D, Duncalf D: The effect of equi-analgesic doses of fentanyl, morphine, merperidine, and pentazocine on common bile duct pressure. Anaesthesist 29:26–29, 1980

206. Jaffe JH: Drug addiction and drug abuse. In Gilman, Goodman, Gilman (eds): The Pharmacological Basis of Therapeutics, 6th ed. New York, Macmillan, 1980

207. Martin WR, Eades CG: Demonstration of tolerance and physical dependence in the dog following a short term infusion of morphine. J Pharmacol Exp Ther 133:262–270, 1961

208. Cox BM, Ginsburg M, Osman OH: Acute tolerance to narcotic analgesic drugs in rats. Br J Pharmacol 33:245–256, 1968

Cardiovascular Effects of Narcotic Analgesics: Morphine

209. Stoelting RK, Gibbs PS: Hemodynamic effects of morphine and morphine-nitrous oxide in valvular heart disease and coronary-artery disease. Anesthesiology 38:45–52, 1973

210. Lowenstein E, Hallowell P, Levine FH et al: Cardiovascular response to large doses of intravenous morphine in man. N Eng J Med 281:1389–1393, 1969

211. Conahan TJ, Ominsky AJ, Wollman H, Stroth RA: A prospective random comparison of halothane and morphine for open-heart anesthesia: One year's experience. Anesthesiology 38:528–535, 1973

212. Arens JF, Benbow BP, Ochsner JL, Theard R: Morphine anesthesia for aortocoronary bypass procedures. Anesth Analg 51:901–909, 1972

213. Krishna G, Paradise RR. Effect of morphine on isolated human atrial muscle. Anesthesiology 40:147–151, 1974

214. Dahlstrom B, Bolme P, Feychting H et al: Morphine kinetics in children. Clin Pharmacol Ther 26:354–365, 1979

215. Hug CC Jr: Pharmacokinetics of morphine during cardiac surgery (abstr) pp 305–306. Chicago, Annual Meeting of the American Society of Anesthesiologists, 1978

216. Eckenhoff JE, Oech SR: The effects of narcotics and antagonists upon respiration and circulation in man. Clin Pharmacol Ther 1:483–524, 1960

217. Marta JA, Davis HS, Eisele JH: Vagomimetic effects of morphine and Innovar in man. Anesth Analg (Cleve) 52:817–821, 1973

218. Zelis R, Flaim SF, Eisele JH: Effects of morphine on reflex arteriolar constriction induced in man by hypercapnia. Clin Pharmacol Ther 22:172–178, 1977

219. Hsu HO, Hickey RF, Forbes AR: Morphine decreases peripheral vascular resistance and increases capacitance in man. Anesthesiology 50:98–102, 1979

220. Zelis R, Mansour EJ, Capone RJ, Mason DT: The cardiovascular effects of morphine: The peripheral capacitance and resistance vessels in human subjects. J Clin Invest 54:1247–1258, 1974

221. Toda N, Hatano Y: Alpha-adrenergic blocking action of fentanyl on the isolated aorta of the rabbit. Anesthesiology 46:411–416, 1977

222. Flaim SF, Vismara LA, Zelis R: The effects of morphine on isolated cutaneous canine vascular smooth muscle. Res Commun Chem Pathol Pharmacol 16:191–194, 1977

223. Flaim SF, Zelis R, Eisele JH: Differential effects of morphine on forearm blood flow: attenuation of sympathetic control of the cutaneous circulation. Clin Pharmacol Ther 23:542–546, 1978

224. Lowenstein E, Whiting RB, Bittar DA et al: Local and neurally mediated effects of morphine on skeletal muscle vascular resistance. J Pharmacol Exp Ther 180:359–367, 1972

225. Kistner JR, Miller ED, Lake CL, Ross WT Jr: Indices of myocardial oxygenation during coronary-artery revascularization in man with morphine versus halothane anesthesia. Anesthesiology 50:324–330, 1979

226. Roizen MF, Horrigan RW, Fraser B: Anesthetic doses blocking adrenergic (stress) and cardiovascular responses to incision: MAC BAR and MAC BCVR. Anesthesiology (in press)

227. Philbin DM, Coggins CH: Plasma antidiuretic hormone levels in cardiac surgical patients during morphine and halothane anesthesia. Anesthesiology 49:95–98, 1978

228. Bailey DR, Miller ED Jr, Kaplan JA, Rogers PW: The renin-angiotensin-aldosterone system during cardiac surgery with morphine-nitrous oxide anesthesia. Anesthesiology 42:538–544, 1975

229. Stanley TH, Gray NH, Stanford W, Armstrong R: The effects of high-dose morphine on fluid and blood requirements in open heart operations. Anesthesiology 38:536–541, 1973

230. Green JF, Jackman AP, Parsons G: The effects of morphine on the mechanical properties of the systemic circulation in the dog. Circ Res 42:474–478, 1978

231. Green JF, Jackman AP, Krohn KA: Mechanism of morphine-induced shifts in blood volume between extracorporeal reservoir and the systemic circulation of the dog under

conditions of constant blood flow and vena caval pressures. Circ Res 42:479–486, 1978

Cardiovascular Effects of Narcotic Analgesics: Fentanyl

232. Lunn JK, Stanley TH, Eisele J et al: High dose fentanyl anesthesia for coronary artery surgery: Plasma fentanyl concentrations and influence of nitrous oxide on cardiovascular responses. Anesth Analg 58:390–395, 1979
233. Stanley TH, Webster LR: Anesthetic requirements and cardiovascular effects of fentanyl-oxygen and fentanyl-diazepam-oxygen anesthesia in man. Anesth Analg 57:411–416, 1978
234. Stanley TH, Philbin DM, Coggins CH: Fentanyl-oxygen anaesthesia for coronary artery surgery: Cardiovascular and antidiuretic hormone responses. Canad Anaesth Soc J 26:168–172, 1979
235. Waller JL, Hug CC Jr, Nagle DM, Craver JM: Hemodynamic changes during fentanyl–oxygen anesthesia for aortocoronary bypass, operation. Anesthesiology 55:212–217, 1981
236. Toda N, Hatano Y: Alpha-adrenergic blocking action of fentanyl on the isolated aorta of the rabbit. Anesthesiology 46:411–416, 1977
237. Goldberg AH, Padget CH: Comparative effects of morphine and fentanyl on isolated heart muscle. Anesth Analg (Cleve) 48:978–982, 1969
238. Strauer BE: Contractile responses to morphine, piritramide, meperidine, and fentanyl: A comparative study of effects on the isolated ventricular myocardium. Anesthesiology 37:304–310, 1972
239. Faulkner SL, Boerth RC, Graham TP Jr: Direct myocardial effects of precatheterization medications. Am Heart J 88:609–614, 1974
240. Bovill JG, Sebel PS: Pharmacokinetics of high-dose fentanyl. Br J Anaesth 52:795–801, 1980
241. Moldenhauer CC, Hug CC Jr: Continuous infusion of fentanyl for cardiac surgery. Anesth Analg (Cleve) 61:(In press), 1982
242. Ostheimer GW, Shanahan EA, Guyton RA et al: Effects of fentanyl and droperidol on canine left ventricular performance. Anesthesiology 42:288–291, 1975
243. Freye E: Cardiovascular effects of high dosages of fentanyl, meperidine, and naloxone in dogs. Anesth Analg (Cleve) 53:40–47, 1974
244. Eisele JH, Reitan JA, Torten M, Miller CH:

Myocardial sparing effect of fentanyl during halothane anaesthesia in dogs. Br J Anaesth 47:937–940, 1975
245. Liu W-S, Bidwai AV, Stanley TH, Isern-Amaral J: Cardiovascular dynamics after large doses of fentanyl and fentanyl plus N₂O in the dog. Anesth Analg (Cleve) 55:168–172, 1976
246. Patschke D, Gethmann JW, Hess W et al: Hamodynamik, koronardurchblutung und myokardialer sauerstoff verbrauch unter hohen fentanyl und peritramiddosen. Anaesthetist 25:309–317, 1976
247. Liu W-S, Bidwai AV, Stanley TH, Loeser EA, Bidwai V: The cardiovascular effects of diazepam and of diazepam and pancuronium during fentanyl and oxygen anaesthesia. Can Anaesth Soc J 23:395–403, 1976
248. van der Vusse GJ, van Belle H, Van Gerven W et al: Acute effect of fentanyl on haemodynamics and myocardial carbohydrate utilization and phosphate release during ischaemia. Br J Anaesth 51:927–935, 1979
249. Rosow CE, Moss J, Philbin DM, Saverese JJ: Histamine in human plasma following administration of morphine or fentanyl (abstr), p. 285. Hamburg, 7th World Congress of Anesthesiologists, September 14–21, 1980
250. Stanley TH: Personal communication
251. Hug CC Jr: Unpublished observations
252. Laubie M, Schmitt H, Canellas J et al: Centrally mediated bradycardia and hypotension induced by narcotic analgesics: dextromoramide and fentanyl. Eur J Pharmacol 28:66–75, 1974
253. Freye E: Die Anwendung hoher Dosen von Fentanyl und Naloxone in der anaesthesie. Anaesthetist 24:145–150, 1975
254. Freye E: Effect of high doses of fentanyl on myocardial infarction and cardiogenic shock in the dog. Resuscitation 3:105–113, 1979
255. Daskalopoulos NT, Laubie M, Schmitt H: Localization of the central smypathoinhibitory effect of a narcotic analgesic agent, fentanyl, in cats. Eur J Pharmacol 33:91–97, 1975
256. Hatano Y, Toda N: Influence of fentanyl on the chronotropic response of isolated rabbit atria to cholinergic and adrenergic stimulation. Jpn J Pharmacol 28:105–114, 1978
257. Takahashi K, Iwatsuki K: Effects of pentazocine and fentanyl on the pulmonary hemodynamics. Tohoku J Exp Med 113:89–95, 1974

258. Freye E: The effect of fentanyl on the resistance and capacitance vessels of the dog's hindlimb. Arzneim-Forsch 27:1037–1039, 1977

259. Stoelting RK, Gibbs PS, Creasser CW, Peterson C: Hemodynamic and ventilatory responses to fentanyl-droperidol, and nitrous oxide in patients with acquired valvular heart disease. Anesthesiology 42:319–324, 1975

260. Zelis R, Flaim SF, Eisele JH: Effects of morphine on reflex arteriolar constriction induced in man by hypercapnia. Clin Pharmacol Ther 22:172–178, 1977

261. de Lange S, Stanley TH, Boscoe MB: Comparison of sulfentanyl–O_2 and fentanyl–O_2 anesthesia for coronary artery surgery. Anesthesiology 53:s64, 1980

262. Mummaneni N, Rao TLK: Awareness and recall with high dose fentanyl-oxygen anesthesia. Anesthesiology (in press)

263. Murphy MR, Olson WA, Hug CC Jr: Pharmacokinetics of ^{3}H-fentanyl in the dog anesthetized with enflurane. Anesthesiology 50:13–19, 1979

264. McClain DA, Hug CC Jr: Intravenous fentanyl kinetics. Clin Pharmacol Ther 28:106–114, 1980

265. Hug CC Jr: Pharmacokinetics of morphine during cardiac surgery, pp 305–306 (abstr). Chicago, American Society of Anesthesiologists Annual Meeting, 1978

266. Murphy MR, Hug CC Jr: Pharmacokinetics of intravenous morphine in patients anesthetized with enflurane-nitrous oxide. Anesthesiology 54:187–192, 1981

267. de Castro J, van de Water A, Wouters L et al: Comparative study of cardiovascular, neurological and metabolic side-effects of eight narcotics in dogs. Acta Anaesthesiol Belg 30:5–99, 1979

268. Kalenda Z, Scheijgrond HW: Anaesthesia with sulfentanil-analgesia in carotid and vertebral arteriography: a comparison with fentanyl. Anaesthetist 25:380–383, 1976

269. Dubois–Primo J, Dewachter B, Massaut J: Analgesic anesthesia with fentanyl (F) and sufentanil (SF) in coronary surgery: a double-blind study. Acta Anaesthesiol Belg 30:113–126, 1979

270. Reddy P, Liu W-S, Stanley TH, Johansen R: Hemodynamic effects of anesthetic doses of alpha-prodine and sufentanil in dogs. Anesthesiology 51:102, 1979

271. Kay B, Pleuvry B: Human volunteer studies of R 39209, a new short-acting narcotic analgesic. Br J Anaesth 52:631–632, 1980

272. Spierdijk J, van Kleef J, Nauta J: Alfentanyl: A new narcotic anesthetic induction agent. Anesthesiology 53:32, 1980

Cardiovascular Effects of Narcotic Analgesics: Other Narcotic Analgesics

273. Neff W, Mayer ED, Perales M de la Luz: Nitrous oxide and oxygen anesthesia with curare relaxation. California Medicine 66:67–69, 1947

274. Bailey P, Gerbode F, Garlington L: An anesthetic technique for cardiac surgery which utilizes 100% oxygen as the only inhalant. AMA Arch Surg 76:437–440, 1958

275. Jaffe JH, Martin WR: Opioid analgesics and antagonists. In Gilman, Goodman, Gilman: The Pharmacological Basis of Therapeutics, 6th ed. New York, Macmillan, 1980

276. Foldes FF, Swerdlow M, Siker ES: Narcotics and Narcotic Antagonists, Springfield (Ill), Charles C Thomas, 1964

277. Eckenhoff JE, Oech SR: The effects of narcotics and antagonists upon respiration and circulation in man. Clin Pharmacol Ther 1:483–524, 1960

278. Strauer BE: Contractile responses to morphine, piritramide, meperidine, and fentanyl: A comparative study of effects on the isolated ventricular myocardium. Anesthesiology 37:304–310, 1972

279. Freye E: Cardiovascular effects of high dosages of fentanyl, meperidine, and naloxone in dogs. Anesth Analg 53:40–47, 1974

280. Mather LE, Tucker GT, Pflug AE et al: Meperidine kinetics in man: intravenous injection in surgical patients and volunteers, Clin Pharmacol Ther 17:21–30, 1975

281. Stanley TH, Bidwai AV, Lunn JK, Hodges MR: Cardiovascular effects of nitrous oxide during meperidine infusion in the dog. Anesth Analg (Cleve) 56:836–841, 1977

282. Stanley TH, Liu W-S: Cardiovascular effects of meperidine-N_2O anesthesia before and after pancuronium. Anesth Analg (Cleve) 56:669–673, 1977

283. Szeto HH, Inturrisi CE, Houde R et al: Accumulation of normeperidine, an active metabolite of meperidine in patients with renal failure or cancer. Ann intern Med 86:738–741, 1977

284. Reddy P, Liu W–S, Stanley TH, Johansen R:

Hemodynamic effects of anesthetic doses of alpha-prodine and sufentanil in dogs. Anesthesiology 51:102, 1979

Narcotic Antagonist Analgesics

285. Lasagna L: The clinical evaluation of morphine and its substitutes as analgesics. Pharmacol Rev 16:47–83, 1964
286. Jaffe JH, Martin WR: Opioid analgesics and antagonists. In Gilman, Goodman, Gilman: The Pharmacological Basis of Therapeutics, 6th ed. New York, Macmillan, 1980
287. Reevaluation of parenteral pentazocine. Med Lett Drugs Ther 18:46–47, 1976
288. Butorphanol (Stadol): a new parenteral analgesic. Med Lett Drugs Ther 20:111–112, 1978
289. Nalbuphine. Med Lett Drugs Ther 21:83–84, 1979
290. Popio KA, Jackson DH, Ross AM et al: Hemodynamic and respiratory effects of morphine and butorphanol. Clin Pharmacol Ther 23:281–287, 1978
291. Lee G, DeMaria AN, Amsterdam EA et al: Comparative effects of morphine, meperidine and pentazocine on cardiocirculatory dynamics in patients with acute myocardial infarction. Am J Med 60:949–955, 1976
292. Romagnoli A, Keats AS: Comparative hemodynamic effects of nalbuphine and morphine in patients with coronary artery disease. Bulletin of the Texas Heart Institute 5:19–24, 1978
293. Fahmy NR: Nalbuphine in "balanced" anesthesia: Its analgesic efficacy and hemodynamic effects. Anesthesiology 53:s66, 1980
294. Sederberg J, Stanley TH, Reddy P et al: Hemodynamic effects of butorphanol-oxygen in anesthesia in dogs. Anesthesiology 53:s70, 1980
295. Murphy MR, Hug CC, Jr: "Ceiling effect" of butorphanol (Stadol) as an anesthetic supplement. Anesthesiology 55:A260, 1981
296. Moldenhauer CC, Hug CC Jr, Nagle DM, Youngberg JA: High-dose butorphanol (Stadol) in anesthesia for aortocoronary bypass surgery. Abstracts, 3rd Annual Meeting, Society of Cardiovascular Anesthesiologists, San Francisco, May 10–13, 1981, pp 59–60
297. Duckworth EN, Lake CL, DiFazio CA, Magruder MR: Cardiovascular effects of nalbuphine in patients with coronary artery disease. Abstracts, 3rd Annual Meeting, Society of Cardiovascular Anesthesiologists, San Francisco, May 10–13, 1981, pp 61–62

Ketamine

298. Marshall BE, Wollman H: General anesthetics. In Gilman, Goodman, Gilman: The Pharmacological Basis of Therapeutics, 6th ed. New York, Macmillan, 1980
299. Zsigmond EK, Domino EF: Ketamine: clinical pharmacology, pharmacokinetics and current clinical uses. Anesthesiology Review 7:13–33, 1980
300. Nettles DC, Herrin TJ, Mullen JG: Ketamine induction in poor-risk patients. Anesth Analg (Cleve) 52:59–64, 1973
301. Barson P, Arens JF: Ketamine as an induction anesthetic for poor-risk patients. South Med J 67:1398–1402, 1974
302. Hirshman CA, Downes H, Farbood A, Bergman NA: Ketamine prevents bronchospasm in asthma: mechanism involved. Anesthesiology 51:363, 1979
303. White PF, Ham J, Way WL, Trevor AJ: Pharmacology of ketamine isomers in surgical patients. Anesthesiology 52:231–239, 1980
304. Slogoff S, Allen GW, Wessels JV, Cheney DH: Clinical experience with subanesthetic ketamine. Anesthesiology 53:354–360, 1974
305. Smith DJ, Westfall DP, Adams JD: Ketamine interacts with opiate receptors as an agonist. Anesthesiology 53:5, 1980
306. Kraynack LL, Gintautas J, Kraynack BJ, Racz G: Antagonism of ketamine induced narcosis by naloxone. Anesthesiology 53:59, 1980
307. Fratta W Casu M, Balestrieri A et al: Failure of ketamine to interact with opiate receptors. Eur J Pharmacol 61:389–391, 1980
308. Liang HS, Liang HG: Minimizing emergence phenomena: subdissociative dosage of ketamine in balanced surgical anesthesia. Anesth Analg (Cleve) 54:312–316, 1975
309. Mattila MAK, Larni HM, Nummi SE, Pekkola PO: A double-blind study: effect of diazepam on emergence from ketamine anesthesia. Anesthetist 28:20–23, 1979
310. Jackson APF, Dhadphale PR, Callaghan ML, Alseri S: Haemodynamic studies during induction of anesthesia for open-heart surgery using diazepam and ketamine. Br J Anaesth 50:375–378, 1978
311. Dhadphale PR, Jackson APF, Alseri S: Comparison of anesthesia with diazepam and ketamine vs. morphine in patients undergo-

ing heart-valve replacement. Anesthesiology 51:200–203, 1979

312. Kumar SM, Kothary SP, Zsigmond EK: Plasma free norepinephrine and epinephrine concentrations following diazepam: ketamine induction in patients undergoing cardiac surgery. Acta Anaesthesiol Scand 22:593–600, 1978

313. Ivankovick AD, Miletich DJ, Reimann C et al: Cardiovascular effects of centrally administered ketamine in goats. Anesth Analg (Cleve) 53:924–931, 1974

314. Goldberg AH, Keane PW, Phear WPC: Effects of ketamine on contractile performance and excitability of isolated heart muscle. J Pharmacol Exp Ther 175:388–394, 1970

315. Dundee JW: Ketamine, Proc R Soc Lond [Biol] 64:1159–1160, 1971

316. Traber DL, Wilson RD, Priano LL: Differentiation of the cardiovascular effects of CI-581. Anesth Analg (Cleve) 47:769–778, 1968

317. Stanley TH: Blood-pressure and pulse-rate responses to ketamine during general anesthesia. Anesthesiology 39:648–649, 1973

318. Chodoff P: Evidence for central adrenergic action of ketamine: Report of a case. Anesth Analg (Cleve) 51:247–250, 1972

319. Traber DL, Wilson RD: Involvement of the sympathetic nervous system in the pressor response to ketamine. Anesth Analg (Cleve) 48:248–252, 1969

320. Tweed WA, Minuck M, Mymin D: Circulatory responses to ketamine anesthesia. Anesthesiology 37:613–619, 1972

321. Reves JG, Lell WA, McCracken LE et al: Comparison of morphine and ketamine anesthetic techniques for coronary surgery: a randomized study. South Med J 71:33–36, 1978

322. Tweed WA, Mymin D: Myocardial force-velocity relations during ketamine anesthesia at constant heart rate. Anesthesiology 41:49–52, 1974

323. Hill GE, Wong KC, Shaw CL et al: Interactions of ketamine with vasoactive amines at normothermia and hypothermia in the isolated rabbit heart. Anesthesiology 48:315–319, 1978

324. Koehntop DE, Liao J-C, Van Bergen FH: Effects of pharmacological alterations of adrenergic mechanisms by cocaine, tropolone, aminophylline, and ketamine on epinephrine-induced arrhythmias during halothane-nitrous oxide anesthesia. Anesthesiology 46:83–93, 1977

325. Dundee JW, Lilburn JK, Moore J: Attempted reduction of the cardiostimulatory effects of ketamine by labetalol. Anesthesia 33:506–511, 1978

Major Tranquilizers (Neuroleptics)

326. Baldessarini RJ: Drugs and the treatment of psychiatric disorders. In Gilman, Goodman, Gilman (eds): The Pharmacological Basis of Therapeutics, 6th ed. New York, Macmillan, 1980

327. Mainzer J Jr: Awareness, muscle relaxants and balanced anaesthesia. Can Anaesth Soc J 26:386–393, 1979

328. Marshall BE, Wollman H: General anesthetics. In Gilman, Goodman, Gilman: The Pharmacological Basis of Therapeutics, 6th ed. New York, MacMillan, 1980

329. Stanley TH, Bennett GM, Loeser EA et al: Cardiovascular effects of diazepam and droperidol during morphine anesthesia. Anesthesiology 44:255–258, 1976

330. Faulkner SL, Boerth RC, Graham TP Jr: Direct myocardial effects of precatheterization medications. Amer Heart J 88:609–614, 1974

331. Ostheimer GW, Shanahan EA, Guyton RA et al: Effects of fentanyl and droperidol on canine left ventricular performance. Anesthesiology 42:288–291, 1975

332. Edmonds–Seal J, Prys–Roberts C: Pharmacology of drugs used in neuroleptanalgesia. Br J Anaesth 42:207–216, 1970

333. Ellis FR, Wilson J: An assessment of droperidol as a premedicant. Br J Anaesth 44:1288–1290, 1972

334. Dangers of Innovar. Medical Lett Drugs Ther 16:42–43, 1974

335. Ferrari HA, Gorten RJ, Talton IH et al: The action of droperidol and fentanyl on cardiac output and related hemodynamic parameters. South Med J 67:49–53, 1974

336. Whitwam JG, Russell WJ: The acute cardiovascular changes and adrenergic blockade by droperidol in man. Br J Anaesth 43:581–591, 1971

337. Muldoon SM, Janssens WJ, Verbeuren TJ, Vanhoutte PM: Alpha-adrenergic blocking properties of droperidol on the isolated blood vessels of the dog. Br J Anaesth 49:211–216, 1977

338. Becsey L, Malamed S, Radnay P, Foldes FF: Reduction of the psychotomimetic and cir-

culatory side-effects of ketamine by droperidol. Anesthesiology 37:536–542, 1972

339. Erbguth PH, Reiman B, Klein RL: The influence of chlorpromazine, diazepam, and droperidol on emergence from ketamine. Anesth Analg (Cleve) 51:693–699, 1972

340. Mainzer J, Jr: Awareness, muscle relaxants, and balanced anesthesia. Canad Anaesth Soc J 26:386–393, 1979

341. Lee CM, Yeakel AE: Patient refusal of surgery following Innovar premedication. Anesth Analg (Cleve) 54:224–226, 1975

342. Bradshaw EG, Pleuvry BJ, Sharma HL: Effect of droperidol on dopamine-induced increase in effective renal plasma flow in dogs. Br J Anaesth 52:879–883, 1980

343. Birch AA, Boyce WH: Effects of droperidol-dopamine interaction on renal blood flow in man. Anesthesiology 47:70–71, 1977

344. Bertolo L, Novakovic L, Penna M: Antiarrhythmic effects of droperidol. Anesthesiology 37:529–535, 1972

345. Johnston RR, Eger EI II, Wilson C: A comparative interaction of epinephrine with enflurane, isoflurane, and halothane in man. Anesth Analg 55:709–712, 1976

Other Drugs

346. Gilman LS, Goodman LS, Gilman AG: The Pharmacological Basis of Therapeutics, 6th ed. New York, Macmillan, 1980

10

The Use of Muscle Relaxants in the Patient with Cardiovascular Disease

RICHARD P. FOGDALL

INTRODUCTION

Often I have been asked why the choice of muscle relaxant or antagonist is of concern to the anesthesiologist or intensivist. In this chapter we will discuss these concerns relative to the patient with cardiovascular (and respiratory) disease, providing the information necessary for safe and effective clinical usage. The emphasis will be a strongly clinical one, and not an exhaustive regurgitation of all known *in vivo* or *in vitro* experimentation. Subjects discussed will be of a clinical nature, with laboratory data injected only where it clarifies mechanism or provides answers not available yet in the human patient. The references have been pared to a minimum, and are provided for background reading or further elaboration of questions of clinical importance.

MUSCLE RELAXANTS

INTRODUCTION

Historical Perspectives

Skeletal muscle relaxant drugs have been used for centuries by primitive peoples.[1] Laboratory experimentation with curare-like poisons began as early as the mid-18th century, providing physiologists of the 18th and 19th centuries with fascinating observations. It later became obvious to investigators and physicians that life could be maintained in the curarized animal if artificial respiration were provided.

The first clinical use of curare is believed to have been on New Year's Day in 1857, in the treatment of a patient with tetanus. This, and other clinical trials, ended in failure because the potion was applied directly to wounds, and was of variable strength and purity.

In the 1930s, investigations by Gill, Holaday, King, West, and Burman separately led to the availability of the pure alkaloid d-tubocurarine chloride, and its clinical trial in spastic children by Burman. The availability of curare for clinical use in anesthesia was promoted by Lew Wright, E. M. Papper, Stuart Cullen, and Harold Griffith, all in 1940. The introduction and use of curare and similar compounds in anesthesia and critical care has provided historians and clinicians with a fascinating series of tales. An excellent review by Betcher covers much of this development, and will provide the reader with some background information necessary to understand the milieu into which these drugs were "injected".[1]

These drugs obviously provide for the relaxation of skeletal muscle, usually administered to facilitate anesthetic and surgical manipulations or to facilitate the more precise control of mechanical respiratory ventilation. They are not meant to be used as alternatives to properly conducted general anesthesia, and are used best only in the fully anesthetized or comatose patient. If used in the awake patient, cardiovascular (as well as psychic) consequences may be substantial.[2]

Importance of Relaxant Choice

The cardiovascular effects of relaxants, as seen by the clinician, are indeed important, but need to be placed into perspective. There are many instances in which a minor alteration in hemodynamics might be evident (*e.g.*, a 15 percent increase in heart rate following pancuronium administration), but in the larger scope of patient care could be without significance. It would be foolish for the clinician to be concerned unduly with a minor hemodynamic change following relaxant administration, while concomitantly demonstrating no concern for a major cardiovascular derangement, produced by a poorly timed, or poorly performed laryngoscopy, intubation, or other manipulation. Unfortunately, such seemingly inconsistent actions occur.

An identical hemodynamic change following relaxant administration may occur in each of two dissimilar patients, yet have profoundly different effects upon each of the two. For instance, a young healthy patient might tolerate easily the inadvertent produc-

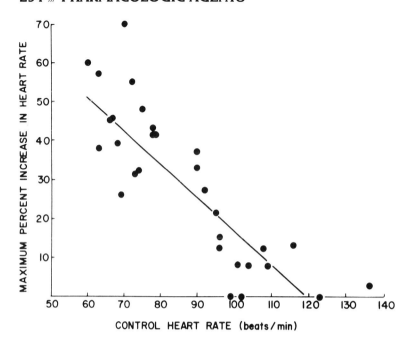

Fig. 10–1 Correlation of heart rate before pancuronium (control heart rate) with maximum percentage increase in heart rate following pancuronium. The line represents analysis of linear regression ($r = 0.85$). The greatest changes occur when control heart rate is lowest. (Miller RD, Eger EI II, Stevens WC: Anesthesiology 42:352–355, 1975)

tion of both tachycardia and hypertension from pancuronium. Yet the same degree of tachycardia and hypertension can provoke myocardial ischemia in a patient with severe coronary artery disease. I have seen examples of both.

On the other hand, two identical patients might demonstrate completely divergent cardiovascular effects from pancuronium only because their initial heart rates, before the relaxant, were different. Miller has illustrated the effect of control heart rate on the subsequent change in heart rate following pancuronium (Fig. 10-1).[3] Patients with low control heart rates have a greater increase in heart rate than those patients who begin with higher heart rates. The milieu into which the relaxant is administered is probably more important than the exact pharmacologic effect of the agent. However, a clear understanding of the pharmacologic effects of a relaxant drug, based upon its known structure, should allow the clinician to predict hemodynamic effects with a fair degree of accuracy.

In this text, it would be tempting to wonder if the anesthesiologist is concerned only with patients undergoing cardiac surgery because this accounts for approximately 75,000 to 100,000 patients per year in the United States. I would remind the reader that abnormalities of the heart or blood vessels account for approximately 1,000,000 deaths annually in the United States, two-thirds of which are from myocardial infarction, and another one-fifth from cerebrovascular accidents (strokes). Cardiovascular disease is present in at least 32 million Americans.* There are no figures for the actual number of these persons who will undergo general anesthesia yearly, but it certainly must be in the millions. Thus each reader of this chapter will probably care for many patients with cardiovascular diseases.

Patients with cardiac disease have either abnormalities of nutrient supply and demand balance (coronary artery disease), valvular dysfunction, ventricular dysfunction (multiple etiologies), intracardiac shunts, rhythm disturbances, or combinations of these. Because relaxant drugs may impact upon any or all of these areas, a thorough knowledge

---

*1979 data from the American Heart Association

of pharmacology, physiology, and pathophysiology is important.

Alterations in Hemodynamics and Patients at Risk

Circulatory alterations which may occur after relaxant administration are not, however, isolated from each other. Changes and interactions which occur often include direct cardiac and vascular alterations, secondary alterations such as a decrease in venous return from a loss of muscle tone, and impairment of cardiac filling because of controlled ventilation. Alterations in electrolyte concentrations, during altered ventilation, may produce cardiovascular effects.

These changes are not always predictable or measurable, and some may occur only under certain circumstances (autonomic imbalance, halothane anesthesia, and the like). None exists in a vacuum, and unfortunately (or, in some cases, fortunately) an alteration in any one of them may lead to changes in another. Reflex mechanisms tend to reregulate the cardiovascular system back to normal, and thus relaxant-induced circulatory effects must be evaluated by looking at changes *over time*. There are no studies of relaxant effects on the pulmonary vasculature.

In the young healthy patient, any of these changes will probably be well tolerated. There are, however, four major hemodynamic alterations which are measured easily in every patient, and which can be used to

define changes which are risks for certain patient groups. These four areas of risk are summarized in Table 10-1.

Obviously, several of the pathological states seen in Table 10-1 may occur together in any one patient, and, thus, evaluation of, and control of, hemodynamic changes will be vitally important. The reader will notice that the patient with coronary artery disease may appear at risk in *all* four of these categories. This patient group constitutes a large number of patients seen in a standard anesthetic or critical care practice.

It is obvious that a patient listed in a specific category should not, as a routine, receive a relaxant expected to produce an effect deemed to place that patient at risk. For instance, the rapid administration of a high dose of pancuronium to a patient with mitral stenosis would be expected to produce tachycardia, left ventricular filling problems, and cardiac output deterioration. Or, the administration of d-tubocurarine (dTc), in high doses over a short period of time, to a patient with aortic stenosis would be expected to produce substantial hypotension, and deterioration of body perfusion.

On the other hand, a patient with coronary artery disease might be treated beneficially by the judicious use of metocurine because of its relative absence of cardiovascular effects. Or, the patient with pure aortic insufficiency would receive benefit from the administration of d-tubocurarine, to augment a decrease in systemic vascular resistance, a lowering of impedance to left ventricular

Table 10-1. Patients at Risk From Cardiovascular Alterations Produced by Relaxants

HYPERTENSION	HYPOTENSION	TACHYCARDIA	BRADYCARDIA
Coronary artery disease	Coronary artery disease	Coronary artery disease	Coronary artery disease
Aortic insufficiency	Low cardiac output	Mitral stenosis	Low cardiac output
Mitral insufficiency	Fixed cardiac output	Aortic stenosis	Fixed cardiac output
Increased intracranial pressure	Aortic stenosis	IHSS	Myocardial ischemia
Recent vascular anastomosis	Mitral stenosis		Small stroke volume
Obstetrical patient	IHSS		Arrhythmia-prone patient
	Increased intracranial pressure		
	Obstetric patient		
	Intracardiac shunts		
	Hypertensive patient		

ejection, and a larger forward cardiac output. One can easily devise additional clinical settings in which physiologic processes could be aided or harmed by pharmacologic interventions. Each relaxant will be discussed in further detail later in this chapter.

Miscellaneous Effects

One area of altered hemodynamics which will not receive further detailed attention is that of the production of hyperkalemia. Occasionally, after the administration of succinylcholine (also decamethonium ?), muscle cells release potassium into the general circulation, producing a level of potassium greater than can be tolerated by electrically conductive cardiac tissue.[4] Such hyperkalemia has produced cardiac arrest after the administration of depolarizing muscle relaxants.[5] The patient with demyelinating nerve injury (e.g., cord transection, polio, amyotrophic lateral sclerosis) or massive thermal burn injury to muscle may respond in such a fashion. These clinical settings are now well recognized, and will not be discussed further here. A thorough presentation of this problem and these clinical conditions is provided by Katz.[6] Obviously, succinylcholine should not be administered to any patient in whom a hyperkalemic response is anticipated.

Neuromuscular Monitoring

Monitoring of cardiovascular function is presently routine intraoperatively and in the critical care setting. Monitoring of neuromuscular function is not, but should be. Because many drugs used in the critical care setting have cardiovascular and neuromuscular effects, their more precise use is possible only with appropriate monitoring. Monitoring might involve clinical observations, measurement of mechanical muscle response to evoked stimulus, measurement of electrical response to evoked stimulus, measurement of end-organ function (e.g., respiratory function testing), or plasma drug levels correlated with clinical situations. If the professional administering a relaxant desires a certain neu-

romuscular end point, preferably avoiding cardiovascular changes from the relaxant, measurement of that neuromuscular endpoint is essential. By doing so, only a minimum amount of relaxant (or antagonist) need be given, thus possibly avoiding hemodynamic side-effects. Thorough reviews of neuromuscular monitoring in adults and infants are provided by Ali,[7] Donlon,[8] and Crumrine,[9] and will allow the reader to gain additional information necessary to evaluate neuromuscular function during relaxant use.

PHARMACOLOGIC AND PHYSIOLOGIC CONSIDERATIONS

Neuromuscular Function

Muscle relaxant drugs exert their primary effects at the neuromuscular junction. While a detailed analysis of this interaction is beyond the scope of this chapter, this detail is provided by Katz.[10] Simplified, the majority of these agents serve as blocking drugs at neuromuscular receptors for acetylcholine (ACh). They may serve also as blocking drugs plus false transmitters to the receptor, such as with succinylcholine. They provide for a failure of muscle response to the stimulus of the innervating nerve. Because of their structure allowing blockade at these nicotinic ACh receptors, they also exhibit effects at muscarinic ACh receptors. These secondary effects may produce alterations in vagal activity (especially cardiac rate), and at autonomic ganglia (control of systemic vascular resistance). These secondary areas also are under the control of catecholamines, anesthetic agents, central nervous system alertness, and so on. Thus, many interactions are possible.

Factors Affecting Relaxant Effects

The effects of any administered drug are affected by many factors. The reader is reminded that these factors need to be considered when a relaxant is studied. Some of these factors have received investigative attention with regard to muscle relaxants. Others (e.g., rate of administration) have not, but should. Any, or all, of them may determine the concentration and/or effectiveness of the relaxant in the vascular compartment, or at some final effector organ. Reviews on relaxant pharmacokinetics are offered.[11, 12]

It must be remembered that a preset dose of relaxant may have extremely variable results from patient to patient (from no measurable response to a maximally measurable response). *Variability is the rule.* For the cardiovascular system, the *state of autonomic balance* is one of the key factors regulating hemodynamic responses from relaxant administration.

The concomitant administration of anesthetic agents and other drugs may have profound effects upon the hemodynamic changes produced by relaxants.[13–20] Such drugs might be halothane, nitrous oxide, enflurane, isoflurane, or narcotics. The dose of the relaxant is also important.[20] On the other hand, the relaxant drug may affect the state of general anesthesia, and thus hemodynamics.[21]

Muscle Relaxant "Side-Effects"

This topic often has been referred to as complications of relaxants, side-effects of relaxants, or adverse relaxant effects. Cardiovascular effects may or may not be adverse. But to evaluate possible mechanisms for side-effects, one could categorize them in the following way:

Anaphylactic: "allergic"
Immunologic
Histamine mediated
Vasoactive polypeptide mediated
Overdose (normal receptor)
Transmitter problems (*e.g.,* succinylcholine)
Receptor problems (blockade, abnormal structure, etc.)
End-organ sensitivity problems (muscle cell disease)

Most cardiovascular side-effects from relaxants will be secondary to dosage relationships, histamine release, or receptor blockade with a subsequent change in autonomic bal-

ance. The blockade of nicotinic cholinoceptive sites yields both neuromuscular blockade and autonomic ganglionic blockade. Muscarinic receptor activity produces postganglionic parasympathetic alterations. The structure of the drug determines the basic receptor effect and most of these can be predicted, if the physiologic circumstances are measured, quantitated, and understood. Thus, for instance, hypotension from histamine release and ganglionic blockade, produced by d-tubocurarine (as expected), will be of little clinical consequence if hemodynamic status is known, patient position and volume status adjusted, and concomitant use of anesthetic agent attenuated.

One should be careful to separate primary effects from secondary ones. For instance, a relaxant might have no direct effect on cardiac output, but yet might indirectly affect cardiac output by its effects on venous return during mechanical ventilation. Because mechanical ventilation is mandatory in the paralyzed patient, such a decrease in cardiac output often would accompany the use of the relaxant. The effect of a relaxant on the reduction of venous return from inactive, paralyzed muscle might be caused by a decrease in the milking action of extremity muscles, and not be a direct effect of the relaxant. By increasing the patient's circulating blood volume (optimizing preload), that effect might no longer occur. Thus, again, we see that the milieu of the patient is a very important determinant of the final effect of the relaxant.

INVESTIGATION OF RELAXANT CIRCULATORY EFFECTS

There are many problems in analyzing hemodynamic effects of relaxants. Some areas in which detailed evaluation or control of the experimental protocol has not occurred include rate of administration, drug–drug interactions, equipotency of doses, nonparallel dose-responses, dissimilar patient groups, primary versus secondary effects, and interventions.

Apart from species differences, one of the major problems in studies comparing circulatory effects of the various relaxants is the failure of some investigators to utilize *equipotent doses* of drugs. One first has to define the dose of each relaxant which provides identical neuromuscular effects, and then use these doses to evaluate the circulatory effects. These doses might be the dose to achieve 50 percent twitch depression (ED_{50}) or 95 percent twitch depression (ED_{95}) or, in some cases, twice the ED_{95} (a dose producing consistently good conditions for laryngoscopy and intubation, without coughing and the like). With parallel dose-response curves, comparing identical portions of the curves will allow potency differences to be assessed accurately, and thus correct potency ratios used to evaluate circulatory effects of *equipotent* relaxant doses. Several investigators have published such comparative curves for the four major nondepolarizing relaxants presently in use in the United States.[22-24] While there are minor differences among them, Figure 10-2 illustrates the relative potency positions of each of these four relaxants, the most potent relaxant (pancuronium) on the left, the least potent (gallamine) on the right.[24] Only if the relaxants are parallel to each other may a dose of one be compared

to an equipotent dose of another for accurate assessment of a secondary effect. In early studies of metocurine (dimethyl tubocurarine) and d-tubocurarine, these equipotent doses were not used. In the early comparative studies of pyridostigmine and neostigmine in humans, equipotent doses were not used. In the case of metocurine versus d-tubocurarine, further investigation using equipotent doses yielded informative comparative data.[25] And using equipotent doses of neostigmine and pyridostigmine, Fogdall and Miller demonstrated similar heart rate responses with the two drugs.[26]

Another method of evaluating some of the circulatory effects of muscle relaxants is to compare several effects on the *same* dose-response curve for *each* relaxant. Such work by Hughes, comparing the neuromuscular, vagolytic, and sympathetic ganglionic activities of the above four relaxants (pancuronium, gallamine, d-tubocurarine, and metocurine) in cats, demonstrates how the two cardiovascular blockades compare with the neuromuscular blockade.[27] These experiments will be referred to later in the text and in a figure below; they contain much information of interest to clinicians, and their

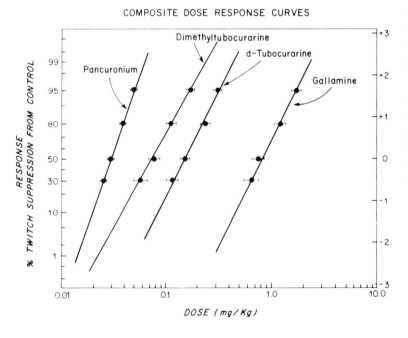

COMPOSITE DOSE RESPONSE CURVES

Fig. 10–2. Composite dose-response curves for four nondepolarized relaxants on log-probit paper. Nine patients in each patient group. Note the relative positions of the four curves. Pancuronium is the most potent, and gallamme the least potent. (Donlon JV Jr., Ali HH, Savarese JJ: Anesth Analg 53:934–939, 1974)

value should not be underestimated; the "meat" of hemodynamic alterations from these four relaxants is demonstrated in this series of experiments.

DEPOLARIZING RELAXANTS

Depolarizing relaxants, such as succinylcholine and decamethonium, act upon nicotinic and muscarinic receptors by design. Succinylcholine is not a naturally occurring compound. In general, succinylcholine has little effect on the cardiovascular system of the average patient. Discussion of the release of potassium seen after succinylcholine administration in the patient with demylinating nerve injury, or in the patient with massive burns is excluded here. Such potassium release and subsequent hyperkalemia can produce cardiovascular consequences.

Succinylcholine

Succinylcholine (diacetylcholine) may mimic acetylcholine at muscarinic and nicotinic receptors (Table 10-2). Thus unchecked, succinylcholine may produce an effective increase in "vagal tone," producing bradycardia. This decrease in heart rate depends upon the balance of sympathetic and parasympathetic activity present at the SA node. It appears to be related both to dose and to rate of administration of succinylcholine.[28–31] Subsequent doses produce greater effects, and high infusion rates of succinylcholine infusion produce a progressive bradycardia. Children appear more susceptible than adults to this effect. Upon discontinuance of succinylcholine, the bradycardia gradually lessens, and the effect is transient. Tachycardia also may occur during succinylcholine use, most likely as a result of stimulation of the nicotinic receptors at sympathetic autonomic ganglia.

The anesthetic agent being administered concomitantly appears to have an influence on this inconsistent response. Thiopental may be protective, as may hexafluorenium, suggesting that hydrolysis of succinylcholine may play a role in the production of bradycardia, as might be postulated. The brady-

Table 10-2. Succinylcholine Hemodynamic Effects

Mimics acetylcholine
Bradycardia
Rate/dose dependent
Blockable
Children > adults
Arrhythmias ±
Histamine release-rare
Hyperkalemia-selected patients

cardia is blocked by atropine, and ganglionic blocking agents such as trimethaphan. Prior administration of nonpolarizing relaxants is said to protect against succinylcholine-induced bradycardia, but did not do so in a healthy adult patient who developed complete asystole after succinylcholine 90 mg IV, after pretreatment with d-tubocurarine 3 mg.[32]

Succinylcholine is reported to protect against arrhythmias induced by epinephrine in dogs.[33] It also is reported to increase the arrhythmias produced by epinephrine in dogs.[34] Obviously this issue has not been settled. Histamine release, while very infrequent, has been reported.[35]

As mentioned previously (and shown in Table 10-1), patients at risk from bradycardia are those with coronary artery disease, low and fixed cardiac output, small ventricular stroke volume, and the patient prone to ventricular escape rhythms at low sinus heart rates. Obviously, the cardiac rate and rhythm should be monitored in such a patient during administration of succinylcholine.

NONDEPOLARIZING RELAXANTS

Gallamine

Gallamine is known widely for its ability to produce tachycardia. A review of the composite dose-response curve measured in cats demonstrates why this should be so (Fig. 10-3A). The vagolytic effects after gallamine begin at lower doses than necessary to produce neuromuscular blockade.[36] In order to achieve effective neuromuscular blockade, vagolytic activity must occur to a considera-

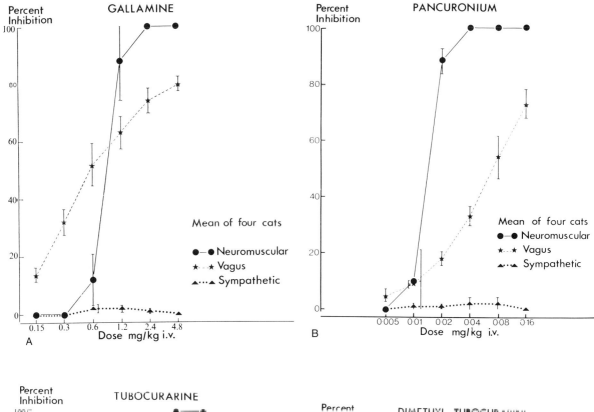

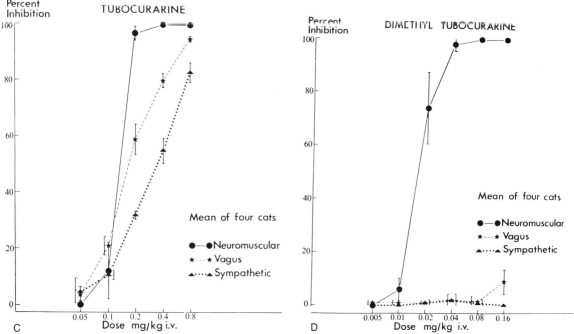

Fig. 10–3. Simultaneous dose-response curves for gallamine (*A*), pancuronium (*B*), d-tubocurarine (*C*), and dimethyl-tubocurarine (metocurine) (*D*), respectively, for neuromuscular, vagal, and sympathetic blockade in cats. See text for discussion. (Hughes R, Chapple DJ: Br J Anaesth 48:59–68, 1976)

ble degree. It is obligatory. Sympathetic ganglionic blockade is not demonstrated, at least in cats (see Fig. 10-3A). Histamine release is said to occur with gallamine, but to a lesser extent than with d-tubocurarine.

When used clinically, vagolytic activity is seen also.[37, 38] Small (subparalyzing) doses of gallamine may produce tachycardia. Whether this pronounced increase in heart rate is detrimental depends upon the cardiovascular status of the patient. In healthy patients, it probably is of little consequence. But if the high heart rate contributes to a decrease in cardiac filling time, and thus a decrease in cardiac output, serious consequences might ensue.

In the patient with coronary artery disease, the tachycardia could produce such an increase in myocardial oxygen consumption that myocardial oxygen availability is exceeded. In the patient with aortic or mitral stenosis, the presence of a stenotic valvular lesion will prevent rapid flow through the stenotic valve. In such instances, a slow heart rate and long flow time are preferred. This allows for maximum blood flow across the stenotic valve before surgical correction. If a patient has a disease process in which tachycardia is to be avoided (see Table 10-1), then so is gallamine. Put another way, if one would not give a large dose of atropine to such a patient whose heart rate is already normal, then one should not give gallamine.

Pancuronium

Pancuronium bromide has achieved widespread clinical use, probably because of its apparent lack of hypotension when administered to a great variety of patients. It is touted for its *cardiovascular stability,* but that term should be used with caution.

Comparing the cumulative dose-response curve for pancuronium (Fig. 10-3B) with that of gallamine (Fig. 10-3A) shows one important difference. While vagolytic activity still occurs in the cat with pancuronium, the vagal dose-response curve is situated to the right

of the neuromuscular curve.[39] Alcuronium behaves in similar fashion.[39, 40] That indicates that while vagolytic activity (and tachycardia) can occur, the dose of pancuronium required to achieve a substantial neuromuscular blockade may *not necessarily* produce tachycardia (at least in the cat). Clinical onditions would confirm that blockade and tachycardia do not necessarily have to occur simultaneously.

Miller and co-workers have described tachycardia at even low doses of pancuronium in adult patients.[41] They could not demonstrate a dose-related effect on heart rate (Fig. 10-4). However, the smallest dose used (1.2 mg/m^2 or about 2.25 mg in an average adult) is not the smallest dose often used clinically. In addition, rate of administration was not evaluated, nor precisely controlled. Many clinicians have noted that very slow administration of pancuronium can achieve neuromuscular blockade without measurable effects on heart rate, or other cardiovascular variables. This relationship deserves further attention.

Miller found that the tachycardia from pancuronium was independent of alveolar halothane concentration (Fig. 10-5) and dependent upon control heart rate as previously discussed (Fig. 10-1).[41] There were no significant changes in systolic blood pressure at any halothane concentration or at any dose of pancuronium.

Other reports of the response of the systemic vasculature to pancuronium are variable. Referring again to Figure 10-3B, an absence of sympathetic ganglionic blockade with pancuronium is noted. Thus one could expect no direct change in systemic vascular resistance. In the absence of major changes in cardiac output, no blood pressure changes would be predicted. Yet investigators have demonstrated increases in cardiac output, blood pressure, and heart rate in healthy patients.[42] Stanley has shown a decrease in systemic vascular resistance from pancuronium during meperidine anesthesia (by reflex?) in patients without cardiovascular disease.[43] Stoelting found no change in systemic vascular resistance, but an increase in cardiac

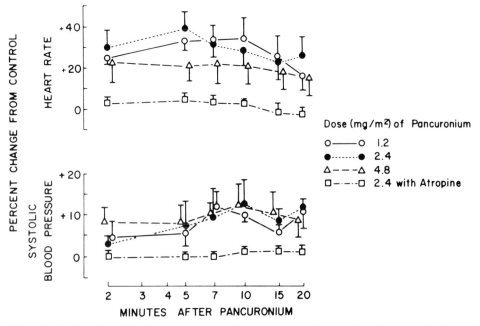

Fig. 10–4. **Relationship between percentage increase in heart rate, systolic blood pressure, and time after pancuronium (1.2, 2.4, or 4.8 mg/m²) administration.** One group of patients received 0.33 mg/m² atropine before pancuronium administration. Each symbol represents the mean ± 1 SE for five patients. No pancuronium dose-response relationship is seen. (Miller RD, Eger EI II, Stevens WC: Anesthesiology 42:352–355, 1975)

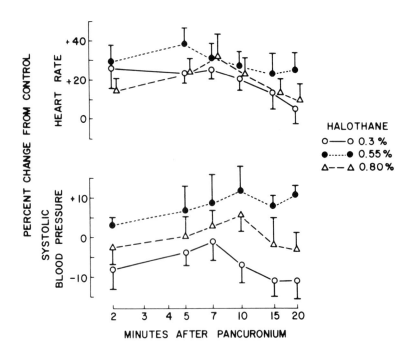

Fig. 10–5. Relationship between percentage increase in heart rate, systolic blood pressure, and time after pancuronium (2.4 mg/m²) administration during three alveolar concentrations of halothane and 60% N₂O. Each symbol represents the mean ±1 SE for five patients. No relationship is seen. (Miller RD, Eger EI II, Stevens WC: Anesthesiology 42:352–355, 1975)

output, heart rate, and mean arterial blood pressure.[44] The usual response, if one is provoked, is an increase in heart rate, cardiac output, and blood pressure.

Arrhythmias are seen often following pancuronium, especially atrial and junctional tachycardia, ventricular extrasystoles, and A-V dissociation. Arrhythmias appear to be more common during halothane anesthesia than during N_2O-barbiturate anesthesia, and probably are related to the vagolytic properties of the relaxant. Whether pancuronium directly alters cardiac muscle cells is unclear. It is possible that it exerts effects on calcium, potassium, or sodium ion membrane fluxes. Despite occasional case reports implying otherwise,[45] pancuronium appears not to release histamine;[46] or if it does, it is very uncommon. It appears as though the stimulating properties of pancuronium would serve to attenuate the circulatory depressant effects of depressive anesthetic agents, if that is the clinician's goal. The hemodynamic effects of pancuronium are summarized in Table 10-3.

As shown in Table 10-1, those patients classified as at risk from tachycardia or hypertension should receive pancuronium at the lowest dose and slowest administration rate as possible, if at all. Alternatives, such as metocurine, may be preferable to pancuronium in some patients, such as those with coronary artery disease, idioathic hypertrophic subaortic stenosis (IHSS), mitral stenosis, or aortic stenosis.

d-Tubocurarine

The most common cardiovascular response seen after administration of d-tubocurarine (dTc) is hypotension. Referring again to one of the cumulative dose-response curves (see Fig. 10-3C), one sees that dTc produces, in cats, *all three* responses at approximately the same dose. That is, neuromuscular blockade occurs hand-in-hand with vagolytic activity and is followed closely by sympathetic ganglionic blockade.[47] Thus tachycardia and decreased systemic vascular resistance (and

Table 10-3. Pancuronium Hemodynamic Effects

Increases A-V conduction
Catecholamine release?
Increases myocardial O_2 demand*
Tachycardia
Hypertension
Cardiac output ↑
Increases myocardial O_2 supply*
Increases diastolic pressure
Increases coronary perfusion pressure?

*Increases in oxygen demand exceed increases in oxygen supply.

possibly hypotension) will occur quite routinely with dTc. These investigative findings confirm clinical impressions.

The degree of hypotension is directly related to the dose of dTc (Fig. 10-6) and to the alveolar concentration of halothane (Fig. 10-7)[48] and is augmented by nitrous oxide. While early reports of myocardial depression from dTc implied cardiac depression from the drug preservatives, this phenomenon has been disproven by Stoelting[49] and by Munger.[48] Doses as large as 18 mg/m² dTc do not depress myocardial function in patients, provided the alveolar halothane concentration is 0.5 percent or less (Fig. 10-6 and 10-7; no change in $1/PEP^2$, a measure of contractility).

Hypotension appears to be related both to a decrease in systemic vascular resistance (see ganglionic blockade in Fig. 10-3C), and to histamine release (Table 10-4).[47, 50] Spontaneous postganglionic sympathetic activity is also reduced.[47] Arrhythmias are uncommon following dTc administration to patients.

Thus, the clinical consequences of increased heart rate and decreased systemic vascular resistance really depend upon the patient's ventricular function and intravascular volume. The hypovolemic patient or the patient who cannot increase cardiac output will become hypotensive. The patient with an increased vascular volume or with good ventricular function may be able to increase cardiac output to compensate for the decrease in systemic resistance, thus avoiding hypotension. In conditions where controlled

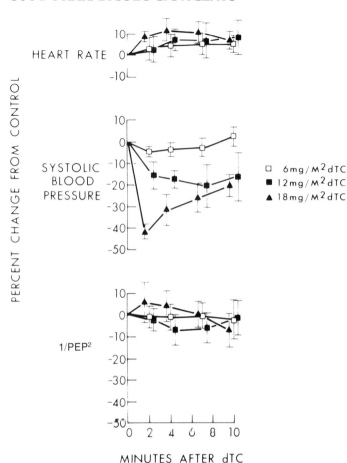

Fig. 10–6. **Effects of three bolus doses d-tubocurarine (dTc) on heart rate, systolic blood pressure, and pre-ejection period (1/PEP²),** **during 0.5% halothane anesthesia with 60% N₂O.** Mean ± 1 SE; five patients each dose. Heart rate and contractility (1/PEP²) are unchanged. Decrease in blood pressure is dose related. (Munger WL, Miller RD, Stevens WC: Anesthesiology 40:442–448, 1974)

hypotension is desirable, dTc can be used as the relaxant of choice to augment the hypotensive effects of other drugs.

Metocurine

Metocurine iodide, formerly known as dimethyltubocurarine (Metubine) has been known to anesthesiologists for over forty years. Overshadowed by dTc, it is now enjoying a clinical revival. The principal reason for the revival in the United States is the desire to utilize a nondepolarizing relaxant with as few side-effects, especially cardiovascular side-effects, as possible. With newly synthesized relaxants not approved at present for clinical use, metocurine appears to have a solid place for the next several years.

McCullough demonstrated cardiovascular stability and lack of histamine release from metocurine 0.4 mg/kg IV in cats.[51] Hughes has confirmed these findings (see Fig. 10-3D) in work in which the entire neuromuscular dose-response curve can be produced without evidence of vagolytic activity or ganglionic blockade.[52] Thus, in essence, a pure neuromuscular response appears to be present.

In patients, while stability appears quite genuine,[53] all is not that pure. Stoelting reported an overall stability in healthy patients, yet some of his patients developed clinical hypotension from metocurine 0.2 mg/kg.[54] In patients with coronary artery disease, Zaidan has shown a slight increase in cardiac output and slight decrease in systemic vascular resistance from metocurine 0.35 mg/kg.[55] He postulates that these effects are secondary to histamine release, yet no investigator has verified increased histamine levels in pa-

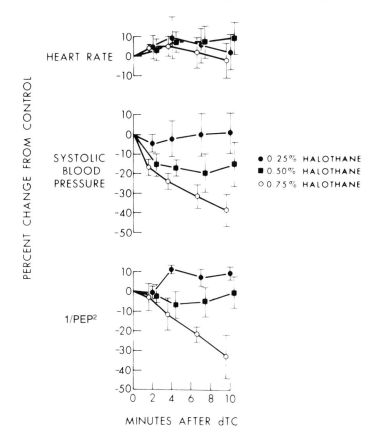

Fig. 10–7. Effects of alveolar halothane concentration on heart rate, systolic blood pressure, and pre-ejection period (1/PEP²), following d-tubocurarine, 12 mg/m², as a bolus. Mean ± 1 SE; five patients at each concentration. All patients received 60% N_2O. Heart rate is unchanged, blood pressure decreased at the highest halothane concentration, and contractility (1/PEP²) unchanged except at the highest halothane concentration. (Munger WL, Miller RD, Stevens WC: Anesthesiology 40:442–448, 1974)

● 0.25% HALOTHANE
■ 0.50% HALOTHANE
○ 0.75% HALOTHANE

Table 10-4. d-Tubocurarine Hemodynamic Effects

Hypotension		
Ganglionic blockade	→	↓ Systemic vascular resistance
Histamine release		↓ Venous tone
Tachycardia		

tients. Savarese states that approximately one-third of patients receiving metocurine 0.4 mg/kg demonstrate clinical evidence of histamine release.[56] At Stanford we have found clinical signs of histamine release to be present in less than 10 percent of patients receiving that dose. Other factors, such as anesthetic drug background, may explain these differences. Arrhythmias are uncommon following metocurine.

We have found no effect of metocurine on the arterial vasculature of morphine-anesthetized patients at doses of less than 0.70 mg/kg IV, doses much higher than are used clinically under normal circumstances (Fig. 10-

8).[57] Under the same conditions, metocurine produces an apparent venodilation, as measured by loss of return to an oxygenator reservoir of venous blood, during total cardiopulmonary bypass (Fig. 10-9).[57] In this instance, both dTc and metocurine produce a reduction in blood volume returning to the oxygenator, at a time when mean arterial pressure is unchanged by metocurine. Metocurine would appear to have venodilating properties under these conditions, but without effect on the arterial vasculature.

It appears that of the four nondepolarizing relaxants herein discussed, metocurine has the least effect upon the circulatory system

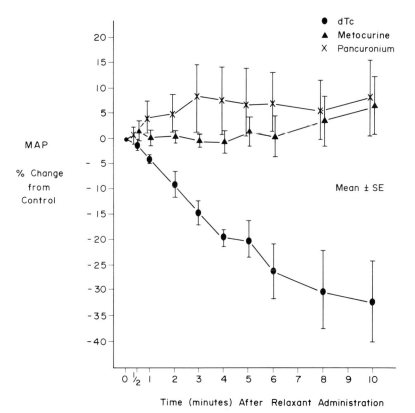

Fig. 10–8. Effect on mean arterial pressure (MAP) of d-tubocurarine (dTc), 0.5 mg/kg; metocurine, 0.35 mg/kg; and pancuronium, 0.1 mg/kg, during fixed cardiac output in patients on total cardiopulmonary bypass. (Equipotent doses for neuromuscular blockade). Both metocurine and pancuronium show no change in MAP, while dTc produces hypotension as expected. (Fogdall RP, DeMaster RJ: Abstracts of Scientific Papers. ASA Annual Meeting, 315–316, 1977)

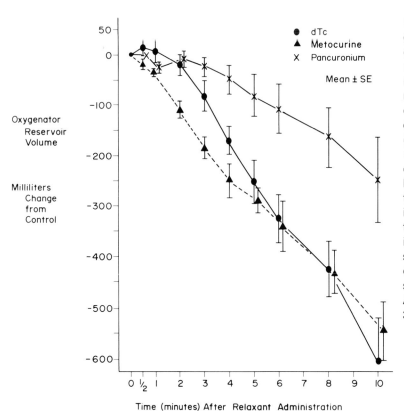

Fig. 10–9. Effect on oxygenator reservoir volume of d-tubocurarine (dTc), 0.5 mg/kg; metocurine, 0.35 mg/kg; or pancuronium 0.1 mg/kg, during fixed cardiac output in patients on total cardiopulmonary bypass. (Equipotent doses for neuromuscular blockade). Loss of reservoir volume occurs because blood is not returned to the reservoir and is being held within the patient. With metocurine (during stable MAP) this would suggest venodilation. (Fogdall RP, DeMaster RJ: Abstracts of Scientific Papers. ASA Annual Meeting, 315–316, 1977)

of humans (Table 10-5). At Stanford, we use it when we wish to avoid the tachycardia (and/or hypertension) from gallamine and pancuronium, or the hypotensive effects of d-tubocurarine. There is still a void of information regarding metocurine's hemodynamic effects in specific patient groups under specific conditions: What are the interactions with inhalation anesthetic agents or with catecholamines such as dopamine or isoproterenol? How should it be used in patients with renal insufficiency[58]? Should it be used, and if so how, in patients with "iodide sensitivity"? Does it indeed release histamine or vasoactive polypeptides, and in whom, under what conditions? There is much to learn about this useful relaxant.

Nondepolarizing muscle relaxants can potentiate each other. Pancuronium-metocurine and pancuronium-dTc have been shown to produce greater than additive neuromuscular blockade (intensity). A metocurine-dTc combination did not have this effect. The duration of blockade was not prolonged longer than expected by additive effect.[59]

INVESTIGATIONAL MUSCLE RELAXANTS

Why New Relaxants?

New muscle relaxants are on the horizon. Some presently are in use in patients in Eu-

Table 10-5. Metocurine Hemodynamic Effects

Histamine release	
Cats:	No
Humans:	Perhaps?
Ganglionic blockade?	
Cats:	No
Humans:	Doubtful
Vagolytic?	No
Vasopressive?	No
A-V conduction changes?	Doubtful

ropean countries, others are in various stages of development. Savarese and Kitz suggested that new neuromuscular blocking agents would be desirable and used in clinical settings.[60] At present, there is no ideal muscle relaxant, devoid of any effects other than pure neuromuscular blockade. Metocurine is the cleanest of the relaxants presently available in the United States.

Savarese and Kitz believe that the ideal relaxant should have a "brief, noncumulative, nondepolarizing neuromuscular blocking action, with rapid onset and recovery," readily reversible, and should lack clinically important hemodynamic side effects.[60] Development of such a drug has been slowed by species differences as demonstrated in Figure 10-10. Species differences between cats and monkeys also is demonstrated by Hughes.[61] In one species, neuromuscular effects may be

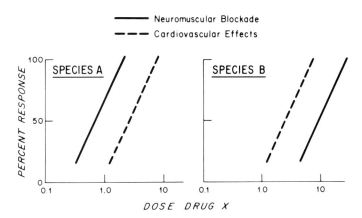

—— Neuromuscular Blockade
--- Cardiovascular Effects

Fig. 10–10. Example of a species difference in relative sensitivities to the neuromuscular and cardiovascular effects of a hypothetical quaternary ammonium compound, Drug X, which has qualitatively similar cardiovascular effects in species *A* and species *B*. In the former, complete neuromuscular blockade is produced by Drug X before any important cardiovascular effect becomes evident. In the latter, the opposite is true. Drug *X* is therefore safe in species *A* but disadvantageous and possibly dangerous in species *B*. (Savarese JJ, Kitz RJ: Anesthesiology 42:236–239, 1975)

A. Short-acting non-depolarizing agent

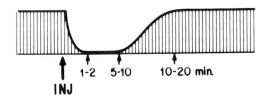

B. Intermediate-duration noncumulative non-depolarizing agent

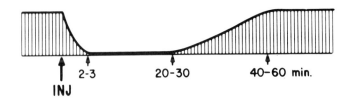

C. Long-duration non-depolarizing agent devoid of cardiovascular side effects

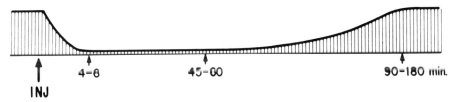

Fig 10–11. Three new nondepolarizing neuromuscular blocking agents for use in clinical anesthesia. *A, B,* and *C* represent hypothetical adductor thumb-twitch tracings of the "typical" effect of each of these drugs in an average anesthetized patient. Numbers beneath tracings represent cumulative times from injection. For example, Drug A, a short-acting agent, would within 1–2 min produce complete paralysis lasting 5–10 min, complete recovery occurring within 10–20 min. Drug B, an intermediate-duration agent, would have a total duration of action approximately twice that of Drug A. Drugs A and B ideally would lack significant autonomic side-effects. Some clinically acceptable autonomic effect such as a mild vagolytic or ganglion-blocking effect resulting in slight tachycardia or hypotension, would not detract from the clinical usefulness of such drugs. Drug C would not offer any advantage over current agents in duration of action. A total lack of cardiovascular effect, even at fully paralyzing doses, might make Drug C the agent of choice for patients who have a variety of cardiovascular disorders. (Savarese JJ, Kitz RJ: Anesthesiology 42:236–239, 1975)

seen without cardiovascular effects, yet in another the dose required for neuromuscular blockade is higher than the dose producing cardiovascular effects. Thus, animal testing may or may not yield a clinically useful relaxant. The *ideal* spectrum of muscle relaxants would have available short, intermediate, and long duration relaxants, all without cardiovascular effects (see Fig. 10-11). If a short-acting drug without hemodynamic effects were available, especially if cumulative effects were absent, it might be a useful addition to the anesthesiologist's or intensivist's armamentarium.

AH 8165 and BW 403C65

Several years ago, AH 8165 received a flurry of attention. While initially the drug appeared short acting, in humans this proved not to be so. In addition, it possessed strong vagolytic activity, even at small doses, producing tachycardia.[62] Another drug, BW 403C65, demonstrated no hemodynamic effects in dogs, but produced vagolytic activity in cats, and tachycardia and hypertension in humans.[63]

Organon NC 45

Organon NC 45 (Org NC 45) appears to be a short-acting (Fig. 10-12),[64] noncumulative (Fig. 10-13),[65] nondepolarizing muscle relaxant in humans. It is antagonized readily by neostigmine, pyridostigmine, and 4-amino-pyridine.[66] In comparison to pancuronium, d-tubocurarine, and metocurine, it produces no hemodynamic alterations in animals.[67–69] Its comparative effects on left-heart filling pressure, systemic vascular resistance, mean arterial pressure, heart rate, and cardiac output are demonstrated in Figures 10-14 to 10-18. At the time of this manuscript's submis-

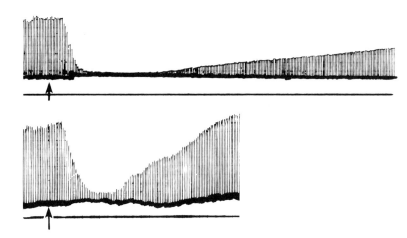

Fig. 10–12. **A.** 94% neuromuscular blockade produced by pancuronium 0.04 mg/kg. **B.** 91% neuromuscular blockade produced by organon NC 45 (Org NC 45) 0.03 mg/kg. (Different patients). Note the shorter duration of action of Org NC 45. (Baird WLM, Herd D: Br J Anaesth 52:61S–69S, 1980.)

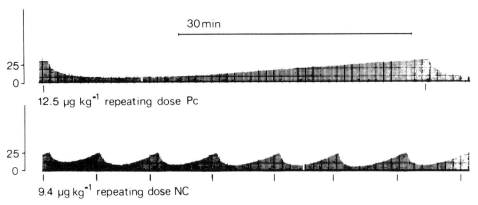

Fig. 10–13. **Time-course of action of first and maintenance doses of pancuronium (Pc) and Org NC 45 (NC) on the ulnar nerve adductor pollicis muscle in humans.** Doses chosen closely imitate the way in which muscle relaxation is maintained in humans. Note also the absence of cumulative effects of Org NC 45 with multiple injections. (Crul JF, Booij LHDJ: Br J Anaesth 52:49S–52S, 1980)

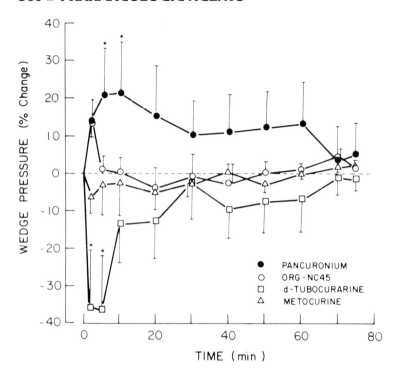

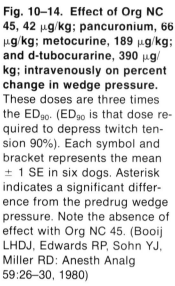

Fig. 10–14. Effect of Org NC 45, 42 μg/kg; pancuronium, 66 μg/kg; metocurine, 189 μg/kg; and d-tubocurarine, 390 μg/kg; intravenously on percent change in wedge pressure. These doses are three times the ED_{90}. (ED_{90} is that dose required to depress twitch tension 90%). Each symbol and bracket represents the mean $\pm$ 1 SE in six dogs. Asterisk indicates a significant difference from the predrug wedge pressure. Note the absence of effect with Org NC 45. (Booij LHDJ, Edwards RP, Sohn YJ, Miller RD: Anesth Analg 59:26–30, 1980)

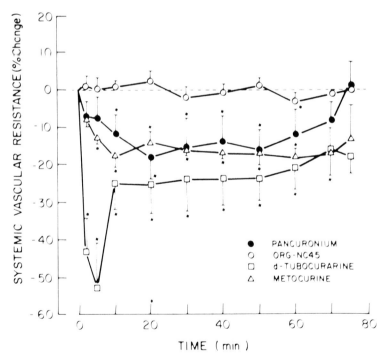

Fig. 10–15. Effect of Org NC 45, 42 μg/kg; pancuronium, 66 μg/kg; metocurine, 189 μg/kg; and d-tubocurarine, 390 μg/kg; intravenously on percent change in systemic vascular resistance. These doses are three times the ED_{90}. Each symbol and bracket represents the mean $\pm$ 1 SE in six dogs. Asterisk indicates a significant difference from the predrug systemic vascular resistance. Note the absence of effect with Org NC 45. (Booij LHDJ, Edwards RP, Sohn YJ, Miller RD: Anesth Analg 59:26–30, 1980)

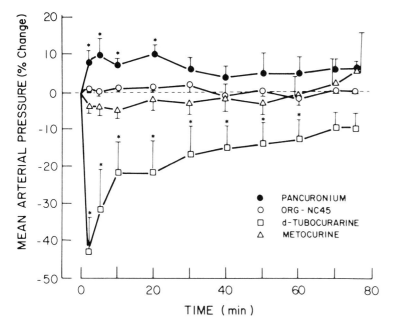

Fig. 10–16. Effect of Org NC 45, 42 μg/kg; pancuronium, 66 μg/kg; metocurine, 189 μg/kg; and d-tubocurarine, 390 μg/ kg; intravenously on percent change in mean arterial blood pressure. These doses are three times the ED_{90}. Each symbol and bracket represents the mean $\pm$ 1 SE in six dogs. Asterisk indicates a significant difference from the predrug mean arterial blood pressure. Note the absence of effect with Org NC 45. (Booij LHDJ, Edwards RP, Sohn YJ, Miller RD: Anesth Analg 59:26–30, 1980)

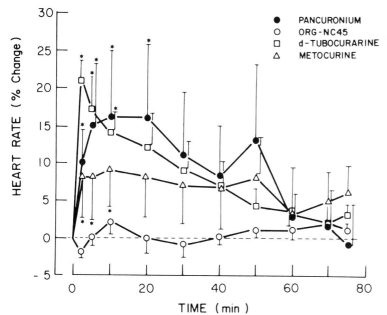

Fig. 10–17. Effect of Org NC 45, 42 μg/kg; pancuronium, 66 μg/kg; metocurine, 189 μg/kg; and d-tubocurarine, 390 μg/ kg; intravenously on percent change in heart rate. These doses are three times the ED_{90}. Each symbol and bracket represents the mean $\pm$ 1 SE in six dogs. Asterisk indicates a significant difference from the predrug heart rate. Note the absence of effect with Org NC 45. (Booij LHDJ, Edwards RP, Sohn YJ, Miller RD: Anesth Analg 59:26–30, 1980)

sion, it is undergoing clinical trials in the United States. If these investigations confirm a lack of hemodynamic effects, Org NC 45 may be in clinical practice within several years. If so, its availability for use in the care of the patient with severe cardiovascular disease will be most welcome.

RELAXANT ANTAGONISTS

BASIC PHARMACOLOGY

The termination of a nondepolarizing muscle relaxant's effects may occur slowly, by natural competitive inhibition between ACh and

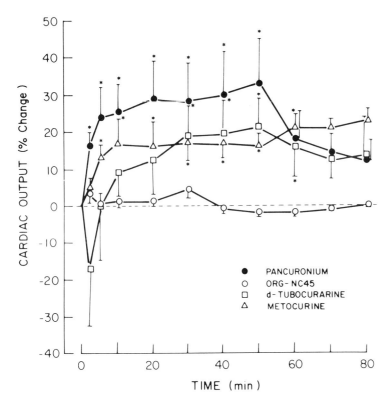

Fig. 10–18. Effect of Org NC 45, 42 μg/kg; pancuronium, 66 μg/kg; metocurine, 189 μg/kg; and d-tubocurarine, 390 μg/kg; intravenously on percent change in cardiac output. These doses are three times the ED_{90}. Each symbol and bracket represents the mean $\pm$ 1 SE in six dogs. Asterisk indicates a significant difference from the predrug cardiac output. Note the absence of effect with Org NC 45. (Booij LHDJ, Edwards RP, Sohn YJ, Miller RD: Anesth Analg 59:26–30, 1980)

the relaxant, or in augmented fashion by increasing the concentration of ACh at the neuromuscular junction with drugs. This increase in ACh concentration may be produced by either increasing ACh production or release, or decreasing ACh destruction (anticholinesterase drugs), or both.

ANTICHOLINESTERASE DRUGS

Neostigmine and pyridostigmine produce an increase in ACh concentration by inhibiting the destruction of ACh by acetylcholinesterase. The resultant increase in ACh concentration at the nicotine receptor is responsible for antagonism of the neuromuscular effects of the relaxant, and thus a return to normal neuromuscular function. The increase in ACh concentration at the muscarinic receptor is responsible for an increase in apparent vagal activity (bradycardia), salivation, and increased gastrointestinal motility. In the dosage required for return to normal of sub-stantial neuromuscular paralysis, both neostigmine and pyridostigmine, given alone, produce profound bradycardia.[70] Used in equipotent dosage (5.5:1) pyridostigmine and neostigmine produce identical effects on heart rate.[70] Edrophonium, effective in large doses, has not received sufficient hemodynamic investigation.[71–73]

4-AMINOPYRIDINE

4-Aminopyridine is an investigational drug producing antagonism of neuromuscular blockade from nondepolarizing muscle relaxants. It acts by facilitating the release of ACh from the nerve terminal, not by affecting acetylcholinesterase. It potentiates neostigmine and pyridostigmine in humans. In animals, it appears free of muscarinic side effects, and may stimulate the sympathetic nervous system. Central nervous system stimulation occurs, which may limit its use in humans. The drug is reviewed by Miller and co-workers.[74]

ADJUVANTS

Because of these undesirable hemodynamic and alimentary effects, a drug such as atropine or glycopyrrolate may be required to counteract the effects of increased ACh concentration at the muscarinic receptor. If a standard clinical dosage of neostigmine (2.5 mg) or equipotent pyridostigmine (14.5 mg) is administered with atropine 0.3 mg, bradycardia ensues with either antagonist (Fig. 10-19).[75] If atropine 1.0 mg is used, initial tachycardia is seen, followed by return to baseline heart rate within approximately 6 minutes (Fig. 10-20).

Glycopyrrolate also can protect against the bradycardia and salivation from neostigmine or pyridostigmine. Its effects on heart rate,

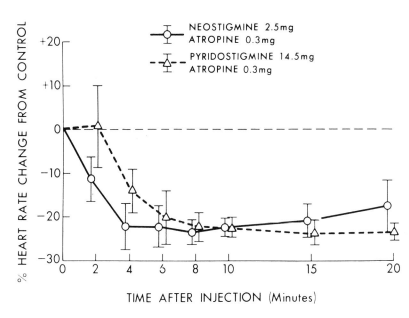

Fig. 10–19. The administration of 0.3 mg atropine with either 2.5 mg neostigmine or equipotent pyridostigmine (14.5 mg) yields identical results on heart rate in anesthetized patients. Moderate bradycardia develops promptly. Mean ± 1 SE. (Fogdall RP, Miller RD: Anesthesiology 39:504–509, 1973)

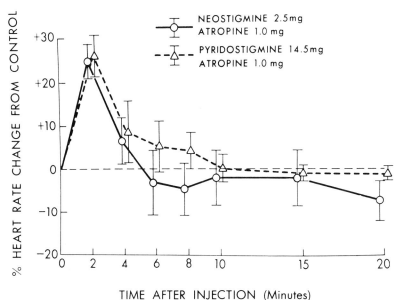

Fig. 10–20. The administration of 1.0 mg atropine with either 2.5 mg neostigmine or equipotent pyridostigmine(14.5 mg) yields identical results on heart rate in anesthetized patients. Initial tachycardia is followed by a return to baseline heart rate within 6 min. (Fogdall RP, Miller RD: Anesthesiology 39: 504–509, 1973)

when administered with identical doses of neostigmine to patients, are dose related.[76] It is an excellent antisialogogue, without central nervous system effects (it does not cross the blood-brain barrier). Clinical dose is approximately 0.20 mg glycopyrrolate per each one mg of neostigmine or per each 5.0 mg of pyridostigmine.

SUMMARY

In choosing a relaxant in a specific patient at a given time, the physiologic processes presently occurring in that patient must be evaluated thoroughly. The hemodynamic changes which would be beneficial or harmful in *that patient at that time* must be foreseen. The relaxant to be administered then can be chosen on the basis of the circulatory effect(s) desired, the duration of action required, and the renal status required for excretion. Slow titration to effect will allow the production of the desired amount of neuromuscular blockade, while minimizing hemodynamic side effects. With appropriate hemodynamic and neuromuscular monitoring, safe relaxant administration is achievable.

REFERENCES*

MUSCLE RELAXANTS

1. Betcher AM: The civilizing of curare: a history of its development and introduction into anesthesiology. Anesth Analg (Cleve) 56:305–319, 1977
2. Mainzer J Jr: Muscle Relaxants and Problems of Surgical Awareness. Anesthesiology Review 8:30–33, 1980
3. Miller RD, Eger EI II, Stevens WC et al: Pancuronium-induced tachycardia in relation to alveolar halothane, dose of pancuronium, and prior atropine. Anesthesiology 42:352–355, 1975
4. Gronert GA, Theye RA: Effect of succinylcho-line on skeletal muscle with immobilization atrophy. Anesthesiology 40:268–271, 1974
5. Wong AL, Brodsky JB: Asystole in an adult after a single dose of succinylcholine. Anesth Analg (Cleve) 57:135–136, 1978
6. Katz RL (ed): Muscle relaxants. Monographs in Anaesthesiology, volume 3. Amsterdam, Exerpta Medica, 1975
7. Ali HH, Savarese JJ: Monitoring of neuromuscular function. Anesthesiology 45:216–249, 1976
8. Donlon JV Jr, Savarese JJ, Ali HH et al: Human dose-response curves for neuromuscular blocking drugs: a comparison of two methods of construction and analysis. Anesthesiology 53:161–166, 1980
9. Crumrine RS, Yodlowski EH: Assessment of neuromuscular function in infants. Anesthesiology 54:29–32, 1981

Pharmacological and Physiological Considerations

10. Katz RL (ed): Muscle relaxants. Monographs in Anaesthesiology, volume 3. Amsterdam, Exerpta Medica, 1975
11. Stanski DR, Sheiner LB: Pharmacokinetics and dynamics of muscle relaxants. Anesthesiology 51:103–105, 1979
12. Brotherton WP, Matteo RS: Pharmacokinetics and pharmacodynamics of metocurine in humans with and without renal failure. Anesthesiology 55:273–276, 1981
13. Waud BE, Waud DR: The effects of diethyl ether, enflurane, and isoflurane at the neuromuscular junction. Anesthesiology 42:275–280, 1975
14. Stoelting RK: Hemodynamic effects of gallamine during halothane-nitrous oxide anesthesia. Anesthesiology 39:645–647, 1973
15. Grossman E, Jacobi A, McNeil A: Hemodynamic interaction between pancuronium and morphine. Anesthesiology 40:299–301, 1974
16. Miller RD, Eger EI II, Stevens WC et al: Pancuronium-induced tachycardia in relation to alveolar halothane, dose of pancuronium, and prior atropine. Anesthesiology 42:352–355, 1975
17. Geha DG, Rozelle BC, Raessler KL et al: Pancuronium bromide enhances atrioventricular conduction in halothane-anesthetized dogs. Anesthesiology 46:342–345, 1977
18. Stanley TH, Liu WS: Cardiovascular effects of meperidine-N_2O anesthesia before and after

*These references have been distilled from a collection of over 500 references. They represent those references thought most appropriate for the clinician.

pancuronium. Anesth Analg (Cleve) 56:669–673, 1977

19. Edwards RP, Miller RD, Roizen MF et al: Cardiac responses to imipramine and pancuronium during anesthesia with halothane or enflurane. Anesthesiology 50:421–425, 1979

20. Munger WL, Miller RD, Stevens WC: The dependence of d-tubocurarine-induced hypotension on alveolar concentration of halothane, dose of d-tubocurarine, and nitrous oxide. Anesthesiology 40:442–448, 1974

21. Savarese JJ: How may neuromuscular blocking drugs affect the state of general anesthesia? Anesth Analg (Cleve) 58:449–451, 1979

Investigation of Relaxant Circulation Effects

22. Donlon JV Jr, Savarese JJ, Ali HH et al: Human dose-response curves for neuromuscular blocking drugs: a comparison of two methods of construction and analysis. Anesthesiology 53:161–166, 1980

23. Ali HH, Savarese JJ: Stimulus frequency and dose-response curves to d-tubocurarine in man. Anesthesiology 52:36–39, 1980

24. Donlon JV Jr, Ali HH, Savarese JJ: A new approach to the study of four nondepolarizing relaxants in man. Anesth Analg (Cleve) 53:934–939, 1974

25. Fogdall RP, DeMaster RJ: Comparative effects of metocurine, d-tubocurarine, and pancuronium on the peripheral circulation during cardiopulmonary bypass (abstr), pp 315–316. New Orleans, ASA Annual Meeting, 1977

26. Fogdall RP, Miller RD: Antagonism of d-tubocurarine and pancuronium-induced neuromuscular blockade by pyridostigmine in man. Anesthesiology 39:504–509, 1973

27. Hughes R, Chapple DJ: Effects of nondepolarizing neuromuscular blocking agents on peripheral autonomic mechanisms in cats. Br J Anesth 48:59–68, 1976

Depolarizing Relaxants

28. Leigh MD, McCoy DD, Belton MK et al: Bradycardia following intravenous administration of succinylcholine chloride to infants and children. Anesthesiology 18:698–702, 1957

29. Craythorne NWB, Turndorf H, Dripps RD: Changes in pulse rate and rhythm associated with the use of succinylcholine in anesthetized children. Anesthesiology 21:465–470, 1960

30. Williams CH, Deutsch S, Linde HW et al: Effects of intravenously administered succinyldicholine on cardiac rate, rhythm, and arterial blood pressure in anesthetized man. Anesthesiology 22:947–954, 1961

31. Williams RT, Gain EA: Electrocardiographic changes following repeated injections of decamethonium and subsequent injections of succinylcholine. Can Anaesth Soc J 9:263–269, 1962

32. Wong AL, Brodsky JB: Asystole in an adult after a single dose of succinylcholine. Anesth Analg (Cleve) 57:135–136, 1978

33. Wong KC, Wyte SR, Martin WE et al: Antiarrhythmic effects of skeletal muscle relaxants. Anesthesiology 34:458–462, 1971

34. Tucker WK, Munson ES: Effects of succinylcholine and d-tubocurarine on epinephrine-induced arrhythmias during halothane anesthesia in dogs. Anesthesiology 42:41–44, 1975

35. Katz RL (ed): Muscle relaxants. Monographs in Anaesthesiology, volume 3. Amsterdam, Exerpta Medica, 1975

Non-depolarizing Relaxants

Gallamine

36. Hughes R, Chapple DJ: Effects of nondepolarizing neuromuscular blocking agents on peripheral autonomic mechanisms in cats. Br J Anesth 48:59–68, 1976

37. Eisele JH, Marta JA, Davis HS: Quantitative aspects of the chronotropic and neuromuscular effects of gallamine in anesthetized man. Anesthesiology 35:630–633, 1971

38. Longnecker DE, Stoelting RK, Morrow AG: Cardiac and peripheral vascular effects of gallamine in man. Anesth Analg 52:931–935, 1973

Pancuronium

39. Hughes R, Chapple DJ: Effects of nondepolarizing neuromuscular blocking agents on peripheral autonomic mechanisms in cats. Br J Anesth 48:59–68, 1976

40. Kennedy BR, Kelman GR: Cardiovascular effects of alcuronium in man. Br J Anesth 42:625–630, 1970

41. Miller RD, Eger EI II, Stevens WC et al: Pancuronium-induced tachycardia in relation to alveolar halothane, dose of pancuronium, and

prior atropine. Anesthesiology 42:352–355, 1975

42. Kelman GR, Kennedy BR: Cardiovascular effects of pancuronium in man. Br J Anesth 43:335–338, 1971

43. Stanley TH, Liu WS: Cardiovascular effects of meperidine-N_2O anesthesia before and after pancuronium. Anesth Analg (Cleve) 56:669–673, 1977

44. Stoetling RK: The hemodynamic effects of pancuronium and d-tubocurarine in anesthetized patients. Anesthesiology 36:612–615, 1972

45. Buckland RW, Avery AF: Histamine release following pancuronium: a case report. Br J Anesth 45:518–521, 1973

46. Dobkin AB, Arandia HY, Levy AA: Effect of pancuronium bromide on plasma histamine levels in man. Anesth Analg (Cleve) 52:772–775, 1973

d-Tubocurarine

47. Hughes R, Chapple DJ: Effects of nondepolarizing neuromuscular blocking agents on peripheral autonomic mechanisms in cats. Br J Anesth 48:59–68, 1976

48. Munger WL, Miller RD, Stevens WC: The dependence of d-tubocurarine induced hypotension on alveolar concentration of halothane, dose of d-tubocurarine, and nitrous oxide. Anesthesiology 40:442–448, 1974

49. Stoetling RK: Blood-pressure response to D-tubocurarine and its preservatives in anesthetized patients. Anesthesiology 35:315–317, 1971

50. Moss J, Rosow CE, Savarese JJ et al: Role of histamine in the hypotensive action of d-tubocurarine in humans. Anesthesiology 55:19–25, 1981

Metocurine

51. McCullough LS, Stone WA, Delaunois AL et al: The effect of dimethyl tubocurarine iodide on cardiovascular parameters, postganglionic sympathetic activity, and histamine release. Anesth Analg (Cleve) 51:554–559, 1972

52. Hughes R, Chapple DJ: Effects of nondepolarizing neuromuscular blocking agents on peripheral autonomic mechanisms in cats. Br J Anesth 48:59–68, 1976

53. Hughes R, Ingram GS, Payne JP: Studies on dimethyl tubocurarine in anaesthetized man. Br J Anesth 48:969–974, 1976

54. Stoetling RK: Hemodynamic effects of dimethyltubocurarine during nitrous oxide-halothane anesthesia. Anesth Analg (Cleve) 53:513 515, 1974

55. Zaiden J, Philbin, Antonio R et al: Hemodynamic effects of metocurine in patients with coronary artery disease receiving propranolol. Anesth Analg (Cleve) 56:255–259, 1977

56. Savarese JJ, Ali HH, Antonio RP: The clinical pharmacology of metocurine: dimethyltubocurarine revisited. Anesthesiology 47:277–284, 1977

57. Fogdall RP, DeMaster RJ: Comparative effects of metocurine, d-tubocurarine, and pancuronium on the peripheral circulation during cardiopulmonary bypass (abstr), pp 315–316. New Orleans, ASA Annual Meeting, 1977

58. Brotherton WP, Matteo RS: Pharmacokinetics and pharmacodynamics of metocurine in humans with and without renal failure. Anesthesiology 55:273–276, 1981

59. Lebowitz PW, Ramsey FM, Savarese JJ et al: Potentiation of neuromuscular blockade in man produced by combinations of pancuronium and metocurine or pancuronium and d-tubocurarine. Anesth Analg (Cleve) 59:604 609, 1980

Investigational Muscle Relaxants

60. Savarese JJ, Kitz RJ: Does clinical anesthesia need new neuromuscular blocking agents? Anesthesiology 42:236–239, 1975

61. Hughes R, Chapple DJ: Cardiovascular and neuromuscular effects of dimethyl tubocurarine in anesthetized cats and rhesus monkeys. Br J Anaesth 48:847–852, 1976

62. Coleman AJ, O'Brien JW, Downing JW et al: AH8165: A new nondepolarizing muscle relaxant. Anesthesia 28:262–267, 1973

63. Hughes R: Evaluation of the neuromuscular blocking properties and side effects of the two new isoquinolinium bisquaternary compounds (BW.252C64 and BW.403C65). Br J Anaesth 44:27–36, 1972

64. Baird WLM, Herd D: A new neuromuscular blocking drug, Org NC 45. Br J Anaesth 52:615–695, 1980

65. Crul JF, Booij LHDJ: First clinical experiences with Org NC 45. Br J Anaesth 52:49S–52S, 1980

66. Booij LHDJ, van der Pol F, Crul JF et al: Antagonism of Org NC 45 neuromuscular blockade by neostigmine, pyridostigmine, and 4-aminopyridine. Anesth Analg (Cleve), 59:31–34, 1980
67. Booij LHDJ, Edwards RP, Sohn YJ et al: Cardiovascular and neuromuscular effects of Org NC 45, pancuronium, metocurine, and D-tubocurarine in dogs. Anesth Analg (Cleve) 59:26–30, 1980
68. Marshall RJ, McGrath JC, Miller RD et al: Comparison of the cardiovascular actions of Org NC 45 with those produced by other nondepolarizing neuromuscular blocking agents in experimental animals. Br J Anaesth 52:21S–32S, 1980
69. Son SL, Waud BE, Waud DR: A comparison of the neuromuscular blocking and vagolytic effects of ORG NC45 and Pancuronium. Anesthesiology 55:12–18, 1981

RELAXANT ANTAGONISTS

70. Fogdall RP, Miller RD: Antagonism of d-tubocurarine and pancuronium-induced neuromuscular blockade by pyridostigmine in man. Anesthesiology 39:504–509, 1973

71. Ferguson A, Egerszegi P, Bevan DR: Neostigmine, pyridostigmine, and edrophonium as antagonists of pancuronium. Anesthesiology 53:390–394, 1980
72. Kopman AF: Edrophonium antagonism of pancuronium-induced neuromuscular blockade in man. Anesthesiology 51:139–142, 1979
73. Morris RB, Cronnelly R, Miller RD et al: Pharmacokinetics of edrophonium and neostigmine when antagonizing d-tubocurarine neuromuscular blockade in man. Anesthesiology 54:399–402, 1981
74. Miller RD, Booij LHDJ, Agoston S, et al: 4-Aminopyridine potentiates neostigmine and pyridostigmine in man. Anesthesiology 50:416–420, 1979

Adjuvants

75. Fogdall RP, Miller RD: Antagonism of d-tubocurarine and pancuronium-induced neuromuscular blockade by pyridostigmine in man. Anesthesiology 39:504–509, 1973
76. Ramamurthy S, Shaker MH, Winnie AP: Glycopyrrolate as a substitute for atropine in neostigmine reversal of muscle relaxant drugs. Can Anaesth Soc J 19:399–411, 1972

11

Inotropic Agonists and Antagonists

CHRIS H. KEHLER
RICHARD P. FOGDALL

ADRENERGIC FUNCTION

INTRODUCTION

Since the classic studies by Dale in 1906, the concept of receptor substances has helped us to understand the function of the sympathetic nervous system in health and disease.[1] Ahlquist studied various sympathomimetic agents and found that each agent had a different potency for each physiologic response observed.[2] On this basis, he proposed the existence of two main types of adrenergic receptor: the α- and the β-receptor. Observing the effects of β-receptor stimulation more closely, Lands and coworkers found that agents which were potent bronchodilators were also potent vasodilators.[3] They proposed that these agents act on β-2 receptors. In addition, they found that the agents with the greatest lipolytic activity gave the greatest stimulation of myocardial contractility. These, they proposed, act upon β1 receptors. More recently, the unique pattern of vasodilation produced by dopamine[4] and the ability to antagonize this with selective agents[5, 6] has led to the recognition of dopaminergic receptors.

With an understanding of the different adrenergic receptors, the clinician is able to use safely adrenergic agonists and antagonists in the treatment of patients with cardiovascular disease. The receptor concept allows us to envision the effect of various drugs and neurotransmitters at the cellular level.

A receptor is defined as a specific cellular structure that interacts with a specific agent or agents to produce a certain cellular response. Agents that produce this response are called agonists and agents that bind to the receptor but which do not produce the response are called antagonists. The adrenergic nervous system has a well-defined group of receptors, agonists, and antagonists.

The adrenergic receptors that have been identified are α, β1, β2, and dopaminergic.* In the cardiovascular system, stimulation of each of these receptors produces a different response (Table 11–1). Alpha1 receptor stim-

---

*A new subtype of α receptor has been identified recently, called the α2 receptor. It is a *presynaptic* autoregulatory receptor that *inhibits* norepinephrine release when *stimulated*, and *enhances* norepinephrine release when *blocked*. The α2 receptor is thought also to exist on the platelet surface. Some alpha agonist drugs may be more selective for α2 receptors (clonidine) than for α1 receptors; and antagonists more selective for α1 receptors (prazosin) than for α2 receptors. For purposes of discussion in this chapter, the term α receptor will refer to the standard postsynaptic α1 receptor. The reader is referred to Hoffman BB, Lefkowitz RJ: Alpha-adrenergic receptor subtypes. N Engl J Med 302:1390–1396, 1980, for further details regarding subdivision of alpha receptor function (Table 11–2.)

Table 11-1. Adrenergic Receptor Response

ORGAN	RECEPTOR*	BASIC RESPONSE
Heart	β1	↑ Heart rate ↑ Contractility ↑ A-V conduction
Bronchial wall	β2	Dilation
Blood vessels	β2	Dilation
Eye	α	Contraction of radial muscle
	β	Pupillary dilation
GI	α′β	↓ Motility
Renal	β Dopaminergic	Renin Release Vasodilation

*A new subtype of α receptor has been identified recently, called the α2 receptor. It is a *presynaptic* autoregulatory receptor which *inhibits* norepinephrine release when *stimulated*, and *enhances* norepinephrine release when *blocked*. For purposes of discussion here, the term alpha receptor refers to the standard postsynaptic alpha1 receptor. Hoffman BB, Lefkowitz RJ: Alpha-adrenergic receptor subtypes. N Engl J Med 302:1390–1396, 1980. (For further details regarding subdivision of α-receptor function, see Table 11-2.)

Table 11-2. Classification of α Adrenergic Receptor Agents

	α_1 POSTSYNAPTIC	α_2 PRESYNAPTIC
Agonists	Methoxamine Phenylephrine Norepinephrine Epinephrine Dopamine	Clonidine Norepinephrine Epinephrine
Antagonists	Phentolamine Prazosin Phenoxybenzamine Phenothiazine Butyrophenones	Phentolamine Yohimbine

(Modified from Maze M: Clinical implications of membrane receptor function in anesthesia. Anesthesiology 55:160–171, 1981

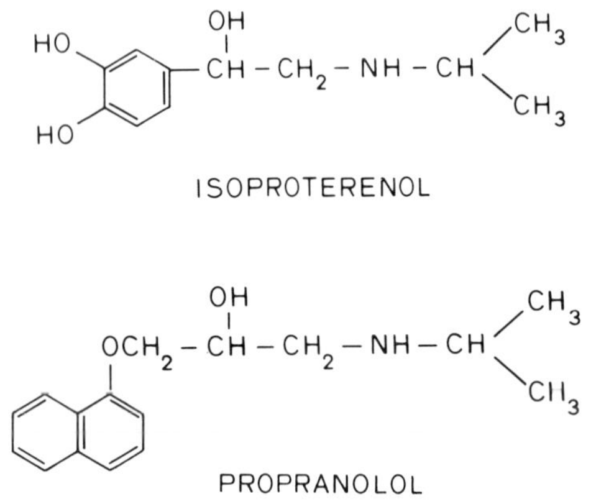

ISOPROTERENOL

PROPRANOLOL

Fig. 11–1. Comparison of the structures of isoproterenol and propranolol.

ulation produces vasoconstriction, β_1 receptor stimulation results in increased myocardial contractility and heart rate, β_2 receptor stimulation causes muscle and skin vasodilation, and dopaminergic stimulation produces renal and mesenteric vasodilation.

In discussing inotropic agonists the emphasis will be placed on the β_1 receptor. Many agonists have a spectrum of action on all the adrenergic receptors, depending on the individual patient and dosage of the agent. Dopamine is a good example of such an agent. Also, the physiologic effect of an agonist may be modified by the reflex cardiovascular responses to its primary action.

Later in this chapter, the β blocking agents will be discussed. As mentioned, these are drugs which have an affinity for the β receptor but produce no cellular response. These antagonists competitively inhibit the inotropic and chronotropic effects of β agonists. An agonist (isoproterenol) and an antagonist (propranolol) may have similar biochemical structures yet behave very differently (Fig. 11–1).

ADRENERGIC RECEPTOR PHYSIOLOGY

Since the discovery of cyclic-AMP (c-AMP) by Sutherland in 1957, a great deal of information has accumulated relating adrenergic receptor activation to the observed cellular response.[7] Two current reviews provide concise summaries of the available information.[8, 9] Tsien, in greater detail, relates the formation of c-AMP to myocardial contractility[10].

The agonist-receptor interaction is the first of many steps leading to a physiologic response (Fig. 11-2). The likelihood of myocardial β receptor activation will depend upon agonist concentration and affinity for the receptor. Once bound, the agonist must be able to initiate adenyl cyclase activity. Evidence exists to support the idea of an intermediate component that links the receptor, on the outer membrane surface, to adenyl cyclase, on the cytoplasmic surface of the membrane. The intermediate component is probably a membrane phospholipid.[11]

Activation of adenyl cyclase results in the conversion of ATP to c-AMP, in the presence of magnesium. Cyclic-AMP activates various intracellular protein kinases which lead to the phosphorylation of specific cellular proteins. This may lead to enhancement of a number of calcium-dependent processes which influence myocardial contraction and relaxation (see Fig. 11–2). The influence of c-AMP on calcium pumping by the sarcoplasmic reticulum and cell membrane is not clearly established. Also, the effect of c-AMP on calcium binding by troponin is still under investigation.

REGULATION OF ADRENERGIC RECEPTORS

Under normal circumstances, myocardial adrenergic activity is controlled by sensitive autonomic reflexes, as well as rapid uptake and metabolism of catecholamines at the sympathetic nerve endings. However, when the receptor is exposed to constant levels of agonist, other regulatory mechanisms occur. Initially, it was unclear whether the observed tachyphylaxis, with constant adrenergic stimulation, was the result of qualitative or quantitative receptor changes. With the relatively recent ability to label β receptors, using radioligands, it has been found that a definite decrease in receptor number occurs during constant exposure to a β agonist (Fig. 11–3). The time course of such desensitization is measured in minutes to hours.[12]

The reverse situation also applies. That is, chronic β blockade or catecholamine depletion results in an increased number of receptors.[12] This has been proposed as one of the mechanisms by which sudden withdrawal of a β blocking agent may precipitate acute myocardial ischemia. An increase in receptor number also explains the hyperdynamic response seen in thyrotoxicosis.[12]

The multistep pathway between β receptor activation and cellular response creates many possible regulatory sites. Calcium may act as an inhibitor of adenyl cyclase, which may provide a negative feedback loop, to control formation of c-AMP.[13] Other sites such as the phosphodiesterase and protein kinase en-

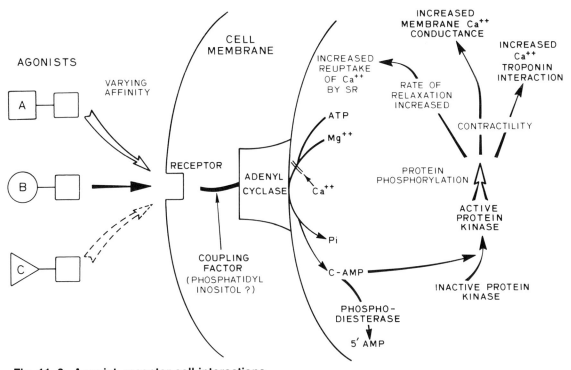

Fig. 11–2. Agonist–receptor-cell interactions.

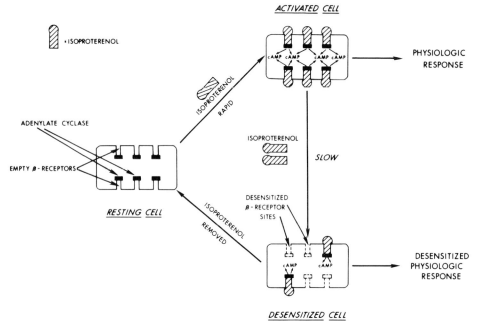

Fig. 11–3. Activation and inactivation of β-adrenergic receptors. *Rapid* refers to processes occurring within a few seconds, whereas *slow* refers to processes requiring minutes to hours for completion. (Lefkowitz RJ, Physiology in Medicine: N Engl J Med 295:327, 1976)

zymes also may provide methods of intracellular β adrenergic regulation.

NONADRENERGIC MECHANISMS OF INOTROPIC STIMULATION

A number of classes of drugs are currently available to stimulate myocardial contractility. Each class has its own basic mechanism of action. The final common step is the binding of intracellular calcium to troponin to allow actinomyosin cross-linking to occur. The greater the rate and extent of actin and myosin interaction, the greater the contractile response.

There are various methods by which intracellular calcium may be increased. The production of c-AMP is a mechanism by which β receptor stimulation increases intracellular calcium. Glucagon also exerts its inotropic effect by activating adenyl cyclase. This stimulation of c-AMP production is unaffected by β receptor blockade.[14, 15]

Cyclic-AMP activity may be maintained by decreasing its rate of destruction by phosphodiesterase. The inotropic and chronotropic effects of the xanthines, such as caffeine and theophylline, are thought to occur by this mechanism.

Digitalis glycosides also are thought to exert their inotropic effects by increasing intracellular calcium. The suggested mechanism by which this occurs involves inhibition of the sodium-potassium ATP-ase system.[16, 17]

INOTROPIC AGONISTS

When using pharmacologic means to support the failing myocardium, it is important for the clinician to understand the pathophysiology of the many causes of heart failure. This subject has been reviewed extensively and will not be discussed in detail in this chapter.[18–20] However, a few basic concepts are reviewed.

Heart failure is generally defined as an inability of the cardiac pump to meet the metabolic requirements of the body. There are numerous ways in which myocardial dysfunction or excessive demands can lead to failure (Table 11–3). In many cases, heart failure is produced by an increased load superimposed upon an already poorly functioning myocardium. An example of this is the common combination of hypertension and ischemic heart disease. Another situation seen often in the intensive care unit is the increased demand of sepsis added to the myocardial dysfunction produced by hypotension, acidosis, and hypoxemia.

In many cases, inotropic agonists are used as an adjunct to other measures directed at the primary disease. Often their use is temporary, designed to assist the failing myocardium through a critical period of the disease process. In other situations, inotropic agents may be used on a long term basis as the primary mode of therapy. In yet other circumstances, an inotropic agent may be contraindicated. Thus, the pathophysiologic process first must be considered before deciding to use inotropic agents.

In addition to physiologic considerations, attention also should be paid to some of the cellular and biochemical aspects of myocardial failure. In Chapter 3 the complex structure and function of the myocardial cell was described. Acid-base and electrolyte disorders accompanying many major physiologic disturbances may contribute to myocardial dysfunction. Thus, an appropriate cellular milieu must exist before relying on inotropic agonists to support the failing myocardium.

The actual subcellular defects associated with myocardial failure are still not defined clearly. Abnormalities have been found in many cellular structures: sarcoplasmic reticulum, sarcolemma, mitochondria, and contractile proteins. The question that still remains is "what is cause and what is effect?" The possible role of these structures in heart failure is summarized in Table 11–4.

The primary site of dysfunction appears to be in the sarcoplasmic reticulum.[21] The result of this abnormality is a change in the cyclical release of calcium in response to the action potential and, therefore, a change in excitation-contraction coupling.

SYMPATHOMIMETIC INOTROPIC AGONISTS

For many years, these agents have been used in the care of the critically ill patient. The primary myocardial actions of these drugs are summarized in Table 11–5. Depending

Table 11-3. Pathogenesis of Heart Failure

UNDERLYING PATHOLOGY	EXAMPLES
Primary myocardial dysfunction (cardiomyopathy)	Ischemia/infarction Metabolic (*e.g.*, acidosis, hypoxia) Nutritional Idiopathic
Increased demand on myocardium	
a. Volume overload	Intracardiac/A-V shunts Mitral/aortic incompetence
b. Pressure overload	Aortic stenosis IHSS Valvular Stenosis Coarctation Hypertension
c. Metabolic overload	Thyrotoxicosis Sepsis Obesity Iatrogenic (drugs) Anemia
Other factors interfering with myocardial function	Pericardial disease Arrhythmias

Table 11-4. Subcellular Myocardial Elements Involved in Heart Failure

Sarcoplasmic Reticulum (SR)
   Source and *Sink* for Ca^{++}
   Early disruption of SR seen in acute heart failure

Damaged SR $\longrightarrow$ $\downarrow$ Ca^{++} uptake

   $\downarrow$ Relaxation $\downarrow$ Ca^{++} available for release during subsequent action potential

Contractile Proteins/Troponin
   Structural changes of actin/myosin $\rightarrow$ $\downarrow$ Rate of tension development
                                                       $\downarrow$ Force of contraction

   Changes in troponin $\rightarrow$ $\downarrow$ Sensitivity to Ca^{++}

Mitochondria
   Normally very little Ca^{++} uptake
   With Abnormal Ca^{++} uptake by SR, mitochondria markedly increases uptake of Ca^{++} to buffer intracellular Ca^{++}. Release from the mitochondria is very slow.

   Result
   Ca^{++} sequestered in mitochondria unavailable for binding to troponin
   Uncoupling of electron transport chain from oxidative phosphorylation with resultant reduction in ATP production

Sarcolemma

   Damage   Altered adrenergic receptor and adenyl cyclase function

           Shortened phase 2 of action potential with $\downarrow$ time for slow Ca^{++} current into the cell

Table 11-5. Effects of Sympathomimetic Agents on the Myocardium

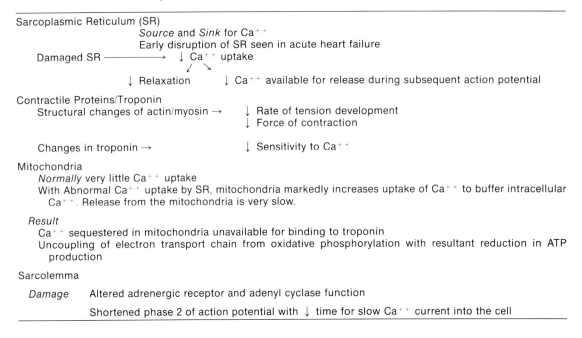

$\uparrow$ Contractility
   $\uparrow$ Rate of Developed Tension
   $\uparrow$ Force of Contraction
$\uparrow$ Conduction Velocity
   Atria
   A-V node
   His-Purkinje
$\uparrow$ Automaticity/rate of discharge
   Sinus node
   A-V junction
   His-Purkinje
Results $\longrightarrow$ $\uparrow$ Heart rate $\Big\}$ $\uparrow$ Cardiac output
             $\uparrow$ Stroke volume
Risks $\longrightarrow$ Tachycardia/arrhythmias
            Myocardial ischemia (demand > supply)

Table 11-6. Factors Determining Organ Response to Sympathomimetic Agonist

Agonist
Effect on receptors α
                             β
                             Dopaminergic
Tissue
Predominance of receptors α
                             β
                             Dopaminergic
Reflex modification of physiologic response
   e.g., norepinephrine $\rightarrow$ vasoconstriction $\rightarrow$ reflex bradycardia
Other modifying factors
   e.g., circulating blood volume

upon the agonist, both inotropic and chronotropic stimulation may occur. In some situations, such as complete heart block, the chronotropic response is desirable. However, in many other situations the added oxygen demand of an increased heart rate is undesirable. A sympathomimetic agent with potent inotropic actions and minimal chronotropic effects is preferred, if available.

The final effect of an adrenergic agonist is the result of a number of factors (Table 11–6). It is not difficult to see how two different sympathomimetic inotropic agonists may have a similar effect on cardiac output but have opposite effects on perfusion of the vital organs. In addition, the same agent may have a different action on the same patient on two separate occasions. If dopamine, for example, is administered to a patient who is hypovolemic, the heart rate may increase considerably. Once the patient's intravascular volume status is corrected, the same dose of dopamine may produce little or no change in heart rate.

It is important to understand the difference between direct- and indirect-acting agents. A direct agonist is one which exerts its effects by acting directly on the adrenergic receptor. An indirect agonist is one which produces its effects by releasing norepinephrine from the postganglionic sympathetic nerve ending. Such an agent would not be expected to have a strong inotropic effect on myocardium in chronic failure, depleted of catecholamines. Long-term administration of an indirect-acting agonist may deplete the sympathetic nerve endings of norepinephrine. Table 11–7 summarizes the site of action and recommended dosage of the sympathomimetic inotropic drugs.

Epinephrine

Physiology. Epinephrine is a naturally occurring catecholamine, released from the adrenal medulla. It serves a major metabolic role, with regulation of blood sugar and free fatty acids via effects on gluconeogenesis, glycogenolysis, glucose uptake, and lipolysis. Only under conditions of extreme stress does it play a role in cardiovascular homeostasis.[22]

The cardiovascular effects of epinephrine are exerted by stimulation of both α and β receptors. A strongly positive inotropic and chronotropic response results from β_1 receptor stimulation. The response of the peripheral vasculature depends upon the status of the end organ as well as the dose administered. Vasoconstriction occurs in the skin and

Table 11-7. Sympathomimetic Inotropic Agonists*

AGENT	RECEPTOR	RECOMMENDED DOSAGE
Epinephrine	β	1–2 μg/min
	α, β	2–10 μg/min
	α	>10 μg/min
Norepinephrine	α, β	1–15 μg/min
Isoproterenol	β	1–4 μg/min: titrate to heart rate
Dopamine	Dopaminergic, β	1–10 μg/kg/min
	α	>10 μg/kg/min
Dobutamine	β	1–10 μg/kg/min
Metaraminol	Indirect (α, β)	1–10 mg IV 5–10 mg IM 25–30 mg PO
Ephedrine	Direct/indirect (α, β)	2.5–20 mg IV 15–50 mg IM 15–50 mg PO

*The response to these agents demonstrates extreme individual variability. If the situation permits, it is safer to start with a low dose of each agent and titrate each drug to the desired physiologic response.

Table 11-8. Effects of Epinephrine on Coronary Blood Flow

Direct effect
  α Mediated vasoconstriction*
Metabolic effect
  Coronary vasodilation
Shortened systolic period
  ↑ Time for diastolic filling
Increased heart rate
  ↓ Time for diastolic filling
Improved ventricular performance
  ↑ Ventricular emptying
  ↓ Wall tension
  Improved subendocardial perfusion

*Anderson et al: Adrenergic α- and β- receptors in coronary vessels in man. Acta Med Scand 191: 241, 1972

kidneys at all doses. Vasodilation, secondary to β$_2$ stimulation, occurs in the splanchnic and skeletal muscle beds at low doses (1–10 μg/min). At higher doses (>10 μg/min), vasoconstriction predominates because of α stimulation. Effects on the coronary circulation are influenced by a number of factors (Table 11–8). The major factor is myocardial metabolic demand, which results in increased coronary blood flow.

Pharmacology. Absorption of epinephrine from subcutaneous and intramuscular sites is slow because of local vasoconstriction. When used in resuscitative circumstances, the recommended route is intravenous. In extreme situations, although this route is no longer recommended by the American Heart Association, the agent may be given by the intracardiac route. Also, in the very rare instance where venous access cannot be obtained, epinephrine may be injected into an endotracheal tube for absorption from the bronchial mucosa.

Although stable in the circulation, the effects of epinephrine are rapidly terminated by tissue uptake and metabolism. The two enzymes responsible for this are monoamine oxidase (MAO) and catechol-O-methyl transferase (COMT). The major metabolite, 3 methoxy-4-hydroxy mandelic acid (incorrectly called vanyll mandelic acid: VMA) is excreted in the urine in conjugated or free form.

Clinical Use. Epinephrine's vasoconstricting effects are used along with local anesthetic drugs to limit local absorption and prolong local duration of anesthesia. It is used extensively as a bronchodilator. The combined bronchodilating and pressor properties make it the agent of choice in anaphylactic shock. It is indicated in ventricular asystole, and in converting fine ventricular fibrillation to a coarse ventricular pattern, more amenable to defibrillation.

In cardiac surgery, epinephrine has been used in relatively small doses (0.01 μg/kg/min) to improve myocardial performance during discontinuance of cardiopulmonary bypass,[23] although dopamine is used for this purpose presently. In this dose range, cardiac index was observed to increase by 30 percent, heart rate 10 percent, and systemic vascular resistance was unchanged.[23] The effect on urine output or duration of use was not reported. With the current availability of agents such as dopamine or dobutamine, epinephrine is usually reserved for those situations where the failing myocardium is unresponsive to these other agents.

The recommended adult doses of epinephrine for cardiovascular use are as follows:

Anaphylaxis	0.5–1.0 ml 1/1000 epinephrine SC (then 1–20 μg/min IV infusion)
Cardiac Arrest	0.5–1.0 ml 1/1000 epinephrine IV or 5.0–10 ml 1/10,000 intracardiac
Low cardiac output states	2–20 μg/min IV infusion

Risks. The two vital organs most in jeopardy from the use of epinephrine are the heart and kidneys. As might be expected, the higher the dose, the greater the potential damage to these organs. The potential for creating an unfavorable myocardial oxygen supply/demand ratio is very high. The favorable increase in contractility and decreased wall tension may be overshadowed by a marked tachycardia. Tachycardia not only increases myocardial oxygen demand but also reduces supply by shortening the duration of diastole. This is especially dangerous when ischemia and infarction are already present.[24] With the ability of epinephrine to increase automaticity and its potential to create ischemia, dysrhythmias may also be a problem.

The peripheral vascular effects of epinephrine also limit its use. With small intravenous doses (0.1 μg/kg) blood pressure may decrease.[22] The reduction in systemic vascular resistance occurs mainly in skeletal muscle. Renal vascular resistance increases at all doses.[22] As the dose in increased, α effects predominate with marked vasoconstriction and venoconstriction, increasing myocardial oxygen demand and worsening preexisting heart failure.[25]

Although it is an excellent inotropic drug, epinephrine's combined potential risks of renal and myocardial ischemia, tachycardia, and dysrhythmias may make it a second line choice to agents such as dopamine.

Norepinephrine

Pharmacology. Norepinephrine is the principal neurotransmitter released from peripheral postganglionic sympathetic nerve endings. Unlike epinephrine, it plays an important role in cardiovascular homeostasis, under normal physiologic conditions.

The peripheral vascular effects of norepinephrine arise from α stimulation. It has a very weak β_2 agonism and does not produce the vasodilation seen with epinephrine and isoproterenol. The direct myocardial effects of norepinephrine arise from β_1 stimulation with positive inotropic and chronotropic responses. In spite of myocardial stimulation,

cardiac output may decrease as a result of reflex slowing of heart rate and an increase in afterload produced by peripheral vasoconstriction.[25] Until the direct effects on the myocardium were studied by Goldberg and coworkers in 1960, norepinephrine was regarded as a pure pressor with no myocardial action.[26] Because of marked venoconstriction, it is recommended that the agent be given through a large central vein.[22]

Metabolism and excretion are the same as for epinephrine. There is rapid tissue uptake with metabolism by MAO and COMT. Excretion of conjugated and unconjugated metabolites occurs in the urine, with only from 4 to 16 percent of administered norepinephrine appearing unchanged.[22]

Clinical Use. Norepinephrine is used in situations in which arterial blood pressure has decreased to levels which acutely jeopardize coronary and cerebral perfusion. By temporarily sacrificing perfusion to other tissues, blood pressure may be increased to levels which will ensure coronary and cerebral blood flow, and prevent infarction of these organs. The inotropic effect of norepinephrine also may help the heart to cope with the resultant increased afterload.[27] Studying critically ill patients in cardiogenic shock, Mueller and coworkers showed an improvement in myocardial metabolism after increasing blood pressure with norepinephrine.[28]

However, a large price is being paid in terms of increased myocardial work and reduced renal perfusion. Thus, the lowest possible dose should be used to attain the blood pressure necessary to ensure coronary and cerebral perfusion. Such a pressure may be from 30 to 40 torr lower than the patient's normal level. Norepinephrine should be used for as short a period of time as possible, while alternative therapeutic measures are being instituted. The recommended adult dosage range is from 2 to 16 μg/min.

Risks. Myocardial oxygen consumption will increase with heart rate, contractility, and wall tension. Ischemia and dysrhythmias may result. The intense vasoconstriction produced by norepinephrine may lead to ischemia of renal and splanchnic beds. Accidental extravasation of the drug into the subcutaneous tissues may lead to skin necrosis and sloughing. If this should occur, immediate infiltration of the area with phentolamine or local anesthetic is recommended, along with the application of hot packs.[22]

Isoproterenol

Pharmacology. Isoproterenol is a synthetic sympathomimetic agonist with essentially pure β activity, studied extensively by Ahlquist in 1948[29] and by others.[22, 30, 31] Isoproterenol acts as a potent stimulant of heart rate and contractility as well as producing a reduction in systemic vascular resistance. Although this reduction occurs in a number of vascular beds, increased skeletal muscle flow may predominate at the expense of renal blood flow.[32, 33] Coronary blood flow increases as a result of increased myocardial metabolic demand[34, 35] and possible direct vasodilatory effects.[36]

For cardiovascular use, the recommended mode of administration is by intravenous infusion. Oral and sublingual preparations are available, but their absorption is erratic and clinical response may be difficult to control. Isoproterenol has a very short duration of action, because of rapid tissue uptake. Excretion is mainly urinary, with greater than 60 percent appearing as unchanged isoproterenol. When given intravenously, the major metabolite is 3-O-methylisoproterenol. When given orally, the major metabolite is the sulfated ester of isoproterenol.

Clinical Uses. In a brief description of eight patients, Morse and coworkers described the successful use of isoproterenol in cardiogenic shock caused by myocardial infarction.[37] Others do not concur.[27, 28] A major difficulty in studying shock arises from the extreme instability of these patients and from the different hemodynamic patterns that may be present.[38] In general, if systemic vascular resistance is already high, and cardiac output is able to compensate for a decrease in resistance, a beneficial effect may be obtained with isoproterenol.[39] In myocardial infarc-

tion, however, the potential risks of using this agent may exceed its benefits.

Isoproterenol has also been used successfully in the early postoperative period following cardiac surgery.[40, 41] A large proportion of the increase in cardiac output, however, arises from an increased heart rate.[30] Alternative agents, such as dopamine, have been shown to achieve comparable increases in cardiac output, without a marked change in heart rate, and may be preferable to isoproterenol.[42] The recently transplanted heart, on the other hand, has been shown to benefit greatly from the combined chronotropic and inotropic effects of isoproterenol.[43]

The potent chronotropic actions of isoproterenol have also been used in the treatment of bradycardia, arising from abnormalities in the sinus or A-V nodes.[44] Although long-term use of isoproterenol has been described, its use is usually temporary, until a pacemaker can be inserted.[45]

The vasodilator effects of isoproterenol are present in the pulmonary circulation as well as the systemic circulation.[46] This effect has been used in an attempt to lower the pulmonary vascular resistance seen in primary pulmonary hypertension,[47, 48] but a favorable response is not seen consistently.[49]

Risks. The primary risk with the use of isoproterenol is the potential for imbalance of myocardial oxygen supply and demand. This applies especially to the heart with preexisting ischemia or infarction.[50–53]

The tachycardia produced by isoproterenol will increase myocardial oxygen consumption in the face of a shortened diastolic filling time. In addition, the reduced systemic vascular resistance may decrease the aortic diastolic pressure to levels that could jeopardize coronary perfusion. The direct coronary vasodilation produced by isoproterenol also may be detrimental in patients with coronary artery disease. An area of ischemia already may be maximally vasodilated, and the addition of a coronary vasodilator may serve only to divert flow to nonischemic areas and extend the area of ischemia and injury.[54]

Mueller and coworkers studied the effects

of isoproterenol on patients in cardiogenic shock, secondary to myocardial infarction,[28] and on postoperative cardiac patients having correction of rheumatic valvular disease.[38] In both groups an increase in anaerobic metabolism was produced, as indicated by a decreased lactate consumption or shift to lactate production.

The potential to produce myocardial ischemia, along with its effects on automaticity, make dysrhythmias another problem with isoproterenol. Also, when used for Mobitz II (2°) A-V block, isoproterenol may increase the degree of block. Thus its use may be limited.

Dopamine

Pharmacology. Dopamine is a naturally occurring sympathomimetic agent. It is produced in postganglionic sympathetic nerve endings and in the adrenal medulla as a precursor of norepinephrine. Dopamine also is an important neurotransmitter in the central nervous system. The cardiovascular effects of dopamine have been reviewed quite extensively by Goldberg in 1972,[55] and excellent, updated reviews of the clinical use of dopamine also are available.[56, 57]

The adrenergically mediated cardiovascular actions of dopamine may involve activation of dopaminergic, β and α receptors, depending upon the dose used (Tables 11–7, 11–9, and 11–10). Activation of dopaminergic receptors results in vasodilation within the renal and mesenteric vasculature.[55] The renal vasodilating effects of dopaminergic stimulation is blocked by phenothiazines,[58, 59] such

as chlorpromazine, and butyrophenones, such as haloperidol[60] and droperidol. Beta blockade does not inhibit dopamine's renal vasodilation.[61, 62]

Stimulation of α and β receptors by dopamine is produced by direct receptor stimulation and by norepinephrine release from postganglionic sympathetic nerve endings. The positive inotropic and chronotropic effects of dopamine are blocked by β-blocking drugs and the α vasoconstriction seen at higher doses is attenuated by α-blocking drugs.[63] The effect of dopamine on different adrenergic receptors may lead to a variety of hemodynamic responses, depending upon the dose used, the individual's response to a given dose, and hemodynamic status.

Infusion of from 1 to 10 μg/kg/min of dopamine will produce a dose-dependent increase in cardiac output,[64] because of increased stroke volume, positive inotropy, and reduced systemic vascular resistance.[57, 64] In addition, venoconstriction may facilitate the increase in stroke volume.[65] As the dose increases, heart rate also may increase.[66] Alpha-mediated reflex vasoconstriction may oppose the increase in heart rate.

Because of its mixed adrenergic receptor

Table 11-9. Classification of Dopamine Receptor Agents

AGONIST	ANTAGONIST
Apomorphine	Phenothiazine
Bromocryptine	Butyrophenone
Dopamine	Metoclopramide
	Sulpiride

(from Maze ML Clinical implications of membrane receptor function in anesthesia. Anesthesiology 55:160–171, 1981

Table 11-10. Hemodynamic Dose Response to Dopamine*

DOSE (μg/kg/min)	PREDOMINANT RECEPTOR	RESPONSE
1–3	Dopaminergic	Renal and mesenteric vasodilation
1–10	β₁	↑ Contractility ↑ Heart rate as dose increases
>10	α	↑ Vasoconstriction as dose increases

*There is considerable receptor overlap within each of these dose ranges and considerable individual variation in response to a given dose.

stimulation, dopamine has a complex effect on the peripheral vasculature. The effects of dopamine on the individual organ perfusion are still not defined clearly, but the most extensively studied organ is the kidney. Early animal studies demonstrated increased renal plasma flow and excretion of sodium and potassium,[67] later confirmed in humans.[68–70] These result from an increase in renal blood flow and redistribution of perfusion within the kidney.[70, 71]

Dopamine produces coronary artery vasodilation in proportion to the increased myocardial oxygen demand.[72] Dopamine has been shown to increase myocardial oxygen consumption, but not to change the myocardial lactate extraction ratio in patients with coronary artery disease.[73] In contrast to isoproterenol, dopamine does not produce *direct* coronary vasodilation, and therefore should not cause a shunting of blood flow away from ischemic areas.[53]

The effects of dopamine on pulmonary vascular resistance are not defined clearly. Doses of from 5 to 20 µg/kg/min, in animals, show an increase in resistance, which is blocked by phentolamine.[74] At doses of from 1 to 10 µg/kg/min, dopamine did not change pulmonary vascular resistance in adults in congestive heart failure[64] and children after congenital heart surgery, with or without pulmonary hypertension.[75] Three out of eighteen patients with coronary artery disease or cardiomyopathy undergoing cardiac catheterization, showed an increase in pulmonary vascular resistance, unrelated to underlying disease or hemodynamic status.[76]

Although investigators have sought an oral form of dopamine, the accepted mode of administration is by intravenous infusion (Tables 11–7 and 11–10).[57] Suggested dose ranges serve as clinical guides for infusion titration.

The pharmacologic effects of dopamine are terminated by rapid tissue uptake and metabolism. Small amounts are converted to norepinephrine and epinephrine. The major metabolites are 3,4-dihydroxyphenylacetic acid and 3-methoxy-4-hydroxyphenylacetic acid, both rapidly excreted in the urine.

Clinical Uses. In the usual inotropic dose range, dopamine has been shown to augment urine output, glomerular filtration rate, renal plasma flow and sodium excretion in patients with congestive heart failure.[64, 69] These variables increase to a greater extent than would be expected from an increased cardiac output alone. Increased renal blood flow, with possible intrarenal redistribution of perfusion, may occur. Also, augmented cardiac output and increased mean arterial blood pressure may attenuate the renin-angiotensin-aldosterone response seen in congestive heart failure.[77] Dopamine also may have a direct diuretic action.[78] The addition of vasodilator therapy to dopamine, in severe congestive heart failure, has been shown to be of considerable benefit.[79] Combined therapy usually allows augmentation of cardiac output at lower filling pressures and therefore contributes to reducing myocardial wall tension and oxygen consumption. In addition, vasodilator therapy allows the use of lower doses of dopamine with concomitant reduction of the potential risks of ischemia, tachycardia, and dysrhythmias.

First described in 1972, dopamine demonstrated reasonable success in postoperative open-heart patients, who were unstable and not responding to other available inotropic drugs.[80] In six patients in cardiogenic shock following cardiac surgery, all recovered from shock, and five were discharged from the hospital.[81] Holloway and coworkers found similar increases in cardiac output with dopamine and isoproterenol in cardiac surgical patients, but no change in heart rate with dopamine.[42] Isoproterenol produced heart rate increases of 18 and 28 percent at doses of 0.0125 and 0.0250 µg/kg/min, respectively. In a comparison of the use of dopamine, dobutamine, and epinephrine in cardiac surgical patients, dopamine produced the greatest increase in cardiac output at comparable dose levels.[82] Heart rate increased slightly with all three agents.

Goldberg and coworkers first described the potential of dopamine in shock in 1969.[83] Loeb and coworkers compared norepinephrine, isoproterenol, and dopamine in patients with shock resulting from various causes.[63] The limiting factors for both norepinephrine and isoproterenol were their marked peripheral vascular effects. In septic shock, isoproterenol increased cardiac output more than dopamine but the already low systemic vascular resistance decreased further, and blood pressure and urine flow decreased. Dopamine increased mean arterial pressure by 30 percent, cardiac output by 37 percent, and increased urine output from 0.5 ml/min to 1.6 ml/min. Norepinephrine resulted in a higher mean arterial pressure but a lower cardiac output, compared with dopamine, in all patients.

In spite of its beneficial effects in shock, patients with marked hypoperfusion and increased lactate levels usually do not respond to therapy with dopamine.[84] In such cases, cardiovascular reserve is totally exhausted and the heart appears unresponsive to any type of sympathomimetic support.

Risks. Although dopamine may be superior to the older sympathomimetic agents for certain cardiovascular derangements, it still shares the same potential risks, including increased myocardial oxygen consumption. In cases of ischemia or infarction, damage may increase in areas of myocardium where demand exceeds supply.[24] Tachycardia may occur with dopamine, especially at higher doses, producing increased oxygen demand. Ventricular dysrhythmias may occur, necessitating a reduction in dose.

Marked vasoconstriction and pedal gangrene have been described with doses as low as 1.5 µg/kg/min.[85] Under these circumstances, predisposing vascular disease or injury is usually present.[86] Because of the potent venoconstricting effects of dopamine, it is best to administer dopamine through a central vein. If it is administered through a peripheral vein and extravasation occurs, the management should be as previously described for norepinephrine—immediate infiltration with local anesthetic agent and phentolamine.

Nausea and vomiting may occur with doses of from 9 to 10 µg/kg/min.[87] Dopamine

should be avoided in those patients taking MAO inhibitors because of its ability to release norepinephrine from sympathetic nerve endings. If used in such a patient, dopamine should be started in doses of about 0.1 µg/kg/min, and increased judiciously.[57]

Dobutamine

Pharmacology. Dobutamine is a synthetic sympathomimetic agonist which has been available for clinical use in the United States since 1978. Although it has a very weak α agonist activity,[88] dobutamine exerts its primary cardiovascular actions through direct β-receptor stimulation. Unlike dopamine, it has no indirect agonist activity.[88, 89]

Dobutamine increases cardiac output by increasing contractility and heart rate. When developed initially, it was hoped that dobutamine would be an agent providing inotropic stimulation with little chronotropic effect.[88] However, heart rate increases by 25 to 30 percent in doses used clinically.[90–92] In addition, electrophysiologic studies have shown that dobutamine has the same effects as isoproterenol on atrioventricular and intraventricular conduction pathways. The potential for dysrhythmias is present, but may be lower.

The peripheral vascular effects of dobutamine resemble those of isoproterenol. Except for minimal α-mediated vasoconstriction at very low doses, the predominant effect is vasodilation.[88] Although this effect is quite marked in patients with severe heart failure,[93] it also occurs in patients without impaired left ventricular function.[91] Similar to isoproterenol, the vasodilation favors redistribution of blood flow to skeletal muscle.[93, 94] Unlike dopamine, the renal vasodilation produced by dobutamine can be blocked with propranolol.[94] Coronary artery blood flow increases concomitantly with the increase in myocardial oxygen consumption.[95, 96] Dobutamine may produce direct coronary vasodilation.

Dobutamine is administered in doses of from 2.5 to 10.0 µg/kg/min by intravenous infusion (Table 11–7). Its plasma half life is approximately two minutes.[89] Dobutamine is rapidly cleared from the circulation and metabolized in the liver. The major products of this metabolism are 3-O-methyldobutamine and glucuronide conjugates, which are excreted in the urine.

Clinical Use. Dobutamine has been used to treat congestive heart failure of various etiologies.[97-101] The patient with nonischemic congestive cardiomyopathy seems to respond better to dobutamine than dopamine.[99, 102]

In congestive heart failure, cardiac output increases and pulmonary artery occluded pressure decreases.[99-102] Systemic and pulmonary vascular resistances decrease.[97-102] A dose related increase in heart rate usually is observed, similar to isoproterenol. In patients with low output cardiac failure, isoproterenol and dobutamine showed no significant differences in observed cardiovascular effects.[103]

The combined myocardial stimulation and reduction of vascular resistance from dobutamine are useful in the patient with severe congestive heart failure, high peripheral vascular resistance, and normal or increased blood pressure. The combination of dobutamine and nitroprusside is beneficial.[102] However, some patients require a high peripheral vascular resistance to compensate for severely depressed myocardial function. If the heart does not respond with an increase in cardiac output, the predominant effect of dobutamine may be to decrease blood pressure acutely by decreasing systemic vascular resistance. Dobutamine is best avoided in the patient who is already hypotensive.

Comparison of dobutamine and isoproterenol in cardiac surgical patients who were hemodynamically stable in the postoperative period demonstrated similar hemodynamic responses to the two agents.[104-106] Heart rate increased, in a dose related fashion, with both drugs.[104, 105] Systemic vascular resistance decreased in similar fashion. A low incidence of ventricular dysrhythmias was observed with both agents.

Steen and coworkers compared dobuta-mine with dopamine and epinephrine to provide inotropic support for patients being separated from cardiopulmonary bypass (CPB).[82] Mean arterial blood pressure and cardiac output increased significantly with all agents. Heart rate increased slightly but no differences were observed between drugs. Systemic vascular resistance did not decrease significantly in response to from 5 to 15 μg/kg/min of dobutamine. During separation from CPB, isoproterenol at 0.02 μg/kg/min produced a 9-percent increase in cardiac output with a 44-percent increase in heart rate.[107] Dobutamine in doses of 5 and 10 μg/kg/min increased cardiac output by 16 and 28 percent with an increase in heart rate of 6 and 15 percent, respectively.

Hilberman and coworkers found a significant increase in heart rate and decrease in systemic vascular resistance with dobutamine in doses of 2.5 to 7.5 μg/kg/min.[78] Dopamine produced greater urine flow and sodium excretion than dobutamine at equal cardiac output. Thus, dobutamine exerts its inotropic actions with variable chronotropic and peripheral vascular effects. The hemodynamic effects of dobutamine thus seem to resemble those of isoproterenol.

Risks. The dose related increase in heart rate may increase myocardial oxygen demand while reducing supply. If systemic vascular resistance decreases, aortic diastolic pressure may decrease and further reduce myocardial oxygen supply. Isoproterenol and dobutamine both produce equivalent increases in anaerobic myocardial metabolism.[105]

Dobutamine produces an increase in the amount of ST segment elevation during experimental myocardial injury, but less than that seen with isoproterenol.[108, 109] Dobutamine has been used in patients following acute myocardial infarction, in spite of the potential to increase ischemia, but no difference was seen between patients receiving or not receiving dobutamine.[109]

Dobutamine has the same effect as isoproterenol on the A-V and ventricular conduction pathways.[92] The potential risk of dysrhythmias is therefore as high with dobutamine as with isoproterenol. Six out of thirty-six patients developed ventricular ectopic beats in response to dobutamine.[91] Patients in atrial fibrillation or flutter also may suddenly increase ventricular rate because of increased A-V conduction.

Even though dobutamine produces systemic vasodilation, subcutaneous infiltration of the drug may cause skin necrosis.[110] Management is the same as for norepinephrine and dopamine; infiltration of the area with local anesthetic and phentolamine.

Ephedrine

Pharmacology. Ephedrine, is an alkaloid obtained from a Chinese herb, and has been used for various disorders for more than 5000 years. Its historical background and physiologic effect were reviewed by Chen and Schmidt in 1930[111] and more recently by Aviado in 1970.[112]

The cardiovascular effects of ephedrine result from direct and indirect stimulation of adrenergic receptors.[112] Depletion of norepinephrine from sympathetic nerve endings will attenuate the effects of ephedrine but not abolish them completely.[112]

The increased blood pressure seen with ephedrine is mainly a result of myocardial stimulation. In normal subjects, and patients with congestive heart failure, an increase in cardiac output occurs with little change in systemic vascular resistance.[113, 114] Both heart rate and stroke volume increase. Although venoconstriction may enhance the increase in cardiac output, Cohn found no significant change in venous tone in normal subjects.[113]

For all routes, except intravenous, the recommended dose range is from 15 to 50 mg, increasing progressively to achieve the desired response. The response to intravenous administration of from 2.5 to 10 mg is immediate, with a duration of 5 to 10 minutes. Intramuscular or subcutaneous ephedrine will produce a cardiovascular response in 10 minutes, lasting about 30 minutes.[112]

Clinical Use. Ephedrine is used to correct acute hypotension in patients who are volume repleted. Such a situation may involve acute myocardial depression from an inhalational or intravenous anesthetic agent. It is also used to correct hypotension caused by spinal or epidural anesthesia, which does not respond to vascular volume administration. The absence of uterine vasoconstriction makes this a popular agent in obstetric anesthesia.[115, 116] In chronic congestive heart failure, in spite of possible myocardial catecholamine depletion,[117] cardiac output increased significantly in response to oral ephedrine.[114]

Ephedrine is used as a bronchodilator, although the more specific β_2 agonists are replacing ephedrine for this use. Nevertheless, ephedrine has favorable properties that have sustained its use for more than 5000 years.

Risks. The predominant risks of ephedrine use are those of increased myocardial oxygen consumption, tachycardia, and dysrhythmias.[112] It should not be used in patients who have been receiving monoamine oxidase inhibitors because the effect of a drug which causes norepinephrine release may produce a dangerous increase in blood pressure.[118, 119]

Norepinephrine depletion has been used to explain the tachyphylaxis that is seen after chronic ephedrine use.[112] Cardiomyopathy also may result from high-dose ephedrine used for long periods.[120]

High doses of ephedrine may cause anxiety and agitation. Addiction also has been described in asthmatic patients receiving ephedrine for prolonged periods.[112]

Metaraminol

Pharmacology. Metaraminol is a synthetic sympathomimetic agent with both direct and indirect adrenergic stimulating actions. The primary cardiovascular effect of metaraminol is to increase peripheral vascular resistance, similar to norepinephrine.[22, 121] Cardiac output usually remains unchanged or decreases as a result of reflex bradycardia. When bradycardia is treated with atropine, cardiac output increases in response to metaraminol. Just as with norepinephrine, the increase in blood pressure occurs at the expense of vasoconstriction in renal, splanchnic, and pulmonary beds.[121, 122]

Table 11-11. Cardiac Glycoside Preparations

AGENT	GASTROINTESTINAL ABSORPTION	ONSET OF ACTION* (min)	PEAK EFFECT (hr)	AVERAGE HALF-LIFE†	PRINCIPLE METABLIC ROUTE (EXCRETORY PATHWAY)	AVERAGE DIGITALIZING DOSE ORAL§	AVERAGE DIGITALIZING DOSE INTRAVENOUS"	USUAL DAILY ORAL MAINTENANCE DOSE‡
Ouabain	Unreliable	5–10	1/2–2	21 hr	Renal; some gastrointestinal excretion		0.3–0.5 mg	
Deslanoside	Unreliable	10–30	1–2	33 hr	Renal		0.8 mg	
Digoxin	55–75%#	15–30	1 1/2–5	36 hr	Renal; some gastrointestinal excretion	1.25–1.5 mg	0.75–1.0 mg	0.25–0.5 mg
Digitoxin	90–100%	25–120	4–12	4–6 days	Hepatic;** renal excretion of metabolites	0.7–1.2 mg	1.0 mg	0.1 mg
Digitalis leaf	About 40%			4–6 days	Similar to digoxin	0.8–1.2 mg		0.1 g

*For intravenous dose
†For normal subject (prolonged by renal impairment with digoxin, ouabain and deslanoside, and probably by severe hepatic disease with digitoxin and digitalis leaf)
‡Average for adult patients without renal or hepatic impairment; varies widely among individual patients and requires close medical supervision
§Divided doses over 12–24 hr at intervals of 6–8 hr
"Given in increments for initial subcomplete digitalization, to be supplemented by further small increments as necessary
#For tablet form of administration (may be less in malabsorption syndromes and in formulations with poor bioavailability)
**Enterohepatic cycle exists
(From Smith TW, Haber E: Digitalis. N Engl J Med 289: 1064, 1973)

While oral, subcutaneous and intramuscular routes may be used, intravenous administration is the most controllable. The recommended single intravenous dose is from 0.5 to 5 mg, with a starting dose of 20 mg/min for continuous intravenous infusion. An intramuscular dose of 5 mg will exert a pressor effect for approximately 1.5 hours.[22] A single intravenous dose will have an immediate onset, with a duration of 5 to 10 minutes or more. Metaraminol may be more difficult to titrate than norepinephrine because of its longer duration of action. Tissue uptake is responsible for the termination of metaraminol's effects.[112]

Clinical Use. The primary use for metaraminol is rapid and temporary restoration of blood pressure during acute hypotension. This increase in blood pressure occurs at the expense of renal and splanchnic blood flow, pulmonary vasoconstriction, and increased myocardial oxygen demand. It should be used only in situations where hypotension is severe enough to jeopardize cerebral or coronary perfusion.

Risks. The risks of metaraminol are similar to those of norepinephrine; the addition of increased afterload to the inotropic effects may further increase myocardial oxygen consumption. the combination of oxygen deficit, ventricular ischemia, and reflex bradycardia may increase the risk of dysrhythmias.

Metaraminol may lead to depletion of norepinephrine from sympathetic nerve endings. This may produce tachyphylaxis, seen with prolonged use. Unlike norepinephrine, metaraminol does not cause skin sloughing if subcutaneous infiltration occurs.

CARDIAC GLYCOSIDES

The cardiac glycosides, derived from plant extracts, have been used for medicinal purposes for centuries.[123] They had been used for many illnesses by the ancient Egyptians and Romans. Records of Welsh physicians, dating back to 1250, describe the medical use of a plant called *foxglove,* now known as *Digitalis purpurea.* Describing its use in dropsy, Withering mentioned the cardiac actions of foxglove, but did not ascribe the beneficial results to these cardiac effects. Shortly afterward, in 1799, Ferriar attributed the primary beneficial effects of digitalis to its action on the heart. At the start of the 20th century, the main clinical use of digitalis was in the treatment of atrial fibrillation. Harrison and coworkers in 1931 examined the use of digitalis in congestive heart failure and provided an interesting review.[124] After more than 50 years of research on digitalis, the clinical indications for this drug remain the same, and so do many of the questions.

Pharmacology

Digoxin, the most commonly used cardiac glycoside, is derived from *Digitalis lanata.* Lanatoside C (Cedilanid), present in the plant's leaves, is subjected to alkaline and enzymatic hydrolysis to produce digoxin. A parenterally available form of lanatoside C, deslanoside (Cedilanid D), is produced by alkaline hydrolysis of lanatoside C. Digitoxin is produced from both *Digitalis purpurea* and *lanata.* Ouabain is derived from *Strophanthus gratus.*

A number of digitalis preparations thus are available for clinical use. Although their physiologic actions are similar, chemical differences give rise to differing pharmacokinetics (Table 11–11). While digoxin is by far the most commonly used cardiac glycoside, the clinician occasionally may treat a patient who is taking one of the less frequently used preparations. This topic has recently been reviewed by Doherty.[125]

Digoxin may be administered by oral, intravenous, or intramuscular routes. Absorption by the oral route is 85 percent for digoxin elixir and from 60 to 75 percent for the tablet form.[126] Peak serum levels are achieved in 45-60 minutes, with a peak pharmacologic response in 1.5 to 5.0 hours. Gastrointestinal absorption of digoxin may be influenced by a number of factors.[127] Administration after a meal has been shown to decrease peak serum drug levels.[128] Concurrent ingestion of nonabsorbable compounds such as antacids, kaolinpectin,[129] and neomycin[130] also reduce digoxin absorption.

Given intravenously, the serum concentration peaks immediately, and redistribution occurs over a 2- to 4-hour period.[126] Intramuscular administration, in addition to being painful, gives rise to a slow increase in serum concentration, and consequent slow distribution to tissues, and is not recommended.

Once in the blood, digoxin exhibits from 20 to 25 percent protein binding. The major tissues that bind digoxin are skeletal and cardiac muscle, kidney, liver, adrenal glands, and pancreas. Because skeletal muscle comprises such a large proportion of the body's mass, it serves as the major depot for digoxin.

The elimination half-life of digoxin is from 30 to 36 hours. The major mode of elimination is by renal excretion of unchanged drug. In a 24-hour period, 33 percent of body stores of digoxin are excreted, presuming normal renal function. Thirty percent is excreted through the kidney and three percent appears in the feces. Approximately 7 percent of body stores of digoxin are recycled by the enterohepatic route.[126]

The adult loading dose of digoxin necessary to produce therapeutic effects has been found to be from 0.010 to 0.015 mg/kg.[123] This dose assumes a normal proportion of skeletal muscle mass to total body weight. If a patient is grossly edematous or obese, lean body mass will have to be estimated. Loading may be achieved rapidly, usually by dividing total loading dose into three equal doses, administered 6 hours apart. Complete digoxin effect can be achieved within 12 hours. This method is not recommended if the patient has received, or is thought to have received, digoxin in the recent past. A slower method of loading is to administer the calculated maintenance dose on a daily basis. For the average adult, with normal renal function, this dose is usually from 0.25 to 0.50 mg/day, with full digoxin effect occurring over approximately seven days.

While determination of loading dose is based upon skeletal muscle mass, maintenance dose is determined by renal function. With normal renal function, one third of the body's digoxin stores are eliminated per day.

Maintenance dose will therefore be one third of the total loading dose. In situations in which reduced renal function is present, maintenance dosage will need to be adjusted accordingly. A scale for adjusting maintenance digoxin dosage, on the basis of creatinine clearance is as follows:

Daily Maintenance Dose (% Total Body Loading Dose)	Creatinine Clearance (ml/min)
33	>100
30	90
27	80
24	60
21	40
18	20
15	0

These loading and maintenance dosage guidelines are based upon digoxin pharmacokinetics. Many individual clinical situations may necessitate modification of these guidelines. Elderly patients[131] and patients with reduced thyroid function[132, 133] should have dosage reduced. Hyperthyroidism may necessitate higher dosage. Patients requiring digoxin for treatment of atrial fibrillation or flutter often need higher doses of digoxin than are needed for congestive heart failure.[134]

Concomitant drug administration may also require adjustment of digoxin dosage. The use of various non-absorbable antacids may reduce the absorption of digoxin. Quinidine also has been shown to increase serum digoxin levels when the two drugs are used together.[135-137] At the present time, however, it is still not clear whether the effect results from a reduced volume of distribution,[135] or from a decrease in renal clearance.[136] Quite likely both mechanisms are involved.

Digitoxin is probably the second most frequently used cardiac glycoside in North America. It is available for oral or intravenous administration. Gastrointestinal absorption is rapid and complete. Digitoxin is 90% protein bound. Tissue distribution is similar to digoxin, but distribution time is much longer, 4 to 10 hours.[126] Elimination half-life is from 4 to 7 days, and the major mode of elimination is by hepatic metabolism. The amounts and routes of excretion of metabolites are not clear.[126]

Deslanoside is used less frequently, and much less information is available. It is very poorly absorbed from the gastrointestinal tract, and thus the recommended route of administration is intravenous. Virtually no protein binding occurs. Elimination half-life is similar to that of digoxin, with the major route of elimination by renal excretion.[125]

Ouabain's proposed advantage over digoxin is its rapid onset of action. However, the differences are not great enough for ouabain to replace digoxin. One advantage of intravenous digoxin is that once the desired effect is achieved, the patient can be given the oral preparation for maintenance.

Cardiovascular Effects

The direct effect of digitalis on the heart is to produce an increase in contractility, occurring in both the failing[138] and nonfailing[139] heart (Table 11–12). The beneficial effects of digitalis in congestive heart failure occur because of this direct inotropic action and the resulting effects on autonomic reflexes. In congestive heart failure, in order to increase cardiac output and to maintain tissue perfusion, the heart must compensate by functioning at a higher preload.[140] In addition, autonomic reflexes result in increased peripheral vascular resistance and increased venous tone. Increases in heart rate and contractility depend

upon the degree of depletion of myocardial catecholamines. As preload and afterload increase, pressures in the left ventricle, left atrium, and pulmonary veins also increase. If pressures above 20 torr persist and lymphatic resorptive capacity is exceeded, pulmonary edema will ensue. Filling pressure may continue to increase without a corresponding increase in cardiac output. Digitalis allows the failing myocardium to move to a more efficient ventricular function curve. The increase in contractility enables the overloaded ventricle to empty more effectively. The increased dP/dt will result in an attenuation of baroreceptor-mediated autonomic reflexes. Decreased vasoconstriction will also allow the left ventricle to empty more effectively, and reduced venous tone will help to decrease the elevated ventricular filling pressure. The final outcome will be a ventricle able to sustain the necessary cardiac output at a lower preload.

The proposed site of action of digitalis is Na-K-ATPase.[132, 141–143] The most important site of Na-K-ATPase inhibition may be within the transverse tubular system of the myocardial cell.[142–144] By inhibiting extrusion of Na^+ by the Na^+-K^+-ATPase system, more intracellular Na^+ is available for exchange with extracellular Ca^{++}. Augmentation of Na^+-Ca^{++} exchange is therefore proposed to be the mechanism by which digitalis produces its positive inotropic response[145] (see also the chapter on myocardial cellular mechanism).

Table 11-12. Physiological Effects of Digoxin

	NORMAL	MYOCARDIAL DYSFUNCTION WITH CHF
Cardiac		
Contractility*	↑, Direct	↑, Direct
Rate	↓, Direct	↓, Indirect
Cardiac output	↓	↑
Improved ventricular emptying	nil	↓ LVEDP
Peripheral Vasculature		
Systemic vascular Resistance	↑, Direct	↓, Indirect
Venous tone	↑, Direct	↓, Indirect

*Myocardial O_2 consumption may increase in the normal heart, but decrease in the heart during CHF, because heart size and end diastolic wall tension may decrease with treatment.

Table 11-13. Electrophysiologic Effects of Digoxin on Myocardium

SITE	EFFECT	COMMENTS
SA node	Normal No effect	Mainly ↓ reflex

	CHF
	    ↓ Sympathetic tone
	    ↑ Vagal tone
	    ↓ Automaticity	

Atria	↑ Conduction velocity	Mainly vagotonic effect
A-V node	↓ Conduction velocity ↑ Refractory period	Combined vagotonic and direct effects
	↑ Automaticity	Seen at toxic levels
Purkinje system	↓ Conduction velocity ↑ Refractory period	Direct effect
Ventricle	↑ Automaticity ↓ Conduction velocity ↓ Refractory period	These effects seen at toxic levels; result in frequent ventricular ectopic beats

Patients in congestive heart failure will usually respond to digitalis with a slowing of heart rate. The major mechanism involved is the reduction in reflex sympathetic activity and increase in vagal activity on the sinus node. Subjects with normal ventricular function show no change in heart rate from digitalis.[146] Patients with sinus tachycardia, for reasons other than myocardial failure, should not receive digitalis in an attempt to slow heart rate.[123]

The electrophysiologic effects of digitalis are quite complex (Table 11–13). Rosen and coworkers[147] and Moe and Farah[123] provide complete reviews. The effect of digitalis on the sinus node results mainly from its influence on autonomic reflexes. The increased atrial conduction velocity, seen with digitalis, is a result of the vagotonic action of this drug. The rate of rise of phase 4 of the action potential is accelerated. The direct effect of digitalis, however, is to cause a reduction of membrane potential. This will antagonize the vagally mediated increase in conduction velocity. The end result will be the balance of these two mechanisms.

Slowing of conduction velocity through the A-V node is a result of both direct and vagotonic effects of digitalis. This effect makes digitalis extremely useful in the control of ventricular response to supraventricular tachyarrhythmias. Digitalis facilitates conduction through aberrant A-V pathways, such as occur in Wolff–Parkinson–White syndrome.[148] At toxic levels, digitalis may increase junctional automaticity. Thus, one of the rhythms seen with digitalis toxicity is a combination of junctional tachycardia with A-V block.

Digitalis slows the conduction velocity through the Purkinje system. Such slowing may predispose the heart to reentrant ventricular dysrhythmias. The added effect of decreased refractory period and increased ventricular automaticity, with toxic levels, explains why ventricular ectopic beats are the most common dysrhythmias seen with digitalis toxicity.

Therapeutic levels of digitalis produce the following effects on the ECG:

PR Interval: Increased but not usually more than 0.25 seconds

QT Interval: Shortened as a result of shortened action potential

ST Segment: Depressed in characteristic "scoop" wave pattern

T Wave: Usually flattened or inverted

The effects of digitalis on myocardial oxygen demand depend upon the state of ventricular function (see Table 11–12). Patients with normal myocardial function demonstrate an increased myocardial oxygen consumption in response to digitalis.[149] Patients with ventricular dysfunction and heart failure may decrease myocardial oxygen consumption in response to digitalis. The primary beneficial effect of digitalis is to reduce heart size and ventricular wall tension. The reduction in myocardial oxygen requirements are therefore greater than the increase produced by increasing contractility.

Significant vascular effects also occur in response to digitalis. Subjects with normal ventricular function demonstrate an increase in systemic vascular resistance, as well as increased venous tone, following digitalis administration.[150] This increase in systemic vascular resistance has been used to explain the lack of rise of cardiac output in normal subjects, despite an increase in contractility.[143] Patients with congestive heart failure, however, demonstrate a decrease in systemic vascular resistance and venous tone in response to digitalis.[150]

In patients with ventricular failure, the main action is reduction of reflex sympathetic tone by improving ventricular contractility. This may be facilitated by enhancement of baroreceptor function.[151] Subjects with normal ventricular function increase vascular tone by a mechanism which is not clear. Digitalis may exert effects at various levels of the sympathetic nervous system.[151] Peripheral vascular resistance increases in animals despite ganglionic blockade.[152] This indicates that digitalis produces at least a portion of its constricting effects by postganglionic sympathetic stimulation or direct action on vascular smooth muscle.

Clinical Uses

The routine use of digitalis in many cases of congestive heart failure is frequently questioned,[153] although its use for certain supraventricular dysrhythmias is undisputed.[154]

This arises mainly from the recognition that congestive heart failure often can be controlled with diuretics and vasodilator therapy.[155, 156]

Probably the most common use of digitalis is in congestive heart failure secondary to chronic ischemic heart disease. The combination of diuretic and digitalis is often beneficial in these patients. However, the hypokalemia produced by diuretics may increase the risk of digitalis toxicity. In addition, such a patient is often elderly and frequently has reduced renal function. This may produce toxicity if digitalis dosage is not adjusted carefully.

Hypertension is a frequent cause of congestive heart failure. In this situation, a favorable response is usually obtained with therapy directed at the increased afterload. Digitalis is reserved for those patients who do not respond completely to control of the hypertension.

Often the severely depressed myocardium with idiopathic cardiomyopathy will show no response to digitalis. Toxicity may occur if the dose is increased in order to obtain a favorable cardiovascular response. The one cardiomyopathy in which digitalis definitely should not be used is idiopathic hypertrophic subaortic stenosis (IHSS). In that situation, increased contractility will increase the gradient across the stenotic area.

In congenital and rheumatic valvular heart disease, the primary problem is usually mechanical in nature. Patients with mitral stenosis in sinus rhythm show no hemodynamic improvement with digitalis.[157, 158] Other lesions, however, impose an increased load on the myocardium and benefit may be gained from inotropic support with digitalis.[153]

The use of digitalis in cor pulmonale is controversial. Although it does improve right ventricular function,[159, 160] digitalis also increases pulmonary vascular resistance.[160] In addition, patients with pulmonary disease show a predisposition to digitalis toxicity. Green and Smith suggest that digitalis may be of benefit in cor pulmonale but should be used after other methods to reduce right ventricular afterload have failed.[160]

Digitalis use in acute ventricular failure is controversial. In cardiogenic shock,[161] despite an increase in contractility as measured by dP/dt, cardiac output increased minimally but clinical status was unimproved.[161] Two patients, following myocardial infarction, demonstrated an acute increase in LVEDP and developed ventricular fibrillation, following the use of digitalis. Da Luz and coworkers recommend that digitalis can be used only in situations in which the heart is enlarged.[162] The myocardium may be too badly damaged to respond to digitalis. If cardiac output does not increase in response to digitalis, the predominant effect may be an increased afterload secondary to the peripheral vascular effects of the drug. In addition, the hypoxemia, electrolyte imbalance, and reduced renal function that frequently accompany shock, may predispose to digitalis toxicity. A titratable inotropic agent, such as dopamine, is more desirable in such an unstable patient.

Digitalis is extremely useful in the treatment of the supraventricular tachyarrhythmias.[154] In atrial fibrillation, the reduction in A-V conduction allows a dose-related control of ventricular response. The same effect occurs in atrial flutter but higher doses of digitalis are often required.[163] In addition, enhanced atrial conduction may increase the rate of flutter or convert it to atrial fibrillation. When atrial flutter is associated with hemodynamic instability, cardioversion should provide the primary mode of therapy.

By slowing A-V conduction velocity and increasing refractory period, digitalis is useful in paroxysmal atrial tachycardia. However, this rhythm may be one of the manifestations of digitalis toxicity.[163] Although slowing of conduction through usual A-V pathways occurs, digitalis enhances conduction through aberrant pathways. For this reason, the drug should be used cautiously in the patient with Wolff–Parkinson–White syndrome. It also may convert atrial fibrillation to ventricular fibrillation.[163]

The prophylactic use of digitalis is still controversial. A lower incidence of supraventricular tachycardia in postoperative patients who were given digitalis before coronary artery bypass surgery is reported.[164] An increase in supraventricular arrhythmias in a similar group of patients given prophylactic digitalis is also reported.[165] Morrison and Killip found that patients developed evidence of digitalis toxicity at much lower serum digoxin levels, following open-heart surgery.[166] Difficulty arises when comparing such studies, because of numerous differences in pre-, intra-, and post-operative management between different centers. Selzer and Cohn caution against the prophylactic use of digitalis because of the low therapeutic ratio of the drug.[167]

Toxicity

In many patients there is little difference between the dose of digitalis which produces the desired clinical effect, and that dose which produces toxicity. Digitalis effects the central nervous, gastrointestinal, and cardiovascular systems. Mild lethargy, anorexia, or nausea may be difficult to interpret because these are often symptoms of congestive heart failure. Central nervous system toxicity produces confusion, psychosis, and seizures. Vomiting and diarrhea may result from stimulation of the chemoreceptor trigger zone and vagal motor centers in the brain stem.[127, 168] Visual disturbances such as transient scotomata and abnormalities of color vision are thought to result from retinal effects of digitalis.[168]

Unfortunately, cardiovascular toxicity may be the first manifestation of digitalis excess.[168] Cardiovascular signs of digitalis toxicity are related to the electrophysiologic actions of digitalis. Although certain dysrhythmias occur more frequently with digitalis toxicity, any known rhythm disturbance is possible (Table 11–14).[127, 168]

A number of factors may predispose to digitalis toxicity, either by potentiating the myocardial effects of the drug or by reducing elimination (Table 11–15). One of the most important predisposing factors is hypokalemia. Because of the frequent concomitant use of digitalis and diuretics, this is common. When correcting severe hypokalemia (occur-

Table 11-14. Rhythm Complications During Digitalis Treatment

SITE	ARRHYTHMIA	COMMENTS
Atria	Atrial fibrillation Atrial flutter	Atrial fibrillation and flutter are usually associated with slow ventricular rate
	Atrial tachycardia*	Usually associated with A-V block
A-V node	Second degree A-V block	Usually Mobitz I
A-V junction	Junctional tachycardia	
Purkinje system and ventricular muscle	Ventricular ectopics* Ventricular tachycardia Ventricular fibrillation	May be unifocal or multifocal: may be very difficult to correct

*Most commonly seen arrhythmias resulting from digitalis toxicity

Table 11-15. Factors Predisposing to Development of Digitalis Toxicity

FACTOR		COMMENTS
Metabolic:	Hypokalemia Hypomagnesemia Hypercalcemia Hypoxemia Acidosis	May all produce digitalis toxicity at lower digitalis tissue concentrations
Electrical cardioversion		If necessary should be started at low level
Renal failure		Causes reduced elimination. Dialysis may produce ↓ K⁺ AND ↓ Mg⁺⁺
Cardiopulmonary bypass		Tissue levels do not change but electrolyte and acid-base changes may occur.

ring with digitalis-induced A-V block), an increase in serum potassium may increase the degree of block. Hypomagnesemia frequently accompanies hypokalemia and may potentiate digitalis toxicity.[169]

Calcium increases digitalis toxicity and should be avoided if toxicity is present. Acidosis will increase the flux of potassium from the myocardial cell and thereby potentiate digitalis toxicity. Hypoxemia, by increasing anaerobic metabolism, will produce a similar effect.

Electrical cardioversion causes transmembrane electrolyte shifts as well as local myocardial catecholamine release, which may account for the potentiation of digitalis toxicity seen after electrical cardioversion.[170]

Renal failure may predispose to digitalis toxicity if dosage is not adjusted for reduced elimination. In addition, during dialysis, acute potassium and magnesium changes may occur, which may potentiate toxicity.

Although changes in serum digoxin level occur during cardiopulmonary bypass,[171] patients receiving digoxin preoperatively show no change in myocardial tissue digoxin levels when pre- and postcardiopulmonary bypass concentrations are compared.[172]

In many cases, the clinical manifestations of digitalis toxicity are the same as those resulting from the underlying disease. Currently available radioimmunoassays for the cardiac glycosides may aid in the diagnosis of digitalis toxicity.[173, 174] The generally accepted digoxin therapeutic range is 1.5 to 3.0 mg/ml.[170] Levels which may be therapeutic in a patient at one time may produce toxicity at another. Also, levels which normally would be considered toxic may be necessary to achieve the desired clinical response in some patients. This applies especially to the use of digitalis for control of supraventricular arrhythmias.[134] The diagnostic value of serum digitalis levels has, therefore, been questioned strongly.[175, 176]

If toxicity is suspected, further administration should be withheld. Any disturbances of electrolyte, acid-base, or blood-gas status should be corrected. Potassium replacement should be withheld in patients with a high degree A-V block unless hypokalemia is very severe. If the rhythm disturbance consists only of occasional ectopic beats, first degree A-V block, or atrial fibrillation with a slow ventricular response, temporary withdrawal of the drug and readjustment of subsequent dosage may be all that is necessary. More ominous or hemodynamically significant dysrhythmias will require further management.

Marked sinus bradycardia, or second or third degree A-V block should be treated with atropine. If this is not successful, temporary transvenous pacing may be necessary. Diphenylhydantoin or lidocaine are useful for digitalis-induced ventricular arrhythmias. In addition, diphenylhydantoin can be used for supraventricular arrhythmias. Propranolol has been used for digitalis toxicity but may cause myocardial depression and further decrease in A-V conduction. Procainamide and quinidine are not recommended for use in digitalis toxicity.[127] Electrical cardioversion should be avoided unless absolutely necessary; if it must be used, a low energy level should be employed.

GLUCAGON

Pharmacology

Glucagon is a polypeptide hormone produced by pancreatic alpha cells. Its cardiac effects were first described by Farah and Tuttle in 1960.[177] Increases in contractility and heart rate occurred following addition of glucagon to a dog heart-lung preparation. Subsequent studies confirmed this action and found that it could not be blocked with propranolol,[178–181] or abolished with reserpine

pretreatment.[178, 180] The mechanism by which glucagon produces this response is unclear, although it may activate membrane adenyl cyclase by binding to a site which is separate from the adrenergic receptor.[182] In this way it can increase intramyocardial c-AMP in spite of β blockade.[182]

The cardiovascular effects of glucagon in humans were first studied by Parmley and coworkers in 1968.[179] Doses of 1 mg given to adult patients increased cardiac index and systolic ejection rate, and decreased systemic vascular resistance. Doses of 3 to 5 mg increased systolic ejection rate and heart rate. No significant change in systemic vascular resistance occurred with the higher dose. A number of patients in this study were fully digitalized, and showed improvements in myocardial contractility with no precipitation of arrhythmias.

Glucagon produces an increase in myocardial oxygen consumption with a corresponding increase in coronary blood flow.[180, 181, 183] The direct effects of glucagon on the coronary circulation are unclear but may produce coronary vasodilation in animals.[182]

Glucagon stimulates S-A and A-V automaticity without increasing ventricular automaticity.[184] However, when administered to subjects in doses of 50 μg/kg over 30 seconds, supraventricular and ventricular extrasystoles were produced.[185]

Glucagon is available for parenteral use only. For cardiovascular effects, the drug may be given as an intravenous bolus of 1 to 5 mg or as an infusion of 2 to 5 mg/hr. Onset of action occurs in 3 to 5 minutes with a duration of 20 to 30 minutes. Glucagon is metabolized by proteolytic enzymes in liver, kidney, tissue receptor sites, and plasma.[186]

Clinical Uses

Vaughn and coworkers found a marked improvement in heart rate, stroke volume, and cardiac output in patients receiving glucagon on the first postoperative day following open heart surgery.[187] Systemic vascular resistance showed a variable response. Glucagon also has been shown to improve myocardial function in patients in cardiogenic shock secondary to acute myocardial infarction.[188]

Patients with chronic myocardial dysfunction do not, however, respond as favorably to the inotropic effects of glucagon.[189] The lack of inotropic response may be caused by an inability of glucagon to bind to its receptor.[182]

Another potential role for glucagon may be to improve myocardial contractility in patients who are taking β-blocking medications. Ward and Jones described the successful use of glucagon in the resuscitation of a man who had received an overdose of oxprenolol.[190]

Risks

Glucagon may produce a significant tachycardia, with resulting detrimental effects on myocardial oxygen supply and demand. Its effects on the A-V node may suddenly increase ventricular rate if given to a patient in atrial flutter or fibrillation. Because glucagon can cause release of catecholamines from pheochromocytomas, it should be avoided in the patient in whom this problem is known or suspected.

Because glycogenolysis is stimulated, hyperglycemia may result from glucagon administration. Insulin release, in response to an increased blood glucose, will cause entry of glucose into cells. The accompanying intracellular shift of potassium may produce hypokalemia.[182] In addition, prolonged use or abrupt discontinuation of a glucagon infusion may result in hypoglycemia.

The most commonly observed side-effect seen with glucagon is nausea and vomiting. While this is not a problem with anesthetized patients, it may cause significant distress in the awake patient. Concomitant administration of an antiemetic may be necessary.

CALCIUM

Pharmacology

Calcium is a divalent cation which plays an important role in cellular function. A detailed discussion of calcium and its effect on the myocardial cell is provided in Chapter 3.

The distribution of calcium in the body is illustrated in Figure 11–4. Ninety percent of the body's calcium is complexed with phos-

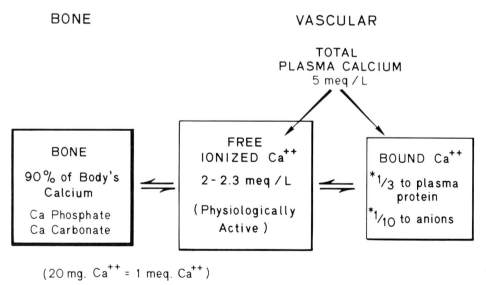

Fig. 11–4. Calcium hemostasis. Physiologically active calcium is in equilibrium with bound calcium and calcium stored in bone. (* indicates fraction of total calcium which is bound)

phate and carbonate in bone. Under the influence of parathyroid hormone, calcitonin, and vitamin D, bone stores exist in an equilibrium with serum calcium. One-third of serum calcium is bound to plasma protein and one-tenth is bound to serum anions.[191] The remainder, free ionized calcium, is the physiologically active form.

Alkalosis increases protein binding of calcium and may decrease free calcium levels. Acidosis has the opposite effect. Rapid blood transfusion, with sudden increases in serum citrate concentration, may reduce free ionized calcium.[192] This reduction is directly related to the rate of blood transfusion. The effect is short-lived, provided that rapid redistribution and hepatic metabolism of citrate occurs.

The positive inotropic effects of calcium have been demonstrated in various experimental preparations[193, 194] as well as in awake[195] and anesthetized[196] human subjects. Calcium also has been shown to reverse the negative inotropic effects of nitrous oxide[197] and halothane[198] in isolated papillary muscle.

Calcium decreases heart rate in healthy human subjects[195, 196] probably by a reflex vagal mechanism. Vagotomy or atropine pretreatment has been shown to abolish calcium-induced bradycardia.[199] The denervated heart increases its rate of contraction in response to calcium.[193, 194] Atrioventricular conduction is delayed by both increased and reduced calcium levels.[199] By shortening phase 2 of the myocardial action potential, calcium produces a shortened QT interval on the ECG. Comparison of the similar electrophysiologic actions of calcium and digitalis illustrates the hazards of giving calcium to a patient with digitalis toxicity.

Sialer and coworkers, using relatively high infusion rates of calcium chloride in pentobarbital-anesthetized dogs, showed a slight increase in peripheral vascular resistance.[199] Awake calves, with artificial hearts, showed a decrease in peripheral vascular resistance in response to calcium chloride, 5 and 10 mg/kg IV.[200] In humans, Denlinger and coworkers demonstrated a decreased systemic vascular resistance, with 7 mg/kg of calcium chloride, during halothane anesthesia.[196] Lappas and coworkers observed a 10 percent increase in systemic vascular resistance, with no change in cardiac output from 5 mg/kg of calcium chloride.[201] Factors such as body temperature, acid-base levels, and electrolyte balance may have influenced this response.

For an immediate cardiovascular response, the recommended dose of calcium chloride is from 5 to 10 mg/kg intravenously over a period of several minutes. The duration of action of such a dose will be approximately fifteen minutes.[196] Calcium gluconate is also available for use but provides significantly less calcium ion on an equal volume basis:

10 ml 10% calcium gluconate = 4.5 meq Ca^{++}
10 ml 10% calcium chloride = 13.6 meq Ca^{++}

Even when doses providing an equivalent amount of calcium ion are administered, the chloride salt provides a more pronounced cardiovascular response.[202]

Clinical Use

Calcium is used commonly in the immediate post cardiopulmonary bypass period after cardiac surgery. Administration of from 0.5 to 2.0 grams of calcium chloride may aid the heart in recovering from hyperkalemic cardioplegia, the period of ischemia during aortic cross-clamping, and overcome the citrate load which may occur during blood administration. If the heart is still failing after rewarming of the heart, optimal oxygenation, and correction of acid-base and electrolyte abnormalities, a continuous infusion of a sympathomimetic agent may be necessary. Occasionally an infusion of an epinephrine and calcium combination (epi-cal) provides inotropic support where dopamine or isoproterenol fails.

Drop and coworkers have found low ionized calcium concentrations in a number of critically ill patients demonstrating low-flow hemodynamic states.[203, 204] These patients frequently required calcium doses as high as 1.5 mg/kg/min to correct ionized calcium levels.[203] In addition, such a poor correlation existed between total serum calcium and ionized calcium that the authors recommended frequent direct measurement of ionized calcium for such patients.[203] In many of their patients, serum calcium levels did not correct until hemodynamic status was improved by infusing isoproterenol. Calcium may be of use in any situation where an inotropic response is required, but an increase in heart rate is to be avoided.

In addition to its use in the cardiac surgical patient, calcium is used also as a cardiac stimulant during cardiopulmonary resuscitation. It may be useful especially for electromechanical dissociation caused by severe myocardial depression. For this purpose a rapid intravenous dose of 0.5–1.0 g is used. Sodium bicarbonate and calcium chloride must not mix in the intravenous tubing; if this occurs, calcium carbonate will form and plug the intravenous tubing. Calcium also is useful as one of the acute pharmacologic measures in the treatment of hyperkalemia.

Risks

The relative safety of calcium makes it a popular agent in situations in which an inotropic response is required, without major effects on heart rate or vascular resistance. Hypercalcemia may result during chronic use.

Calcium should be administered slowly. Lloyd in 1928 described vividly the effect of rapid injection of 4 ml of 10 percent calcium chloride into his own circulation.[205] The result was profound S-A block with cardiorespiratory arrest, requiring his assistant to provide almost five minutes of cardiopulmonary resuscitation. This caution is emphasized by Howland with respect to the routine use of calcium with blood transfusions.[206] The risks include S-A and A-V block as well as increased ventricular irritability.

A major risk of calcium administration is in the patient with digitalis toxicity. Eliot and coworkers demonstrated the ability to reverse digitalis-induced dysrhythmias by chelating ionized calcium with sodium ethylene diamine tetraacetate (EDTA).[207] In this same study, ventricular fibrillation occurred immediately after calcium gluconate was given

to a 9-month-old, digitalis-toxic baby, in the treatment of tetany. Administration of a digitalis glycoside to hypercalcemic dogs also demonstrated toxic dysrhythmias at much lower digitalis doses.[208] Calcium should be avoided in any patient where digitalis toxicity is suspected. A summary of the inotropic agonists and their clinical uses is provided in Table 11–16.

INOTROPIC ANTAGONISTS

Armed with the knowledge presented earlier in this chapter, the reader now is ready to evaluate the blockade of β-receptors and the clinical effects which occur secondary to the use of β-blocking drugs. The early understanding of receptors occurred because of Ahlquist in 1948.[209] With the discovery of dichloroisoprenaline (dichloroisoproterenol or DCI) by Powell and Slater 10 years later, β-receptor blockade was demonstrated.[210] Since that time, many compounds have been shown to exert blocking activity at the β₁ and β₂ receptors. Some of the available drugs with such activity are shown in Figure 11–5. Some of these are now available within the United States for clinical use. Practolol and alprenolol are not available in the United States because of carcinogenicity and other adverse effects.[211]

PHARMACOLOGY

Many of these drugs enjoy a wide spectrum of activity, while others behave in a "selective" manner. Obviously, drug structure is responsible for the position of the drug within the spectrum. From the clinician's viewpoint, the arbitrary categorization of each drug into "cardioselective" or "nonselective" categories serves a useful purpose. A "cardioselective" drug is one which, in the ideal sense, exhibits only β₁ cardiac blocking effects. All of these drugs exhibit competitive activity at the β receptor(s), and thus, the same effect may be provided by several different drugs if each is used at its own individual dose for that effect. Since selectivity

Table 11-16. Inotropic Agonists—Summary

CLINICAL DISORDER	THERAPEUTIC AIM	INOTROPIC AGONIST	ALTERNATIVE	COMMENTS
Chronic CHF secondary to ischemia/hypertension	Reduce ventricular size and wall tension ($\downarrow MVO_2$)	Digoxin	New oral agents being tested but not available	Should be used after primary measures have failed: Ischemia: nitrates $\downarrow$Preload: nitrates, diuretics $\downarrow$Afterload: antihypertensives
Acute myocardial infarction with cardiogenic shock	1 Maintain organ perfusion 2 Reduce ventricular wall tension	Dopamine	Dobutamine	1. Very high risk of increasing ischemia or injury 2. Risk of arrhythmias
Septic shock	Enable cardiac output to keep up with very low peripheral resistance	Dopamine	1. $CaCl_2$ 2. Norephinephrine (occasionally)	Adjunct: to other therapeutic measures: 1. Antibiotics 2. Optimize volume status 3. Steroids
Rheumatic or congenital cardiac disease	Enable myocardium to cope with increased load, until mechanical defect is corrected	Dopamine (acute) Digoxin (chronic)		Primary therapy is correction of mechanical lesion
Idiopathic congestive cardiomyopathy	Assist primary dysfunctional myocardial cells	Vasodilator and dopamine (acute) Digoxin (chronic)	Dobutamine	Response to inotropic therapy is extremely variable
Postcardiopulmonary bypass	Enable myocardium to recover from 1. ischemia 2. hypothermia 3. hyperkalemic cardioplegia 4. surgical manipulation	1. $CaCl_2$ 2. Dopamine	1. Epinephrine 2. Dobutamine if peripheral resistance is very high	Other factors must be optimized 1. Temperature 2. Rhythm 3. Oxygenation 4. Acid-base balance 5. Electrolyte balance 6. Volume status
Postcardiac transplant	1. As above 2. Inotropic and chronotropic support of denervated heart	Isoproterenol	Dopamine	1. As above 2. Dose is titrated to heart rate
Anesthetic-induced myocardial depression Volatile agents N_2O	Help to restore myocardial function while agent is being eliminated	$CaCl_2$	1. Ephedrine 2. Dopamine	Sympathomimetics should be avoided with violatile agent, if possible, because of potential for arrhythmias

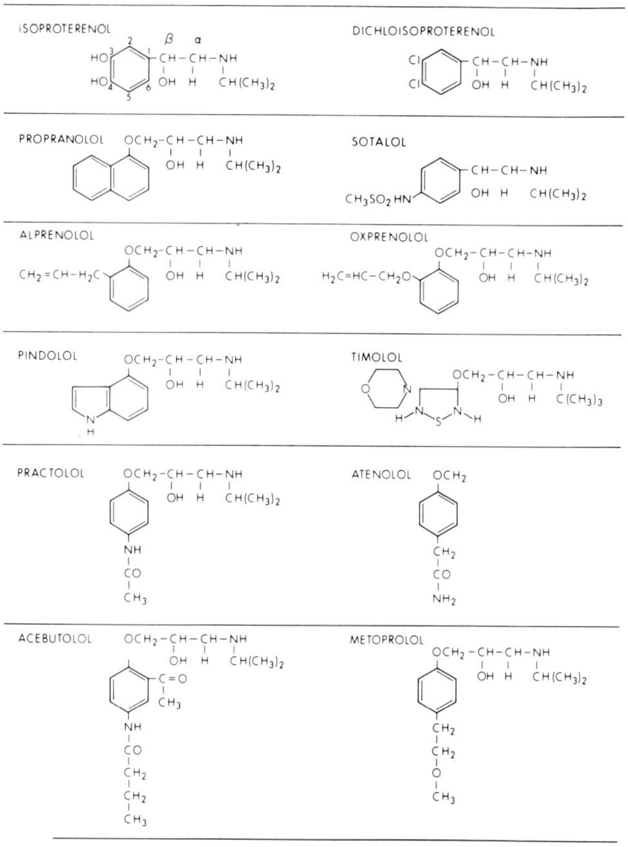

Fig. 11–5. Structural formulas of available beta-blocking drugs. (Frishman W: Clinical pharmacology of the new beta-adrenergic blocking drugs. Part I. Am Heart J 97:663–670, 1979)

thus may be *dose-dependent,* such categorization is, at best, a rough one, and is useful *only* if the dose is specified. The dose specified for purposes here is usually an average dose used in human patients, and should not be extrapolated either to other species, nor to dramatically different doses. Virtually all β-blocking drugs exhibit a spectrum of selective versus nonselective functions.

In addition to the above two categories, each drug may be subcategorized further into categories of those drugs which have membrane stabilizing effects (MSE) or intrinsic sympathomimetic activity (ISA), or both. Those drugs exhibiting MSE decrease the rate of rise of a cell membrane action potential, but do not alter either the resting potential or the spike duration. Those drugs exhibiting MSE act independently of β-receptor competitive inhibition.[211] ISA implies direct agonist activity of the drug on the β receptor, even in the absence of the usual agonist for

that receptor. Those drugs exhibiting ISA should counteract some or all of the effects of β blockade. For example, pindolol has ISA, compared to propranolol which does not and should produce a lesser decrease in heart rate than propranolol when each is administered in a dose producing equivalent β-receptor blockade.[211] Figure 11–6 and Table 11–17, demonstrate further the comparative properties and categories of each of these drugs.

Potency is determined by comparing the β-blocking action of each drug to the heart rate effects of isoproterenol, yielding a rough potency scale in the following order: pindolol (most potent), timolol, propranolol, atenolol, metoprolol, oxprenolol, acebutolol, alprenolol, practolol, and sotalol (see Table 11–17).

Potency with respect just to β_1 activity demonstrates that acebutolol, atenolol, metoprolol, and practolol are 50 to 100 times more potent at β_1 receptors than at β_2 receptors. These four antagonists thus would be

Fig. 11–6. Categorization of the available beta-blocking drugs by nonselective and cardioselective categories. Further breakdown by intrinsic sympathomimetic activity (ISA) and membrane stabilizing effects (MSE) provides a convenient method of displaying spectrum of activity. Roman numerals depict the grouping as provided by Fitzgerald. (from Prichard BNC: Beta-adrenergic receptor blockade in hypertension, past, present, and future. Br J Clin Pharm 5:379–399, 1978)

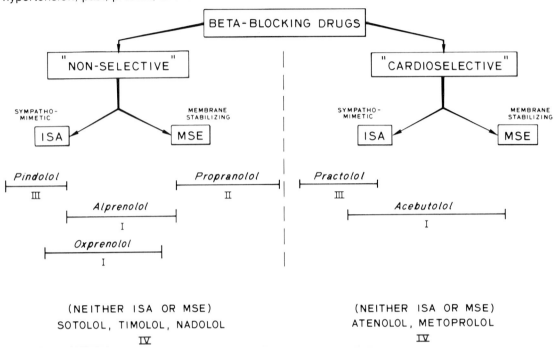

Table 11-17. Basic Properties of β-Blocking Drugs

ORAL DRUG	BRAND	SELECTIVE/ NONSELECTIVE	AGONIST OR SYMPATHOMIMETIC ACTIVITY (ISA)	MEMBRANE STABILIZING EFFECTS (MSE)	COMMENTS
Propranolol	Inderal Avlocardin	NS	No	Yes	The prototype drug; most experience
Practolol	Eraldin	Sel	Yes	No	First Cardioselective drug developed; withdrawn 2° toxic effects
Oxprenolol	Trasicor	NS	Yes	Minimal	Equal potency with propranolol
Alprenolol	Aptin Betaptin Betacard	NS	Yes	Yes	No special advantages
Pindolol	Visken	NS	Yes (strong)	Minimal	Most potent β-blocker; longer duration of action
Sotalol	Betacardone Sotacor	NS	No	No	Half-life = 10 hr; twice daily dose
Timolol	Blocadren	NS	No	No	≈ 6× more potent than propranolol; 15–45mg/d (not for oral use in US)
Acebutolol	Sectral	? (Sel in animals)	Yes	Yes	—
Atenolol	Atenol Tenormin	Sel	No	No	Half-life 7 hours
Metoprolol	Betaloc Lopresor	Sel	No	±	Approved for hypertension Rx. Best drug for asthmatic or COPD patient
Nadolol	Corgard	NS	?	?	Approved for hypertension and angina Long half-life; once daily dose

likely candidates for selective cardiac β_1 blockade, with minimum β_2 blockade. The patient with pulmonary asthma requiring beta blocking for cardiovascular control (hypertension, angina pectoris, etc.) *might* be treated more optimally with an approved drug exhibiting cardioselective β_1 blockade at clinical doses. Presently, metoprolol would be the approved drug of choice.

ABSORPTION AND METABOLISM

Individual variability is the rule. All of these drugs (see Figure 11–5), except atenolol and nadolol, are well absorbed from the gastrointentinal tract (see Table 11–18), and reach peak plasma concentrations in 2 to 4 hours. The presence of food within the stomach enhances the absorption of propranolol and metoprolol (see Fig. 11–7).[212] Many other factors will determine the plasma concentration of β-blocking drugs, especially the hepatic deactivation of drugs which occurs after portal vein absorption. In very high doses, hepatic alteration may be less effective, so that deactivation may not be related linearly to dose. Because of this first-pass phenomenon, a large oral dose may be required to produce the same effect as a very small intravenous

dose. For instance, a patient receiving orally several hundred milligrams of propranolol to decrease heart rate to 60 beats per minute may require only from 0.5 to 1.0 mg propranolol IV to produce the same effect. Practolol (and perhaps nadolol) is the least affected by hepatic metabolism, whereas propranolol and metoprolol are greatly affected (see Table 11–18). The elderly patient may exhibit higher plasma concentrations than the young patient, unrelated to degree of concomitant hypertension (Fig. 11–8).[213]

Drugs with high lipid solubility (propranolol, alprenolol) may cross the blood-brain (and placental?) barrier and produce central nervous system effects. Those with low lipid solubility (practolol, metoprolol) do not. Protein binding is less well understood, but seems to parallel roughly lipid solubility. Alprenolol is bound to plasma protein approximately 85 percent, while metoprolol is bound 12 percent. It is reported that the administration of heparin to a patient may increase the availability of free propranolol.[214] It has been speculated that the presence of heparin increases the level of free fatty acids because of heparin's lipoprotein lipase activity. Additional free fatty acids then might serve to displace propranolol from plasma

Table 11-18. Potency, Plasma Elimination, Absorption, and Metabolism of β-Blocking Drugs

DRUG	BRAND	POTENCY (PROPRANOLOL = 1)	PLASMA ONE-HALF LIFE (HOURS)	ORAL USE ABSORPTION	METABOLISM ORAL DOSE
Propranolol	Inderal Avlocardin	1	3–6	>90%	99%
Practolol	Eraldin	0.3	6–8	>95%	<10%
Oxprenolol	Trasicor	0.5–1	2	70–95%	
Alprenolol	Aptin Betaptin Betacard	0.3	2–3	>90%	99%
Pindolol	Visken	6	3–4	>90%	≈60%
Sotalol	Betacardone Sotacor	0.3	5–13		≈40%
Timolol	Blocadren	6	4–5	>90%	≈80%
Acebutolol	Sectral	0.3	8		
Atenolol	Atenol Tenormin	1	6–9		≈60%
Metoprolol	Betaloc Lopressor	1	3–4	>95%	≈97%
Nadolol	Corgard	?	14–17	≈33%	10–20%?

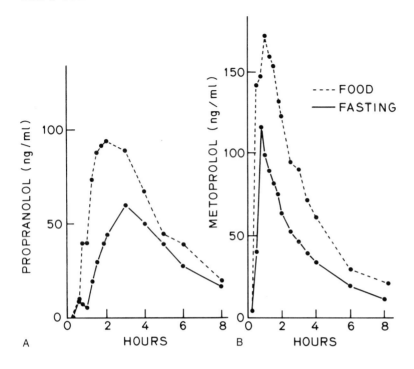

Fig. 11–7. Concentrations of (A) propranolol (serum) and (B) metoprolol (plasma) in two healthy volunteers following ingestion of single doses (80 and 100 mg, respectively) of the drugs on an empty stomach (solid line) and together with a standardized breakfast (broken line). The concentrations were higher when the drugs were ingested during nonfasting conditions. (from Melander A, Danielson K, Schersten B et al: Clin Pharmacol Ther 22:108–112, 1977)

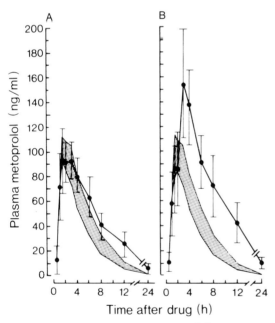

Fig. 11–8. Mean plasma metoprolol concentrations (± s.e. mean) in (A) hypertensive and (B) elderly subjects. The shaded area represents the mean values for young volunteers (± s.e. mean). (Kendall MJ, Brown D, Yates RA: Plasma metoprolol concentrations in young, old, and hypertensive subjects. Br J Clin Pharm 4:497–499, 1977)

proteins, increasing the concentration of free propranolol. Assay selectivity and specificity have been questioned. This effect remains controversial, and has not been confirmed by others at the time of submission of this manuscript.

PHARMACOKINETICS

Beta-blocking drugs are distributed rapidly, but with individual differences. The average plasma half-life is from 2 to 4 hours and is related to lipid solubility (see Table 11–18) and renal excretion.[215] Half-life can be decreased by hemodialysis. The use of a β-blocking drug with a long half-life (nadolol; see Table 11–18) offers a reduced dosage schedule, but increases the risk of accumulation and toxicity, especially if renal or hepatic function is impaired. Hepatic disease or dysfunction will increase the half-life of those beta-blocking drugs substantially metabolized in the liver.[215] In the patient with decreased hepatic or renal function, or both, monitoring of plasma levels of β-blocking drug(s) is advised.

The relationship between plasma concentration of a β-blocking drug and a therapeutic effect may be quite variable. Sympathetic tone may alter therapeutic effect without regard to plasma concentration. Active metabolites of a β-blocking drug may alter therapeutic effect, but be unmeasured by drug assay; 4-hydroxypropranolol is such a compound.[216] In general, however, a reasonable fit occurs between the log plasma level and the β-blocking effects of most β-blocking drugs to isoproterenol-induced, or exercise-induced, tachycardia in patients. A thorough review of this relationship is presented by Johnsson and Regàrdh.[215]

MAJOR PHYSIOLOGICAL AND METABOLIC EFFECTS

Hypertension

Beta-blocking drugs are used presently in the treatment of hypertension from whatever cause[217] (Fig. 11–9). If cardiac output is above normal, the effect of a beta-blocking drug in decreasing ventricular contractility and thus cardiac output, will result in a decrease in blood pressure, all other variables remaining constant. The ability of systemic vascular resistance to increase will determine the final effect on blood pressure with changes in cardiac output (Fig. 11–10).[217] A nonselective β-blocking drug, such as propranolol, will block the β_2 vasodilating effects of catecholamines, leaving unopposed α effects and a resultant increase in systemic vascular resistance. A cardioselective drug is preferred.

It is thought that some of the blood pressure lowering effects of β-blocking drugs are caused by central nervous system depression, but this is poorly understood. Both the l and the d,l forms of propranolol cause a decrease in blood pressure if present in the cerebral ventricles.[218] d-Propranolol, however, causes an increase in blood pressure when present in the cerebral ventricles.[218]

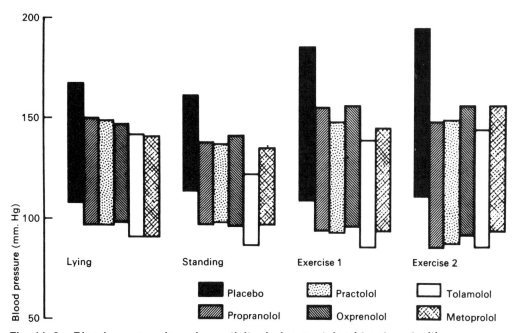

Fig. 11–9. **Blood pressure lowering activity during sustained treatment with beta-adrenoreceptor antagonists possessing different ancillary pharmacological properties.** Data from a double-blind randomized crossover study in 25 patients with stable, uncomplicated essential hypertension. Shown in the figure are the blood pressure values (determined 1 hour after an oral dose) at the end of 8 weeks' treatment. (Gross F (ed): The cardioprotective action of beta-blockers, p 84. Berne, Hans Huber)

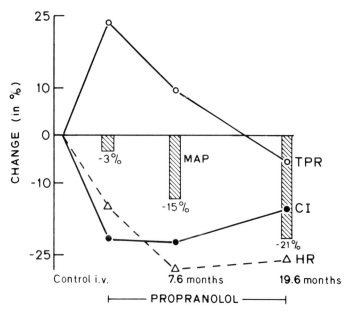

Fig. 11–10. Changes recorded in ten hypertensive patients in response to intravenous injection of propranolol and to long-term oral treatment with this beta-blocker. The changes in cardiac index (CI), total peripheral resistance (TPR), and heart rate (HR), as well as the decrease in mean arterial pressure (MAP), are all expressed in percentages of the pretreatment values. (From Gross F (ed): The cardioprotective action of beta-blockers, p 30. Berne, Hans Huber)

Lipid soluble β-blocking drugs would be more likely to exert central nervous system effects.

Beta-blocking drugs are associated with a decrease in renin release from the kidney during sympathetic stimulation.[218] The l form of propranolol, but not the d form, is active at the renin release site, in both hypertensive and non-hypertensive patients. Some β-blocking drugs, such as pindolol, have demonstrated *increased* renin release in animals,[219] probably caused by agonist ISA properties. Renin release likely is mediated by β receptors in humans. Blood pressure control with β-blocking drugs may be unrelated to renin release in some patients; however, the patient with high renin responds more faborably to propranolol than the patient with low renin.[218]

If a β-blocking drug is used without an α-blocking drug, the resultant increase in systemic vascular resistance (SVR) following decreased cardiac output may leave blood pressure unchanged. The addition of one or more drugs that can block an increase in SVR (by any method) will augment the blood-pressure-lowering effects of the β-blocking agent. In addition, the use of a cardioselective β-blocking drug will leave β2 vasodilating activity intact.

Propranolol does not affect the ability of insulin to decrease plasma glucose concentrations or change resting plasma glucose or insulin levels. The β receptor for insulin release is probably a β2 receptor, requiring substantial blockade.[218] Release of glucose by glycolytic mechanisms in muscle is blocked by β-blocking drugs. Propranolol decreases free fatty acid levels at rest, or in fasting and exercise states, and blocks the lipolytic effects of isoproterenol. Because glycolysis is impaired, propranolol (or other nonselective β-blocking drugs) should be used with caution in the diabetic patient. A cardioselective drug appears to be a better choice for treatment of angina or hypertension in the diabetic patient.

Angina Pectoris

Coronary heart disease produces symptoms when myocardial oxygen demand exceeds supply and local or systemic regulatory mechanisms fail to correct perfusion imbalance. Beta-blocking drugs are used to decrease those variables which promote increased oxygen utilization. Thus, if a β-blocking drug can decrease heart rate, contractile force and velocity, and promote cardiac efficiency (longer diastolic coronary artery perfusion time and greater ejection fraction), symptoms of ischemia may decrease or cease. Beta-blocking drugs decrease heart rate, left ventricular pressure rate of rise (dp/dt), and ventricular systolic pressure. The l form of propranolol is more potent than the d form in producing a decrease in myocardial oxygen consumption. As myocardial oxygen demand decreases, local regulatory mechanisms may lead to a decrease in coronary blood flow. This is thought to be an indirect effect during β-blocking drug therapy.[218] During such alterations in coronary artery flow and resistance, subendocardial blood flow appears to be maintained.[220]

Even though exercise tolerance may improve, the rate-pressure product (heart rate times systolic blood pressure) at which angina occurs may be *less* during β-blockade.[218] This may occur if left ventricular size increases with β blockade, producing an increase in myocardial oxygen demand based upon an increase in muscle fiber stretching.

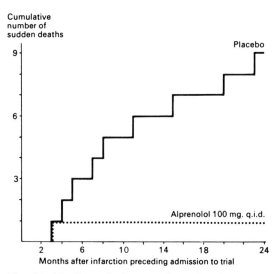

Fig. 11–12. Cumulative number of sudden deaths in the group treated with alprenolol and the placebo group during the 2-year follow-up period. (Gross F (ed): The cardioprotective action of beta-blockers, p 62. Berne, Hans Huber)

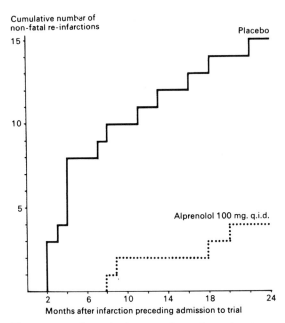

Fig. 11–11. Cumulative number of nonfatal reinfarctions in the group treated with alprenolol and the placebo group during the 2-year follow-up period. (Gross F (ed): The cardioprotective action of beta-blockers, p 62. Berne, Hans Huber)

Beta-blocking drugs without agonist properties (ISA), such as propranolol and metoprolol, may produce greater decreases in heart rate, for equal β receptor blockade, than drugs with ISA. The patient who requires β-blocking drug therapy for the control of angina pectoris, should receive a dose titrated to produce the asymptomatic state. This often is a heart rate of approximately 60 beats per minute (resting), with 80 to 90 beats per minute during moderate exercise.

All β-blocking drugs tested in humans have been found effective in the treatment of angina, although doses and side-effects vary. Chronic administration of alprenolol, as compared to placebo, has been shown to decrease the incidence of nonfatal myocardial reinfarction[217] (Fig. 11–11), and decrease the incidence of sudden death (Fig. 11–12).[217]

In the presence of asthma or chronic obstructive pulmonary disease, a cardioselective drug, such as approved metoprolol, should be preferable to a nonselective drug. (See Tables 11–17 and 11–19, and Fig. 11–6). The cardioselective drug will be *less likely* to be associated with increased bronchial or airway tone, but not necessarily free of that

Table 11-19. Practical Use of Available β-Blocking Drugs

	β_1	β_2	IV DOSE RANGE	AVERAGE DAILY ORAL DOSE RANGE	COMMENTS
Propranolol	√	√	0.25 mg increments	20–600 mg	May exacerbate asthma, AV block, or CHF Potent IV Titrate to HR or contractility ↓
Metoprolol	√		?	50–300 mg	Cardioselective at average dose; best for asthmatic or COPD patient
Nadolol	√	√	?	80–300 mg	Long acting: once a day dose; May exacerbate asthma, AV block, or CHF
Timolol	√	√	?	Not used orally in US	Opthalmic use for glaucoma May ↓ HR if sufficient dosage absorbed systemically

potential. Beta$_2$ agonist treatment (such as with salbutamol) still may be required in the asthmatic patient, and will be tolerated better and demonstrate pulmonary improvement if the patient is receiving a cardioselective drug for angina or hypertension.

Arrhythmia Treatment

Beta-blocking drugs produce a decrease in the slope of the action potential in pacemaker tissue. The membrane stabilizing effects (MSE) are quinidine-like or local anesthetic-like on cardiac cells. Very large doses of propranolol are needed for this effect. Practolol has no MSE, but is effective at arrhythmia control. d-Propranolol has MSE, but no β_1 blocking action, and is only weakly effective at arrhythmia control. Thus, arrhythmia control is most likely related to the β_1 blocking activity of these drugs, and not to MSE.

Beta blockade decreases the rate of S-A node discharge, decreases the rate of ectopic pacemaker activity, and increases the A-V refractory period. Thus, all β-blocking drugs in clinical use today have the potential of producing substantial A-V block. Beta-blocking drugs with agonist properties (ISA), such as pindolol, practolol, and alprenolol, help protect from complete A-V block. There are no ISA drugs approved for clinical use presently. Because of the decrease in S-A node discharge activity, β-blocking drugs should not be used in the patient with sick sinus syndrome unless a working pacemaker is in place. Specific differences between the various β-blocking drugs use for arrythmia treatment are not documentable. In general, *all* drugs available for clinical use have been found effective.

Beta blockade in the treatment of supraventricular arrhythmias may show variable results. Beta blockade in the treatment of digitalis toxicity is effective, along with potassium therapy. Because of effects on the A-H interval, and refractory periods of reentry pathways, β blockade may be useful in forms of supraventricular tachycardia. Atrial fibrillation and atrial flutter may respond to β blockade, because of decreased A-V conduction, but digitalis preparations are the drugs of choice. Treatment of ventricular arrhythmias by beta blockade is most effective if digitalis toxicity or catecholamines are the cause of ventricular irritability. In the patient with intractable ventricular tachycardia or ventricular fibrillation, β-blocking drugs having MSE properties may be effective prophylaxis or treatment.

Miscellaneous Effects

Propranolol and alprenolol (but not practolol or α-blocking drugs) block the exercise-induced increase in plasma levels of coagulation factor VIII. Exercise-induced fibrinolytic activity is blocked by propranolol but not by practolol. Propranolol has been shown to interfere with platelet aggregation produced by ADP, epinephrine, or exposure of platelets to collagen and thrombin.[218] Both d- and l-propranolol exhibit similar effects.

Practolol does not appear to inhibit platelet aggregation. These findings would suggest that the membrane stabilizing effects of β-blocking drugs are responsible for inhibition of platelet aggregation. If so, this side-effect upon platelet aggregation might serve a useful function during β-blocking treatment for angina pectoris.

Beta$_2$ agonist activity produces uterine muscle relaxation. Beta$_2$ antagonism produces an increase in uterine tone, inhibiting uterine relaxation between contractions. Beta$_2$ antagonism makes uterine muscle more sensitive to oxytocin.[221] The pregnant patient receiving a β-blocking drug may deliver a high enough concentration of β blocker to the fetus to produce fetal cardiovascular effects. Fetal bradycardia and an attenuation of the ability of the fetus to increase heart rate in response to intrauterine stress may accompany β blockade.[222] Propranolol antagonizes the release of renin by the uterus; clinical implications of this effect are unclear.

CLINICAL IMPLICATIONS

Beta-blocking drugs are used for treatment of many diseases. Hypertension, angina pectoris, and cardiac arrhythmias have been presented above. Additional diseases in which β blockade may be useful (or necessary) included IHSS, hyperthyroidism, and pheochromocytoma. These drugs have been tried in the treatment of migraine headaches, anxiety states, schizophrenia, tremors, narcotic and alcohol withdrawal, and open-angle glaucoma, but are not approved presently by the FDA for some of these conditions.[223]

Timolol has FDA approval for ophthalmic use in chronic open-angle glaucoma.[224–226] It is a potent nonselective β-blocking drug when administered orally, intravenously, or as an ophthalmic solution. It does not have local anesthetic properties when administered onto the surface of the eye, and is five to ten times more potent than propranolol at reducing intraoccular pressure. The use in one eye is effective in both eyes. Absorption

into the systemic circulation may produce bradycardia, and possibly hypotension.[227, 228] Its use *may* be contraindicated in the patient with asthma, congestive heart failure, or A-V block. Dosage should be kept to the lowest concentration effective in the eye, and cardiac rate and blood pressure monitored.

Complications from β blockade treatment occur in approximately 9% of patients,[229] and can include bradycardia, A-V block, hypotension, congestive heart failure, and an exacerbation of asthma. Symptoms occur often within the first 24 hours of treatment, and may be seen at low dose in half of the patients exhibiting symptoms.[229] Cautious therapy, along with monitoring, will minimize complications.

Withdrawal of a β-blocking drug should occur slowly, unless a complication from β blocker therapy is present. Abrupt withdrawal of a β-blocking drug may be associated with significant signs and symptoms of myocardial ischemia. As has been mentioned previously, myocardial infarction may result from sudden withdrawal of β blockade in the patient who requires the drug for treatment of angina or hypertension, or both.

A β-blocking drug need not be discontinued before surgery or anesthesia. If a patient is asymptomatic and comfortable, and if resting heart rate is 55 to 70 beats per minute, the β-blocking drug should be continued to within 5 to 6 hours of the beginning of anesthesia. If anxiety or mild exercise or both produce a heart rate greater than 100 beats per minute, the β-blocking drug should be increased in the preoperative period (in the absence of CHF or A-V block). If heart rate is less than 55 beats per minute, the drug should be reduced to one-half the usual dose during the 12 hours of the immediate preoperative period.

The availability of newer cardioselective β-blocking drugs, such as metoprolol, should allow treatment with fewer complications and a greater margin of safety. An excellent review of metoprolol is available.[230] Table 11–19 summarizes the basic information needed for clinical use of the approved β-blocking drugs.

SUMMARY

Inotropic agonists and antagonists are used often in the critical care setting. The activity of agonists and antagonists can be anticipated if an understanding of pharmacology and pathophysiology is coupled with appropriate monitoring. Most physiologic effects are dose-related, and may vary from patient to patient, and from minute to minute in the same patient. The availability of newer drugs, such as dopamine, dobutamine, and metoprolol, increases drug selectivity, and thus increases the margin of safety.

Additional agonists and antagonists will be developed in the near future, and some may receive approval for clinical use. There are plenty of "me-too" drugs. Care must be taken to choose new drugs wisely because of real, not imagined, improvements.

REFERENCES

ADRENERGIC FUNCTION

Introduction

1. Dale HH: On some physiological actions of ergot. J Physiol 34:163, 1906
2. Ahlquist RR: A study of the adrenergic receptors. Am J Physiol 153:586, 1948
3. Lands AM, Arnold A, McAuliff JP et al: Differentiation of receptor systems activated by sympathomimetic amines. Nature 214:597, 1967
4. Goldberg LI: Cardiovascular and renal actions of dopamine: Potential clinical applications. Pharmacol Rev 24:1, 1972
5. Yeh BK, McNay JL, Goldberg LI: Attenuation of dopamine renal and mesenteric vasodilation by haloperidol: Evidence for a specific receptor. J Pharmacol Exp Ther 168:303, 1969
6. Goldberg LI, Yeh BK: Attenuation of dopamine induced renal vasodilation in the dog by phenothiazines. Eur J Pharmacol 15:36, 1971

Adrenergic Receptor Physiology

7. Sutherland EW, Rall TW: Fractionation and characterization of a cyclic adenine nucleo-

tide formed by tissue particles. J Biol Chem 232:1077, 1958
8. Lefkowitz RJ: β-adrenergic receptors: Recognition and regulation. N Engl J Med 295:323, 1976
9. Steer ML: Adrenergic receptors. Clin Endocrinol Metab 6:577, 1977
10. Tsien RW: Cyclic AMP and contractile activity in heart. Adv Cyclic Nucleotide Res 8:364, 1977
11. Levey GS: Restoration of norepinephrine responsiveness of solubilized myocardial adenylate cyclase by phosphatidylinositol. J Biol Chem 246:7405, 1971

Regulation of Adrenergic Receptors

12. Lefkowitz RJ: β-adrenergic receptors: Recognition and regulation. N Engl J Med 295:323, 1976
13. Steer ML, Atlas D, Levitzki A: Inter-relations between β-adrenergic receptors, adenylate cyclase and calcium. N Engl J Med 292:409, 1975

Nonadrenergic Mechanisms of Inotropic Stimulation

11. Lucchesi BR: Cardiac actions of glucagon. Circ Res, 22:777, 1968
15. Ward DE, Jones B: Glucagon and beta-blocker toxicity. Br Med J 2:151, 1976
16. Lee KS, Klaus W: The subcellular basis for the mechanism of inotropic action of cardiac glycosides. Pharmacol Rev 23:193, 1971
17. Langer GA: Effects of digitalis on myocardial ionic exchange. Circulation 46:180, 1972

INOTROPIC AGONISTS

18. Braunwald E: Heart failure. In Isselbacher, KJ, Adams, RD, Braunwald, E et al (eds): Harrison's Principals of Internal Medicine, 9th ed, pp 1035–1044. New York, McGraw–Hill, 1980
19. Schlant RC: Altered physiology of the cardiovascular system in heart failure. In Hurst, JW et al (eds): The Heart, 4th ed, pp 532–550. New York, McGraw–Hill, 1978
20. Braunwald E: The Myocardium, Failure and Infarction. New York, HP 1974
21. Hess ML: Concise review: Subcellular function in the acutely failing myocardium. Circ Shock 6:119, 1979

Sympathomimetic Inotropic Agonists

22. Innes IR, Nickerson M: Norepinephrine, epinephrine, and the sympathomimetic amines. In Goodman LD, Gilman A (eds): The Pharmacological Basis of Therapeutics, pp 483–504. New York, Macmillan, 1975
23. Steen PA, Tinker JH, Pluth JR et al: Efficacy of dopamine, dobutamine, and epinephrine during emergence from cardiopulmonary bypass in man. Circulation 57:378, 1978
24. Lesch M: Inotropic agents and infarct size. Am J Cardiol, 37:508, 1976
25. Lucchesi BR: Inotropic agents and drugs used to support the failing heart. In Antonaccio M (ed): Cardiovascular Pharmacology, p 337–375. New York, Raven Press, 1977
26. Goldberg LI, Bloodwell RD, Braunwald E, Morrow AG: The direct effects of norepinephrine, epinephrine, and methoxamine on myocardial contractile force in man. Circulation 22:1125, 1960
27. Gunnar RM, Loeb HS, Pietras RJ, Tobin JR: Ineffectiveness of isoproterenol in shock due to acute myocardial infarction. JAMA 202:1124, 1967
28. Mueller H, Ayres SM, Gregory JJ et al: Hemodynamics, coronary blood flow, and myocardial metabolism in coronary shock: Response to 1-norepinephrine and isoproterenol. J Clin Invest 49:1885, 1970
29. Ahlquist RR: A study of the adrenergic receptors. Am J PHysiol 153:586, 1948
30. Krasnow N, Rolett EL, Yurchak PM et al: Isoproterenol and cardiovascular performance. Am J Med 37:514, 1964
31. Allwood MJ, Cobbold AF, Ginsburg J: Peripheral vascular effects of noradrenaline, isopropylnoradrenaline and dopamine. Br Med Bull 19:132, 1963
32. McNay JL, Goldberg LI: Comparison of the effects of dopamine, isoproterenol, norepinephrine and bradykinin on canine renal and femoral blood flow. J Pharmacol Exp Ther 151:23, 1966
33. Rosenblum R, Berkowitz WD, Lawson D: Effects of acute intravenous administration of isoproterenol on cardiorenal hemodynamics in man. Circulation 38:158, 1968
34. Krasnow N, Rolett EL, Yurchak PM et al: Isoproterenol and cardiovascular performance. Am J Med 37:514, 1964
35. Mueller H, Giannelli S, Ayres SM et al: Effect of isoproterenol on ventricular work and myocardial metabolism in the postoperative heart. Circulation [Suppl 2] 37:146, 1968
36. Anderson R, Holmberg S, Svedmyr N, Aberg G: Adrenergic α- and β-receptors in coronary vessels in man. Acta Med Scand 191:241, 1972
37. Morse BW, Danzig R, Swan HJC: Effect of isoproterenol in shock associated with acute myocardial infarction. Circulation [Suppl 2] 35:192, 1967
38. Talley RC, Goldberg LI, Johnson CE, McNay JL: A hemodynamic comparison of dopamine and isoproterenol in patients in shock, Circulation 39:361, 1969
39. Smith HJ, Oriol A, Morch J, McGregor M: Hemodynamic studies in cardiogenic shock: Treatment with isoproterenol and metaraminol. Circulation 35:1084, 1967
40. Beregovich J, Reicher–Reiss H, Hunstadt D, Grishman A: Hemodynamic effects of isoproterenol in cardiac surgery. J Thorac Cardiovasc Surg 62:957, 1971
41. Harrison DC, Kerber RE, Alderman EL: Pharmacodynamics and clinical use of cardiovascular drugs after cardiac surgery. Am J Cardiol 26:385, 1970
42. Holloway EL, Stinson EB, Derby GC, Harrison DC: Action of drugs in patients early after cardiac surgery. I. Comparison of isoproterenol and dopamine. Am J Cariol 35:656, 1975
43. Stinson EB, Caves PK, Griepp RB et al: Hemodynamic observations in the early period after human heart transplantation. J Thorac Cardiovasc Surg 69:264, 1975
44. Lee W: The rational use of drugs in the management of heart block. Ration Drug Ther 9:1, 1975
45. Hatle L, Saeterhaug A, Rokseth R: Long term conservative therapy of chronic A-V block. Acta Med Scand 196:411, 1974
46. Mentzer RM, Alegre CA, Nolan SP: The effects of dopamine and isoproterenol on the pulmonary circulation. J Thorac Cardiovasc Surg 71:807, 1976
47. Shettigar UR, Hultgren HN, Specter M et al: Primary pulmonary hypertension. Favorable effect of isoproterenol. N Engl J Med 295:1414, 1976
48. Pantano JA: Isoproterenol in primary pulmonary hypertension. N Engl J Med 302:919, 1980
49. Daoud FS, Reeves JT, Kelly DB: Isoproterenol as a potential pulmonary vasodilator in pri-

mary pulmonary hypertension. Am J Cardiol 42:817, 1978

50. Maroko PR, Kjekshus JK, Sobel DB et al: Factors influencing infarct size following experimental coronary artery occlusion. Circulation 43:67, 1971

51. Vatner SF, Ritchie JM, Maroko PR et al: Effects of catecholamines, exercise, and nitroglycerin on the normal and ischemic myocardium in conscious dogs. J Clin Invest 54:563, 1974

52. Schwartz DA, Grover FL, Horwitz LD: Effect of isoproterenol on regional myocardial perfusion and tissue oxygenation in acute myocardial infarction. Am Heart J 97:339, 1979

53. McClenathan JH, Guyton RA, Breyer RH et al: The effects of isoproterenol and dopamine on regional myocardial blood flow after stenosis of circumflex coronary artery. J Thorac Cardiovasc Surg 73:431, 1977

54. Cohen MV, Sonnenblick EH, Kirk ES: Coronary steal: Its role in detrimental effect of isoproterenol after acute coronary occlusion in dogs. Am J Cardiol 38:880, 1976

55. Goldberg LI: Cardiovascular and renal actions of dopamine: Potential clinical applications. Pharmacol Rev 24:1, 1972

56. Goldberg LI: Dopamine: Clinial uses of an endogenous catecholamine. N Eng J Med 291:707, 1974

57. Goldberg LI, Hsieh Y, Resnekov L: Newer catecholamines for treatment of heart failure and shock: An update on dopamine and a first look at dobutamine. Prog Cardiovasc Dis 19:327, 1977

58. Goldberg LI, Yeh BK: Attenuation of dopamine induced renal vasodilation in the dog by phenothiazines Eur J Pharmacol 15:36, 1971

59. Brotzu G: Inhibition by chlorpromazine of the effects of dopamine on the dog kidney. J Pharm Pharmacol 22:664, 1970

60. Yeh BK, McNay J., Goldberg LI: Attenuation of dopamine renal and mesenteric vasodilation by haloperidol: Evidence for a specific receptor. J Pharmacol Exp Ther 168:303, 1969

61. Brotzu G: Inhibition by chlorpromazine of the effects of dopamine on the dog kidney. J Pharmacol 22:664, 1970

62. McNay JL, Goldberg LI: Comparison of the effects of dopamine, isoproterenol, norepinephrine and bradykinin on canine renal and femoral blood flow. J Pharmacol Exp Ther 151:23, 1966

63. Loeb HS, Winslow EBJ, Rahimtoola SH et al: Acute hemodynamic effects of dopamine in patients with shock. Circulation 44:163, 1971

64. Beregovich J, Bianchi C, Rubler S et al: Dose related hemodynamic and renal effects of dopamine in congestive heart failure. Am Heart J 87:550, 1974

65. Wheeler RC, Marquardt JF, Ayers CR, Wood JE: Peripheral vascular effects of dopamine. Circulation [Suppl] 26:269, 1967

66. McDonald RH, Goldberg LI: Analysis of the cardiovascular effects of dopamine in the dog. J Pharmacol Exp Ther 140:60, 1963

67. Meyer MB, McNay JL, Goldberg LI: Effects of dopamine on renal function and hemodynamics in the dog. J Pharmacol Exp Ther 156:186, 1967

68. Breckenridge A, Orme M, Dollery CT: The effect of dopamine on renal blood flow in man. Eur J Clin Pharmacol 3:131, 1971

69. Rosenblum R, Tai AR, Lawson D: Dopamine in man: Cardiorenal hemodynamics in normotensive patients with heart disease. J Pharmacol Exp Ther 183:256, 1972

70. Hollenberg NK, Adams, DF, Mendell P et al: Renal vascular responses to dopamine: Haemodynamic and angiographic observations in normal man. Clinical Science and Molecular Medicine 45:733, 1973

71. Hardaker WT, Wechsler AS: Redistribution of renal intracortical blood flow during dopamine infusion in dogs. Circ Res 33:437, 1973

72. Mueller HS: Effects of dopamine on hemodyhamics and myocardial energetics in man: Comparison with effects of isoprenaline and L-noradrenaline. Resuscitation 6:179, 1978

73. Crexells C, Bourassa MG, Biron P: Effects of dopamine on myocardial metabolism in patients with ischemic heart disease. Cardiovasc Res 7:438, 1973

74. Mentzer RM, Alegre CA, Nolan SP: The effects of dopamine and isoproterenol on the pulmonary circulation. J Thorac Cardiovasc Surg 71:807, 1976

75. Stephenson LW, Edmunds LH, Raphaely R et al: Effects of nitroprusside and dopamine on pulmonary arterial vasculature in children after cardiac surgery. Circulation [Suppl 1] 60:104, 1979

76. Polumbo RA, Harrison DC: Response of the pulmonary circulation to dopamine infusion in man. Circulation [Suppl 2] 46:220, 1972

77. Cannon PJ: The kidney in heart failure. N Engl J Med 296:26, 1977

78. Hilberman M, Maseda J, Spencer R et al: A comparison of the hemodynamic and renal

functional effects of dopamine and dobutamine following open cardiac operations. (Personal communication)

79. Stemple DR, Kleiman JH, Harrison DC: Combined nitroprusside-dopamine therapy in severe chronic congestive heart failure. Am J Cardiol 42:267, 1978
80. Rosenblum R, Frieden J: Intravenous dopamine in the treatment of myocardial dysfunction after open heart surgery. Am Heart J 83:743, 1972
81. Holzer J, Karliner JS, O'Rourke RA et al: Effectiveness of dopamine in patients with cardiogenic shock. Am J Cardiol 32:79, 1973
82. Steen PA, Tinker JH, Pluth JR et al: Efficacy of dopamine, dobutamine, and epinephrine during emergence from cardiopulmonary bypass in man. Circulation 57:378, 1978
83. Goldberg LI, Talley RC, McNay JL: The potential role of dopamine in the treatment of shock. Prog Cardiovasc Dis 12:40, 1969
84. Ruiz DE, Weil MH, Carlson RW: Treatment of circulatory shock with dopamine: Studies on survival. JAMA 242:165, 1979
85. Greene SI, Smith JW: Dopamine gangrene. N Engl J Med 294:114, 1976
86. Alexander CS, Sako Y, Mikulic E: Pedal gangrene associated with the use of dopamine. N Engl J Med 293:591, 1975
87. Hollenberg NK, Adams DF, Mendell P et al: Renal vascular responses to dopamine: Haemodynamic and angiographic observations in normal man. Clinical Science and Molecular Medicine 45:733, 1973
88. Tuttle RR, Mills J: Dobutamine. Development of a new catecholamine to selectively increase cardiac contractility. Circ Res 36:185, 1975
89. Koch–Weser J: Dobutamine: A new synthetic cardioactive sympathetic amine. N Engl J Med 300:17, 1979
90. Beregovich J, Bianchi C, D'Angelo R et al: Hemodynamic effects of a new inotropic agent (dobutamine) in chronic cardiac failure. Br Heart J 37:629, 1975
91. Loeb HS, Khan M, Klodnycky ML et al: Hemodynamic effects of dobutamine in man. Circ Shock 2:29, 1975
92. Loeb HS, Sinno MZ, Saudye A et al: Electrophysiologic properties of dobutamine. Circ Shock 1:217, 1974
93. Akhtar N, Mikulic E, Cohn JN, Chaudhry MH: Hemodynamic effect of dobutamine in patients with severe heart failure. Am J Cardiol 36:202, 1975
93A. Robie NW, Goldberg LI: Comparative systemic and regional hemodynamic effects of dopamine and dobutamine. Am Heart J 90:340, 1975
94. Vatner SF, McRitchie RJ, Braunwald E: Effects of dobutamine on left ventricular performance, coronary dynamics, and distribution of cardiac output in conscious dogs. J Clin Invest 53:1265, 1974
95. Vatner SF, McRitchie RJ, Braunwald E: Effects of dobutamine on left ventricular performance, coronary dynamics, and distribution of cardiac output in conscious dogs. J Clin Invest 53:1265, 1974
96. Stephens J, Ead H, Spurrell R: Hemodynamic effects of dobutamine with special reference to myocardial blood flow: A comparison with dopamine and isoprenaline. Br Heart J 42:43, 1979
97. Leier CV, Webel J, Bush CA: The cardiovascular effects of the continuous infusion of dobutamine in patients with severe cardiac failure. Circulation 56:468, 1977
98. Andy JJ, Curry CL, Ali N, Mehrotra PP: Cardiovascular effects of dobutamine in severe congestive heart failure. Am Heart J 94:175, 1977
99. Leier CV, Heban PT, Huss P et al: Comparative systemic and regional hemodynamic effects of dopamine and dobutamine in patients with cardiomyopathic heart failure. Circulation 58:466, 1978
100. Stoner JD, Bolen JL, Harrison DC: Comparison of dobutamine and dopamine in treatment of severe heart failure. Br Heart J 39:536, 1977
101. Loeb HS, Bredakis J, Gunnar RM: Superiority of dobutamine over dopamine for augmentation of cardiac output in patients with chronic low output cardiac failure. Circulation 55:375, 1977
102. Mikulic E, Cohn JN, Franciosa JA: Comparative hemodynamic effects of inotropic and vasodilator drugs in severe heart failure. Circulation 56:528, 1977
103. Loeb HS: Acute hemodynamic effects of dobutamine and isoproterenol in patients with low output cardiac failure. Circ Shock 3:55, 1976
104. Kersting F, Follath F, Moulds R et al: A comparison of cardiovascular effects of dobutamine and isoprenaline after open heart surgery. Br Heart J 38:622, 1976
105. Lewis GRJ, Poole Wilson PA, Angerpointer TA et al: Measurement of the circulatory effects of dobutamine, a new inotropic agent,

in patients following cardiac surgery. Am Heart J 95:301, 1978

106. Sakamoto T, Yamada T: Hemodynamic effects of dobutamine in patients following open heart surgery. Circulation 55:525, 1977

107. Tinker JH, Tarhan S, White RD et al: Dobutamine for inotropic support during emergence from cardiopulmonary bypass. Anesthesiology 44:281, 1976

108. Maroko PR, Swain J, Vatner S: Effect of dobutamine on myocardial injury after coronary occlusion. Circulation [Suppl 3] 49/50:189, 1974

109. Gillespie TA, Ambos HD, Sobel BE, Roberts R: Effects of dobutamine in patients with acute myocardial infarction. Am J Cardiol 39:588, 1977

110. Hoff JV, Beatty PA, Wade JL: Dermal necrosis from dobutamine. N Engl J Med 300:1280, 1979

111. Chen KK, Schmidt CF: Ephedrine and related substances. Medicine 9:1, 1930

112. Aviado DM: Direct and indirect stimulants of α and β receptors. In Sympathomimetic Drugs, pp 95–192. Springfield (Ill), Charles C Thomas, 1970

113. Cohn JN: Comparative cardiovascular effects of tyramine, ephedrine, and norepinephrine in man. Circ Res 41:174, 1965

114. Franciosa JA, Cohn JN: Hemodynamic effects of oral ephedrine given alone or combined with nitroprusside infusion in patients with severe left ventricular failure. Am J Cardiol 43:79, 1979

115. James FM, Greiss FC, Kemp RA: An evaluation of vasopressor therapy for maternal hypotension during spinal anesthesia. Anesthesiology 33:25, 1970

116. Ralston DH, Shnider SM, deLorimor AA: Effects of equipotent ephedrine, metaraminol, mephenteramine, and methoxamine on uterine blood flow in the pregnant ewe. Anesthesiology 40:354, 1974

117. Chidsey CA, Braunwald E, Morrow A: Catecholamine excretion and cardiac stores of norepinephrine in congestive heart failure. Am J Med 39:442, 1965

118. Hirsch MS, Walter RM, Hasterlik RJ: Subarachnoid hemorrhage following ephedrine and MAO inhibitor. JAMA 194:201, 1965

119. Elis J, Laurence DR, Mattie H, Prichard BNC: Modification by monoamine oxidase inhibitors of the effect of some sympathomimetics on blood pressure. Br Med J 2:75, 1967

120. Van Mieghem W, Stevens E, Coseman J: Ephedrine induced cardiopathy. Br Med J 1:816, 1978

121. Zaimis E: Vasopressor drugs and catecholamines. Anesthesiology 29:732, 1968

122. Aviado DM: Cardiovascular effects of some commonly used pressor amines. Anesthesiology 20:71, 1959

Cardiac Glycosides

123. Moe GK, Farah AE: Digitalis and allied cardiac glycosides. In Goodman LS, Gilman A (eds): Pharmacological Basis of Therapeutics, pp 653–682. New York, Macmillan, 1975

124. Harrison TR, Calhoun JA, Turley FC: Congestive heart failure. XI. The effect of digitalis on the dyspnea and on the ventilation of ambulatory patients with regular cardiac rhythm. Arch Intern Med 48:1203, 1931

125. Doherty JE: Digitalis glycosides: Clinical pharmacology. Adv. Intern Med 24:287, 1979

126. Doherty JE, de Soyza N, Kane JJ et al: Clinical pharmacokinetics of digitalis glycosides. Prog Cardiovasc Dis 21:141, 1978

127. Smith TW, Haber E: Digitalis (in four parts). N Engl J Med 289:945, 1019, 1063, 1125, 1973

128. White RJ, Chamerlain DA, Howard M, Smith TW: Plasma concentrations of digoxin after oral administration in the fasting and postprandial state. Br Med J 1:380, 1971

129. Brown DD, Juhl RP: Decreased bioavailability of digoxin due to antacids and kaolin-pectin. N Engl J Med 295:1034, 1976

130. Lindenbaum J, Maulitz RM, Saha JR et al: Impairment of digoxin absorption by neomycin. Clin Res 20:410, 1970

131. Ewy GA, Kapadia GG, Yao L et al: Digoxin metabolism in the elderly. Circulation 39:449, 1969

132. Lee KS, Klaus W: Subcellular basis for the mechanism of inotropic action of cardiac glycosides. Pharmacol Rev 23:193, 1971

133. Croxson MS, Ibbertson HK: Serum digoxin in patients with thyroid disease. Br Med J 3:566, 1975

134. Goldman S, Probst P, Selzer A, Cohn K: Inefficacy of "therapeutic" serum levels of digoxin in controlling the ventricular rate in atrial fibrillation. Am J Cardiol 35:651, 1975

135. Hager WD, Fenster P, Mayersohn M et al: Digoxin quinidine interaction: Pharmacokinetic evaluation. N Engl J Med 300:1238, 1979

136. Doering W: Quinidine-digoxin interaction: Pharmacokinetics, underlying mechanism and clinical implications. N Engl J Med 301:400, 1979

137. Bigger JT: The quinidine-digoxin interaction: What do we know about it? N Engl J Med 301:779, 1979

138. Ferrer MI, Conroy RJ, Harvey RM: Some effects of digoxin upon the heart and circulation in man. Circulation 21:372, 1960

139. Braunwald E, Bloodwell RD, Goldberg LI, Morrow AG: Studies on digitalis. IV. Observations in man on the effects of digitalis preparations on the contractility of the nonfailing heart and on total vascular resistance. J Clin Invest 40:52, 1961

140. Mason DT: Regulation of cardiac performance in clinical heart disease: Interactions between contractile state mechanical abnormalities and ventricular compensatory mechanisms. Am J Cardiol 32:437, 1973

141. Schwartz A, Allen JC, Harigaya S: Possible involvement of cardiac Na^+, K^+-adenosine triphosphatase in the mechanism of action of cardiac glycosides. J Pharmacol Exp Ther 168:31, 1969

142. Sonnenblick EH, Spotnitz HM, Spiro D: Role of the sarcomere in ventricular function and the mechanism of heart failure. Circ Res [Suppl 2] 15:70, 1968

143. Mason DT: Digitalis pharmacology and therapeutics: Recent advances. Ann Intern Med 80:520, 1974

144. Smith TW, Wagner H, Markis JE, Young M: Studies on the localization of the cardiac glycoside receptor. J Clin Invest 51:1777, 1972

145. Langer GA: Digitalis: Effects of digitalis on myocardial ionic exchange. Circulation 46:180, 1972

146. Rodman T, Gorczyca CA, Pastor BH: The effect of digitalis on the cardiac output of the normal heart at rest and during exercise. Ann. Intern Med 55:620, 1961

147. Rosen MR, Wit AL, Hoffman BF: Electrophysiology and pharmacology of cardiac arrhythmias. IV. Cardiac Antiarrhymic and toxic effects of digitalis. Am Heart J 89:391, 1975

148. Chung EK: Tachyarrhythmias in Wolff–Parkinson–White Syndrome. JAMA 237:376, 1977

149. Covell JW, Braunwald E, Ross J, Sonnenblick EH: Studies on digitalis. XVI. Effects on myocardial oxygen consumption. J Clin Invest 45:1535, 1966

150. Mason DT, Braunwald E et al: Studies on digitalis. X. Effects of ouabain on forearm vascular resistance and venous tone in normal subjects and in patients in heart failure. J Clin Invest 43:532, 1964

151. Gillis RA, Helke CJ, Kellar KJ, Quest JA: Autonomic nervous system actions of cardiac glycosides. Biochem Pharmacol 27:849, 1978

152. Daggett WM, Weisfeldt ML: Influence of the sympathetic nervous system on the response of the normal heart to digitalis. Am J Cardiol 16:394, 1965

153. Cohn, JN: Indications for digitalis therapy. JAMA 229:1911, 1974

154. Warner H: Therapy of common arrhythmias. Med Clin North Am 58:995, 1974

155. Cohn JN, Franciosa JA: Vasodilator therapy of cardiac failure. N Engl J Med 297:27, 1977

156. Chatterjee K, Parmley WW: The role of vasodilator therapy in heart failure. Prog Cardiovasc Dis 19:301, 1977

157. Capone RJ, Mason DT, Amsterdam EA, Zelis R: Digitalis in mitral stenosis with normal sinus rhythm: Studies of left atrial contractility and cardiac hemodynamics. Circulation [Suppl 2] 46:75, 1972

158. Beiser GD, Epstein SE, Stampfer M, et al: Studies on digitalis. XVII. Effects of ouabain on the hemodynamic response to exercise in patients with mitral stenosis in normal sinus rhythm. N Engl J Med 278:131, 1968

159. Ferrer MI, Conroy RJ, Harvey RM: Some effects of digoxin upon the heart and circulation in man. Circulation 21:372, 1960

160. Green LH, Smith TW: The use of digitalis in patients with pulmonary disease. Ann Intern Med 87:459, 1977

161. Cohn JN, Tristani FE, Khatri IM: Cardiac and peripheral vascular effects of digitalis in clinical cardiovenic shock. Am Heart J 78:318, 1969

162. da Luz PL, Weil MH, Shubin H: Current concepts on mechanisms and treatment of cardiogenic shock. Am Heart J 92:103, 1976

163. Hayward R, Hamer J: Digitalis. In Hamer J (ed): Drugs for Heart Disease, pp 244–317. Chicago, Year Book Medical Publishers, 1979

164. Johnson LW, Dickstein RA, Fruehan CT et al: Prophylactic digitalization for coronary artery bypass surgery. Circulation 53:819, 1976

165. Tyras DH, Stothert JC, Kaiser GC et al: Supraventricular tachyarrhythmias after myocardial revascularization: A randomized trial of prophylactic digitalization. J Thorac Cardiovasc Surg 77:310, 1979

166. Morrison J, Killip T: Serum digitalis and arrhythmia in patients undergoing cardiopulmonary bypass. Circulation 47:341, 1973

167. Selzer A, Cohn JN: Some thoughts concerning the prophylactic use of digitalis. Am J Cardiol 26:214, 1970

168. American Hospital Formulary Service: Current drug therapy: Cardiac glycosides. Am J Hosp Pharm 35:1495, 1978

169. Seller RH: The role of magnesium in digitalis toxicity. Am Heart J 82:551, 1971

170. Lucchesi BR: Inotropic agents and drugs used to support the failing heart. In Antonaccio M (ed): Cardiovascular Pharmacology p 337–375. New York, Raven Press, 1977

171. Morrison J, Killip T: Serum digitalis and arrhythmia in patients undergoing cardiopulmonary bypass. Circulation 47:341, 1973

172. Carruthers SG, Cleland J, Kelly JG et al: Plasma and tissue digoxin concentrations in patients undergoing cardiopulmonary bypass. Br Heart J 37:313, 1975

173. Smith TW: Digitalis toxicity: Epidemiology and clinical use of serum concentration measurements. Am J Med 58:470, 1975

174. Smith TW: Digitalis: Ions, inotropy and toxicity. N Engl J Med 299:545, 1978

175. Ingelfinger JA, Goldman P: The serum digitalis concentration: Does it diagnose digitalis toxicity? N Engl J Med 294:867, 1976

176. Lasagna L: How useful are serum digitalis measurements? N Engl J Med 294:898, 1976

Glucagon

177. Farah A, Tuttle R: Studies on the pharmacology of glucagon. J Pharmacol Exp Ther 129:49, 1960

178. Glick G, Parmley WW, Wechsler AS, Sonnenblick EH: Glucagon: Its enhancement of cardiac performance in the cat and dog and persistence of its inotropic action despite beta-receptor blockade with propranolol. Circ Res 22:789, 1968

179. Parmley WW, Glick G, Sonnenblick EH: Cardiovascular effects of glucagon in man. N Engl J Med 279:12, 1968

180. Manchester JH, Parmley WW, Matloff JM et al: Effects of glucagon in man and dog. Circulation 41:579, 1970

181. Rowe GG: Systemic and coronary hemodynamic effects of glucagon. Am J Cardiol 25:670, 1970

182. Lucchesi BR: Inotropic agents and drugs

used to support the failing heart. In Antonaccio M (ed): Cardiovascular Pharmacology, pp 337–375. New York, Raven Press, 1977

183. Goldschlager N, Robin E, Cowan CM et al: Effect of glucagon on the coronary circulation in man. Circulation 40:829, 1969

184. Katz RL, Hinds L, Mills CJ: Ability of glucagon to produce cardiac stimulation without arrhythmias in halothane anesthetized animals. Br J Anesth 41:574, 1969

185. Markiewicz K, Cholewa M, Gorski L: Cardiac arrhythmias after intravenous administration of glucagon. Eur J Cardiol 6:449, 1978

186. Larner J, Haynes RC: Insulin and oral hypoglycemic drugs: glucagon. In Goodman LS, Gilman A (eds): The Pharmacological Basis of Therapeutics, pp 1527–1529. New York, Macmillan, 1975

187. Vaughn CC, Warner HR, Nelson RM: Cardiovascular effects of glucagon following cardiac surgery. Surgery 67:204, 1970

188. Vander Ark CR, Reynolds EW: Continuous infusion of glucagon in cardiogenic shock Circulation [Suppl 3] 40:206, 1969

189. Nord HJ, Fontanes AL, Williams JF: Treatment of congestive heart failure with glucagon. Ann Intern Med 72:649, 1970

190. Ward DE, Jones B: Glucagon and beta-blocker toxicity. Br Med J 2:151, 1976

Calcium

191. Peach MJ: Cations: Calcium, magnesium, barium, lithium, and ammonium. In Goodman LS, Gilman A (eds): The Pharmacological Basis of Therapeutics, pp 782–787. New York, Macmillan, 1975

192. Denlinger JK, Nahrwold ML, Gibbs PS, Lecky JH: Hypocalcemia during rapid blood transfusion in anesthetized man. Br J Anaesth 48:995, 1976

193. Feinberg H, Boyd E, Katz LN: Calcium effect on performance of the heart. Am J Physiol 202:643, 1962

194. Seifen E, Flacke W, Alper MH: Effects of calcium on isolated mammalian heart. Am J Physiol 207:716, 1964

195. Shiner PT, Harris WS, Weissler AM: Effects of acute changes in serum calcium levels on the systolic time intervals in man. Am J Cardiol 24:42, 1969

196. Denlinger JK, Kaplan JA, Lecky JH, Wollman H: Cardiovascular responses to calcium ad-

ministered intravenously to man during halothane anesthesia. Anesthesiology 42:390, 1975

197. Price HL: Myocardial depression by nitrous oxide and its reversal by Ca^{++}. Anesthesiology 44:211, 1976

198. Price HL: Calcium reverses myocardial depression caused by halothane. Anesthesiology 41:576, 1974

199. Sialer S, McKenna DH, Corliss RJ, Rowe GR: Systemic and coronary hemodynamic effects of intravenous administration of calcium chloride. Arch International Pharmacodyn Ther 169:177, 1967

200. Stanley TH, Isern–Ameral J, Liu W et al: Peripheral vascular versus direct cardiac effects of calcium. Anesthesiology 45:46, 1976

201. Lappas DG, Drop LJ, Buckley MJ et al: Hemodynamic response to calcium chloride during coronary artery surgery. Surg Forum 26:234, 1975

202. Hempelmann G, Pipenbrock S, Frerk C, Schleussner E: Effects of calcium gluconate and calcium chloride on cardiocirculatory parameters in man (English abstr). Anaesthesist 27:516, 1978

203. Drop LJ, Laver MB: Low plasma ionized calcium and response to calcium therapy in critically ill man. Anesthesiology 43:300, 1975

204. Drop LJ, Laver MB, Williams W: Persistant hypocalcemia during low flow states following cardiac surgery. Circulation [Suppl 4] 7/8:99, 1973

205. Lloyd WDM: Danger of intravenous calcium therapy. Br Med J 1:662, 1928

206. Howland WS, Jacobs RG, Goulet AH: An evaluation of calcium administration during rapid blood replacement. Anesth Analg (Cleve) 39:557, 1960

207. Eliot RS, Blount SG: Calcium, Chelates, and digitalis: A clinical study. Am Heart J 62:7, 1961

208. Nola GT, Pope S, Harrison DC: Assessment of the synergistic relationship between serum calcium and digitalis. Am Heart J 79:499, 1970

INOTROPIC ANTAGONISTS

209. Ahlquist RP: A study of the adrenotropic receptors. Am J Physiol 153:586, 1948

210. Powell CE, Slater IH: Blocking of inhibitory adrenergic receptors by a dichloro-analog of isoproterenol. J Pharm Exp Ther 122:480, 1958

211. Frishman W: Clinical pharmacology of the new beta-adrenergic blocking drugs. Part 1. Pharmacodynamic and pharmacokinetic properties. Am Heart J 97:663–670, 1979

Absorption and Metabolism

212. Melander A, Danielson K, Scherstein B et al: Enhancement of the bioavailability of propranolol and metoprolol by food. Clin Pharmacol Ther 22:108–112, 1977

213. Kendall MJ, Brown D, Yates RA: Plasma metoprolol concentrations in young, old, and hypertensive subjects. Br J Clin Pharm 4:497–499, 1977

214. Wood M, Shand DG, Wood AJJ: Propranolol binding in plasma during cardiopulmonary bypass. Anesthesiology 51:512–516, 1979

Pharmacokinetics

215. Johnsson G, Regårdh C–G: Clinical pharmacokinetics of β-adrenoreceptor blocking drugs. Clin Pharmacokinet 1:233–263, 1976 (a thorough review of studies relating plasma concentrations to β-block effects)

216. Frishman W: Clinical pharmacology of the new beta-adrenergic blocking drugs. Part 1. Pharmacodynamic and pharmacokinetic properties. Am Heart J 97:663–670, 1979

Major Physiological and Metabolic Effects

217. Gross F (ed): The cardioprotective action of beta-blockers, p 84. Baltimore, University Park Press, 1976

218. Frishman W, Silverman R: Clinical pharmacology of the new beta-adrenergic blocking drugs. Part 2. Physiologic and metabolic effects. Am Heart J 97:797–807, 1979

219. Weber MA, Stokes GS, Gain JM: Comparison of the effects of renin release of beta-adrenergic antagonists with differing properties. J Clin Invest 54:1413, 1974

220. Becker LC, Fortuin NJ, Pitt B: Effects of ischemia and anti-anginal drugs on the distribution of radio-active microspheres in the canine left ventricle. Circ Res 28:263, 1971

221. Diaz JH, McDonald JS: Propranolol and induced labor: Anesthetic implications. Anesthesiology Review pp 29–32, 1979 (a good review of the subject)

222. Renou P, Newman W, Wood C: Autonomic control of fetal heart rate. Am J Obstet Gynecol 105:949–953, 1969

Clinical Implications

223. Engelman F: Beta blocker cardioselectivity: What is its clinical significance? Hospital Physician (Primary Cardiology Supplement) 1:59–72, 1981 (a good summary)

224. Heel RC, Brogden RN, Speight TM et al: Timolol: A review of its therapeutic efficacy in the topical treatment of glaucoma. Drugs 17:38–55, 1979 (an excellent review)

225. Zimmerman TJ, Kaufman HE: Timolol, a β-adrenergic blocking agent for the treatment of glaucoma. Arch Ophthalmol 95:601–604, 1977

226. Zimmerman TJ, Kaufman HE: Timolol, dose response and duration of action. Arch Ophthalmol 95:605–607, 1977

227. Zimmerman TJ, Harbin R, Pett M: Timolol and facility of outflow. Invest Ophthalmol Vis Sci 16:623–624, 1977

228. Samuels SI, Maze M: Beta-receptor blockade following the use of eye drops. Anesthesiology 52:67–68, 1980

229. Greenblatt DJ, Koch–Weser J: Adverse reactions to β-adrenergic receptor blocking drugs: A report from the Boston Collaborative Drug Surveillance Program. Drugs 7:118–129, 1974

230. Koch–Weser, J: Metoprolol (drug therapy). N Eng Med 301:698–703, 1979 (an excellent review of metoprolol)

12

Vasoactive Drugs

JOHN R. AMMON
RICHARD P. FOGDALL

This chapter discusses the drugs which are primarily vasoactive agents. In general, these either relax or constrict the peripheral vasculature (vasodilators or vasopressors). Drugs which exert primarily cardiac effects are discussed in the previous chapter, although a precise division of vasoactive and cardioactive drugs cannot be made easily; this separation is based upon therapeutic utility.

Section I: Vasodilators

These drugs are valuable particularly in acute and chronic cardiac failure associated with ischemic heart disease, aortic and mitral valve regurgitation, and cardiomyopathy.[1-3] In the postoperative cardiac surgical patient, myocardial depression and resultant low cardiac output can be a major cause of morbidity or mortality. Vasodilator therapy, frequently combined with inotropic support and intraaortic balloon counterpulsation, has been a significant advance. Deliberate (induced) hypotension during surgical procedures with large anticipating blood losses (*e.g.*, major reconstructive, orthopedic, or cancer surgery) can benefit significantly appropriately selected patients. The use of vasodilators in the treatment of elevated systemic blood pressure was well recognized by 1961, when sodium nitroprusside was listed as a useful drug in hypertensive emergencies.[4]

A prerequisite to the rational use of vasodilator drugs is adequate hemodynamic monitoring. The expanding use of vasodilator therapy has coincided with the development of catheter monitoring techniques which quantify the hemodynamic effects of a given drug or intervention. Baseline cardiovascular variables must be known before initiating vasodilator therapy. These include arterial and pulmonary blood pressure, left and right ventricular filling pressures (PA$_0$ or pulmonary capillary wedge pressure [PCWP], and central venous pressure [CVP], respectively), cardiac output, and vascular resistance in the systemic and pulmonary circulations. Thus, knowledge of each patient's hemodynamic profile will enable the clinician to choose the appropriate vasodilator regimen for the specific circulatory abnormality and to safely titrate therapy.

MECHANISM OF ACTION

Peripheral vasodilation can be pharmacologically induced by at least four mechanisms:

1. Direct vascular smooth muscle relaxation
2. Alpha-receptor blockade
3. Ganglionic blockade
4. Central nervous system sedation

Direct vascular smooth muscle relaxation is the most common mechanism of vasodilation in the acute setting. Nitroglycerin and sodium nitroprusside are the notable examples of direct-acting vasodilators. It is believed that the interaction of the active nitrate metabolite, or the parent nitroprusside molecule with sulfhydryl (—SH) groups on or within the vascular smooth muscle membranes, is responsible for relaxation vasodilation.[5, 6]

Alpha-receptor blockade is an effective method of eliminating or reducing smooth muscle tone. The autonomic control of the peripheral circulation is predominantly adrenergic, the vast majority of adrenergic receptors being alpha in nature. The neurohumoral transmitter for adrenergic regulation of the circulation is norepinephine. Its action on the alpha receptor causes contraction and increased tone of vascular smooth muscle. Alpha blockade is caused by a direct action of blocking drugs on alpha-adrenergic receptors in a competitive type of reaction with norepinepine. Phenoxybenzamine, chlorpromazine, and phentolamine are the major clinical examples of alpha-blocking drugs.

Ganglionic blocking drugs act by competing with acetylcholine for intraganglionic postsynaptic receptor sites. They prevent the action of acetylcholine on the postsynaptic membrane, hence blocking autonomic ganglionic transmission. Interruption of sympathetic ganglionic transmission blocks adrenergic control of arterioles and veins, resulting in decreased systemic vascular resistance and increased venous capacitance, respectively. In addition, because the predominant control of heart rate is vagal (parasympathetic), significant antonomic ganglionic blockade will result in tachycardia. Also, sympathetically mediated vasomotor reflexes may be inhibited or abolished by ganglionic blockade. Trimethaphan camsylate is the major ganglionic blocking agent in clinical use today.

Finally, a central nervous system (CNS) site of action for drug-induced vasodilation is known. If the efferent sympathetic neural traffic originating in the vasomotor areas of the brainstem is blocked pharmacologically, diminished arteriolar resistance, increased venous capacitance, and negative effects on the inotropic and chronotropic state may result. The only commonly used drugs with vasodilator properties which appear to have predominantly central actions are clonidine and alpha-methyldopa. Both drugs are useful in the management of mild to moderate essential hypertension.

It must be appreciated that in addition to different mechanisms for drug induced vasodilation, there is a specificity to the type of vasodilation obtained by various drugs. The arterial (resistance) and venous (capacitance) portions of the circulation are differentially affected by the various vasodilator drugs, as well as exerting quantitative effects on pulmonary vascular tone. These differential effects shall be discussed with each drug below.

Regardless of the specific mechanism (*i.e.,* direct smooth muscle relaxation, alpha-blockade, ganglionic blockade, or CNS site) of each vasodilator drug, the effects on circulatory and myocardial physiology are predictable, if we know the initial state of the heart and peripheral circulation, and the different sites of action (arterial, venous, pulmonary, and so on) of each agent. The use of a pulmonary artery (Swan–Ganz) catheter has greatly facilitated the appropriate application of these drugs, both in establishing baseline circulatory and myocardial states and in defining and measuring the therapeutic effects of the various drugs.

PHYSIOLOGIC BASIS OF VASODILATOR THERAPY

Ventricular performance reflects a complex interaction of both central and peripheral circulatory factors. Central factors include the cardiac rate and rhythm, valvular competency, and the intrinsic quality of the myocardium (*i.e.,* inotropic state or contractility) and the compliance or filling characteristics of each ventricle.

Peripheral factors include the effective circulating blood volume and its distribution; the state of the arterial, venous, and pulmonary circulations; and the level of autonomic activity in these circulations. Altered ventricular performance and overall hemodynamic changes result from manipulation of smooth muscle size and tension in the arterial (resistance), venous (capacitance), and pulmonary vascular beds with the various vasoactive drugs.

The choice of a vasodilator drug must be based on known and anticipated hemodynamic alterations. The effects of a vasodilator on the determinants of myocardial function (preload, afterload, contractility, and heart rate) and the ratio of myocardial oxygen supply and demand are in large measure the way we judge a vasodilator's benefit and efficacy. The reader is referred to Chapter 2 for a complete discussion of hemodynamics and myocardial energy balance. Preload is defined by the pressure in the ventricle just before the start of systole, the ventricular end diastolic pressure (left—LVEDP; right—RVEDP). The compliance of the ventricle must be considered in assessing preload, for it is an important factor in determining end diastolic volume. The end diastolic volume in turn, affects stroke volume on the basis of Starling's Law. At the bedside, LVEDP and RVEDP are approximated by the pulmonary

Table 12-1. Classification of the Continuously Administered Intravenous Vasodilators

DRUG	ARTERIAL ACTIVITY 0-4	VENOUS ACTIVITY 0-4	COMMENTS
Sodium nitroprusside	3	2	Excessive dosage (>5 μg/kg/min) prone to produce cyanide toxicity; reflex tachycardia common
Nitroglycerin	1	4	Tachycardia rare;
Phentolamine	4	1	↓ Pulmonary vascular resistance greater than ↓ systemic vascular resistance? (Data controversial)
Trimethaphen	3	2	Tachycardia expected; sympathetic and parasympathic blockade; pupillary dilatation and cycloplegia

Table 12-2. Clinical Use of the Continuously Administered Vasodilators

DRUG	SUGGESTED CONCENTRATION FOR CONTINUOUS INTRAVENOUS INFUSION	USUAL BEGINNING DOSE	USUAL DOSE RANGE
Sodium Nitroprusside	50 mg/250 ml; 200 μg/ml	0.3–1.0 μg/kg/min	0.5–5.0 μg/kg/min* (35–350 μg/min)
Nitroglycerin	50 mg/250 ml; 200 μg/ml	0.5–1.5 μg/kg/min	0.5–5.0 μg/kg/min (35–350 μg/min)
Phentolamine	25 mg/250 ml; 100 μg/ml	50 μg/min	50–500 μg/min
Trimethaphen	500 mg/250 ml; 2 mg/ml	0.2 mg/min	0.2–6.0 mg/min

*Infusion at a higher rate should be of concern; see text for discussion of cyanide toxicity

artery occluded pressure (PA$_0$, PCWP) and the CVP, respectively, in the absence of significant mitral or tricuspid valvular dysfunction.

Afterload is the pressure in the aortic root at the opening of the aortic valve. *Afterload* and *impedance* are terms that describe the resistance to ejection of ventricular blood during systole.[7] In concert with ventricular chamber size (by the Law of LaPlace) and wall thickness, afterload determines ventricular wall tension, affecting myocardial oxygen demand.

Vasodilator drugs are used for control of preload and of afterload, and as an adjunct to the control of vascular volume, all with the implicit purpose of improving the myocardial oxygen supply and demand ratio or increasing cardiac output or both. Preload control, by vasodilator effects on venous capacitance, is usually in conjunction with more standard manipulations of volume loading with fluids and transfusion or volume depletion by diuretics and blood loss. It is usually not an isolated therapeutic endpoint. Optimizing preload then allows afterload manipulation to enhance forward flow

in the failing, low-output ventricle or to relieve myocardial ischemia or both. This stage is of particular importance in the anesthetic management of the cardiovascular and open-heart surgical patient. Control of vascular volume by vasodilator therapy permits higher cardiac output and improved perfusion in systemic capillary beds. With lower afterload, lesser myocardial oxygen demand and enhanced systemic perfusion increases safety in the compromised cardiac patient.

Specific application of each vasodilator drug is discussed in the following sections. Regardless of the differences in usage, sites, and mechanisms of action, it is essential to define the patient's baseline hemodynamic state before commencing vasodilator therapy. In choosing a specific vasodilator drug, it is important to know the degree of arterial vasodilation versus venodilation produced by each agent (see Table 12-1 for the continuously administered vasodilators). The hemodynamic profile of a particular vasodilator will ultimately depend upon the relative effects of the drug on the venous and arterial circulation at a given dose or rate, more than on the basic mechanism of action (direct, alpha-blockade, ganglionic blockade, or central). Table 12-2 summarizes the clinical use of the four continuously administered vasodilators.

SPECIFIC VASODILATORS*

DIRECT SMOOTH MUSCLE RELAXATION

Sodium Nitroprusside

Sodium nitroprusside has been well-known for over 100 years. Its application was first suggested in 1929 by Johnson, who recommended its use in severe hypertension.[8] It was introduced into clinical usage for hypertensive emergencies in the late 1950s,[9] but it was 1974 before the drug was approved and made widely available (Nipride). Since then, the application of continuous intravenous nitroprusside infusion has become a much used therapy in a variety of clinical settings.

The hemodynamic effects of sodium nitroprusside have been carefully studied in humans and animals over the past two and one-half decades.[10-15] Nitroprusside dilates both the resistance (arteriolar) and capacitance (venous) vessels, generally in a balanced manner. The effects on arterial blood pressure and cardiac output are dependent largely on the subject's myocardial function, volume status, and sympathetic tone before nitroprusside therapy.

In the presence of ventricular dysfunction and an elevated filling pressure, reduction of afterload with nitroprusside lessens impedance to ejection, thereby increasing stroke volume and improving ventricular performance. The rapid and reliable effects of afterload reduction has been the basis of widespread usage.

The use of nitroprusside for hypertension during coronary surgery is based on the acute reduction of systemic vascular resistance. The rapid lowering of myocardial oxygen demand by afterload reduction in this setting is

---

* Grouped by mechanism of action.

beneficial.[16] Investigation of the differential effects of nitroprusside and nitroglycerin in the coronary circulation, however, suggest the superiority of nitroglycerin in the ischemic myocardium.[17-20] Nitroprusside has been implicated in a coronary steal syndrome, with possible enhancement of myocardial ischemia. Nitroglycerin increases flow to an ischemic zone by dilator effects on large, conducting vessels and collateral circulation. In addition, a brisk cardiac rate response from nitroprusside in the presence of ischemic heart disease, may be deleterious in terms of an unfavorable myocardial oxygen supply and demand ratio (see chapter two on physiology).

The major uses of nitroprusside are presented below. Each area will be discussed under *Therapeutic Applications of Vasodilator Drugs.*

1. Hypertensive emergencies
2. Deliberate intraoperative hypotension
3. Perioperative management in cardiac and peripheral vascular surgery (including aneurysm resection)
4. Myocardial failure accompanying myocardial infarction
5. Myocardial failure from causes other than #4
6. Acute mitral and aortic valvular insufficiency

Nitroprusside is administered only intravenously (see Table 12-2). Because the drug is characterized by rapid action, immediate reversibility, high potency, and basically linear dose-response relationship, it is very useful in clinical settings in which moment-to-moment, reliable, and titratable vasodilation is required. Nitroprusside is supplied as a 50 mg lyophylized powder; 50 mg are dissolved in 250 ml of D5W, resulting in a concentration of 200 µg/ml. Usual infusion rates range from 25 to 200 µg/min, although a higher dose range may be necessary. It is best to begin at a low infusion rate increased gradually until the desired hemodynamic improvement is achieved. Relative hypovolemia will be quickly unmasked by the use of nitroprusside, and volume expansion (preload restoration) may be necessary. Severe hypotension is the major side effect of nitroprusside, an extension of its physiologic use: vasodilation. It is dose-dependent and is reversible by decreasing or stopping the infusion and positioning the patient with the legs above heart level.

Recently, reports of rebound hypertension with adverse hemodynamic effects after abrupt discontinuation of nitroprusside have appeared.[21, 22] Activation of vasoconstrictive reflexes and enhanced renin-angiotension activity have been implicated. Of particular concern is abrupt cessation in the setting of deliberate hypotension for surgical correction of intracranial aneurysms and in afterload reduction therapy for severe left ventricular failure, especially with underlying ischemic heart disease.

To understand the potential toxicity of nitroprusside, its metabolism must be understood. Nitroprusside has five cyanide groups on each parent molecule. These are released by reaction with free and intracellular hemoglobin in which the hemoglobin ion (Fe^{++}) is oxidized to Fe^{+++} or methemoglobin. An unstable nitroprusside radical results which quickly breaks down, releasing all five cyanide ions.[23] One of the five cyanide groups combines with methemoglobin to form cyanmethemoglobin. The remaining cyanide groups undergo conversion to thiocyanate in the liver and kidneys, mediated by the enzyme system rhodanase, and an endogenous sulfur source, usually thiosulfate. The toxicity of sodium nitroprusside relates to potentially incomplete cyanide conversion with acute cyanide binding to, and inactivation of, the intracellular cytochrome oxidase system. Many investigators have presented evidence to support tissue cyanide binding as the basis for acute nitroprusside toxicity.[23–25] They have suggested using measurements of increased anaerobic metabolism to detect its onset and severity, including base deficit, elevated blood lactate and lactate:pyruvate ratios, and elevation of mixed venous blood oxygen content.[26] Maximum dosage recommendations for short-term administration of nitroprusside are from 1.0 to 1.5 mg/kg total

over several hours[25, 27] and 10 μg/kg/min for a maximum of 300 minutes.[28] Longer term maximum administration (up to 48 hours), with regard to potential cyanide toxicity, has been suggested at a rate not to exceed 0.5 mg/kg/hr (8 μg/kg/min).[29]

Therapy for suspected cyanide poisoning, secondary to nitroprusside therapy, is a controversial clinical problem. Several antidotes have been recommended for both prophylaxis and treatment.[28–30] Sodium nitrite is used to form methemoglobin ($Hb\text{–}Fe^{++} + NaNO_2 \rightleftharpoons Hb\text{–}Fe^{+++}$), which then competes with cytochrome oxidase for the cyanide ion ($Hb\text{–}Fe^{+++} + Cyt\ FeCN \rightleftharpoons Hb\text{–}FeCN + Cyt\text{–}Fe^{+++}$). The adult dose is 0.3 to 0.5 g in 10 to 15 ml solution, infused over 3 to 4 minutes. Sodium thiosulfate, 150 to 200 mg/kg in 50 ml, administered over a 10-minute period, is then useful for the conversion of cyanide to thiocyanate. Hydroxocobalamin (vitamin B_{12a}) has been investigated in baboons as a cyanide antidote.[28] The authors suggested 22.5 mg B_{12a} per milligram of nitroprusside.

Chronic toxicity of nitroprusside is a result of thiocyanate accumulation. As stated above, thiocyanate is the product of cyanide detoxification with thiosulfate and the rhodanase enzyme system in liver and kidney. Thiocyanate is excreted largely unchanged through the kidney. Accumulation of thiocyanate can cause fatigue, nausea and anorexia, miosis, toxic psychosis, hyperreflexia, and convulsions.[31] Hypothyroidism has been reported with prolonged nitroprusside therapy, presumably the result of the antithyroid action of thiocyanate.[32] Toxicity from thiocyanate accumulation begins to appear at plasma level of from 5 to 10 mg/dl, with fatalities reported at levels of 20 mg/dl and above.

Nitroglycerin and Related Organic Nitrates

Nitroglycerin (glyceryl trinitrate) has been in clinical use for over 100 years. It is the most commonly used drug in the therapy of angina pectoris. In fact, angina pectoris constitutes the only currently approved indication for its use. More recently, sustained-release capsules of nitroglycerin for oral use, and an ointment preparation for continual cutaneous absorption into the circulation, have been made available for the management and prophylaxis of angina pectoris. Other nonparenteral organic nitrates of clinical importance include isosorbide dinitrate, erythrityl tetranitrate, and pentaerythrityl tetranitrate. Several, or all, of the nitrate drugs will be encountered in the preanesthetic work-up of most patients with coronary artery disease.

More recently, nitroglycerin has been used as an intravenous infusion to produce a sustained hemodynamic effect.[33–36] The application of intravenous nitroglycerin in left ventricular failure with acute myocardial infarction has been the subject of intense investigation in recent years.[37, 38]

Nitroglycerin has a more selective effect on the venous capacitance vessels, although arterial vascular resistance is reduced, particularly at higher infusion rates. With enhanced venous capacitance, effective circulating blood volume and LVEDP are reduced. A failing ventricle benefits from this preload reduction by a decrease in size, filling pressure, and myocardial oxygen demand. Afterload reduction also reduces myocardial oxygen demand and additionally, enhances forward flow. This latter effect, in combination with the various clinical modalities of maintaining optimal preload (volume, diuretics, and so on), is a major benefit with intravenous nitroglycerin in the early postoperative coronary surgical patient with depressed myocardial function. In patients with only mild ventricular dysfunction, cardiac output may be unchanged or reduced.

The mechanism of smooth muscle relaxation by the organic nitrates is an interaction between the active nitrate and a nitrate receptor, involving sulfhydryl groups capable of reducing the nitrate molecule. It is this interaction or the nitrite ion formed locally that causes smooth muscle relaxation. Depletion of tissue sulfhydryl produces tolerance to the organic nitrates, but not to the nitrite ion.

The clinical use of nitroglycerin and the organic nitrates is usually for sublingual and oral antianginal therapy. With newer applications of these agents in the areas of angina prophylaxis and the treatment of chronic congestive heart failure, nitroglycerin ointment offers significant effects lasting several hours.

As with nitroprusside, the use of intravenous nitroglycerin must be guided by adequate hemodynamic monitoring, including measurements of left- and right-sided filling pressures and systemic arterial pressure. The use of intravenous nitroglycerin in the management of the patient undergoing coronary artery bypass surgery has been investigated by Kaplan and coworkers.[19, 39] Their studies involved the treatment of intraoperative hypertension and the resultant ischemic ST-segment changes. They concluded that nitroglycerin can be safely administered intravenously during anesthesia, decreasing myocardial oxygen demand, relieving myocardial ischemia and offering several advantages over nitroprusside in this setting. Fahmy investigated intravenous nitroglycerin and nitroprusside for use in deliberate hypotension.[40] He concluded that nitroglycerin better supports the coronary perfusion pressure because of its lesser effect on aortic diastolic pressure compared to nitroprusside. Blood loss was less with nitroglycerin as compared to nitroprusside, a fact he attributed to the lower systemic venous pressure attained with nitroglycerin. It produces a smooth and gradual decrease in blood pressure with minimal danger of producing severe hypotension.

A convenient concentration for the intravenous administration of nitroglycerin is 200 μg/ml (see Table 12-2). The initial infusion rate should begin at approximately 30 μg/min (0.5 μg/kg/min), titrating the infusion to the desired hemodynamic endpoint (i.e., decreased LVEDP, RVEDP, PA_0 or CVP); until there is improvement in ischemic signs; until there is decrease in ventricular arrhythmias; or until there is improvement in cardiac output. As with nitroprusside, the importance of baseline measurements must be stressed. A fundamental aspect of the use of intravenous nitroglycerin is knowledge of the patient's ventricular function and volume status. Hypotension is possible in patients who are hypovolemic as the drug shifts volume into the capacitance vessels.

Complications, other than hypotension in the hypovolemic patient, resulting from the use of intravenous nitroglycerin, are few. Reflex tachycardia occurs less frequently, and less severely, than with nitroprusside. A rare, but dangerous, complication of both sublingual and intravenous nitroglycerin, occurring in patients during the first 24 hours after acute myocardial infarction, has been reported by Come and Pitt.[41] They described simultaneous bradycardia and hypotension in that setting, possibly used by acute reflex changes in heart rate and changes in central blood volume induced by nitroglycerin. Their report underscores the need for careful observation and hemodynamic monitoring during its use.

Isosorbide Dinitrate

Isosorbide dinitrate is an organic nitrate in common usage today for the acute and prophylactic management of angina pectoris. It is encountered frequently in patients undergoing coronary artery bypass surgery. More recently, its use in the management of acute and chronic congestive heart failure has been shown to be beneficial, with resultant decreases in pulmonary capillary wedge pressure and a slight increase in cardiac index after sublingual administratin.[42, 43]

The hemodynamic effects of isosorbide dinitrate are very similar to those of nitroglycerin. It acts predominantly on the venous circulation and changes in cardiac output are related to the initial ventricular filling pressures. Systemic vascular resistance decreases only slightly or not at all. In the absence of left ventricular dysfunction, systemic arterial pressure may decrease, possibly accompanied by a reflex tachycardia.

The drug is administered orally for prophylactic therapy and sublingually (or by chewing tablet) for relief of anginal pain. In the management of angina, propanolol is used frequently with isosorbide dinitrate, the two drugs being complementary in that they reduce cardiac work by different mechanisms.

Erythrityl Tetranitrate and Pentaerythritol Tetranitrate

These organic nitrates are encountered occasionally in the patient undergoing coronary artery bypass surgery. Neither drug is intended for the acute management of anginal pain, but rather for prophylaxis and long-term treatment of patients with frequent or recurrent angina. Both are available in oral form, with erythrityl tetranitrate also used sublingually for anticipated physical or emotional stress and at bedtime for patients subject to nocturnal angina.

Hydralazine

Hydralazine is an acute and chronic antihypertensive drug that has been in use for over 25 years.[44] Its application in the treatment of chronic hypertension has increased in recent years, used with the beta-blockade of propranolol.[45] Available in parenteral form, it is particularly well suited for the treatment of acute hypertensive problems in various anesthetic and surgical settings. The use of oral hydralazine in patients with chronic left ventricular failure has been recent, but promising. Several studies demonstrate clearly improved cardiac output and diminished systemic and pulmonary vascular resistance.[46, 47] The combination use of hydralazine and an organic nitrate—the former for enhancement of cardiac output, the latter for its ability to increase venous capacitance and decrease ventricular filling pressures—has been advocated in chronic congestive heart failure.[48]

Hydralazine acts predominantly on the arteriolar sites in the peripheral circulation with little effect on the venous capacitance side. Reduction of systemic and pulmonary vascular resistance is the main hemodynamic effect, with a resultant increase in cardiac output and stroke volume. The vasodilating effects of hydralazine are not uniform. The decrease in resistance is greatest in the cerebral, coronary, splanchnic, and renal vasculature. Direct effects in the muscle and cutaneous vascular beds are minor. In the normal or nonfailing heart, activation of the baroceptor reflex with tachycardia and increased inotropy can offset the hypotensive effect of the drug. The resultant hyperdynamic state of the circulation may precipitate myocardial ischemia in the patient with the coronary artery disease and a nonfailing left ventricle. It has long been known that hydralazine in the patient with mitral valve disease can increase pulmonary artery pressure because of the resultant enhancement of cardiac output and venous return.[49] In patients with left ventricular failure there is a lack of change in heart rate and little decrease in arterial pressure, but an increase in stroke volume. It is this last effect that has recently been applied in the use of hydralazine in patients with chronic heart failure, as mentioned above.

Several important contraindications and side effects should be noted. As stated, angina may be precipitated or worsened by hydralazine. The addition of beta-blockade to hydralazine therapy will be protective, allowing hydralazine to exert its hypotensive action without activation of sympathetic reflexes. An unopposed hyperdynamic state resulting from hydralazine therapy in the management of dissecting aneurysm is to be avoided. Despite an increase in renal blood flow, sodium and water retention may occur as is common with most antihypertensive drugs, necessitating the use of a diuretic with chronic therapy. Prolonged use of hydralazine at daily doses exceeding 400 mg may precipitate an acute rheumatoid state, some patients actually demonstrating a lupus syndrome. Peripheral neuropathy is a well-known toxic effect of hydralazine. It results from pyridoxine's (vitamin B_6) condensation with a metabolite of hydralazine and its subsequent elimination.

Parenteral use of hydralazine is indicated in the acute management of elevated systemic blood pressure. It is a particularly effective drug for the hypertension of acute glomerulonephritis and toxemia of pregnancy. In the anesthetic setting, it is a useful adjunct. Marked elevation of blood pressure may be seen in the early postoperative phase of intracranial surgery, repair of coarctation of the aorta and surgery of any nature in the chronicly hypertensive patient. Intravenous administration should be cautious, starting with from 5 to 10 mg, allowing 10 to 15 minutes for peak action before repeating the dose. Intramuscular dosage should start at from 10 to 20 mg, with a slower peak action of 10 to 80 minutes. Effective circulating blood volume should be corrected before administration. An excessive sympathetic response to blood pressure lowering may be blocked by propanolol.

Diazoxide

Diazoxide is an intravenous vasodilator used almost exclusively for hypertensive emergencies. It is a benzothiadiazine derivative, similar in structure to the thiazide diuretics, but devoid of any direct diuretic properties. Its main physiologic activity is direct relaxation of arteriolar smooth muscle tone with a consequent reduction in peripheral vascular resistance. Diazoxide exerts no significant effect on venous capacitance vessels.[50] As a result of these physiologic effects, the drug lends itself particularly well to the treatment of most hypertensive emergencies.

The main hemodynamic effect, a direct and rapid reduction in peripheral vascular resistance, causes baroreceptor reflex activation, resulting in tachycardia and increased myocardial contractility. Increased stroke volume, left ventricular ejection velocity, and cardiac output result from these unloading and chronotropic effects, with a greater reduction in peripheral vascular resistance than in arterial blood pressure. Consequently, reduction of arterial blood pressure below normotensive levels is uncommon. Left ventricular performance improves because of the acutely reduced afterload.[51] Propranolol inhibits the increase in myocardial contractility and heart rate attendant to diazoxide administration, and augments its antihypertensive effect. Patients treated with propranolol initially should receive a lower than usual dose of diazoxide to prevent an exaggerated response. Propranolol inhibits the elevation of plasma renin activity, also seen with diazoxide therapy.[52]

Diazoxide is bound extensively to serum albumin, explaining the need for rapid infusion (total dose over 10–30 seconds) to obtain maximum hypotensive effect,[53, 54] The primary route of excretion of diazoxide is through glomerular filtration, with hepatic transformation accounting for a small degree of elimination.

The major advantage of diazoxide in the severely hypertensive patient is that it rapidly and consistently lowers arterial pressure toward normal but rarely to dangerous levels, with the antihypertensive effect lasting several hours. It is used most commonly in the setting of accelerated or malignant hypertension. The bolus administration of diazoxide at 5 mg/kg (usual dose approximately 300 mg) acutely lowers blood pressure within 1 to 3 minutes, with a gradual increase in blood pressure over 10 to 20 minutes, as reflex cardiovascular responses occur, and then a slower increase to pretreatment levels within 3 to 15 hours.[54] Oral antihypertensive therapy should be started early after diazoxide administration to stabilize and continue its therapeutic benefit. Diazoxide is not felt to be a suitable agent in the anesthetic setting because of its steep and prolonged blood pressure lowering effects. With the availability of tritratible drugs such as nitroprusside and trimethaphan and the requirement for minute-to-minute control of blood pressure, diazoxide has found little application in the perioperative period.

Major problems with diazoxide include its tendency for salt and water retention, and hyperglycemia[54] necessitating concomitant diuretic therapy. Because of reflex increases in left ventricular ejection velocity and stroke volume, it should not be used in patients with dissecting aortic aneurysm, subarachnoid, subdural, or intracerebral hemorrhage or the patient with coronary artery disease demonstrating ischemia.

ALPHA-ADRENERGIC BLOCKING DRUGS

Phentolamine

Phentolamine is described classically as an alpha-blocking drug. It is also known to act by direct vascular smooth muscle relaxation.[53–57] Phentolamine has been used in various perioperative settings. These include the control of intra- and postoperative hypertension, reduction of pulmonary vascular resistance,[58] intraoperative treatment of paroxysmal hypertension associated with manipulation and removal of pheochromocytoma, and for pre- and afterload reduction during open-heart surgery.[59] Phentolamine is useful in the reduction of systemic vascular resistance and control of perfusion pressure during cardiopulmonary bypass.[60] In the medical setting, phentolamine has been used in patients with acute myocardial infarction with left ventricular failure.[61–63]

Phentolamine reduces tone in both the resistance and capacitance vessels, and hence can reduce both afterload and preload. Pulmonary vascular resistance is decreased also by both alpha-blockade and direct smooth muscle relaxation. The relative degree of changes in systemic vs. pulmonary vascular resistance remains controversial. Phentolamine is reported to have an indirect positive inotropic effect on the myocardium, probably involving endogenous norepinephrine.[64] Reflex tachycardia is seen, though a chronotropic response may again be partly related to endogenous release of norepinephrine. This tachycardia may be quite significant. The inotropic and chronotropic effects of phentolamine may be reduced by beta-blockade with propranolol.[65]

Phentolamine is administered predominantly as an intravenous bolus or constant infusion (see Table 12-2). It has a rapid onset of action, within 2 to 3 minutes of intravenous injection, and lasts for 15 to 30 minutes. It may be given as from 1 to 3 mg increments for short or intermittent effects, or by constant infusion in the range of from 50 to 500 µg/min for sustained activity; 100 or 120 µg/ml are convenient concentrations for infusion. Most of the administered phentolamine is metabolized in the liver, with little of the original active drug excreted in the urine.

The major and most disturbing side-effects of phentolamine are tachycardia and cardiac stimulation, as previously mentioned, and occasionally the appearance of arrhythmias. Myocardial ischemia can be precipitated or enhanced. This is a distinct disadvantage when attempting to use the drug in the setting of acute myocardial infarction and left ventricular dysfunction. It has been shown experimentally that the area of ischemic injury can actually be increased during administration of phentolamine.[66] Gastrointestinal stimulation also may occur, with nausea, vomiting, diarrhea, abdominal pain, and exacerbation of peptic ulcer disease.

Phenoxybenzamine

Phenoxybenzamine is a long-acting alpha-adrenergic blocker of the haloalkylamine series. The alpha blockade is the result of a direct competition at alpha-adrenergic receptors, a stable covalent bond being formed between drug and receptor.[67, 68] It is much longer-acting than phentolamine, and a more complete blocker. Blockade by a single dose of phenoxybenzamine can be detected for three to four days. Phenoxybenzamine is used in both oral and intravenous forms for the preoperative management of patients with pheochromocytoma,[69, 70] and orally in the prolonged treatment of pheochromocytoma not amenable to surgery.[71] The use of phenoxybenzamine during cardiopulmonary bypass has been described in relation to renal blood flow[72] and for control of perfusion pressures.[73] Its routine use in this setting is not presently recommended.

The vasodilating effect of phenoxybenzamine is primarily on resistance and pulmonary vessels. The magnitude of change in pressure or flow will depend upon the preexisting level of adrenergic vasomotor control. Heart rate may increase on a reflex basis and cardiac output may increase subsequent to the decrease in vascular resistance.

The alpha-blocking action of phenoxybenz-

amine is responsible for the untoward effects. Postural hypotension, reflex tachycardia, and marked hypotension in the hypovolemic patient may occur. With alpha blockade, compensatory peripheral vasoconstriction may be impaired or eliminated, greatly exaggerating the effects of commonly used drugs such as thiopental, halothane, enflurane, and morphine.[74] Miosis, nasal stuffiness, inhibition of ejaculation, and gastrointestinal stimulation are additional reported complications.

Chlorpromazine

Chlorpromazine is a phenothiazine with well-known, alpha-adrenergic blocking properties. Its major use today is as an oral antipsychotic, but intravenous administration may be useful in the cardiovascular anesthetic setting because of its alpha-blocking effect.

The mechanism of chlorpromazine's vasodilation and blood pressure lowering effects is threefold. In addition to alpha-blockade, the drug depresses hypothalamic and brainstem-mediated vasomotor reflexes in relatively low doses, and has a direct relaxant action on blood vessels. Coronary blood flow may increase with chlorpromazine.[75] Chlorpromazine also has a weak peripheral cholinergic blocking action. In the cat papillary muscle, chlorpromazine has been shown to have a direct depressant action on the heart at relatively low concentrations.[76] An antiarrhythmic effect of chlorpromazine is known, caused by either a quinidine-like action or to local anesthetic effect.[76] Chlorpromazine can block the dopaminergic receptors in the renal and mesenteric vasculatures.[77]

In the setting of cardiac anesthesia, chlorpromazine is used intravenously in small doses for the control of hypertension. Increased peripheral vascular resistance during cardiopulmonary bypass and the early postoperative period can be treated with initial intravenous doses of from 1 to 2 mg. A rather marked, even profound, decrease in arterial pressure may result if vascular tone is high or blood volume low or both. If systemic pressure remains high or returns to excessive levels after multiple incremental doses, a more titratable drug such as nitroprusside may be added. Stinson and coworkers, comparing several vasodilator drugs immediately after open-heart surgery, found incremental doses of chlorpromazine hemodynamically similar to nitroprusside, except for a significant increase in heart rate.[78] They attributed the tachycardia to the vagolytic (anticholinergic) effect of chlorpromazine and reflex response. Systemic and pulmonary vascular resistances declined significantly, as did mean arterial pressure and ventricular filling pressure. Cardiac index increased, but was related to heart rate.

Chlorpromazine is metabolized extensively in the liver, with metabolites excreted in feces and urine. It is bound extensively to plasma protein (>90%) and can interact with other drugs. It can enhance the effects of other CNS depressants, especially the respiratory depression produced by narcotics. One major problem with intravenously administered chlorpromazine in the acute care setting is its potential to cause rapid and excessive degrees of hypotension if used initially in more than small, conservative (1–2 mg) doses.

Droperidol

Droperidol is a butyrophenone which is used either alone or in combination with fentanyl (Innovar) to produce the neuroleptic state. Droperidol and haloperidol, another commonly used butyrophenone, are both known to cause alpha-adrenergic blockade.[79, 80] Droperidol, alone or with fentanyl, is used in both the preinduction and induction phases of anesthesia. Droperidol is classified as a major tranquilizer. The clinical response to droperidol and fentanyl administration is the neuroleptic state, characterized by a suppression of affect and a slowing of motor function, with the preservation of the ability to follow simple commands.[81] Neuroleptic drugs cause general quiescence and a state of psychic indifference to environmental stimuli.[82]

The alpha-blocking and CNS sedative effects of droperidol are responsible for hypotension in patients with low blood volume or high systemic vascular resistance or both. Decreased arteriolar tone and increased venous capacitance result from droperidol. Several studies employing intravenous droperidol, administered in total divided doses of from 10 to 17.5 mg, have demonstrated a transient lowering of systemic vascular resistance and venous pressure.[83–85] Droperidol has an antiarrhythmic effect felt to be caused by local anesthetic properties or the blood pressure lowering effect on pressure-sensitive arrhythmias or both.[86, 87] The butyrophenones are known to cause selective blockade of dopaminergic receptors.[88, 89] Droperidol has a potent antiemetic effect, a useful property in the perioperative setting.

Droperidol is employed intravenously in 2.5 mg doses or in a fixed 50:1 combination with fentanyl (2.5 mg/ml:0.05 mg/ml, respectively) as Innovar. Droperidol is a long-acting tranquilizer with a half-life of from 2 to 3 hours. Its effects can be prolonged markedly in the aged patient. The major side-effect of droperidol is excessive hypotension. Extrapyramidal movements occur in a small percentage of patients. A feeling of anxiety and inner discomfort has been described when droperidol is used alone without a narcotic analgesic.[90] With the droperidol-fentanyl mixture, bradycardia may be seen in addition to arterial hypotension. Chest wall rigidity (from the fentanyl), associated with generalized muscular rigidity, can be a significant problem for ventilation, but is treated readily with neuromuscular paralysis.

Prazosin

Prazosin is a new oral antihypertensive drug in use since 1976. It was thought to act by direct, vascular smooth muscle relaxation until recently.[91, 92] Its alpha-blocking action is now firmly established.[93, 94] Prazosin is used generally in concert with other antihypertensive drugs. The combination of a diuretic, beta-blocker, and prazosin has been found to be particularly effective.[95] Recently, prazosin has been found also to be effective in the management of severe acute and chronic congestive heart failure, with improvement in cardiac index, lowering of ventricular filling pressures, and minimal change in heart rate.[96, 97]

Hemodynamically, prazosin's actions are similar to nitroprusside, producing a balanced reduction in arterial and venous tone.[98] As a result, arterial pressure is decreased secondary to a diminished systemic vascular resistance. Preload is decreased as venous capacitance is increased.

Prazosin is used orally for control of hypertension in doses beginning at 2 to 3 mg, and up to 20 to 30 mg per day. In the therapy of congestive heart failure, initial doses of from 2 to 7 mg a day are administered with maintenance dosages of from 8 to 28 mg a day. Prazosin is metabolized primarily in the liver with a plasma half-life of 3 to 4 hours.[99] The half-life of the drug's antihypertensive effect is considerably longer. Postural hypotension, when seen, is usually an early side-effect of prazosin, but can be a chronic problem in a small percentage of patients. Although tachycardia is mild or absent, it may occur and may worsen preexisting angina.[100]

GANGLIONIC BLOCKADE

Trimethaphan

Trimethaphan is a potent ganglionic blocking drug in clinical use since 1953. It is a sulfur containing monoquarternary molecule which, in addition to its ganglionic blocking activity, is known to release histamine[101] and directly relax vascular smooth muscle.[102, 103] Trimethaphan produces ganglionic blockade by occupying intraganglionic, postsynaptic receptor sites, preventing the action of acetylcholine liberated from presynaptic nerve endings. Trimethaphan is administered as a continuous intravenous infusion. Its major uses have been in producing controlled hypotension during surgery and in the management of hypertensive emergencies. Its application has diminished over recent years with the widespread use of nitroprusside.

The hemodynamic properties of trimeth-

aphan are complex. As with any vasodilator drug, the existing background autonomic activity and blood volume determine the extent of decrease in arterial blood pressure. The awake, unpremedicated patient will have a lesser and more limited hypotensive response than the anesthetized patient. Most clinical studies demonstrate a reduced systemic vascular resistance (SVR) with trimethaphan. Hypotension is a result of both decreased SVR and a loss of venous tone, with resulting increased peripheral pooling. Postural effects, blood volume, and positive airway pressure all impact upon the venous pooling effects of trimethaphan. Scott and coworkers studied trimethaphan-induced hypotension in man during nitrous oxide/halothane anesthesia. Systemic vascular resistance and mean arterial pressure decreased, with heart rate and cardiac output remaining unchanged.[104] Stinson and coworkers studied patients with relatively well-preserved left ventricular function in the immediate post-cardiac surgical period for the control of hypertension.[105] Trimethaphan caused decreases in mean arterial pressure, left and right ventricular filling pressures, systemic vascular resistance, and cardiac index. Heart rate was unchanged. Thus, in the nonfailing heart, trimethaphan appears to produce myocardial depression.

The different circulatory beds may have variable and specific responses to trimethaphan administration. In both humans and animals the effects of ganglionic blockade on cerebral hemodynamics and metabolism have been studied. It does not alter the autoregulatory mechanism or the cerebrovascular response to $PaCO_2$ in conscious humans.[106] In awake humans, Moyer and coworkers showed that cerebral blood flow and metabolic rate decreased when trimethaphan-induced hypotension occurred below levels of from 35 to 60 torr.[107] Magness and coworkers, using a dog model, suggested an adverse cerebral metabolic effect by trimethaphan, separate from the hemodynamic changes, that may potentiate neurologic damage.[108] Michenfelder and Theyer studied cerebral hemodynamics and metabolic parameters in dogs during induced hypotension produced by several methods.[109] Trimethaphan was not desirable because of a greater reduction in cerebral blood flow at the level of mean arterial pressure studied (40–50 torr), increased cerebral lactate levels, and greater postoperative neurologic deficits.

It is well-known that as mean arterial pressure is lowered below approximately 70 torr, the limits of renal autoregulation are exceeded and glomerular filtration decreases.[110] Several investigators have shown that glomerular filtration may diminish or cease with trimethaphan-induced hypotension.[102, 111] The kidney's metabolic needs are met with continued renal perfusion. Glomerular filtration returns as systemic blood pressure is restored.

Redistribution of blood away from the pulmonary circulation during trimethanphan administration has been found to be the basis for a decreased effective pulmonary capillary bed[112] and an increased Vd/Vt and altered V/Q relationships.[113] Changes in pulmonary arterial pressure and vascular resistance are variable, depending upon the variable response of cardiac output to trimethaphan administration. Blood flow to skeletal muscle and skin increases with ganglionic blockade in anesthetized dogs, while mesenteric blood flow decreased significantly.[102]

There are several important aspects to be noted in the clinical pharmacology of trimethaphan. Pupillary dilation and cycloplegia are the result of blockade of the ciliary ganglion. The cycloplegia may persist for several hours postinfusion, and obscure clinical neurologic evaluation.[114] Tachyphylaxis is common, particularly in the young, requiring increasing dosage for a sustained hypotensive effect. A sensitization of the receptors to epinephrine and norepinephrine, induced by trimethaphan, has been postulated.[115] Tachycardia usually accompanies tachyphylaxis, and is attributed to increased catecholamine sensitivity, baroreceptor reflex activation, and blockade of vagal ganglionic traffic. Both halothane[116] and beta-blockade by propranolol[117] have been advocated to suppress the heart rate response and to promote a greater

hypotensive effect from trimethaphan. It is suggested that propranolol be administered before the initiation of ganglion blockade[117] and that the concomitant use of belladonna drugs should be avoided or reduced.

Trimethaphan infusions should be prepared freshly (see Table 12-2). Infusion rates are highly variable but generally are in the range of from 0.2 to 6.0 mg/min. Trimethaphan has a rapid onset of action, with hypotension effects lasting approximately from 10 to 30 minutes after discontinuation of the infusion. Trimethaphan is thought to be metabolized by pseudocholinesterase. Patients with low levels of pseudocholinesterase, such as in severe hepatic disease or cachexia, or abnormal pseudocholinesterase, should not receive trimethaphan. Because of known histamine release by trimethaphan, it is felt best to avoid trimethaphan in the asthmatic or highly allergic patient. Theoretically, histamine release also might be of concern in certain neurosurgical patients because of potential direct cerebral vasodilation and a possible increase in intracranial pressure.[118]

Pentolinium Tartrate

Pentolinium is a bisquaternary ganglionic blocking drug. It was introduced by Enderby in 1954 for deliberate hypotension.[119] It remains in clinical practice today as a useful drug for the production of deliberate hypotension, particularly in major orthopedic surgery.

The major hemodynamic properties of pentolinium have been studied well.[120] Significant reduction in systemic vascular resistance is noted approximately 10 minutes after administration, with a greater decrease seen in approximately at 60 minutes. The decrease in mean arterial pressure may lag behind the decrease in SVR because of increases in cardiac output secondary to tachycardia but the heart rate tends to return to initial levels. The deliberate hypotension produced by pentolinium is felt by some to be advantageous because of its slower, more gradual onset and lack of tachyphylaxis, commonly seen with trimethaphan. Of course, once pentolinium's effects are established, they are not dissipated readily.

Pentolinium is administered intravenously to a total dose of from 0.1 to 0.3 mg/kg, depending on age. Initially, 3 mg is usually given, the response observed, and the remainder of the dose then given incrementally over 5 to 10 minutes.[121] Peak effect is seen in approximately 30 to 40 minutes, with the duration variable at 1 to 6 hours. Pentolinium is manufactured in 10-ml vials containing 10 mg/ml.*

CENTRAL NERVOUS SYSTEM SITE OF ACTION

Methyldopa (Alpha-Methyldopa)

Methyldopa is one of the major drugs used in the treatment of essential hypertension, usually with a diuretic. Methyldopa's mechanism of action has been in dispute for many years, but the current, generally accepted interpretation is that the major antihypertensive action of methyldopa is on the CNS.[122] It originally was felt to be a peripheral adrenergic blocking agent because of its inhibition of dopa decarboxylase and consequent reduction of norepinephrine stores in sympathetic nerves. Methyldopa is metabolized to alpha-methylnorepinephrine and its role as a false transmitter originally was considered the basis of its action. Alpha-methylnorepinephrine, as a metabolite of methyldopa in the CNS is now thought to be the active agent in the antihypertensive action of this drug.[123]

Hemodynamic effects include reduction of peripheral vascular resistance and cardiac output. Heart rate is decreased, though less so with chronic administration. Autonomic competence is not compromised severely and exercise hypotension and postural hypotension are not major problems. Renal blood flow is not restricted with the hypotensive action of methyldopa.

Methyldopa can be used when control of the blood pressure over several hours is the therapeutic goal. Intravenous infusion of from 0.5 to 1.0 g over 20 minutes will produce a hypotensive effect in 1 to 2 hours. In the previously hypertensive postoperative patient, blood pressure control is frequently necessary but difficult. After major vascular surgery, avoidance of excessive arterial pressures is essential. While nitroprusside is very effective, intravenous methyldopa is useful in reestablishing the longer term control of the patient's hypertension. Intravenous administration is well-suited for the presurgical stabilization of patients with dissection aneurysms of the aortic arch and in the medical management of DeBakey type III dissections. Both a hypotensive effect and a diminished inotropic state will be helpful in limiting further dissection (see discussion in *Therapeutic Applications of Vasodilators*).

Methyldopa is excreted mostly unchanged in the urine, a significant concern in the patient with renal impairment. Sedation is a major side-effect of the drug. When administered parenterally for control of blood pressure after craniotomy, the CNS sedative effects may interfere with clinical assessment of the patient. A positive direct Coomb's test occurs in from 10 to 20 percent of patients on chronic methyldopa therapy, with a rare patient exhibiting a hemolytic anemia.

Clonidine

Clonidine is a potent antihypertensive drug introduced in recent years. Its mechanism of action is by stimulation of alpha-adrenergic receptors in the cardiovascular control center of the medulla oblongata. This in turn inhibits efferent sympathetic activity.[124] It is used orally in combination with a diuretic in the control of moderate to severe essential hypertension. Dosage is from 400 µg to 2.0 mg per day.

The hemodynamic effects of clonidine resulting from central suppression of efferent sympathetic activity include diminished systemic vascular resistance, cardiac output, and heart rate. Postural hypotension is not a se-

---

* Wyeth Laboratories reports that pentolinium tartrate (Ansolysen) is no longer available. Their drug source, May and Baker (England), has not manufactured nor distributed the agent since January 1977.

vere problem and cardiovascular responses to exercise remain largely intact.

Sedation and dry mouth are the most frequent and annoying side effects. Of concern is the potential for a sharp rebound to pretreatment hypertensive levels or beyond (with the possible triggering of a hypertensive crisis) if clonidine is abruptly stopped. Overreactivity of the sympathetic nervous system is the etiology, indicated by elevated urinary and blood catecholamines.[125] This acute withdrawal syndrome has been described in the perioperative period.[126, 127] It is recommended that clonidine be continued throughout the patient's surgical experience, including oral administration on the morning of operation.

THERAPEUTIC APPLICATIONS

SURGICAL APPLICATIONS

Open-Heart Surgery

The vasodilator drugs are important in the treatment of intra- and postoperative myocardial depression and hypertension. Myocardial depression and its consequences, pump failure and low cardiac output, are seen not infrequently after cardiopulmonary bypass and occasionally in the cardiac patient undergoing noncardiac surgery. Low cardiac output contributes significantly to postoperative morbidity and mortality. The cardiac index has been used as a prognostic factor determining survival in the postcardiac surgical patient.[128]

Many patients with ischemic heart disease or valvular disease or both come to cardiac surgery with chronic dysfunction of one or both ventricles. A hypertensive response to airway instrumentation, skin incision, or sternotomy may cause a compensated or hemodynamically normal heart to decompensate acutely. Increased impedance to left ventricular ejection resulting from increased systemic resistance has been shown to reduce stroke volume and left ventricular stroke work in patients with diseased myocar-

dium.[129] Intravenous vasodilators have been found useful for lowering increased left ventricular filling pressure and improving ventricular function, in terms of improved stroke index and relief of ischemia.

Lappas and coworkers evaluated the hemodynamic response to nitroprusside administered intraoperatively in patients undergoing coronary artery operation.[130] They demonstrated significantly improved left ventricular performance in patients with chronic left heart dysfunction and elevated filling pressures. Sodium nitroprusside effectively controlled acute intraoperative hypertension with restoration to normal of elevated filling pressures and ischemic electrocardiographic changes attendant to raised systemic blood pressure. The resolution of ischemia was attributed to diminished myocardial oxygen demand as the acutely raised left ventricular filling pressure (LVFP) and systemic pressure were lowered with sodium nitroprusside. Kaplan and coworkers studied and compared the use of intravenous nitroglycerin and nitroprusside for intraoperative hypertension in patients with ischemic heart disease undergoing coronary artery surgery.[131, 132] The study suggested the superiority of nitroglycerin infusion to nitroprusside in patients with acute intraoperative ischemia, on the basis of better maintained coronary perfusion pressure, redistribution of coronary blood flow, and resolution of ischemic ECG changes.

Valvular defects, including mitral regurgitation and aortic insufficiency, are common causes of perioperative pump failure. These hemodynamic abnormalities, and subsequent myocardial dysfunction, are often amenable to vasodilator therapy.

Reduction of systemic vascular resistance and impedance to left ventricular ejection with nitroprusside can produce marked improvements in patients with severe mitral regurgitation from either ischemic heart disease (papillary muscle dysfunction)[133] or of purely valvular origin.[134] A decreased regurgitant volume was correlated to a reduction in the magnitude of the peak V wave in the PCWP tracing. Nitroglycerin, as a preload reducing agent, has been shown to decrease regurgitant volume and LVEDV (volume) in severe mitral regurgitation, without the accompanying marked increase in forward stroke volume seen with nitroprusside and hydrazaline.[135]

Aortic regurgitation is marked by volume overloading of the left ventricle. In severe chronic aortic regurgitation, LVEDP is elevated with increased pulmonary venous pressure. If acute, aortic regurgitation can quickly result in refractory pulmonary edema, inadequate forward cardiac output and death. Vasodilator therapy can be beneficial for both chronic and acute aortic regurgitation. As seen with mitral regurgitation, increased impedance to left ventricular ejection enhances the degree of regurgitation and lessens forward output. In severe chronic aortic regurgitation, nitroprusside decreased LVEDV, LVEDP, and regurgitant fraction, with an increase in forward stroke volume.[136] Afterload reduction with nitroprusside in severe acute aortic regurgitation improved cardiac performance with greatly decreased left ventricular volume and aortic regurgitant volume.[137] In vasodilator drug therapy of aortic regurgitation, extra caution is needed if coronary artery disease is present. Excessive reduction of aortic diastolic pressure from an already lower-than-normal level can compromise coronary perfusion pressure and result in, or enhance, myocardial ischemia.

Vasodilator therapy is used frequently in the early postoperative period in cardiac surgical patients to increase cardiac output when depressed from ventricular dysfunction and elevated systemic vascular resistance. Kouchoukous and coworkers demonstrated the benefit of trimethaphan camsylate in enhancing low cardiac output after mitral valve replacement.[138] Stinson and coworkers compared trimethaphan, nitroprusside, nitroglycerin, and chlorpromazine in the early cardiac surgical postoperative period.[139] All four drugs caused significant reductions of systemic arterial pressure and left and right atrial pressures. Nitroprusside, though, was the only agent to demonstrate a significant decrease in systemic vascular resistance and increase in stroke volume as left atrial pressure was reduced. They judged nitroprusside to be particularly favorable early after cardiac operation because of its ability to reduce left ventricular stroke and minute work while simultaneously enhancing cardiac pumping performance. In a later study, Stinson and coworkers again demonstrated the benefit of nitroprusside-induced afterload reduction during mild-to-moderate low cardiac output immediately postoperatively, but demonstrated the need for optimal preload maintenance (i.e., volume augmentation to base-line left atrial pressure) to achieve maximal hemodynamic benefit.[140]

Vasodilation in the immediate, intraoperative, post-cardiopulmonary bypass period is also helpful. One application of sodium nitroprusside intraoperatively is the transferring to the patient of all the remaining perfusate from the oxygenator reservoir, thereby diminishing requirements for additional units of homologous bank blood.[140] Vasodilation can be used in concern with inotropic support of the myocardium, frequently dopamine, or with intraaortic balloon counterpulsation. It has been shown, in acute myocardial infarction and severe pump failure, that combined sodium nitroprusside and intraaortic balloon counterpulsation causes a greater increase in cardiac output than intraaortic balloon counterpulsation alone.[141]

Induced Hypotension

Induced hypotension is the deliberate lowering of systemic blood pressure to improve operating conditions and to minimize overall blood loss. Introduced in 1946 by means of arteriotomy and controlled hemorrhage, induced hypotension has led to much controversy and reassessment through the years.[142] Today, induced hypotension is a useful and safe adjunct when managed by an anesthesiologist with sufficient experience and knowledge of its physiologic and pharmacologic principles, and with adequate hemodynamic monitoring.

Induced hypotension is beneficial for tumor surgery in the cranium (meningioma), head, neck, and pelvis, during intracranial surgery for AV malformation and aneurysm clipping, and major orthopedic surgery including total hip replacement and scoliosis correction. This last indication is controversial because of potential disruption of spinal cord blood flow. Patients undergoing extensive plastic surgical and skin-grafting procedures, mammoplasty, thoracoplasty, and portacaval shunt operations can benefit by deliberate lowering of blood pressure. Patients refusing transfusion because of religious persuasion or with difficult cross-matching problems also can benefit from induced hypotension.

Appropriate patient selection is fundamental to the safe application of induced hypotension. The anesthesiologist must judge the patient's ability to tolerate the physiologic manipulations involved. Contraindications may include documented ischemic heart disease, congestive heart failure, respiratory failure, gross anemia, evidence of hypovolemia, previous cerebrovascular accident, clinical or angiographic evidence of cerebrovascular disease, severe hypertension, and significant renal or hepatic disease.[143] Because of pupillary dilation, ganglionic blocking drugs are contraindicated in narrow-angle glaucoma. Advanced age alone is not a contraindication to the technique.[143]

The safe conduct of induced hypotension demands attention to several important technical details. In addition to adequate experience and proper patient selection, careful patient positioning must be observed. Postural changes can be significant, resulting in excessive peripheral pooling or potential cerebral vascular congestion. Mechanical ventilation with a $PaCO_2$ of from 35 to 40 torr, confirmed with arterial blood gas analysis, is required to avoid cerebral vasoconstriction and possible cerebral hypoxia in the face of a lowered perfusion pressure. With vasodilators, sympathetic vasoconstriction in response to hypovolemia is impaired or lost, necessitating strict and precise vascular volume replacement. Continuous monitoring of systemic blood pressure by direct arterial can-

nula and a pressure transducing system, is considered standard today.

Regardless of the specific pharmacologic means employed for blood pressure lowering, tissue perfusion is of utmost concern. The critical (minimal) arterial pressure and specific organ blood flow should be considered. In young, healthy patients (American Society of Anesthesiologists class I or II), systolic pressure should not be below 60 to 70 torr. Elderly patients should have a minimum systolic pressure of 80 torr. Specific investigations of organ perfusion have been reported regarding blood flow to brain,[144–146] myocardium,[146, 147] lung,[148, 149] kidney,[146, 150] and liver.[146, 151] Cerebral autoregulation is preserved above a mean arterial pressure of approximately 60 torr, below which perfusion may become pressure dependent. An interesting and important observation by Eckenhoff and coworkers during investigation of the adequacy of cerebral blood flow during induced hypotension, was that the jugular bulb $P_{jb}O_2$ depended more on the level of $PaCO_2$ than on arterial blood pressure, stressing the need for close monitoring and control of ventilation and subsequent gas exchange.[152] This effect of increased $PaCO_2$ increasing jugular bulb $P_{jb}O_2$ is most likely a shunting or "steal" phenomenon, and does *not* necessarily signal cerebral well-being.

Coronary perfusion is dependent in large measure on aortic diastolic pressure, and must be adequate to meet oxygen demand. Myocardial work and $M\dot{V}O_2$ are decreased with induced hypotension. This helps to maintain the oxygen supply greater than demand if pressure is not decreased too rapidly or to less than a mean pressure of 50 torr, and providing the coronary arteries are free of obstructive lesions. In the lung, a reduction in pulmonary artery pressure and blood volume may result in a decreased perfusion of well-ventilated alveoli, causing an increase in both $\dot{V}/Q$ ratio and physiologic deadspace. With changes in both lung volume and deadspace, mechanical ventilation and blood gas analysis are mandatory. Renal perfusion is maintained at low systemic pressure because of autoregulation. Glomerular filtration, though, does diminish and may cease at systolic pressures less than 70 torr. Urine output also may diminish or cease, but renal metabolic needs appear to be met. Urine flow may occur as systolic pressure is increased above 70 torr.

Today, vasodilator drugs commonly used for induced hypotension include nitroprusside, nitroglycerin, trimethaphan, and pentolinium (if available). Nitroprusside is the most commonly used agent, with advantages of potent action and immediate control. Infusion should begin with a low dose (*e.g.*, 0.3 μg/kg/min) titrated to a predetermined endpoint. Lowering of systemic pressure should be gradual, over approximately several minutes, with careful monitoring and complete replacement of blood loss. Continuous infusion of nitroglycerin has been used more recently for induced hypotension. Infusion is begun at 0.5 μg/kg/min and titrated to the desired hypotensive level. Lowering of blood pressure is smoother and more gradual than with nitroprusside. It is effective, easily reversible and may have a more favorable effect on the coronary circulation during induced hypotension than nitroprusside.[151] Trimethaphan was used extensively in the 1950s and 1960s, but is being replaced by the direct-acting vasodilators nitroprusside and nitroglycerin. It is used in a concentration of 1 to 2 mg/ml, at a dose range of 0.2 mg to 6 mg/min. Like nitroprusside, onset of action is rapid and initial dosage should be low. Its effects are absent after 10 to 30 minutes of drug discontinuation. Tachycardia and tachyphylaxis may limit the usefulness of this agent, particularly in the young. Pentolinium, given in intravenous bolus form, has a gradual onset of from 5 to 30 minutes and a long duration of action, variable at 1 to 6 hours. Dosage is from 0.1 to 0.3 mg/kg. An initial 3 mg dose is given to observe the circulating response. The remaining dose is given over 5 to 10 minutes.

Complications of induced hypotension are a result of compromised tissue perfusion, sometimes occurring in the postoperative period. They include renal failure, ischemic injury or death of myocardium, and cerebral infarction. Reactionary hemorrhage beyond termination of the period of induced hypotension can occur, but is minimized when blood pressure gradually is allowed to return to normal and adequate surgical hemostasis is assured.[153]

Major Vascular Surgery

Abdominal and thoracic aortic aneurysms and occlusive disease of the aorta and its major branches are common surgical problems seen frequently by the anesthesiologist. Patients present either electively for repair and reconstruction or occasionally on an emergency basis with aortic and major vessel dissection, rupture, or occlusion. Both elective and emergency aortic surgery present major anesthetic and surgical challenges. In this patient population, there is frequently concomitant hypertension and coronary artery disease, with and without left ventricular dysfunction and failure. Myocardial infarction in the perioperative period is a major cause of mortality among these patients. Vasodilator therapy is a particularly useful adjunct in the perioperative management of these patients.

During surgical resection of an abdominal aortic aneurysm and aortofemoral bypass, cross-clamping of the aorta causes an acute increase in afterload. In patients with significant ischemic heart disease or left ventricular dysfunction or both, myocardial ischemia and acute increases in LVFP are reported.[154–156] Attia and coworkers effectively treated the afterload-related ischemia with nitroprusside, initiating treatment at from 10 to 15 μg/min, with a dose range from 15 to 40 μg/min.[154] Another potentially critical point during repair is at the time of release of the aortic cross-clamp. This can be characterized by profound hypotension and is often referred to as declamping shock. Multiple etiologies have been proposed for its occurrence.[157–159] Volume loading during aortic resection and the cross-clamp period in anticipation of cross-clamp release has been found to be the most effective therapy in preventing or minimizing declamping shock.[160, 164] Vasodilator therapy and measurement of mean pulmonary artery occluded pressure ($\overline{PA}_0$) allows optimal volume loading before unclamping, maintaining $\overline{PA}_0$ in the 10 to 20 torr range.[160] Discontinuation of the vasodilator infusion shortly before cross-clamp release contributes to hemodynamic stability and avoidance of profound hypotension. Postoperative hypertension is a frequent problem, necessitating the transient use of a vasodilator to protect the newly placed aortic graft, to diminish bleeding, and to maintain a favorable oxygen supply and demand balance for the heart. Nitroprusside is the most commonly used drug. Hydralazine, chlorpromazine, and propranolol also are useful adjuncts.

Vasodilator therapy plays a fundamental role in the management of thoracic aneurysms. In managing dissecting aneurysms of the thoracic aorta, prompt surgical therapy is usually the treatment of choice for dissection in the ascending aorta (DeBakey type I and II), whereas medical therapy is usually superior in patients with dissection limited to the descending aorta (DeBakey type III).[162] Whether in the ascending or descending aorta, the first step in therapy is to decrease systolic blood pressure to 110 to 130 torr and decrease myocardial contractility, thereby stopping the process of dissection and pain.[162, 163] Vasodilator drugs recommended are trimethaphan, nitroprusside, reserpine, methyldopa, and guanethadine. The latter three drugs or propranolol will diminish myocardial contractility, thus lessening the impact of ventricular systole against the aortic wall.[164] During surgery for thoracic aneurysm, partial cardiopulmonary bypass (femoral-femoral or left atrial-femoral) may be employed. The placement of a high aortic cross-clamp can increase proximal mean arterial pressure in excess of 200 torr. Cerebral edema is possible as the upper limits of autoregulation are exceeded. Nitroprusside is useful, but an excessive decrease in blood pressure can jeopardize spinal cord perfusion. Arterial systolic pressure in the upper part of the body should be kept at approximately 150 torr. Postoperatively, mean arterial blood pressure should be maintained in the 70 to 80 torr range to avoid excessive tension within the aortic suture line.[165] (Please see Chapter 22 for further details.)

Pheochromocytoma

Pheochromocytoma is a catecholamine-producing tumor of chromaffin tissue, usually occurring in or around the region of the adrenal glands. It is occasionally bilateral. The resultant high levels of circulating epinephrine and norepinephrine are responsible for the signs and symptoms of pheochromocytoma, particularly paroxysmal or persistent hypertension and arrhythmias. Surgical removal of the tumor is a major anesthetic challenge, with extreme swings in blood pressure, and potentially lethal arrhythmias.

Vasodilators constitute an essential part of perioperative therapy. Alpha-blockade of catecholamine-induced hypertension in the preoperative period prevents hypertensive episodes and permits expansion of the contracted plasma volume commonly seen in these patients. Oral phenoxybenzamine is administered, 10 mg three times a day for two weeks before surgery. Phenoxybenzamine is replaced by short-acting phentolamine, 5 mg intramuscularly every 6 hours for 48 hours before surgery, to avoid prolonged hypotension after tumor removal.[166] Beta-adrenergic mediated cardiac arrhythmias and excessive cardiac rate are treated or prevented effectively by propranolol.

The intraoperative manipulation of the tumor and certain anesthetic maneuvers, such as laryngoscopy and intubation, can precipitate severe hypertension and arrhythmias, even if preoperative preparation has been aggressive. Sodium nitroprusside has been acknowledged as a useful drug in the intraoperative setting.[166-168] It is well suited for these problems because of its quick onset, short duration, and ease of titration. It is effective in the presence of high plasma catecholamine levels.[166] Infusion rates may be markedly higher than in other settings (*e.g.,* cardiac surgery, left ventricular failure) because of the competing vasoconstrictive effects of the increased plasma catecholamines. After tumor removal, the loss of intense catecholamine stimulation can result in hypotension, if vascular volume replacement is inadequate or if vasodilator administration is not adjusted.

MEDICAL APPLICATIONS

Angina Pectoris

Vasodilator therapy with nitroglycerin has been used in angina pectoris for over 100 years. The application of nitroglycerin and the related organic nitrates has been discussed in detail. Nitroglycerin's efficacy in the relief of angina pectoris is related primarily to its peripheral vascular action, although direct coronary effects have been documented and may contributed to improvement of myocardial oxygenation during ischemia.[169] With enhanced venous capacitance from a more selective effect on venous smooth muscle tone, nitroglycerin reduces venous return, and hence, preload. Thus, myocardial oxygen demand is lessened, and as filling pressures are decreased, endocardial blood flow may be increased. In addition, the mild arterial dilating effect may reduce afterload, further decreasing myocardial oxygen demand.

Congestive Heart Failure

The use of vasodilator drugs in congestive heart failure (CHF) has had increasing interest and application over the past decade. Benefits to the failing heart, in both the acute and chronic setting, result from increased venous capacitance with lower ventricular filling pressures (preload reduction), and decreased systemic vascular resistance enhancing left ventricular ejection (afterload reduction).

Nitroprusside has been shown to improve cardiac output and to decrease LVFP in patients with left ventricular failure during

acute myocardial infarction.[170–172] Intravenous and sublingual nitroglycerin have also been found effective in this setting.[173, 174] A consistent decrease in LVFP has been found, but if initially below 15 torr, stroke volume and cardiac output may decrease.[175] Symptoms of acute pulmonary edema can be relieved by vasodilators by a reduction in ventricular filling pressure and pulmonary vascular pressure, and by an increase in cardiac output.[176, 177]

In the management of chronic CHF, vasodilator drugs have been added to more standard regimens of digitalis and diuretic therapies, especially when chronic CHF is severe and refractory. Both ischemic and nonischemic chronic CHF have benefited from vasodilator therapy.[178] With chronic failure, both parenteral[177, 179] and nonparenteral drugs have been used, the latter including isosorbide dinitrate,[180] hydralazine,[181, 182] and prazosin.[183] Because of the selective arteriolar and venous dilator responses of the various vasodilator drugs, it is possible to select a regimen tailored to the patient's individual hemodynamic profile (*i.e.*, relief of pulmonary and ventricular congestion by preload reduction or reduction of impedance to ejection and increased cardiac output by afterload reduction or both).

Hypertensive Emergencies

Uncontrolled blood pressure increase may occur in several settings, all of which demand immediate and intensive treatment. Accelerated hypertension, hypertensive encephalopathy, hypertension complicated by acute left ventricular failure, intracranial hemorrhage, aortic dissection, or postoperative bleeding are the usual situations encountered clinically.[184] Vasodilator drugs are central to the management of hypertensive emergencies.

Parenteral administration of vasodilator agents is important in initial management. The particular drug employed will depend on the duration of action and the specific hemodynamic effects desired.[185] After initial control of blood pressure and amelioration of symptoms, it is important to convert to oral antihypertensive therapy as early as possible. Rapid control is obtained by a bolus injection of diazoxide (5 mg/kg in 10–20 seconds) or a constant infusion of nitroprusside or trimethaphan. Nitroprusside is particularly valuable in treating malignant hypertension refractory to standard antihypertensive drugs.[186] Hydralazine has been used in hypertensive emergencies, though by itself rarely controls blood pressure satisfactorily and is rarely desirable in the presence of coronary artery disease because of its ability to increase cardiac work (by reflex).[184] Propranolol is very useful as an adjunct to hydralazine and diazoxide by virtue of its action in blocking adrenergic reflex induced increases in cardiac output and heart rate. Methyldopa is useful in the patient whose blood pressure need not be controlled immediately. It reduces peripheral vascular resistance without decreasing cardiac output.

Section II: Vasopressors

A vasopressor increases blood pressure above the existing level. Most vasopressors are sympathomimetics. They stimulate adrenergic receptors (direct-acting) or stimulate the nerve terminals of the sympathetic nervous system to release the neurotransmitter, norepinephrine (indirect-acting). The drugs discussed in this section have specific vasoconstrictor properties. Isoproterenol, dopamine, and dobutamine, in therapeutic ranges, have vasopressor or vasodilator activity in addition to their inotropic properties and have been discussed in the previous chapter.

Classification of the vasopressors (and all sympathomimetics) by the type of receptor(s) they stimulate is useful for vasopressor selection and for evaluation of the receptor and end-organ response (Table 12-3).[187] Adrenergic receptors are classified as alpha, beta[1], and beta[2].* Dopaminergic receptors, more recently described, are found in the renal and mesenteric vascular beds, and mediate vasodilation in response to dopamine. Alpha receptors mediate increased smooth muscle tone in the peripheral vasculature, increasing

---

* A new subtype of alpha receptor has been identified recently, called the alpha[2] receptor. It is a *presynaptic* autoregulatory receptor which *inhibits* norepinephrine release when *stimulated,* and *enhances* norepinephrine release when *blocked*. The alpha[2] receptor is thought also to exist on the platelet surface. Some alpha-agonist drugs may be more selective for alpha[2] receptors (clonidine) than for alpha[1] receptors, and antagonists more selective for alpha[1] receptors (prazosin) than for alpha[2] receptors. For purposes of discussion in this chapter, the term alpha receptor will refer to the standard postsynaptic alpha[1] receptor. The reader is referred to Hoffman BB, Lefkowitz RJ: Alpha-adrenergic receptor subtypes. N Engl J Med 302:1390–1396, 1980, for further details regarding subdivision of alpha receptor function and to Table 12-4.

Table 12-3. Major Clinical Characteristics of the Vasopressors

DRUG	HEART	TARGET ORGAN PERIPHERAL CIRCULATION Vasoconstriction	Vasodilation	TYPE OF ACTION Direct	Indirect	RECEPTOR SPECIFICITY Alpha	Beta[1]	Beta[2]
Epinephrine	+ + + +	+ + + +	+ + +	yes	no	yes	yes	yes
Norepinephrine	+ +	+ + + +	0	yes	no	yes	yes	no
Phenylephrine	0	+ + + + +	0	yes	no	yes	no	no
Methoxamine	0	+ + + + +	0	yes	no	yes	no	no
Ephedrine	+ + +	+ +	+	yes	yes	yes	yes	yes
Metaraminol	+	+ + +	+ +	yes	yes	yes	yes	yes
Mephentermine	+ +	+	+ + +	yes	yes	yes	yes	yes

resistance to blood flow. Beta$_1$ receptors are responsible for chronotropic, inotropic, and arrhythmogenic effects, while beta$_2$ receptors cause vasodilation in skeletal muscle and relaxation of bronchial smooth muscle. Table 12-3 summarizes the major clinical characteristics of the vasopressors by target organ, type of pharmacologic action (direct or indirect), and receptor specificity. Table 12-5 lists suggested concentrations for intravenous infusion, infusion rates, and dose.

Reflex adjustments determine to some degree the circulatory effect of a particular sympathomimetic drug. With phenylephrine, a pure alpha agonist, vasoconstriction activates the carotid baroreceptor reflex, with a subsequent vagal slowing of the heart and diminished endogenous sympathetic tone. A drug with predominantly beta action will significantly dilate blood vessels in skeletal muscle. If arterial blood pressure is decreased, reflex-induced sympathetic tone may enhance the inotropic and chronotropic actions of the beta-agonist drug.

Use of the vasopressors has undergone much reassessment in the past decade. Emphasis has shifted appropriately to total and regional tissue perfusion as a measure of circulatory integrity rather than simply the level of arterial blood pressure. Monitoring of left ventricular function and cardiac output, new intravenous vasodilator drugs, and newer sympathomimetics such as dopamine and dobutamine have revamped vasoactive drug therapy in patients undergoing open-heart surgery, acute myocardial infarction with ventricular failure, and various forms of circulatory shock. The vasopressors retain an important role in the management of regional anesthesia and cardiopulmonary resuscitation.

Epinephrine

Epinephrine, an endogenous catecholamine produced in the adrenal medulla, is considered the prototype of the sympathomimetic drugs. It is direct-acting, capable of stimulating alpha, beta$_1$, and beta$_2$ receptors. Beta$_1$ receptor activation produces both inotropic and chronotropic action. The arrhythmogenic effect of epinephrine also results from beta$_1$ stimulation and is one of the more troublesome side-effects. Beta$_2$ stimulation produces relaxation of bronchial smooth muscle, vasodilation in skeletal muscle vessels and, to

Table 12-4. Classification of Alpha-adrenergic Receptor Agents

	ALPHA$_1$ POSTSYNAPTIC	ALPHA$_2$ PRESYNAPTIC
Agonists	Methoxamine Phenylephrine Norepinephine Epinephrine Dopamine	Clonidine Norepinephrine Epinephrine
Antagonists	Phentolamine Prazosin Phenoxybenzamine Phenothiazine Butyrophenones	Phentolamine Yohimbine

(Maze M: Clinical implications of membrane receptor function in anesthesia. Anesthesiology 55:160-171, 1981)

Table 12-5. Clinical Use of the Vasopressors

DRUG	SUGGESTED CONCENTRATION FOR CONTINUOUS INTRAVENOUS INFUSION	IV INFUSION RATE	IV BOLUS DOSE	IM DOSE
Epinephrine	1 mg/250 ml; 4 μg/ml	2–20 μg/min	0.3–1.0 mg*	†
Norepinephrine	4 mg/250 ml; 16 μg/ml	2–16 μg/min		
Phenylephrine	10 mg/250 ml; 40 μg/ml	10–50 μg/min	100–400 μg	
Methoxamine			2–10 mg	10–20 mg
Ephedrine			5–25 mg	25–50 mg
Metaraminol	100 mg/250 ml; 400 μg/ml	50–500 μg/min	0.5–5.0 mg	2–10 mg
Mephentermine	30 mg/250 ml; 120 μg/ml	?	5–15 mg	15–30 mg

*For user in the management of cardiac arrest during cardiopulmonary resuscitation
†Also used subcutaneously in the treatment of acute, severe bronchospasm; 0.1–0.5 mg

a lesser degree, vasodilation in the pulmonary circulation. Alpha effects, predominating with increased dosage, produce widespread vasoconstriction, particularly in the renal, splanchnic, pulmonary, and cutaneous circulations. The relative degree of receptor activation changes through the clinical range of intravenous epinephrine infusion (2–16 μg/min). At low dose, beta effects predominate. Both alpha and beta effects are seen at a moderate dose. There is a predominance of alpha vasoconstrictor effect at the higher range, although a positive inotropic effect is achieved throughout the entire range of 2 to 20 μg/min.[188] An increase in systemic blood pressure is produced by a threefold mechanism: direct myocardial stimulation, an increase in heart rate, and widespread vasoconstriction in both resistance and capacitance vessels.[189]

The diverse clinical usefulness of epinephrine is the result of its cardiocirculatory and bronchial smooth muscle actions. Epinephrine is a primary drug used in the management of cardiac arrest, capable of restoring electrical activity in ventricular asystole, and enhancing defibrillation in ventricular fibrillation.[190] The principal use of epinephrine in cardiovascular anesthesia is to increase cardiac output by increasing contractility of the failing heart.[191] Newer methods of myocardial preservation during bypass and aortic cross-clamping, newer inotropic agents (dopamine and dobutamine), and vasodilator therapy have decreased the use of epinephrine in treating the post-cardiopulmonary bypass low-output syndrome. Epinephrine has broad clinical application in the treatment of bronchospasm and pulmonary hypersensitivity reactions to drugs and allergens. When mixed in local anesthetic solutions, epinephrine causes local vasoconstriction, delaying absorption of the anesthetic drug, and prolonging the duration of the local anesthetic.

Ventricular ectopic beats, particularly in the presence of halothane, may occur commonly during epinephrine administration. The potential for a severe reduction in renal blood flow (and thus possible renal failure) subsequent to alpha vasoconstrictor activity on the renal arterioles should be considered whenever epinephrine is used. The increase in all determinants of myocardial oxygen demand by epinephrine can jeopardize seriously the ischemic myocardium. Ischemia may be produced quickly. Extension of a recently infarcted zone of myocardium is a reported possibility.[192]

Norepinephrine

Norepinephrine is the neurotransmitter of the peripheral autonomic nervous system. Its role in the regulation of the heart and peripheral circulation is central. This catecholamine, like epinephrine, is direct-acting and has a mixture of alpha and beta effects, differing mainly in the ratio of their effectiveness in stimulating alpha and beta receptors.[189] Norepinephrine's dominant actions are marked peripheral vasocontriction (alpha), and inotropic and chronotropic effects on the heart (beta$_1$). Beta$_2$-mediated peripheral vasodilation is negligible. In the intact circulation, cardiac output is unchanged or decreased, the latter effect secondary to an increase in left ventricular afterload. Heart rate may decrease because of baroreceptor reflex activation.

The current application of norepinephrine is limited. Its infusion for various shock states or cardiac failure is no longer justified because newer modalities exist which avoid or minimize the intense vasoconstriction and excessive myocardial oxygen demand produced by norepinephrine.

Phenylephrine

Phenylephrine is a direct-acting, noncatecholamine sympathomimetic. It is almost completely alpha-stimulating in its action. Phenylephrine's dominant hemodynamic effect is an increase in systemic vascular resistance. Cardiac effects are indirect; they occur through baroreceptor reflex activity and increased preload with venoconstriction. Phenylephrine may be used as an intravenous bolus or infusion to support arterial blood pressure in the early period during cardiopulmonary bypass, during carotid or aortic surgery, and during regional anesthesia. Its ability to enhance vagal tone through reflex activity is sometimes useful in the management of supraventricular tachycardia with hypotension.

Methoxamine

Methoxamine is an almost pure alpha-receptor agonist. It is a direct-acting noncatecholamine sympathomimetic, devoid of cardiac and peripheral beta effects. Its vasoconstrictor properties account for its use in the management of hypotension during spinal anesthesia and supraventricular tachycardia. It should be stressed that methoxamine's effect on the resistance vessels is marked. The resultant increases in afterload and myocardial oxygen demand can be detrimental to the dysfunctional or ischemic left ventricle.[193] In addition, renal blood flow is reduced. Methoxamine is reported to have a mild antiarrhythmic action, perhaps due to a weak beta-blocking effect on cardiac adrenergic receptors.[194]

Ephedrine

Ephedrine is a mixed sympathomimetic, having both alpha- and beta-receptor agonist activity, and acting both directly and indirectly. The cardiovascular effects of ephedrine are similar to epinephrine, with both vasoconstriction and cardiac stimulation, the latter effect predominating. The peripheral vascular actions are both alpha and beta$_2$, the alpha receptor effect being more potent. Bronchial smooth muscle relaxation also occurs. Ephedrine differs significantly from epinephrine in its lesser potency and longer duration of action. It is effective orally, intramuscularly, and intravenously.

Both peripheral and cardiac effects of ephedrine are well applied in treating the sympathetic blockade produced by spinal and epidural anesthesia.[195] Small intravenous doses of ephedrine (5–15 mg) may be useful if halothane-induced myocardial depression is significant, while the inspired halothane concentration is being reduced. This occurs not infrequently after anesthetic induction and stimulation by endotracheal intubation, but before surgical stimulation commences. Hypotension associated with nodal bradycardia is effectively treated with ephedrine and may contribute to the restoration of sinus rhythm. Oral ephedrine is useful in the management of chronic asthma and mild acute exacerbations. Epinephrine is used more correctly during a severe asthmatic attack for its more potent bronchial smooth muscle beta$_2$ effect.

Mephentermine

Mephentermine is a noncatecholamine sympathomimetic used as a pressor agent. It acts directly and indirectly and has both alpha and beta agonist activity. Its predominant cardiocirculatory effects are increased inotropy and peripheral vasoconstriction. Venoconstriction is prominent, enhancing veous return and preload. An antiarrhythmic effect has long been known, secondary to decreased conduction time in the AV junction, bundle of His, and Purkinje system, and a decrease in the refractory period of the atrium.[196] Mephentermine's predominant clinical application has been to counteract hypotension during regional anesthesia.

Metaraminol

Metaraminol is a noncatecholamine vasopressor that acts both directly and indirectly. Although much less potent, metaraminol resembles norepinephrine in its hemodynamic actions. Potent vasoconstriction occurs, with a subsequent reflex decrease in heart rate. The drug possesses some beta-agonist activity, although alpha stimulation is predominant. Cardiac output may increase secondary to this beta-activity, particularly if atropine is administered or if used during hypotensive states. Increased venous tone, decreased renal and cerebral blood flow, and pulmonary vasoconstriction may occur.[189] Metaraminol has been used in the treatment of hypotension associated with spinal anesthesia.

Summary

We have presented the pharmacology of drugs which act primarily on the peripheral vasculature. These agents have many clinical applications. The choice of vasodilator or vasopressor should be based upon the baseline hemodynamic state, the physiologic alterations desired, and the characteristics of the specific drug under consideration. Ideally, each of these drugs should be used only if the benefit to be derived exceeds the risks of each drug. Optimal use should occur concomitantly with safe and effective hemodynamic monitoring.

REFERENCES

Section I: Vasodilators

1. Parmley WW, Chatterjee K: Vasodilator therapy. Curr Prob Cardiol 2(12), 1978
2. Cohn JN, Franciosa JA: Vasodilator therapy of cardiac failure. N Engl J Med 297:254, 1977
3. Parmley WW, Chatterjee K: The role of vasodilator therapy in heart failure. Prog Cardiovasc Dis 19:301, 1977
4. Gifford RW Jr: Hypertensive emergencies and their treatment. Med Clin North Am 45:441, 1961

MECHANISM OF ACTION

5. Nickerson M: Vasodilator drugs. In Goodman LS, Gilman A (eds): The Pharmacological Basis of Therapeutics, p 727. New York, Macmillan, 1975
6. Palmer RF, Lasseter KC: Sodium nitroprusside. N Engl J Med 292:294, 1975

PHYSIOLOGIC BASIS OF VASODILATOR THERAPY

7. Cohn JN: Blood pressure and cardiac performance. Am J Med 55:351, 1973

Direct Smooth Muscle Relaxation

8. Johnson CC: The actions and toxicity of sodium nitroprusside. Arch Int Pharmacodyn Ther 35:489, 1929
9. Gifford RW Jr: Current practices in general medicine. 7. Treatment of hypertensive emergencies including the use of sodium nitroprusside. Proc Mayo Clin 34:387, 1959
10. Page IH, Corcoran AC et al: Cardiovascular effects of sodium nitroprusside in animals and hypertensive patients. Circ. 11:188, 1955
11. Schlant RC, Tsagaris TS, Robertson RJ: Studies on the acute cardiovascular effects of intravenous sodium nitroprusside. Am J Cardiol 9:51, 1962
12. Styles M, Coleman AJ, Leary WP: Some hemodynamic effects of sodium nitroprusside. Anesthesiology 38:173, 1973
13. Rowe GG, Henderson RH: Systemic and coronary hemodynamic effects of sodium nitroprusside. Am Heart J 87:87, 1974
14. La Jemtal TH, Nelson RG et al: Preload and afterload changes induced by nitroprusside: beneficial and detrimental effects on ischemia. Circulation 54:69, 1976
15. Miller RR, Vismara LA et al: Pharmacological mechanisms for left ventricular unloading in clinical congestive heart failure: differential effects of nitroprusside, phentolamine, and nitroglycerin on cardiac function and peripheral circulation. Circ Res 39:127, 1976
16. Lappas DG, Lowenstein E et al: Hemodynamic effects of nitroprusside infusion in coronary artery operation in man. Circulation 54:4, 1976
17. Chiariello M, Gold HK et al: Comparison between the effects of nitroprusside and nitroglycerin on ischemic injury during acute myocardial infarction. Circulation 54:766, 1976
18. Hillis LD, Braunwald E: Myocardial ischemia. N Engl J Med 296:1093, 1977
19. Kaplan JA, Jones EL: Vasodilator therapy during coronary artery surgery: comparison of nitroglycerin and nitroprusside. J Thorac Cardiovasc Surg 77:301, 1979
20. Cohn PF, Maddox D et al: Effect of sublingually administered nitroglycerin on regional myocardial blood flow in patients with coronary artery disease. Am J Cardiol 39:672, 1977

21. Packer M, Meller J et al: Rebound hemodynamic events after the abrupt withdrawal of nitroprusside in patients with severe chronic heart failure. N Engl J Med 301:1139, 1979
22. Khambatta HJ, Stone JG, Kahn E: Hypertension during anesthesia on discontinuation of sodium nitroprusside—induced hypotension. Anesthesiology 51:127, 1979
23. Smith RP, Kruszyna H: Nitroprusside produces cyanide poisoning via a reaction with hemoglobin. J Pharmacol Exp Ther 191:557, 1974
24. Daris DW, Kadar D et al: A sudden death associated with the use of sodium nitroprusside for induction of hypotension during anesthesia. Can Anaesth Soc J 22:547, 1975
25. Michenfelder JD: Cyanide release from sodium nitroprusside in the dog. Anesthesiology 46:196, 1977
26. Tinker JH, Michenfelder JD: Sodium nitroprusside. Anesthesiology 45:340, 1976
27. Vesey CJ, Cole PV, Simpson PJ: Cyanide and thiocyanate concentrations following sodium nitroprusside infusion in man. Br J Anaesth 48:651, 1976
28. Posner MA, Rodkey FL, Tobey RE: Nitroprusside-induced cyanide poisoning: antidotal effect of hydroxycobalamia. Anesthesiology 44:333, 1976
29. Michenfelder JD, Tinker JH: Cyanide toxicity and thiosulfate protection during chronic administration of sodium nitroprusside in the dog: correlation with a human case. Anesthesiology 47:441, 1977
30. Davies DW, Greiss L et al: Sodium nitroprusside in children: observation on metabolism during normal and abnormal responses. Can Anaesth Soc J 22:553, 1979
31. Deichmann WB, Gerarde HW: Toxicology of Drugs and Chemicals. New York, Academic Press, 1969
32. Novrok DS, Glassock RJ et al: Hypothyroidism following prolonged sodium nitroprusside therapy. Am J Med Sci 248:129, 1964
33. Cohn JN, Franciosa JA: Vasodilator therapy of cardiac failure. N Engl J Med 297:254, 1977
34. Flaherty JT, Reid PR et al: Intravneous nitroglycerin in acute myocardial infarction. Circulation 51:132, 1975
35. Armstrong PW, Walker DC et al: Vasodilator therapy in acute myocardial infarction: a comparison of sodium nitroprusside and nitroglycerin. Circulation 52:1118, 1975
36. Kötter V, Leitner ER et al: Comparison of hemodynamic effects of phentolamine, sodium nitroprusside, and glyceryl trinitrate in acute myocardial infarction. Brit Heart J 39:1196, 1977
37. Chiariello M, Gold HK et al: Comparison between the effects of nitroprusside and nitroglycerin on ischemic injury during acute myocardial infarction. Circulation 54:766, 1976
38. Epstein SE, Kent KM et al: Reduction of ischemic injury by nitroglycerin during acute myocardial infarction. N Engl J Med 292:29, 1975
39. Kaplan JA, Dunbar RW, Jones EL: Nitroglycerin infusion during coronary artery surgery. Anesthesiology 45:14, 1976
40. Fahmy NR: Nitroglycerin as a hypotension drug during general anesthesia. Anesthesiology 49:17, 1978
41. Come PC, Pitt B: Nitroglycerin-induced severe hypotension and bradycardia in patients with acute myocardial infarction. Circulation 54:624, 1976
42. Mantle JA, Russel RO et al: Isosorbide dinitrate for the relief of severe heart failure after acute myocardial infarction. Am J Cardiol 37:329, 1976
43. Gray R, Chatterjee K et al: Hemodynamic and metabolic effects of isosorbide dinitrate in chronic congestive heart failure. Am Heart J 90:346, 1975
44. Koch–Weser J: Hydralazine. N Engl J Med 295:320, 1976
45. Zacest R, Gilmore et al: Treatment of essential hypertension with combined vasodilation and beta-adrenergic blockade. N Engl J Med 286:617, 1972
46. Chatterjee K, Parmley W et al: Oral hydralazine therapy for chronic refractory heart failure. Circulation 54:879, 1976
47. Franciosa JA, Cohn JN: Hemodynamic improvement with hydrazaline in left heart failure. Clin Res 25:217, 1976
48. Massie B, Chatterjee K, et al: Hemodynamic advantage of combined oral hydrazaline and nonparenteral nitrates in the vasodilator therapy of chronic heart failure. Am J Cardiol 40:794, 1977
49. Aitchison JD, Cranston WI et al: The effects of l-hydrazinophthalazine on the pulmonary circulation in mitral valve disease. Br Heart J 17:425, 1953
50. Thirwell MP, Zsoter TT: The effect of diazoxide on the veins. Am Heart J 83:512, 1972

51. Limbourg P, Fregel P et al: Effect of diazoxide on left ventricular performance in hypertension. Eur J Clin Pharmacol 8:387, 1975

52. Baer L, Goodwin FJ, Laragh JM: Diazoxide-induced renin release in man: dissociation from plasma and extracellular fluid volume changes. J Clin Endocrinol Metab 29:1107, 1969

53. Sellers EM, Koch–Weser J: Protein binding and vascular activity of diazoxide. N Engl J Med 281:1141, 1969

54. Koch–Weser J: Diazoxide. N Engl J Med 294:1271, 1976

Alpha-Adrenergic Blocking Drugs

55. Taylor SM, Sutherland GR et al: The circulatory effects of phentolamine in man with particular respect to changes in forearm blood flow. Clin Sci Mol Med 28:265, 1965

56. Gould L, Reddy CVR: Phentolamine. Am Heart J 92:397, 1976

57. Nickerson M, Collier B: Drugs inhibiting adrenergic nerves and structures innervated by them. In Goodman LS, Gilman A (eds): The Pharmacological Basis of Therapeutics, 5th ed, pp 553–564. New York, Macmillan 1975

58. Lappas DG, Buckley MJ et al: Left ventricular performance and pulmonary circulation following addition of nitrous oxide to morphine during coronary artery surgery. Anesthesiology 43:61, 1975

59. Laver MB: Coronary artery disease and anesthesia. 1976 Annual Refresher Course Lectures, American Society of Anesthesiologists Annual Meeting, San Francisco, CA, October 9–13, 1976

60. Finlayson DC, Kaplan JA: Cardiopulmonary bypass. In Kaplan JA (ed): Cardiac Anesthesia, New York, Grune & Stratton, 1979

61. Kelly DT, Delgado CE et al: Use of phentolamine in acute myocardial infarction associated with hypertension and left ventricular failure. Circulation 47:729, 1973

62. Gould L, Reddy CVR et al: Use of phentolamine in acute myocardial infarction. Am Heart J 88:144, 1974

63. Perret CL, Gardaz JP et al: Phentolamine for vasodilator therapy in left ventricular failure complicating acute myocardial infarction: hemodynamic study. Br Heart J 37:640, 1975

64. Das PK, Parrat JR: Myocardial and haemodynamic effects of phentolamine. Br J Pharmacol 41:437, 1971

65. Singh JB, Hood WB, Abelman WH: Beta-adrenergic mediated inotropic and chronotropic actions of phentolamine. Am J Cardiol 26:660, 1970

66. Ramanathan KB, Bodenheimer MM: Contrasting effects of nitroprusside and phentolamine in experimental myocardial infarction. Am J Cardiol 39:994, 1977

67. Nickerson M: Nonequilibrium drug antagonism. Pharmacol Rev 9:246, 1957

68. Nickerson M, Hollenberg NK: Blockade of alpha-adrenergic receptors. In Roof WS, Hoffman FG (eds): Physiological Pharmacology, vol 4, pp 243–305. New York, Academic Press, 1967

69. Crout JR, Brown BR Jr: Anesthesia management of pheochromocytoma: the value of phenoxybenzamine and methoxyflurane. Anesthesiology 30:29, 1969

70. Ross EJ, Prichard BNC et al: Preoperative and operative management of patients with pheochromocytoma. Br Med J 1:191, 1967

71. Engleman K, Sjoerdsoma A: Chronic medical therapy for pheochromocytoma: a report of four cases. Ann Intern Med 61:229, 1964

72. Mandelbaum I, Silbert N, Berry J: Phenoxybenzamine and renal blood flow during extracorporeal circulation. J Thorac Cardiovasc Surg 8:73, 1967

73. Finlayson DC, Kaplan JA: Cardiopulmonary bypass. In Kaplan JA (ed): Cardiac Anesthesia, p 423. New York, Grune & Stratton, 1979

74. El–Etr AA, Glisson SN: Alpha-adrenergic blocking agents. In Ivankovich AD (ed): Nitroprusside and other short-acting hypotensive agents. Int Anesthesiol Clin 16:244, 1978

75. Byck R: Drugs and the treatment of psychiatric disorders. In Goodman LS, Gilman A (eds): The Pharmacological Basis of Therapeutics, 5th ed, pp 160–162. New York, Macmillan, 1975

76. Byck R: Drugs and the treatment of psychiatric disorders. In Goodman LS, Gilman A (eds): The Pharmacological Basis of Therapeutics, 5th ed, pp 160–162. New York, Macmillan, 1975

77. Hug CC Jr, Kaplan JA: Pharmacology: cardiac drugs. In Kaplan JA (ed): Cardiac Anesthesia, p 43. New York, Grune & Stratton, 1979

78. Stinson EB, Holloway EL, Derby G et al: Comparative hemodynamic responses to chlorpromazine, nitroprusside, nitroglyc-

erin, and trimethaphan immediately after open-heart operations. Circulation 51, 52:26, 1975

79. Prys–Roberts C, Kolman GR: The influence of drugs used in neuroleptanalgesia on cardiovascular function. Br J Anaesth 39:134, 1967

80. Whitwan JG, Russel WJ: The acute cardiovascular changes and adrenergic blockade by droperidol in man. Br J Anaesth 43:58, 1971

81. Fox JWC, Fox EJ, Cromdell DL: Neuroleptanalgesia for heart and major surgery. Arch Surg 94:102–106, 1967

82. Price HL: General anesthetics: intravenous anesthetics. In Goodman LS, Gilman A (eds): The Pharmacological Basis of Therapeutics, 5th ed, pp 97–101. New York, Macmillan, 1975

83. Farari HA, Gorten RJ et al: The action of droperidol and fentanyl on cardiac output and related hemodynamic parameters. South Med J 67:49–53, 1974

84. Graves CL, Downs NH, Browne AB: Cardiovascular effects of minimal analgesic quantities of innovar, fentanyl, and droperidol in man. Anesth Analg (Cleve) 54:15, 1975

85. McDonald HR, Baird DP et al: Clinical and circulatory effects of neuroleptanalgesia with dehydrobenzperidol and phenoperidine. Br Heart J 28:654, 1966

86. Long G, Dripps RD, Price HL: Measurement of anti-arrhythmic potency of drugs in man: effects of dehydrobenzperidol. Anesthesiology 28:318, 1967

87. Bertolo L, Novakovic L, Penna M: Antiarrhythmic effects of droperidol. Anesthesiology 37:529, 1972

88. Yeh BK, McNay JL, Goldberg LI: Attenuation of domamine renal and mesenteric vasodilation by haloperidol: evidence for a specific receptor. J Pharmacol Exp Ther 168:303, 1969

89. Goldberg LI: Dopamine: clinical user of an endogenous catecholamine. N Engl J Med 291:707, 1975

90. Clark MM: Droperidol in preoperative anxiety. Anaesthesia 24:36, 1969

91. Kosman ME: Evaluation of a new antihypertensive agent: prazosin hydrochloride (Minipres). JAMA 238:157–159, 1977

92. Gross F (ed): Handbook of Experimental Pharmacology: Antihypertensive Agents. Heidelberg, Springer–Verlag, 1977

93. Graham RM, Oates MF et al: Alpha blocking action of the antihypertensive agent, prazosin. J Pharmacol Exp Ther 201:747–752, 1977

94. Oates ME, Graham RM et al: Haemodynamic effects of prazosin. Arch Int Pharmacodyn Ther 224:239–247, 1976

95. Marshall AJ, Barrit DW et al: Evaluation of beta blockade, bendroflurazide, and prazosin in severe hypertension. Lancet 1:271–274, 1977

96. Miller RR, Awan NA et al: Sustained reduction of cardiac impedance and preload in congestive heart failure with the antihypertensive vasodilator prazosin. N Engl J Med 297:303–307, 1977

97. Awan NA, Miller RR et al: Clinical pharmacology and therapeutic application of prazosin in acute and chronic refractory congestive heart failure: balanced systemic venous and arterial dilation improving pulmonary congestion and cardiac output. Am J Med 65:146–154, 1978

98. Awan NA, Miller RR, Mason DT: Comparison of effects of nitroprusside and prazosin of left ventricular function and the peripheral circulation in chronic refractory congestive heart failure. Circulation 57:152–159, 1978

99. Wood AJ, Boll P, Simpson FO: Prazosin in normal subjects: plasma levels, blood pressure and heart rate. Br J Clin Pharmacol 3:199–201, 1976

100. Stokes GS, Oates HF: Prazosin: new alpha-adrenergic blocking agent in the treatment of hypertension. Cardiovasc Med 3:41–57, 1978

Ganglionic Blockade

101. Payne JP: Histamine release during controlled hypotension with Arfonad. Proceeding of the World Congress of Anesthesiologists, pp 180–181. Minneapolis, Burgess Publishing Co, 1955

102. Wang HH, Liu LMP, Katz RL: A comparison of the cardiovascular effects of sodium nitroprusside and trimethaphan. Anesthesiology 46:40, 1977

103. Mendolowitz M, Naftch NE et al: The effect of trimethaphan on the human digital circulation. Clin Pharmacol Ther 9:50, 1968

104. Scott DB, Stephan GW et al: Circulating effects of controlled arterial hypotension with trimethaphan during N_2O/halothane anaesthesia. Br J Anaesth 44:523, 1972

105. Stinson EB, Holloway EL, Derby G et al: Comparative hemodynamic responses to

chlorpromazine, nitroprusside, nitroglycerin, and trimethaphan immediately after open-heart operations. Circulation 51, 52:26, 1975

106. Stone HH, MacKrell FN, Wechsler RL: The effect on cerebral circulation and metabolism in man of acute reduction in blood pressure by means of intravenous hexamethonium bromide and head-up tilt. Anesthesiology 16:168, 1955

107. Moyer JH, Morris G: Cerebral hemodynamics during controlled hypotension induced by the continuous infusion of ganglionic blocking drugs. J Clin Invest 33:1081, 1954

108. Magness A, Yashon D et al: Cerebral function during trimethaphan-induced hypotension. Neurology 23:506, 1973

109. Michenfelder JD, Theye RA: Canine systemic and cerebral effects of hypotension induced by hemorrhage, trimethaphan, halothane, or nitroprusside. Anesthesiology 46:188, 1977

110. Pitts RF: Physiology of the Kidney and Body Fluids, p 167. Chicago, Year Book Medical Publishers, 1974

111. Parrish AE, Kleh J, Fazekas JF: Renal and cerebral hemodynamics with hypotension. Am J Med 32:35, 1957

112. Krumholz RA, Brashear RE et al: Physiological alterations in the pulmonary capillary bed at rest and during exercise: the effect of body position and trimethaphan camphorsulfonate. Circulation 33:872, 1966

113. Eckenhoff JE, Enderby GE et al: Pulmonary gas exchange during deliberate hypotension. Br J Anaesth 35:750, 1963

114. Eckenhoff JE: The use of controlled hypotension for surgical procedures. Surg Clin North Am 45:1579, 1955

115. Zaimis E: The interruption of ganglionic transmission and some of its problems. J Pharm Pharmacol 7:497, 1955

116. Adams AP: Techniques of vascular control for deliberate hypotension during surgery. Br J Anaesth 47:777, 1975

117. Salem MR, Ivankervich AD: The place of beta-adrenergic blocking drugs in the deliberate use of hypotension. Anesth Anal (Cleve) 49:427, 1970

118. Larson AG: Deliberate hypotension. Anesthesiology 25:682, 1964

119. Enderby GEM: Pentolinium tartrate in controlled hypotension. Lancet 11:1097, 1954

120. Fahmy NR, Laver MB: Hemodynamic response to ganglionic blockade with pentolinium during N₂O-halothane anesthesia in man. Anesthesiology 44:6, 1976

121. Fahmy NR: Arterial hypotension: deliberate and unwanted, p 229. American Society of Anesthesiologists Refresher Course, 1975

Central Nervous System Site of Action

122. Nickerson M, Ruedy J: Antihypertensive agents and the drug therapy of hypotension. In Goodman LS, Gilman A (eds): The Pharmacological Basis of Therapeutics, 5th ed, pp 705–726. New York, Macmillan, 1975

123. Day MD, Roach AG, Whiting RL: The mechanism of the antihypertensive action of alpha-methyldopa in hypertensive rats. Eur J Pharmacol 21:271, 1973

124. Lowenstein J: Clonidine. Ann Int Med 92:74, 1980

125. Hansson L, Hunyor SN et al: Blood pressure crisis following withdrawal of clonidine, with special reference to arterial and urinary catecholamine levels, and suggestions for acute management. Am Heart J 85:605, 1973

126. Brodsky JB, Bravo JJ: Acute postoperative clonidine withdrawal syndrome. Anesthesiology 44:519, 1976

127. Bruce DL, Croley TF, Lee JS: Postoperative clonidine withdrawal syndrome. Anesthesiology 51:90, 1979

Surgical Applications

128. Benzig G III, Hemswork JA et al: Human myocardial performance during surgical treatment of cardiac defects. J Thorac Cardiovasc Surg 59:809, 1970

129. Ross J Jr, Braunwald E: The study of left ventricular function in man by increasing resistance to ventricular ejection with angiotensin. Circulation 29:739, 1964

130. Lappas DG, Lowenstein E et al: Hemodynamic effects of nitroprusside infusion in coronary artery operation in man. Circulation 54(III):4, 1976

131. Kaplan JA, Jones EL: Vasodilator therapy during coronary artery surgery: comparison of nitroglycerin and nitroprusside. J Thorac Cardiovasc Surg 77:301, 1979

132. Kaplan JA, Dunbar RW, Jones EL: Nitroglycerin infusion during coronary artery surgery. Anesthesiology 45:14, 1976

133. Chatterjee K, Parmley WW et al: Beneficial effects of vasodilator agents in severe mitral regurgitation due to dysfunction of subvalvular apparatus. Circulation 48:684, 1973
134. Harshaur MD, Grossman W et al: Reduced systemic vascular resistance as therapy for severe mitral regurgitation of valvular origin. Ann Intern Med 83:312, 1975
135. Sniderman AD, Marpole DG et al: Response of the left ventricle to nitroglycerin in patients with and without mitral regurgitation. Br Heart J 36:357, 1974
136. Bolen JL, Alderman EL: Hemodynamic consequences of afterload reduction in patients with chronic aortic regurgitation. Circulation 53:879, 1976
137. Miller RR, Vismara LA et al: Afterload reduction therapy with nitroprusside in severe aortic regurgitation: improved cardiac performance and reduced regurgitant volume. Am J Cardiol 38:564, 1976
138. Kouchoukos NT, Sheppard LC, Kirkland JW: Effect of alterations in arterial pressure on cardiac performance early after open intracardiac operations. J Thorac Cardiovasc Surg 64:563, 1972
139. Stinson EB, Holloway EL, Derby G et al: Comparative hemodynamic responses to chlorpromazine, nitroprusside, nitroglycerin, and trimethaphan immediately after open-heart operations. Circulation 51, 52:26, 1975
140. Stinson EB, Holloway EL et al: Control of myocardial performance early after open heart operations by vasodilator treatment. J Thorac Cardiovasc Surg 73:523, 1977
141. Chatterjee K, Swan HC et al: Vasodilator therapy for pump failure complicating acute myocardial infarction. Cardiology Digest 10:10, 1975
142. Gardner WJ: The control of bleeding during operation by induced hypotension. JAMA 132:572, 1946
143. Fahmy NR: Indications and contraindications for deliberate hypotension with a review of its cardiovascular effects. In Philbin D (ed): International Anesthesiology Clinics, p 178. Boston, Little, Brown & Co, 1979
144. Slack WK, Walther WW: Cerebral circulation studies during hypotensive anesthesia using radioactive xenon. Lancet 1:1082, 1963
145. Stone HH, MacKrell TN, Wechsler RL: The effect on cerebral circulation and metabolism in man of acute reduction in blood pressure by means of intravenous hexamethonism bromide and head up tilt.
146. Thompson GE, Miller RD et al: Hypotensive anesthesia for total hip arthroscopy: a study of blood loss and organ function (brain, heart, liver and kidney). Anesthesiology 48:91–96, 1976
147. Fahmy NR, Laver MB: Hemodynamic response to ganglionic blockade with pentolinium during N2O-halothane anesthesia in man. Anesthesiology 44:6, 1976
148. Askrog VF, Pender JW, Eckenhoff JE: Changes in physiological dead space during deliberate hypotension. Anesthesiology 25:744, 1964
149. Stone JG, Khambatta MJ et al: Pulmonary shunting during anesthesia with deliberate hypotension. Anesthesiology 45:508–515, 1976
150. Hugosson R, Hogstrom S: Factors disposing to morbidity in surgery of intracranial aneurysms with special regard to deep controlled hypotension. J Neurosurg 38:561–567, 1973
151. Fahmy NR: Nitroglycerin as a hypotension drug during general anesthesia. Anesthesiology 49:17, 1978
152. Eckenhoff JE, Enderby GE et al: Human cerebral circulation during deliberate hypotension and head-up tilt. J Appl Physiol 18:1130, 1963
153. Salem MR, El–Etr AA: Management of hemorrhage following induced hypotension. Anesthesiology 28:1104, 1967
154. Attia RR, Murphy JD et al: Myocardial ischemia due to infrarenal aortic cross-clamping during aortic surgery in patients with severe coronary artery disease. Circulation 53:961, 1976
155. Carrol RM, Laravuso RB, Schauble JF: Left ventricular function during aortic surgery. Arch Surg 111:740, 1976
156. Dunn E, Pragen RL et al: The effect of abdominal aortic cross-clamping on myocardial function. J Surg Res 22:463, 1971
157. Strandness DE, Parrish DG, Bell JW: Mechanisms of declamping shock in operations on the abdominal aorta. Surgery 60:488, 1961
158. Brant B, Armstrong RP, Vetto RM: Vasodepressor factor in declamp shock production. Surgery 67:650, 1970
159. Rittenhouse EA, Maixner W et al: The role of prostaglandin E in the hemodynamic re-

sponse to aortic clamping and declamping. Surgery 80:137, 1976

160. Silverstein PR, Caldera DL et al: Avoiding the hemodynamic consequences of aortic cross-clamping and unclamping. Anesthesiology 50:462, 1979

161. Bush HL, LoGerto FW et al: Assessment of myocardial performance and optimal volume loading during elective abdominal aortic aneurysm resection. Arch Surg 112:1301, 1977

162. Dalen JE, Alpert JS et al: Dissection of the thoracic aorta, medical or surgical therapy? Am J Cardiol 34:803, 1974

163. Dalen JE, Howes JP: Dissection of the aorta: current diagnostic and therapeutic approaches. JAMA 242:1530, 1979

164. McFarland J, Willerson JT et al: The medical treatment of dissecting aortic aneuryms. N Engl J Med 286:115–119, 1972

165. Dunbar RW: Thoracic aneurysms. In Kaplan JA (ed): Cardiac Anesthesia, pp 369–376. Grune and Stratton, 1979

166. Daggett P, Verner I, Carruthers M: Intraoperative management of pheochromocytoma with sodium nitroprusside. Br Med J 2:311, 1978

167. Darby S, Prys-Roberts C: Unusual presentation of phaeochromocytoma. Management of anaesthesia and cardiovascular monitoring. Anaesthesia 31:913, 1976

168. Katz RL, Wolf CE: Pheochromocytoma. In Mark LE , Ngai SM (eds): Highlights of Clinical Anesthesiology, pp 55–65. New York, Harper and Row, 1971

Medical Applications

169. Likoff W, Kasparian H et al: Evaluation of coronary vasodilators by coronary arteriography. Am J Cardiol 138:7, 1964

170. Franciosa JA, Guiha NH et al: Improved left ventricular function during nitroprusside infusion in acute myocardial infarction. Lancet 1:650, 1972

171. Chatterjee K, Parmley WW, et al: Hemodynamic and metabolic responses to vasodilator therapy in acute myocardial infarction. Circulation 48:1183, 1973

172. Chatterjee K, Swan MJC et al: Effects of vasodilator therapy for severe pump failure in acute myocardial infarction on short term and late term prognosis. Circulation 53:797, 1976

173. Gold HK, Leinbach RC, Sanders CA: Use of sublingal nitroglycerin in congestive heart failure following acute myocardial infarction. Circulation 46:839, 1972

174. Flaherty JT, Reid RR et al: Intravenous nitroglycerin in acute myocardial infarction. Circulation 51:132, 1975

175. Chatterjee K, Parmley WW: The role of vasodilator therapy in heart failure. Prog Cardiovasc Dis 19:301, 1977

176. Guiha NM, Cohn JN: Treatment of refractory heart failure with infusion of nitroprusside. N Engl J Med 291:587, 1974

177. Miller RR, Vismara LA et al: Clinical use of sodium nitroprusside in chronic ischemic heart disease: effects on peripheral vascular resistance and venous tone and on ventricular volume, pump, and mechanical performance. Circulation 51:328, 1975

178. Pierpont GL, Cohn JN, Franciosa JA: Congestive cardiomyopathy: pathophysiology and response to therapy. Arch Intern Med 138:1847, 1978

179. Cohn JN, Mathew KJ et al: Chronic vasodilator therapy in the management of cardiogenic shock and intractable left ventricular failure. Ann Intern Med 81:777, 1974

180. Franciosa JA, Mikulic E et al: Hemodynamic effects of orally administered isosorbide dinitrate in patients with congestive heart failure. Circulation 50:1020, 1974

181. Franciosa JA, Pierpont GL, Cohn JN: Hemodynamic improvement after oral hydralazine in left ventricular failure: a comparison with nitroprusside infusion in sixteen patients. Ann Intern Med 86:388, 1977

182. Pierpont GL, Cohn JN, Franciosa JA: Combined oral hydralazine-nitrate therapy in left ventricular failure: hemodynamic equivalency to sodium nitroprusside. Chest 73:8, 1978

183. Miller RR, Awan NA et al: Sustained reduction of cardiac impedance and preload in congestive heart failure with the antihypertensive vasodilator prazosin. N Engl J Med 297:303–307, 1977

184. Koch-Weser, J: Hypertensive emergencies. N Engl J Med 290:211, 1974

185. Bhatin SK, Frohlich ED: Hemodynamic comparison of agents useful in hypertensive emergencies. Am Heart J 85:367, 1973

186. Ahearn DJ, Grim CE: Therapy of malignant hypertension with sodium nitroprusside. Arch Intern Med 133:187, 1974

Section II: Vasopressors

187. Tarazi RC: Sympathomimetic agents in the treatment of shock. Ann Intern Med 81:364, 1974

188. Steen PA, Tinker JM et al: Efficiency of dopamine, dobutamine, and epinephrine during emergence from cardiopulmonary bypass in man. Circulation 57:378, 1978

189. Innes IR, Nickerson M: Norepinephrine, epinephrine, and the sympathomimetic amines. In Goodman LS, Gilman A (eds): The Pharmacological Basis of Therapeutics, 5th ed, pp 477–515. New York, Macmillan, 1975

190. Standards for cardiopulmonary of emergency cardiac care (ECC). JAMA 227 [suppl]:833–868, 1974

191. Hug CC Jr, Kaplan JA: Pharmacology: cardiac drugs. In Kaplan JA (ed): Cardiac Anesthesia, pp 39–69. New York, Grune and Stratton, 1979

192. Lesch M: Inotropic agents and infarct size: theoretical and practical considerations. Am J Cardiol 37:508, 1976

193. Smith NT, Whitcher C: Acute hemodynamic effects of methoxamine in man. Anesthesiology 28:735, 1967

194. Imai S, Shigoi T, Hashimoto K: Cardiac actions of methoxamine, with special reference to its antagonistic action to epinephrine. Circ Res 9:552, 1961

195. Smith NT, Corbascio AN: The use and misuse of pressure agents. Anesthesiology 33:58, 1970

196. Oppenheimer MJ, Lynch PR, Barrera F: Antiarryhthmic actions of mephentermine. Am J Physiol 187:620, 1956

Part IV ADULT CARDIAC SURGERY

13

The Prebypass Period

J. KENT GARMAN
RICHARD P. FOGDALL

INTRODUCTION

This chapter guides the reader through the details of preoperative evaluation, the anesthetic management of specific cardiovascular disease entities, and the essentials of a smooth transition onto cardiopulmonary bypass.

PREOPERATIVE EVALUATION

The anesthesiologist must collect methodically sufficient information to allow safe management of the patient scheduled for cardiac surgery, usually on the day before surgery. Good cooperation from the surgical team is essential to ensure the availability of all patient information, such as referring letters, catheterization reports, old hospital records, and complete history, physical, and laboratory evaluation.

It is helpful to study all the accumulated data before seeing the patient. If this is not done, much valuable time is wasted in gathering information already available. After the chart is reviewed, the patient is approached. With knowledge of old and present records, a pertinent history and physical examination is performed. The American Heart Association, in its five booklet series of Examination of the Heart, has summarized the essentials of data collection and interpretation in the cardiac patient.[1] The series consists of *The Clinical History, Inspection and Palpation of Venous and Arterial Pulses, Precordial Pulsations, Auscultation,* and *The Electrocardiogram.* Those interested in reviewing the essentials of history taking and physical examination in more detail should read these five paperback booklets and also chapters 12 through 24 in *The Heart.*[2]

It is useful to utilize the problem-oriented progress note method in collecting preoperative information.[3] This requires organizing a preanesthetic note under the following headings (modified from Hurst):[4]

S *Subjective*—historical data and review of systems

O *Objective*—data from physical and laboratory examination

A *Assessment*—interpretation of subjective and objective data

P *Plan*—further work-up if necessary, planned anesthetic management, anesthetic risk, and patient consent.

SUBJECTIVE—HISTORICAL DATA AND REVIEW OF SYSTEMS

History and Exercise Tolerance

The patient should be questioned regarding symptoms of cardiovascular disease as outlined in the list below. The patient's exercise tolerance should be determined. This determination is important because it enables the physician to predict the patient's response to the stress of upcoming procedures. At one extreme is the bedridden patient, unable to perform any activity without symptoms (and who often has symptoms while at rest). The other extreme is the patient who continues to work, who is very infrequently (if at all) limited by symptoms, and who may even have a regular program of exercise.

Drug History

The patient's drug history should be examined in detail. Specific information concerning drugs, especially the following, should be obtained:

Digitalis Is digitalization adequate? This can be checked best in patients who are in atrial fibrillation by subjecting them to a short walk in the hallway and observing the change in pulse rate. If well digitalized, the ventricular rate will remain below 100 beats per minute. If the rate increases to above 120 beats per minute after brief exercise, digitalization is inadequate.

In general, it is safer to have a patient under-digitalized than close to digitalis toxicity. If tachycardia in a patient with atrial fibrillation is a problem, small intravenous doses of a short-acting digitalis preparation such as ouabain or digoxin can be administered intraoperatively.

In a patient who is fully or over-digitalized, intraoperative arrhythmias will be more difficult to interpret because the specter of possible digitalis toxicity always exists. Alterations in the serum potassium level or acid-base status may unmask digitalis toxicity in the fully digitalized patient. Hypokalemia (low serum potassium), alkalosis (caused by hyperventilation or bicarbonate administration),[5] and calcium potentiate the effects of digitalis. Therefore, it is important to know the serum potassium level in the digitalized patient. (Is the patient receiving potassium supplementation? Has the patient been depleted of potassium because of diuretic therapy?) In general, except in the patient with a combination of atrial fibrillation and tachycardia, digitalis should be discontinued in the 12-hour immediate preoperative period. Also, the patient should arrive in the operating suite with a serum potassium level greater than 3.5 to 4.0 meq/liter. It may be necessary to give oral or even intravenous KCl the day before surgery to accomplish this goal. If necessary, intravenous KCl may be administered intraoperatively. A good rule of thumb is to administer intravenous potassium no faster than 1–2 meq/min in the monitored adult patient, although this depends upon many factors, such as the patient's cardiac output, body size, and total body potassium stores.[6]

β-Blocking Agents The current thinking concerning β-blocking drugs is to maintain a patient on at least a reduced dosage of the drug if the patient requires it for control of angina, hypertension, or arrhythmias.[7-18] This applies especially to the patient with coronary artery disease, exhibiting normal ventricular function, who often will tolerate an anesthetic induction much better with adequate β-blockade. It is better to discontinue or greatly reduce the drug in a patient who has a history (or signs) of heart failure, and who does not require the drug to control angina, hypertension, or arrhythmias. If necessary, the anesthesiologist may administer

---

Symptoms of Cardiovascular Disease

Chest discomfort or pain
Dyspnea
Paroxysmal nocturnal dyspnea
Orthopnea
Edema
Nocturia
Phlebitis
Dizziness
Syncope
Palpitations/tachycardia
Fatigue
Cough
Hemoptysis
Claudication
Cyanosis
History of heart failure or myocardial infarction

---

halothane, enflurane, or isoflurane during anesthetic induction (and vasodilating drugs and propranolol), to control heart rate and blood pressure in selected patients.

Nitrates The patient may be taking long-acting nitrate preparations, or supplemental sublingual nitroglycerin (NTG) to control angina. Determine whether the requirement for NTG has changed since hospitalization. The patient should continue to receive nitrates (especially NTG) up to the time of anesthetic induction. In fact, we frequently begin anesthetic induction concomitantly with a NTG infusion. The patient who requires NTG for control of angina, should have an order written to send a small bottle of NTG tablets with the patient to the operating room, and the patient should be instructed to take them whenever needed. NTG ointment is an alternative method of administering the drug in the preoperative period. Some physicians write a routine order for NTG ointment to be applied at the same time as the preoperative medications. The usual dose is 2 inches every 3 to 4 hours.

Anticoagulants Aspirin and all aspirin-containing medications should be discontinued one week before operation. The patient also should have coumadin derivatives discontinued as far in advance of surgery as safely possible and, if anticoagulation is necessary, should be started on heparin therapy. Heparin can be continued up until the time of surgery because it is a simple matter to evaluate coagulation status intraoperatively and antagonize heparin with protamine, if necessary. In the patient who has long-standing heart failure or hepatic congestion or both, modified factors II, VII, IX, and X may be deficient. It is rarely effective to attempt to increase these clotting factors using vitamin K or fresh frozen plasma (FFP) before surgery. This patient will require coagulation factor administration (FFP) after bypass. Therefore, we do not administer FFP or platelets until the patient has completed cardiopulmonary bypass, at which time coagulation deficiencies are treated aggressively. Evaluation and treatment of coagulation disorders is discussed in more detail in Chapter 15 and Chapter 24.

Antiarrhythmic Drugs Antiarrhythmic drugs should be continued up until the time of surgery. There are several exceptions to this suggestion: digitalis (as mentioned above), and in mapping procedures (see Chapter 8). Disopyramide (Norpace) has been implicated in the precipitation of acute cardiac failure and probably should be discontinued.[19] We rarely see a decrease in inotropy connected with the continued administration of the commonly used clinical doses of the antiarrhythmic drugs.

Preoperative Physical Examination

Weight and height on chart
Blood pressure measurement in both arms
Current pulse rate and cardiac rhythm
Auscultation of the heart and lungs (murmurs, thrills, rubs, rales, and so on)
Radial and ulnar artery patency (Allen's test)
Condition of veins (for cannulation sites)
Mandible, airway, neck, bruits over carotids
Venous pulses? Neck vein distention? Hepatic enlargement?
Presence or absence of peripheral edema
Patient response to exercise during examination (heart rate, blood pressure, angina, and so on)

Antihypertensive Drugs The person who is receiving antihypertensive drugs should be maintained on these drugs, with rare exceptions, up until the time of surgery. The patient in whom these drugs have been discontinued preoperatively becomes hypertensive, and tends to be much more difficult to control during anesthetic induction and maintenance.[20]

Diuretic Drugs Usually, the patient receiving diuretics can have these drugs discontinued several days before surgery because with hospital-induced bedrest, this patient tends not to accumulate fluid. It is safer and easier to induce anesthesia in a patient who is not severely volume depleted. And with diuretics discontinued, potassium depletion can be corrected more easily in the several days before surgery.

Prior Anesthetic Experience

In addition, the patient's prior experience with anesthetic drugs should be determined, especially any allergic, hypersensitivity, or hyperthermic history. A brief review of systems with emphasis on hypertension, diabetes, steroid dependence, arrhythmias, and renal, pulmonary, hepatic, and hematologic problems should be completed.

OBJECTIVE—DATA FROM PHYSICAL AND LABORATORY EXAMINATION

Physical Examination

An abbreviated, pertinent physical examination should be performed. Without fail, the items listed below should be examined, and abnormalities noted. These items should be correlated with examinations by other physicians, and correlated with cardiac catheterization results. Discrepancies should be addressed.

Laboratory Studies

The laboratory studies outlined below are essential to the complete preoperative evaluation. Abnormalities should be explainable by patient history, and corrected preoperatively if possible. Uncorrectable abnormalities may dictate a change in anesthetic plan (drug use, application of PEEP, and so on).

Cardiac Catheterization

Perhaps the most important data are contained in the report from the cardiac catheterization laboratory.[21, 22] With the data outlined below and in Table 13-1, a more precise determination of diagnosis, response to stress, cardiac reserve, and prognosis can be made.

Especially important are the ejection fraction (fraction of end diastolic volume ejected during systole, or stroke volume/end diastolic volume), the left ventricular filling pressure (end diastolic pressure, LVEDP), and the presence or absence of dyssynergy (abnormal ventricular wall motion) on ventriculography. An ejection fraction of less than 0.5 and the presence of significant ventricular dyssynergy are good predictors of ventricular dysfunction. Normal ventricular function can be inferred if no ventricular wall dyssynergy is evident on the ventriculogram.[23]

Often, the left ventricular end diastolic pressure (LVEDP) will increase after dye injection into the coronary arteries. This is the result of low $[Ca^{++}]$ in the dye causing inotropic failure, an increase in the preload because of the hyper-osmolar nature of the dye, an increase in the peripheral resistance (probably caused by a pain reflex), and ventricular ischemia produced by the infusion of anoxic dye. New dyes are being developed which may avoid the problem of inotropic failure. There are no data available on the prognostic significance of this LVEDP increase after dye injection.[24]

Electrocardiography

The ECG should be examined with emphasis on rhythm, rate, electrical axis, chamber enlargement, bundle-branch block or other conduction system disease, reentry phenomenon, ischemic or infarction patterns, and drug effects, especially digitalis (see also

---

Preoperative Laboratory Studies

Complete blood count (CBC): hemoglobin, hematocrit (PCV), white blood cell count
Blood chemistry: electrolytes (especially serum potassium), BUN and creatinine, blood glucose, liver enzymes, cardiac enzymes if indicated
Urinalysis
Coagulation studies: bleeding time, platelet count, prothrombin time, partial thromboplastin time
Arterial blood gases (if indicated)
Pulmonary function studies (if indicated)

Chapter 6). If an artificial pacemaker is present, the degree of actual pacing dependence must be determined. Also, the thresholds and security of the lead system are critical in a pacemaker-dependent patient. The type of pacemaker should be known (*e.g.*, ventricular-inhibited, fixed rate, atrial-triggered, A-V sequential, and so on). If the pacemaker has programming capability, the appropriateness

---

Important Cardiac Catheterization Information

Cardiac output and index
Peripheral and pulmonary vascular resistances
Gradients (pressure decreases) across diseased cardiac valves
Intracardiac and Extracardiac Shunts
Ventriculography (presence or absence of dyssynergy)
Cardiac pressures (especially PA_o and LVEDP)
Coronary arteriography
Pulmonary angiography
Ejection and regurgitant fractions

Table 13-1. Abnormal Findings—Cardiac Catheterization

Ejection Fraction	< 0.50
Dyssynergy	2 or more segments with < 20% contraction
Stroke Work Index	< 30 g • m/m²
End Systolic Volume	> 34 ml/m²
End Diastolic Volume	> 90 ml/m²
Cardiac Index	< 2.5 l/min/m²
End Diastolic Pressure	> 12 torr

(From Mangano DT: Preoperative assessment of cardiac catheterizatioin data: which parameters are the most important? Anesthesiology 53: S106, 1980)

Table 13-2. New York Heart Association Guidelines

CARDIAC STATUS	PROGNOSIS
I. Uncompromised	I. Good
II. Slightly compromised	II. Good with therapy
III. Moderately compromised	III. Fair with therapy
IV. Severely compromised	IV. Guarded despite therapy

(Criteria Committee of the NYHA: Nomenclature and Criteria for Diagnosis of Diseases of the Heart and Great Vessels, 7th ed. Boston, Little, Brown and Co, 1973)

of the present programming in relation to the upcoming stress should be determined. Thought should be given to the availability of a programmer for the particular brand of pacemaker during induction and surgery. For example, it is relatively simple to convert a ventricular-inhibited mode to a fixed rate mode during surgery with a magnet or a programming unit. This may be necessary because of electrocautery interference with pacemaker function (see also Chapter 7).

Stress Testing

The patient's cardiovascular responses to an exercise stress test can be a useful predictor of how the stress of anesthetic induction and surgery will be tolerated. The presence of anginal pain during exercise is a good predictor of significant coronary artery disease.

Exercise stress tests are evaluated by observing changes in ST segments on the ECG, heart rate and blood pressure, and presence or absence of angina during the test.[25, 26] Although any ST segment depression is pathologic during exercise, depression greater than 2 mm has a very significant correlation with coronary artery disease. Down-sloping ST segments have worse prognostic significance than horizontal or up-sloping ST segments.

The normal response to exercise is to increase heart rate to an age-related peak. The inability to reach this age-related peak value correlates with poor left ventricular function and severe coronary artery disease.

The development of hypotension during exercise has grave prognostic significance. This is probably caused by ischemic ventricular failure secondary to the exercise, and indicates a lack of cardiac reserve.

ASSESSMENT—INTERPRETATION OF ALL SUBJECTIVE AND OBJECTIVE DATA

After all of the data have been gathered, the patient should be classified to aid in the formation of an anesthetic management plan. The following classifications are suggested.

The New York Heart Association Status

The Criteria Committee of the New York Heart Association discusses in great detail the terms of classification of patients with cardiovascular disease.[27] A major change occurred in the recommended New York Heart Association classification in 1973. At this time, the "functional and therapeutical classification" system was abandoned and a new classification system was adopted based upon cardiac status and prognosis. The term *cardiac status* is meant to represent a total assessment of the etiologic, anatomic, and physiologic diagnoses. The term *prognosis* is based on an assessment of the potential effects of optimal current medical and surgical therapies. Patients should be classified according to the New York Heart Association guidelines as seen in Table 13-2.

American Society of Anesthesiologists Physical Status Classification

The classification system used by the American Society of Anesthesiologists is shown in Table 13-3.[28] It was designed originally only as a descriptive analysis of patient status. It often is used as means of classifying the patient's status relative to the risks of the proposed operative intervention.

Cardiac Risk Index

Although Goldman's Cardiac Risk Index does not refer specifically to the patient undergoing cardiac surgery, it is still a useful tool in assessing the degree of risk present in the cardiac surgical patient.[29] The cardiac risk index was the result of a study of 1001 patients over 40 years of age. The study attempted to determine which preoperative factors might affect the development of cardiac complications after major *non*cardiac operation. Nine independent significant correlates of serious cardiac complications were identified. *Points* accumulate depending upon the degree of significance of each variable. The total possible points are 53, as shown in Table 13-4.

After computation of the total points, the patient can be applied to one of four risk classes. As can be seen in Table 13-5, there

Table 13-3. American Society of Anesthesiologists Physical Status Classifications

Class 1	The patient has no organic, physiologic, biochemical or psychiatric disturbance. The pathologic process for which operation is to be performed is localized and does not entail a systemic disturbance.
Class 2	Mild to moderate systemic disturbance caused either by the condition to be treated surgically or by other pathophysiologic processes
Class 3	Severe systemic disturbance or disease from whatever cause, even though it may not be possible to define the degree of disability with finality
Class 4	Indicative of the patient with severe systemic disorders which are already life-threatening, not always correctable by operation
Class 5	The moribund patient who has little chance of survival but is submitted to operation in desperation
Emergency Operation (E)	Any patient in one of the classes listed previously who is operated upon as an emergency is considered to be in less optimal physical condition. The letter *E* is placed after the numerical classification.

(Dripps RD, Eckenhoff JE, Vandam LD: Introduction to Anesthesia, 5th ed. Philadelphia, WB Saunders, 1977)

Table 13-4. Goldman Cardiac Risk Index

CRITERIA*	POINTS
History	
Age > 70 yr	5
MI in previous 6 mo	10
Physical examination	
S_3 gallop or JVD	11
Important VAS	3
ECG	
Rhythm other than sinus or PACs on last preoperative ECG	7
>5 PVCs/min documented at any time before operation	7
General Status	
PO_2 < 60 or PCO_2 > 50 torr	3
K < 3.0 or HCO_3 < 20 meq/l	
BUN > 50 or Cr > 3.0 mg/dl	
abnormal SGOT, signs of chronic liver disease or patient bedridden from noncardiac causes	
Operation	
Intraperitoneal, intrathoracic or aortic operation	3
Emergency operation	4
Total Possible	53 points

*MI denotes myocardial infarction; *JVD*, jugular-vein distention; *VAS* valvular aortic stenosis; *PACs*, premature atrial contractions; *ECG*, electrocardiogram; *PVCs*, premature ventricular contractions; PO_2, partial pressure of oxygen; PCO_2, partial pressure of carbon dioxide; *K*, potassium; HCO_3, bicarbonate; *BUN*, blood urea nitrogen; *Cr*, creatinine; and *SGOT*, serum glutamic oxalacetic transaminase.
(Goldman L et al: Multifactorial Index of Cardiac Risk in Noncardiac Surgical Procedures. N Engl J Med 297:845, 1977)

Table 13-5. Cardiac Risk Index

CLASS	POINT TOTAL	NO OR ONLY MINOR COMPLICATIONS	LIFE-THREATENING COMPLICATIONS*	CARDIAC DEATHS
I (N = 537)	0–5	532 (99)†	4 (0.7)	1 (0.2)
II (N = 316)	6–12	295 (93)	16 (5)	5 (2)
III (N = 130)	13–25	112 (86)	15 (11)	3 (2)
IV (N − 18)	≥ 26	4 (22)	4 (22)	19 (56)

*Documented intraoperative or postoperative infarction, pulmonary edema, or ventricular tachycardia without progression to cardiac death.
†Figures in parentheses denote %.
(Goldman et al: Multifactorial Index of Cardiac Risk in Noncardiac Surgical Procedures. N Engl J Med 297:845, 1977)

Table 13-6. Coronary Artery Disease: Normal or Hyperdynamic Ventricle— Important Considerations

Pathophysiology
  Potential for decreased myocardial oxygen supply to various areas of the myocardium
  Deeper layer (subendocardium) tends to be relatively more ischemic because of back pressure effects of LV diastolic filling pressure
  Tendency for failure or arrhythmias when ischemic
  Ventricular compliance probably normal
  Elements of coronary artery spasm may be present

Management
  Minimize myocardial oxygen demand as follows:
    Continue preoperative β-blocking therapy until time of surgery
    Minimize preinduction anxiety
    Keep heart rate low
    Adequate levels of anesthesia/analgesia
    Intratracheal lidocaine
    Use of myocardial depressant drugs when indicated
  Maximize myocardial oxygen supply as follows:
    Keep diastolic blood pressure normal or increased
    Keep heart rate low
    Oxygen during critical periods (F_IO_2 1.0)
    Use NTG to reduce preload and relieve coronary artery spasm
    Ensure adequate blood oxygen carrying capacity (Hb over 10–12, cessation of smoking to decrease carboxyhemoglobin at least 8–12 hours preoperatively)

Table 13-7. Coronary Artery Disease: Hypodynamic Ventricle—Important Considerations

Pathophysiology
  May have congestive heart failure
  Little or no cardiac reserve
  Hypokinetic or dyskinetic areas of left ventricle (dyssynergy)
  History of myocardial infarction and ventricular aneurysm
  May have recurrent ventricular arrhythmias

Management
  Monitor pulmonary artery pressures, perform cardiac output determinations, and calculate resistances
  Avoid myocardial depressants (no inhalation anesthetic or β-blocking agents)
  Use afterload reduction
  Use inotropic drugs
  Maintain preinduction filling pressures

is a progression from class 1 to class 4 of the percentage of both life-threatening complications and cardiac deaths.

Left Ventricular Function

Another important determination to make, from an anesthetic standpoint, is whether the patient has normal or dysfunctional ventricles. A hyperdynamic patient, or one who has a normal or almost normal left ventricle usually has the following characteristics: little or no myocardial damage (perhaps no history of myocardial infarction), a normal cardiac reserve, no history of cardiac failure, a normal sized heart on chest film, a LVEDP less than 12 torr, an ejection fraction greater than 0.50, no left ventricular aneurysm, no dyssynergy (abnormal wall motion) on ventriculogram, a tendency to have hyperdynamic or labile responses to anxiety or pain stimuli, and can tolerate the administration of β-blocking agents. The patient with a hypodynamic ventricle, on the other hand, may have suffered previous major cardiac damage (e.g., myocardial infarction), ventricular aneurysm, mitral or aortic valvular dysfunction, a history of cardiac failure, a LVEDP greater than 18 torr, significant dyssynergy (abnormal wall motion) on ventriculogram, an ejection fraction less than 0.50, a tendency not to tolerate the administration of β-blocking agents, and compromised cardiac reserve.

It is important to decide whether a patient is hyperdynamic or normal, or hypodynamic because anesthetic management during induction and the prebypass period will differ markedly. The hyperdynamic patient tends to respond to anxiety, preoperative stimuli, and anesthetic manipulations with hypertension, tachycardia, and lability of cardiovascular variables. Therefore, management should include adequate preoperative discussion and sedation, adequate anesthesia, β-adrenergic blockade (both preoperatively and intraoperatively), use of intravenous nitroglycerin or sodium nitroprusside or both, intratracheal spray with lidocaine before tracheal intubation, and the possible use of metocurine instead of pancuronium. The use of enflurane or halothane, either as a major anesthetic agent or as an adjunct to a narcotic technique, is desirable. All of the above measures tend to minimize an increase in myocardial oxygen demand in the hyperdynamic patient.

The hypodynamic patient, on the other hand, may develop heart failure if myocardial depressants are used. Therefore, propranolol, potent inhalation anesthetic agents, and thiopental must be used cautiously if at all.

Generally, the patient in the hypodynamic group will benefit from monitoring of pulmonary artery pressure, cardiac output, and calculation of vascular resistances. The patient in the hyperdynamic (or normal) group may or may not, depending upon the severity and anatomic location of the coronary artery lesions.

Patients with significant disease of the left-main coronary artery are at special risk during induction and should be treated accordingly. The use of preinduction hemodynamic monitoring (direct arterial pressure, central venous pressure, pulmonary arterial pressure), cardiac output determinations, and pharmacologic interventions to manipulate preload, afterload, heart rate, and contractility reduced intraoperative mortality in one study from 20 to 3.5 percent.[30]

The disease entities which bring patients

Table 13-8. Aortic Stenosis—Important Considerations

Pathophysiology
  Outflow obstruction with LV pressure overload; essentially fixed cardiac output
  LV hypertrophy, not dilation
  Decreased LV compliance
  Thickened ventricular wall with relative subendocardial ischemia (even with normal coronary arteries)
  High myocardial oxygen demand

Management
  Keep mean systemic pressure at or above awake baseline; use vasopressors if necessary
  Assure that patient is full but *not* over full
  Avoid inotropic stimulation unless below inotropic baseline
  Avoid bradycardia; low stroke volume requires higher heart rate to maintain coronary perfusion
  Avoid tachycardia; faster ejection increases oxygen demand and increases gradient
  Deterioration can occur with loss of atrial kick; be prepared to cardiovert if loss of sinus rhythm

Table 13-9. Aortic Insufficiency—Important Considerations

Pathophysiology
  LV volume overload
  LV hypertrophy and dilation
  Low aortic diastolic pressure (with decreased coronary flow)
  Increased LV output and work

Management
  Hypertension increases regurgitation; avoid hypertension
  Decreased peripheral resistance decreases regurgitation (beneficial)
  Avoid bradycardia
    Lower diastolic pressure during regurgitation
    Increased intraventricular volume and pressures
    Decreased coronary flow
  Keep "full"!

Table 13-10. Mitral Stenosis—Important Considerations

Pathophysiology
  Obstruction to LV filling; essentially fixed cardiac output
  LA pressure and volume overload
  Backward transmission of increased pressures
  Pulmonary hypertension
  RV failure (pressure overload)
  Atrial fibrillation

Management
  Tachycardia to be avoided; decreased LV filling
  Bradycardia may be dangerous, lower cardiac output
  A narrow range of acceptable right-sided pressures and fixed low cardiac output require *slow* changes, even in correct direction (as rate of induction, rate of fluid infusion)
  Inotropic stimulation rarely helpful unless contractility is below awake baseline and may be harmful
  Rarely, vasopressors may be necessary to assure adequate aortic root diastolic pressure for coronary perfusion
  Control fast atrial fibrillation with digoxin
  Keep full but not to point of pulmonary edema
  May require prolonged ventilatory assistance
  May be *very* sensitive to postural changes (Trendelenberg, turning on side)

to cardiac surgery have been covered in previous chapters and will not be repeated here. Tables 13-6 through 13-11 summarize important considerations which the anesthesiologist should keep in mind during patient evaluation, and during planning for anesthetic management. These considerations

Table 13-11. Mitral Insufficiency—Important Considerations

Pathophysiology
  LV volume overload
  LA enlargement
  Backward transmission of high pressures
  Right heart failure and pulmonary edema
  Atrial fibrillation
  LV used to low afterload

Management
  Hypertension increases regurgitation. Decreased peripheral resistance decreases regurgitation (use nitroprusside).
  Keep full
  Bradycardia increases regurgitation—avoid
  LV may need inotropic support

and concepts should be reviewed in other chapters if the reader is unsure of any of the concepts presented here in brief table form.

PLAN

DISCUSSION WITH PATIENT

It is appropriate to discuss the plans for anesthetic management with the patient. It is our practice not to routinely discuss great detail concerning risks of the procedure, yet we are very careful to ensure that the patient understands the degree of overall risk. The patient should be asked whether he or she wishes to be informed in detail concerning risk and, if so, time should be taken to ensure that this is done. The very nature of severe

Preoperative Patient Discussion

NPO instructions
Details of planned preinduction vascular cannulation
Positive suggestions regarding degree of relaxation before surgery, amnesia during and after surgery, and postoperative discomfort and ventilation
Type of anesthetic induction planned (slow, fast, intravenous, inhalation, and the like)
Consent
Discussion with family

coronary artery disease often contraindicates any discussion which could precipitate undue anxiety, subsequent angina, and risk of ischemia or infarction. Therefore, the discussion should be calm and designed to establish good rapport and to reassure the patient regarding anesthetic management. Medicolegal considerations regarding informed consent tend to require more detailed discussions than are medically justified in the sick cardiac patient. Therefore, one must try to inform the patient as thoroughly as possible without creating anxiety.

The details outlined in the list above should be communicated to the patient and to family members, if indicated. At Stanford, an information class with slide presentations is provided to the patient (and family) the night before surgery, by the cardiovascular intensive care nursing staff. This class has always received an enthusiastic response from patients and family, and provides excellent supporting information which otherwise might not be transmitted to the patient by busy anesthesiologists and surgeons.

In a teaching institution, the house officer and faculty attending should discuss fully the patient and the anticipated procedure, ascertain if important data are missing, and formulate a complete anesthesia plan. All problems requiring additional assistance, information, or work-up should be addressed at the earliest possible time. This will avoid last minute "problem-chasing."

PREOPERATIVE DRUG THERAPY

A decision regarding preoperative sedation also must be made. The sick, hypodynamic patient should be given little or no preoperative medication because the depressive effects of most premedicant drugs may be profound. On the other hand, the anxious hyperdynamic patient with coronary artery disease requires substantial doses of preoperative medications, including narcotics, sedatives (such as diazepam),[31] NTG (tablets or ointment), and β-blocking drugs. The type and dose of "premed" drug may be chosen based upon the anesthesiologist's familiarity with specific agents and the patient's condition. There is little indication for the administration of atropine because it only serves to make the patient uncomfortable (dry mouth) and may be associated with a significant increase in heart rate and arrhythmias during induction.[32–35] However scopolamine, in low dose, may be useful because of its amnesic and sedative properties.

MONITORING

Planning should include the degree of hemodynamic monitoring required in the specific patient. In general, *every* patient should have a direct arterial pressure cannula and a central venous pressure cannula placed. At Stanford, the only optional monitoring line is the flow-directed pulmonary arterial (Swan–Ganz) catheter. Indications and contraindications for pulmonary arterial pressure monitoring are shown in Table 13-12 (see also Chaps. 4, 5).

PREPARATION FOR INDUCTION

On the day of surgery the patient should arrive in the operating room appropriately premedicated. Even though the premedication will have been ordered so as not to either overly depress the patient or leave the patient in an anxious state, it is important to assess the actual effect of the premedication when the patient arrives. This is done best by measuring blood pressure and pulse rate immediately upon the patient's arrival, talking to the patient to assess whether anxiety or angina or both are present, and observing the degree of sedation and respiratory depression present. If the patient has coronary artery disease and is known to develop angina when anxious, he or she should be sedated adequately, and oxygen should be available. If a patient demonstrates angina, treatment with oxygen, intravenous narcotic or sedative, and NTG should commence, in addition to ECG monitoring and personal observation.

Table 13-12. Pulmonary Arterial Pressure Monitoring

Relative Indications
  Severe congestive heart failure
  Severe, high-grade coronary artery disease (especially left main disease)
  Aortic aneurysm surgery with severe coronary artery disease
  Combined coronary artery and carotid artery disease
  Poor left ventricular function, hypodynamic circulation
  Pulmonary hypertension/emboli
  Sepsis with an unstable circulation

Relative Contraindications
  Unfamiliarity with procedure
  Inadequate monitors or equipment
  Severe coagulation disorder
  History of recurrent ventricular arrhythmias, irritable myocardium
  Abnormal cardiac anatomy (VSD, ASD)
  Tricuspid or pulmonic valvular disease (especially if surgical procedure planned for tricuspid or pulmonic valves)
  Cardiac transplant recipient or donor

Drugs for patient care and resuscitation should be available during patient preparation (see list below).

Drugs to be Drawn into Syringes Before Every Adult Cardiac Surgical Procedure

Morphine 1% (10 mg/ml)—obtained in 300 mg vials (15 mg/cc), should be diluted to 1% strength before use for convenience; or *fentanyl* (50 µg/ml)—total dose for case = 30–80 µg/kg; or *Dilaudid* (1–2 mg/ml). *Approximately* 1 mg Dilaudid is equivalent to 6 mg of morphine.

Diazepam 0.5% (5 mg/ml)—approximately 30 mg drawn up.

Thiopental 2.5% (25 mg/ml)—1000 mg drawn up.

Pancuronium 0.1% (1 mg/ml)—usual intubation dose is 0.10 mg/kg; or *Metocurine* 0.2% (2 mg/ml)—usual intubation dose is 0.3–0.4 mg/kg; or *d-Tubocurarine* 0.3% (3 mg/ml)—usual intubation dose 0.5–0.6 mg/kg.

Ephedrine 0.5 (5 mg/ml)—dilute 50 mg ampule to 10 ml.

Atropine (0.8 mg/ml)—1–2 mg.

Chlorpromazine 0.2% (2 mg/ml)—dilute ampule (25 mg) to 12.5 ml.

Lidocaine 1% (10 mg/cc)—available in prefilled 100 mg syringes.

Lidocaine for laryngeal spray—4% (40 mg/ml) attach LTA sprayer to syringe containing 160 mg lidocaine.

Heparin flush—1000 units heparin (1 ml of heparin-1000) in 250 ml NSS (thus 4 µg/ml).

Calcium chloride 10% (100 mg/ml)—comes in 10 ml (1-gram) ampule.

Neosynephrine 0.1% (1 mg/ml)—dilute 10-mg ampule to 10 ml, and 0.01% (100 µg/ml)—dilute 1 ml of 0.1% mix to 10 ml.

Propranolol 0.02% (0.2 mg/ml)—dilute 1 mg to 5 ml.

At Stanford monitoring lines are introduced in a preinduction room which is adjacent to the operating rooms. Lines are placed in this room in order to facilitate turnover time between cases, and to provide house officers with sufficient time to place lines without hurrying. This room is equipped with ECG and pressure monitors, defibrillator, self-inflating bag-mask ventilation system, wall suction, wall oxygen, good lighting, resuscitative drugs, intubation equipment, intercom system, and an emergency call button to summon help if necessary. Although the pressure-monitoring capabilities in this room are sufficient to place a flow-directed pulmonary artery catheter, this catheter is usually placed in the operating room. Patients can be observed by nursing personnel after lines are placed in this area.

LINE PLACEMENT

All the details regarding placement of intravenous, direct arterial, central venous, and pulmonary artery cannulae have been discussed in the chapter on monitoring. The following is a brief review of a logical sequence for placement of these lines and the rationale for this sequence.

1. Reestablish rapport with the patient and discuss NPO status, presence or absence of angina, and any other problem.
2. Determine a cuff blood pressure and pulse rate.
3. Place a large bore (#14) intravenous catheter using local anesthesia.
4. Administer additional medication as necessary through this intravenous route, and adjust intravenous flow rate.
5. Place a direct arterial pressure cannula using local anesthesia.
6. With the patient in a slightly head-down position, and while continuously observing the arterial pressure and the effects of Trendelenberg's position on the patient, place a central venous pressure line (internal or external jugular approach) using satisfactory local anesthesia.
7. With continuous electrocardiographic and pressure monitoring, and with the patient in the Trendelenberg position, place a pulmonary artery (Swan–Ganz) catheter. This line may be optional as discussed earlier.

One of the most common problems which occurs during this sequence is the development of angina if local anesthesia is not satisfactory and the patient becomes anxious and frightened during line placement. This usually can be treated with more IV sedation and satisfactory local anesthesia. Also, the effect of placing the patient in the head-down position for central line placement may precipitate angina because increased preload increases myocardial oxygen demand. This can be discovered by the patient's subjective complaints of angina and also the effects of anxiety on blood pressure and pulse rate. The major complications which can occur during pulmonary artery line placement include arrhythmias, angina, air embolism, cardiac or vascular damage, hematoma formation, and bleeding.

It has been reported that the placing of monitoring lines (especially pulmonary artery lines) can increase blood pressure and heart rate in susceptible patients.[36] This has not been the common experience, if sufficient local anesthesia, appropriate skill, and substantive verbal communication are employed.[37, 38] We feel strongly that all monitoring lines deemed necessary for patient care should be placed in the adult patient before induction. Exceptions to this are young children and the hyperdynamic patient with coronary artery disease who demonstrates angina during attempted line placement.

The potential for harm does exist during line placement. The anesthesiologist must never focus so narrowly on the procedure that he or she forgets to observe vital signs and signs of anxiety or angina. Most often this is best accomplished by carrying on a continual conversation with the patient while the lines are being placed. This patient contact provides feedback, so that problems are apparent and treatment is instituted.

Rarely, in a hyperdynamic patient with coronary artery disease, it is necessary to move immediately to the operating room and begin anesthetic induction as treatment for angina. In general, it is better to stabilize the patient's circulatory system, using adequate doses of IV narcotic, diazepam, and NTG before attempting to move the patient. A precipitous trip to the operating room may further increase the patient's anxiety and increase angina. If angina occurs, one person should be delegated to remain at the patient's head with an oxygen mask (preferably a system capable of delivering an F_IO_2 of 1.0) and a precordial stethoscope. This person's only function should be to maintain communication with the patient and to monitor the state of consciousness and ventilation.

In the severely ill patient with severe myocardial dysfunction, it may be desirable to place all lines in the operating room. Should serious problems develop, there is no delay in fully effecting ventilation, tracheal intubation, drug administration, and rapid sternotomy, if necessary. Special precautions and techniques used in patients with intractable arrhythmias, or scheduled for cardiac mapping, are discussed in Chapter 8.

Preinduction Criteria

1. The patient's chart should be checked for recent progress and nursing entries, laboratory results, and blood availability, and all found satisfactory.
2. The anesthesia record should be prepared with times and drugs to be used, already written on the chart. Preinduction hemodynamic control values should be recorded.
3. All planned vascular cannulations should be completed and secured.
4. All electronic monitoring should be established (transducers properly flushed and connected, pressure amplifiers zeroed and calibrated, oscilloscope calibrated, and the ECG connected and functioning).
5. Any infusion drugs should be labeled clearly, connected, and readied for infusion into the central venous line.
6. The patient's position on the operating room table should be checked before starting drugs which have vasodilating properties.
7. Qualified surgeons and a perfusionist should be available.
8. A fully primed and operational cardiopulmonary bypass pump should be in the operating suite.
9. The operating room nursing staff is ready to initiate maximal surgical support.

INDUCTION

Anesthetic induction should not begin until the criteria listed above are met. These criteria will allow a smooth, coordinated induction to begin. Drugs which are in use, or are to be used, need to be connected to a central venous line as close to the patient as possible. (See tables in Chapters 11 and 12 on drug dilutions for inotropic, chronotropic, and vasoactive drugs.) Thus during continuous infusion, potent drugs such as dopamine or nitroprusside will reach the circulation at steady rates and not accumulate in long fluid-filled lines. We prefer to avoid mechanical infusion pumps (because of their cost, complexity, and inconvenience), in favor of simple flow-restricting devices such as the Dial-a-flow and a drip-counting stopwatch (Concept AccuRate Meter). Inotropic and chronotropic agents should be ready for use in the patient with ventricular dysfunction, antiarrhythmic agents in the patient with arrhythmias, and vasodilators and β-blocking drugs in the hyperdynamic patient.

There are many different induction techniques and methods. Commonly used drug combinations are narcotics and sedatives (such as *morphine/diazepam*), with the addition of potent inhalation agents such as *enflurane* or *halothane* in hyperdynamic patients who require myocardial depression. *Isoflurane* currently is undergoing clinical investigation in patients with cardiovascular disease. Other narcotics such as *hydromorphone (Dilaudid)* or *fentanyl* (Sublimaze) are available. Both of these narcotics appear to have the advantage of less (or no) histamine release, and less (or no) vasodilation than morphine. Both of these narcotics are undergoing current hemodynamic investigation. *Thiopental* is a useful adjunct to gain quick circulatory control in a hyperdynamic patient. *Ketamine* should be used only in very specialized conditions, such as severe pericardial effusion, cardiac tamponade, or hypovolemic shock. It may be useful in the patient with a severely depressed heart, in whom bradycardia might compromise cardiac output. It should not be used routinely in the patient with coronary artery disease because it increases myocardial oxygen demand.[39, 40] The details of the cardiovascular effects of anesthetic drugs have been presented in Chapter 9. At Stanford, the most common anesthetic technique, as of this writing, is either fentanyl (30–80 µg/kg) or hydromorphone (0.3–0.5 mg/kg) combined with diazepam (0.3–0.5 mg/kg), supplemented with enflurane or isoflurane as needed.

The use of intravenous, intratracheal, or both forms of lidocaine during induction serves several purposes. Lidocaine (1) decreases the MAC of inhalation anesthetics,[41] (2) attenuates the heart rate and blood pressure responses to laryngoscopy and intubation,[42–49] and (3) reduces the chance of ventricular arrhythmias by decreasing ventricular irritability. It is safe because its major toxic effect of cerebral irritability is not a problem in the anesthetized patient. It has virtually no deleterious hemodynamic ef-

fects. Lidocaine is omitted in the patient undergoing cardiac mapping (see Chapter 8).

The choice of relaxant has been discussed in a previous chapter. One relaxant used at Stanford is pancuronium (Pavulon) because of its lack of ganglionic blockade and histamine release. If administered slowly, and in doses not exceeding 0.1 mg/kg total dose, tachycardia is uncommonly a problem. Metocurine (Metubine) often is used in hyperdynamic patients with coronary artery disease who cannot tolerate an increase in heart rate and myocardial oxygen demand. We do not use gallamine. d-Tubocurarine may be used occasionally if a decrease in blood pressure is desired. We rarely use succinylcholine when a long-acting nondepolarizing muscle relaxant is to be used during maintenance. (Why use two drugs when only one is necessary?)

The major determinants of myocardial oxygen consumption are discussed in Chapter 2. None of the principles mentioned in that chapter should be compromised, if possible. The patient should be managed in such a way as to maximize myocardial oxygen supply, minimize myocardial oxygen demand, facilitate cardiac efficiency, and provide sufficient cardiac output for all total-body needs. Each patient will have individual limits for each hemodynamic variable.

The anesthesiologist must consider known information based upon physiologic and pharmacologic studies,[50, 51] patient history, cardiac catheterization data, and direct patient response. A patient may know the heart rate above which he or she develops angina. Clearly this rate should not be exceeded. The cardiac catheterization report may indicate the limits of heart rate or blood pressure associated with ischemia in a particular patient, at a particular time, under specific conditions. These limits should serve as *guidelines* for that patient.

Because the anesthesiologist is trained to conduct anesthesia based upon patient *response*, the limits for blood pressure, heart rate, and the like intraoperatively should be established by patient response (see also Chap. 5). ECG signs of ischemia (ST segment depression, arrhythmias), cardiac failure, hypotension, and so on should direct the anesthesiologist to alter the course of induction.

Heart rate is *generally* maintained in the 50 to 80 beats/minute (bpm) range. A heart rate lower than 50 bpm may predispose to ventricular escape rhythms or inadequate cardiac output. Heart rate above approximately 80 bpm may predispose to ischemia. Each patient will be different, but in general a slow heart rate is preferred.

Blood pressure below 60 torr diastolic may be inadequate to provide optimal coronary perfusion, yet blood pressure greater than 100 to 120 torr systolic may produce myocardial ischemia. *In general,* most cardiac anesthesiologists maintain mean arterial pressure at approximately 65 to 85 torr, diastolic arterial pressure greater than 50 to 60 torr, and systolic arterial pressure less than 120 torr. Modest hypertension is relatively inexpensive for the heart because an increase in diastolic arterial pressure will augment coronary artery perfusion. In the failing heart, however, hypertension may be damaging. Exceptions to these guidelines will be dictated by specific patient needs.

The rate-pressure-product (RPP; heart rate times systolic arterial pressure) is a *crude* index, at best, of myocardial oxygen demand. It does not take into consideration contractility, the intrachamber pressures (LVEDP, RVEDP) which oppose subendocardial perfusion, nor examine diastolic coronary perfusion pressure, nor differentiate between a low heart rate and high heart rate with equal RPP values. If all other variables are maintained constant, *in general,* as RPP increases, so does myocardial oxygen consumption. Thus an increasing RPP should signal the anesthesiologist to evaluate other indices of cardiac performance and cardiac well-being, and provide treatment to decrease heart rate or systolic blood pressure, if indicated.

Anesthetic induction should never be performed so rapidly that a large dose of any drug is administered without waiting to see the effect of a previously administered dose. The induction should be titrated over a period of time appropriate to the patient's con-

dition. Continuous infusion (drip) is preferred over bolus drug administration. If morphine is used, it should be administered at rates less than 10 mg/min, with the initial increments administered more slowly. Some patients will react adversely to morphine with marked histamine release, manifested by flushing, particularly evident over the neck and upper thorax, and subsequent hypotension. This is treated with incremental doses of ephedrine (or phenylephrine if heart rate is increased), head-down table tilt, and IV fluid administration. Other narcotics, such as fentanyl (Sublimaze) or hydromorphone (Dilaudid) may be administered at faster rates (in equipotent doses) and are preferred to morphine. Ventilatory assistance should commence before obviously inadequate ventilation occurs to prevent significant carbon dioxide retention and hypoxemia. Upon patient unresponsiveness, a relaxant may be given. This is usually performed over a 1 to 4 minute period, with either pancuronium 0.1 mg/kg, or metocurine 0.4 mg/kg. Intubation then may be performed in 3 to 5 minutes. If muscle relaxation is delayed, laryngospasm, chest wall rigidity, or coughing may occur, and all of these have adverse effects.

The larynx and trachea should be sprayed with 4 percent lidocaine before intubation unless the patient is to receive a cardiac mapping procedure. We perform a double laryngoscopy in order to judge the level of anesthesia before intubation. This is accomplished in the following manner. An assistant watches the monitors continuously while the first laryngoscopy is performed. If blood pressure or heart rate begins to increase after placement of the blade in the mouth, laryngoscopy is discontinued and anesthesia deepened. If blood pressure and heart rate are stable, a commercially available 4 percent lidocaine spray (LTA–Abbott) is administered. Then the blade is removed from the mouth and mask ventilation with 100 percent oxygen continued. If a precipitous increase in either blood pressure or heart rate after this procedure is observed, anesthesia is deepened, usually with thiopental or an inhalation agent or both. After blood pressure and heart rate are controlled, or if no precipitous increase is seen, a second laryngoscopy is performed. The trachea is then intubated as smoothly as possible. The amount of time that the laryngoscope blade is in the mouth should be minimized, and intubation performed by skilled personnel. In other words, the patient with coronary artery disease should not be used to teach intubation techniques to the novice!

If the guidelines listed below are followed, cardiovascular complications of laryngoscopy and intubation should be rare. We prefer oral intubation using a soft cuff disposable endotracheal tube and no longer use high-pressure cuff endotracheal tubes. Nasal intubation has no short-term advantage over oral intubation, and carries the risks of bacteremia, nasal bleeding, other nasal trauma, and is used rarely in the adult.

After the patient's trachea is intubated, mechanical ventilation may begin, the endotracheal tube secured with tape, and a chest roll placed to elevate the chest. An esophageal stethoscope is placed so that continuous monitoring of breath and heart sounds can continue. We place a urinary catheter post-induction in all patients, except cardiac transplant recipients, to monitor urine output. An arterial blood gas determination should be performed before the beginning of surgery. The surgical prep is generally started after tracheal intubation, and the surgeons' presence requested.

The following items should always be plotted on the anesthesia record along with the routine variables: heart rate and rhythm; arterial pressures; central venous or pulmonary artery pressures or both, temperatures (rectal and nasal); urine output (incremental and cumulative); aortic cross-clamp and cardiopulmonary bypass times; bypass pump flow; time and dose(s) of heparin administration; activated coagulation times (ACT);[52] all blood gas tensions; and laboratory results. An accurate and up-to-date record should be kept during induction. This can be difficult for the novice, but becomes easy with experience. A record composed one-half hour after the fact may bear little resemblance to what actually occurred. A continuously written display of each pressure channel and ECG/heart rate is instructive.

Generally, during the prep, one can expect blood pressure to decrease because the patient is not being stimulated and is adequately anesthetized. It may be necessary to increase arterial blood pressure during this period with inotropic drugs or vasopressors, until the time of surgical incision.

START OF SURGERY AND TRANSITION TO CARDIOPULMONARY BYPASS

Most often the patient should receive a supplemental dose of anesthetic drug(s) just before surgical incision. If this is not done, an increase in blood pressure and heart rate may occur. This should be done also just before sternotomy, which is a strong, painful stimulus, and which may produce an increase in myocardial oxygen demand. During sternotomy, the anesthesiologist must observe the field for hemorrhage, and be prepared to infuse fluid or blood rapidly if the heart or great vessels are damaged. This occurs infrequently, but is more common in the patient who has had previous cardiac surgery. The airway should be open to atmospheric pressure during sternotomy because this allows the lungs, heart, and great vessels to fall away from the sternum (dorsally), lessening the chances for accidental cardiotomy.

A control ACT should be performed and

Avoidance of Complications Associated With Intubation

1. Adequate monitoring
2. Enough anesthesia
3. Laryngotracheal topical anesthesia
4. Double laryngoscopy
5. Preoxygenation
6. Use of propranolol, NTG, nitroprusside when indicated
7. Fast, smooth laryngoscopy by skilled personnel

then heparin administration recorded on the anesthesia record (dose and time). We administer the dose of heparin necessary to increase the ACT by four to five times the control value. This is often a dose of 300 to 400 units/kg (3.0–4.0 mg/kg; see also Chapters 14 and 24). Bypass cannot commence until the anesthesiologist is absolutely certain that heparin has been administered *and effect verified* by appropriate testing (ACT).[52] The anesthesiologist is just as responsible as the surgeon if bypass commences without adequate heparinization!

The transition from patient self-sufficiency to total cardiopulmonary bypass should be performed smoothly and in a controlled manner. A **pre-bypass check list,** provided below, should **always** be performed before bypass. Upon institution of bypass, an **immediate on-bypass check list** should be reviewed to ensure patient safety and adequate equipment function (see list below). Within the **first 4 minutes of the institution of bypass,** another check should commence as listed below, to ensure proper patient-equipment functioning. If all checks are performed, and any corrections appropriate instituted, bypass will be safely and carefully performed. The next chapter will cover in detail the history, pathophysiology, and management of cardiopulmonary bypass.

Prebypass Check List

1. All IV infusion drugs off
2. All inhalation anesthetic agents off
3. Has heparin been given and recorded on the chart? Has this been checked with an activated coagulation time?
4. Give supplemental relaxant and IV anesthetic agents.
5. Empty urimeter.
6. Are transducers properly zeroed and calibrated?
7. Prepare and debubble cardioplegic infusion.
8. Check patient's pupils.
9. Are all patient-equipment connections satisfactory, free of air bubbles, and ready for bypass?
10. Are all personnel ready to institute bypass (anesthesiologist, perfusionist, surgeons, nurses, technicians?)

Immediately "On-Bypass" Checklist

1. Check connections of cardiopulmonary equipment, verify adequate function, and ensure that perfusionist is satisfied with patient-equipment interface.
2. Ventilator off.
3. Check venous drainage from head and neck, observe face and eyes for swelling.
4. Reset alarm limits on arterial pressure monitor.
5. Adjust operating table to level pericardial sac, and facilitate venous drainage from lower extremities.
6. Prepare to infuse cardioplegic solution.
7. Double-check function of all equipment.

Checklist for the First 4 Minutes of Cardiopulmonary Bypass

1. Repeat immediate "on-bypass" checklist.
2. Perform an ACT. Correct low ACT with heparin.
3. Perform an arterial blood gas.
4. Check pupils for size and equality.
5. Check face and eyes for swelling.
6. Adjust arterial blood pressure if indicated.

REFERENCES

PREOPERATIVE EVALUATION

1. Examination of the Heart (5 Booklets). American Heart Association, Dallas, 1975
2. Hurst JW: The Heart, Arteries and Veins, 4th ed. New York, McGraw-Hill, 1978
3. Hurst JW, Walker HK: The Problem-Oriented System. New York, Medcom, 1972
4. Hurst JW, Walker HK: The Problem-Oriented System. New York, Medcom, 1972

Subjective—Historical Data and Review of Systems

5. Lawson NW, Butler GH, Ray CT: Alkalosis and cardiac arrhythmias. Anesth Analg (Cleve) 52:951, 1973
6. Tanaka K, Pettinger WA: Pharmacokinetics of bolus potassium injections for cardiac arrhythmias. Anesthesiology 38:587, 1973
7. Klinke WP, Christie LG, Nichols WW et al: Use of catheter-tip velocity-pressure transducer to evaluate left ventricular function in

man: effects of intravenous propranolol. Circulation 61:946–954, 1980

8. Kopriva CJ, Brown ACD, Pappas G: Hemodynamics during general anesthesia in patients receiving propranolol. Anesthesiology 48:28 33, 1978

9. Editorial: Should propranolol be stopped before surgery? Med Lett Drugs Ther 18:41–42, 1976

10. Slogoff S, Keats AS, Hibbs CW et al: Failure of general anesthesia to potentiate propranolol activity. Anesthesiology 47:504–508, 1977

11. Leaman DM, Levenson LW, Shiroff RA et al: Persistence of biologic activity after disappearance of propranolol from the serum. J Thorac Cardiovasc Surg 72:67–72, 1976

12. Viljoen JF, Estafanous GF, Kellner GA: Propranolol and cardiac surgery: J Thorac Cardiovasc Surg 64:826–830, 1972

13. Miller RR, Olson HG, Amsterdam EA et al: Propranolol-withdrawal rebound phenomenon. N Engl J Med 293:416–418, 449–451, 1975

14. Shand DG: Editorial: Propranolol withdrawal. N Engl J Med 293:449–450, 1975

15. Danilevicius Z: Editorial: Caution in propranolol withdrawal. JAMA 237:53, 1977

16. Faulkner SL, Hopkins JT, Boerth RC et al: Time required for complete recovery from chronic propranolol therapy. N Engl J Med 289:607–609, 635–636, 1973

17. Alderman EL, Coltart DJ, Wettach GE et al: Coronary artery syndromes after sudden propranolol withdrawal. Ann Intern Med 81:625–627, 1974

18. Slogoff S, Keats AS, Ott, E: Preoperative propranolol therapy and aortocoronary bypass operation. JAMA 240:1487–1490, 1978

19. Podrid PJ, Schoeneberger A, Loun B: Congestive heart failure caused by oral disopyramide. N Engl J Med 302:614, 1980

20. Brown BR: Anesthesia and Essential Hypertension Refresher Courses in Anesthesiology, vol 7, pp 41–50. Philadelphia, JB Lippincott, 1979

Objective—Data from Physical and Laboratory Examination

21. Yang SS et al: From Cardiac Catheterization Data to Hemodynamic Parameters, 2nd ed. Philadelphia, FA Davis, 1978

22. Grossman W: Cardiac catheterization and angiography. Philadelphia, Lea & Febiger, 1975

23. Mangano DT: Preoperative assessment of cardiac catheterization data: which parameters are the most important? Anesthesiology 53:S106, 1980

24. Mason J: Personal communication, 1980

25. Cooke BM, Ellestad MH: Using stress testing to identify the severity of coronary artery disease. CVP p 14, 1979

26. Ellestad MH: Stress Testing. Philadelphia, FA Davis, 1976

Assessment—Interpretation of All Subjective and Objective Data

27. Criteria Committee of the New York Heart Association: Nomenclature and Criteria for Diagnosis of Diseases of the Heart and Great Vessels, 7th ed. Boston, Little, Brown & Co, 1973

28. Dripps RD, Eckenhoff JE, and Vandam LD: Introduction to Anesthesia, 5th ed. Philadelphia, WB Saunders, 1977

29. Goldman L et al: Multifactorial index of cardiac risk in noncardiac surgical procedures. N Engl J Med 297:845, 1977

30. Moore CH et al: Left main coronary artery stenosis: hemodynamic monitoring to reduce mortality. Ann Thorac Surg 26:445–451, 1978

PLAN

31. Lyons SM et al: The premedication of cardiac surgical patients. A clinical comparison of four regimens. Anaesthesia, 30:459–470, 1975

32. Mirakhur RK, Clarke RSJ, Elliott J et al: Atropine and glycopyrronium premedication: a comparison of the effects on cardiac rate and rhythm during induction of anesthesia. Anesthesia 33:906–912, 1978

33. Mirakhur RK, Dundee JW: Cardiovascular changes during induction of Anesthesia: influence of three anticholinergic premedicants. Ann R Coll Surg Engl 61:463–469, 1979

34. Viby–Mogensen J et al: Halothane anesthesia and suxamethonium: the significance of preoperative atropine administration. ACTA Anaesthesiol Scand, 20(2):129–140, 1976

35. Eikard B: Arrhythmias during halothane anesthesia: The influence of atropine. Acta Anaesthesiol Scand 21(3):245–251, 1977

LINE PLACEMENT

36. Lunn JK, Stanley TH, Webster LR et al: Arterial blood-pressure and pulse-rate responses to pulmonary and radial arterial catheterization prior to cardiac and major vascular operations. Anesthesiology 51:265–269, 1979
37. Waller JL, Zaidan JR, Kaplan JA et al: Hemodynamic responses to vascular cannulation before coronary bypass surgery (abstr). Presented at the annual meeting of the International Anesthesia Research Society, 1980
38. Waller JL, Zaidan JR, Kaplan, JA et al: Hemodynamic effects of vascular cannulation by residents (abstr). Anesthesiology 53:S114, 1980

INDUCTION

39. Spotoft H, Korshin JD, Sorensen MB et al: The cardiovascular effects of ketamine used for induction of anaesthesia in patients with valvular heart disease. Can Anaesth Soc J 26:463–467, 1979
40. Stanley TH: Blood-pressure and pulse-rate responses to ketamine during general anesthesia. Anesthesiology 39:648–649, 1973
41. Himes RS Jr, DiFazio CA, Burney RG: Effects of lidocaine on the anesthetic requirements for nitrous oxide and halothane. Anesthesiology 47:437–440, 1977
42. Abou–Madi MN, Keszler H, Yacoub JM: A method for prevention of cardiovascular reactions to laryngoscopy and intubation. Can Anaesth Soc J 22:316–329, 1975
43. Abou–Madi MN, Keszler H, Yacoub JM: Cardiovascular reactions to laryngoscopy and tracheal intubation following small and large intravenous doses of lidocaine. Can Anaesth Soc J 24:12–19, 1977
44. Bassel GM, Lin YT, Oka Y et al: Circulatory response to tracheal intubation in patients with coronary artery disease and valvular disease. Bull NY Acad Med 54:842–848, 1978
45. Denlinger JK, Ellison N, Ominsky AJ: Effects of intratracheal lidocaine on circulatory responses to tracheal intubation. Anesthesiology 41:409–412, 1974
46. Denlinger JK, Messner JT, D'Orazio DJ et al: Effect of intravenous lidocaine on the circulatory response to tracheal intubation. Anesthesiology Review, pp 13–15, 1976
47. Fox EJ, Sklar GS, Hill CH et al: Complications related to the pressor response to endotracheal intubation. Anesthesiology 47:524–525, 1977
48. Scott DB, Littlewood DG, Covino BG et al: Plasma lignocaine concentrations following endotracheal spraying with an aerosol. Br J Anaesth 48:899–902, 1976
49. Smith RB: Letter: Uptake of lidocaine from the trachea. Anesthesiology 44:269, 1976
50. Loeb HS, Saudye A, Croke RP, et al: Effects of pharmacologically induced hypertension of myocardial ischemia and coronary hemodynamics in patients with fixed coronary obstruction. Circulation 57:41–46, 1978
51. Rowe GG: Response of the coronary circulation to physiologic changes and pharmacologic agents. Anesthesiology 41:182–196, 1974
52. Fischbach DP, Fogdall RP: Coagulation: The Essentials. Baltimore. Williams & Wilkins, 1981

14

Cardiopulmonary Bypass

ALLEN K. REAM

HISTORY*

Although many believe that the history of cardiopulmonary bypass began with the efforts of Charles Lindbergh and Alexis Carrel in 1930, efforts go back nearly 200 years.[6] LeGallois is believed to be the first to predict that support could be provided by an appropriately constituted and pumped perfusate in 1812.[7] The first artificial oxygenation of blood is credited to Ludwig in 1869; accomplished by shaking the blood with gas in a balloon during circulation.[8] Bunge used a similar technique in 1876 to accomplish the first isolated organ perfusion.[9] The first bubble oxygenator for organ perfusion was built in 1882, but failed because of foaming.[10] An isolated organ perfusion system using a blood film spread on a rotating cylinder was first reported in 1885.[11] At that time organ perfusion was usually accomplished by cross circulation with another animal. Hooker reported the forerunner of the modern disk oxygenator in 1910.[12]

American workers reported the first film oxygenator using a perforated silk screen suspended from a glass ring in 1915;[13] the same year that heparin was discovered.[14,15] Hooker

---

*Because of the breadth of material available, this chapter can provide only an introduction to the literature. The reader is strongly encouraged to read further, and the general references are suggested.[1-5]

investigated the effect of pulsatile flow in the kidney in 1910,[16] but pulsatile perfusion of a fully isolated organ was not reported until 1928.[17] It would appear that the real contribution of Lindbergh and Carrel was the recognition of the need for bacterial filtering.[18]

The development of modern bypass techniques began in 1934 with DeBakey's invention of the roller pump.[19] Gibbon accomplished the first total cardiopulmonary bypass in cats in 1937.[20] The modern disc oxygenator was invented by Bjork in 1948[21, 22] and the first modern bubble oxygenator, incorporating defoaming agents, by Clark in 1950.[23] The first surgical attempt in man using total cardiopulmonary bypass was by Dennis in 1951,[24] but failed because a presumed atrial septal defect was actually an endocardial cushion defect not susceptible to simple closure.[25] Gibbon reported the first clinical success in 1954 with one survivor out of four operations for atrial septal defect.[26] Finally, in 1956 the disposable bubble oxygenator was invented[27, 28] and the first clinical application of a membrane oxygenator was reported.[29] These developments are summarized in Table 14–1.

It would appear that the critical discoveries in this chain of events were the discovery of heparin, the development of an adequate pump, the development of an acceptable antifoaming technique, the gradual appreciation of the crucial role of aseptic technique in protecting patients against progressive septicemia, and mastering the technical problem of accomplishing adequate oxygenation without blood trauma. Many early clinical complications appear related to the difficulty in separating the problems of gram-negative sepsis from those of unacceptable blood trauma associated with oxygenation.

It was by no means clear in the early 1950s that mechanical extracorporeal oxygenation was the most promising approach. Lewis reported in 1953 the first success in open-heart surgery using only hypothermia,[30] and his results seemed quite promising. Lillehei reported the first of a series of human survivors using cross circulation with living human subjects in 1954.[31] Dogliatti reported the first successful human surgery involving organ

Table 14-1. History of Cardiopulmonary Bypass

1812	Prediction of support with injection of arterial blood (LeGallois)
1869	Artificial oxygenation of blood (Ludwig)
1876	Isolated perfusion of kidney (Bunge)
1882	Bubbler for organ perfusion; foaming problems (Schröder)
1885	Oxygenation via film on cylinder (Frey)
1910	First disk-type oxygenator (Hooker)
1915	Improved film oxygenator (Richards and Drinker)
1915	Discovery of heparin (McClean)
1928	Pulsatile perfusion of dog's head, using piston pump (Dale and Schuster)
1930	Organ perfusion, bacterial filtering (Lindbergh and Carrel)
1934	Roller pump for blood infusion (DeBakey)
1937	Support of cats on total cardiopulmonary bypass (Gibbon)
1948	Invention of disc oxygenator (Bjork)
1950	First modern bubbler, first application effective defoaming (Clark)
1951	Successful organ bypass in man; direct bubble injection (Dogliatti)
1951	First attempt, total bypass in man (Dennis)
1953	Success in open heart surgery using only hypothermia (Lewis)
1954	First human survivors, total bypass (Gibbon)
1954	Successful bypass, using human lung in cross circulation (Lillehei)
1956	Invention of disposable bubbler design (DeWall)
1956	First clinical use of membrane oxygenator (Clowes)

bypass and oxygenation by direct bubble injection in 1951.[32]

Considerable uncertainty existed at that time regarding the most appropriate technique for oxygenation. Competing techniques included direct chemical reaction as by injection of peroxide, bubble oxygenation both in its modern form and as direct bubble injection with limited defoaming techniques, and membrane oxygenation, the most direct imitation of the natural physiologic mechanism.

Out of this confusion three oxygenator designs survived. The surface oxygenator was the first, and depended on a thin film of blood moving over a solid surface. Oxygen diffused into the film from the surrounding gas. This was supplanted by the bubble oxygenator in the early 1960s as disposable systems were developed and defoaming techniques were improved. Modern research is centered on the membrane oxygenator because of the recognition that avoidance of a direct blood-gas interface reduces blood trauma, and would therefore permit longer periods of perfusion.

MODERN DESIGN

In this section we will discuss the general design concepts of modern oxygenators. The reader is referred to the literature for a more detailed review[33] and for discussion of specific proprietary designs.[34-97]

The diagram of Figure 14-1 shows a typical arrangement of the cardiopulmonary bypass apparatus. The oxygenator is shown in Figure 14-2. In the major circuit, blood is accepted through cannulae usually placed in the vena cavae, passed through the oxygenator and is returned via a roller pump to the patient's arterial system. A filter is placed in the line close to the return to the patient to trap any emboli. Typical modern filters are also inverted, with a bleed back to the oxygenator, so that should air embolism occur, it can be trapped in the filter and passed to the oxygenator to be eliminated. The bleed flow when fluid filled can be quite slow because, should the bleed line fill with gas, flow will increase. A filter is also placed on the input to the oxygenator for closed circulation before the patient is perfused, to remove inorganic emboli shed by system components.

A second circuit consists of the so-called coronary or clean suction. Originally a return for blood obtained through a cannula placed in the coronary sinus (to prevent distention), it is now used for blood removed from the operative field that may be suitable for reinfusion. Blood is passed by a roller pump to a reservoir and is then returned to the oxygenator via a filter to remove contaminants. The additional reservoir is important because this return fluid may be diluted by significant amounts of extravascular fluid used to cool the heart. Use of a reservoir and filter with intermittent return to the system allows operator quantification of the extent of dilution and contamination. External supplies to the oxygenator customarily include controlled temperature water for the heat exchanger, and oxygen with selection of carbon dioxide concentration between 0 and 5 percent.

OXYGENATOR

At the gas-blood interface, the rate of gas moving into the blood is directly affected by

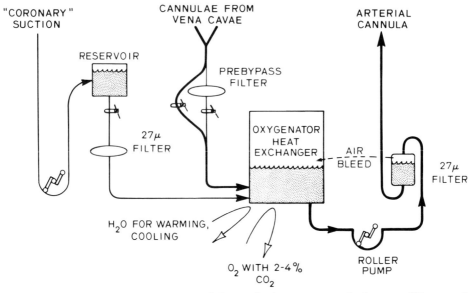

Fig. 14-1. A schematic diagram of the typical arrangement of pump, filters and oxygenator during cardiopulmonary bypass.

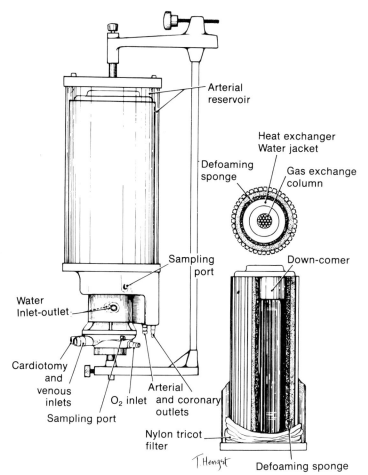

Arterial
reservoir

Heat exchanger
Water jacket

Defoaming
sponge

Gas exchange
column

Sampling
port

Down-comer

Water
Inlet-outlet

Cardiotomy
and
venous
inlets

O_2 inlet

Arterial
and coronary
outlets

Sampling port

Nylon tricot
filter

T Hengst

Defoaming sponge

Fig. 14–2. The Harvey oxygenator. Shown at left in the operating position. Shown at lower right in cross section. The down-comer distributes the oxygenated blood foam evenly to the defoaming sponges. Top view at upper right. (Reed CC, Clark DK: Cardiopulmonary Perfusion. Houston, Texas Medical Press, 1975)

the thickness of the blood film. Transfer of oxygen is limited by the diffusion resistance of oxygen across plasma and within the red cell (approximately four times greater). This diffusion resistance and the relatively small plasma solubility and large binding capacity within the red cell mean that diffusion beyond the first echelon of red cells is quite slow. Thus the rate of gas transfer to blood is much greater in a system where the diffusion path in blood is very short. In the organic lung, the capillaries are so small that only a single red cell can pass at a time. Designing an artificial lung to this tolerance is physically impossible. Other techniques for increasing the rate of oxygen uptake are employed, including slowing the transit time of the red cell in the lung from the normal 100 to 300 msec by 3 to 20 times, increasing the oxygen tension to increase the driving gra-

dient, thinning the blood to reduce transport capacity and thereby increase the rate of equilibration, and stirring to increase gas exchange.

Stirring may also increase erythrocyte destruction. Erythrocytes are destroyed when the shear rate (force tangential to the cell membrane) exceeds a threshold value in the fluid. A much lower shear rate is destructive if associated with wall contact. Wall contact also activates or denatures many blood proteins. The bubble oxygenator has proven simple and successful partly because wall contact is reduced. The small bubbles released into the blood promote turbulence, mixing blood and gas, and increasing the effective surface area exposed to the blood. While blood is also denatured by contact with a gas interface (some blood components going into surface solution within milliseconds), the degree of injury is acceptable for the normal bypass duration.

However, the blood components which go into surface solution stabilize the foam which develops. The discovery of silicon antifoaming agents is the key to modern application of the bubble oxygenator. After gas mixing, the blood must pass sufficiently treated filtration surfaces to insure bubble removal before returning to the patient.

Excretion of carbon dioxide is not a practical problem. On theoretical grounds, it can be shown that to achieve the normal A-V CO_2 difference of 4 ml/dl, about 76 ml of ventilating gas per 100 ml of blood must be provided. A higher gas flow is required to assure adequate oxygenation in the typical bubble oxygenator, thus it is necessary to add carbon dioxide to the gas mixture to slow exchange, and prevent hypocarbia. Sampling of arterial gases during bypass is customarily employed to assure an acceptable partial pressure of CO_2. A typical concentration in the supply gas is 3 percent.

The priming volume is sensitive to gas exchange efficiency and usually, greater efficiency permits a smaller priming volume. Many of the design subtleties of modern oxygenators relate directly to attempts to reduce the priming volume.

While the film oxygenators reduced the trauma associated with the blood-gas interface, the surface interaction posed other problems. Material accumulated on the exchange surfaces, requiring aggressive and caustic cleaning. The cleaning caused surface etching and erosion, increasing surface reactivity with repeated use. The cleaning process was demanding and construction requirements made a disposable version economically impractical. The simplicity, economy and ease of use have favored the bubble oxygenator where duration of bypass was not unacceptably long.

Membrane oxygenators represent a separate class of problems and are discussed under *Long-Term Cardiopulmonary Bypass.*

PUMPS

The most commonly used pump is a roller pump first developed by DeBakey in 1934 (Fig. 14–3). The blood passes through tubing compressed by a roller at the end of a rotating arm. The tubing lies in a semicircular trough, and is compressed between the trough and the roller. The rollers are spaced 180 degrees apart so that a second roller begins occlusion as the first is reaching the end of the compression arc, preventing backflow. The pump

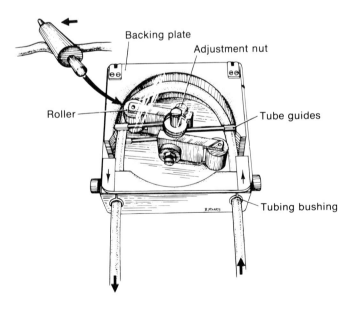

Fig. 14–3. A typical roller pump. The tubing bushings are sized to the tubing used, and keep the tubing from creeping. Various arrangements are provided for setting tubing occlusion under the roller. In this example, an adjustment nut permits the rollers to be moved toward or away from the backing plate. The drawing of the rolling pin at upper left illustrates the basic principle of all roller pumps. (Reed CC, Clark DK: Cardiopulmonary Perfusion. Houston, Texas Medical Press, 1975)

occlusion is set so it leaks with a back pressure higher than 30 cm of water, because with full occlusion hemolysis is significant. Occlusive hemolysis is due to the red cell-tubing wall interaction, associated with the high shear rate. Flow is almost constant, with a small pressure pulse each half revolution. Bladder type valved pumps have been employed for artificial heart research (see Chap. 27), but have not achieved popularity in this application because of their increased complexity. They do, however, permit more physiologic pulsatile flow.

In recent years two impeller type pumps have been developed and are being marketed. The Biomedicus is a series of concentric rotating cones within a matching housing which expels the blood by entrainment against the smooth surface of the spinning cones. The second (Medtronics) uses a bladed impeller (nicknamed the "Waring blender"). It was believed for many years that this type of pump would not work. However, Blackshear and Bernstein demonstrated in 1969 that red cell hemolysis occurs in bulk solution at much higher shear rates than when liquid-solid contact is involved. This pump is designed so that little red cell contact with the rotating blades occurs.

It is claimed that both pumps can provide pulsatile flow as well. However, while both appear to be effective under steady state flow conditions, running them in a pulsatile mode results in less stable flow patterns and increased materials contact. The resulting change in rate of hemolysis is still a matter of dispute. Also, in the event of a power failure there is no impediment to reverse flow. Air entrainment is then possible through the patient, or a check valve must be installed.

HEAT EXCHANGER

While not evident in many cardiopulmonary bypass systems, a heat exchanger is an essential component. Typical designs are illustrated in Figure 14–4. The need for a heat exchanger to maintain patient temperature is twofold. First, heating prevents the temperature gradient between the patient and the room from cooling the patient. Second, heat loss occurs in bubble oxygenators as a result of evaporative fluid loss. It is not customary to prehumidify oxygenator gases.

An additional incentive is the practice of moderately cooling the patient to enhance tissue preservation. Cooling also permits lower bypass flow, because oxygen demand is reduced. Fewer blood transits through the oxygenator reduces the severity of blood trauma. The heat exchanger speeds cooling. In disposable bubble oxygenators, the heat exchanger is usually integrated into the oxygenator. In theory this permits increased heat exchanger efficiency, but efficiency varies widely from one commercial device to another and should be individually investigated if, in the contemplated application, this is a matter of concern.

When significant cooling (*e.g.*, below 25°C) is contemplated, an external heat exchanger should be added to the circuit. Cooling rarely presents unusual delay or risk because the bypass blood can be considerably cooler than the desired patient temperature, without unacceptable blood trauma. However on warming, the margin of safety is considerably smaller. First, gas solubility in blood decreases with rising temperature. When warming the patient, one must be sure that the heat exchanger is placed in the circuit before the debubbler so that gas bubbles formed consequent to decreased gas solubility are removed. Secondly, on warming, the maximum blood temperature which can be tolerated without significant injury lies below 42°C. This means that a very small gradient is permitted between the end-stage temperature desired in the patient and the maximum temperature achievable in the blood. Not so commonly appreciated is that this maximum temperature is not the bulk blood temperature exiting the heat exchanger, but the temperature at any point in the blood. Thus, the blood temperature in the film closest to the heat exchanger surface is of critical interest.

In calf studies with implanted heat exchangers, it was noted that significant hem-

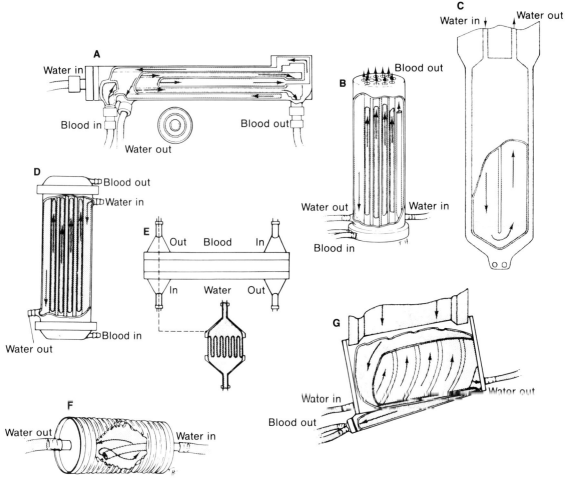

Fig. 14–4. Cutaway drawing of heat exchangers. *A:* Sarns. *B.* Harvey integral unit. *C.* Optiflow integral unit. *D.* Brown–Harrison, *E.* Miniprime, *F.* TMP Venotherm, *G.* Benthy integral unit. (Reed CC, Clark DK: Cardiopulmonary Perfusion. Houston, Texas Medical Press, 1975)

olysis occurred when the temperature contour of 42°C passed the cell-free layer (skimming layer) of the passing blood (*i.e.,* deep enough in the flowing blood to warm the outermost red cells as they passed).[98] Under these circumstances, counter-current design is essential so that the entering warming fluid can be held below 42°C, and the exiting blood can be brought as close to this temperature as is practically possible. In many modern installations, this is the least carefully controlled parameter. Water circulating through the heat exchanger is often controlled manually and temperature calibration may not be adequately monitored.

FILTERS

The use of filters in cardiopulmonary bypass is a relatively recent development. The development of effective blood filters of 20 to 30 μ was originally believed to be impractical because of potential red cell damage associated with the necessary material contact. In recent years, such filters have been made available and demonstrated to be satisfactory and effective. Acceptance of filters, particularly those used to filter the primed system before cardiopulmonary bypass, has been stimulated by the observation that use appears to correlate with a marked decrease in post bypass neurologic dysfunction. This is discussed further under *Complications.*

SENSORS AND CONTROLS

System complexity has regressed since the early days of cardiopulmonary bypass. Many of the early systems included automated techniques to assure an adequate fluid reservoir level, adequate flows, and appropriate system response in the event of mechanical or electrical failure. The modern cardiopulmonary bypass system, aside from the details of oxygenator construction, is a remarkably simple system. In most centers, automatic controls are entirely lacking, with the exception of a low-level alarm on the oxygenator reservoir. Even here, operator response is the final assurance that the pump is stopped before air is transmitted to the patient.

The reasons for this trend appear to be twofold. First, it has been found that there is very little which can be monitored on the unit during cardiopulmonary bypass that helps define the quality of individual patient status. Hence, most bypass protocols, in most major institutions, follow a precise schema derived from experience with a large number of patients over a long period of time. Second, the number of possible failures which can occur with cardiopulmonary bypass are so large as to make it virtually impossible to protect against them by purely automatic means. Systems which seriously address this issue become quite complicated, and until very recently were probably not technologically feasible. Increasing complexity decreases reliability.

Monitoring does include the most significant variables. Pressure in the line returning to the patient is rarely monitored because it is recognized that the cannula used by most centers is small enough to result in artificially high pressures on the pump side of the cannula. When flow is known, the pressure in

the aortic root can be estimated; the pressure in the perfusion system is not directly relevant, though too large a pressure drop increases blood trauma.[99] Aortic pressure is monitored directly through the radial artery. Flow is usually monitored by counting revolutions of the occlusive roller pump. If one of the modern rotor pumps is used, a flow meter must be added to the circuit. The blood level in the oxygenator reservoir is usually monitored visually with a photocell threshold alarm as backup because of the simplicity and ease with which it is accomplished. Similarly, operator controlled return of the coronary suction reservoir blood to the oxygenator makes monitoring easy to perform at the operator's convenience. Gas flows are easily monitored through gas regulators. Electronic gas sensors do not appear to be advantageous until equipment of greater reliability and more reasonable cost is available.

INITIATING CARDIOPULMONARY BYPASS

PUMP PRIME

A typical priming solution for cardiopulmonary bypass is shown in Table 14–2. Three primary considerations affect the composition of pump prime. These are the requirements for iso- or modest hypertonicity, electrolyte balance, and appropriate hemodilution.

Table 14-2. Typical Oxygenator Priming Solution

Lactated Ringer's solution	2000 ml*
Heparin	4400 units/l of prime
NaHCO$_3$	50 mEq/l
Mannitol	12.5 g/l†/hour of bypass
KCl	20–40 mEq‡
CaCl$_2$	4.5 mEq (0.5 g)/unit of blood in prime

* Total solution volume 2000 to 2200 ml; if whole blood added to adjust hematocrit on bypass, reduce R/L by equivalent amount.

† Mannitol is sometimes added after perfusion begins (see text).

‡ Less potassium is added if cardioplegic solution containing potassium is administered

The pump priming solution must be isotonic or slightly hypertonic to both facilitate equilibration with intravascular fluids without rapid, excessive extravascular shifts, and to avoid hemolysis or other injuries associated with hypotonic solutions or excessive gradients.

The solution customarily chosen is Ringer's lactate because of its buffered pH and balanced content of the most significant electrolytes.

Potassium chloride is customarily added to the bypass prime because serum potassium declines continuously during cardiopulmonary bypass. Sodium bicarbonate is added to the prime solution. It appears this is primarily for historical reasons because acidosis frequently occurred during the early years. The buffering capacity of the bicarbonate is useful during the initial minutes of perfusion when the perfusate is not oxygenated. It has become customary in many centers to add an osmotic diuretic to the perfusate to ensure continued urine flow and thus facilitate assessment of renal function during bypass, and because some believe osmotic diuresis may have a beneficial effect on renal blood flow.

Anticoagulation is maintained during cardiopulmonary bypass by heparinization. Thus it is customary to add an adequate amount of heparin to the prime to ensure anticoagulation of the blood used in the prime. Originally, only heparin was added to the blood prime but the use of citrated blood now appears almost universal.[100] Calcium chloride is added in a quantity estimated to be sufficient to balance the citrate.

A major controversy in recent years has been the question of the most appropriate red cell content in the pump prime. Originally it was felt that whole blood must be used in order to adequately support tissue oxygenation. However, several factors have encouraged testing this assumption. Blood is a scarce commodity and any reduction in priming requirements will stretch it further. Stored blood exhibits increased red cell fragility; fragility is also increased by exposure to the oxygenator during cardiopulmonary bypass. Thus survival of transfused blood is materially reduced by bypass. Some suggest that withdrawal of patient blood with postbypass reinfusion is helpful, but the results are equivocal, and the risk of error is increased.[101,102]

Cooling the patient during cardiopulmonary bypass also supports the desire to hemodilute for two reasons. First, with falling blood temperature, blood viscosity increases. Both clinical experience with patients having increased blood viscosity under preoperative conditions, and experience during surgery suggests that a rise in viscosity is undesirable. It is believed that this both increases perfusion resistance (reducing flow) and also increases the probability of sludging with stasis at the capillary level. Secondly, with a fall in temperature, tissue oxygen requirements are reduced. Thus, a lower oxygen-carrying capacity is required, given normal flows, to maintain a normal arterial-venous oxygen difference. See Chapter 26.

At present a tentative consensus appears to have developed suggesting that a hematocrit near 25 is acceptable under most circumstances.[103,104] A variety of evidence supports this view.[105] Patients with chronic renal failure typically have hematocrits of 18 to 22 and no apparent perfusion difficulties. Intraoperative experience with Jehovah's Witnesses, in whom transfusion was entirely avoided for religious reasons, has been very encouraging[106] although a slight increase in morbidity and mortality has been reported.[107] Despite the concern that use of crystalloid in preference to plasma and whole blood products would result in increased tissue edema and impaired oxygen transfer, a number of recent studies have suggested that such postoperative differences are minimal and may favor crystalloid.[108] It has also been suggested that increased hemodilution may have a beneficial effect on post operative gas exchange despite evidence of increased lung water. Some esoteric problems may also be avoided, such as abnormally high blood carbon monoxide levels associated with old stored blood.[109]

The relationship of oxygen transport and blood flow during cardiopulmonary bypass is discussed in the next section.

PATIENT ANTICOAGULATION

The reader should refer to Chapter 24 for a detailed discussion of coagulation mechanisms and therapy. This section is confined to a discussion of practical techniques.

The patient is heparinized immediately prior to placement of the cannulae. Customarily we use 300 units/kg. Because of the extreme risk associated with failure to give the proper dose or inadequate uptake, an intraoperative procedure for verification of heparin administration should always be used. In Stanford's operating rooms, the surgeon always gives the heparin and the anesthesiologist always verifies that it was given. Approximately 5 minutes after the heparin is given a blood sample is withdrawn through the central venous line and an activated clotting time (ACT) is obtained in the operating room. No heparin is ever added to this line's fluids. This result is plotted, together with the control ACT obtained previously, using the graph shown in Figure 14-5.

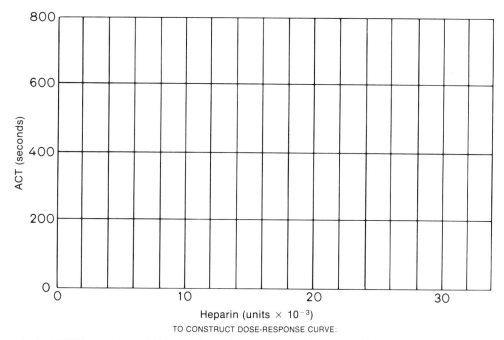

TO CONSTRUCT DOSE-RESPONSE CURVE:

1. Plot ACT before heparin is administered (control value); get sample from non heparinized line.
2. Plot ACT done 3–4 min after administration of pre-bypass heparin dose.
3. Draw line between these 2 points—extrapolate if value is below 450 seconds (ideal for total heparinization during bypass).
4. Additional heparin needed to reach ACT of 450 seconds can be calculated from graph.
5. Do another ACT during bypass—if below 400 seconds, think about adding heparin.
6. Protamine dose needed for complete reversal to control value can be calculated by using protamine/heparin ratio of 1.3 (using ACT done at end of bypass and graph).
7. 1 ml heparin—1000 IU: 1 ml. protamine = 10 mg

Ref: Bull et al: Evaluation of tests used to monitor heparin therapy during extracorporeal circulation. Anesthesiology 43:3436, 1975.

Note: The pump prime contains 4400 units of heparin per liter. The routine patient dose is approximately 300 units per kilogram. If the patient's blood volume is approximately 7% of body weight, the heparin concentrations are roughly equal in blood and prime.

Fig. 14–5. Instruction sheet for calculating heparin dose used at Stanford.

While the ACT dose response curve is non-linear, over this range a linear approximation is reasonable, and this simple graphic technique assures rapid calculation of the dose of additional heparin should it be required. The test should not be performed through the clinical laboratory service because of the unacceptable delay in reporting the result.

The same curve may be used to estimate additional heparin requirements with prolonged bypass. The ACT is performed at appropriate intervals, usually every ½ to 1 hours. When the ACT is too low, below 400 sec, the supplementary dose is estimated from the curve in identical fashion.

At the end of bypass and after protamine reversal, the ACT is measured. The immediate prereversal and postreversal ACTs may be used to construct a dose-response curve. This may also be used to estimate dosage, should additional protamine be required.

An older technique, the titration *in vitro* of protamine dosage by serial dilution at the end of bypass was once relatively popular but has fallen into disuse. There appear to be several reasons for this. The technique is tedious and requires more time and attention than the ACT. The result gives the instantaneous balance required, neglecting the fact that heparin and protamine clear from the serum at different rates. Thus, an arbitrary factor must be used to estimate the additional protamine required, or the titration must be repeated at intervals dependent on when and how fast the protamine is administered. And in the control sense the technique is not as effective because it measures an intermediate (or anticipated) rather than final (or actual) result. Automated protamine titration is available, reducing the professional time required, but the objections of accuracy and control stability remain and the device is quite expensive.

Control of anticoagulation by the ACT has proven markedly superior to control by formula, with heparin and protamine dosage based solely on patient weight and time on bypass.[110] In a recent study, it was noted that the use of the ACT in contrast to the standard heparin-protamine protocol reduced postoperative blood loss by 48 percent.[111] The protective benefit does not relate solely to balanced reversal. An inadequately prolonged clotting time can lead to significant depletion of clotting factors without gross clot in the surgical field or oxygenator. Excessive heparinization has been associated with histologic evidence of pulmonary injury in membrane oxygenator studies. Yet it is clear that this method of anticoagulant monitoring is crude and we expect better techniques to be developed.

CANNULATION

After heparinization of the patient, the surgeon proceeds with cannulation. In the early days of cardiopulmonary bypass, it was customary to cannulate the femoral vein and artery to establish control before entering the mediastinum. In recent years, it has become common practice to cannulate through the right atrium after sternotomy, threading cannulae into the superior and inferior venae cavae. This technique results in lower postoperative morbidity and eliminates one surgical incision. Many surgeons put tapes around the superior and inferior vena cavae so that no blood can leak past the cannulae into the right atrium. However, at Stanford, tapes are not placed unless the right heart will be entered; this appears to have the advantage of permitting the cannulae to accept blood entering the right heart by other routes, avoiding cardiac distention. Capture of this additional return would also appear to assist in cooling the heart. Return to the patient from the oxygenator is accomplished by placing a cannula in the ascending aorta. A reported complication is dissection caused by failure to place the tip of the cannula in the true lumen of the aorta. With modern surgical techniques and experience this is now an unlikely event.

GOING ON BYPASS

A checklist for going on cardiopulmonary bypass is shown in Table 14-3. Flow is started slowly, coming up to full flow over a period of 30 seconds to 3 minutes. The ventilator is turned off. At this time, the anesthesiologist should turn off all drips containing drugs required for prebypass pharmacologic support, and reduce fluid infusion to "keep-open" status. The surgeon may want the patient tilted slightly into the head-up position, in order to level the chest so that cooling fluids surrounding the heart will not be lost. This should be accomplished by raising the back rather than by lifting the entire table because making the legs dependent increases the static pressure across the leg vessels, decreasing flow resistance. Because flow on cardiopulmanary bypass is always kept as low as possible, it is desirable to encourage preferential perfusion of the viscera and brain.

The patient response to beginning bypass is determined by the perfusate. Because no anesthetic drug is present in the perfusate initially, the patient may respond unless a supplemental dose of anesthetic and muscle relaxant is given several minutes before starting. Because there has been no circulation through the pump immediately before bypass, flow during the first few seconds has a low oxygen content, stimulating vasodilation and increasing the probability of a transient hypotensive episode. The lowered hematocrit of the perfusate, with its attendant drop in viscosity, means that the flow through the vascular bed will be higher before peripheral resistance has an opportunity to adapt, also increasing the probability of initial hypotension.[112] Giving potent vasopressors at this stage is undesirable if it can be avoided because vasoconstriction sufficient to raise perfusion pressure will preferentially include the kidneys, one of the organs in which it is essential to maintain perfusion. In some cases, it may be necessary to increase flow transiently, but with experience this is rarely necessary. Mannitol added to the prime may be associated with an accentuated hypotensive dip, and can instead be added after bypass pressures have stabilized.[113]

The first few minutes of bypass are a dangerous time because conditions are rapidly changing. If any deficiencies exist, they can

Table 14-3. Check List: Going on Bypass

Anticoagulation	Heparin given ACT
Positioning	Legs level or up
	Chest up
Ventilation	Inhalation agents off, O_2 on, PEEP 1–2 cm H_2O
	Ventilator off
Fluids	Drips—keep open rate only
	Cardioplegia solution ready, if used
	Empty urine collector
Drugs	Drips initially off (as nitro-prusside, isoproterenol, dopamine, dobutamine, lidocaine)
	Bolus of anesthetics just before bolus of muscle relaxant
	Set bypass vaporizer, if used
Immediate Checks	Blood color, then blood gas ACT systemic arterial pressure

rapidly produce serious patient injury. Thus the anesthesiologist must be confident that the ACT is adequately prolonged or take steps to correct it. An arterial blood gas should be drawn approximately 5 to 7 minutes after going on bypass, long enough to ensure that equilibrium values with the bypass unit have been achieved, soon enough to detect significant problems before patient injury. *All* monitored variables and anesthetic equipment should then be systematically reviewed, and appropriate settings verified. Use the monitors' alarms!

CARDIOPULMONARY BYPASS

A typical schema of surgical activities during cardiopulmonary bypass is presented in Figure 14–6. Bypass may be initiated well before opening the heart if cardiac support is necessary to complete cardiac exposure. Typically, as in coronary artery bypass grafting, the aortic cross-clamp is applied and the heart is fibrillated shortly after going on bypass. If local cooling is employed, the heart is allowed to warm and perfuse passively after the aortic cross-clamp is removed before defibrillation is attempted. An additional period, which I call the "idling time," is usually allowed to elapse between defibrillation and

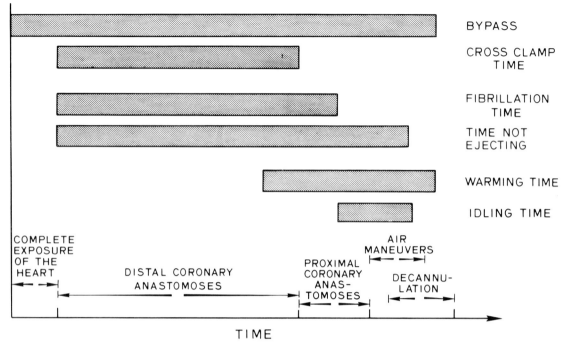

Fig. 14–6. Surgical activities during cardiopulmonary bypass for coronary artery bypass.

discontinuation of cardiopulmonary bypass. Doing the distal grafts first increases the idling time, and appears to enhance recovery from bypass.

SURGICAL TECHNIQUES

Left ventricular venting is of interest to the anesthesiologist because left ventricular distention can result in seriously compromised myocardial contractility at termination of bypass. Distention is caused by excessive blood collecting in the left ventricle, as a result of aortic insufficiency, thebesian drainage into the left ventricle or atrium, congenital lesions, and drainage from the right heart by coronary sinus drainage or bronchial return through the pulmonary vessels. Injury is caused by three effects: (1) rising intracavitary pressure decreases endocardial flow during coronary perfusion, (2) excessive myocardial stretch results in impaired ability to contract; and (3) with local myocardial cooling, the return of warm blood to the ventricle

decreases the acceptable duration of interrupted coronary artery flow.

Venting through the left ventricle at the apex is the only reliable way to prevent the first two effects; but if aortic insufficiency is not significant, it is not necessary in the majority of cases. Current practice appears to support this view. Miller noted that the majority of surgeons still recommend left ventricular venting but that surgeons performing more than 200 cases per year were less likely to vent than those performing fewer.[114,115] Nonetheless, the majority of the busiest surgeons continue to vent. Venting through the left atrium or pulmonary artery will usually prevent the return of significant quantities of warm blood in patients without aortic insufficiency, and is useful if direct myocardial cooling is employed. Limited venting may be done through the cardioplegia arteriotomy. If a vent is not used, the caval tapes should be left open to allow retrograde flow and drainage into the cardiopulmonary bypass cannulae.[116]

Cardiac cooling is employed to reduce myocardial oxygen demand and increase acceptable cross clamp time. This is accomplished in several ways. The pericardium is opened to form a well, and the heart is continuously bathed in 4°C saline solution during the period of ischemia. When aortic cross-clamping is initiated, the aortic root is perfused with cold solution to improve endocardial cooling. When possible, the interior of the heart is also lavaged with cold solution. The rationale and details of this technique and alternatives are discussed in Chapter 26.

PERFUSION FLOWS AND PRESSURES

Considerable controversy exists about the appropriate range of perfusion flows and pressures. A survey conducted in 1975 by Garman[117] indicated that, of 19 centers polled, the preferred flows varied from 1.2 to 3.5 l/min/m^2 of body surface. The rationale for high flow is based on the presumption that normal resting cardiac output is an indicator of necessary perfusion. Proponents of low flow recognize that injury to the blood increases with each passage through the oxygenator and presume reduced cummulative injury with lower flow for the same time on bypass.

A similar controversy centers around acceptable perfusion pressures. Some feel that pressures as high as 80 torr are necessary to assure adequate cerebral and renal perfusion. It has been claimed that urine output effectively ceases below a mean blood pressure of 60 torr. This is obviously untrue at Stanford, where mean blood pressure often falls to 30 torr, but many patients make significant quantities of urine. Continued urine output is more common with mannitol in the perfusate. Available data indicates that below approximately 30 torr, critical opening pressures in the capillaries may not be achieved. This implies 30 torr may be the minimum acceptable pressure. However, experimental data to support this assertion is still incomplete.

Controversy also exists as to whether pressors are appropriate. Some use pressors to maintain a mean pressure as high as 80 torr; others are reluctant to use them at all, because renal blood flow is one of the first components affected.

Several years ago Stockard proposed a perfusion index which was the product of torr less than 50, and minutes at that pressure, and suggested that when this index exceeded 50 to 100 torr-minutes, serious injury to the patient was much more likely to result.[118] At Stanford, where flows are typically 1.6 l/min/m^2, a prospective study of 204 consecutive patients divided into equal groups (with the dividing line the median of 560 torr-minutes perfusion) demonstrated no significant difference in neurologic dysfunction.[119] This occurred despite the fact that a number of patients satisfied the proposed index for injury. It should be noted that vasopressors were only rarely used.

With low flow perfusion on cardiopulmonary bypass and no administration of pressors, pressures will commonly fall initially to 30 to 40 torr then rise gradually throughout bypass. This rise may be associated with a rise in serum catecholamines. At Stanford, pressure above 60 to 70 torr is reduced with a vasodilator to ensure a reasonable distribution of blood flow, and to avoid excessive return of blood to the heart.

Urine output can be a useful estimate of perfusion during bypass, but low output does not clearly indicate renal injury. If the advantages of low flow in facilitating surgical intervention appear to outweigh the inability to maintain urine output, the anesthesiologist should not blindly resist.

Low flow can confer another advantage. Forming a well with the pericardium and bathing the heart in 4°C saline provides significant metabolic protection while maintaining body temperatures above 30°C so that clotting factors are less likely to be impaired. However, as Conti has noted, when using a flow of 2.2 l/min/m^2 and above, the cardiac temperature may not be maintainable at a low value because of warming by coronary collateral flow to the myocardium.[120] Thus the selection of pressure and flow criteria, and the approach to venting may have significant effects on the efficacy of the cooling technique employed.

PULSATILE FLOW

At the present time, flow during cardiopulmonary bypass in most centers is not pulsatile. However, arguments for adding pulsation are increasing. The issue seems to be whether adequate benefits offset the added effort and complexity.[121, 122]

The first known quantitative study of the effects of pulsatile perfusion was performed by Hooker in 1910.[123] He built an oxygenator and perfusion system to study the performance of the isolated kidney. He concluded that, with a constant mean perfusion pressure, urine formation and blood flow through the kidney varied directly with the pulse pressure, and the amount of protein in the urine varied inversely with the pulse pressure. Gesell reported the same results 2 years later, but the first animal perfusion systems were nonpulsatile, presumably because of technical difficulties.[124]

Then in 1951 and 1952, several investigators attempted to duplicate these results and failed, reporting no difference with pulsatile flow.[125, 126] By the time Wesolowski's study in 1955 had been widely reviewed, interest in pulsatile flow had markedly diminished. In 2-hour and 6-hour perfusions in animals, he noted that in comparing nonpulsatile and pulsatile flows, mean blood pressure, pump minute flow, and blood volume remained constant. Neither the rate of recovery postoperatively nor the function of crucial organs was significantly different from control to pulsatile flow.[127] It appears that concerned clinicians concluded from these data that while pulsatile flow did offer some advantages, they were not significant for the perfusion times usually employed.

However, a number of studies suggest that this conclusion is not correct. A series of reports published more than 10 years later documented the fall in urine output with decreased pulse pressure,[128] also showing increased vascular resistance,[129] decreased creatinine clearance and increased levels of lactic acid,[130] and histologic evidence of pathologic changes in renal structure.[131] Other reports from the 1960s included evidence of progressive slowing of flow and finally stasis at the capillary level,[132] increased blood levels of lactate, pyruvate and the ratio of lactate to pyruvate,[133] tissue edema,[134] and ischemic changes in the central nervous system.[135]

It has been suggested that these conflicting reports can be reconciled by reference to experimental differences.[136] Those reporting no benefit from pulsatile flow employed pulse pressures of a different contour. Pressure fell as rapidly as it rose, leaving little time for perfusion during the period of elevation. When a more physiologic contour was employed, differences were reported. In practical terms, pulsatile pressure and flow are not the same. Pulsatile pressure of such short duration as to result in steady flow appears to produce little benefit.

There are many proposed mechanisms by which pulsatile flow may improve perfusion. The shaking present at the cellular level may assist in diffusion of metabolites between capillary and tissue. Lymph and interstitial fluid movement is enhanced, increasing transport. Pulsatile flow appears more effective in reopening capillaries which open and close in cyclic fashion during normal perfusion. And the rise in systemic vascular resistance with nonpulsatile flow may be baroreceptor mediated, reducing flow inappropriately. All of these mechanisms appear valid.[137]

The previous discussion has centered on the advantages of pulsatile flow in supporting body tissue. The effect on the heart is more complex. During fibrillation, the results have been equivocal. Perhaps because of the metabolic responsiveness of coronary autoregulation, pulsatile benefit has been difficult to demonstrate at higher flows. However, Steed demonstrated enhanced endocardial perfusion during fibrillation when autoregulation was inhibited.[138] In the beating heart, it appears that muscular contraction is more important than pulsatile pressure in the aortic root, so long as mean pressure is adequate. Thus the heart is likely to benefit from pulsatile bypass only during fibrillation.

Recent clinical studies suggest that pulsatile flow may also confer patient benefit during typical bypass procedures. Maddoux noted that in a series of 40 patients the ejection fraction decreased from 52 to 39 percent with nonpulsatile perfusion, but increased from 51 to 62 percent with pulsatile perfusion during the first postoperative day. In a series of 235 patients, he found that the incidence of intraoperative infarction was reduced in the series with pulsatile flow (p < .05).[139] Pappas also found that the ejection fraction increased with pulsatile flow, but decreased with nonpulsatile flow in the postoperative period.[140] Bregman noted a significant increase in urine output during bypass.[141] And Taylor noted that normal cortisol levels are maintained with pulsatile flow, but fall markedly with nonpulsatile flow during bypass.[142] It would appear that as the technical problems associated with generating pulsatile flow become more tractable, it will be employed more frequently.

Recent clinical interest does appear to be related to technical considerations. Much of the work done in the 1960s used artificial heart apparatus[143] or specially constructed equipment.[144] More recently, the widespread acceptance of the intraaortic balloon has made suitable equipment clinically available and at least one manufacturer has made a special adapter specifically for use during bypass (in which the balloon is in the bypass system, removing the need for further surgical insult to the patient).[145, 146] Variations on these themes continue to appear.[147] See also Chapter 27.

ELECTROLYTES

Electrolyte shifts also occur during bypass. Progressive hypokalemia is well documented,[148–151] and has been suggested to result from hemodilution, urinary loss, and intracellular shift of potassium. This problem can clearly be exacerbated by preoperative hypokalemia caused by diuretic therapy. In one study of patients without significant urine output, muscle biopsies were performed and have demonstrated that intracellular potassium falls as well.[152] However, this may be a problem of interpretation; intracellular stores are much larger than serum stores, and the decrease is in the range of experimental error. Balancing the pump prime solution to physiologic values does not significantly reduce the fall in serum levels. It seems clear that potassium is sequestered, almost certainly intracellularly, but the mechanism remains to be elucidated. However, intrabypass potassium replacement must be provided. Typical amounts are 20 to 60 mEq, in order to assure normal serum values and myocardial stability in the immediate postbypass period. Hyperkalemia should be avoided. The well-known rhythm disturbances may be preceded by tachycardia, increasing myocardial oxygen consumption.[153]

Recently it has been noted that both calcium and magnesium ions are depleted unless the pump prime contain physiologic concentrations.[154, 155] Administration of proteins as fresh frozen plasma or particularly salt-poor albumin can also bind calcium and magnesium. If acidosis corrected with alkalinizing agents occurs, additional calcium may be required even though the correction of acidosis is complete.[156] Some anesthesiologists add calcium to remove dependence on citrate metabolism for a blood prime.[157]

Because calcium is the common pathway for all inotropic effects on the heart, this can be of considerable concern in weaning from cardiopulmonary bypass (see Chapter 3). Many clinicians now give 1 g or more of calcium chloride near the end of cardiopulmonary bypass to assure adequate blood levels, an inappropriate therapy with a hyperdynamic heart. Controversy exists as to whether hyopcalcemia during bypass is undesirable; many feel it is not because it helps reduce myocardial oxygen consumption.[158]

The magnesium ion has received less attention. However, an increased incidence in sudden death associated with low magnesium in community water supplies has been reported,[159] and several authors have suggested that hypomagnesemia may relate to an increased incidence of spontaneous ventricular fibrillation and difficulties in defibrillation at the end of bypass.[160, 161] One paper reported three patients in which ventricular fibrillation was not resolved until shock was preceded by administration of magnesium sulfate.[162] Magnesium is involved in all the enzymes associated with metabolism of adenosine triphosphate (ATP), and would appear to be essential, as is calcium, to normal myocardial inotropic response.[163] It appears advisable to add magnesium to the pump prime. If body stores are normal, some suggest that raising the prime to physiologic levels is adequate.[164] We suggest 10 to 20 mEq. Some investigators feel that a *majority* of normal subjects may have a dietary magnesium deficiency;[165] diuretic therapy can also produce magnesium deficiency.[166] If body depletion is suspected, it is appropriate to give additional magnesium.

VENTILATION

The majority of cardiac anesthesiologists, according to the survey cited above,[167] do not ventilate during total bypass. However, the majority do apply a few centimeters of positive end expiratory pressure (PEEP) in order to assure apneic oxygenation. As a general rule, whenever the left heart begins ejecting, implying that blood flow through the lungs has resumed, ventilation should also be resumed.

TEMPERATURE

Management of patient temperature is discussed in the chapter on myocardial preservation and hypothermia. We commonly cool (rectal) to 30 to 31°C, and warm to terminate bypass at 34 to 36°C. Many centers cool to 26 to 27°C, in practice associated with greater bypass flows which reduce the effectiveness of myocardial cooling.

ENDING CARDIOPULMONARY BYPASS

Ending cardiopulmonary bypass transiently increases patient risk because it is a time of change. In addition, the heart and lungs must resume function after physiologic injury. The transfer may be divided into three categories: preparation, transition, and post-transition evaluation and support. We shall concentrate our attention on the events leading up to the termination of bypass; the reader is referred to the following chapter for a discussion of post-bypass management.

Preparation for ending bypass is a dual concept; assuring both the required information and resources for adequately monitored management are at hand. The critical factors are summarized in Table 14–4 and briefly discussed in the following sections.

TEMPERATURE

Rewarming should continue until the rectal temperature has returned to a minimum of 35°C. A lower temperature indicates that the low blood flow areas of the body (*vessel-poor group*) are not yet warm enough, and gradually will release cold blood into the circulation as these areas thermally equilibrate after bypass. Nasopharyngeal temperature is measured in an area of high blood flow (posterior nasal turbinates); it represents the best measurement of blood temperature as received from the extracorporeal system, and is also a good estimate of blood temperature to the brain. It should be normal before bypass is discontinued.

Post-bypass, all blood, blood products, and intravenous fluids will need to be warmed to approximately 37°C, to assist in the last stage of warming. If necessary, a warming blanket can be used to help maintain patient temperature, but warming must not involve excessive thermal gradients between the patient and the heat source.

LABORATORY VALUES

In addition to urinary loss, serum potassium decreases in a roughly linear fashion with time on bypass, and must be checked near the end to assure normal values during weaning. The well-recognized syndrome of intracellular depletion, associated with chronic diuretic therapy, suggests a desirable serum value near the upper limits of normal. Calcium should be checked if abnormalities are suspected. The causes are predictable, and many do not order this test routinely, once typical clinical patterns have been documented. Ionized calcium is the active agent, but total calcium is helpful and may be more easily obtained.

As the patient warms, the oxygen transport capacity of the red cell becomes more important. We feel that the packed cell volume should be above 23 percent at termination of bypass, and adjust infusions during bypass accordingly.

We do not recommend routinely sampling arterial gas tensions at the end of bypass because the vast majority of problems develop early and should have been detected from an earlier sample. But, if difficulty in management of gas tensions is experienced, additional determinations should be made. Venous tension is also useful to assess oxygen extraction. Weaning is difficult and dangerous if the oxygen tension and pH are not within normal limits.

CALIBRATION OF MONITORS

While a seemingly obvious step, calibration is often overlooked. Accurate quantitative information is essential for safe and rapid weaning; this step should never be omitted.

DRUGS AND FLUIDS

Ideally, all myocardial depressants should be avoided during this period. Even modest depression can compromise the transition because of the increased stress and changing physiologic state. Halothane or other inhalation agents should be discontinued well in advance of termination if a vaporizer is employed on the bypass unit. None should be given by the pulmonary route. Halothane may also contribute to arrhythmias. Even the modest depressant effects of small doses of thiopental can be transiently evident if administered shortly before or during weaning.

Essential drugs should be checked, or drawn up and labelled. Syringes can be in-

Table 14-4. Early Preparations for Ending Bypass

Data
 Temperature
  Rectal $\geq 35°C$
  Nasopharyngeal $\geq 36.5°C$
  Infusion warmer(s) functioning properly
 Laboratory
  K ≥ 4.5
  Ca ≥ 9.5
  PCV $\geq 23\%$
  ACT: checked (if indicated)
  Arterial blood gas tensions: checked (if indicated)
 Equipment
  Monitors calibrated (*zero* and *gain*)
Responses
 Drugs
  Discontinue cardiac depressants (*e.g.*, halothane, thiopental)
  Vasoactive agents available
  Anticipated infusions prepared (*e.g.*, dopamine, isoproterenol, nitroprusside, dobutamine, lidocaine)
  Protamine dose prepared and checked
 Volume
  Sufficient blood and crystalloid available
  Coagulation products ready (if need anticipated)
 Equipment
  Special equipment ready (*e.g.*, intraaortic balloon)

terchanged; protamine should be kept in a separate spot. Potent infusions should be prepared ahead of time, to reduce the opportunity for errors in content or dilution because of other distractions. The most important drugs and dosages are always checked by two individuals, typically the anesthesiologist and the circulating nurse.

If coagulation products are required, preparation and transmit time from the blood bank should be anticipated. Even the availability of infusion fluids should be verified; if matters go awry the circulating nurse may not be available during a critical period.

OTHER PREPARATIONS

Any specialized equipment should be checked if possible. Uncommon devices, as the intraaortic balloon (IAB) pump may not otherwise be ready when needed, and these requirements should be carefully reviewed with the responsible parties. If the decision to use an IAB is made early, early preparation both speeds the procedure and permits pulsation during bypass; improving urine output and the rate of warming.

VENTILATION

Insufflation of the lungs toward the end of bypass accomplishes two goals. First, the removal of trapped intravascular air is aided by ventilation and Valsalva maneuvers. Second, any blood passing through the lungs from the vena cavae will enhance oxygenation and carbon dioxide removal. Little is gained by ventilating the lungs if the heart is empty, even if beating; the lungs should be left quiet to facilitate surgery. The lungs should be ventilated with an appropriate tidal volume and rate if the arterial pressure tracing indicates that the aortic valve is opening.

The pleural spaces should not contain fluid or blood. Direct inspection is most effective. If the lungs seem unusually full on direct inspection, or a free lung in an open pleural space is situated higher (ventral) in the chest upon adequate exhalation, or a confined lung (closed pleural space) appears less compliant than prebypass, trapped fluid or air should be suspected. Surgical evacuation of trapped air, fluid, or blood is mandatory. The absence of cold fluids in the pleural spaces also permits more efficient warming of the patient.

Arterial blood gases should be evaluated toward the end of bypass if abnormalities of oxygenation, carbon dioxide removal, or acid-base status are suspected, and appropriate correction accomplished. Ventilation should now be stable, at a level suitable for maintenance after ending bypass.

THE HEART AND SYSTEMIC PERFUSION

Resuming cardiac support of the circulation begins with removal of the aortic cross-clamp. The heart is first passively perfused, until it is warm enough to support coordinated contraction. One can often observe the sequence of quiescence, fine-slow and finally coarse-fast fibrillation, occasionally with spontaneous defibrillation in the healthier heart. If a circus rhythm occurs, it is an indication that the heart is warm enough to permit successful defibrillation. *Look* at the heart!

Active cardiac contraction improves coronary blood flow, even in the absence of ejection. This idling time from defibrillation to ending bypass is essential to permit washout of air and ischemic byproducts. The aortic root pressure is permitted to rise during this time to facilitate washout, unless ventricular distention is a problem.

A preliminary evaluation of contractility can be obtained by direct observation of the heart: contraction is uniform throughout the ventricles, "snappy," and at an adequate rate, typically above 80 beats per minute. The monitors provide little assistance at this stage because pulmonary flow will remain low until filling pressures are returned to normal by returning perfusate from the bypass reservoir.

Before transferring circulatory support to the heart, all air must be removed. Surgical venting of the aortic root, if the left heart or aorta are opened, and of bypass grafts, is standard practice. The heart is often lifted and massaged to encourage passage of air through the chambers. Significant coronary air embolism is often easy to demonstrate: contraction is not uniform, there is discoloration of the flaccid areas, and air can sometimes be observed passing through the larger vessels. If severe, the washout can be hastened by transient elevation of the arterial pressure, as with 200 μg of neosynephrine administered intravenously. Remember that once active cardiac ejection begins, any air still present may be carried to the brain. The origin of the cephalic vessels at the aortic root must be kept below the venting site(s) by keeping the operating table tilted head-down until the surgeon is satisfied that removal is complete.

Cardiac rate and rhythm should also be evaluated during the idling time. While arrhythmias may appear shortly after defibrillation, they should have diminished substantially or disappeared by the end of bypass if cardiac recovery is adequate. Possible causes of continued arrhythmias include inadequate potassium replacement, hypomagnesemia, myocardial edema (particularly associated with valvular surgery), and escape beats associated with a low heart rate.

However, the primary cause of premature ventricular contractions after adequate washout, with a normal serum potassium, is continued myocardial ischemia. Another indicator is persistent S-T segment elevation or depression, which usually returns the majority of the distance to baseline within 15 to 45 minutes after removal of the aortic cross-clamp. Typically it is easy to corroborate this diagnosis by direct observation, but occasionally the conduction pathways are the primary area of dysfunction, and contractility will appear adequate. If it is possible to wean the patient from bypass, it should always be possible to produce effective cardiac contraction at this stage because myocardial oxygen consumption is below the minimum required to sustain systemic perfusion.

After perfusion time for myocardial recovery has been allowed, usually 15 to 30 minutes of idling time after defibrillation with a cross-clamp time of an hour, the final process of developing adequate cardiac output while maintaining myocardial function is initiated. Increments of blood are transferred to the patient from the oxygenator reservoir, while observing the heart and arterial pressure waveform. A heart with good mechanical function will increase contractility with increasing end diastolic pressure, increasing arterial pulse pressure, and cardiac output. The increased contractility is evident both in the snap of the contracting ventricle, and the rate of rise of arterial pressure with each systole.

Appropriate filling pressures are dependent on the specific situation, but a number of useful general rules can be stated. Because of the recent period of myocardial ischemia, myocardial edema reduces ventricular compliance, and ideal filling pressures are always higher than those appropriate later. At Stanford, the use of left atrial catheters is extremely rare, and pulmonary artery catheters are not ordinarily used unless there is evidence of right heart or pulmonary decompensation. In the more usual situation, the

central venous pressure is monitored, with values at termination of bypass in the range of 12 to 16 torr.

Direct observation of the heart is a useful adjunct during the critical period. Experienced observers agree on the appearance of a full or empty heart, and this result can then be correlated with the value of central venous pressure in an individual patient. This is not a frivolous activity; careful studies in large animals have demonstrated the difficulty of achieving accurate measurement in the low pressure systems. Even agreeing on the reference level for measurement can be difficult in some patients, and direct observation of the heart can appreciably improve the determination of appropriate filling pressures in the individual patient.

Further, visual observation of the heart is not a rejection of the concept of quantitative measurement. Strict evaluation of contractility requires both measurement of dp/dt (only partially assessed by monitoring arterial pressure), and heart size. Direct observation permits integrating these data to estimate myocardial contractile element velocity directly.

With resumption of cardiac output, aortic root pressure should always be returned to normal values (in the range of 70–85 torr mean). Initially the anesthesiologist must establish adequate filling pressure, then control aortic root pressure with a vasodilator if necessary. If the aortic root pressure is low, attention must be given to myocardial contractility. Sustained use of a vasopressor at this stage is normally contraindicated.

As previously mentioned, the heart rate should usually be in the range of 80 to 100 beats/minute. Lower rates usually result in an inadequate output, and increase the incidence of arrhythmias. Higher rates are associated with increased myocardial oxygen consumption, without a matching increase in output, unless stroke volume is small and cannot be adequately increased. Heart block is common in patients undergoing valve surgery, and most centers routinely place pacemaker leads in these patients. Block from this cause usually appears a minimum of several hours after ending bypass, but within the first 1 to 3 days, and is often temporary. Atrial fibrillation should never be tolerated unless chronic atrial fibrillation existed preoperatively or repeated shocks are ineffective because the negative effect on cardiac output can be large.

A failing heart can prove to be exquisitely difficult to manage if adequately applied routine measures are ineffective. More often, a required step has been compromised or overlooked. Some common approaches to exceptions follow, but virtually every conceivable mode of failure has been encountered, and should be considered when the more obvious approaches fail.

If the underlying disease is not surgically correctable, such as extensive muscle loss secondary to chronic ischemia or severely compromised coronary perfusion not susceptible to surgical correction, only marginal improvement may be possible acutely. In such cases, inotropic support is mandatory to prevent cardiac distention while increasing output to an acceptable level; however, the concomitant increase in oxygen demand must be carefully considered (see Chap. 2).

Low-dose inotropic agents may be quite useful in the unstable patient, only modestly increasing oxygen consumption while improving minimum performance. Higher dosages should be employed only if there is evident improvement, such as increased cardiac output or diminished cardiac size. In rare cases, a vasopressor may adequately improve cardiac perfusion during this period, particularly if there is good reason to presume that cardiac output cannot be significantly increased. Calcium is a necessary adjunct to inotropic agents, and may be deliberately elevated (though doses above 3 g of $CaCl_2$ are difficult to justify). Acidosis substantially reduces inotropic response and must be corrected. The anesthesiologist must be confident that he can distinguish between the transient acidosis associated with washout after a period of ischemia, and continuing acidosis—signifying an unrecognized condition which must be corrected before bypass can be safely ended.

When a persistent arrhythmia results in inadequate function, and appears clearly associated with ischemia (such as an increased incidence when myocardial work is increased), occasionally magnesium sulfate (9–18 mEq or 2–4 ml of 50% solution) can produce a dramatic improvement. As previously noted, the use of magnesium supplements during bypass produced a statistically significant decrease in the number of shocks required for effective defibrillation and may resolve episodes of intractable fibrillation.

Except for mild forms of ventricular outflow obstruction and mild valvular regurgitation, valvular abnormalities during weaning are usually obvious to the skilled anesthesiologist and surgeon. Direct palpation of the atrium as well as the presence of V waves on the occluded pulmonary artery (wedge) or left atrial pressure tracings will demonstrate mitral insufficiency. Aortic insufficiency will most commonly be evident by a wide pulse pressure on the arterial pressure waveform, with a low diastolic arterial pressure. The left ventricle will rapidly distend in diastole (especially with low filling pressures), and the surgeon may palpate a diastolic thrill at the left ventricular apex. If a left ventricular vent is in place and the left atrium is empty, the most obvious origin for a large amount of blood flowing through the vent is a regurgitant aortic valve. While acute post-bypass tricuspid insufficiency is common, it is rarely of clinical significance.

Valvular stenosis must be suspected whenever ventricular filling or emptying is impaired. Direct pressure measurement across the suspected stenotic area is the only way to precisely determine the nature and extent of obstructive valvular lesions. Obviously, significant valvular defects require surgical correction before ending bypass.

Finally, one must base expectations for performance on the nature of the lesion. A seeming paradox is that the sicker patient may demonstrate greater improvement on ending bypass. If a patient is severely compromised before surgery, such as when there is severe valvular inadequacy or coronary insufficiency at rest, surgery may provide immediate functional improvement. But if the patient is undergoing coronary artery bypass for ischemia occurring only with exercise, the primary immediate effect is intraoperative ischemia, and the heart will be transiently compromised. This does not mean that an untoward event has occurred.

If the preparations summarized in Table 14–5 for ending bypass are adequate and assessment is accurate, termination is rapid and simple. Flow is reduced over 15 to 45 seconds to zero, with intermediate supplementation of fluid from the pump as necessary to maintain previously established filling pressures. The heart will easily assume the work load, and bypass is safely terminated.

However, if the heart begins to fail during termination or immediately afterward, particularly if distention (on *direct* observation) occurs, bypass must be immediately resumed. The injury associated with acute myocardial distention can be severe, and can occur with surprising rapidity. Once injured, no immediate remedy is available, and the chance of subsequent successful termination is substantially reduced.

Weaning from bypass should not be attempted until adequate reperfusion time has been allowed; the resulting post-bypass course is obviously improved. Termination should not be attempted during persistent signs of ischemia, unless all alternatives have been eliminated. Examples of particular concern are impaired contractility in a patient with coronary artery disease showing no other cardiac abnormality, sudden and unexplained hypotension during attempts to discontinue bypass, and occurrence of supraventricular arrhythmias.

COMPLICATIONS

The list of possible complications is almost overwhelming. Mortenson and coworkers, in a study funded by the Food and Drug Administration, reviewed the world literature and reported on the findings of nearly 400 published reports.[166, 167] Their summary of the most common complications along with estimates of frequency, severity, and possible

Table 14-5. Ending Bypass

Ventilation
  Establish
  Set appropriate values
  Evacuate air/fluid from pleural cavities
Heart
  Early
    Remove cross-clamp
    Defibrillate after adequate warming
    Air maneuvers
    Observe rate, rhythm
  Volume Loading (repeat previous steps as necessary when subsequent step alters them)
    Add incrementally to adequate filling pressures
    Observe
      arterial waveform (increased pulse pressure and rise rate)
      heart (uniform contraction; neither empty nor distended)
      rate and rhythm
    Establish appropriate filling pressure
    Establish appropriate aortic root pressure
    Review ventilator setting
    Assess cardiac output
    Adjust vascular resistance as necessary
    Add inotropic support if indicated
  Weaning
    Reduce bypass flow over 15–45 seconds
    Transfuse from oxygenator as necessary to maintain filling pressures
    Return to bypass with
      progressive distention
      progressive dysfunction (as arrhythmias)
Observe the effects of each intervention, adjusting one variable at a time.

value of device standards is shown in Table 14–6. It is apparent that in the vast majority of situations an oxygenator cannot be designed so that it can operate safely and reliably without significant user skill. This study documents the reason for the move away from early oxygenator designs with redundant fail-safe instrumentation and monitoring systems. The remainder of the discussion will concentrate on physiologic mechanisms accessible to control by the medical professional.

BLOOD TRAUMA

Significant trauma to blood occurs with the bubble oxygenator during relatively short perfusion times.[170] A typical sequence was reported by Galletti in 1962 noting initial thrombocytopenia and leukopenia.[171] Later, he noted increased mechanical fragility of red

Table 14-6. Clinical Problems in Safety and Efficacy Observed During Use of Blood Oxygenators, Subjectively Rated as to Frequency, Seriousness, and Amenability to Correction by Standards (+ = minimal or least; + + + + = maximal or most)

MECHANICAL FAILURES/ERRORS IN OXYGENATOR OR ITS CONNECTIONS

	FREQUENCY	SERIOUSNESS	AMENABILITY TO CORRECTION BY STANDARDS
Leaks or disruptions			
Gas lines, connections, containers	+	+ +	+ +
Blood lines, connections, containers	+ +	+ +	+ +
Heat exchanger water lines, connections, containers	+ + +	+ + +	+ + +
Membranes, reservoirs	+ + +	+ + +	+ + +
Obstructions (Resulting in impaired flow or increased pressure)			
Gas lines	+ + +	+ + +	+ + +
Blood lines	+	+	+ + +
Heat exchanger water or blood lines	+ +	+ + +	+ + +
Excessive foaming	+ + +	+ +	+
Water loss from blood			
Into oxygenator spaces or membranes	+ +	+	+ +
Into effluent gases	+ +	+	+ +
Water transfer to blood			
From gases	+ + +	+ + +	+ + +
From heat exchange	+ + +	+ + +	+ + +
Migration or slippage of membranes	+ + +	+ + +	+ + + +
Errors in assembly and operation	+ + +	+ + + +	+ + +

CONTAMINATION OF BLOOD AT BLOOD OXYGENATOR INTERFACES

	FREQUENCY	SERIOUSNESS	AMENABILITY TO CORRECTION BY STANDARDS
Viable contaminants (bacteria, fungi, yeasts, viruses)	+ +	+ + + +	+ +
Chemical contaminants	+ +	+ +	+ + +
Toxic eluants			
Sterilizing agents	+	+ +	+ + +
Anesthetic gases	+	+	+ +
Surface contaminants	+ +	+ +	+ + +
Sodium Chloride	+ +	+ +	+ + +
Antifoam Leached toxicants	+	+ +	+ + +
Pyrogens	+ +	+ +	+ + +
Particulate debris	+ + + +	+ + +	+ + +

ALTERATIONS IN BLOOD FLOWING THROUGH OXYGENATOR

	FREQUENCY	SERIOUSNESS	AMENABILITY TO CORRECTION BY STANDARDS
Hemolysis of RBC	+ + +	−	+ +
Destruction of platelets	+ + +	+ +	+ + +
Alteration of platelet function	+ + +	+ +	+ + +
Destruction of WBC	+ + +	+	+ + +
Reduced phagocytosis	+ +	+ +	+ +
Changes in blood viscosity	+ + +		+ +
Formation of fibrin	+ + +	+ +	+ +
Loss of fibrinogen	+ + +	+ +	+ + +
Denaturation of serum proteins	+ + + +	+	+
Thrombosis (impaired gas transfer, obstruction to flow emboli)	+ +	+ + +	+ +
Introduction of air bubbles (micro or macro emboli; air lacks)	+ + +		+ + +
Changes in blood pH	+ + +	+ + +	+ + +

ALTERATIONS IN PHYSIOLOGIC STATE

	FREQUENCY	SERIOUSNESS	AMENABILITY TO CORRECTION BY STANDARDS
Anemia	+ +	+ +	+ +
Pulmonary parenchymal injury (bypass lungs)	+ +	+ + +	+ + +
Low flow (hemodynamic syndrome)	+ +	+ +	+ +
Systemic arterial hypotension	+ + +		+
Intervascular compartmentalization	+ + + +		
Sludging (impaired capillary flow, increased blood viscosity)	+ + + +	+ +	+ +
Hemorrhage	+ +	+ + +	+ + +
Impaired renal function	+	+ + +	+ + +
Increased peripheral vascular resistance		+ + +	+ + + +
Increased capillary fragility	+ +		+
Sepsis		+ + + +	+ + + +
Impaired renal function			
Unexplained death		+ + +	

IMPROPER GAS TRANSFER FUNCTION

	FREQUENCY	SERIOUSNESS	AMENABILITY TO CORRECTION BY STANDARDS
Erratic or inadequate oxygen transfer	+ + +	+ + +	+ +
Erratic or inadequate carbon dioxide transfer	+ + +	+ + +	+ + +
Exessive CO_2 transfer	+ +	+ + +	+
Introduction of bubbles into patient (micro or macro air emboli)	+	+ + +	+

cells, compensatory leukocytosis with a shift to the left, leveling off of platelet counts, and the appearance of nucleated red blood cells. Damage to the blood can be divided into two categories: damage to the formed or cellular elements and damage to the unformed elements.

Cellular damage appears to be a combination of mechanical trauma and physical interaction with adjacent surfaces. Osmotic fragility is not a useful predictor.[172] It has been demonstrated that red cells can withstand considerably higher shear rates if not exposed to a foreign surface at the same time. A major cause of red cell injury and hemolysis is interaction with foreign surfaces accompanied by high shear. Examples are inadequate roller pump tubing clearance, small cannulae with high shear rates and wall contact at the tips, and materials interaction during the oxygenation process, such as in the early disc oxygenators in which rotation increased the shear rate as well as surface contact. Red cell hemolysis increases with time on bypass, and continues for many hours after bypass.

The reader should be aware of the technical difficulty of measuring red cell injury. The classical approach has been to measure the serum hemoglobin. But, serum hemoglobin is the difference between hemolysis and clearance, not an absolute measure of the rate of hemolysis. Clearance capacity varies from one individual to another. And red cell injury associated with clearance over many hours through the reticuloendothelial system may not result in increased serum hemoglobin.

For example, Coburn has shown that systemic carbon monoxide production is stochiometrically related to hemoglobin clearance.[173] In one well-performed but unpublished study, he examined the rate of hemolysis by this technique after a period of bypass using a properly adjusted roller pump (without oxygenator), and demonstrated elevated red cell clearance for many hours. Serum hemoglobin measurements failed to document post-bypass hemolysis.

Platelet counts fall abruptly on initiation of bypass and usually continue to fall during the first one to two hours. The decrease can persist for several days.[174] Values can increase immediately after bypass is discontinued. Some suggest that this is caused by platelet sequestration with consequent release after bypass.[175] Others suggest that fall is the result of platelet elimination after surface interaction.[176] However, while counts increase following bypass, it has been shown that platelet viability is decreased and effectiveness in supporting clot formation is diminished.[177–179] Platelet decreases may be more moderate with hemodilution.[180] Platelet replacement is not ordinarily necessary.[181]

Labile clotting factors V and VIII are particularly vulnerable to bypass with bubble oxygenation. This appears related to the fact that many of the more labile blood proteins go into surface solution within milliseconds after being exposed to a blood-air interface. Many of these proteins are irreversibly denatured on exposure to such an interface.

The fall in leukocyte count observed during cardiopulmonary bypass appears to be a result of sequestration because the leukocytes are not found in significant numbers within the bypass unit.[182] Most studies of coagulation are conducted in a bulk solution which is not flowing. Studies in recent years, in *in vivo* perfusing systems, suggest that leukocytes play a larger role in the normal coagulation process than is generally appreciated. Thus, the injury to plasma proteins, and diminished function of both leukocytes and platelets has a direct and broad-based effect on coagulation.

Hypothermia negatively affects coagulation. The degree and duration of lower temperatures both appear to diminish coagulation capacity. It would appear, although it has not been documented, that the association of direct air-blood interaction with low temperatures enhances this effect.

A major source of toxic materials and direct blood trauma is the blood returned through the auxiliary suction. While filtration may reduce the embolic complications, trauma to unformed elements is not inhibited, and this source may need to be better controlled.[183]

Other nonspecific factors have been difficult to quantify. It is generally agreed that exposure of blood to a bubble oxygenator results in the release of vasoactive substances which can have profound effects. Whether this is a direct result of blood trauma or a blood trauma-mediated release of vasoactive agents is not known. It is clear, however, that the reaction is blood mediated. In a classic experiment, Dobell in 1965 took blood that had been circulated through a pump oxygenator for a fixed time period and exchange transfused it into a second animal. The blood circulated in the oxygenator for 15 hours; 22 out of 26 animals died within 24 hours, exhibiting progressive acidosis and initial or gradual loss of consciousness. When plasma only was circulated through the pump, mortality remained near 100 percent. The air-fluid interaction appears to be a significant component; when the experiment was repeated with circulation through a membrane oxygenator, mortality decreased to 10 percent.[184]

In a recent study commissioned for the Food and Drug Administration on development of standards for evaluation of blood trauma, it was concluded that the variables which influence the degree of blood trauma included the perfusion time, blood flow rate, gas flow rate, temperature, blood-glucose concentration, clotting time, perfusion pressure, and gas line pressure.[185]

EMBOLI

Emboli can enter the perfusate from a variety of sources. Air can be entrained through leaks or inadequate defoaming. The antifoam coating has been implicated as a source of embolization.[186] Fibrin and fibrin products associated with inadequate anticoagulation or unusual blood materials interactions can be observed. Platelet and white blood cell aggregates have been reported in significant numbers[187] and can be increased by foaming.[188] Fat embolism was reported early,[189] presumably in association with the cardiotomy suction or other contaminants. In the mid1970s it was noted that particulate embolization from the materials comprising the oxygenator was also a significant source of contamination.[190] Studies demonstrated that

filtration of the blood was effective in removing these particles, but that the original 200 μ filter was too large. Present filters are in the 27 μ range and will remove most significant particulate matter.[191-193] The primary side effect is a reduced platelet count.[194, 195] Concomitant with this development, a number of centers have reported a significant reduction in postoperative neurologic complications. Ideally three filters are used, two during bypass, as shown in Figure 14–1, and a third for prebypass filtration of the prime to remove shed particles.

TRANSPORT PROBLEMS

Additional problems relating to transport have been discussed in other sections of this chapter. Hypoxemia, inadequate flow or pressure, inappropriate cannulation or assembly of the bypass can all create serious difficulties. One cannot rule out reactions present under other conditions, such as increasing metabolic demand with malignant hyperthermia, but such events are rare.

Mechanical failures also occur and are usually of a straightforward nature. The most common problems are failure of system integrity, permitting gas to enter the system and be pumped to the patient, and rupture of the tubing associated with the roller pump, causing embolism and pump failure. Most pump systems include apparatus for manual pumping in the event of power failure. Backflow should always be considered and steps taken to prevent it if necessary. The user should be aware that overfilling many bubble oxygenators can, with a small volume increase, produce an abrupt desaturation of arterial blood. Blood gas tensions should be measured immediately if this complication is suspected.

TARGET ORGANS

The heart is discussed in Chapter 26. Renal complications are discussed in Chapter 25.

Postoperative confusion and psychosis has been described since the early days of open-heart surgery. Initially it was suggested that this was a psychiatric response to the fear of surgery for a lesion recognized by the patient as life-threatening.[196] It was then pointed out that the incidence was unusually high after bypass[197] and that many of these psychoses are associated with demonstrable ischemic lesions in the central nervous system.[198] At least one source of injury appears to be the blood-material interaction, with consequent protein denaturation. As one might expect, the disc provides a greater[199] and the membrane a lesser[200] insult than the bubble oxygenator.

However, in the last 10 years a general consensus has developed that a major source of neurologic deficits is microemboli.[201–203] Reports from many centers have shown that adequate filtration using 27 μ filters has substantially reduced the incidence of postoperative psychosis and neurologic deficit. The use of these filters appears to be far more important than any subtlety in the bypass protocol or psychiatric management, yet the discussion of psychiatric management of post cardiotomy delerium persists.[204, 205]

Pulmonary injury has long been associated with cardiopulmonary bypass,[206, 207] though some continue to dispute its significance.[208] This injury was called the *postperfusion pulmonary congestion syndrome* or *pump lung.*[209] On autopsy the lungs are dark red and congested, with focal zones of collapse and parenchymal hemorrhage. Causes suggested included blood trauma, foreign proteins on the oxygenator screen from past use and possible endotoxin injury. It is clear that the degree of dysfunction relates to the time of bypass.[210, 211] Cigarette smoking and other pulmonary trauma also predispose to injury.[212] The advent of blood filters suggested a common etiology. Early lung biopsy in surviving patients demonstrated extensive occlusion of the capillary beds by aggregates of leukocytes. Filtration substantially reduced the incidence of these findings and the degree of pulmonary dysfunction.[213, 214] The use of hypothermia to reduce bypass flow and duration also appears beneficial.[215]

It was also claimed in early publications that the use of an electrolyte prime increased lung water and impaired gas exchange, but recent studies suggest that significant increases in lung water may occur *after* cardiopulmonary bypass.[216] Some suggest that a dilute prime may improve gas exchange.[217] A number of centers suggest that exposure to high oxygen tensions on cardiopulmonary bypass, particularly with hypothermia, leads to increased pulmonary dysfunction. However, no study has yet been published clearly documenting this presumption. One study suggests that pulmonary dysfunction is minimized by maintaining intact pleura, suggesting that part of the dysfunction may be related to mechanical factors and expulsion of surfactant. Vascular hypertension may also be an unrecognized cause.[218, 219] Nonpulsatile flow does not appear to affect postoperative gas exchange.[220]

The implication remains that damage to the unformed elements of the blood is a component of pulmonary insult.[221] It has been demonstrated, for example, that substituting heparinized fresh blood for stored blood in the pump prime leads to increased pulmonary dysfunction,[222] suggesting that vasoactive factors are released from fully competent blood constituents. High doses of heparin have also accentuated pulmonary injury. The increase in pulmonary dysfunction with time on bypass using modern techniques also suggests that blood trauma is still a significant etiologic factor, but its exact nature remains to be elucidated. The primary incentive for development of membrane oxygenators has been reduction of pulmonary, renal and cerebral injury secondary to blood trauma.

The reader should remember that many other factors contribute to postoperative pulmonary dysfunction. These are discussed in Chapter 16 and many excellent references.

LONG-TERM CARDIOPULMONARY BYPASS

The advent of the membrane oxygenator, based on the invention of membrane dialysis by Kolff, first clinically applied in 1956,[221] was greeted with special interest because of the implication that it would be less traumatic to blood during cardiopulmonary bypass. It is now generally agreed that, with extended perfusion, blood trauma associated with a blood-gas interface becomes unacceptable. The membrane permits gas exchange without a free blood-gas interface. The problem in membrane oxygenator design is that the blood-material contact substituted for the blood-gas contact is extensive. Materials with unusually good blood compatibility must be used. These requirements are far more strict than for any other current clinical application, including vascular protheses.

A second problem relates to the requirement of minimum blood film thickness for gas exchange. Because of fabrication problems, this has meant a substantial increase in priming volume in most membrane oxygenators. It has also created severe practical problems in stability because the pressure drop across a membrane oxygenator is usually higher. With higher perfusion pressures, deformation of the membranes occurs, changing the size of the blood channels, blood film thickness, and gas exchange efficiency. These fabrication problems and the relatively scarcity of adequate materials have made membrane oxygenators more expensive and more difficult to use. The higher flow resistance also increases the required pumping pressure, and the opportunity for blood trauma associated with flow across the significant pressure gradient.

The primary application of membrane oxygenators in bypass procedures of typical duration (1–2 hours) is in infants and young children, in whom blood trauma is greater for the same flow and duration, because of the greater priming volume and surface area of the support system relative to the patient. The membrane design is unlikely to displace the bubble design in routine use until costs are reduced and the apparatus is simplified, despite measurable advantages.[222]

Studies of support of patients with traumatic injuries have produced criteria for extended use given the present state of the art. Typically, the target organ for initial injury is the lung, often through fat embolism secondary to trauma and fracture of large bones. If oxygenation can be sustained for a period of days in a person otherwise young and healthy, it is presumed that full recovery can be achieved. Because the heart is usually normal, the primary function of bypass is to assure oxygenation. However, membrane oxygenators are still not sufficiently atraumatic to permit extended total pulmonary bypass. A careful perusal of available survivor reports strongly suggests that when extracorporeal membrane oxygenation is undertaken, survivors are rare when diversion through the membrane oxygenator exceeds 70 percent of systemic flow for a period of days. This is still a substantial improvement over the percent shunt which could be tolerated with a bubble oxygenator.

SUMMARY

Cardiopulmonary bypass techniques and equipment are probably the single most important group of developments underlying modern cardiovascular surgery. As can be seen in this discussion, an understanding of the underlying mechanisms is essential to successful patient management. There are far too many opportunities for difficulty and error to permit memory to substitute for understanding. Equally, it is clear that many of the underlying mechanisms are not understood and that much work remains to be done. Although few anesthesiologists were involved in the early development of cardiopulmonary bypass, our central role in life support has fostered continuing professional growth and development in this area.

REFERENCES

GENERAL REFERENCES

1. Ionescu MI, Wooler GH (eds): Current Techniques in Extracorporeal Circulation. Boston, Butterworths, 1976
2. Reed CC, Clark DK: Cardiopulmonary Perfusion. Texas Medical Press, Houston, 1975
3. Allen JG (ed): Extracorporeal Circulation. Springfield Ill, Charles C Thomas, 1958

4. Rendell–Baker L: History of thoracic anesthesia. In Mushin WW (ed): Thoracic Anesthesia, pp 643–661. Oxford, Blackwell Scientific Publications, 1963
5. Curtis LE: An early history of extracorporeal circulation. J Cardiovasc Surg 7:240–247, 1966

HISTORY

6. Edwards WS, Edwards PD: Alexis Carrel-visionary surgeon, p 91. Charles C Thomas, Springfield, Ill, 1975
7. Nelson RM: Era of extracorporeal respiration. Surgery 78:685–693, 1975
8. Ludwig C, Schmidt A: Das verhalten der gase, welche mit dem blut durch die reizbaren saugethiermuskelz stromen. Arb Physiol Annst Leipz 3:1–61, 1869
9. Bunge G, Schmiedeberg O: Über die bildung der hippursaure. Arch Path Pharm 6:233–255, 1869
10. Schroder WV: Über die bildungsstatte des harnstoffes. Arch F Exp Path M Pharm 15:364, 1882
11. von Frey M, Gruber M: Untersuchungen über den stoffwechsel isolierter organe. Ein respirations-apparat für isolierted organe. Arch F Physiol 9:519, 1885
12. Hooker DR: The perfusion of the mammalian medulla: the effect of calcium and of potassium on the respiratory and cardiac centers. Am J Physiol 38:200–208, 1910
13. Richards AN, Drinker CK: An apparatus for the perfusion of isolated organs. J Pharmacol Exp Ther 7:467–483, 1915
14. Howell WH, Holt E: Two new factors in blood coagulation—heparin and proantithrombin. Am J Physiol 47:328–341, 1918
15. McLean J: The discovery of heparin. Circulation 19:75–78, 1959
16. Hooker DR: A study of the isolated kidney: the influence of pulse pressure upon renal function. Am J Physiol 27:24–44, 1910
17. Dale HH, Schuster EHJ: A double perfusion pump. J Physiol 64:356–364, 1928
18. Carrel A, Lindbergh CA: The culture of whole organs. Science 81:621–623, 1935
19. DeBakey M: New Orleans Med Surg J 87:386–389, 1934
20. Gibbon JH Jr: Artificial maintenance of circulation during experimental occlusion of pulmonary artery. Arch Surg 34:1105–1131, 1937
21. Björk VO: Brain perfusions in dogs with artificially oxygenated blood. Acta Chir Scand [Suppl] 96:1, 1948
22. Björk VO: Brain perfusions in dogs with artificially oxygenated blood. Acta Chir Scand 117:27–30, 1957
23. Clark LC Jr, Gollan F, Gupta VB: The oxygenation of blood by gas dispersion. Science 111:85–87, 1950
24. Dennis C, Spreng DS Jr, Nelson GE et al: Development of a pump oxygenator to replace the heart and lungs: an apparatus applicable to human patients and application to one case. Ann Surg 134:709–721, 1951
25. Nelson RM: Era of extracorporeal respiration. Surgery 78:685–693, 1975
26. Gibbon JH Jr: Application of a mechanical heart and lung apparatus to cardiac surgery. Minn Med 37:171–185, 1954
27. DeWall RA, Warden HE, Read RC et al: A simple expendable artificial oxygenator for open heart surgery. Surg Clin North Am, 36:1025–1034, 1956
28. DeWall RA, Warden HE, Gott VL et al: Total body perfusion for open cardiotomy utilizing the bubble oxygenator. J Thorac Cardiovasc Surg 32:591–603, 1956
29. Clowes GHA Jr, Hopkins AL, Neville WE: An artificial lung dependent upon diffusion of oxygen and carbon dioxide through plastic membranes. J Thorac Cardiovasc Surg 32:630–637, 1956
30. Lewis FT, Mansar T: Closure of atrial septal defects with the aid of hypothermia: experimental accomplishments and the report of one successful case. Surgery 33:52–59, 1953
31. Lillehei CW, Cohen M, Warden HE et al: The direct vision intracardiac correction of congenital anomalies by controlled cross-circulation. Surgery 38:11–29, 1955
32. Dogliotti AM, Costantini A: Primo caso di applicazione all'uomo apparecchio di circolazione sanguinea extracorporea. Minerva Chir 6:657–659, 1951

MODERN DESIGN

General References

33. Galletti PM: Advances in heart lung machines. In Levine SN (ed): Advances in Biomedical Engineering and Medical Physics, vol 2, pp 121–165. New York, Interscience, 1968
34. Galletti PM: Advances in heart lung machines. In Levine SN (ed): Advances in

Biomedical Engineering and Medical Physics, vol 2, pp 121–165. New York, Interscience, 1968

35. Mortensen JD: Prolonged open-chest total cardiopulmonary bypass in calves. Med Instrum 10:22–26, 1976

36. Mortensen JD et al: Safety and efficacy of blood oxygenators, vol I: Summary; vol II: Report of Testing, Vol. III: Literature Review. Report: FDA Contract 223-74-5253, Task Order 10, May 1976 (The major source of references 35–79)

37. Friedman LI, Richardson PD, Galletti PM: Observations of acute thrombogenesis in membrane oxygenators. Trans Am Soc Artif Intern Organs 17:369–375, 1971

38. Peirce EC II: The theory and function of the membrane lung. Mt Sinai J Med 40:119–134, 1973

Becton–Dickinson

39. McCullough NJ, Falke K, Lowenstein E et al: Respiratory gas exchange with spiral coil membrane lungs: total cardiopulmonary bypass in adult sheep and clinical experience with long-term perfusion in adult patients. Mt Sinai J Med 40:207–221, 1973

Bentley

40. Andersen MN, Duchiba K: Blood trauma produced by pump oxygenators. J Thorac Cardiovasc Surg 57:238–44, 1969

41. Becker RM, Smith MR, Dobell ARC: Effect of platelet inhibition on platelet phenomena in cardiopulmonary bypass in pigs. Ann Surg 179:52–57, 1974

42. Douglas M, Birnbaum D, Eiseman B: Biological evaluation of a disposable membrane oxygenator. Arch Surg 103:89–91, 1971

43. Dutton RL, Edmunds LH Jr: Measurement of emboli in extracorporeal perfusion systems. J Thorac Cardiovasc Surg 65:523–530, 1973

44. Kessler J, Patterson RH Jr: The production of microemboli by various blood oxygenators. Ann Thorac Surg 9:221–228, 1970

45. Mielke CH Jr, de Leval M, Hill JD et al: Drug influence on platelet loss during extracorporeal circulation. J Thorac Cardiovasc Surg 66:845–854, 1973

46. Palmer AS, Clark RE, Mills M: The low pressure rocking membrane oxygenator: An infant model. Ann Thorac Surg 9:13–20, 1970

47. Reed CC, Romagnoli A, Taylor DE et al: Particulate matter in bubble oxygenator. J Thorac Cardiovasc Surg 68:971–974, 1974

48. Simmons MD, McGuire C, Lichti E et al: A comparison of the microparticles produced when two disposable-bag oxygenators and a disc oxygenator are used for cardiopulmonary bypass. J Thorac Cardiovasc Surg 63:613–621, 1972

49. Subramanian VA, Wright WL, Berger RL: A new efficient disposable rotating disc membrane oxygenator versus Bentley bubble oxygenator. Surg Forum 25:132–134, 1974

50. Visudh–arom K, Miller ID, Castaneda AR: Hematological studies following total cardiopulmonary bypass in infant puppies. Trans Am Soc Artif Intern Organs 15:161–164, 1969

Bramson (see also References 37, 38, 45, 46)

51. Bramson ML, Hill JE, Osborn JJ et al: Partial veno-arterial perfusion with membrane oxygenation and diastolic augmentation. Trans Am Soc Artif Intern Organs 15:412–416, 1969

52. Gerbode F, Osborn JJ, Bramson ML: Experiences in the development of a membrane heart-lung machine. Am J Surg 114:16–23, 1967

53. Hill JD, de Leval, Meilke CH et al: Clinical prolonged extracorporeal circulation for respiratory insufficiency: hematological effects. Trans Am Soc Artif Intern Organs 18:546–552, 1972

54. Hill JD, Bramson ML, Hackel A et al: Laboratory and clinical studies during prolonged partial extracorporeal circulation using the Bramson Membrane Lung. Circulation 37:139, 1968

55. Hill JD, Bramson ML, Kleinhenz R et al: Lung Morphology Following Prolonged Venovenous Perfusions with the Bramson Membrane Lung. In Norman JC (ed): Organ Perfusion and Preservation, New York, Appleton–Century Crofts, 1968

Dorson

56. Dorson WJ Jr, Baker E, Hull H et al: A long term partial bypass oxygenation system. Ann Thorac Surg 8:297–311, 1969

Dow (see also References 38, 43)

57. Dutton RC, Mather FW III, Walker SN et al: Development and evaluation of a new hol-

low-fiber membrane oxygenator. Trans Am Soc Artif Intern Organs 17:331–335, 1971

58. Kaye MP, Pace JB, Blatt SJ et al: Use of a capillary membrane oxygenator for total cardiopulmonary bypass in calves. J Surg Res 14:58–63, 1973

59. Rawitscher RE, Dutton RC, Edmunds LH Jr: Evaluation of hollow fiber and spiral coil membrane oxygenators designed for cardiopulmonary bypass in infants. Circulation [Suppl] 48:105–111, 1973

60. Ward BD, Hood AG: Comparative performance of clinical membrane lungs. J Thorac Cardiovasc Surg 68:830–836, 1974

Galen (see also Reference 47)

61. Chopra PS, Dufek JH, Droncke GM et al: Clinical comparison of the General Electric-Peirce Membrane Lung and bubble oxygenator for prolonged cardiopulmonary bypass. Surgery 74:874–879, 1973

Peirce GE (see also References 37, 38, 60)

62. Gille JP, Trudell J, Snider MT et al: Capability of the microporous membrane lined capillary oxygenator in hypercapnic dogs. Trans Ann Soc Calif Int Organs 16:365, 1970

63. Joseph WL, Giordano JM, Gedlock GW: Clinical use of the membrane lung oxygenator for acute respiratory insufficiency. Mt Sinai J Med 40:222, 1973

64. Peirce EC II, Corrigan JJ, Kent BB et al: Comparative trauma to blood in the disc oxygenator and membrane lung. Trans Am Soc Artif Intern Organs 15:33–39, 1969

65. Peirce EC II: A comparison of the Lande–Edwards, the Peirce, and the General Electric–Peirce Membrane Lungs. Trans Am Soc Artif Intern Organs 16:358, 1970

66. Rawlings CA, Bisgard JH, Dufek DD et al: Prolonged perfusion with a membrane oxygenator in awake ponies. J Thorac Cardiovasc Surg 69:539–550, 1975

67. Timmons EH, Lindsey ES, Woolverton: Long term veno-venous perfusion with a membrane oxygenator in puppies. Trans Am Soc Artif Intern Organs 16:339–343, 1970

Gomes

68. Gomes OM, Conceicao DS, Nogueira D Jr et al: Variable column bubble oxygenator. J Thorac Cardiovasc Surg 69:606–614, 1975

Harvey (see also Reference 47)

69. Page PA, Haller AJ: Clinical evaluation of the new Harvey H200 Disposable Bood Oxygenator. J Thorac Cardiovasc Surg 67:213, 1974

Hirose

70. Hirose Y, Everett HF, Marshall DV et al: The single-pass oxygenator. Ann Thorac Surg 9:313–320, 1970

Lande–Edwards (see also References 38, 60, 64)

71. Baffes T, Patel K, Jegathesan S: Total cardiopulmonary bypass with the Lande–Edwards Membrane Oxygenator. Am J Cardiol 29:672–677, 1972

72. Bartlett RH, Gassaniga AB, Fong SW et al: Prolonged extracorporeal cardiopulmonary support in man. J Thorac Cardiovasc Surg 68:918–932, 1974

73. Carlson RG, Lande AJ, Subramanian VA et al: The Lande–Edwards Disposable Membrane Oxygenator for aorto-coronary artery-vein bypass graft operations. J Cardiovasc Surg (Torino) 13:333–345, 1972

74. Carlson RG, Lande AJ, Twichell J et al: Prolonged cardiopulmonary support with disposable membrane oxygenator during aortocoronary bypass grafts. NY State J Med 72:2513–2520, 1972

75. Carlson RG, Lande AJ, Ivey LW et al: Total cardiopulmonary support with disposable membrane oxygenator during aortocoronary artery-vein graft operations. Chest 62:424–432, 1972

76. Houseman LB, Braunwald NS: Experimental evaluation of the Travenol and Lance–Edwards membrane oxygenators for use in neonate perfusions. Ann Thorac Surg 14:150–158, 1972

77. Lande AJ, Bloch JH, Edwards L et al: Clinical experience with emergency use of prolonged cardiopulmonary bypass with a membrane pump-oxygenator. Ann Thorac Surg 10:409–423, 1970

78. Lande AJ, Fillmore SJ, Subramanian V et al: 24 hours venous-arterial perfusions of awake dogs with a simple membrane oxygenator. Trans Am Soc Artif Intern Organs 15:181–186, 1969

79. Lande AJ, Carlson RG, Patterson RH et al: Cardiac surgery with disposable membrane

lungs. Trans Am Soc Artif Intern Organs 18:532–536, 1972

80. Lande AJ, Edwards L, Bloch JH et al: Prolonged cardiopulmonary support with a practical membrane oxygenator. Trans Am Soc Artif Intern Organs 16:352–356, 1970

81. Vervloet AFC, Edwards MJ, Edwards ML. Minimal apparent blood damage in Lande–Edwards Membrane Oxygenator at physiologic gas tensions. J Thorac Cardiovasc Surg 60:774–780, 1970

Medical Monitors (see also References 44, 47)

82. Benn JA, Drinker PA, Milkie B et al: Predictive correlation of oxygen and carbon dioxide transfer in a blood oxygenator with induced secondary flows. Trans Am Soc Artif Intern Organs 17:317–322, 1971

83. Katsuhara K, Yokosuka T, Sakakibara S: The swing-type membrane oxygenator. J Surg Res 8:245–252, 1968

Rugg-Kyusgaard (see References 39, 40, 47, 59, 60)

Sci Med (See also References 37, 42, 61)

84. Kolobow T, Zapol WM, Sigman RL et al: Partial cardiopulmonary bypass lasting up to seven days in alert lambs with membrane lung blood oxygenation. J Thorac Cardiovasc Surg 60:781–788, 1970

85. Kolobow T, Zapol W, Pierce J: High survival and minimal blood damage in lambs exposed to long term (1 week) veno-venous pumping with a polyurethane chamber roller pump with and without a membrane blood oxygenator. Trans Am Soc Artif Intern Organs 15:172–176, 1969

86. Kolobow T, Spragg RC, Pierce JE et al: Extended term (to 16 days) partial extracorporeal blood gas exchange with the spiral membrane lung in unanesthetized lambs. Trans Am Soc Artif Intern Organs 17:350–354, 1971

87. White JJ, Andrews HG, Risemberg et al: Prolonged respiratory support in newborn infants with a membrane oxygenator. Surgery 70:288–296, 1971

88. White JJ, Leenders E, Andrews HG et al: Studies of a membrane oxygenator for prolonged respiratory support. J Pediatr Surg 5:610–619, 1970

89. Zapol W, Pontoppidan H, McCullough N et al: Clinical membrane lung support for acute respiratory insufficiency. Trans Am Soc Artif Intern Organs 18:553–559, 1972

90. Zapol WM, Qvist J, Pontoppidan H et al: Extracorporeal perfusion for acute respiratory failure. J Thorac Cardiovasc Surg 69:439–449, 1975

Travenol (see also References 38, 40, 42, 44, 47, 48, 76)

91. Birnbaum D, Eiseman B: Laboratory evaluation of a new silicone membrane oxygenator. J Thorac Cardiovasc Surg 64:441–451, 1972

92. Boyd JC, Moran JF, Clark RE: An analysis of the operating characteristics of the 0.25 M² Travenol infant membrane oxygenator. Surgery 71:262–269, 1972

93. Eiseman B, Birnbaum D, Leonard R et al: A new gas permeable membrane for blood oxygenators. Surg Gynecol Obstet 135:732–736, 1972

94. Karlson KE, Murphy M, Kakvan P et al: Total cardiopulmonary bypass with a new microporous Teflon membrane oxygenator. Surgery 76:935–945, 1974

95. Murphy W, Trudell LA, Friedman LI et al: Laboratory and clinical experience with a microporous membrane oxygenator. Trans Am Soc Artif Intern Organs 20:278–285, 1974

96. Trudell LA, Friedman LI, Kakvan M et al: Evaluation of a disposable membrane oxygenator. Trans Am Soc Artif Intern Organs 18:538–543, 1972

97. Wildevuur J, Kuipers RG, Spaan JAE et al: The use of a membrane oxygenator for treatment of respiratory insufficiency. Trans Am Soc Artif Intern Organs 17:362–368, 1971

Heat Exchanger

98. A study on the effects of additional endogenous heat relating to the artificial heart. Annual Report of the Battelle Memorial Institute Pacific Northwest Laboratories, June 1973, PB 224-973/AS (available from NTS, 5285 Port Royal Road, Springfield, VA 22161)

Sensors and Controls

99. Mortensen JD: Prolonged open-chest total cardiopulmonary bypass in calves. Med Instrum 10:22–26, 1976

INITIATING BYPASS

Pump Prime

100. Bigelow JE, Dobbs JL, Fogdall RP: Acid-citrate-dextrose vs. heparinized whole blood prime. Arch Surg 96:65–70, 1968
101. Cohn LH, Fosberg AM, Anderson WP et al: The effects of phlebotomy, hemodilution and autologous transfusion on systemic oxygenation and whole blood utilization in open heart surgery. Chest 68:283–287, 1975
102. Sherman MM, Dobnik DB, Dennis RC et al: Autologous blood transfusion during cardiopulmonary bypass. Chest 70:592–595, 1976
103. Yeh T Jr, Shelton L, Yeh TJ: Blood loss and bank blood requirement in coronary bypass surgery. Ann Thorac Surg 26:11–16, 1978
104. Nadjmabadi MH, Rastan H, Saidi MT et al: Haemodynamic effects of acute intra-operative haemodilution in open heart surgery. Anaesthesist 27:364–369, 1978
105. Schorr JB, Marx GJ: New trends in intra-operative blood replacement. Anesth Analg (Cleve) 49:646–651, 1970
106. Ott DA, Cooley DA: Cardiovascular surgery in Jehovah's Witnesses: report of 542 operations without blood transfusion. JAMA 238:1256–1258, 1977
107. Dor V, Mermet B, Kreitmann P et al: Cardiac surgery in Jehovah's Witnesses. Apropos of 47 cases. Arch Mal Coeur 70:549–554, 1977
108. Hallowell P, Bland JH, Dalton BC et al: The effect of hemodilution with albumin or Ringer's lactate on water balance and blood use in open-heart surgery. Ann Thorac Surg 25:22–29, 1978
109. Subramanian VA, Berger RL: Carbon monoxide accumulation during extracorporeal membrane oxygenation for acute respiratory failure. Ann Thorac Surg 22:195–198, 1976

Patient Anticoagulation

110. Mattox KL, Guinn GA, Rubio PA et al: Use of the activated coagulation time in intraoperative heparin reversal for cardiopulmonary operations. Ann Thorac Surg 19:634–638, 1975
111. Verska JJ: Control of heparinization by activated clotting time during bypass with improved postoperative hemostasis. Ann Thorac Surg 24:170–173, 1977

Going on Bypass

112. Gordon RJ, Ravin M, Daicoff GR et al: Effects of hemodilution on hypotension during cardiopulmonary bypass. Anesth Analg (Cleve) 54:482–488, 1975
113. Coté CJ, Greenhow DE, Marshall BE: The hypotensive response to rapid intravenous administration of hypertonic solutions in man and the rabbit. Anesthesiology 50:30–35, 1979

CARDIOPULMONARY BYPASS

Surgical Technique

114. Miller DW Jr: The Practice of Coronary Artery Bypass Surgery, p 237. New York, Plenum Medical Book Co, 1977
115. Miller DW Jr, Hessel EA II Winterscheid LC et al: Current practice of coronary artery bypass surgery: results of a national survey. J Thorac Cardiovasc Surg 73:75–83, 1977
116. Arom KV, Vinas JF, Fewel JE et al: Is a left ventricular vent necessary during cardiopulmonary bypass? Ann Thorac Surg 24:566–573, 1977

Flow and Pressure

117. Garman JK: Personal communication.
118. Stockard JJ, Bickford RG, Schauble JF: Pressure dependent cerebral ischemia during cardiopulmonary bypass. Neurology 23:521–529, 1973
119. Kolkka R, Hilberman M: Neurological dysfunction following cardiac surgery with low flow, low pressure cardiopulmonary bypass. J Thorac Cardiovasc Surg 79:432–438, 1980
120. Conti VR, Bertranou EG, Blackstone EH et al: Cold cardioplegia versus hypothermia for myocardial protection. J Thorac Cardiovasc Surg 76:577–589, 1978

Pulsatile Flow

121. Mavroudis C: To pulse or not to pulse. Ann Thorac Surg 25:259–271, 1978
122. Milnor WR: Pulsatile blood flow. N Engl J Med 287:27–34, 1972
123. Hooker DR: A study of the isolated kidney: the influence of pulse pressure upon renal function. Am J Physiol 27:24–44, 1910
124. Gesell RA: On the relation of pulse pressure

to renal secretion. Am J Physiol 32:70–93, 1913

125. Goodyer AVN, Glenn WWL: Relation of arterial pulse pressure to renal function. Am J Physiol 167:689–697, 1951

126. Ritter ER: Pressure/flow relations in the kidney: alleged effects of pulse pressure. Am J Physiol 168:480–489, 1952

127. Wesolowski SA, Sauvage LR, Pinc RD: Extracorporeal circulation: the role of the pulse in maintenance of the systemic circulation during heart-lung bypass. Surgery 37:663–682, 1955

128. Many M, Soroff HS, Birtwell WC et al: The physiologic role of pulsatile and nonpulsatile blood flow. III. Effects of unilateral renal artery depulsation. Arch Surg 97:917–923, 1968

129. Mandelbaum I, Burns WH: Pulsatile and nonpulsatile blood flow. JAMA 191:657–660, 1965

130. Jacobs LA, Klopp EH, Seamone W et al: Improved organ function during cardiac bypass with a roller pump modified to deliver pulsatile flow. J Thorac Cardiovasc Surg 58:703–712, 1969

131. Dalton ML, Mosley EC, Woodward KE et al: The effect of pulsatile flow on renal blood flow during extracorporeal circulation. J Surg Res 5:127–131, 1965

132. Ogata T, Ida Y, Nonoyama A et al: A comparative study on the effectiveness of pulsatile and non-pulsatile blood flow in extracorporeal circulation. Nippon Geka Hokan 29:59–66, 1960

133. Ida Y: Experimental studies on carbohydrate metabolism during heart lung bypass, with special reference to a comparison of pulsatile flow with non-pulsatile flow. Nippon Geka Hokan 31:181–196, 1962

134. Takeda J: Experimental study of peripheral circulation during extracorporeal circulation, with a special reference to a comparison of pulsatile flow with non-pulsatile flow. Nippon Geka Hokan 29:1407–1430, 1960

135. Sanderson JM, Wright G, Sims FW: Brain damage in dogs immediately following pulsatile and non-pulsatile blood flows in extracorporeal circulation. Thorax 27:275–286, 1972

136. Mavroudis C: To pulse or not to pulse. Ann Thorac Surg 25:259–271, 1978

137. Mavroudis C: To pulse or not to pulse. Ann Thorac Surg 25:259–271, 1978

138. Steed DL, Follette DM, Foglia R et al: Effects of pulsatile assistance and nonpulsatile flow in subendocardial perfusion during cardiopulmonary bypass. Ann Thorac Surg 26:133–141, 1978

139. Maddoux G, Pappas G, Jenkins M: Effect of pulsatile and nonpulsatile flow during cardiopulmonary bypass on left ventricular ejection fraction early after aortocoronary bypass surgery. Am J Cardiol 37:1000–1006, 1976

140. Pappas G, Winter SD, Kopriva CJ et al: Improvement of myocardial and other vital organ functions and metabolism with a simple method of pulsatile flow (IABP) during clinical cardiopulmonary bypass. Surgery 77:34–44, 1975

141. Bregman D, Bowman FO Jr, Parodi EN et al: An improved method of myocardial protection with pulsation during cardiopulmonary bypass. Circulation 56:II, 1157–1160, 1977

142. Taylor KM, Bain WH, Maxted J et al: Comparative studies of pulsatile and nonpulsatile flow during cardiopulmonary bypass. J Thorac Cardiovasc Surg 75:569–584, 1978

143. Dalton ML, McCarty RT, Woodward KE et al: The Army artificial heart pump. II. Comparison of pulsatile and nonpulsatile flow. Surgery 58:840–845, 1965

144. Trinkle JK, Helton NE, Wood RE et al: Metabolic comparison of a new pulsatile pump and a roller pump for cardiopulmonary bypass. J Thorac Cardiovasc Surg 58:562–569, 1969

145. Bregman D, Bowman FO Jr, Parodi EN et al: An improved method of myocardial protection with pulsation during cardiopulmonary bypass. Circulation 56:II, 1157–1160, 1977

146. Bregman D, Bailin M, Bowman FO Jr et al: A pulsatile assist device (PAD) for use during cardiopulmonary bypass. Ann Thorac Surg 24:574–581, 1977

147. Kaplitt MJ, Tamari Y, Frantz SL et al: Clinical experience with Tamari–Kaplitt Pulsator. New device to create pulsatile flow or counterpulsation during open-heart surgery. NY State J Med 78:1090–1094, 1978

Electrolytes

148. Dieter RA, Nevill WE, Pifarre R: Hypokalemia following hemodilution cardiopulmonary bypass. Ann Surg 171:17–23, 1969

149. Henney PR, Riemenschneider TA, Deland EC et al: Prevention of hypokalemic cardiac arrhythmias associated with cardiopulmonary bypass and hemodilution. Surg Forum 21:145–147, 1971

150. Abrahams N, Johnston AE, Taylor J et al: A comparison of the effects of two haemodiluents on monovalent and divalent cations in children undergoing cardiopulmonary bypass and open heart surgery. Can Anaesth Soc J 20:153–169, 1973

151. Pacifico AD, Digerness S, Kirklin JW: Acute alterations of body composition after open heart intracardiac operations. Circulation 41:331–341, 1970

152. Mandal AK, Callaghan JC, Sterns LP: Changes in intracellular potassium resulting from extracorporeal circulation. Surg Forum 19:137–138, 1968

153. Beal AM: Changes in arterial blood pressure, heart rate and haematocrit during acute hyperkalemia in conscious sheep. J Exp Physiol 61:297–308, 1976

154. Romero EG, Castillo–Olivares JL, O'Connor F et al: The importance of calcium and magnesium ions in serum and cerebrospinal fluid during cardiopulmonary bypass. J Thorac Cardiovasc Surg 66:668–672, 1973

155. Schaer H: Effects on ionized calcium of a correction of acidosis with alkalinizing agents. Br J Anaesth 48:327–332, 1976

156. Moffitt EA, Tarhan S, Goldsmith RS et al: Patterns of total and ionized calcium and other electrolytes in plasma during and after cardiac surgery. J Thorac Cardiovasc Surg 65:751–757, 1973

157. Fuchs C, Brasche M, Spieckermann PG, et al: Divalent ions and myocardial function during cardiopulmonary bypass (CPB): changes in total calcium, ionized calcium and magnesium in plasma. J Cardiovasc Surg (Torino) 16:476–483, 1975

158. Garcia–Romero E, Castillo–Olivares JL, Figuera D: Prevention of hypomagnesemia and hypocalcemia in open-heart surgery. J Cardiovasc Surg (Torino) 18:257–260, 1977

159. Chipperfield B, Chipperfield JR: Magnesium and the heart. Am Heart J 93:679–682, 1977

160. Scheinman NM, Sullivan RW, Hutchinson JC et al: Clinical significance of changes in serum magnesium in patients undergoing cardiopulmonary bypass. J Thorac Cardiovasc Surg 61:135–140, 1971

161. Calverley RK, Jenkins LC, Griffiths F: A clinical study of serum magnesium concentrations during anesthesia and cardiopulmonary bypass. Can Anaesth Soc J 20:499–518, 1973

162. Sala A, Ferrozzi G, Biglioli P et al: Changes in the plasma magnesium content in patients subjected to cardiopulmonary bypass. Minerva Chir 30:513–515, 1975

163. Langer GA, Brady AJ: Ionic movement and the control of contraction. In The Mammalian Myocardium, p 214. New York, John Wiley and Sons, 1974

164. Abrahams N, Johnston AE, Taylor J et al: A comparison of the effects of two haemodiluents on monovalent and divalent cations in children undergoing cardiopulmonary bypass and open heart surgery. Can Anaesth Soc J 20:153–169, 1973

165. Turnier E, Osborn JJ, Gerbode F et al: Magnesium and open heart surgery. J Thorac Cardiovasc Surg 64:694–705, 1972

166. Holden MP, Ionescu MI, Wooler GH: Magnesium in patients undergoing open-heart surgery. Thorax 27:212–218, 1972

Ventilation

167. Garman JK: Personal communication

COMPLICATIONS

General

168. Mortensen JD et al: Safety and efficacy of blood oxygenators, vol I: Summary; vol II: Report of Testing, Vol. III: Literature Review. Report: FDA Contract 223-74-5253, Task Order 10, May 1976. (The major source of references 35–79).

169. Mortensen JD: Safety and efficacy of extracorporeal blood oxygenators. A review. Med Instrum 12:128–132, 1978

Blood Trauma

170. Hewitt WC Jr, Brown LW Jr, Eadie AS et al: The ultimate *in vivo* survival of erythrocytes which have circulated through a pump oxygenator. Surg Forum 7:271, 1956

171. Brinsfield DE, Hopf MA, Geering RB et al: Hematological changes in long-term perfusion. J Appl Physiol 17:531–534, 1962

172. Yarborough KA, Mockros LF, Lewis FJ: Hydrodynamic hemolysis in extracorporeal machines. J Thorac Cardiovasc Surg 52:550–557, 1956

173. Coburn RF: Endogenous carbon monoxide production. N Engl J Med 282:207–209, 1970

174. Moriau M, Masure R, Hurlet A et al: Hae-mostasis disorders in open heart surgery with extracorporeal circulation. Importance of the platelet function and the heparin neutralization. Vox Sang 32:41–51, 1977

175. Gollan F: Physiology of Cardiac Surgery: hypothermia, extracorporeal circulation and extracorporeal p 37. Springfield Ill, Charles C Thomas, 1959

176. Ward BD, Berry GL: Comparative platelet function during prolonged extracorporeal bubble and membrane oxygenation. Am SECT Proceedings, 1975

177. Bailey Y, Sicard–Desnuelles MP, Gallet de Santerre G JR et al: Direct action of extracorporeal circulation on platelets and coagulation factors. Ann Anesthesiol Fr 18:43–50, 1977

178. Belleville J, Paul J, Ollat G et al: Coagulation deficits and hemorrhagic consequences after cardiac surgery under ECC. Ann Anesthesiol Fr 18:51–61, 1977

179. McKenna R, Bachmann F, Whittaker B et al: The hemostatic mechanism after open-heart surgery. II. Frequency of abnormal platelet functions during after extracorporeal circulation. J Thorac Cardiovasc Surg 70:298–308, 1975

180. Lilleaasen P: Moderate and extreme haemodilution in open-heart surgery. Blood requirements, bleeding and platelet counts. Scand J Thorac Cardiovasc Surg 11:97–103, 1977

181. Harding SA, Shakoor MA, Grindon AJ: Platelet support for cardiopulmonary bypass surgery. J Thorac Cardiovasc Surg 70:350–353, 1975

182. Gollan F: Physiology of Cardiac Surgery: hypothermia, extracorporeal circulation and extracorporeal p 37. Springfield, Ill, Charles C Thomas, 1959

183. Okies JE, Goodnight SH, Litchford B et al: Effects of infusion of cardiotomy suction blood during extracorporeal circulation for coronary artery bypass surgery. J Thorac Cardiovasc Surg 74:440–444, 1977

184. Dobell ARC, Mitri M, Galva R et al: Biologic evaluation of blood after prolonged recirculation through film and membrane oxygenators. Ann Surg 161:617–622, 1965

185. Mortensen JD: Evaluation of ASAIO blood damage test. Final Report to FDA on Contract # 253-74-5253, Task order 17, two vols, June 8, 1977

Emboli

186. Frick R, Bauer L, Leutschaft R: Antifoam coating of the bubble oxygenator as a possible cause of capillary silicone embolism. Chirurg 45:410–412, 1974

187. Dutton RD, Edmunds LH Jr, Hutchinson JC et al: Platelet aggregate emboli produced in patients during cardiopulmonary bypass with membrane and bubble oxygenators and blood filters. J Thorac Cardiovasc Surg 67:258–265, 1973

188. Kessler J, Patterson RH Jr: The production of microemboli by various blood oxygenators. Ann Thorac Surg 9:221–228, 1970

189. Owens G, Adams JE, Scott HW Jr: Embolic fat as a measure of adequacy of various oxygenators. J Appl Physiol 15:999–1000, 1960

190. Reed CC, Romagnoli A, Taylor DE, et al: Particulate matter in bubble oxygenators. J Thorac Cardiovasc Surg 68:971–974, 1974

191. Loop FD, Szabo J, Rowlinson RD et al: Events related to microembolism during extracorporeal perfusion in man: effectiveness of in-line filtration recorded by ultrasound. Ann Thorac Surg 21:412–20, 1976

192. Buley R, Lumley J: Some observations on blood microfilters. Ann R Coll Surg Engl 57:262–267, 1975

193. Patterson RH Jr, Twichell JB: Disposable filter for microemboli; use in cardiopulmonary bypass and massive transfusion. JAMA 215:76–80, 1971

194. Cullen DJ, Ferrara L: Comparative evaluation of blood filters. Anesthesiology 41:568–575, 1974

195. Dunbar RW, Price KA, Cannarella CF: Microaggregate blood filters: effect of filtration time, plasma hemoglobin, and fresh blood platelet counts. Anesth Analg (Cleve) 53:577–583, 1974

Target Organs

196. Blacher RS: The hidden psychosis of open-heart surgery. JAMA 222:305–308, 1972

197. Lee WH, Miller W, Rowe J et al; Effects of extracorporeal circulation on personality and cerebration. Ann Thorac Surg 7:562–570, 1969

198. Rufo HM, Ostfeld AM, Shekelle R: Central nervous system dysfunction following open-heart surgery. JAMA 212:1333–1340, 1970

199. Aberg T, Kihlgren M: Cerebral protection during open heart surgery. A comparison be-

tween a disk oxygenator and two bubble oxygenators. Thoraxchir Vask Chir 25:146–151,
1977

200. Foliguet B: Pulmonary complications after
extracorporeal circulation. ECC Lung syndrome. Ann Anesthesiol FR 18:134–149, 1977
201. Sachdev NS, Carter CC, Swank RL et al: Relationship between postcardiotomy delirium,
clinical neurological changes, and EEG abnormalities. J Thorac Cardiovasc Surg 54:557–
563, 1967
202. Branthwaite MA: Prevention of neurological
damage during open-heart surgery. Thorax
30:258–261, 1975
203. Aberg T, Kihlgren M: Cerebral protection
during open-heart surgery. Thorax 32:525–
533, 1977
204. Vasquez E, Chitwood WR Jr: Postcardiotomy
delirium: an overview. Int J Psychiatry Med
6:373–383, 1975
205. Meyendorf R; Mental and neurological disorders associated with heart operations. Pre-
and postoperative studies. Fortschr Med
94:315–320, 1976
206. McClenahan JB, Young WE, Sykes MK: Respiratory changes after open-heart surgery.
Thorax 20:454–554, 1965
207. Rea HH, Harris EA, Seelye ER et al: The
effects of cardiopulmonary bypass upon pulmonary gas exchange. J Thorac Cardiovasc
Surg 75:104–120, 1978
208. Laver MB: Lung function following open
heart surgery. In Litwack RS (ed): Care of the
Cardiac Surgical Patient. New York, Appleton–Century Crofts, 1980
209. Baer DM, Osborn JJ: The postperfusion pulmonary congestion syndrome. Am J Clin
Path 34:442–445, 1960
210. Andersen NB, Ghia J: Pulmonary function,
cardiac status, and postoperative course in
relation to cardiopulmonary bypass. J Thorac
Cardiovasc Surg 59:474–483, 1970
211. Hewson JR: Perfusion characteristics during
cardiopulmonary bypass and subsequent
changes in alveolar-arterial oxygen tension
gradients. Anesth Analg (Cleve) 57:298–302,
1978
212. Llamas R, Forthman HJ: Respiratory distress
syndrome in the adult after cardiopulmonary
bypass. JAMA 225:1183–1186, 1973
213. Connell RS, Page VS, Bartley TD et al: The
effect on pulmonary ultrastructure of dacron
wool filtration during cardiopulmonary bypass. J Thorac Cardiovasc Surg 15:217–229,
1973
214. Reul GJ Jr, Greenberg SD, Lefrak EA et al:
Prevention of post-traumatic pulmonary insufficiency. Arch Surg 106:386–394, 1973
215. Barash PG, Berman MA, Stansel HC Jr et al:
Markedly improved pulmonary function after open heart surgery in infancy utilizing
surface cooling, profound hypothermia, and
circulatory arrest. Am J Surg 131:499–503,
1976
216. Byrick RJ, Kay C, Noble WH: Extravascular
lung water accumulation in patients following coronary artery surgery. Can Anaesth Soc
J 24:332–345, 1977
217. Lilleaasen P, Stokke O: Moderate and extreme hemodilution in open-heart surgery:
fluid balance and acid-base studies. Ann
Thorac Surg 25:127–133, 1978
218. Kopman EA, Ferguson TB: Pulmonary
edema following cardiopulmonary bypass.
Anesth Analg (Cleve) 57:367–371, 1978
219. Byrick RJ, Finlayson DC, Noble WH: Pulmonary arterial pressure increases during
cardiopulmonary bypass: a potential cause of
pulmonary edema. Anesthesiology 46:433–
435, 1977
220. Clarke CP, Kahn DR, Dufek JH et al: The
effects of nonpulsatile blood flow on canine
lungs. Ann Thorac Surg 6:450–457, 1968
221. Dobell ARC, Mitri M, Galva R et al: Biologic
evaluation of blood after prolonged recirculation through film and membrane oxygenators. Ann Surg 161:617–622, 1965
222. Brismar B, Gullbring B, Olsson P: Effects of
stored and fresh blood transfusions on postoperative pulmonary function. A clinical
study on patients following extracorporeal
circulation in association with aortic valve
surgery. Eur Surg Res 10:153–164, 1978

LONG TERM CARDIOPULMONARY BYPASS

References

223. Kolff WJ, Effler DB, Groves LK et al: Disposable membrane oxygenator (heat-lung machine) and its use in experimental surgery.
Cleve Clin Q 23:69–97, 1956
224. Bregman D (ed): Mechanical Support of the
Failing Heart and Lungs. New York, Appleton–Century Crofts, 1977

15

The Post-Bypass Period

RICHARD P. FOGDALL

INTRODUCTION

The post-bypass period is the increment of time between cessation of cardiopulmonary bypass (CPB) and the end of the operative stay. It represents only a portion of the operative and peripoerative continuum. In the previous chapter, there is a detailed discussion of the preparations necessary for successful discontinuation of cardiopulmonary bypass. The reader is referred again to the previous chapter, especially Tables 14–4 and 14–5, in order to comprehend fully the orderly transition from mechanical cardiopulmonary function, to the patient's own total cardiovascular and pulmonary function. This transition must be carefully controlled because a poorly performed transition can injure the patient. The pump is not just turned off, hoping for full and optimal patient performance! A myriad of variables must be examined continuously during this transition, and all changes performed gradually and deliberately, consistent with the patient's ability to adjust to them. Coordination between the members of the surgical team (anesthesiologist, surgeons, perfusionist, and surgical nurses) assures an orderly and successful transition into the post-bypass period.

Because both augmentation of cardiac function and alteration of vascular resistance are often desirable, a variety of cardioactive and vasoactive infusion drugs need to be available for post-bypass use. The choice and type will be individually determined by the nature and degree of cardiovascular disease and the desired cardiovascular alterations desired in the post-bypass period. For example, the 40-year-old "healthy" patient with good ventricular function, undergoing coronary artery bypass grafting, may need little cardiovascular drug manipulation post-bypass, usually limited to vasodilator therapy and propranolol. On the other hand, the 70-year-old patient with severe mitral and aortic stenosis and insufficiency, severe ventricular dysfunction, arrhythmias, digitalis toxicity, and elevated systemic vascular resistance might require treatment with every drug presented in this chapter. Each anticipated drug infusion should be readily available, and administered as indicated during discontinuance of bypass. Again the reader is reminded that simplicity in infusion equipment makes the anesthesiologist's (or critical care specialist's) job easier, and thus is safer for the patient. Post-bypass infusion drugs may be administered safely and adequately utilizing flow-restrictor devices (Dial-a-Flow), in place of costly, electrically driven, and bulky infusion pump systems.

PHILOSOPHY OF TRANSITION

The transfer of cardiopulmonary work and function from the mechanical pump to the patient depends upon the individual patient and upon the goals and principles for post-bypass management (Table 15–1). Myocardial oxygen supply must always exceeed, or at least equal, myocardial oxygen demand. Those factors affecting myocardial oxygen supply should be altered in such a way as to maximize myocardial oxygen supply (Table 15–2). Those factors affecting myocardial oxygen demand should be minimized consistent with optimal cardiac function (Table 15–3). Cardiac output should be high enough to supply sufficient blood flow and pressure to meet the total body requirements, but not beyond the heart's ability to sustain it or at the expense of optimizing efficiency by movement on the Starling curve.

Ventricular filling pressures should be adjusted with volume transfer from the pump reservoir to optimize preload. These will be individually determined endpoints, initially estimated, and then realized by trial-and-error for each patient. Renal function should be maintained by providing adequate cardiac

Table 15-1. Guiding Principles and Goals for Post-Bypass Patient Management

General
  Maintain all variables to where benefit exceeds risk, through effective monitoring.

Cardiovascular
  Maintain myocardial oxygen supply > demand.
  Maintain cardiac output sufficient for total body needs.
  Maintain heart rate 80–100 b p m—sinus rhythm.
  Optimize preload for best cardiovascular function.
  Maintain cardiac output by adjusting vascular volume, vascular resistance, and then contractility.
  Maintain systemic blood pressure first by adjusting vascular resistance.
  Maintain renal function by adequate CO and volume status, diuretics only as a secondary concern.

Respiratory
  Maintain PaO_2 125–150 torr.
  Maintain $PaCO_2$ and bicarbonate within normal ranges.
  Minimize reductions in FRC; prevent atelectasis.
  Maintain sufficient anesthesia and relaxation to match postoperative ventilatory plans.

Miscellaneous
  Maintain coagulation status within normal limits.
  Plan to have PCV in early postop period above 30%.
  Return rectal temperature to normal if possible.
  Maintain serum K^+ 5.0–5.5 mEq/l.
  Maintain serum ionized calcium in normal range.
  Anticipate the conceivable and plan.

Table 15-2. Factors Affecting Myocardial Oxygen Supply

Oxygen Availability of Coronary Perfusate
  Hemoglobin concentration
  Hemoglobin oxygen saturation
    PaO_2
    Hemoglobin type
    Acid-base status
    Temperature
    2,3-DPG concentration

Coronary Perfusion
  Diastolic arterial pressure ⎱ Coronary
  Intracardiac chamber pressures ⎰ Perfusion
    (LVEDP and RVEDP) ⎰ Pressure

  Percent of cardiac cycle in diastole (heart rate, contractility)
  Natural caliber of coronary vessels
  Obstructive lesions
  Viscosity of perfusate
  Regional and local vascular flow control mechanisms

Myocardial Tissue Function
  Metabolic factors controlling regional blood flow
  Drug toxicity

Table 15-3. Factors Affecting Myocardial Oxygen Demand

Ventricular Wall Tension
 Preload: end diastolic ventricular pressure
 Afterload: aortic root pressure when aortic value
  opens

Ventricular Contracility
 $\Delta P/\Delta t$ during ejection

Heart Rate
 Through effects on wall tension, contractility

Efficiency
 Position on starling curve
 Arrhythmias

output (and thus renal blood flow) and volume status, not just by driving urinary output with dopamine or diuretics or both. Control of afterload should be provided by decreasing systemic vascular resistance with vasodilating agents, rather than by withholding blood volume to lower blood pressure.

GENERAL SEQUENCE OF TRANSITION

The sequence of events *generally* followed in the cardiovascular transition is outlined in Table 15–4. First, cardiac rhythm is optimized, and then cardiac rate adjusted to between 80 and 100 beats per minute by chronotropic support, volume corrections, or beta adrenergic blockade, as needed. Ventricular filling pressures are then adjusted based upon direct measurement of mean central venous pressure ($\overline{\text{CVP}}$) (for the right ventricle) and mean pulmonary artery occluded pressure ($\overline{\text{PA}}_o$), or pulmonary artery diastolic pressure (PAD), or mean left atrial pressure ($\overline{\text{LAP}}$) (for the left ventricle).* Each patient's preload is optimized, based upon ventricular function at that specific moment, as determined by individual response. Mean arterial pressure (MAP; and hence "afterload") is then adjusted both with volume and ino-

tropic support, if lower than desired, or by decreasing systemic vascular resistance, if higher than desired. All of the above variables are then readjusted one by one, to further fine-tune the cardiovascular system. By adjusting only *one* variable at a time, each variable can be brought to optimal status. An excellent review is offered.[6]

CARDIOVASCULAR MANAGEMENT

CARDIAC RHYTHM

In order to optimize cardiac output, cardiac rhythm should be the best achievable for that patient; usually this means sinus rhythm. Loss of the atrial contraction (atrial kick), with the loss of sinus rhythm, can decrease cardiac output by at least 15 percent.[7] In some patients, however, sinus rhythm may not be obtainable (*e.g.*, chronic atrial fibrilla-

Table 15-4. Cardiovascular Adjustments Post-Bypass

Cardiac Rhythm
 Sinus rhythm preferred

Cardiac Rate (bpm)
  80–100 Preferred
  < 80 ⟶ Chronotropic Support
  >120 ⟶ Volume corrections or
    β-adrenergic blockade, or both

Adequate Ventricular Filling Pressures and Volumes
 Measure and individualize
 Optimize preload for patient's own ventricular
  function curve
 Change gradually

Adequate Mean Arterial Pressure
  < 60 torr ⟶ Volume and inotropic support
  60–90 torr ⟶ 1. If cardiac output OK:
     vasodilation
     volume infusion
    2. If cardiac output low:
     volume infusion
     vasodilation
     inotropic support
  > 90 torr ⟶ Reduce systemic vascular resistance

Readjust each of the above as needed, one variable
 at a time.

Consider Mechanical Assistance
 Intraaortic counterpulsation balloon or other

*Indications, contraindications, identity, and nonidentity of these various pressure recordings have already been covered in the monitoring chapters and elsewhere.[1-5] I shall not debate their relative values here. At Stanford, however, the use of the LAP catheter is extremely rare.

tion, complete heart block). Table 15–5 outlines the steps which can be taken to correct rhythm disturbances during the post-bypass period and in which order these corrections should occur. (For details of specific arrhythmias and treatment, see Chap. 6 and a separate review.[8])

PRELOAD (VOLUME ADMINISTRATION)

The *amount* of volume to infuse will depend upon the state of ventricular function, the use of vasoactive agents, renal status, and the level of hemostasis. The *type* of fluid will depend upon the coagulation status of the patient, the volume administered, the PCV (hematocrit) on bypass and desired PCV, and the availability of blood and blood products in an institution.

The initial infusion for vascular volume expansion ordinarily begins with transfer of volume from the pump oxygenator. Typically, the surgeon will have removed one of the two vena caval cannulae before discontinuing bypass. After bypass is discontinued and the patient is stable, the arterial cannula is then removed and inserted into the removed vena caval cannula. The return line to the oxygenator remains clamped, and the pump is then used to infuse through the arterial cannula and through the remaining vena cava cannula to the patient (Fig. 15–1).

We customarily reinfuse all of the remaining perfusate. Nitroprusside is used to provide vasodilation, while maintaining systemic arterial pressure at the originally desired value. When done properly, CVP slowly increases while MAP is held constant. The rate of infusion depends upon the state of myocardial contractility. In a failing or weak heart, too rapid an infusion can result in ventricular failure in the face of left-sided hypovolemia. By watching the pressures on both right and left sides, the progression of the infused volume through the patient's vascular system can be observed and the infusion rate adjusted. When the oxygenator volume is safely transferred to the patient, the remaining vena cava cannula is removed,

Table 15-5. Arrhythmia Management Post-Bypass

RHYTHM CONDITION	TREATMENT
Sinus rhythm ⟶	0
Nodal rhythm ⟶	0
Sinus bradycardia ⟶	Atropine Isoproterenol or dopamine Atrial pacemaker
Sinus tachycardia ⟶	Decrease chronotropic drugs Increase vascular volume Evaluate anesthetic status Switch to dobutamine (?) Consider cardiac glycosides/propranolol Atrial pacemaker overdrive (?)
PACs ⟶	0
PNCs ⟶	0
PVCs* ⟶	Check ventilation (and ABGs) Check K^+ (administer KCl 1–2 mEq/min) Consider magnesium sulfate (1–2g; 8–16 mEq) Lidocaine 1 mg/kg IV; infusion 2 mg/min Bretylium (?) Procainamide Quinidine
AV Dissociation 2° AV Block ⟶ 3° AV Block	Isoproterenol A-V sequential pacemaker Ventricular pacemaker
SVT Atrial fibrillation ⟶ Atrial flutter	Cardioversion Digitalis glycosides Verapamil Atrial pacemaker overdrive? A-V sequential pacemaker

Recurrent
  Ventricular
    fibrillation ⟶
  Ventricular
    tachycardia
	Look for treatable cause of ischemia!
	Lidocaine 2 mg/kg IV; infusion 3–4 mg/min
	KCl 2 mEq/min until $K^+ \geq$ 6.0 mEq/l
	Intraaortic counterpulsation balloon (IACPB)
	Magnesium sulfate 1–2g IV (8–16 mEq)
	Bretylium 8–10 mg/kg IV
	Procainamide
	Quinidine
	Propranolol (?)
	Experimental antiarrhythmic agents (?)
	Defibrillation

*Treat PVCs only if hemodynamically significant, or if runs of PCVs.

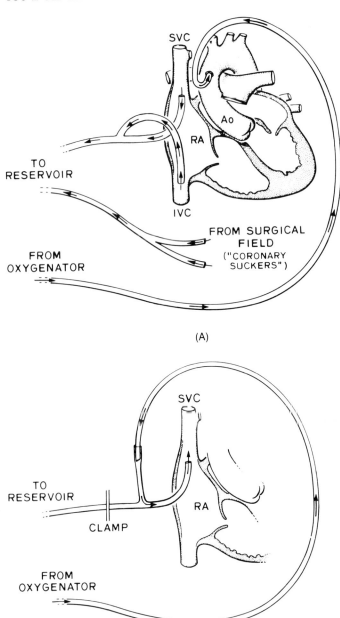

SVC

Ao

RA

IVC

TO
RESERVOIR

FROM
OXYGENATOR

FROM SURGICAL
FIELD
("CORONARY
SUCKERS")

(A)

SVC

RA

TO
RESERVOIR

CLAMP

FROM
OXYGENATOR

(B)

Fig. 15–1A, B. Volume Transfer from oxygenator to patient post-bypass. Note that flow in aortic in-flow line can move in one direction only; the pump cannot flow in reverse. Thus the aortic line is connected to one of the venous lines and the flow reversed in the remaining caval line for infusion.

and the patient thus totally disconnected from the bypass equipment.

Additional volume is then administered intravenously, and the patient is vasodilated to assure an adequate circulating blood volume and a normal or decreased systemic vascular resistance. The anesthesiologist thus is transferring the patient from a state of lower flow (CPB) to one of higher flow (post-CPB). Va-

sodilation and administration of warmed IV solutions and blood products facilitate patient warming.

Renal effects of fluid balance and cardiovascular performance are discussed in the chapter on renal function. The optimizing of preload has already been covered, based upon the response of the patient regarding ventricular function. Assuming a patient temperature greater than approximately 34°C, viscosity considerations related to blood temperature are not significant. Electrolyte replacement must be such that the venous serum K^+ is maintained between 5.0 and 5.5 mEq/l.[9] Serum total and ionized calcium should be normal, as should serum sodium and chloride. Potassium can be administered safely to the monitored adult patient at 2 mEq/min, and calcium at 200 mg/min. Calcium chloride, 1000 mg per each three units of CPD blood, should be administered to assure adequate Ca^{++} concentrations.

The controversy regarding vascular volume replacement with crystalloid versus colloid will not be resolved in this chapter.[10-13] Several points are without much controversy, however. Colloid solutions are vastly more expensive than crystalloid solutions (as high as 50 times the dollar cost). Patients receiving crystalloid, to equal the hemodynamic values of those receiving colloid, will receive higher volumes (two times) and gain more weight. Even though patients receiving crystalloid show a greater decrease in the colloid osmotic pressure than those receiving colloid, these changes are transient and not related to differences in patient outcome nor postoperative pulmonary status.

Thus the use of colloid (*i.e.,* albumin) in the post-bypass period must be considered as yet of unproven value. Certainly the use of salt-poor albumin, mixed with 0.9 percent sodium chloride solutions cannot be defended rationally. The cost of such a mixture approaches $250.00 per liter of 5 percent albumin mixture, and thus is markedly more expensive than a liter bottle of Ringer's lactate solution at approximately $2.00. We rarely use colloid solutions in the post-bypass period. Virgilio has nicely outlined this controversy for the reader.[13]

The PCV ideally should be maintained between 35 and 40 percent. This allows some margin for loss by bleeding or hemolysis, yet provides sufficient hemoglobin to provide substantial oxygen content to peripheral tissues (assuming optimal saturation). A lower PCV usually requires a higher cardiac output to deliver the same amount of oxygen to the periphery, which may place excessive demands on cardiac performance. A PCV above 40 percent is associated with a higher viscosity and thus peripheral sludging. A PCV greater than 40 percent also wastes precious blood products. The only patient in whom the PCV should be increased specifically above 40 percent is one in whom continued intracardiac shunting and desaturation necessitates a higher than normal hemoglobin concentration. The choice of post-bypass volume replacement is summarized in Table 15–6.

AFTERLOAD (CONTROL OF RESISTANCE AND PRESSURE)

For control of systemic vascular resistance and venous tone, intravenous vasodilating drugs of various arterial or venous activity are available. These drugs have already been discussed in Chapter 12. Table 15-7 compares the most useful of these drugs, their relative arterial and venous activities, and *usual* infusion dosages. Drugs with predominantly arterial effects are useful in treating high systemic vascular resistance, and thus produce afterload reduction. Those with predominantly venous activity are useful for reducing venous tone or to produce preload reduction. Trimethaphan, in addition to arterial and venous activity, provides sympathetic and parasympathetic ganglionic blockade, and is often limited in its use by the

Table 15-6. Choice of Replacement Fluids for Deficient Vascular Volume

PCV < 25%	PCV 25–35%	PCV 35–40%	PCV > 40%
Packed red cells (or whole blood)	Whole blood 2 parts to crystalloid 1 part (fresh frozen plasma can substitute for crystalloid in a ratio of 1:2)	Crystalloid 2 parts to whole blood 1 part (fresh frozen plasma can substitute for crystalloid in a ratio of 1:2)	Crystalloid (fresh frozen plasma can subsitute for crystalloid in a ratio of 1:2)

Table 15-7. Intravenous Vasodilator Drugs

DRUG	ARTERIAL ACTIVITY 0–4	VENOUS ACTIVITY 0–4	INFUSION PREPARATION	INFUSION CONCENTRATION	INFUSION DOSAGE	COMMENTS
Hydralazine (Apresoline)	4	1	*	*	2–3 mg*	Vascular smooth muscle relaxation
Phentolamine (Regitine)	4	1	25 mg/250 ml	100 μg/ml	1–10 μg/kg/min	α Blockade ↓ Pulmonary vascular resistance (?)
Chlorpromazine (Thorazine)	3	2	†	†	1–2 mg†	α Blockade CNS sedation
Trimethaphan (Arfonad)	3	2	500 mg/500 ml	1000 μg/ml	5–20 μg/kg/min	Tachycardia common Sympathetic and parasympathetic blockade
Nitroprusside (Nipride)	3	2	50 mg/250 ml	200 μg/ml	0.5–3 μg/kg/min	Excessive dosage > 5 μg/kg/min prone to → cyanide toxicity Reflex tachycardia common
Nitroglycerin	1	4	50 mg/250 ml	200 μg/ml	1–5 μg/kg/min	Tachycardia less common

*Hydralazine used rarely as continuous infusion; usually administered in 2–3 mg IV increments. Time from injection to maximum activity approximately 30 minutes
†Chlorpromazine used rarely as continuous infusion; usually administered in 1–2 mg IV increments
(See also Chapter 12)

severe tachycardia which may accompany its vagal blockade. By controlling resistance in either or both arterial and venous vascular beds, and then restoring preload to higher levels with further volume administration, cardiac output *may* be optimized without the use of inotropic or chronotropic drugs.

INOTROPIC MANAGEMENT

For ease of discussion, diagnosis, and treatment, the status of cardiac output post-by-pass can be categorized into *lower-than-normal* or *higher-than-normal*. The most disturbing of these is the low cardiac output state, for it indicates profound circulatory problems and is associated with higher postoperative morbidity and mortality. Certainly, the major organ systems (CNS, cardiac, pulmonary, renal, and hepatic) will be in jeopardy during low cardiac output states. It should go without saying that the only way to *know* what the cardiac output is, is to *directly measure* it. Indirect measures *estimating* cardiac output are employed by many physicians: warming, blanching, width of pulse pressure, visual observations of the heart and great vessels, and so on. Under conditions of hemody-

namic stability and relatively good health, these serve well. Under conditions of extreme hemodynamic instability and severe pathophysiology, more direct and precise measures are necessary.

In order to understand and use relationships between end diastolic pressure and volume and measures of cardiac performance, the use of a ventricular function curve is imperative. It might not actually be constructed during the care of a patient (although to do so is most informative and useful), but its principles should be utilized. Such a curve is demonstrated in Figure 15-2. While it is only one such curve, it uses variables of a clinical, and thus useful, nature.

During normal ventricular function, an increase in the filling pressure provides an increase in output. If ventricular function is depressed, a given filling pressure will provide a lower output, and a flatter curve with a smaller slope will be seen. Such a depression might be caused by propranolol, halothane, ischemia, or nitrous oxide. In order to obtain a higher output, a greatly increased filling pressure would be required.

If ventricular function is enhanced above normal, for instance by endogenous or exogenous catecholamines, or occasionally by afterload reduction, the output for a given filling pressure will be higher than normal. The slope of the curve will be steeper. It is important that the entire triad of relationships shown in Figure 15-2 (filling pressure, cardiac performance, and inotropic state) be considered during manipulations of the cardiovascular system. All are irrevocably interrelated. (See Chapters 2, 11, and elsewhere[14] for further study.)

If inotropic drug support is required, the choice of drug to be infused should be based upon the known pathophysiology presently confronting the physician, and the known pharmacologic aspects of the various drugs. The drug should be tailored to produce only those effects desired. For an inotropic drug, obviously positive inotropism is desired, but chronotropic activity may or may not be. If one also desires to increase heart rate or A-V conduction, then a drug such as isoproterenol may be useful. On the other hand, if an increase in heart rate or A-V conduction is undesirable, then perhaps dobutamine would be a better choice[15, 16]. If dopaminergic renal effects are desired, dopamine in moderate dose could be chosen. Table 15-8 compares the presently useful intravenous

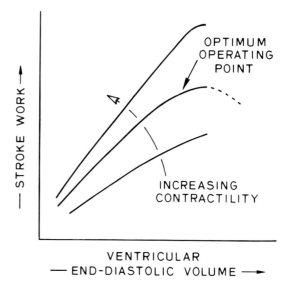

Fig. 15–2. One type of ventricular function curve. Basic relationship is one comparing changes in end diastolic fiber length and a measure of ventricular performance. Horizontal axis is the filling volume of each ventricle. The vertical axis represents cardiac work, usually correlating with stroke work. End-diastolic pressure and MAP may serve as rough substitutes in some cases. Interpretations and limitations are explained in text.

Table 15-8. Intravenous Intotropic Drugs*

INOTROPIC DRUG	CHRONOTROPIC ACTIVITY 0–4	INFUSION PREPARATION	INFUSION CONCENTRATION	INFUSION DOSAGE	COMMENTS
Isoproterenol (Isuprel)	4	1 mg/250 ml	4 μg/ml	1–4 μg/min	Tachycardia expected Arrhythmias likely
Epinephrine (Adrenaline)	3	1 mg/250 ml	4 μg/ml	1–4 μg/min	Tachycardia likely Arrhythmias likely
Dopamine (Intropin)	2	200 mg/250 ml	800 μg/ml	1–20 μg/kg/min	Renal effects from 1–10 μg/kg/min Alpha predominates above 10 μg/kg/min Arrhythmias uncommon
Dobutamine (Dubutrex)	1–2	250 mg/250 ml	1000 μg/ml	1–20 μg/kg/min	Arrhythmias rare Increases blood flow to skeletal muscle
Calcium Chloride	0	2.5 g/50 ml	50 mg/ml	1–2 mg/kg/min	ECG abnormalities shortened QT interval Enhances digitalis effect and toxicity Hazardous in hypokalemic conditions Short-acting

*See also Chapter 11.

Table 15-9. Etiology of Low Cardiac Output Post-Bypass

CARDIAC ORIGIN
  Arrhythmias
    Tachyarrhythmias
    Bradyarrhythmias
    A-V block
    Multiple premature beats
  Failure of supply
    Ischemia
    Emboli
  Myocardial dysfunction
    2° Hx CPB ischemia
    Cardiomyopathy
  Mechanical dysfunction
    Valvular
    Surgical technical error
    Direct cardiac or coronary injury

EXTRACARDIAC ORIGIN
  Myocardial depression
    Inhalation anesthetics
    β-Blocking drugs
    Calcium binding
    Electrolyte abnormalities
    Acid-base abnormalities
    Hypoxemia
    Sepsis
  Low preload or poor filling or both
    Volume depletion
    Pericardial tamponade
    Pneumothorax (left heart)
  High Afterload
    High systemic vascular resistance
    Pneumothorax (right heart)
    Poorly timed intraaortic counterpulsation balloon

inotropic drugs. The reader will note the absence of norepinephrine, a drug rarely used in modern cardiac anesthesia because of its many undesirable potent alpha effects.

It is common for us to combine the use of an inotropic drug with a vasodilating drug, thus achieving an improvement in ventricular function both by inotropic enhancement and by concomitant afterload reduction. Dopamine-nitroprusside, dobutamine-nitroprusside, dopamine-nitroglycerin, and dobutamine-nitroglycerin are favorite combinations. When used in this manner, the vasodilating drug is administered in a dose necessary to achieve optimal afterload or preload or both. This dose is often found to be in the range of 1 to 3 µg/kg/min. Then the inotropic drug is administered at a rate producing an optimal heart rate, often at a dose of from 2 to 10 µg/kg/min.

LOW CARDIAC OUTPUT

The causes of low cardiac output can be divided into cardiac and extracardiac (Table 15-9). Some causes can be measured, some must be suspected, and some may or may not be treatable. Persistent cardiac arrest may follow cardioplegic solution.[17] Arrhythmias should be treated according to Table 15-5. Myocardial ischemia should be treated by increasing coronary perfusion (maximizing myocardial oxygen supply; see Table 15-2) and decreasing myocardial oxygen demand (see Table 15-3). Residual valvular abnormalities or surgical technical errors will require direct surgical intervention. Preexisting cardiomyopathy may not be treatable, but instead will require substantial inotropic support, afterload reduction, and perhaps mechanical assistance to achieve even marginal ventricular function.

Two common extracardiac causes of a low cardiac output are an abnormally low ventricular filling pressure for that patient and an abnormally high systemic vascular resistance (> 1200 dynes-sec-cm^{-5}). The treatment of low filling pressures is restoration of preload to achieve greater ventricular end-diastolic fiber stretching. If venodilating agents are being administered (such as nitroglycerin), these may need concomitant dose reduction to achieve optimal preload restoration. The treatment of an abnormally high systemic vascular resistance is the judicious use of vasodilating agents which act on the arterial circulation, such as chloropromazine, hydralazine, or sodium nitroprusside. Nitroglycerin does not serve as well to accomplish pure afterload reduction (see Chapter 12 for details).

Electrolyte abnormalities contributing to reduced ventricular contractility include hypocalcemia, hyperkalemia, and hypermagnesemia. Obviously, hypoxemia and acidosis reduce optimal ventricular function. Pericardial tamponade, or other space-occupying compression (e.g., pneumothorax) may impair cardiac filling or emptying and thus reduce cardiac output. Sepsis also may contribute to decreased ventricular performance.

The detailed treatment of low cardiac out-

Hemodynamic Conditions   Initial Treatment

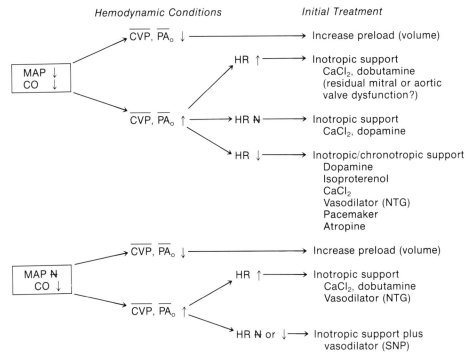

Fig. 15–3. Treatment of low cardiac output.

put is outlined in Figure 15-3. If obvious left ventricular failure occurs or insufficient cardiac output or both cannot be obtained with the sequence of treatment outlined above, mechanical assistance with an intraaortic counterpulsation balloon may be indicated.

INTRAAORTIC BALLOON ASSISTANCE

The detailed understanding and use of the intraaortic counterpulsation balloon (IACPB) is discussed in Chapter 27. However its greatest use in cardiac surgery is in the post-bypass period. Patients most likely to benefit from its use are those with ischemic ventricular dysfunction, secondary to coronary artery disease. It is the only present method by which myocardial perfusion can be increased, concomitant with a reduction in myocardial work. There is presently no pharmacologic counterpart. Simply, its basic design is that of an elongated gas-filled balloon surgically placed in the descending aorta. Immediately before left ventricular ejection, it rapidly deflates, lowering aortic pressure during ejection and thus reducing left ventricular work and increasing stroke volume. During diastole, it reinflates, increasing coronary and systemic perfusion pressure.

There are various sizes and types of balloons. The device must be triggered and coordinated with the cardiac cycle, from either the ECG or the arterial waveform, and thus requires a nonchaotic cardiac rhythm and a rate of preferably less than 130 beats per minute. It performs poorly during the use of electrocautery equipment, if triggering is provided by the ECG signal. It can be triggered by a pacemaker, if the pacemaker is not operating on a demand mode during electrocautery. It also requires an intact (nonregurgitant) aortic valve, and an aorta acceptable in structure to receive the device. At present, there is no right ventricular counterpart balloon useful for successful implantation into the pulmonary artery, although aortic implantation has been reported to improve right ventricular function.[18] An example of a radial

INTRAORTIC COUNTERPULSATION
BALLOON FUNCTION

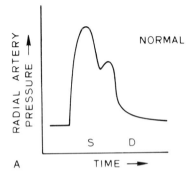

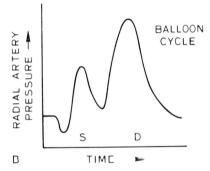

Fig. 15–4. Intraaortic counterpulsation balloon function. *A.* Normal; *B.* Balloon cycle. Schematic diagram of the effect of an intraaortic counterpulsation balloon on radial artery pressure. *S* = systole (LV ejection); *D* = diastole (LV filling and coronary artery filling). Note the reduction of systolic pressure during balloon deflation, providing easier left ventricular ejection into a lower pressure area. Note also an increase in the diastolic pressure, and a larger pressure-time area during diastole, enhancing coronary perfusion.

artery pressure waveform during use of the IACPB is demonstrated in Figure 15-4. Excellent coordination between the anesthesiologist and the specialist operating the IACPB is mandatory for optimal cardiovascular function. (See Chaps. 16 and 27 for a complete discussion.)

HIGH CARDIAC OUTPUT

The presence of a high cardiac output, or a hyperdynamic state, is seen occasionally post-bypass. The most common instance is seen in a healthy young patient after uncomplicated coronary artery bypass grafting, aortic valve replacement, or other procedures (*e.g.,* sinus of Valsalva aneurysm resection, uncomplicated ASD or VSD repair). The cardiac output should be high enough for total body needs and some reserve, but not so high as to be detrimental to myocardial oxygen supply and demand relationships. Often, the excessive use of arterial vasodilators (SNP) and inotropic agents, hypervolemia, or inadequate anesthesia, contributes to such a hyperdynamic state. In addition, many of these patients are in a state of acute drug withdrawal from preoperative antihypertensive and β-blocking drugs.

The etiology should be explored, and the cause treated (Fig. 15-5). There should be little hesitation to treat such a patient with *judiciously* administered increments (0.20–0.40 mg) of intravenous propranolol, as indicated, until tachycardia and hypertension are controlled. Vasodilators, such as nitroglycerin, which have less effect on arterial vasomotor tone (and thus less reflex tachycardia) should be used. Trimethaphan does not offer any advantages in this setting, because of vagal blockade-induced tachycardia. Regional anesthesia (stellate-ganglion block) has been used successfully as well.[19]

Rarely, a patient is seen with a high cardiac output but a low MAP. Calculated systemic vascular resistance is almost always very low. This patient is markedly arterially vasodilated (*e.g.*, sepsis, histamine release, hyperthyroid) and may be treated by fluid administration or by a judicious increase in systemic vascular resistance, or both, usually with an α drug, such as a phenylephrine infusion. Management of such a patient is summarized in Figure 15-6.

RESPIRATORY MANAGEMENT

Postoperative respiratory abnormalities or hypoxemia may be of cardiac or noncardiac origin.[20-23] The control of ventilatory function and resulting respiratory effectiveness should be governed by the principles and goals of respiratory management (see Table 15-1). Accurate and complete assessment of ventilatory function cannot be achieved without arterial blood gases, even if volume or pressure respiratory measurements are made. End-tidal CO_2 measurement is invaluable in minute-to-minute assessment of CO_2 elimination, dead-space changes, pulmonary artery emboli, and airway disconnection.

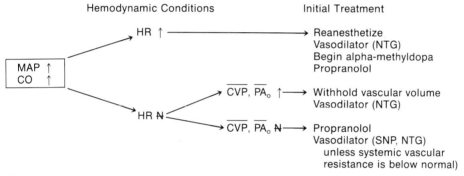

Fig. 15–5. Treatment of the hyperdynamic patient. Catecholamines and $CaCl_2$ are withheld.

Fig. 15–6. Treatment of the high cardiac output, low resistance state. Isoproterenol, $CaCl_2$ and dobutamine should be withheld. Sepsis, hyperthyroid state, and other noncardiac problems should be treated.

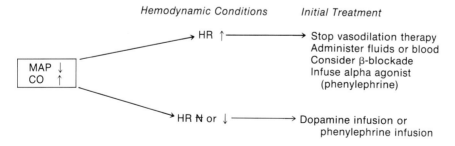

Table 15-10. Respiratory Management of PaO₂

	F_IO_2 = 1.0		
< 100 torr	100–300 torr	> 300 torr
↑ V_T	↑ V_T to maximum 18 ml/kg	↓ F_IO_2
PEEP	PEEP	PEEP
Suction if needed	Inflation hold	
Inflation hold	(Non-pulmonary shunting?)	
↑ Vascular Volume?		
(Nonpulmonary shunting?)		

	F_IO_2 = 0.5		
< 100 torr	100–200 torr	> 200 torr
Same as above and ↑ F_IO_2	V_T ≥ 15 ml/kg PEEP	↓ F_IO_2 to 0.4 PEEP

Table 15-11. Respiratory Management of PaCO₂

< 35 TORR	35–40 TORR	> 40 TORR
Decrease minute ventilation ↓ respiratory frequency and/or Add deadspace	No changes	Increase minute ventilation ↑ V_T ↑ respiratory frequency CO_2 being administered? Hyperthermia present? PaO₂ OK?

Measurement of airway pressure at the level of the endotracheal tube allows calculation of pulmonary compliance if tidal volume is measured concomitantly, and also confirms the correct application of positive end expiratory pressure (PEEP) devices.[24]

In the adult patient, the PaO₂ should be maintained in the range of from 125 to 150 torr. This will ensure as completely as possible the oxygen saturation of hemoglobin, even if changes in intracardiac or pulmonary shunting occur to lower the PaO₂ by 20 to 30 percent. There is no need to maintain the PaO₂ at greater than 150 torr (which usually requires an F_IO_2 greater than 0.4). A prolonged exposure to an F_IO_2 greater than 0.5 may contribute to pulmonary oxygen toxicity. In the operative setting, the desired F_IO_2 can be provided by dilution of oxygen with air or nitrous oxide, if there are no contraindications to the use of nitrous oxide in a specific patient. If the PaO₂ decreases below 100 torr, the likelihood of reduced hemoglobin saturation is increased. Such a reduced hemoglobin saturation might necessitate an increase in cardiac output in order to provide suffi-

cient oxygen delivery to the tissues. This would be detrimental to a patient whose cardiac output could not be increased without damagingly high myocardial oxygen consumption. Adjustment of the PaO₂ under various circumstances is detailed in Table 15-10.

The PaCO₂ and bicarbonate should be maintained within, or near, normal ranges, so that the arterial pH remains within its normal limits. In that manner, no acid-base shifting of the oxyhemoglobin dissociation curve will occur. In addition, a normal pH will prevent shifting of various cations, such as K^+ and Ca^{++}, as a result of acid-base abnormalities. In addition, catecholamines are less effective under conditions of acidosis. Tables 15-11 and 15-12 describe the basic management plan for controlling PaCO₂ and bicarbonate levels post-bypass.

Post-bypass, the patient's functional residual capacity (FRC) should be at least as high as in the preoperative state. The supine position, and effects of nonventilation during bypass already will have decreased the FRC. The prevention of airway closure and resulting atelectasis is a prime respiratory post-bypass goal. This can be accomplished with the aid of a relatively high tidal volume (12–15 ml/kg), slow inhalation gas flow, and after chest closure, the application of PEEP (commonly 5–8 cm H_2O)[25-28] and inspiratory hold (inflation hold or inflation pause).[29] (See Table 15-10 and Fig. 15-7.) PEEP must be adjusted for optimal effect,[30, 31] realizing that possible PEEP-induced alterations in hemodynamic variables may occur.[32] Hand ventilation, with Valsalva maneuvers, also will aid in reducing or correcting atelectasis. The most commonly used respiratory variables are V_T = 12–15 ml/kg; f = 7–8 breaths/minute; PEEP = 5–8 cm H_2O; F_1O_2 as indicated; inflation hold (if available) 0.5–0.8 seconds.

The respiratory management plan selected for the first several hours of the postoperative period will determine (and be determined by) the level of anesthesia provided by the anesthesiologist in the post-bypass period. It must be remembered that the prebypass, bypass, post-bypass, and early postoperative periods are all parts of a continuum. If the postoperative plan in a specific practice routinely employs early extubation (for purposes here meaning endotracheal extubation in the first several hours) for uncomplicated, non-critical patients, then the use of long-acting, high-dosage intravenous anesthetic agents (*e.g.,* morphine, fentanyl, diazepam) must be minimized, especially in the post-bypass period. Anesthesia then must be supplied by low-dose, short-acting intravenous drugs, or inhalation anesthetic agents such as nitrous oxide, halothane, enflurane, or isoflurane.

Table 15-12. Respiratory Management of Bicarbonate

< 21 mEq/l	21–26 mEq/l	> 26 mEq/l
Correct circulatory status and PaO_2 HCO_3^- administration [(24 − value) × 0.3 × kg body weight] (in mEq)	No changes	Stop bicarb/lactate administration if $PaCO_2$ normal ↓ Respiratory frequency and/or Add deadspace

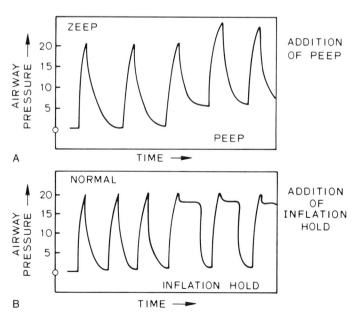

Fig. 15–7. Schematic diagram of the changes in airway pressure with two patterns of controlled ventilation. *A.* Addition of PEEP increases end-expiratory pressure and all subsequent pressures in airway. *B.* Addition of inflation hold (inspiratory hold) increases time at near-peak (*plateau*) pressure, allowing for better distribution of gas to distal airways.

On the other hand, if the postoperative plan is to maintain the patient intubated for longer periods (*e.g.*, 6–12 hours or more, overnight routinely), then post-bypass anesthetic management should include longer-acting drugs such as morphine, hydromorphone, high-dose fentanyl, and diazepam, to provide a smooth introduction into the postoperative period. I shall not debate here all of the pros and cons of each end of the spectrum. Points of view on both ends are held strongly, with "scientific" data supporting each.[33, 34] If the patient is hemodynamically unstable or shivering, is bleeding, is a "redo," or has a history of respiratory dis-

ease, early extubation is not recommended. With sedation and adequately monitored controlled ventilation, full attention can be paid to early cardiovascular and hemostatic management, unhampered by patient struggling, shivering, moving, coughing, and the like. What is most important is that the post-bypass anesthesia plan be coordinated with the early postoperative ICU plan, consistent with patient status, and found successful in practice.

MANAGEMENT OF HEMOSTASIS AND COAGULATION

A thorough discussion of hemostasis and coagulation is provided in Chapter 24 and in a clinically-oriented coagulation textbook.[35] The discussion here focuses on the evaluation and treatment of post-bypass bleeding.

THEORY

The intent of the hemostatic system is the prevention of blood loss from the vascular compartment without hindrance to blood flow. Hemostasis depends upon the interplay of four components: maintenance of vascular integrity, platelet function, the coagulation cascade production of fibrin, and the eventual removal of fibrin by fibrinolysis. Derangements of each of these four components may exist in the patient post-bypass and are summarized in Table 15-13. The problem is in the identification of the exact cause of bleeding, especially if multiple causes are possible. *Usually* a single cause is preeminent. However, multiple abnormalities may be present, especially if bleeding is long-term or if blood component therapy has already begun. In addition, multiple abnormalities may coexist independently (*e.g.*, an open blood vessel within the patient's chest along with continued heparin effect).

There are many reasons why precise identification is important. Death may ensue if bleeding is profound. Sublethal organ injury may result from prolonged hypoten-

Table 15-13. Hemostatic Abnormalities Which May Occur After Cardiopulmonary Bypass

Vascular Integrity Defect
  Surgical holes
  Hypertension: arterial or venous
  Intimal vascular damage from atherosclerosis
  Inflammatory process (endocarditis, vasculitis)

Platelet Dysfunction or Deficiency
  Quantitative disorder from sequestration, dilution, or destruction
  Qualitative disorders
    Drugs: ASA, dextran, aminoglycosides, or protamine
    Effects of fibrin split products
    Storage defects in transfused platelets
    Presence of uremic plasma

Coagulation Cascade
  Hypothermia (decreased enzymatic reaction rates)
  Inactive factor deficiencies
    Dilution, destruction, consumption (V, VIII, I, AT-3)
    Coumadin therapy ⎫
    Hepatic dysfunction ⎬ (II, VII, IX, X)
    Dilution ⎭
  Active factor deficiencies
    Heparin effect (II, VII, IX, X, XI)
    Inhibition by fibrin split products

Increased Fibrinolysis
  DIC with increased fibrinolysis, secondary to inadequate heparinization, deficiency of AT-3, circulating tissue phospholipids, sepsis, and so on.
  Fibrinolysis secondary to streptokinase therapy
  Hemolytic anemia secondary to transfusion reaction
        (Combinations of any of the above)

(Modified from Fischbach DP, Fogdall RP: Coagulation: The Essentials. Baltimore, Williams and Wilkins 1981.

sion. Drug and blood therapy are expensive and some drugs and blood products carry hazards. Treatment with the wrong therapy delays curative therapy. "Shotgun" therapy (the administration of every possible treatment mode simultaneously) is expensive, hazardous, and wasteful of valuable human blood components, and is *rarely* indicated.

What is important, then, is the learning of a systemic approach to the bleeding patient, such that rapid and correct diagnosis will lead to proper treatment. Unless the exact cause is *clearly* obvious, a learned systematic approach will produce greatest success. Remember that horses are more common than zebras (unless one lives in the zoo). Improper use of heparin and protamine (especially if give by formulas) is more common than hemophilia. Untied and uncauterized blood vessels are more common than fibrinolysis with hemolytic anemia. The reader is referred to Figure 15-8 for a flow chart summary of analysis and treatment of bleeding.[35]

Maintenance of vascular integrity post-bypass is the primary responsibility of the surgeon. The likelihood of a surgical vascular defect is inversely proportional to surgical skill, care, and experience. A thorough post-bypass closure of all bleeding sites, or potential bleeding areas, is imperative. Open blood vessels, or failed surgical sutures, will allow bleeding without regard to the status of the other three hemostatic components. Suspicion is needed. Indirect evaluations such as angiography may be helpful, but direct surgical inspection, with corrective surgical therapy, will be necessary if the cause is a vascular defect.

Platelet function requires an adequate number of circulating normal platelets. Platelets serve as an initial plug for small vascular defects, and also as the substrate upon which the enzymatic reactions of the coagulation cascade occur. They may be deficient in number (dilution, destruction, or sequestration), or deficient in function (drugs, presence of fibrin split products, uremic plasma, von Willebrand's disease), or both. The platelet count measures only platelet number. The bleeding time evaluates both number and function. If the bleeding time is normal, platelet administration is not required. If the bleeding time is prolonged, platelet therapy will be required during bleeding, along with other adjunctive therapies (see Fig. 15-8). If cardiopulmonary bypass has been prolonged, post-bypass platelet administration is likely. Platelets are administered as indicated by testing, usually at the dose of 1 platelet pack unit per 10 kg body weight if platelet count is less than $60,000/mm^3$, or bleeding time is greater than approximately 15 minutes, or both. After administration, several hours may be required for normal function of the transfused platelets because of storage defects.[35]

A precise determination of the location of an abnormality in the coagulation cascade is important. If the abnormality is one produced by inhibitors (heparin activated antithrombin, or presence of uremic plasma or fibrin split products), the treatment will be aimed at the removal or correction of the inhibitor. If the abnormality is caused by a factor deficiency, the factor will require replacement with administered blood products. Administration of blood products will not cure heparin effect. Administration of protamine will not cure bleeding from hypofibrinogenemia. The reader is referred to the coagulation cascade section of Figure 15-8.

The performance of an activated clotting time (ACT) or activated partial thromboplastin time (aPTT) screens effectively virtually all of the coagulation cascade except factor VII. The endpoint of all tests for evaluation of the coagulation cascade is the production of a fibrin clot. Sample contamination by heparin must be avoided.[36] If the clot is formed effectively (normal ACT or aPTT), neither inhibitors nor factor deficiencies have been demonstrated. If the ACT or aPTT is abnormal, either inhibitors or deficiencies exist. The reactions of the coagulation cascade are enzymatic; hypothemia will reduce the speed to formation of fibrin and prolong clinical bleeding. The tests are run at 37°C, which may speed up the reactions to normal in the

SUMMARY
ANALYSIS AND TREATMENT OF POST-BYPASS BLEEDING

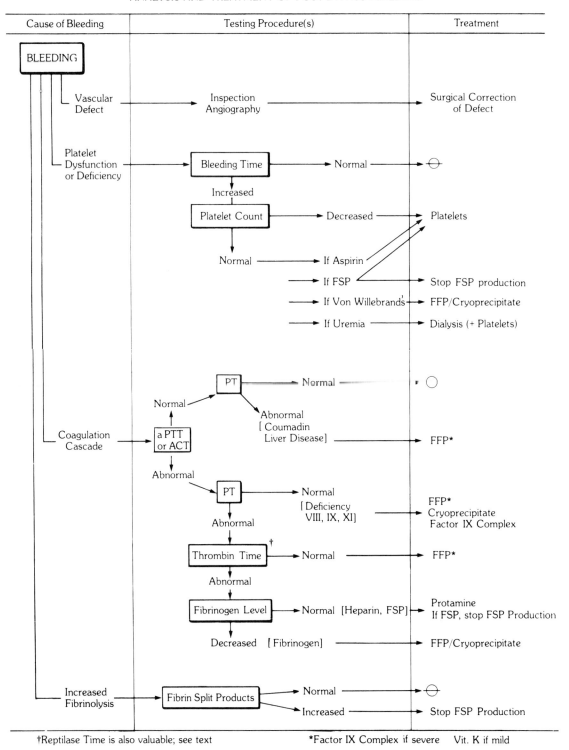

†Reptilase Time is also valuable; see text   *Factor IX Complex if severe   Vit. K if mild

laboratory. The thrombin time (TT) is a sensitive test for inhibitors and fibrinogen deficiency. If the thrombin time is normal, there is *no* significant heparin effect! If the thrombin time is abnormal, either heparin is present, fibrinogen is abnormal or low, fibrin split products are inhibiting fibrin cross-linking, or uremic plasma is present. The Reptilase time is similar to the thrombin time, but this enzyme (Reptilase-R) is not affected by heparin (or antithrombin). Thus if the ACT and thrombin time are abnormal and the reptilase time is normal, heparin is most likely the coagulation cascade cause of bleeding. Factor deficiencies are treated usually with fresh frozen plasma or cryoprecipitate (factors VIII, I, von Willebrand's). A more thorough discussion is offered.[35]

Increased fibrinolysis is rarely a cause for bleeding post-bypass. If heparinization during bypass has been inadequate, and fibrin formation has occurred in large amounts because of exposure of inadequately heparinized blood to artificial surfaces, increased fibrinolysis may be present. If so, the production of fibrin split products (FSP) will be increased and, unless cleared rapidly by the reticuloendothelial system, FSP levels will be elevated. A test for FSP will confirm this if positive. A negative test for FSP indicates a low level of FSP, either because of little fibrinolysis or because of depleted fibrin or fibrinogen. Presence of FSP in this clinical setting is treated by stopping the cause of FSP production, and by allowing time for hepatic and reticuloenthelial FSP clearance.

PRACTICE

In practice, the sequence offered above is altered slightly in the immediate 10 to 20 minutes post-bypass. Because heparin was used during bypass to prevent coagulation during mechanical support, its effects must be antagonized. Protamine sulfate is the preferred antagonist. Its dose must be *calculated* from the *effect* of heparin at the end of bypass, not estimated from some arbitrary formula. The protamine dose can be calculated readily from the ACT simply and inexpensively performed by the anesthesiologist. It requires no laboratory nor extraneous personnel, to perform a clinically useful ACT. The goal is to administer enough protamine to antagonize the effects of heparin, but not excessive amounts, which may produce hemodynamic problems. The actual technique employed in determining the protamine dosage and measuring the effects of either heparin or protamine on the ACT are covered in Chapter 24 and elsewhere.[35] Once the dose has been calculated (often 300–400 mg), it is administered after bypass has been *completely* terminated, at the administered rate of approximately 25 to 50 mg (2.5–5.0 ml) per minute. Protamine should not be administered until the surgeons are satisfied that *surgical* bleeding is controlled and that myocardial function is adequate, removing the risk of returning to bypass. When protamine is begun, it is the anesthesiologist's responsibility to ensure that the perfusionist is aware of protamine administration and has turned off the coro-

---

Fig. 15–8. Analysis and treatment of Post-Bypass bleeding. Analysis of a bleeding patient post-bypass requires an evaluation of abnormalities in each of the four major components of hemostasis: vascular integrity defect, platelet dysfunction, coagulation factor inhibition or deficiency, and increased fibrinolysis. If tests for platelet function, coagulation cascade, and fibrinolysis are all normal, and the patient is still bleeding, one of three problems exists: the tests are incorrect, the patient is substantially hypothermic, or there is surgical bleeding requiring reoperation. *FSP* = fibrin split products; *FFP* = fresh frozen plasma; *PT* = prothrombin time; *aPTT* = activated partial thromboplastin time; *ACT* = activated clotting time. See text and reference below for more detail. (Modified from Fischbach DP, Fogdall RP: Coagulation: The Essentials. Baltimore, Williams & Wilkins, 1981)

nary suction. *No blood containing protamine should be returned to the oxygenator!* This would make the oxygenator and CPB circuit useless if a return to CPB were required.

Excessively high protamine administration rates produce myocardial depression or vasodilation and resultant hypotension, seen on the arterial pressure waveform.[37-40] Rapid protamine administration at this point may bind calcium and magnesium.[41] In addition, protamine may produce histamine release in susceptible patients, leading to abrupt hypotension.[42] These are usually patients with fish allergies because protamine is produced from salmon semen. Protamine has been reported to alter plasma-free propranolol levels.[43] If excessive myocardial depression occurs, filling pressures will tend to increase, as opposed to decreased filling pressures seen with abrupt vasodilation. Excessive myocardial depression from protamine responds to administration of calcium chloride (7–15 mg/kg). Excessive vasodilation responds to the judicious use of positioning and α vasopressors (such as phenylephrine, 10–40 microgram increments IV).

Other coagulation blood products (*e.g.,* platelets, fresh frozen plasma) should not be administered until the ACT has been returned to normal or to its lowest obtainable value with protamine. It does little good to waste valuable platelets or plasma products in the still heparinized, bleeding patient.

Administration of blood and blood products carries risks, specifically those of hepatitis and transfusion reaction.[35] The risk of hepatitis is also of concern to those who handle, prepare, or administer blood products. The risk of hepatitis is inversely proportional to the quality of the blood donors available to each institution. The risk of transfusion reaction relates to the care provided in type and cross-matching of each unit and the care taken in administration to the correct patient. Micro filters (20 μ) may minimize the hazard of IV debris administration but are controversial. All blood or plasma should be warmed to 37°C unless the patient is hyperthermic.

If cardiopulmonary bypass has exceeded 2 hours in duration, if the platelet count is less than 100,000/mm^3, if the bleeding time is greater than 8–10 minutes, if the patient has been administered aspirin within 3-5 days, or if the patient is a "redo," platelets usually are administered. If bleeding is mild, two to three platelet packs are infused; if severe, five to eight platelet packs are infused through a platelet filtration administration set. Platelets should *not* be administered through a blood microfilter (20 μ). The platelet count should increase in the adult by approximately 10,000/mm^3 for each platelet pack unit administered, but normal platelet function will be delayed.[35]

Fresh frozen plasma (FFP) should be reserved for those patients who are bleeding, in whom the ACT has been reduced to its lowest obtainable value post-bypass with protamine, and in whom the platelet function is normal (or has been normalized by platelet administration). FFP or concentrated plasma factors (factor IX concentrates) should be given *only* if their constituents have been shown to be deficient or defective in the bleeding patient, by appropriate coagulation testing. Each FFP unit of approximately 250 ml replaces approximately 8 percent of an adult's normal circulating plasma factors. FFP is administered to the bleeding patient (after protamine treatment above) based upon the prothrombin time (PT) as follows:

PT	> 60%	0
PT	40–60%	10 ml/kg IV
PT	20–40%	20 ml/kg IV
PT	< 20%	30 ml/kg IV (+ factor IX concentrates)

Vasodilation with drugs such as nitroprusside or nitroglycerin may be required to increase vascular space to accommodate such blood products.

If the bleeding time, ACT, PT, and TT are all within normal limits and the patient is still bleeding, one of three circumstances exists: (1) the tests are in error; (2) the patient is substantially hypothermic and the tests (run at 37°C) are not representative of the patient's *in vivo* slow coagulation status; or (3) there are leaks in the operative field. The treatment for the first circumstance is to repeat the test(s). The cure for the second circumstance is to warm up the patient or to run the coagulation tests at the patient's temperature for confirmation, or both. The only cure for the third will be a return to the operating room for control of surgical bleeding. The reader is referred again to Figure 15-8 and further reading.[35]

TRANSPORT OF PATIENT TO INTENSIVE CARE

PREPARATIONS

Once stability of the cardiovascular, respiratory, and the hemostatic systems has been achieved, and the surgical wounds are being closed, preparations for transport to the ICU should be underway. A checklist for such preparations is shown below. Advance notice to the postoperative ICU should be given 30 to 45 minutes before leaving the operating suite. A suggested advance information sheet is provided in Figure 15-9.

In order for the patient to be a candidate for leaving the operating room, the cardiovascular system must be stable. If an external pacemaker is in use, it should be set on *demand* mode (*synchronous*) if there is an underlying competing rhythm. Vascular volume status should be optimal for that particular patient, as judged by the left or right-sided filling pressures or both, and by the ventricular responses. Drugs being administered by continuous infusion should be reviewed, and the administration rates and cardiovascular responses confirmed to be appropriate. The cardiac rate, rhythm, and mean arterial pressure should be monitored during transport, and appropriate equipment, including a defibrillator made available if appropriate.

Arterial blood gases (ABGs) should be stable, if not optimal, and the endotracheal tube fully patent and secured to the patient. A device for providing controlled ventilation for

Checklist—Ready to Leave OR?

Is ICU fully notified, and ready to receive patient?*

Cardiovascular
Stable before and after transfer to bed?
If pacemaker is in use—on *demand* mode?
Is volume status optimal?
Is cardiac output adequate?
Is MAP in correct range?
Are drugs appropriate?
(types, administration rate, *response*)
Are electrolytes (K^+, Ca^{++}) normal?
Monitoring during transport? (rate, rhythm, MAP)
Adequate fluid or blood available for administration during transport?

Ventilation
Are ABGs OK?
Airway (ETT) patent and stabilized?
Ventilation device working? Enough O_2 in tank?
Monitoring? (esophageal stethoscope)

CNS
Is patient adequately anesthetized?
Is patient adequately relaxed?

Coagulation
Is ACT normalized?
Are factor levels normal?
Have laboratory specimens been sent?
(coagulation screen, PCV, platelets)

Miscellaneous
Are all catheters moved or disconnected?
Are chest tubes functioning adequately and sealed?
Are all lines untangled and functioning and injection ports covered?
Is extra blood (or crystalloid) accompanying patient?
Is the bed fully functional?
Are all records with patient?
Are there enough personnel to help?
If IACPB in use—do batteries work?

*Send postoperative ICU information Sheet 45 minutes before expected arrival (see Fig. 15-9).

the patient, with an F_IO_2 of 1.0, should be made available. We prefer a modification of the Rees-modified Ayre's t-piece, with a Norman elbow, using a flow rate of oxygen of 10 to 12 l/min (Fig. 15-10). It is a simple, virtually fool-proof device requiring no valves nor moving mechanical parts (such as a Bird ventilator or demand-valve system might have). PEEP can be provided readily to the patient with such a device. A sufficient supply of oxygen should be available, remembering

Stanford Cardiovascular Anesthesia Service
Postoperative ICU Advance Information Sheet

Age ________ Weight ________

Diagnoses ____________________

Surgical Procedure(s) ____________________

Operative Problems ____________________

- -

- -

(Check or Complete Where Appropriate)

A. Respiratory (Please notify Respiratory Therapy):

1. Ventilator Requested? _____; PEEP? _____ cm H_2O
2. Pediatric "Q-Circle" requested? ________
3. T-piece System requested (no ventilator needed) ________
4. Patient will be extubated on arrival ________
5. Humidified mask oxygen requested ________

B. Monitoring in place:

Arterial catheter? ________ location ____________
CVP catheter? ________ location ____________
PA ("Swan-Ganz") Catheter? ________ location ____________
Surgical PA line? ________ Surgical LA line? ________

C. Intravenous Infusions Presently in Use:

Isoproterenol ____ Epinephrine ____ Nitroprusside ____
Dopamine ____ $CaCL_2$ ____ Nitroglycerin ____
Dobutamine ____ "Epi-cal" ____ Lidocaine ____
Other ____________________

D. Please prepare a fresh drip of _____ (standard ___, double ___, other ___)

E. Laboratory studies drawn in OR (Time ______)

coagulation panel ☐ PCV ☐ K^+ ☐ Platelets "Enzymes" ☐ Blood Gases ☐ Other: ________

F. Special Information:

1. Left ventricular Assist device in use:
Intra-aortic balloon ______ Other type ____________
2. Request cardiac outputs early postoperatively ____________
3. Miscellaneous ____________________

Estimated time of Arrival in ICU: _____AM _____PM

THANK YOU ____________________
(Anesthesiologist)

Fig. 15–9. Stanford Cardiovascular Anesthesia Service postoperative ICU advance information sheet. This sheet is completed by the anesthesiologist intraoperatively and forwarded to the cardiovascular ICU approximately 45 minutes before the patient leaves the operating suite. With such advance information, a smooth transition into the postoperative period is more likely.

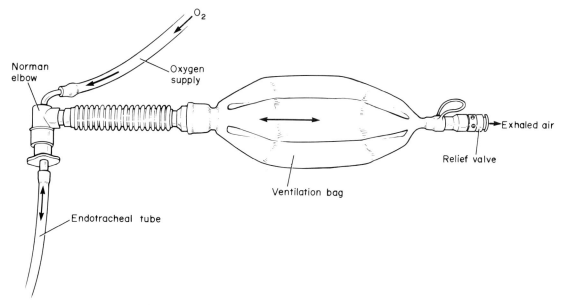

Fig. 15–10. Portable ventilation system for OR-ICU transport. The device is a modification of the Ayre's T-piece, using a Norman elbow and a flow rate of oxygen of 10–12 l/minute. It is simple, without valves or mechanical working parts, and allows the application of PEEP by hand.

that a completely full *E* tank of oxygen contains enough gas to supply 10 to 12 l/min for approximately 50 minutes. Monitoring of ventilation should be provided both by visual chest inflation inspection and by an esophageal stethoscope. If the patient is not to be extubated in the immediate future, proper anesthesia and muscle relaxation should be provided.

Coagulation status should be normal, or as nearly normal as possible. All products to treat coagulation abnormalities should have been administered if possible. We prefer to send blood specimens to the laboratory from the operating room for the determination of coagulation status (aPTT, PT, TT, fibrinogen), platelet count, PCV, serum potassium, and ABGs. The results of these determinations thus will be available to the ICU personnel within moments of the patient's ICU arrival.

An ICU bed should be available for direct patient transfer. All records should be collected in order to be transported with the patient. If an IACPB is in use, the unit should be checked for proper battery function.

TRANSPORT

We prefer to move the patient only once, directly to the ICU bed from the operating table. The move should be performed slowly, smoothly, and as carefully as possible to minimize vascular volume shifts or changes in cardiac rhythm. Chest tubes should be applied to underwater seal. A carefully coordinated move by a sufficient number of personnel should prevent accidents such as disconnected IVs, tubes pulled out or malpositioned,[44] infusion drugs discontinued, and the like. The anesthesiologist is responsible *only* for ventilation and monitoring, not moving, fetching, nor adjusting parts of the bed.

Monitoring during transport should include at least an esophageal stethoscope for respiratory and cardiovascular sounds. In addition, we monitor routinely the MAP with a sterile Tycos anaeroid gauge directly connected to the arterial line by a 50-cm segment of sterile IV tubing. If the patient is exceptionally critical, ECG and an oscillographic display of the arterial pressure by a portable monitor (presently a Tektronix) are also monitored. A defibrillator also accompanies the exceptionally critical patient. The longer and more complex the route to the ICU, the more care must be exercised in planning and execution of this transport. If an elevator separates the operating room from the ICU, it should be equipped with a separate reserve oxygen system, electrical power outlet, phone communication system, and if possible, suction equipment (what would one want available in a jammed elevator for 2 hours?).

ICU ARRIVAL

Upon arrival in the ICU, an immediate mental checklist should begin (see list below). Priorities should be the same as in a cardiac resuscitation: *ABC*—airway, breathing, and circulation. Ventilatory function is assessed as the patient's airway is connected to a ventilator, set initially with an F_1O_2 of 1.0. Initial ventilator settings should duplicate those

---

ICU Arrival Checklist

Priorities
  Ventilation: hand → ventilator
    Assess ventilator function and airway connections
    Confirm F_1O_2
    Auscultate chest bilaterally
  Vital signs
    ECG: rhythm and rate
    $\overline{MAP}$
    $CVP/PAD/\overline{PA}_0$
  Infusion rates of potent drugs and responses
  Coagulation status and blood availability
  Transmission of important data to ICU team

Lesser Importance
  Chest tube(s) drainage
  Urine output
  Other hemodynamic monitoring
  Fine-tuning the ventilator
  Patient CNS status

Laboratory Work on Arrival
  ABGs
  Serum K^+
  PCV
  Coagulation screen (if applicable)
  Chest film
  ECG. 12 lead

---

found optimal in the post-bypass period in the operating room. The chest must be seen and heard to move bilaterally. Vital signs of immediate importance are cardiac rate and rhythm (ECG), MAP, and CVP. Infusion rates of potent drugs are verified, and desired cardiovascular responses confirmed. Blood or crystalloid should be available at the bedside and coagulation status ascertained as soon as possible. Transmission of important data to the postoperative care team is a high priority. Endpoints for cardiovascular variables should be given to the most senior nurse actually providing *direct* patient care (*e.g.*, desired MAP, $\overline{CVP}$, $\overline{PA}_0$, PAD, heart rate, drugs).

Items of lesser importance can be transmitted as time permits, and are covered in the list above. Laboratory and other diagnostic procedures should be performed as soon as practical (chest film, ABGs, serum K^+, PCV, 12-lead ECG, and coagulation screen if indicated). Before the anesthesiologist leaves the ICU, he or she should ascertain the present status of the patient, confirm cardiovascular and respiratory stability, be assured that no problems of an acute nature exist, and confirm that the ICU nurses are satisfied with the patient's status. A brief early postoperative note, as well as a copy of the anesthetic record, should be placed in the patient's chart.

SUMMARY

The post-bypass period is a critical period in the operative-perioperative continuum. Preparations for all possible problems prevent or minimize them. Priorities must be established and followed. Hemodynamic variables should be changed in specific sequence, one at a time, utilizing appropriate monitoring. Drug therapy should be planned based upon measured physiologic and known pharmacologic data. Hemostatic control should be organized, using a logical, methodical analysis and treatment, not "shotgun" therapy.

If the anesthesiologist has performed all procedures necessary, and adjusted the patient's various systems to peak performance, the patient's status will be reflected in a smooth, coordinated ICU arrival. If the patient has been appropriately "tuned-up" by the anesthesiologist, the early postoperative course should be uneventful. And, while the anesthesiologist's work is now mostly completed, the work of other professionals has just begun.

REFERENCES*

GENERAL SEQUENCE OF TRANSITION

1. Risk C, Rudo N, Falltrick R et al: Comparison of right atrial and pulmonary capillary wedge pressures. Crit Care Med 6:172–175, 1978
2. Sharefkin JB, MacArthur JD: Pulmonary arterial pressure as a guide to the hemodynamic status of surgical patients. Arch Surg 105:699–704, 1972
3. Toussaint GP, Mac L, Burgess JH, Hampson LG: Central venous pressure and pulmonary wedge pressure in critical surgical illness. Arch Surg 109:265–269, 1974
4. Bouchard RJ, Gault JH, Ross J Jr: Evaluation of pulmonary arterial end-diastolic pressure as an estimate of left ventricular end-diastolic pressure in patients with normal and abnormal left ventricular performance. Circulation 19:1072–1079, 1971
5. Rice CL, Hobelman CF, John DA et al: Central venous pressure or pulmonary capillary wedge pressure as the determinant of fluid replacement in aortic surgery. Surgery 437–440, 1978
6. Lappas DG, Powell WMJ, Daggett WM: Cardiac dysfunction in the perioperative period: pathophysiology, diagnosis, and treatment. Anesthesiology 47:117–137, 1977

CARDIOVASCULAR MANAGEMENT

7. Samet P, Castillo C, Bernstein WH: Hemodynamic consequences of atrial and ventricular pacing in subjects with normal hearts. Am J Cardiol 18:522–525, 1966
8. Abramowicz M (ed): Treatment of cardiac arrhythmias. Med Lett Drugs Ther 20:113–120, 1978

Preload (Volume Administration)

9. Ward CF, Arkin DB, Benumof JL: Arterial versus venous potassium: clinical implications. Crit Care Med 6:335–336, 1978
10. Carrico CJ, Canizaro PC, Shires GT: Fluid resuscitation following injury: rationale for the use of balanced salt solutions. Crit Care Med 4:46–54, 1976
11. Boutros AR, Ruess R, Olson L et al: Comparison of hemodynamic, pulmonary, and renal effects of use of three types of fluids after major surgical procedures on the abdominal aorta. Crit Care Med 7:9–13, 1979
12. Skillman JJ: The role of albumin and oncotically active fluids in shock: Crit Care Med 4:55–61, 1976
13. Virgilio RW, Rice CL, Smith DE et al: Crystalloid vs. colloid resuscitation: is one better? Surgery 85:129–139, 1979

Inotropic Management

14. Lappas DG, Powell WMJ, Daggett WM: Cardiac dysfunction in the perioperative period: pathophysiology, diagnosis, and treatment. Anesthesiology 47:117–137, 1977
15. Sonnenblick EH, Frishman WH, LeJemtel TH: Dobutamine: a new synthetic cardioactive sympathetic amine. Medical intelligence. N Engl J Med 300:17–22, 1979
16. Sakamoto T, Yamada T: Hemodynamic effects of dobutamine in patients following open heart surgery. Circulation 55:525–533, 1977

Low Cardiac Output

17. Kopman EA, Ramirez–Inawat RC: Persistent electromechanical cardiac arrest following administration of cardioplegic and glucose-insulin-potassium solutions. Anes Analg (Cleve) 59:69–71, 1980

Intraaortic Counterpulsation Balloon (IACPB)

18. Kopman EA, Ramirez–Inawat RC: Intra-aortic balloon counterpulsation for right heart failure. Anes Analg (Cleve) 59:74–76, 1980

---

* References listed here are those relevant only to direct clinical application post-bypass. Hundreds of references are provided in other sections (*e.g.,* vasodilators, inotropic agonists and antagonists, anesthetic drugs, physiology, electrocardiographic monitoring). The reader is referred to those sections for exhaustive reference coverage.

High Cardiac Output

19. Bidwai AV, Rogers CR, Pearce M et al: Preoperative stellate-ganglion blockade to prevent hypertension following coronary-artery operations. Anesthesiology 51:345–347, 1979

RESPIRATORY MANAGEMENT

20. Prakash O, Meij S, Bos E et al: Lung mechanics in patients undergoing mitral valve replacement: the value of monitoring of compliance and resistance. Crit Care Med 6:370–372, 1978
21. Rackow EC, Fein IA: Fulminant noncardiogenic pulmonary edema in the critically ill. Crit Care Med 6:360–363, 1978
22. Tonneson AS, Gabel JC, McLeavey CA: Relation between lowered colloid osmotic pressure, respiratory failure, and death. Crit Care Med 5:239–240, 1977
23. Morthy SS, Losasso AM, Gibbs PS: Acquired right-to-left intracardiac shunts and severe hypoxemia. Crit Care Med 6:28–31, 1978
24. Fogdall RP: Exacerbation of Iatrogenic hypercarbia by PEEP. Anesthesiology 51:173–175, 1979
25. Dammann FL, McAslan TC: PEEP: its use in young patients with apparently normal lungs. Crit Care Med 7:14–19, 1979
26. De Campo T, Civetta JM: The effect of short-term discontinuation of high-level PEEP in patients with acute respiratory failure. Crit Care Med 7:47–49, 1979
27. Garrard CS, Shah M: The effects of expiratory positive airway pressure on functional residual capacity in normal subjects. Crit Care Med 6:320–322, 1978
28. Downs JB, Mitchel LA: Pulmonary effects of ventilatory pattern following cardiopulmonary bypass. Crit Care Med 4:295–300, 1976
29. Dammann JF, McAslan TC, Maffeo CJ: Optimal flow pattern for mechanical ventilation of the lungs: the effect of a sine versus square wave flow pattern with and without an end-inspiratory pause on patients. Crit Care Med 6:293–310, 1978
30. Gallagher TJ, Civetta JM, Kirby RR: Terminology update: optimal PEEP. Crit Care Med 6:323–326, 1978
31. Suter P, Fairly HB, Isenberg MD: Optimum end expiratory airway pressure in patients with acute pulmonary failure. N Engl J Med 292:284, 1975
32. Berryhill RE, Benumof JL: PEEP-induced discrepancy between pulmonary arterial wedge pressure and left atrial pressure: the effects of controlled vs. spontaneous ventilation and compliant vs. noncompliant lungs in the dog. Anesthesiology 51:303–308, 1979
33. Delooz HH: Factors influencing successful discontinuance of mechanical ventilation after open heart surgery: a clinical study of 41 patients. Crit Care Med 4:265–270, 1976
34. Klineberg PL, Geer RT, Hirsh RA et al: Early extubation after coronary artery bypass graft surgery. Crit Care Med 5:272–274, 1977

MANAGEMENT OF HEMOSTASIS AND COAGULATION

35. Fischbach DP, Fogdall RP: *Coagulation: The Essentials.* Baltimore, Williams & Wilkins, 1981
36. Palermo LM, Andrews RW, Ellison N: Avoidance of heparin contamination in coagulation studies drawn from indwelling lines. Anesth Analg (Cleve) 59:222–224, 1980
37. Goldman BS, Joison J, Austen WG: Cardiovascular effects of protamine sulfate. Ann Thorac Surg 7:459–471, 1969
38. Gourin A, Streisand RL, Stuckey JH: Total cardiopulmonary bypass, myocardial contractility, and the administration of protamine sulfate. J Thorac Cardiovasc Surg 61:160–166, 1971
39. Gourin A: Protamine sulfate administration and the cardiovascular system. J Thorac Cardiovasc Surg 62:193, 1971
40. Jastrzebski J: Cardiorespiratory effects of protamine after cardiopulmonary bypass in man. Thorax 29:534–538, 1974
41. Denlinger JK: The effects of heparin and protamine infusion on serum ionized calcium in anesthetized man. Anesthesiology Review, August, 1976
42. Moorthy SS, Pond W, Rowland RG: Severe circulatory shock following protamine: an anaphylactic reaction. Anesth Analg 59:77–78, 1980
43. Wood M, Shand DG, Wood AJJ: Propranolol binding in plasma during cardiopulmonary bypass. Anesthesiology 51:512–516, 1979

TRANSPORT OF PATIENT TO INTENSIVE CARE

44. Conrardy PA, Goodman LR, Lainge F et al: Alteration of endotracheal tube position. Crit Care Med 4:8–12, 1976

16

Management of the Adult Cardiac Patient in the Intensive Care Unit

ROBERT N. SLADEN

HEMODYNAMIC MANAGEMENT

GOALS

Intensive care is a continuation of the hemodynamic weaning that begins at the end of cardiopulmonary bypass (Fig. 16-1). The patient is anesthetized, potentially unstable, and requires mechanical ventilation after arrival in the intensive care unit. The overall goal is to restore hemodynamic and pulmonary independence. It is convenient to subdivide this task into three phases as summarized in Table 16-1.

In the first phase, absolute or relative hypovolemia is the most important problem. The duration and severity of this phase is influenced by the degree of preoperative dysfunction, the duration of bypass, and the nature of the surgical insult. The goal is to provide optimum intravascular volume to prevent cardiac and renal failure.

For the relatively young patient undergoing coronary artery bypass surgery with normal ventricular function and short bypass time, this phase may last from 6 to 8 hours. In the elderly patient with combined mitral regurgitation, ischemic heart disease and left ventricular failure, this phase may last from 24 to 48 hours and be associated with profound fluid requirement, leading to a weight gain of up to 15 kg. Full rewarming and cessation of the capillary leak syndrome ends this phase; administered fluid remains within the intravascular space, preload is easily maintained and the patient is hemodynamically stable.

In phase II, the patient mobilizes interstitial fluid gained during phase I. Weaning from positive pressure ventilation permits increased venous return and exacerbates the effects of increased pulmonary extravascular water. These include pulmonary congestion or edema or both, caused by atelectasis and intrapulmonary shunting, and a predisposition to pulmonary infection. Therapy should reduce pulmonary extravascular water by (1) improving cardiac function to allow the lowest preload requirement possible, (2) careful fluid restriction, and (3) diuresis.

THE CONTINUOUS SPECTRUM OF POST-OPERATIVE SUPPORT

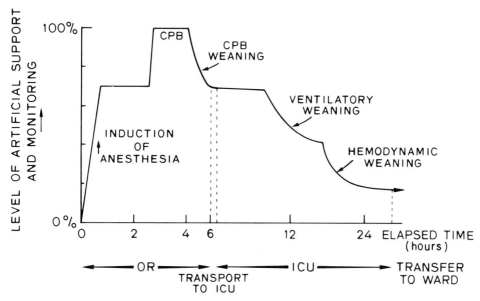

Fig. 16–1. Postoperative support in the ICU is initially an extension of intraoperative care. Later, mechanical and pharmacologic support are withdrawn in a graded manner.

Table 16-1. Goals of Hemodynamic Management

Phase 1:	Restoration of Intravascular Volume *Optimal cardiac output and renal perfusion* *Prevention of acute renal failure*	0–12 hr
Phase 2:	Mobilization of Interstitial Fluid *Ventilatory weaning* *Prevention of respiratory failure*	12–72 hr
Phase 3:	Supraventricular Arrhythmias *Prevention and management*	2–7 days

The duration and difficulty of this phase depends on the duration and difficulty of phase I. The young patient with normal cardiac function can be safely extubated within 12 hours of surgery, and can mobilize interstitial fluid without diuretic therapy over a period of from 36 to 48 hours. The elderly patient may require days or weeks, even with aggressive diuresis. This patient may require prolonged mechanical support with a tracheostomy to facilitate slow, careful weaning.

In the third phase, supraventricular arrhythmias are a major concern. Atrial and junctional tachycardia, multifocal premature atrial contractions, atrial flutter, and atrial fibrillation may all occur. The patient in chronic atrial fibrillation who has converted to sinus rhythm at the end of cardiopulmonary bypass is most likely to revert to fibrillation. These arrhythmias may, in the borderline patient, precipitate cardiac failure, pulmonary edema, hypotension, or syncope, and in the patient with mitral valve disease, mural thromboembolism.

The physician has three constant goals in the postoperative period: (1) restoration of

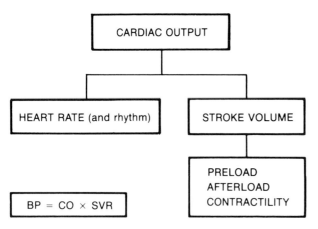

Fig. 16–2. The primary determinants of cardiac function, as discussed in the text. Blood pressure (*BP*) reflects the interaction of cardiac output (*CO*) and systemic vascular resistance (*SVR*); normal blood pressure does not assure adequate cardiac output.

blood volume and prevention of acute renal failure; (2) mobilization of accumulated interstitial fluid to facilitate ventilatory weaning and avoid pulmonary complications, and (3) prevention and management of supreventricular arrhythmias.

PHYSIOLOGY

Enhancement of cardiac output requires manipulation of its determinants (Fig. 16-2).[1] Cardiac output is the product of heart rate and stroke volume. The latter in turn depends on the interrelationship between (1) *preload* (or, in Starling's terms, the ventricular end-diastolic volume), (2) *afterload* (intramyocardial systolic wall tension),* and (3) *contractility* (the contractile state of the heart). Afterload depends on chamber radius, stroke volume, heart rate, anatomic impedance to ventricular outflow, and systemic vascular resistance (see also Chap. 2).

Systemic vascular resistance (SVR) may be used as an indication of patient status. It provides a better guide to therapeutic manipulations of cardiac output than blood pressure alone. A fall in cardiac output may result in no change in blood pressure if systemic vascular resistance is increased, and vice versa. Referencing to normal values of resistance suggests whether pressure, cardiac output, or both must be manipulated.

The determination of a satisfactory cardiac output, however, is not provided by a single quantitative measurement, but by evaluation of the overall clinical status of the patient. In other words, the desired cardiac output is that which provides hemodynamic stability (without excessive myocardial work) and adequate vital organ perfusion.

Cardiac Physiology

Preload The deficit in intravascular volume is fixed in the early postoperative period (Table 16-2). Blood loss may vary greatly. Insensible loss during open thoracotomy is significant. Extracorporeal circulation activates the complement and kinin systems and induces a capillary leak syndrome that results in sequestration of fluid from intravascular into the interstitial space (third-space sequestration).

Up to 1.5 liters of fluid may be left in the oxygenator circuit at the end of bypass if efforts are not made to allow its return to the patient. (We customarily empty the oxygenator.) Mannitol, 12.5 g per hour is added to the perfusate during bypass to preserve renal tubular flow and reduce myocardial edema. The resulting osmotic diuresis can produce 1 to 3 liters of urine in the first 4 hours following bypass.

---

*The term *preload* may be interpreted as filling pressure of the left ventricle when discussing its contribution to myocardial efficiency and oxygen demand. *Afterload* may be expressed clinically by measurement of the tension–time index, *i.e.*, the mean aortic root pressure × duration of aortic valve opening. These concepts are discussed more fully in Chapter 2.

Right and left ventricular filling pressures may not truly reflect intravascular volume because of vasoconstriction induced by hypothermia and other factors. It may not be clear that fluid replacement has been inadequate until rapid rewarming and vasodilation occur 2 to 4 hours after return to the ICU. This fall in systemic vascular resistance may be anticipated by the use of vasodilator therapy after bypass to ensure adequate early fluid replacement. This maneuver has substantially improved postoperative hemodynamic stability.

The functional intravascular volume deficit is exacerbated by increased preload requirement caused by decreased myocardial compliance and function after surgery.[2] It may require more than 24 hours for the benefit of the surgical procedure to be realized (Fig. 16-3).[3]

Underlying myocardial disease may not be corrected by surgery (*e.g.,* ischemia, fibrosis or conduction defects). Notable exceptions include tight aortic stenosis without ventricular failure and myocardial dysfunction sec-

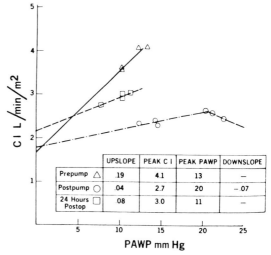

	UPSLOPE	PEAK C I	PEAK PAWP	DOWNSLOPE
Prepump △	.19	4.1	13	—
Postpump ○	.04	2.7	20	− .07
24 Hours Postop □	.08	3.0	11	—

Fig. 16–3. Myocardial function curves determined by thermodilution cardiac output estimations before, during and after coronary artery bypass grafting (prepump, postpump, 24 hours postop). Performance after extracorporeal circulation is markedly impaired; it returns towards normal after 24 hours. *CI* = cardiac index, PAWP = pulmonary artery wedge pressure. (Berger RL et al: Ann Thorac Surg 21:46, 1976)

Table 16-2. Altered Preload

INADEQUATE PRELOAD (INTRAVASCULAR VOLUME DEFICIT)

1. Excessive fluid losses
   Blood loss
   Insensible loss
   "Third spacing"
   CPB residual
   Osmotic diuresis
2. Inadequate fluid replacement (Masked by ↑ SVR)
3. Positive pressure ventilation   ± PEEP

INCREASED PRELOAD REQUIREMENT (MYOCARDIAL DEPRESSION)

1. Residual myocardial disease not corrected by surgery
2. Cardiopulmonary bypass
   a. Inadequate myocardial protection
      edema
      ischemia
      ventricular irritability
   b. Side-effects of cold cardioplegia
      hypothermia
      conduction defects
3. Anesthesia
   halothane, enflurane
4. Acid-base/electrolyte imbalance
   pH, K, Ca, Mg
5. Complications of surgery
   Coronary air embolism, trauma
   Cardiac tamponade
   Perioperative infarction

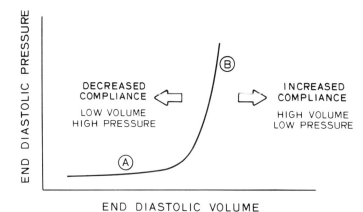

Fig. 16–4. The relationship of end diastolic pressure (EDP) to end diastolic volume (EDV) is exponential rather than linear. Although a normal ventricle may have high compliance at normal levels of EDV (A), excessive distension will ultimately result in rapid fall in compliance (B). Pathologic states may shift the curve to the left or right and alter the response of the ventricle to a given EDV (see Table 16–3).

ondary to critical ischemia. In these instances valve replacement or revascularization is often followed by a lower postoperative preload requirement.

Myocardial edema is always present after cardiopulmonary bypass.[4, 5] Inadequate myocardial protection may result in subendocardial ischemia or ventricular irritability. Cold cardioplegia provides superior protection against ischemia but is associated with decreased ventricular compliance at the end of bypass due to myocardial hypothermia. Myocardial depression by volatile anesthetic agents such as halothane and enflurane is avoided if intravenous narcotic agents are used and the volatile agents are withdrawn by the start of bypass. Acid-base and electrolyte balance has been discussed in Chapters 14 and 26. Extracellular hypokalemia (ventricular irritability), hypocalcemia, and hypomagnesemia (myocardial depression) occur frequently (see Table 16-2).

The physician must anticipate reduced intravascular volume associated with an increased preload requirement in the early postoperative period. The optimal preload for *maximum efficiency of the heart* is just below that resulting in maximum stroke volume. (See the discussion of Starling's Law in Chaps. 2 and 3.) However, the increased capillary leakage and reduced plasma oncotic pressure following cardiopulmonary bypass increase the probability of pulmonary edema at the same value of left ventricular preload.[6]

Optimal preload

1. Is generally increased above normal immediately after surgery. ($\overline{PA}_o$ or $\overline{LAP}$ > 12 torr)*
2. Returns toward normal 24–48 hours after surgery in uncomplicated cases.
3. Is *not* that which provides maximal cardiac output, but that which provides hemodynamic stability and adequate renal function. It reflects a compromise between cardiac and pulmonary needs.
4. Must be individualized for a particular patient at a particular time. Frequent reassessment and adjustment is necessary.

Interpretation of the pulmonary artery wedge or left atrial *pressure* as a guide to the ventricular end-diastolic *volume* may be misleading unless ventricular diastolic compliance is considered. The relationship between ventricular pressure and volume is exponential rather than linear (Fig. 16-4). Many factors exist that alter ventricular compliance and shift the response curve to the left (stiff) or right (compliant), thereby affecting preload management[7, 8] (Table 16-3). In mitral valve disease, wedge or left atrial pressures reflect the degree of stenosis or regurgitation rather than ventricular filling pressure.

Excessive preload has many adverse effects. In the presence of severe myocardial

*$\overline{LAP}$ = mean left atrial pressure
$\overline{PA}_o$ = mean pulmonary artery occluded (wedge) pressure

dysfunction, high filling pressures (occasionally as much as 30–35 torr) are unavoidable and edema will be exacerbated (Fig. 16-5). After prolonged bypass, the capillary leak is severe. Increased pulmonary extravascular water leads to shunting, hypoxemia, decreased compliance (thus increased work of breathing and O_2 demand), delayed ventilatory weaning, and increased postoperative pulmonary complications. Increased left ventricular end diastolic pressure increases myocardial work and decreases myocardial oxygen supply (Table 16-4). If generalized, interstitial edema affects renal, hepatic, and cerebral function (the postperfusion syndrome).

Systemic Vascular Resistance and Afterload

Factors Causing Altered SVR. Arterial vasoconstriction causing increased afterload is common in the early postoperative phase.[9-11] Circulating catecholamine levels are elevated in response to hypotension, reduced

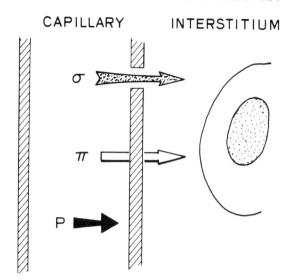

Fig. 16–5. Increased capillary hydrostatic pressure (*P*) exacerbates formation of pulmonary extravascular water (PEVW) due to reduced plasma oncotic pressure (π) and capillary leak (σ).

Table 16-3. Ventricular Diastolic Compliance

INCREASED COMPLIANCE	DECREASED COMPLIANCE
Little change in pressure with large change in volume	Large change in pressure with little change in volume
PA$_o$/LAP underestimates EDV	PA$_o$/LAP overestimates EDV
Regurgitant Lesions 　Aortic regurgitation 　Mitral regurgitation	Acute Dilation 　Pulmonary edema
Shunts (high flow) 　Atrial septal defect 　Ventricular septal defect 　Patent ductus arteriosus	Ventricular Hypertrophy 　Aortic stenosis 　IHSS 　Coarctation 　Hypertension
	Abnormal Ventricle 　Acute ischemia (including AXC) 　Hypothermia (CPB) 　Edema (CPB) 　Necrosis, scarring, infiltrates 　post-aneurysmectomy
	Restriction 　Pericardial disease/tamponade
	Right Ventricular Distension 　(Septal projection into LV) 　Pulmonary hypertension 　RV outflow tract disease

Compliant ventricle may become noncompliant after prolonged CPB. EDV = end diastolic volume; AXC = aortic cross-clamp; CPB = cardiopulmonary bypass; LV = left ventricle; RV = right ventricle

Systemic Vascular Resistance (SVR)

$$\text{Resistance} = \frac{\text{Pressure Gradient}}{\text{Flow}}$$

$$\text{SVR} = \frac{(\text{MAP} - \text{RAP})}{\text{CO}} \times 80 \text{ dyne-sec} \cdot \text{cm}^{-5}$$

(MAP = mean arterial pressure, RAP = right atrial or central venous pressure, 80 = conversion factor)

1. Normal SVR is 800–1500 dyne-sec·cm^{-5}. However, the normal range of SVR is more accurately expressed as an index, *i.e.*, using cardiac index (CI) rather than cardiac output (CO).
2. SVR contributes to, but is not the same as, afterload.
3. The definition of afterload is ventricular wall tension at aortic valve opening, not SVR. It is directly related to transmural pressure and internal chamber radius, and inversely related to wall thickness.
4. The correlation between SVR and afterload in states of left ventricular outflow tract obstruction (aortic stenosis; IHSS) is impaired proportional to the degree of obstruction. (High intraventricular pressures exist with low aortic pressures and low calculated SVR)
5. SVR reflects *total* body vascular resistance; it does not reflect vital organ resistance or perfusion. In the presence of shunts (*e.g.*, gravid uterus, arteriovenous fistula) calculated SVR is very misleading.
6. SVR is a *calculated* variable, and is less accurate than the directly measured indices whence it is derived.

perfusion, surgical stimulation, pain, extracorporeal circulation, and hypothermia. The renin-angiotenin system is activated by renal hypoperfusion during CPB.[12] There may be preexisting essential hypertension. Elevated systemic vascular resistance is often not reflected by increased blood pressure because cardiac output is decreased. In states of severe myocardial dysfunction with elevated resistance, vasodilator therapy is essential to assure an adequate cardiac output.

There is good evidence that extracorporeal circulation causes activation of the kinin and complement-histamine systems, both of which cause vasodilation. Also, splanchnic hypoperfusion during and after bypass may allow absorption of endotoxins despite the local defense mechanisms of the gut. Usually this effect is outweighed by the factors causing vasoconstriction. Very occasionally a patient will have hypotension associated with low systemic vascular resistance in which these mechanisms are assumed to have become dominant. A noteworthy cause of lowered resistance in the early postoperative period is vasodilation secondary to anaphylactic shock (drug allergy, *e.g.*, protamine, or incompatible blood transfusion). The patient who is septic at the time of surgery (*e.g.*, valve replacement for bacterial endocarditis) is more likely to have a persistently low sys-

Table 16-4. Adverse Effects of Excessive Preload

IMPAIRED MYOCARDIAL OXYGEN SUPPLY/DEMAND RATIO	
Decreased TMG (TMG = DAP − LVDP)	
Myocardial distension ⟶ ↑ Systolic work	
EXCESSIVE INTERSTITIAL EDEMA (POSTPERFUSION SYNDROME)	
Lungs	Increased work of breathing (↑ $\dot{V}O_2$)
	Hypoxemia
	Delayed ventilatory weaning
	↑ Postoperative pulmonary complications
Brain	Prolonged obtundation
	Increased perioperative morbidity
Kidneys	Tendency to azotemia
Liver	Jaundice
	Impaired drug metabolism
Skin	Impaired acral perfusion

TMG = transmyocardial gradient; DAP = diastolic aortic pressure; LVDP = left ventricular diastolic pressure; P = pressure; VO_2 = oxygen utilization; ↑ = increased

Table 16-5. Factors Affecting SVR

INCREASED SVR (COMMON: MAY NOT BE ASSOCIATED WITH INCREASED BP.)	
Catecholamines	Hypotension
	Nonpulsatile perfusion on CPB
	Surgical stimulation, pain
	Hypothermia
	Extracorporeal circulation
Renin-Angiotensin	Nonpulsatile renal perfusion
Preexisting Hypertension	
DECREASED SVR (RARE)	
Anaphylactic Shock	Incompatible blood transfusion
	Protamine allergy
Sepsis	Bacterial endocarditis
Vasoactive Amines (unpredictable)	

temic vascular resistance throughout (Table 16-5).

Consequences of Elevated SVR. If myocardial function is normal, a primary increase in resistance provokes compensatory mechanisms that maintain cardiac output: increased blood pressure, increased contractility, and elevated preload. These increase the risk of myocardial ischemia in the postoperative period because they all increase myocardial oxygen consumption. Elevated preload (left ventricular end diastolic pressure) also decreases myocardial oxygen supply because it compromises endomyocardial perfusion (see Chap. 2). Attempts to correct low cardiac output-high resistance states with inotropic agents further increases myocardial oxygen demand. A vicious cycle is set up which can result in myocardial ischemia, infarction or cardiogenic shock. It is no surprise, therefore, that these states correlate with increased morbidity and mortality after cardiac surgery.[13]

Elevated systemic vascular resistance also masks underlying hypovolemia. Because of venoconstriction, right or left-sided filling pressures may be misleadingly high. Unless vasodilator therapy is used to overcome this and allow fluid loading, hypotension and tachycardia will manifest when the resistance falls as the patient warms. This may occur suddenly, and is catastrophic in the patient with incipient cardiac failure or persistent myocardial ischemia.

Table 16-6. Excessive Myocardial Contractility

Preexisting Hyperdynamic Myocardium
Hypertension
Aortic Stenosis
IHSS
Iatrogenic
Narcotic anesthesia in face of above
Excessive inotropism: Calcium, dopamine and others
Excessive afterload reduction: Nitroprusside

Hypertension caused by elevated systemic vascular resistance increases wound bleeding, endangers suture sites, and increases the risk of a cerebrovascular accident.[14]

Contractility Depression of myocardial contractility is always anticipated after cardiac surgery (Table 16-2B). *Excessive* myocardial contractility also occurs (Table 16-6). This response is particularly common in patients with preexisting left ventricular hypertrophy (*e.g.*, systemic hypertension, aortic stenosis, and idiopathic hypertrophic subaortic stenosis [IHSS]). By the time these patients reach the intensive care unit, depression secondary to surgery has often receded and there is return to the previous hyperdynamic state. Pure narcotic anesthetic techniques do not decrease contractility but impair central control. Excessive use of inotropic agents or vasodilators may provoke hypercontractility.

Increased ventricular contractility requires treatment because it increases myocardial oxygen demand and reduces myocardial oxygen supply. The associated systemic hypertension results in unnecessary bleeding and may endanger coronary graft integrity.

Oxygen Balance The factors governing myocardial oxygen supply and demand have been discussed in detail in Chapter 2. A brief review applicable to the postoperative period is provided here.

The clinical determinants of myocardial oxygen demand ($M\dot{V}O_2$) are (1) heart rate,* (2) afterload, (3) contractility, and (4) preload. The rate-pressure product (systolic blood pressure × heart rate) has been used to estimate the effects of afterload on myocardial oxygen demand. However, it is not a reliable indicator of myocardial ischemia[15, 16] (See Chapter 2). Increasing heart rate increases oxygen demand while decreasing supply. Increasing systolic pressure may increase both supply and demand. A rate-pressure product of 12,000 caused by a heart rate of 75 and a systolic pressure of 160 would appear to be more desirable than a heart rate of 160 and systolic pressure of 75. Indeed, a *decrease* in the rate-pressure product is not always beneficial.

Therapy that increases heart rate or contractility should be given with due consideration to its effect on $M\dot{V}O_2$. Pain, hypovolemia, hypothermia, and hypoxia liberate catecholamines and increase afterload and should be aggressively managed in the patient with myocardial ischemia. Unnecessary fluid loading and excessive preload will also increase $M\dot{V}O_2$.

Because 98 percent of net coronary artery inlet flow normally occurs during diastole, diastolic pressures directly affect myocardial oxygen supply. The perfusion gradient across the coronary arteries depends upon the difference between the pressure head (aortic diastolic pressure) and the pressure opposing coronary flow (left ventricular diastolic pressure). Because a measure of left atrial pressure is usually obtained through the mean pulmonary artery occluded pressure ($\overline{PA}_o$) or pulmonary artery diastolic pressure, the clinical expression of the transmyocardial gradient is given by subtracting the $\overline{PA}_o$ from the systemic diastolic pressure.

In patients with myocardial ischemia, vasodilator drugs must be used with due consideration of their effects on the transmyocardial gradient. Vasodilators which decrease aortic diastolic pressure with equal or little effect on ventricular diastolic pressure (nitroprusside, hydralazine) can worsen the gradient and exacerbate ischemia. Nitroglycerin is the vasodilator of choice in this situation because it can be used to decrease ventricular diastolic pressure with little effect on aortic diastolic pressure (Fig. 16-6).

Because the endomyocardium is subjacent to ventricular pressure, it is at the greatest risk from ischemia. The endomyocardial viability ratio (EVR) is derived by comparing the systolic pressure time index (SPTI) with the diastolic pressure time index (DPTI) as illustrated in Figure 16-7. Normally, the ratio between myocardial oxygen supply (DPTI)[17] and demand (SPTI) should approach 1.0 (see Chap. 2).

The critical EVR below which subendocardial ischemia occurs in normal individuals is probably 0.45.[18] However, this value is increased by ventricular hypertrophy, edema or dilation, increased contractility, and coronary artery disease. Although initially defined by intraventricular pressure measurements, the EVR may be accurately obtained with the use of arterial and pulmonary artery (or left atrial) catheters.[19, 20]

Anatomic patency of the coronary arteries remains the limiting factor for coronary perfusion. Predictors of postoperative myocardial ischemia include subocclusive stenosis (manifesting as unstable angina preoperatively), requirement for three or more grafts, and an inability to successfully bypass significant lesions.

---

* If the appropriate measures of a wall tension (tension–time index) and contractility (dP/dt) are used (per beat × heart rate = per minute), the separate contribution of heart rate to oxygen consumption becomes negligible. However, it is also true that increasing heart rate increases oxygen consumption (by increasing contractility per minute, tension–time index per minute, or both). For this reason, when discussing clinical management, we talk about heart rate as though it were a separate effect. See Chapter 2.

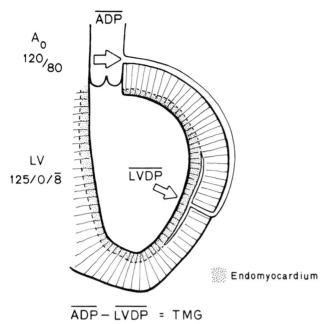

$$\overline{ADP} - \overline{LVDP} = TMG$$

	$\overline{ADP}$	$\overline{LVDP}\,(PA_0)$	TMG
NORMAL	80	8	72
PUL. ED.	↓ →	↑ ↑	↓
SNP.	↓ ↓	↓	↓
HYD.	↓	→	↓
NTG.	→	↓	↑

Fig. 16–6. The transmyocardial gradient of coronary perfusion pressure (*TMG*) is the difference between mean aortic diastolic pressure (*ADP*) in the proximal coronary artery and mean left ventricular diastolic pressure (*LVDP*). During ischemia coronary dilation is maximal and flow becomes directly proportional to the *TMG*. Directional effects in pulmonary edema (*PEd*) and with the use of the vasodilators sodium nitroprusside (*SNP*), hydralazine (*HYD*) and nitroglycerin (*NTG*) are summarized in the table.

Oxygen delivery (ml O_2/min) is the product of cardiac output and arterial oxygen content. Consideration must be given to all factors which influence the latter: hematocrit, arterial oxygen tension, and the P_{50} of the Hb-O_2 dissociation curve. The P_{50} in its turn depends on pH, $PaCO_2$, temperature, and the level of 2,3-DPG. Measures that shift the O_2 dissociation curve to the left will impede release of O_2 from Hb to the tissues. Some suggest incorporating oxygen content into the EVR (*i.e.*, DPTI × Ca_{O_2}/SPTI). A critical ratio is less than 10:1.[21]

In summary, a sound understanding of the factors controlling myocardial oxygen balance is essential for appropriate management in the postoperative period. Measures which improve one modality, such as blood pressure, may do so by adversely affecting myocardial oxygen demand or supply elsewhere;

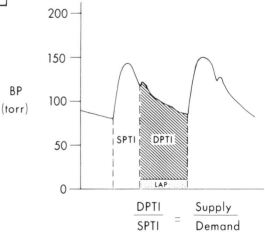

$$\frac{DPTI}{SPTI} = \frac{Supply}{Demand}$$

Fig. 16–7. Endomyocardial viability ratio (EVR) of supply and demand (DPTI/SPTI) derived from an arterial pressure trace and a left atrial catheter. Note that the dichrotic notch (closure of aortic valve) is used to separate SPTI and DPTI. Each index may be derived by planimetry or by multiplying the mean pressure by the respective time interval. (Hoar PF et al: J Thorac Cardiovasc Surg 71:860, 1976)

Table 16-7. Pathogenesis of Postoperative Arrhythmias

SINUS TACHYCARDIA

Sympathetic reflex
   Pain, hypovolemia, anxiety, hypercarbia, hypoxemia, low cardiac output, hyperdynamic response

CONDUCTION DEFECTS

Residual conduction disease
Cardiopulmonary bypass
   Myocardial edema
   Cold hyperkalemic cardioplegia
Surgical procedures
   AVR, MVR, septal myotomy, reconstruction around A-V node
Drugs
   Digitalis, propranolol

VENTRICULAR ARRHYTHMIAS

Sympathetic reflex
   Pain, hypovolemia
Acid-base imbalance
   Acute respiratory alkalosis, acidosis
Electolyte imbalance
   $\downarrow K^+ \downarrow Mg^{++}$
Myocardial ischemia or hypoxia
Drugs
   Sympathomimetics, aminophylline, digitalis, calcium

SUPRAVENTRICULAR ARRHYTHMIAS

Sympathetic reflex
   Pain, hypovolemia
Residual disease
   Chronic pulmonary disease (MAT)
   Chronic atrial fibrillation
   Sick sinus, preexcitation syndromes
Surgical trauma
   Atrial edema
   Rapid atrial distension/contraction
Hypoxemia (atelectasis)
Drugs
   Sympathomimetics, aminophylline, digitalis

the overall effect may not be beneficial to the patient.

Rhythm A brief resume of the pathogenesis of rhythm disorders relevant to the postoperative period is given here (Table 16–7). The subject is covered in depth in Chapters 6, 7, and 8.

Cold cardioplegia with hyperkalemic arrest is thought to improve myocardial preservation and decrease ischemia during cardiopulmonary bypass. Residual cold and myocardial edema has led, however, to an increased incidence of *conduction system defects.* Direct trauma with or without edema is a cause of conduction problems in mitral or aortic or both valve replacement and other reconstructive procedures adjacent to the A-V node. There may be residual conduction system disease not improved by the surgical proce-

dure. Digitalis toxicity can be precipitated by uncontrolled hypokalemia.

For these reasons, sinus arrest and varying degrees of atrioventricular block are common and may necessitate artificial pacing for a period of from 6 to 48 hours after bypass.

In the postoperative period, *ventricular escape rhythms* must be differentiated from *ventricular ectopy.* Suppression of the former with lidocaine will expose the potentially dangerous bradyarrhythmia. Instead, the underlying conduction problem should be treated, using electrical or pharmacologic pacing.

The most common cause of ventricular ectopy in the early postoperative period is *acid-base imbalance* and *hypokalemia.* Many patients come to surgery with low total body potassium induced by chronic diuretic therapy. Acute potassium loss is initiated by the profound osmotic diuresis that follows the routine use of mannitol on the pump. Extracellular hypokalemia is further exacerbated by the alkalosis commonly present on admission to the intensive care unit. Metabolic alkalosis is caused by the addition of sodium bicarbonate to the CPB prime and by the metabolism to bicarbonate of the citrate contained in transfused blood. The low CO_2 production of the cold patient ($\dot{V}CO_2$ decreases approximately 10% for each 1°C decrease below 37°C) is often not acknowledged when ventilatory parameters are set on admission of the patient to the intensive care unit, so that respiratory alkalosis is common. Hypomagnesemia occurs pari passu and will also promote ventricular irritability.

Acute alkalosis (pH > 7.5) can cause a supraventricular tachycardia that is corrected only by return to normal pH.

Residual *myocardial ischemia* may remain despite the surgical procedure. New myocardial ischemia might have occurred as a complication of the surgical procedure (*e.g.,* inadequate preservation, coronary embolization) or myocardial oxygen imbalance might be induced by therapeutic measures, as discussed in the previous section. If removal of an intraaortic balloon has been premature (in that it has played an important role in improving myocardial oxygen balance) the first sign of myocardial ischemia is frequently the onset of ventricular irritability and tachyarrhythmias.

Ventricular irritability may result from the use of agents such as epinephrine, dopamine, calcium, aminophylline, and digitalis. These drugs should be used with due caution in the early postoperative period.

As discussed in the introduction, supraventricular irritability is the most important problem after the first 2 to 3 days following surgery. Supraventricular arrhythmias occurring *early* in the ICU course are often escape rhythms secondary to underlying conduction defects.

Patients with chronic atrial fibrillation who are converted to sinus rhythm at the end of surgery tend to revert to atrial fibrillation after about 12 hours. Patients with severe chronic obstructive lung disease have a high incidence of multifocal atrial tachycardia and this rhythm disorder may return in the postsurgical situation. Primary disorders associated with atrial tachyarrhythmias, may be present. Atrial irritability may be enhanced by excessive stretch or by vigorous diuresis and hypovolemia.

Supraventricular irritability may be the initial manifestation of hypoxemia in the patient who has developed atelectasis after extubation. This will occur particularly if respiratory therapy has been skimpy, and the importance of oxygen therapy ignored. Hypoxemia during sleep should be anticipated. Drugs such as epinephrine, dopamine, and aminophylline should always be suspected as the offender when supraventricular arrhythmias occur during their use.

In patients receiving β-blocker therapy preoperatively, failure to restore β-blockade after surgery is associated with a significantly increased incidence of postoperative arrhythmias.[22] The mechanism is now known to be due to withdrawal hypersensitivity of the adrenergic receptors which are subject to stress stimuli after surgery.[23]

In summary, postoperative arrhythmias may be caused by conduction defects or may arise from ventricular or supraventricular foci. Conduction defects persisting into the early postoperative period have become more common with the advent of cold cardioplegia and ventricular or supraventricular arrhythmias may be escape phenomena. In the early postoperative period, sinus tachycardia suggests pain or hypovolemia. Ventricular arrhythmias are usually caused by hypokalemia or respiratory alkalosis or both, but if associated with acidosis, they are more likely to progress. After 2 or 3 days, an increased incidence of supraventricular arrhythmias should be anticipated, especially in patients on preoperative β-blocker therapy.

Metabolism

Surgical and anesthetic stress provokes the release of catecholamines, cortisol, and glucagon which oppose the action of insulin. Insulin resistance results in hyperglycemia and glycosuria, which may require parenteral insulin for control. The body is unable to utilize fat and becomes dependent on the breakdown of amino acids and the formation of glucose by the process of gluconeogenesis in the liver. Vital protein resources are thus used for energy supply; this includes the structural protein of the myocardium itself. During starvation, the myocardium is able to utilize ketone bodies and fatty acids for energy, but with stress and cellular hypoxia, this ability is lost and it becomes dependent on glucose for energy metabolism. Usually the catabolic hormonal response subsides after 2 to 3 days. Sudden return of hyperglycemia or glycosuria suggests sepsis: insulin antagonism may appear 24 to 48 hours before infection becomes overt.

The rise in plasma norepinephrine levels during CPB has been well documented. Probably the most potent stimulus to its secretion apart from surgical stimulation and stress is hypothermia. Renal hypoperfusion during bypass releases renin which activates angiotensin, the most potent naturally occurring vasoconstrictor. Angiotensin further decreases renal perfusion, and thus a vicious cycle is set up that must be broken by restoring intravascular volume and renal perfusion at the end of bypass. Acute renal failure after cardiac surgery may be related to a progressive rise in renin levels after bypass.[24]

Catecholamines and renin-angiotensin release have several adverse affects: (1) decreased renal perfusion; (2) increased systemic vascular resistance, causing decreased cardiac output and increased afterload and myocardial oxygen demand; (3) systemic hypertension, risking increased surgical bleeding and graft dehiscence; and (4) increased hydrostatic pressure, exacerbating capillary leak and interstitial and pulmonary edema in the postoperative period.

Aldosterone secretion is stimulated during cardiac surgery by (1) renin-angiotensin release, (2) hypovolemia, and (3) hyponatremia (induced by giving low-salt and salt-free dextrose infusions). This causes retention of sodium, which exacerbates interstitial and pulmonary edema, and excretion of potassium, which compounds the loss of this electrolyte and promotes postoperative hypokalemic alkalosis. Aldosterone secretion can best be prevented by *adequate salt loading* before induction of anesthesia. In view of the already described glucose intolerance existing in the perioperative period, the most rational fluid therapy before, during, and after surgery would appear to be *physiologic saline solution.*

ADH secretion is stimulated by many factors during cardiac surgery: previous thazide diuretics, surgical stimulation, anesthetic agents such as halothane and morphine, and positive pressure ventilation. Water retention promotes interstitial and pulmonary edema and oliguria, and is exacerbated by the liberal use of dextrose solutions, which essentially provide free water. After the initial phase of capillary leak and hypovolemia, oliguria in the face of adequate circulating blood volume is usually caused by inappropriate ADH secretion, and may be overcome with the appropriate use of salt-containing fluids and diuretic agents.

Vasoactive Compounds and the Postperfusion Syndrome

Hagemann factor (Factor XII) is activated by contact with foreign surfaces in the oxygenator and in turn triggers the kinin pathway. Moreover, bradykinin accumulates during bypass because its primary site of breakdown, the pulmonary circulation, is bypassed. Our studies indicate that activation of kinins occurs without necessarily manifesting as a change in SVR. Apart from vasodilation, the action of bradykinin is to induce capillary leak.[25] Complement activation occurs on CPB, either through the denaturation of plasma proteins (classic pathway) or through breakdown of white cells (alternate pathway). This results in the liberation of histamine, which also promotes capillary leak.[26, 27] Finally there may be absorption of endotoxins and other vasoactive amines directly from the gut through impairment of local defense mechanisms during splanchnic hypoperfusion during and after bypass.[28] Systemic manifestations in terms of vasodilation are usually masked by other causes of vasoconstriction, except with massive release such as in anaphylactic shock or with an incompatible blood transfusion. However, they probably cause some degree of capillary leak to occur in every instance.

The clinical manifestations of this syndrome (see Table 16–4) depend on (1) the duration of bypass and the extent of activation of vasoactive amines; (2) other factors promoting their activation, such as massive transfusion, acidosis or disseminated intravascular coagulation; and (3) preload levels required by the postoperative myocardium. The patient with a short bypass time and normal ventricular function will have little interstitial and pulmonary edema. The patient with difficult and protracted surgery, often with hemorrhage requiring return to the operating room, and who subsequently requires the maintenance of high intravascular pressures to optimize preload and cardiac function, will have a profound capillary leak syndrome. Maintenance of filling pressures is difficult because fluid challenges given seem to disappear into the third space and wedge pressures are always sinking. Widespread pitting edema with cheimosis appears early, sometimes on admission to the intensive care unit. Weight gain during the perioperative period is awesome, and interstitial pulmonary edema necessitates difficult and prolonged weaning from mechanical ventilation.

Older studies suggest that the use of an antikallikrein agent such as aprotonin (Trasylol) might prevent the activation of bradykinin and its circulatory effects.[29] This approach has not gone beyond the experi-mental stage and remains an interesting avenue for exploration.

Heat Exchange

Changes in body temperature and distribution of heat are important in the response of patients to cardiac surgery. Arterial tone is inversely proportional to temperature; during hypothermia on bypass, systemic vascular resistance becomes markedly elevated and with rewarming it falls. CO_2 production ($\dot{V}CO_2$) and O_2 consumption ($\dot{V}CO_2$) are directly proportional to temperature; $\dot{V}CO_2$ changes 10 percent for every 1°C change. The redistribution and metabolism of drugs, especially muscle relaxants, are profoundly altered by changes in temperature.

The ability to follow temperature changes accurately depends upon the site used. The best measure of central core temperature is nasopharyngeal; it is closest to the cerebral circulation, and reflects changes in $\dot{V}CO_2$ most accurately.[30] Rectal temperature is outside the core during hypothermia, and esophageal temperature often reflects the temperature of the inspired gas. Skin temperature (e.g., the great toe) provides an indication of distribution of heat to the periphery and is useful in estimating overall circulatory status.[31]

The characteristic nasopharyngeal temperature curve is illustrated in Figure 16–8. With the institution of cardiopulmonary bypass, *rapid cooling* of blood to approximately 28°C

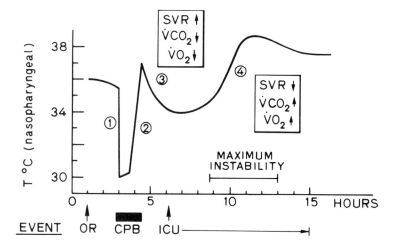

Fig. 16–8. Temperature changes during and after cardiac surgery. 1. Hypothermia on bypass. 2. Rewarming on bypass. 3. Redistribution of heat to periphery after bypass. 4. Rewarming after surgery. Systemic vascular resistance (*SVR*), CO_2 production ($\dot{V}CO_2$) and oxygen consumption ($\dot{V}O_2$) vary markedly with temperature changes. Their effects must be anticipated and vigorously treated.

occurs. At removal of aortic cross-clamp, *gradual warming* is started and the nasopharyngeal temperature usually reaches 37°C by the end of bypass. Over the next hour, the bolus of heat delivered to the blood is *redistributed* to the colder periphery, and the nasopharyngeal temperature decreases to about 34.5°C. This is the temperature at which most patients are admitted to the intensive care unit. The elevated systemic vascular resistance obscures underlying hypovolemia and often provides a false sense of security in that the patient appears to be hemodynamically stable when in actual fact the cardiac output is markedly reduced. CO_2 production is reduced, and minute ventilation should be adjusted accordingly to avoid respiratory alkalosis. After a latent period that varies from 2 to 4 hours, body temperature increases rapidly. This may not be associated with shivering, depending on sedative drugs used, temperature, and the use of neuromuscular blockade. There is usually an overshoot characteristic of the servo mechanisms involved in body homeostasis. Nasopharyngeal temperature typically increases from 34°C to a peak of around 38.5 to 39°C over 8 hours before stabilizing.[32] The first manifestation of body rewarming, which may precede a noticeable increase in nasopharyngeal temperature, is an increase in CO_2 production. Minute ventilation must be increased accordingly to avoid respiratory acidosis. If the patient is on an intermittent mechanical ventilation circuit at this stage, the increasing $\dot{V}CO_2$ should stimulate spontaneous ventilation so that $PaCO_2$ is maintained without increasing ventilator rate. However, residual narcosis and muscle relaxation impair the response to hypercapnia and the patient must be followed closely with serial arterial blood gases.

As body temperature increases, systemic vascular resistance decreases. The phase of *maximum hemodynamic instability*, therefore, commences about *2 to 3 hours after admission to the ICU*. Systemic vascular resistance continues to decrease for hours after nasopharyngeal or even rectal temperature has reached its plateau (Fig. 16–9). Myocardial ischemia may be unmasked at this stage because the decreasing resistance requires an increased cardiac output to maintain blood pressure. Also, $M\dot{V}O_2$ increases progressively with increasing temperature. Over the next 6 to 12 hours nasopharyngeal temperature gradually settles back to normal, although a slight servo wobble continues for 1 or 2 days.

A study presented by Noback and Tinker in 1979 demonstrated that the use of sodium nitroprusside on cardiopulmonary bypass to provide vasodilation through the rewarming phase promotes distribution of heat to the periphery.[33] When cardiopulmonary bypass was discontinued, the temperature decrease over the next 80 minutes was significantly less than controls: about 1.5°C as opposed to 2.6°C. Early use of vasodilator therapy thus not only facilitates adequate fluid loading, blood pressure control, and improved cardiac output, but also modifies the profound

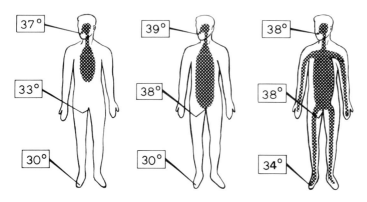

Fig. 16–9. **During rapid rewarming, the core temperature slowly extends to the rectum, with rapid decrease in systemic vascular resistance.** However, the core temperature continues to extend after nasopharyngeal or rectal temperatures have reached a plateau, and vascular resistance continues to decrease for some time. These circulatory changes may be revealed if toe skin temperature monitoring is used.

changes in temperature that occur after surgery and effect ventilatory and hemodynamic function. In this regard, vasodilatory therapy is superior to external measures such as increased ambient air temperature and warming blankets.

MANAGEMENT

Phase I: Restoration of Blood Volume

Assessment The receiving physician should learn as much as possible about the clinical state of the patient before his admission to the ICU. The patient should be visited preoperatively and the cardiac catheterization data reviewed with the surgeon. If the procedure is particularly difficult or prolonged, the ICU attendant should visit the operating room and discuss progress with the anesthesiologist and surgeon. The nursing and ancillary staff should be appraised of any particular problems (*e.g.*, use of IABP) and given some idea of the general clinical approach (routine, difficult, and so on).

On admission to the ICU, details of technique, problems, and results should be sought from the surgeon and anesthesiologist. The anesthesia record should be appraised for the type of anesthesia (short-acting volatile anesthetic or long-lasting narcotic), amount of muscle relaxant used, hemodynamic problems, ventilatory problems, cardiopulmonary bypass time (a guide to the incidence of coagulation problems), and aortic clamp time (a guide to the degree of myocardial ischemia).

Proper hemodynamic assessment begins with careful clinical examination of the patient. Talk to the patient and attempt to get an immediate appraisal of level of consciousness and muscle strength. Pupillary constriction after narcotic anesthesia suggests adequate analgesia; pupillary dilation, tachycardia, hypertension, sweating, lacrimation, or all of these suggest that the patient is in pain or discomfort and requires immediate sedation (nitroprusside is not analgesic). Check color centrally (tongue) and peripherally (nailbeds), temperature (warm and well

Table 16-8. Hemodynamic Evaluation (Checklist)

PREOPERATIVE
Indications for surgery
Examination of patient
Catheterization data
Medication; associated diseases

INTRAOPERATIVE
Anesthetic, surgical problems
CPB, AXC time
Success of procedure (revascularization, valve replacement)
Weaning from CPB
Arrhythmias
Filling pressures
Inotropic status
Vasoactive drugs
Pulmonary function
Hemostasis
Renal function, fluid, electrolytes

ADMISSION TO ICU
Anesthetic depth—need for sedation
Circulatory status
Pulmonary status
Bleeding (wounds, chest tubes)
Urine (volume, nature)
Temperature
Monitoring lines (site, calibration, problems, values)

perfused or cold and vasoconstricted), capillary fill time, and peripheral pulses. Heart sounds are often soft because of background noise, but seek inappropriate murmurs or friction rubs. Check the endotracheal tube position, quality and nature of breath sounds, and equality of chest movement. Examine the abdomen for inappropriate distension and the legs for bleeding if saphenous vein grafts have been taken. Check the urinary catheter and the quantity and quality of urine production. Chest tubes may be mediastinal or pleural; check with the attending surgeon as to their nature and as to whether there was any unusual reason for their insertion (*e.g.*, inadvertent lung puncture). Having examined the patient, evaluate temperature and arterial, central venous, and pulmonary artery pressures. Check that all lines are functioning properly and calibrated to your satisfaction (Table 16–8).

Routine Management The basic principles of early postoperative management involve anticipation of the factors discussed previously:

Table 16-9. Routine Hemodynamic Management

1. Routine monitoring
   ECG, arterial line, CVP
   Urinary catheter, chest tubes
   NP/rectal temperature

2. Stabilize
   heart rate and rhythm (Fig. 16-11)

3. Aggressive fluid therapy
   Restore intravascular volume
      (HR, BP, CVP, urine, skin perfusion)
   Restore hematocrit

4. Vasodilator therapy
   SNP 0.5–3.0 μg/kg/min
      (restoration of volume, heat distribution,
      pressure
      control, afterload reduction)

5. Inotropic support
   Calcium chloride 1 g IV   } When
   Dopamine 3–5 μg/kg/min   } Indicated

hypovolemia, hypoanalgesia, and hypothermia. In general the approach is to deal with any rate or rhythm problems that exist and to use careful vasodilator therapy with adequate fluid loading before spontaneous vasodilation commences with rewarming (Table 16-9).

Routine monitoring at Stanford University Hospital consists of ECG, arterial blood pressure, central venous pressure, chest tube drainage, urine output, and blood gases. The mean arterial pressure is commonly used because it is a convenient single parameter. Because systolic pressure reflects afterload, diastolic pressure coronary perfusion, and pulse pressure shearing stress on fresh suture lines, the mean arterial pressure is a convenience to be used with discretion. Therapeutic manipulations based solely on the mean arterial pressure may be self-defeating. A thermodilution pulmonary artery catheter is usually inserted at induction of anesthesia if postoperative ventricular dysfunction is expected. Rarely, a left atrial (LA) catheter is placed during surgery instead. Indications for insertion of the pulmonary artery catheter in the ICU are summarized in Table 16–10. Data is entered into a large flow chart, illustrated in Figure 16–10.

Arrhythmias. A clear priority is to stabilize

heart rate and rhythm so that further hemodynamic therapy may be instituted in as steady a state as possible. Conduction problems are treated by pharmacologic and electrical pacing, as appropriate, with efforts made to retain atrial contraction if possible. Ventricular irritability is often resolved by due attention to control of pain, hypokalemia, and respiratory acidosis or alkalosis, but lidocaine is used if necessary. The same factors should be considered when supraventricular irritability occurs; digoxin should be used with consideration of potassium flux (see Fig. 16–11).

Sinus tachycardia is the most common postoperative arrhythmia. Inadequate analgesia and hypovolemia must always be suspected and treated first. Inadequate oxygenation or ventilation, acute cardiac failure, or hyperdynamic responses may also reveal themselves via tachycardia.

Conduction disturbances. Sinus bradycardia should be treated if it causes hypotension or escape beats or rhythms or both. It is preferable to maintain the atrial kick because this contributes 25 percent of cardiac output (in idiopathic hypertrophic subaortic stenosis and aortic stenosis, up to 40%). Ideal management would be atrial pacing or isoproterenol infusion. Isoproterenol is made up as 1

Table 16-10. Indications for Insertion of Pulmonary Artery Catheter in ICU

EMERGENT
1. Any hemodynamic instability when CVP measurements not helpful in defining therapy
   (*i.e.,* inappropriately high, low or constant)
2. Low cardiac output syndrome
3. Capillary leak syndromes
4. Diagnosis of suspected cardiac tamponade

ELECTIVE
(when subsequent instability is suspected)
1. Monitoring of preload-dependent states
   Ventricular hypertrophy and stiffness (IHSS, AS with ischemia, aneurysmectomy)
   Poor preoperative ventricular function (ischemic cardiomyopathy, mitral regurgitation)
2. Specific preload/afterload reduction (nitroglycerin, hydralazine)
3. Facilitate ventilatory weaning (manipulation of preload)
   Cachexia, elderly, debilitated patient
   Severe preoperative pulmonary edema (mixed mitral valve disease)

mg in 250 ml D5W (4 μg/ml) and titrated to increase the sinus rate to that which abolishes escape beats or which supports blood pressure, usually about 80/min. Dose requirements are small, often about 0.5 μg/min, and at this level the chronotropic effects of isoproterenol mask the concomitant modest vasodilation. If ventricular pacing is used, the rate must be pushed to 100 to 110/min to obtain the same increase in cardiac output because of loss of the atrial kick; this significantly increases myocardial oxygen demand compared to the other methods.

Junctional rhythms at 40 to 60/min are usually escape rhythms associated with SA depression. Treatment is by atrial pacing; isoproterenol may stimulate return of SA node function. If an intraatrial block exists, ventricular or sequential AV pacing will be required.

With atrioventricular block, isolated atrial pacing is clearly ineffective. The alternatives are sequential AV pacing, a trial of isoproterenol, or ventricular pacing. Mobitz I (Wenckebach) block is benign but requires treatment if associated with hypotension. (It may be associated with digitalis effect.) Mobitz II block is rare but much more serious. Prophylactic pacing is necessary.

Ventricular arrhythmias. It is important to distinguish ventricular escape beats from true ectopy because abolition of the former by an antiarrhythmic will allow the underlying bradycardia to manifest without compensation. The correct approach is to treat the bradycardia. The most common cause of ventricular irritability in the early period is *hyperkalemia.* However, the first step is to exclude pain. Hypertension and catecholamines cause ventricular irritability. Lidocaine and nitroprusside do not provide analgesia and are no substitute for morphine. Respiratory alkalosis should be sought and corrected as well because this is the most rapid way in which extracellular potassium levels can be increased. Ventricular ectopy will frequently abate when potassium levels are pushed into the 4.5 to 5.0 mEq/l range. The approach we use is to (1) add 20 to 40 mEq KCl/l to the maintenance fluid and (2) check serum potassium q.4 h and adjust it to a set level,

routinely 4.5 mEq/l. By protocol, 2 mEq of KCl is given for every 0.1 mEq that the serum level is less than 4.5 q.4 h., at a rate not faster than 0.5 mEq/min. For example, if the serum potassium is 4.0 mEq/l, the patient is given 5 × 2 = 10 mEq KCl over 20 minutes. Because this is a catch-up scale, there is little danger of hyperkalemia unless the patient has renal dysfunction; the *K scale* is not used if urine output is less than 30 ml/hr. When ventricular irritability exists with a serum potassium of less than 4.0 mEq/l, the K scale is increased to 5.0 or even 5.5 mEq/l in an effort to elevate serum potassium to the high-normal range.

Although not routinely measured, hypomagnesemia also predisposes to ventricular irritability, and magnesium replacement should be considered when arrhythmias do not respond to conventional therapy. In most instances, correction of pain, pH, and serum potassium is all that is required to abolish ventricular ectopic activity.

Lidocaine is reserved for the following situations: (1) ectopic activity not responding to the above, (2) ventricular tachycardia, (3) high-risk patient (*i.e.,* where residual myocardial ischemia is suspected as a cause or where hemodynamic stability is essential), and (4) suspicious ventricular ectopics (R on T, multifocal). Lidocaine is given in the usual way (a loading dose of about 1 mg/kg slowly), followed by an infusion of 1 to 2 mg/min. Lidocaine levels should be followed closely because the patient may already have received lidocaine in the operating room (100–200 mg of lidocaine is often added to the pump prior to defibrillation), and because many patients have impaired hepatic perfusion and metabolize the drug slowly.

Drowsiness and confusion may be induced by lidocaine, even at normal therapeutic levels. The patient who is on lidocaine and who has been recently extubated should be closely observed for this side effect. In the vast majority of cases the infusion can be weaned and discontinued within 36 to 48 hours. Discussion of the management of ventricular arrhythmias resistant to lidocaine is beyond the scope of this section and is found in Chapter 6.

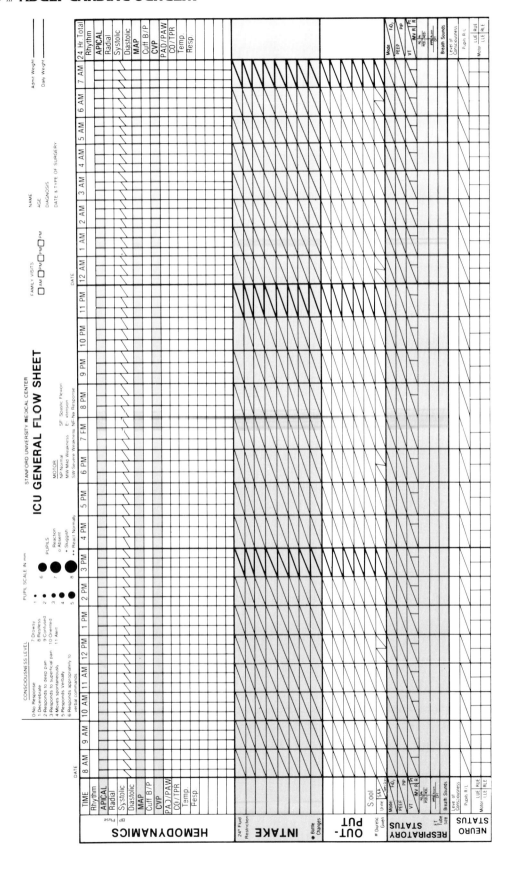

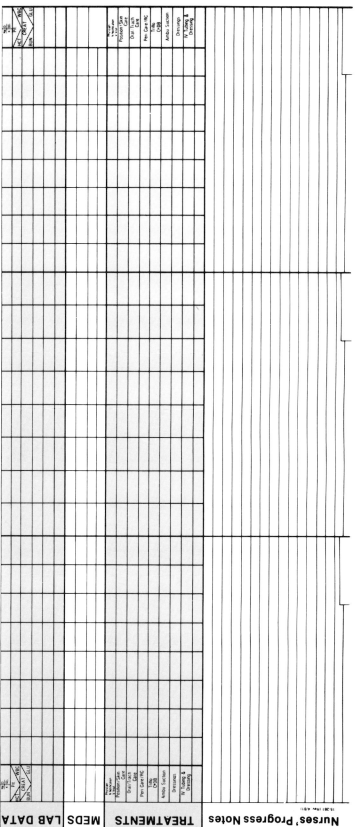

Fig. 16–10. The ICU flow chart is maintained by the ICU nurse. Data are entered at 20 min intervals.

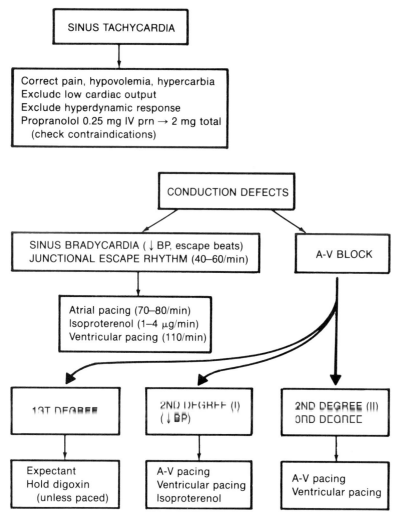

Fig. 16–11. Decision-making in management of postoperative arrhythmias. (Modified from Wynne J, Alpert JS, Koster JK: Medical/surgical treatment of myocardial ischemia. In Cohn LH (ed): The Treatment of Acute Myocardial Ischemia: An integrated Medical/Surgical Approach. Futura, NY, pp 173–197, 1979)

As discussed, supraventricular arrhythmias are common after the second day. When they occur earlier, escape rhythms should be excluded and metabolic problems, especially hypokalemic alkalosis, should be corrected. Their detailed management is discussed in phase III.

Fluid therapy. Vigorous fluid therapy is given to reverse intravascular hypovolemia in the early postoperative phase. The volume administered depends on the overall hemodynamic status of the patient, and is guided by the CVP, which is usually maintained between 8 and 15 cmH$_2$O. Maintenance fluid consists of 5 percent dextrose in 1/4 strength saline with 40 mEq/l KCl at 80 ml/hour. Fluid

challenges are given if CVP decreases below the given limits or if there is hypotension, because this is considered to be secondary to hypovolemia until proven otherwise. Packed red cells are given until the PCV reaches 36 percent.* Fluid challenges are then given in the form of normal saline or human albumin or both.

Albumin continues to be used at Stanford, largely because it is traditional therapy; it reduces the total fluid load but does not confer any distinct advantage in terms of cardiac or pulmonary function to justify its expense. It

---

*If a cell saver device is used, autotransfusion of packed red blood cells may result in a high PCV (40–50%).

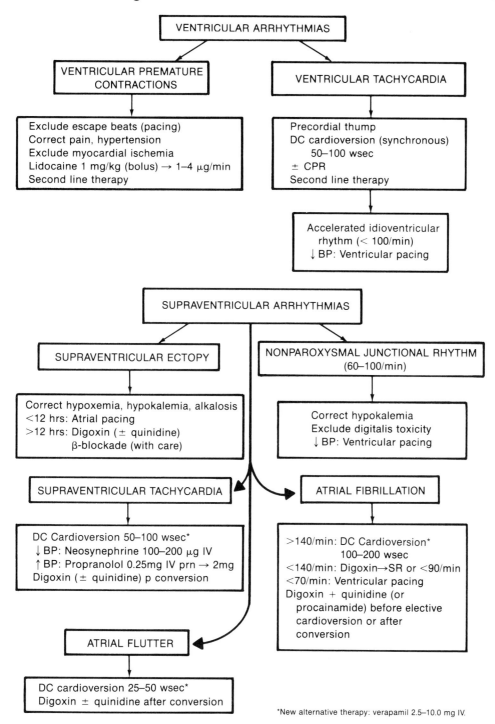

Fig. 16–11. *(continued)*

Fig. 16–11. Decision-making in management of postoperative arrhythmias. (Modified from Wynne J, Alpert JS, Koster JK; Medical/surgical treatment of myocardial ischemia. In Cohn LH (ed): The Treatment of Acute Myocardial Ischemia: An integrated Medical/Surgical Approach. Futura, NY, pp 173–197, 1979)

is excluded if the capillary leak syndrome is thought to exist. Other blood products (*e.g.*, fresh frozen plasma, platelets) are given as indicated. Plasmanate is avoided because of possible hypotension secondary to kinin activation associated with this product.[31] The diuresis induced by mannitol on cardiopulmonary bypass lasts 3 to 4 hours with an average urine flow of 150 to 400 ml/hour. Thereafter, a urine flow of ≥ 0.5 ml/kg/hour is considered acceptable.

Vasodilator therapy. Sodium nitroprusside is started soon before cardiopulmonary bypass weaning to facilitate return of pump volume to the patient. It is continued in the ICU to overcome the vasoconstriction of hypothermia[35] and to allow adequate blood and fluid replacement before spontaneous rewarming. The infusion of sodium nitroprusside (50 mg in 250 ml D5W, or 200 μg/ml) is titrated according to the mean arterial pressure; a typical order will read: "Titrate SNP to keep mean arterial pressure between 75 and 85 torr." The dose ranges from 0.5 to 3.0 μg/kg/min. As the patient warms up and vasodilates, less and less sodium nitroprusside is required to keep the mean arterial pressure in the desirable range, and it is usually weaned within 6 to 8 hours. Apparent tachyphylaxis (dose requirements above 3 μg/kg/min) suggests the hyperdynamic left ventricle syndrome. Intravenous nitroglycerin is being used as an alternate general vasodilator in some centers, based on low toxicity and potentially better myocardial oxygen balance.[36, 37]

Inotropic support. The majority of patients with normal ventricular function do not require inotropic support during intensive care.

Ionized calcium levels are frequently subnormal after cardiopulmonary bypass. This is exacerbated by the decrease that occurs through chelation with citrate during rapid blood transfusion.[38] Hypotension occurring during rapid transfusion is treated with a bolus of 250 mg $CaCl_2$ followed by 750 mg over 10 to 15 minutes. The response may be dramatic. Because calcium is the final common pathway of all muscle contraction, its use as a first-line inotrope is logical. It acts synergistically to increase the effectiveness of all inotropic agents, including dopamine and epinephrine.

Dopamine is usually started in the operating room because of direct observation of impaired myocardial contractility after cardiopulmonary bypass. Sodium nitroprusside is then added to provide vasodilation in the usual way. In the ICU, dopamine is infused at a *constant* rate (usually between 3–5 μg/kg/min) and the sodium nitroprusside infusion is varied to adjust mean arterial pressure. If one allows the nursing staff to manipulate both dopamine and sodium nitroprusside, a juggling match usually ensues that leaves the RN in a state of baffled frustration. Dopamine is often not discontinued with hemodynamic improvement, but merely decreased to low levels (1 μg/kg/min) through ventilatory weaning and extubation, to promote renal perfusion and mobilization of third space fluid. Some patients first demonstrate a requirement for inotropic support during rapid rewarming. Systemic vascular resistance decreases, and increased cardiac output is required to maintain blood pressure; dopamine is helpful in reducing the requirement for volume challenges and avoiding cardiac failure.

Isoproterenol is used routinely after cardiac transplantation for its chronotropism, to pace the denervated heart at 100 to 110/min and maintain stable cardiac output for 24 to 48 hours after operation. Dobutamine, epinephrine, and digoxin are not used as first-line inotropic agents.

Writing of hemodynamic orders. In order to simplify hemodynamic management, as many modalities as possible should be kept constant. In addition, clear-cut guidelines should be given as to the desired range of parameters allowed. For example, this would be typical of a hypothetical clinical situation:

1. Maintain heart rate 110/min with ventricular pacing.
2. Maintain dopamine infusion constant at 5.0 μg/kg/min.
3. Maintain $\overline{PA}_o$ 16–20 torr with fluid challenges as required.

4. Titrate sodium nitroprusside to keep mean arterial pressure 70–75 torr.
5. Repeat cardiac output estimations q2h and calculate hemodynamic profile.
6. Notify physician if heart rate > 130/min, pacer failure, mean arterial pressure < 70 or > 110, $\overline{PA}_o$ < 18 or > 26, urine output < 30 ml/hr.

If other infusions, such as epinephrine/calcium are added, they are kept constant as well. In this way, the RN has only to manipulate the sodium nitroprusside infusion and to give fluid challenges when indicated. The physician is easily able to assess hemodynamic status and is alerted to changes which may require direct intervention or a change in course.

Low Cardiac Output Syndrome *Clinical assessment.* The vast majority of patients have an uneventful postoperative course requiring little modification of the routine management outlined above. This section deals with the patient who is unstable and presents with severe myocardial dysfunction. Postoperative dysfunction should be anticipated if the surgical procedure has proven difficult, if aortic cross-clamp time (ischemia) or total bypass time (bleeding) have been prolonged, or if there have been intraoperative complications (see Table 16–2B). The most meaningful information is difficulty in weaning from cardiopulmonary bypass, and the surgeon and anesthesiologist should be directly questioned in this regard. Requirements for pacing, antiarrhythmic agents or high-dose inotropic support (dopamine > 7.5 µg/kg/min, or epinephrine infusion) are obvious clues that one is dealing with an unstable patient. Insertion of an intraaortic balloon pump (IABP), whether elective or mandatory, is an automatic indication for close hemodynamic monitoring and careful therapeutic manipulation. Clinical evaluation should seek manifestations of a low cardiac output state: persistent obtundation; central cyanosis; cold, poorly perfused extremities despite return to normal core temperature; hypotension (with or without inotropic support); tachycardia and tachyarrhythmias; inappropriately ele-

vated CVP; and oliguria (urine flow less than 0.5 ml/kg/hr).

Management. Management is summarized in the list below.

Optimize rate and rhythm. The initial step is to stabilize rate and rhythm, as discussed in the previous section.

Optimize preload. In a steady state, baseline $\overline{PA}_o$ (an indicator of preload), heart rate, mean arterial pressure, and central venous pressure (CVP) are documented. A cardiac output determination is performed, and cardiac index, stroke index, and systemic vascular resistance are calculated by the usual formula. The systemic vascular resistance is used as a guide to afterload. A fluid challenge is given and the $\overline{PA}_o$ is pushed to a higher level. When a steady state is achieved (usually after 30 minutes or so), the stroke index and systemic vascular resistance are again calculated. In this way a Frank–Starling curve for preload response is constructed. The ideal $\overline{PA}_o$ is that which achieves hemodynamic stability.

Improve contractility. Because ventricular dysfunction invariably declares itself at the time of weaning from cardiopulmonary by-

---

Management of Low Cardiac Output Syndrome

1. Exclude complications (bleeding, tamponade, infarction)
2. Optimize rate and rhythm (see Table 16–10)
3. Optimize preload
   a. Serial fluid challenges → CO determinations (myocardial function curve)
4. Improve contractility
   a. Dopamine 3–12 µg/kg/min
   b. CaCl$_2$ 1 g IV prn
   c. Epinephrine + CaCl$_2$ ("Epical") 1–4 µg/min (Dopamine > 12 µg/kg/min)
   d. Digoxin
5. Reduce afterload
   a. Non-specific: Sodium nitroprusside (SNP) 0.5–3 µg/kg/min
   b. Specific: Hydralazine 2.5–5.0 mg IV q4–6h
6. Restore preload to former level
   Correct decrease in $\overline{PA}_o$ caused by SNP to achieve benefit of afterload reduction (not necessary with hydralazine).
7. Intraaortic balloon support
   If above measures insufficient or if myocardial ischemia suspected

pass, inotropic agents are usually already in use by the time the patients are admitted to the ICU. Management is simplified if infusion of inotropic agents are kept constant during manipulations of preload and afterload. Dosage of inotropic agents should be increased or decreased in quanta and thereafter kept steady. Acidosis impairs catecholamine response and should be corrected.

Dopamine is a first-line agent. It is started at a rate of 3 μg/kg/min; at this level some dopaminergic enhancement of renal perfusion probably still exists. If contractility appears deficient, the rate is increased in quanta of 2 to 3 μg/kg/min, to a maximum of 12 μg/kg/min. Above this level increasing α-adrenergic activity negates the inotropic effect.

Calcium is frequently used in synergy with dopamine. Ionized calcium levels fall after cardiopulmonary bypass and during rapid blood transfusion. Restoration of calcium concentration enhances the inotropic action of all catecholamines. $CaCl_2$ (1000 mg in a volutrol over 10 minutes) should be considered whenever there is an apparent lack of response to dopamine.

Epinephrine is used when myocardial depression is severe. It is made up as 1 mg in 250 ml D5W (4 μg/ml) and infused at 1 to 4 μg/min to augment dopamine and allow use of the latter in the 3 to 8 μg/kg/min range. $CaCl_2$ (1 g in 250 ml) is frequently added to the epinephrine mixture (Epical Drip) to provide synergy.

Dobutamine has a theoretic advantage over dopamine in that it is a direct-acting inotropic agent. Long-standing ventricular dysfunction is associated with depletion of norepinephrine stores, which hampers the indirect action of dopamine. Occasionally we have used a combination of dobutamine (10 μg/kg/min) and low dose dopamine (1–2 μg/kg/min) in patients with a long history of prior cardiac failure. However, in our experience dobutamine appears to have no less effect on heart rate compared with dopamine, it does not selectively improve renal blood flow, and at higher dose ranges its vasodilator activity can be disturbing, especially in the hypovolemic patient. We prefer to use dopamine and to

manipulate systemic vascular resistance independently with sodium nitroprusside.

Digoxin may be given to enhance contractility as long as it is noted that (1) several hours pass before its effect is manifest and (2) digitoxicity is possible when potassium balance and renal function are unstable. It is particularly useful in states of rapid heart rate and atrial dysrhythmias. Digoxin-induced A-V block is not a contraindication to its use as an inotropic agent as long as ventricular pacing is available to maintain an adequate heart rate.

The vigorous use of any or all of these measures increases myocardial oxygen demand and the incidence of ventricular irritability. Inotropic support should never replace restoration of intravascular volume. It is most effective when used for short periods to deal with self-limited myocardial depression (*e.g.*, hypothermia following cardiopulmonary bypass) and should not be relied upon to provide support for periods longer than 12 hours. Continued use of epinephrine or high-dose dopamine, apart from being a poor prognostic sign, predisposes to myocardial, renal, and splanchnic ischemia. Requirement for this amount of support for a longer period than 12 hours may indeed be an indication for the institution of IABP in the postoperative period.

Reduce afterload and adjust preload. It is axiomatic that the more damaged the myocardium, the less responsive it is to inotropy and the more dependent it becomes on afterload reduction to increase stroke volume. Clinically, this situation exists when the cardiac index remains < 2.5 l/m²/min and systemic vascular resistance > 1100 dyne·sec·cm⁻⁵, despite preload augmentation and inotropic support.

Afterload reduction with sodium nitroprusside is preferred because of its rapid onset and short action; it is easily titrated to effect. Furthermore, the use of sodium nitroprusside and dopamine together produce a greater increase in stroke index than either agent used separately.[39] Phentolamine (tachycardia), Chlorpromazine (tachycardia, sedation, fixed vasodilation), trimethaphan (sympathetic blockade), and nitroglycerin (predominant preload reduction) are not used for afterload reduction in this situation.[40]

The clinical endpoint for sodium nitroprusside effect is a reduction in mean arterial pressure by 5 to 15 torr. Once a steady state is achieved, cardiac index, stroke index, and systemic vascular resistance are calculated. There will invariably be a decrease in $\overline{PA}_o$ as well as systemic vascular resistance, because sodium nitroprusside causes balanced venodilation and arterial dilation. Further afterload reduction may be achieved by increasing the dose of sodium nitroprusside as long as $\overline{PA}_o$ remains above ideal levels and mean arterial pressure does not decrease below 65 torr. This is usually associated with a progressive increase in stroke index.

Restore preload to its former level. Although afterload reduction allows lower preload, the decrease in $\overline{PA}_o$ with sodium nitroprusside may be so brisk that stroke index (and mean arterial pressure) may decrease instead. In order to achieve the benefit of afterload reduction, $\overline{PA}_o$ must be restored to (or near to) its previous level by further fluid challenges.[41] This sequence of events (optimize preload, reduce afterload, restore preload) is illustrated in Figure 16–12.

Specific afterload reduction. In certain situations, afterload reduction with sodium nitroprusside either is not tolerated at all because of hypotension, or requires excessive fluid challenges. This occurs in states of severe ventricular dysfunction (cardiac index < 2 l/m²/min) associated with requirement for high preload ($\overline{PA}_o$ > 20 torr)—in particular, mitral regurgitation with left ventricular failure. The failing left ventricle has been chronically off

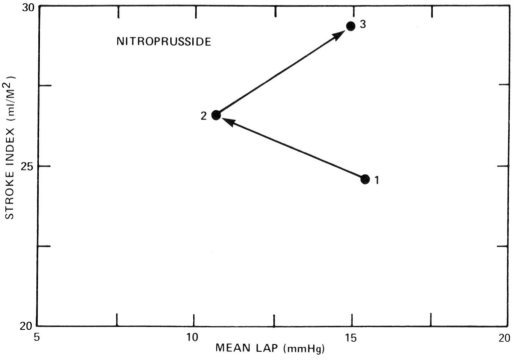

Fig. 16–12. Schematic representation of afterload reduction with sodium nitroprusside. Stroke index is increased while mean left arterial pressure (*LAP*) is reduced from 15 to 10 torr (1→2). Restoration of *mean LAP* (preload) to its former level with a fluid challenge results in a further, marked increase in stroke index (2→3). Preload augmentation allows the full benefit of nitroprusside-induced afterload reduction. (Stinson EB et al: J Thorac Cardiovasc Surg 73:527, 1977)

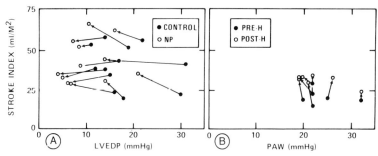

Fig. 16–13. *Nonspecific* (sodium nitroprusside [*NP*]) versus *specific* (hydralazine [*H*]) reduction of afterload. *A.* Relation between left ventricular end diastolic pressure (*LVEDP*) and stroke index (*SI*) before and during nitroprusside therapy in patients with congestive heart failure. *LEVDP* high, reduced to normal; SI increased. LVEDP normal, reduced to low; SI unchanged or decreased. (Miller RR et al: Circulation 51:328, 1975) *B.* Relation between pulmonary artery wedge (*PAW*) pressure and stroke index before and after hydralazine. Note the striking difference of the directional change of stroke index compared to *A.* Specific afterload reduction increases stroke index without change in preload. (Sladen RN, Rosenthal MH: J Thorac Cardiovasc Surg 78:199, 1978)

loaded by the incompetent mitral valve. Mitral valve replacement may actually increase impedance to left ventricular outflow if the systemic vascular resistance remains unchanged or elevated after surgery. We recently reported a series of eight patients with severe ventricular dysfunction and high preload requirement after cardiac surgery who benefited from the intravenous use of the arterial dilator, hydralazine.[42] Reduction in systemic vascular resistance and increase in cardiac index was greater than that achieved by highest tolerable doses of sodium nitroprusside, without decrease in $\overline{PA}_o$ (Fig. 16–13). The drug is given as a test dose of 2.5 mg IV, followed by maintenance doses of from 2.5 to 7.5 mg IV q4 to 6h. Measurement of cardiac output at frequent intervals to assess effect is mandatory. The parenteral dose of the drug is about one-tenth the oral dose because first-pass hepatic metabolism is excluded. This does not preclude conversion from the IV to the PO route at a later stage. An important drawback to hydralazine is that its onset of action takes about 20 to 30 minutes and it lacks the easy titratability of sodium nitroprusside. It is not used during the first 12 hours of relative hemodynamic instability (or at least until temperature has reached its plateau). Wider application of specific afterload reduction awaits further prospective studies.

Intraaortic Balloon Pump (IABP). A detailed account of the indications, actions and complications of the IABP is given in Chapter 27. In general, the IABP is placed under the following circumstances: (1) before surgery in patients with progressive ischemia or mitral regurgitation or septal rupture complicating acute myocardial infarction; (2) during bypass for patients with severe ventricular dysfunction; and (3) after bypass if weaning attempts have failed. IABP insertion in the ICU is indicated if a low cardiac output state persists despite the hemodynamic manipulations outlined above. If acute myocardial infarction is suspected as the cause of pump failure, IABP support should be provided as soon as possible (see *Complications*, below). Insertion is either performed by direct arteriotomy in the OR, or, if an emergency, by transcutaneous insertion by the Seldinger technique in the ICU. Heparinization is not necessary.

The IABP is adjusted to provide optimal afterload reduction and diastolic augmentation; thereafter support is kept constant at 1:1 (every beat) as other hemodynamic changes are made (Figs. 16–14, 16–15).

Weaning should be considered only when hemodynamic stability has been established for at least 12 hours. It is contraindicated during the rapid rewarming phase; with increased heat production, myocardial work increases and oxygen balance becomes more precarious. Inotropic support should be in

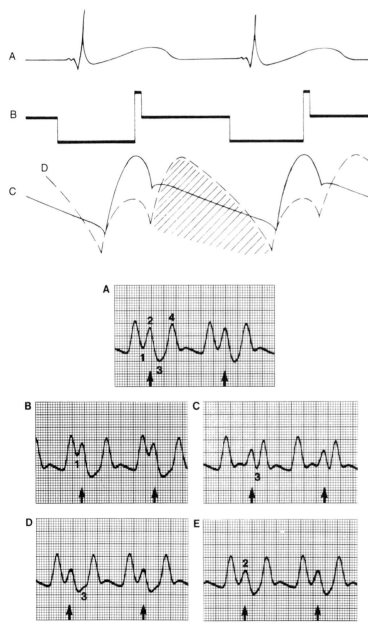

Fig. 16–14. The intraaortic balloon inflation is triggered by the _R_ wave of the ECG (_A_). Inflation and deflation cycles can be demonstrated on the oscilloscope for visual adjustment and timing (_B_). The unassisted arterial trace (_C_) changes its form (_D_) to demonstrate the cumulative effects of diastolic augmentation and afterload (peak systolic pressure) reduction. Shaded area is diastolic augmentation.

Fig. 16–15. Pump timing may be manipulated by adjustment of inflation time, deflation time or balloon filling volume. Tracings illustrate 1:2 support for the sake of clarity. _A. Normal tracing._ Augmentation commences after the dichrotic notch (1), augments diastole (2), and reaches its nadir just before the next systolic contraction (3). Peak systolic pressure in the next (nonaugmented) beat is decreased (4). _B. Early inflation._ Augmentation commences before aortic valve closure (1), thereby increasing afterload and possibly inducing aortic regurgitation. _C. Late inflation._ Diastolic augmentation is inadequate, and end-diastolic pressure is no different from unassisted cycle (3). _D. Early deflation._ Diastolic augmentation and afterload reduction are impaired. _E. Inadequate filling volume._ Timing is satisfactory, but diastolic augmentation is impaired.

the process of being withdrawn or be constant at a low level (*e.g.*, dopamine less than 3 µg/kg/minute). Arrhythmias possibly caused by myocardial ischemia must be absent. In most cases, it is possible to start IABP weaning 12 to 24 hours after surgery. Complications such as thrombosis, ischemia and infection increase with duration of support; it is desirable to limit IABP insertion to not more than 4 days.

The rate of IABP weaning depends on the patient's clinical progress. However, at least 6 hours should be spent at each level of support (*i.e.*, at 1:2 and 1:3). The cardiac output may not decrease when balloon support is reduced from 1:1 to 1:2 to 1:3 over a period of several minutes; however, it is being maintained by increased myocardial work and reduced diastolic coronary perfusion pressure. The effects on myocardial oxygen balance (ST changes, ventricular irritability, pump failure) may not be manifest for several hours. A typical pattern of postoperative IABP support is 1:1 for 24 hours, 1:2 for 12 hours, 1:3 for 12 hours, with balloon removal scheduled for the second postoperative day.

Table 16-11. Intraaortic Balloon Pump (IABP)

FEATURES OF GOOD AUGMENTATION
1. Inflates at dicrotic notch (after aortic valve closure)
2. Upstrokes equal (*i.e.*, rate of rise of augmentation roughly equal to that of natural systolic upstroke)
3. Amplitude of diastolic augmentation greater than or equal to systolic peak
4. Presystolic dip
5. Systole following assisted beat is lower than that following unassisted beat (afterload reduction)
6. Mean arterial pressure increases if previously low

INDICATIONS FOR WEANING
1. Restoration of intravascular volume (phase I) and rewarming (↑ MVO₂) completed
2. Hemodynamic stability
   a. No ischemic arrhythmias (*e.g.*, VPCs)
   b. Inotropic therapy at low levels (*e.g.*, dopamine < 5 µg/kg/min)
3. No evidence of active myocardial ischemia (ST changes)

WEANING PROCEDURE
1. Continue ventilatory support (IMV > 4/min)
2. Spend at least 6 hours at each ratio (1:1 → 1:2 → 1:3) to exclude myocardial ischemia
3. Schedule OR time for removal

Because the presence of the IABP interferes with proper respiratory therapy, ventilatory weaning is stopped at low IMV rates, and extubation is deferred. This also facilitates the provision of general anesthesia for balloon removal, should it be necessary.

Although the percutaneous IABP may be removed at the bedside (with manual compression of the femoral artery for 30 minutes to secure hemostasis), the incidence of bleeding, hematoma, and arterial injury has led most surgeons at Stanford to perform removal in the operating room with primary closure under direct vision. The patient is transported to and from the operating room in the intensive care unit bed by the cardiac anesthesia team in the same manner as the initial transport from the operating room (Table 16–11).

Hyperdynamic Left Ventricle Syndrome
States of excessive (unwanted) ventricular contractility should be recognized as a potential problem after cardiac surgery. Iatrogenic exacerbation is likely to occur when blood pressure control is attempted with a pure vasodilator, such as sodium nitroprusside. Apparent tachyphylaxis to sodium nitroprusside results with little change in mean arterial pressure, despite increasing doses of the drug. Excessive postoperative contractility is more likely to occur in the setting of preexisting ventricular hypertrophy (*e.g.*, aortic stenosis or essential hypertension; see Table 16–6). Narcotic anesthetic techniques currently in vogue cause little myocardial depression, and if cardiopulmonary bypass and aortic cross-clamp times have been short, difficulty in controlling mean arterial pressure with sodium nitroprusside may be noticed soon after weaning from cardiopulmonary bypass.

Manifestations and dangers. As a routine, sodium nitroprusside is infused at 0.5 to 3 µg/kg/min to maintain the mean arterial pressure between 70 and 90 torr. In this situation, despite doses of sodium nitroprusside above 3 µg/kg/min, the mean arterial pressure remains unchanged in the 90 to 110 torr range. The patient appears to be insensitive to so-

dium nitroprusside, and supplementary analgesia has no effect. This apparent tachyphylaxis may or may not be associated with
a progressive increase in heart rate.

If systolic and diastolic arterial pressures
are recorded, it is noted that despite the fixity
of the mean arterial pressure there has been
marked increase in pulse pressure, with a
rise in systolic and fall in diastolic pressure.
If concurrent thermodilution cardiac output
and systemic vascular resistance are measured, the underlying mechanism becomes
clear (Fig. 16–16). When sodium nitroprusside is used for afterload reduction for the
failing myocardium (high systemic vascular
resistance, low stroke volume), stroke volume increases toward normal with little
change in heart rate. When sodium nitroprusside is used for pressure control of the
hyperdynamic myocardium (high systemic
vascular resistance, normal stroke volume),
the underlying excessive inotropism is unmasked, with progressive increase in stroke
volume, pulse pressure, and heart rate.

These changes directly impair myocardial
oxygen balance: demand increases (↑ systolic pressure, ↑ heart rate) in the face of
decreased supply (↓ diastolic pressure, ↑
heart rate).

In the case which first drew this syndrome
to our attention, a fatal cardiac arrest occurred during the administration of high (>
6 µg/kg/min) doses of sodium nitroprusside.
Cyanide toxicity was considered but there
was no metabolic acidosis. Instead, retrospective analysis revealed progressive tachycardia and widening pulse pressure before
the event. Cardiac arrest is presumed to have
occurred because of fulminating myocardial
ischemia. We frequently see this hyperdynamic response to sodium nitroprusside and
have managed many patients in the manner
outlined below.

Management. Recognition of the existence
of the hyperdynamic ventricular response is
an essential prerequisite. Patients with preexisting concentric hypertrophy who have little
intraperative myocardial depression are particularly vulnerable.

Withdrawal from aggressive antihyperten-

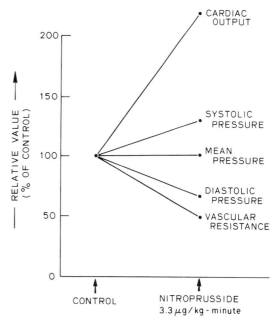

Fig. 16–16. Hemodynamic changes in the hyperdynamic response to sodium nitroprusside
(*SNP*) infusion. Mean data is from four patients
whose response was documented by pulmonary artery catheterization. At moderately high
levels of *SNP* (3.3 µg/kg/min) mean arterial
pressure (*MAP*) remained virtually unchanged
despite a dramatic widening of the pulse pressure. Systolic pressure rose while diastolic
pressure fell. Cardiac output (*CO*) doubled and
systemic vascular resistance halved. (Rosenthal MH, Sladen RN: Abstracts of American Society of Anesthesiologists Annual Meeting,
1978, p 143)

sive therapy (*i.e.*, allowing the mean arterial
pressure to rise to levels of 100–105 torr) will
break the vicious cycle. As the dose of sodium nitroprusside is lowered, pulse pressure and heart rate return to their former
levels, with little change in mean arterial
pressure.

If this approach is not effective, infusion of
a ganglion blocker trimethaphan camsylate
(Arfonad), aborts the sympathetic response
to vasodilation. The infusion is made up as
250 mg in 250 ml D5W. Rates of 250 to 500
µg/min are invariably successful in lowering
of mean arterial pressure to desired levels
with narrowing of pulse pressure. Simulta-

Management of Hyperdynamic Left Ventricle Syndrome

1. Identify widening pulse pressure (± tachycardia) with increasing dose of SNP (> 3 μg/kg/min)
2. Allow MAP to rise to 100–110 torr (*i.e.*, wean SNP)
3. If state persists, add trimethaphan camsylate (Arfonad) 250–500 μg/min, and wean SNP
4. If state persists, or heart rate > 120/min, add propranolol 0.25 mg IV prn to a total of 2.0 mg

neously, sodium nitroprusside can be reduced to a safe dosage (< 3 μg/kg/min).

If wide pulse pressure and tachycardia persist despite trimethaphan, β- blockade is begun using propranolol 0.25 mg IV. The dose is repeated every 5–10 minutes until satisfactory reduction of heart rate and arterial pressure is achieved, to a maximum dose of 2.0 mg. Overzealous use may hamper the response to rewarming or even precipitate frank cardiac failure. If necessary, however, dopamine or isoproterenol will reverse the block.

Phase II: Mobilization of Interstitial Fluid

Recognition The end of the first postoperative phase is heralded by (1) full vasodilation after rewarming, (2) replacement of all losses incurred during and after surgery, and (3) cessation of capillary leak. Fluid given remains within the intravascular space, and $\overline{PA}_o$ and $\overline{CVP}$ tend to rise and stay elevated after fluid challenges. At this stage, there has been a gain in total body water, most if not all to the interstitial space. This must be mobilized because of the diffuse organ dysfunction caused by interstitial edema. In particular, the presence of high hydrostatic pressures and interstitial fluid hamper ventilatory weaning and predispose to postoperative pulmonary complications.

The therapeutic approach required at this stage depends entirely on the duration and severity of phase I. The degree of postoperative weight gain is a helpful indicator. With normal ventricular function, phase II commences about 6 to 8 hours after return to the

ICU. Weight gain is slight (1–2 kg), the excess fluid is mobilized with ease, and the patient can be extubated early. On the other hand, when the first 24 hours has been stormy, the physician is often faced with a patient who, although hemodynamically stable, is 15 kg overweight and in incipient pulmonary edema. In this situation there is little to be gained by aggressive ventilatory weaning and early extubation. Pulmonary edema and (potentially traumatic) reintubation are almost invariable. Ventilatory support, even if modest (*e.g.*, IMV 2–4/min with 5 cm PEEP) should be continued until body weight approaches the preoperative range. This may take several days.

Routine Management Hemodynamic monitoring is continued after extubation as indicated. Careful and frequent clinical examination of the chest for signs of interstitial edema (crackles) or atelectasis (decreased breath sounds, bronchial breathing) is important. Chest films should be obtained daily while the patient is in the ICU.

Patients with good muscle strength are able to cope with the effects of interstitial fluid overload far better than those who are elderly, or cachectic. The margin for error is much smaller in the latter group. After extubation, reassumption of the upright position and walking are most helpful in maintaining good pulmonary function, decreasing venous return to the thorax, and overcoming antidiuretic hormone effects.

Fluid intake is restricted to 2000 ml/24 hours unless otherwise indicated. If tube feedings are required, care should be taken to decrease intravenous intake as enteral intake increases. Strict assessment of daily intake, output, and weight is essential.

Fluid mobilization proceeds spontaneously in most cases. However, oliguria may occur secondary to inappropriate antidiuretic hormone secretion rather than inadequate renal perfusion. A small dose of furosemide (10 mg IV) can overcome this effect. Subsequent doses depend on assessment of filling pressures, chest exam, roentgenographs, and blood gases (Table 16–12).

The Unstable Patient For the first 6 to 12 hours after surgery, diuretic therapy should be restricted to instances of obvious pulmonary edema. Indiscriminate use of loop diuretics to make urine or improve hematocrit will simply exacerbate hypovolemia and predispose to renal failure. Oliguria should *always* be treated first by normalization of cardiac output and renal perfusion. Relative intravascular hypovolemia may exist despite marked interstitial overload. Moreover, intravenous furosemide causes transient but brisk venodilation. Aggressive diuresis thus results in hypotension and tachycardia. Because renal perfusion is decreased, urine output increases only transiently. Attempts at diuresis are frustrated by the necessity for subsequent fluid challenges. The initial fall in filling pressure is rapidly restored by movement of interstitial fluid back into the intravascular space and repeated doses of diuretic must be given. Negative fluid balance may be achieved at a frustratingly slow pace in the complicated patient. However, there are other measures that facilitate management during this phase.

Low-dose dopamine (1–2 µg/kg/min) has the advantage of increasing urine output by increasing renal perfusion; diuresis is induced continuously rather than intermittently and the hemodynamic instability associated with large doses of furosemide is avoided. When no longer needed for inotropic support, dopamine is continued at low dose through weaning and extubation and for several days thereafter, if necessary.

In the patient with severe ventricular dysfunction, a $\overline{PA}_o$ high enough to provide adequate cardiac output may also induce pulmonary edema. Preload management becomes very difficult. Reduction of $\overline{PA}_o$ enough to improve pulmonary function reduces cardiac index. Use of a venodilator such as nitroglycerin, whether by absorption (nitro paste 0.5–1 inch q4h) or by intravenous infusion (nitroglycerin, 50 mg in 250 ml D5W, at 0.5–5.0 µg/kg/min) allows careful titration of preload. Pulmonary function is improved, facilitating extubation, and furosemide may be given in smaller doses, improving stabil-

Table 16-12. Mobilization of Interstitial Fluid

ROUTINE
1. Daily evaluation for pulmonary congestion/edema
2. Fluid restriction < 2000 ml/day
3. Respiratory therapy, ambulation
4. Diuresis, if indicated: furosemide 10–20 mg IV prn

UNSTABLE PATIENT
1. Slow ventilatory weaning
2. Low-dose dopamine (1–2 µg/kg/min)
3. Nitroglycerin (reduce excessive preload)
   IV: 0.5–5.0 µg/kg/min
   Paste: 0.5–1.0 inch q4h

ity. $\overline{PA}_o$ may not remain controlled without nitroglycerin until almost all excess interstitial fluid has been mobilized. Nitroglycerin is especially indicated where high preload is a cause or result of myocardial ischemia. On occasion, the combination of nitroglycerin with hydralazine is particularly useful to allow individual titration of preload and afterload.

The end of phase II is accomplished by return to preoperative weight, adequate mobilization, normal physical and radiographic exam, and normal pulmonary function.

Phase III: Late Arrhythmias

Management is summarized in Fig. 16–11.

Prophylaxis Supraventricular arrhythmias may occur at any time. However, once hemodynamic stability and ventilatory weaning have been achieved, these arrhythmias emerge as the most important clinical problem faced by the attending physician. Their incidence is greatest about 2 to 7 days after surgery, at a time when there might be a reduced concern about the need for close monitoring or when the physician is distracted by the constant supervision required of more recent postoperative patients. Clinical evidence of the benefit of prophylactic postoperative digitalization is conflicting.[43, 44] On the other hand, there is now abundant clinical evidence to indicate that postoperative arrhythmias in patients on preoperative β-blockade can be significantly reduced. Withdrawal hypersensitivity of adrenergic receptors can be prevented by continuing propranolol dosage to the morning of surgery and reinstituting low dose propranolol (1 mg IV every 4 hours or 5 mg PO every 6 hours) immediately after surgery. This therapy has been successful in prophylaxis of postoperative arrhythmias without causing myocardial depression.[45, 46]

Ectopic Beats Isolated atrial ectopic and escape beats are usually innocuous and do not require treatment. Occasionally frequent atrial or junctional ectopic beats will so disturb the rhythm that it becomes advantageous to override them with ventricular pacing; this is especially so when an IABP is being triggered. Supraventricular irritability of this nature is often a harbinger of atrial fibrillation, and may be an indication to start or resume digitalis. If there is no history of digitalis treatment, the patient is fully digitalized (1.0–1.5 mg digoxin over 24 hours). At the same time, potassium therapy is increased to protect against digitalis toxicity.

Supraventricular Tachycardia Supraventricular tachycardia is dangerous and must be managed aggressively. Rapid rate and hypotension may induce myocardial ischemia. Hypoxemia should always be sought as a cause of supraventricular tachycardia. It may occur acutely (*e.g.,* kinked endotracheal tube, pneumothorax) or more insidiously (*e.g.,* unrecognized atelectasis). Carotid massage is undesirable in atherosclerotic patients. A bolus of neosynephrine (200 µg IV) should be given if hypotension is significant; the increased vagal tone caused by rise in pressure may abort the arrhythmia. However, DC cardioversion is the most rapid and predictable treatment and should be used immediately in the sedated, intubated patient. Edrophonium, propranolol or verapamil may be useful if blood pressure is normal or elevated.

Nonparoxysmal junctional tachycardia is a slower regular rhythm (60–100/min) that commonly occurs. Digitalis toxicity should be excluded and hypokalemia treated. Override ventricular pacing is used if cardiac output falls.

The following clinical situation recently encountered by the authors illustrates the problems that may arise in the management of postoperative supraventricular tachycardia. An obese patient, known to have chronic bronchitis, developed increasing bronchospasm 4 days postextubation after cardiac surgery. An aminophyllin infusion was started, during which atrial tachycardia developed at 180/min. Blood pressure was elevated and the surgical attendant was anxious to abort the tachycardia because of the potential for myocardial ishemia. DC cardioversion was the obvious choice in the face of severe bronchospasm, but the patient was wide awake, acutely distressed, and had a full stomach. Awake, oral intubation was achieved with topical anesthesia, and diazepam and thiopental were given once the patient's airway was protected. A single DC shock of 50 watt-seconds converted the rhythm back to sinus and the patient awoke and was uneventfully extubated within 15 minutes.

Atrial Flutter If atrial flutter occurs early on, direct cardioversion with 25 to 50 watt-seconds is the therapy of choice. If the arrhythmia is resistant, digoxin may be helpful in slowing ventricular response. Repeat cardioversion is often successful if quinidine or procameamide is added as well. Override atrial pacing is an attractive alternative, if available.

Atrial Fibrillation Acute atrial fibrillation occurring for the first time in the postoperative period will frequently respond to DC cardioversion with 100 to 200 watt-seconds, which should be considered when ventricular rate exceeds 140/min or hemodynamic instability occurs. Otherwise digitalization in the usual fashion is undertaken, with 0.25 mg given IV q2 to 4h until there is either spontaneous reversion to sinus rhythm (as often happens) or until the ventricular response has been brought down to an acceptable rate, 90 to 100/min. The indications for adding procainamide or quinidine are necessity to avoid return of atrial fibrillation because of hemodynamic consequences, and failure to convert with digoxin. DC cardioversion may also be more successful after combined therapy has been established. (see Fig. 16–11).

Special Considerations

In this section some considerations for the postoperative management of certain specific operative procedures are given.

Aortic Valve Replacement The young patient with tight aortic stenosis and well-preserved ventricular function usually does very well after valve replacement. However, ventricular compliance is reduced because of hypertrophy, so that filling pressures may rise or fall rapidly with little change in ventricular volume. The atrial kick remains important after operation and maintenance of sinus rhythm and adequate preload are desirable. These patients are particularly likely to develop the hyperdynamic left ventricle syndrome. Myocardial oxygen balance is critical when ventricular hypertrophy is combined with coronary artery disease.

The patient with aortic regurgitation and good ventricular function also does well. Compliance is increased so that large changes in ventricular volume are associated with little change in pressure, thus limiting the usefulness of wedge pressure monitoring. If, however, the ventricle is failing and dilated, it stiffens and left-sided pressure monitoring becomes mandatory. IABP support or afterload reduction with hydralazine may be required after surgery.

Mitral Valve Replacement In pure tight mitral stenosis without significant preoperative pulmonary edema the outcome is usually excellent; ventricular function is normal and the postoperative course short. However, patients with a long-standing history of pulmonary edema have markedly increased extravascular lung water which is further increased by fluid loading through the operation. They have a high incidence of postoperative pulmonary complications such as edema, atelectasis, and infection. Most of these patients will either be in or return to atrial fibrillation after surgery, which may cause hemodynamic instability or risk thromboembolism.

In compensated mitral regurgitation ventricular compliance is markedly increased and, like aortic regurgitation, large changes

in intraventricular volume are associated with small changes in pressure. Repeated fluid challenges given simply to treat numerical $\overline{PA}_o$ values may result in little increases in $\overline{PA}_o$ until compliance is decreased by ventricular overdistension and acute pulmonary edema results. The patient with mitral regurgitation and ventricular failure presents the greatest postoperative challenge. Specific afterload reduction with intravenous hydralazine is particularly helpful in this situation.

Cardiomyotomy for Idiopathic Hypertrophic Subaortic Stenosis (IHSS) Cardiomyotomy may by no means fully reverse outlet obstruction; even if it is relieved, the ventricle is still hypertrophied and stiff. Maintenance of adequate preload and sinus rhythm is essential because cardiac output is still greatly dependent on the atrial kick. Vasoactive drugs can readily upset oxygen balance in the hypertrophied ventricle. Inotropic drugs should be used with great care and then only after vigorous fluid loading. Afterload reduction with vasodilator drugs will increase any residual gradient across the left ventricular outflow tract while decreasing coronary perfusion pressure. Nitroprusside is still used to facilitate restoration of intravascular volume before rewarming but with care. There is a high incidence of atrioventricular block after septal myotomy; this is an indication for sequential atrioventricular pacing to maintain atrial kick and ventricular filling.

Aneurysmectomy Results after this procedure are variable, depending on the condition of the residual ventricle. If resection is extensive the plicated ventricle is very stiff; a pulmonary artery catheter is essential to define the elevated filling pressures that may be required for adequate cardiac output. These patients not infrequently require IABP and inotropic support for 48 hours after surgery to allow edema to settle down and contractility to improve.

Pericardiectomy Not infrequently a fibrotic cardiomyopathy develops when constriction has been long-standing; this may be on the basis of chronic ischemia. Remnants of pericardium adhering to the ventricular wall interfere with contractility.[47] Inotropic support is often obligatory for these patients for at least 48 hours; digitalis may have to be continued indefinitely. In addition, thinning of the right ventricular wall is common. Overzealous fluid administration can lead to acute right ventricular failure.

Complications

Bleeding *Etiology.* Postoperative bleeding is usually *overt;* it is obvious from the degree of chest tube drainage or direct loss from wound sites. Not infrequently, however, it is *covert,* and is detected only when it causes complications such as hemothorax, cardiac tamponade, and cardiovascular instability. From a clinical point of view, decision-making depends on determining whether the primary cause of bleeding is medical (*i.e.,* caused by coagulopathy) or surgical (*i.e.,* caused by rapid blood loss from an open vessel). In general, disorders of coagulation are sought and treated first; surgical bleeding becomes a diagnosis of exclusion.

Factors predisposing to postoperative coagulation disorders. Preoperative assessment of bleeding during previous surgery is vital.[48] An abnormal *prothrombin time* (PT) may be caused by anticoagulants or liver dysfunction (primary, or secondary to cardiac failure). Fresh frozen plasma should be used electively after cardiopulmonary bypass in these cases. Abnormal *platelet function* should be expected if the patient is receiving drugs with intended or secondary antiplatelet activity.[49] Acetyl salicyclic acid is particularly important, because platelet function is impaired for a full generation time (7–10 days) after a single tablet. The *bleeding time* is helpful in defining qualitative platelet dysfunction before surgery, but even if it is not done platelets should be given electively at the end of cardiopulmonary bypass. Other bleeding disorders may exist and should be defined before operation.

There are many *intraoperative* factors which interfere with postoperative coagulation.[50] Reversal of *heparin* by protamine may be inadequate. Excessive *protamine* itself acts as an anticoagulant. *Qualitative platelet dysfunction* after bypass is well described. Electron microscopy reveals that after cardiopulmonary bypass, serotonin and ADP granules have been extruded. Bleeding time may be markedly abnormal despite a normal platelet count. Drugs used in the operating room, such as heparin and nitroprusside, may interfere with platelet function. *Thrombocytopenia* is caused by destruction or adsorption in the bypass machine, absorption onto intravascular catheters and the intraaortic balloon device, or by consumption in DIC (see below) triggered by extracorporeal circulation. Dilutional thrombocytopenia results when a massive blood transfusion (more than eight units) is given. Factors V and VIII may also become depleted in this way.[51]

Disseminated intravascular coagulation (DIC) may occur along with extracorporeal circulation. Contact with foreign surface activates Factor XII (intrinsic pathway) and release of thromboplastin from denatured platelets and white cells activates Factor VII (extrinsic pathway.)[52] The degree of DIC may depend on duration of bypass. DIC may also be activated by the presence of widespread bleeding surfaces (from the adhesions in "re-do" patients), by shock and low cardiac output states, by massive blood transfusion, and by anaphylactic reactions. *Fibrinolysis* may be triggered by cardiopulmonary bypass because Factor XII also activates the plasminogen-plasmin pathway.[53]

Risk factors for postoperative coagulation disorders are summarized in Table 16-13. Prevention of unnecessary bleeding depends on their recognition and early elective correction by appropriate factor replacement in the operating room. Routine tests are shown in Figure 16-17.

Clinical approach to postoperative bleeding (see also Chap. 24).

1. Overt bleeding is defined by (1) chest tube

Table 16-13. Factors Predisposing to Postoperative Coagulation Disorders

PREOPERATIVE

Anticoagulant therapy
  Coumadin (PT↑)
Abnormal liver function
  Cirrhosis, congestive heart failure (PT↑, capillary fragility)
Antiplatelet drugs (bleeding time ↑)
  Acetylsalicylic acid (ASA)
  Sulfinpyrazone (Anturane)
  Dipyridamole (Persantine)
  Nonsteroidal antiinflammatory drugs
  Propranolol, clofibrate
Bleeding disorders
  Hemophilia (PTT↑)
  von Willebrand's disease (bleeding time ↑)

INTRAOPERATIVE

Anticoagulant therapy
  Inadequate reversal of heparin (PTT, TT↑)
  Excessive protamine
Redo surgical procedures
  Widespread adhesions, bleeding surface ↑
Prolonged Cardiopulmonary Bypass
  DIC
  Fibrinolysis
  Platelet dysfunction and destruction
Antiplatelet Drugs
  Heparin, protamine
  Sodium nitroprusside
Intravascular catheters (adsorption thrombocytopenia)
  CPB, CVP, PA lines, and IABP
Massive blood transfusion
  Dilutional coagulopathy (I, V, VII, platelets)
  DIC
Hypothermia
  Generalized impairment of coagulation cascade
Low cardiac output (shock, acidosis) *DIC*
Anaphylaxis (drug transfusion reaction) *DIC*

(See also Chap. 15 and Fischbach DP, Fogdall RP: Coagulation: The Essentials. Baltimore, Williams & Wilkins, 1981)

drainage that is persistently greater than 150 ml/hour and (2) profuse wound bleeding with or without clot formation.

The following step-wise approach to management is taken (Fig. 16-18):

a. *Check extrinsic pathway function.* The prothrombin-proconvertin time (P&P) is used to dilute out heparin interference with the PT. If the P&P is abnormal (< 60% of control at Stanford; see Fig. 16-17), fresh frozen plasma is given, 2–4 units at a time, until the P&P is corrected.

b. *Check intrinsic pathway function.* The partial thromboplastin time (PTT) is nonspecific but sensitive. A more reliable clinical indicator is the thrombin time (TT). If the TT is normal, bleeding is probably not the result of heparin effect. If the TT is abnormal, a reptilase time (RT) is performed.[54] Reptilase, a thrombin-like compound obtained from snake serum, is resistant to heparin. A normal RT therefore indicates intrinsic pathway dysfunction due to heparin. Protamine sulfate is given in 50 mg aliquots IV until the TT is corrected.

CHART

COAGULATION - LAB REPORT
STANFORD UNIVERSITY HOSPITAL, STANFORD, CA 94305

CHRISTINA B HARBURY, M.D. Director of Laboratory

- ☐ ROUTINE ☐ NO BLD RT. ARM
- ☐ STAT ☐ PT ISOL.
- ☐ URGENT

LAB USE - TIME CLOCK

WARD OR CLINIC
REQUEST DATE

☐ CLINIC ☐ O.P. ☐ E.D. ☐ DAY CARE

DR. NO.

COLLECTION TIME

☐ **CHECK THIS BOX FOR ANTICOAGULANT DOSAGE CONTROL. TESTS WILL BE EXPEDITED.**
(ORDER 7-9 A.M. DAILY)

☐ **CHECK THIS BOX FOR HEPARIN THERAPY DOSAGE CONTROL. TESTS WILL BE RUN STAT.**
(ORDER 7-8 A.M., 2-3 P.M., 8-9 P.M. DAILY)

☐ PROTHROMBIN TIME 100% _____ sec
  PATIENT _____ sec _____ % (NORMAL 60→100)

① PROTHROMBIN & PROCONVERTIN 100% _____ sec
  PATIENT _____ sec _____ % (NORMAL 60→100)

② ACTIVATED PARTIAL THROMBOPLASTIN TIME (NORMAL 25-37)
  Normal Control _____ sec Patient _____ sec.

TECH

SURGICAL COAGULATION SCREEN

PHASE I: Includes Platelet Count, PTT and Prothrombin Time

PHASE II: Includes Thrombin Time, Prothrombin & Proconvertin, and Fibrinogen.

ORDER PLATELETS ON HEMATOLOGY I

☐ FIBRINOGEN (SEMI-QUANT) (160-350) _____ mgs/100ml

☐ THROMBIN TIME Normal Control ③ _____ sec. Patient _____ sec.
  IF THROMBIN TIME 17.0 sec. a Reptilase Time will be done)

☐ ④ REPTILASE TIME _____ sec (normal 13.8-21 sec)

☐ FIBRIN SPLIT PRODUCTS (NORMAL <10µgm/ml) _____ µ gm/ml)

☐ ANTITHROMBIN III _____ % (NORMAL 88-150%)

☐ OTHER

S08.01 (9/80)

Fig. 16-17. The routine coagulation panel used by ICU team at Stanford University Hospital. 1. Extrinsic pathway. 2. Intrinsic pathway. 3. and 4. Final common pathway. See text.

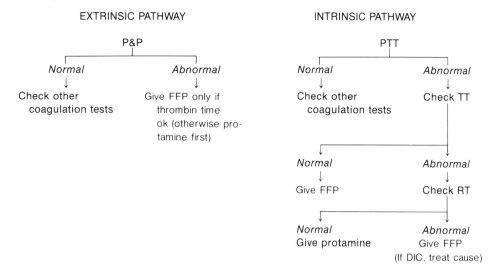

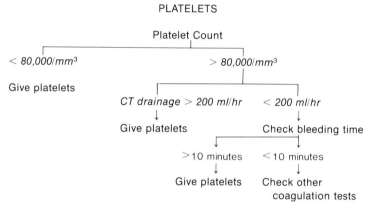

Fig. 16–18. Therapeutic decision-making in the management of postoperative bleeding. This simplified approach is discussed in the text. (See also Fischbach DP, Fogdall RP: Coagulation: The Essentials. Baltimore, Williams & Wilkins, 1981, and Chap. 15.)

c. *Check final common pathway function.* If the TT is abnormal and the RT is also abnormal, there is a defect in fibrinogen, circulating anticoagulants, or ongoing DIC. Cryoprecipitate may reverse hypofibrinogenemia, but treat-treatment of DIC essentially consists of reversing the underlying cause.

d. *Check platelet count.* If the platelet count is less than 80,000/mm³, platelet transfusions with 4 to 6 packs at a time are given to correct it. If the platelet count is greater than 80,000/mm³ but there is a history of antiplatelet therapy or prolonged cardiopulmonary bypass time,

platelet transfusions should be given empirically. If bleeding persists, serial bleeding times may be helpful in defining persistent platelet dysfunction.

e. *If bleeding persists* despite correction of measured coagulation functions, it is probably true surgical bleeding. We do not routinely measure clot lysis time and there is a small group of patients, especially where bleeding is by diffuse oozing, where fibrinolysis undoubtedly exists. However antifibrinolytic agents such as ε-aminocaproic acid (EACA) can cause diffuse clotting and are rarely used. At this stage the empiric use of pooled plasma preparations of activated clotting factors II, VII, IX, and X (Proplex) can be dramatically effective in providing hemostasis. Because of a significant incidence of hepatitis after their use, their use is restricted to situations where bleeding is so great as to be immediately life-threatening, or where surgical reexploration is deemed to be extremely hazardous because of the tenuous condition of the patient.[55]

f. *If bleeding still persists* despite Proplex administration, the patient is taken back for surgical reexploration. In general, chest tube drainage of greater than 400 ml/hour for 2 consecutive hours despite initial factor replacement is taken as a reliable indication of surgical bleeding warranting reexploration.

2. Covert bleeding requires more aggressive surgical intervention because of the mechanical complications. Hemomediastinum and cardiac tamponade are discussed in the next section. Hemothorax may not present as increased chest tube drainage; indeed it is usually caused because drainage is inadequate. Physical examination may reveal unequal chest excursion, dullness to percussion, and diminished breath sounds on the affected side. Ventilator pressures are inordinately high and blood-gas analysis demonstrates ventilatory failure. A chest film will confirm the diagnosis and should be done as soon as there is any suspicion of hemothroax. Management consists of immediate chest tube drainage, followed by surgical exploration if profuse bleeding persists.

Cardiac Tamponade *Etiology.* The most devastating complication after cardiac surgery is cardiac tamponade. Its incidence is variously reported as between 3 and 6 percent; it occurs despite the laying open of the anterior and lateral pericardium at the time of surgery.[56] Onset may be insidious or dramatic, depending on the rate of fluid accumulation. Bleeding occurs directly into the posteroinferior portions of the pericardial sac, or into the surrounding mediastinal space.

Early bleeding, within the first 6 hours, may be a diffuse ooze secondary to coagulopathy (see previous section.) Common sites of direct surgical bleeding include graft suture lines, vein graft side branches, and small arterial bleeders behind the sternum. Less commonly, tamponade may be caused by bleeding after pacing wires or left atrial lines are removed 1 to 2 days following surgery. Late tamponade (*i.e.,* after one week) is rare. It may be caused by hemorrhage associated with anticoagulation or a postpericardiotomy syndrome.[57]

Pathophysiology. Cardiac tamponade is defined as impaired ventricular diastolic filling secondary to increased intrapericardial pressure.[58] However, two separate mechanisms are at work.

Impaired Diastolic Ventricular Filling. An increase in intrapericardial fluid leads to increased pressure because the pericardium has low compliance. The hemodynamic consequences depend largely on the *rate* of fluid formation. Large quantities of fluid up to a liter—may be tolerated if they build up slowly enough, such as uremic pericardial effusion. If it accumulates very rapidly, as little as 100 ml fluid may have devastating effects.[59] At the same time, because the compliance curve of the pericardium exhibits hysteresis, withdrawal of small amounts of fluid may result in dramatic relief.

Increased intrapericardial pressure restricts ventricular diastolic expansion and causes a rapid rise in end diastolic pressure (EDP). This results in early atrioventricular valve closure, poor ventricular filling, and progressive diminution of stroke volume.

When stroke volume and blood pressure fall, a reflex sympathetic response is triggered. Catecholamines are released which increase myocardial contractility and heart rate and cause arterial and venous constriction. The so-called *compensated phase* of cardiac tamponade is thus manifested by cold clammy extremities, narrow pulse pressure, tachycardia, elevated central venous pressure and elevated systemic vascular resistance (Fig. 16-19).

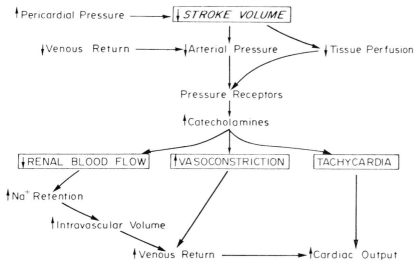

Fig. 16–19. Pathogenesis of the low cardiac output syndrome of cardiac tamponade and the reflex sympathetic mechanisms that ensue to maintain cardiac output. Subendocardial ischemia is an important result of these interactions. (Pores WJ, Gaudiani VA: Surg Clin North Am 55:576, 1975)

Impaired Coronary Perfusion. The alterations which occur cause profound changes in myocardial oxygen balance. Stroke volume, cardiac output, and diastolic pressure fall in the face of elevated left ventricular end diastolic pressure (LVEDP). This compromises the transmyocardial gradient of coronary perfusion pressure (DAP − LVEDP). Shortened diastolic time and elevated diastolic wall tension further impede myocardial oxygen supply, while increased contractility and systolic wall tension increase myocardial oxygen demand.

Using radionuclide-labelled microspheres in iatrogenic tamponade in dogs, Weschler and coworkers showed that, at an early stage, the impaired coronary perfusion affects the subendocardial bed, but that later subepicardial vessels are affected as well.[60] The transition to the decompensated stage (low output shock) is associated with increasing subendocardial necrosis and loss of myocardial contractility. Ischemia in turn increases ventricular stiffness, exacerbates poor filling, and creates a vicious cycle of progressive pump failure.

The above sequence of events explains how a fairly long period of compensation can be followed by abrupt and catastrophic decompensation. Ischemic damage may also explain the persistent myocardial depression (postpericarditis cardiomyopathy) that may be seen after tamponade has been released.

Diagnosis. Not infrequently, cardiac tamponade presents with rapid onset of cardiovascular collapse; indeed the diagnosis may be made when the sternum is opened to allow internal cardiac massage at the time of cardiac arrest. More commonly, the onset is heralded by slow but progressive deterioration over a period of hours (compensated phase) and usually presents a puzzling differential diagnosis. Because decompensation is so swift when it occurs and because ischemia may be progressive throughout the compensated phase, a high degree of suspicion and an aggressive therapeutic approach are mandatory (Table 16-14).

1. Physical Examination. Beck's triad of decreasing arterial pressure, increasing venous pressure, and a small, quiet heart may be different to interpret in the postsurgical patient. Kussmaul's sign (jugular venous distention) and pulsus paradoxus (decrease in systolic pressure by more

Table 16-14. Cardiac Tamponade

DIAGNOSIS
1. Suspicion!
2. Physical examination
   Rapid, thready pulse (paradoxus ↑)
   Jugular venous distension
   Low cardiac output syndrome
3. Chest tube drainage
   Profuse (but may be scanty)
4. ECG
   Low voltage (nonspecific)
   Electrical alternans (rare)
5. Chest film
   Widening mediastinum (serial films)
6. Hemodynamic monitoring
   Rapidly rising CVP
   Plateau pressure
   (RAP = RVEDP = PAD = PA_O)

DIFFERENTIAL DIAGNOSIS
1. Hypovolemia
2. Primary myocardial failure
   Fluid overload (edema, RV distension)
   RV ischemia/infarction
3. Pulmonary embolism
4. Pseudotamponade
   Myocardial swelling (edema)
   Hyperinflation of lungs
   Fulminant pulmonary edema

than 20 torr during inspiration) may both be caused by positive-pressure ventilation; the latter is very common in the presence of hypovolemia. Heart sounds need not be distant if the anterior pericardium has been removed.

Manifestations of a low cardiac output syndrome have to be distinguished from those caused by hypovolemia, myocardial failure, or pulmonary embolism.

Profuse bleeding from chest tubes is suggestive of intramediastinal bleeding but not diagnostic of tamponade; absence of chest tube drainage does not exclude tamponade and may simply reflect inadequate decompression of mediastinal bleeding.

2. ECG. Diffuse low voltage or S-T changes are common but nonspecific. Ventricular electrical alternans is virtually diagnostic when it is present (it is thought to be caused by torsion of the heart from beat-to-beat), but unfortunately occurs rarely.

3. Echocardiogram. This is really a waste of time. It is technically difficult in the emergent situation and is helpful only if the tamponade is caused by a reasonably

large, anterolateral effusion (it is usually caused by a small, posterior effusion). The presence of an effusion is suggestive but not diagnostic of tamponade as a cause of the low output state.

4. Chest Film. When serial chest films demonstrate progressive widening of the mediastinum, there is little doubt of the diagnosis. However, portable roentgenographs are often equivocal unless the changes are dramatic; the mediastinal shadow may not bear a direct relationship to the degree of tamponade.

5. Hemodynamic Monitoring. Equalization of right- and left-sided intracardiac pressures because of restriction of cardiac filling is the single most helpful sign in the confirmation of the diagnosis of tamponade.

The right ventricle is initially far more compliant than the left. When RV restriction occurs, the CVP rises much more rapidly and to a greater degree than does the $\overline{PA}_O$. Close observation of the CVP may in fact be more helpful in making the diagnosis.[61] Ultimately, however, a pressure plateau is reached with matching of right atrial, right ventricular diastolic, pulmonary artery diastolic, and pulmonary artery occluded (*i.e.*, left atrial) pressures (Fig. 16-20).[62]

Early elective insertion of a pulmonary artery catheter is very helpful, therefore, in determining diagnosis in equivocal cases. During insertion, a print-out of right atrial and right ventricular pressures should be obtained so that the pressure plateau between right- and left-sided filling pressures is documented. Insertion of the catheter should not delay specific therapy if the diagnosis is not in doubt and the patient is unstable.

Differential diagnosis. The differential diagnosis is essentially that of the low cardiac output syndrome. *Hypovolemia* should be ruled out by fluid challenges (the CVP may be falsely elevated if the patient is venoconstricted), which result in further increase in CVP without change in blood pressure. *Primary myocardial failure* may occur because of ischemia or overzealous use of fluid or β-blockers in the postoperative period. A de-

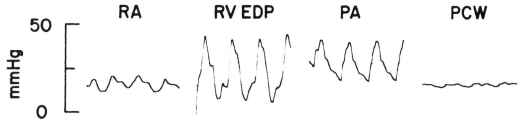

Fig. 16–20. The *pressure plateau* in tracings taken from a patient with cardiac tamponade. Right atrial (*RA*), right ventricular end diastolic pressure (*RVEDP*), pulmonary artery diastolic (*PA*), and pulmonary capillary artery wedge (*PCW*) pressures are virtually identical. (Weeks DR et al: J Thorac Cardiovasc Surg 71:251, 1976)

crease in blood pressure may be associated with a rapid increase in CVP. Very rarely, right ventricular infarction may be present without diagnostic ECG changes but with a rapid increase in CVP. However, right ventricular diastolic pressures will be singularly elevated. *Pulmonary embolism* may be present with sudden onset of hypotension and elevation of the CVP; again there will be a marked increase in right ventricular and pulmonary diastolic pressures relative to $\overline{PA}_o$. *Pseudotamponade,* tamponade not caused by blood in the pericardial sac or mediastinum, occurs occasionally. We have seen an example of myocardial edema so exacerbated by fluid overload as to cause profound swelling; hypotension was dramatically relieved once the sternum was reopened. Compression may be caused by lungs overdistended with air or fluid, as in fulminant pulmonary edema. In the patients reported by Culliford and coworkers, attempts to close the sternum after reexploration were marked by profound hypotension; the heart was being tamponaded by the solid, distended lungs.[63] Patients were returned to the intensive care unit with the sternum laid open and secondary closure was performed once the edema had resolved.

Management. Early diagnosis is paramount; a high degree of suspicion, rapid rise in CVP, and plateau pressure response on pulmonary artery catheterization are the most reliable aids to decision-making. Definitive decompression by reopening the sternal wound and evacuation of the hemopericardium or hemomediastinum is treatment of choice. In the elective situation, the patient is returned to the operating room and anesthesia is in-

duced with ketamine (2.5 mg/kg IV) with local infiltration of the sternum with xylocaine.[64] Once tamponade has been relieved, anesthesia can be maintained in the standard manner: 100 percent oxygen, intravenous narcotics with or without diazepam, pancuronium, and controlled ventilation. In an emergency situation (often presenting as full cardiac arrest), the sternal wires are cut and tamponade relieved in the intensive care unit. After further resuscitation, the patient is taken to the operating room so that the bleeding site can be properly identified, hemostasis achieved, and formal closure completed in an aseptic environment.

Diagnostic or therapeutic pericardiocentesis has its advocates, especially because the removal of as little as 25 to 50 ml of fluid can provide dramatic relief of tamponade. However, the effusion is frequently beyond the reach of the needle. The procedure is not without hazard (myocardial puncture, coronary artery laceration, pneumothorax) and the bleeding site will still have to be found by direct intervention. Definitive therapy is delayed.

Supportive therapy with fluid infusion and isoproterenol may buy time to allow elective surgical decompression.[65] Elevation of the $\overline{CVP}$ above 20 torr may increase intramyocardial pressure above intrapericardial pressure and thereby improve cardiac output. Isoproterenol increases heart rate and drops vascular resistance. However, these measures also exacerbate myocardial ischemia (increased diastolic wall tension, heart rate) and may delay specific treatment while myocardial injury progresses.

Summary. Cardiac tamponade is a potentially fatal complication of cardiac surgery. A low cardiac output syndrome is caused by impeded ventricular filling. Hemodynamic compensation occurs through tachycardia and increased vascular resistance, but progressive myocardial ischemia results in ultimate cardiovascular collapse. The clinical signs of tamponade are difficult to interpret. The most helpful are a falling pulse pressure with tachycardia, a rapidly rising CVP, and equalization of right- and left-sided filling pressures. Early, direct surgical decompression is the treatment of choice.

Perioperative Myocardial Infarction (PMI)

The true incidence of perioperative myocardial infarction (PMI) is extraordinarily difficult to define. Criteria for the definition of PMI vary; in some series, ST changes are included;[66] in others they are not.[67-69] In recent years, there have been several developments that may have markedly influenced the occurrence of PMI. Surgery is being performed on an emergent basis in states of severe myocardial ischemia; the advent of electrophysiologic mapping procedures involves long bypass times without ideal myocardial preservation.[70] On the other hand, cold cardioplegia is now accepted as being superior to previous methods of myocardial preservation. The IABP is being used to support situations of myocardial ischemia. The clinical sequela of PMI vary from silence (discovered at autopsy) to perioperative death from pump failure or ventricular arrhythmias. Some factors, such as unstable angina, are unequivocally associated with an increased incidence of PMI; with many others, data conflicts from one report to another. In this section, an attempt will be made to give an overview of the problem of PMI in order to establish a clinical approach.

Risk Factors for Perioperative Myocardial Infarction

1. Preoperative Factors
   Unstable angina (*i.e.*, angina at rest or increasing in severity), is uniformly accepted as the single most important predisposing factor to PMI.[71-73] This patient group is also exposed to an increased risk if β-blockade is suddenly withdrawn before surgery.[74] Because this competitive block can be reversed by calcium and isoproterenol if necessary, we make it a practice to continue propranolol right up to the morning of surgery to decrease the likelihood of infarction during anesthetic induction. Emergency coronary artery bypass grafting is being performed with increasing frequency for unstable angina following *subendocardial infarction.* The risk of transmural infarction is as high, but not higher, than that for unstable angina alone.[75] Another high-risk setting occurs with the patient who develops chest pain or ischemia during coronary angiography. The incidence of transmural infarction and ultimate outcome after emergency revascularization is improved by (1) as short an interval as possible (ideally, less than 4 hours) between insult and operation; (2) hypokalemic cold cardioplegia; and (3) the use of IABP support after surgery. If collateral flow is deficient or revascularization is delayed more than 24 hours, the procedure can result in reperfusion hemorrhagic infarction.[76] Although other variables, such as diffuse or left main coronary artery disease and poor preoperative ventricular function (low ejection fraction, high LVEDP), would seem to have logical associations with PMI, data in clinical reports is conflicting; in most series they do not seem to increase the risk significantly.

2. Intraoperative Factors
   Anesthetic Techniques. Induction of anesthesia is the most hazardous moment of the perioperative course. Uncontrolled hypotension, hypertension, tachycardia and tachyarrhythmias greatly increase the risk of PMI, as does unappreciated hypoxemia. Elevated CPK isoenzymes have been reported before CPB.[77] Inadequate anesthesia and inappropriate use of vasoactive drugs during induction and maintenance are hazardous. In the patient with severe myocardial ischemia, sodium nitroprusside or hydralazine should not be

used to control hypertension before revascularization. In the first place, hypertension may be the result of inadequate autonomic anesthesia; the supplementation of narcotic techniques with low concentrations of enflurane or halothane is useful and protective in this situation. Sodium nitroprusside and hydralazine decrease diastolic perfusion pressure and reduce the transmyocardial pressure gradient in the face of unchanged or increased myocardial oxygen demand. If hypertension persists in the face of adequate anesthesia, intravenous nitroglycerin is preferred for pressure control in the high-risk patient. Indeed, nitroglycerin is extremely useful in reversing chest pain or ischemic ST changes in the periinduction period. After cardiopulmonary bypass, reliance on excessive inotropic support rather than restoration of intravascular volume increases the risk of myocardial ischemia and PMI.

Surgical Techniques. An increased incidence of PMI has been reported to be associated with incomplete or inadequate revascularization, requirement for multiple grafts, prolonged cross-clamp and bypass times, and coronary endarterectomy.[78] Complications such as coronary air embolism may directly cause infarction. Techniques of myocardial preservation during cardiopulmonary bypass most certainly influence the incidence of PMI; exactly how they do so is not well defined. Selective coronary artery perfusion, normothermic ventricular fibrillation, and intermittent ischemia have been largely superceded by hypokalemic cold cardioplegia. Although the latter is considered by most authorities to offer superior myocardial preservation, current retrospective studies on PMI do not define or differentiate between the technique used during bypass. Atrial and ventricular mapping procedures require prolonged bypass times without hypothermia and predispose toward a higher risk of PMI.

Postoperative Factors. The prevention of myocardial ischemia in the postoperative period is essential. Inadequate analgesia,

Table 16-15. Factors Predisposing to Perioperative Myocardial Infarction (PMI)

PREOPERATIVE
1. Unstable angina ($\pm$ abrupt withdrawal of propranolol)
2. Subendocardial infarction
3. Diffuse coronary artery disease
4. Left main coronary disease
5. Severe ventricular dysfunction ($\uparrow$ LVEDP, $\downarrow$ EF)

INTRAOPERATIVE
Anesthesia
1. Unstable induction
2. Inadequate anesthesia
3. Inappropriate use of vasodilators or inotropic drugs
Surgery
1. Incomplete revascularization
2. Coronary endarterectomy
3. Prolonged CPB/AXC time
4. Technique of myocardial preservation
5. Complications (*e.g.*, coronary air embolism)

POSTOPERATIVE
1. Inadequate analgesia (hypertension, tachycardia)
2. Hypovolemia
3. Arrhythmias
4. Hyperdynamic left ventricle syndrome
5. Hypoxemia

hypovolemia (especially during rewarming), inappropriate use of inotropic drugs and vasodilators, hyperdynamic ventricular function, arrhythmias, and hypoxemia should be anticipated and treated energetically (Table 16-15).

Diagnosis. The search for the ideal marker of PMI continues. Diagnosis is usually made on a combination of the factors presented below; in many cases it is only made at autopsy. Buckley and Hutchins found operation-related myocardial necrosis in 46 of 53 patients dying within one month of surgery; only 18 had had ECG changes suggestive of PMI.

1. *Chest pain* may be atypical, masked by analgesia, confused with wound pain, or absent altogether. The latter is thought to occur when previously ischemic tissue necroses completely; indeed, this mechanism is suggested by some skeptics to be the means by which revascularization relieves angina. Symptoms probably occur in less than 50% of patients with PMI.

2. *The ECG* has been the mainstay of diagnosis. New Q waves after surgery are a specific sign, but probably underestimate the true incidence of PMI.[79] Confusion is caused by preexisting Q waves, intraventricular conduction defects, LBBB, and Q waves caused by aneurysmectomy or infarctectomy. ST changes are nonspecific, and subendocardial infarction may be confused with pericardial inflammation or electrolyte imbalance.

3. *Creatine Phosphokinase MB fraction (CPK-MB)* is sensitive but nonspecific, and if used alone greatly overestimates PMI. Almost all patients undergoing cardiac surgery will sustain some degree of elevation of CPK-MB. In their series, Fennell and coworkers were able to define three broad patient groups.[80] Those without evidence for PMI had CPK levels two to three times normal, peaking on day 2, but CPK-MB fractions less than 6%. Those with definitive evidence of PMI by ECG had CPK levels three to six times normal with CPK-MB fractions of 8–15%. Patients with uncertain evidence of PMI had levels between the first two groups. The authors concluded that despite the apparent separation, the overlap of distribution limits the usefulness of CPK-MB in any individual case.

4. *Scintiscan* with Tc^{99m} technetium pyrophosphate is being used with increasing frequency as an adjunct in the diagnosis of PMI.[81–84] New onset of well-defined, localized uptake of the isotope is highly suggestive of myocardial necrosis. The technique is less specific in defining diffuse ischemia or subendocardial infarction; calcified ventricular aneurysms or valves may provide false positives.[85] Ideally, a preoperative control is required; postoperative scanning must be done early because the test may become negative within 5 days of infarction.

5. *Vectorcardiography* is a specialized diagnostic tool which is especially useful in defining multiple sites of infarction, but is otherwise no more specific than the previous tests.

6. *Combined techniques* are much more useful than any of the studies used alone. Most authorities now diagnose PMI on the presence of new Q waves associated with significant and sustained elevation of CPK-MB (*e.g.*, more than 8% for more than 24 hours) or a positive scintiscan. Some authors also accept the presence of diffuse ST depression associated with CPK-MB or scintiscan changes as being diagnostic of subendocardial infarction.[86]

Sequelae. PMI may be completely uncomplicated. Pump failure is less likely if the circumflex or right systems are involved: conduction defects are prominent. Left main or anterior descending obstruction is associated with acute complications that include ventricular arrhythmias and cardiogenic shock. Mechanical complications may also occur, such as mitral regurgitation or ventricular septal rupture. Delayed complications include congestive heart failure and unstable angina; the latter is associated with a high postoperative mortality.[87] Overall, the majority of patients dying in the perioperative period have autopsy findings of PMI; even so, there is some suggestion that PMI may be better tolerated when it occurs during anesthesia or hypothermia because of obtundation of sympathetic reflex responses that ordinarily occur.[88]

Management. The management of PMI really depends on the sequelae. All patients should be closely monitored for several days; supportive care should include the avoidance of fluid overload or hypovolemia and the vigorous prevention of hypoxemia (elective reintubation should be considered if pulmonary edema or atelectasis are increasing). Invasive monitoring with arterial lines and pulmonary artery catheters should be instituted or continued as indicated by the patient's clinical condition.

Ventricular arrhythmias are managed in the usual way (see also Chap. 6) with two added considerations. We use prophylactic lidocaine infusion for 24 to 48 hours. Mechanical ventilatory support is continued to maintain oxygenation and facilitate repeated

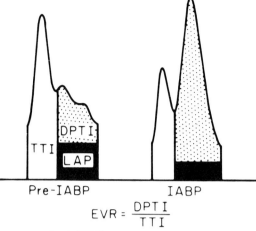

$$EVR = \frac{DPTI}{TTI}$$

1. ↓ TTI
2. ↓ LAP
3. ↑ DPTI
4. ↓ Heart Rate (∴ ↑DPTI)

Fig. 16–21. The beneficial effects of the intraaortic balloon pump (*IABP*) on myocardial oxygen balance (*EVR*) result from a marked increase in diastolic pressure and lengthening of diastolic time (↑ *DPTI*, supply), associated with reduced afterload (↓ *SPTI*, demand), and therefore reduced preload requirement (↓ *LAP*). (The term *SPTI* is preferable to tension time index (*TTI*) because the latter presupposes knowledge of ventricular thickness and radius.) (Philips PA et al: Ann Thorac Surg 23:50, 1977)

cardioversion if necessary. Early use of the intraaortic balloon can dramatically alter myocardial oxygen balance and thereby control arrhythmias induced by ischemia.

Left ventricular dysfunction may be present as a state of increased stiffness rather than decreased contractility. Intravenous nitroglycerin infusion (50 mg in 250 ml saline = 200 µg/ml) at doses of 0.5 to 5.0 µg/kg/min is extremely useful in reducing elevated filling pressures and relieving acute pulmonary edema in this situation. In unstable angina, ischemia may manifest as ST changes with intermittent elevation of $\overline{PA}_o$ rather than chest pain; intravenous nitroglycerin is then titrated to provide control. In less acute situations, nitroglycerin is provided as a paste

(Nitrol), 0.5 to 1 inch every 4 hours; it can be wiped off if hypotension occurs.

Acute pump failure is a definitive indication for emergency insertion of the IABP. Efforts to increase cardiac output with inotropic agents or afterload reduction with vasodilators serve mainly to worsen ischemia; fluid loading is poorly tolerated and quickly results in pulmonary and even myocardial edema. Only the IABP provides a combination of afterload reduction (decreased work) with increased diastolic perfusion pressure (increased supply; Fig 16-21). The balloon can facilitate emergency surgical procedures such as revascularization, repair of mitral regurgitation, or septal rupture; in most cases IABP support for 48 hours is sufficient to control ischemia and allow for enough recovery to sustain adequate pump function. Complete dependence of IABP support for more than 48 hours augurs very poorly for survival.

Summary. PMI is an entity that has a variable presentation and uncertain incidence.

Table 16-16. Perioperative Myocardial Infarction

DIAGNOSIS
1. Chest pain (may be atypical, absent)
2. ECG changes
   a. New Q waves (specific, insensitive)
   b. ST-T changes (nonspecific)
3. Enzyme changes (CPK-MB); (sensitive, nonspecific)
4. Vector cardiography (sensitive, nonspecific)
5. Scintiscan (Tc^{99m} pyrophosphate; nonspecific)
PMI: New Q waves + ↑ ↑ CPK-MB or Scintiscan

MANAGEMENT
1. Prophylaxis: Recognize, avoid risk factors
2. Diagnosis: High index of suspicion
3. Monitoring
   Progression of PMI
   Arrhythmias
   Pump failure
4. Treatment
   Supportive
      Adequate analgesia
      Fluid balance
      Pulmonary function and care
   Definitive
      Arrhythmia prophylaxis (lidocaine)
      Nitroglycerin IV (chest pain, ↑$\overline{PA}_o$, pulmonary edema)
      IABP (pump failure, ventricular arrhythmias, revascularization)

The most important risk factor is unstable angina before surgery. Diagnosis is based upon the association of new Q waves with significant elevation of CPK-MB fraction or positive scintiscan. The incidence of PMI is changing as new indications for cardiac surgery are found and as new means of myocardial support are developed. Sequelae may be minimal or fatal. Management depends on careful diagnosis, monitoring and support, and definitive treatment of complications. In this regard intravenous nitroglycerin is particularly useful for ventricular stiffness and IABP support is mandatory for pump failure (Table 16-16).

PULMONARY MANAGEMENT

GOALS

Rational management of pulmonary function is based on the same fundamental pathophysiologic principles as are applied to hemodynamic therapy. Again, the postoperative period is divided into three phases. Phase I, the restoration of intravascular volume during rapid rewarming, has as its goals the maintenance of adequate gas exchange in the face of increasing O_2 consumption and CO_2 production, and the restoration of the functional residual capacity (FRC) lost during surgery. The second phase, that of mobilization of accumulated interstitial fluid, coincides with ventilatory weaning. Finally, once extubation has been achieved, the primary goal is to avoid further reduction in FRC and to restore normal pulmonary function with careful respiratory care (Table 16-17).

Table 16-17. Goals of Postoperative Pulmonary Management

Phase 1 Restoration of functional residual capacity (FRC)
Maintenance of adequate gas exchange in face of rising VO_2 and VCO_2
Phase 2 Ventilatory weaning and extubation
Phase 3 Postextubation respiratory care

PHYSIOLOGY

Reduction in FRC is the most uniformly constant pathophysiologic process occurring after thoracotomy.[89] It occurs because of progressive closure of small airways and alveoli, resulting in diffuse microatelectasis. Factors responsible come from a wide variety of sources.[90] They are summarized in Table 16-18. Reduction in FRC is associated with an inversely proportional increase in intrapulmonary shunt ($\dot{Q}s/\dot{Q}t$) and ventilation/perfusion mismatching (V_A/Q). This in turn widens the alveolar-arterial oxygen gradient ($AaDO_2$), resulting in hypoxemia.

In the early postoperative period, unrecognized and untreated hypoxemia exacerbates myocardial ischemia and predisposes to arrhythmias. Mechanical ventilation neither impedes nor resolves underlying atelectasis because of the monotonous tidal volumes delivered. If the FRC is still low at the time of extubation, the withdrawal of positive pressure support facilitates alveolar collapse so that gross atelectasis and hypoxemia become manifest. Once alveolar collapse occurs, surfactant is lost and reexpansion is not provided by normal tidal volumes. Lung stiffness and work of breathing increase, and a vicious cycle may result. In addition, lung defense mechanisms are hampered in regions of collapsed lung; this predisposes to infection.

Significant microatelectasis may exist without overt clinical signs such as bronchial breathing or radiographic consolidation, although these usually become more prominent after extubation.

The above mechanisms provide the basis for the therapeutic approach we use in postoperative pulmonary care. From Table 16-18, it is seen that many factors that reduce FRC exist pre- and intra-operatively. Indeed, 70 percent of atelectasis is already established by the time the patient reaches the intensive care unit.[91] Postoperative management starts with appropriate preoperative work-up, and is continued by giving attention to potentially reversible intraoperative factors. Once the patient returns to the intensive care unit, the

Table 16-18. Factors Promoting Postoperative Atelectasis ($\downarrow$ FRC)

MONOTONOUS VENTILATORY PATTERN

Progressive microatelectasis if not interrupted by sighs or PEEP
1. Mechanical ventilation (fixed tidal volume) ⎫
2. Spontaneous ventilation: Anesthesia ⎬ absence
                        Narcotic medication ⎭ of sighs

INCREASED PULMONARY EXTRAVASCULAR WATER (PEVW)

Interstitial edema → small airway closure
1. Preexisting pulmonary edema (cardiac failure)
2. Capillary leak syndrome: CPB induced injury
                       Hypersensitivity reactions
                       Idiopathic
3. Fluid loading: Requirement for high preload
PEWV = Preexisting edema × duration of CPB × preload required

DECREASED SURFACTANT

Increased surface tension → alveolar collapse
1. Cigarette smoking (toxic suppression)
2. Chronic bronchitis (sheets of mucus replace surfactant)
3. Abnormal lung volumes (excessive or deficient)
4. Regional pulmonary hypoperfusion (CPB)

INADEQUATE CLEARANCE OF SECRETIONS

Obstruction of small airways → alveolar collapse
1. Smoking, chronic bronchitis (bronchorrhea, especially with intubation)
2. Tracheal intubation (suppression of ciliary cascade)
3. Blind endotracheal suctioning: Selective right lung clearance mucosal
                       damage and "damming"
4. Inadequate humidification and warming (viscid secretions)

ALVEOLAR HYPOVENTILATION (V_A/Q mismatching)

1. Obesity
2. Passive ventilation of paralyzed diaphragm (dependent hypoventilation)
3. Surgical wound (splinting)

LOCAL FACTORS

Direct pressure → alveolar collapse
1. Pleural fluid: Blood, transudate
2. Chest tubes
3. Heart (passive compression of left lung during CPB)

primary goal is active restoration of FRC. We believe that this can be effectively achieved only by ventilating the patient for at least 6 hours, with manipulations of tidal volume and positive-end expiratory pressure (PEEP) designed to allow extubation from a situation of best FRC. There are other cogent reasons for routine postoperative mechanical ventilation, summarized in Table 16-19. Ventilatory weaning is managed with continued attempts to maintain FRC. After extubation, aggressive respiratory care is essential to restore FRC to normal levels. It has been repeatedly demonstrated that FRC and arterial oxygen tension reach their nadir 24 hours after surgery; normal values may not be reached even up to 7 days later (Fig. 16-22).[92,93] In a busy ICU, nursing staff tend to pay most attention to the patient on a ventilator with multiple monitoring lines. In fact, the extubated, unmonitored patient next door may be the one who requires closer observation and active care. Physicians and nurses alike should guard against complacency after extubation.

MANAGEMENT

Prevention of Postoperative Pulmonary Problems

The intensive care unit attendant should be involved in the preoperative work-up of patients with a high risk of postoperative prob-

Table 16-19. Advantages of Postoperative Mechanical Ventilation

LOGICAL EXTENSION OF CURRENT ANESTHETIC TECHNIQUES

Smoothes transition from OR to ICU; allows use of high-dose narcotic anesthesia; avoids hazards of reversal agents

REDUCES NUMBER OF VARIABLES

Allows aggressive hemodynamic support (including loading) without excessive concern for its effect on pulmonary function

IMPROVED HOMEOSTASIS AND MYOCARDIAL OXYGEN BALANCE

During rewarming, ensures normal pH and oxygen supply in face of increased VCO_2 and VO_2; reduces work of breathing and thereby MVO_2

PATIENT COMFORT

Allows adequate sedation and analgesia without concern for depression of respiration; avoids aggressive respiratory therapy in exhaused, stressed patient

RESTORATION OF FRC

Use of IMV with PEEP facilitates restoration of FRC before extubation and reduces risk of pulmonary complications thereafter.

SUPPORT DURING COMPLICATIONS

Facilitates return to OR if there are surgical complications

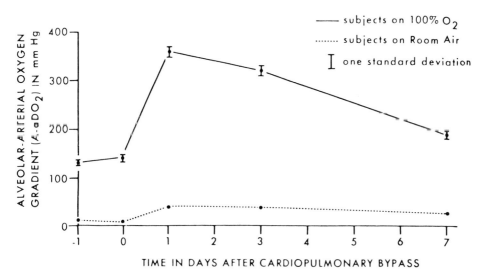

Fig. 16–22. Alveolar arterial oxygen gradient (AaDO₂) increases markedly up to 24 hours after cardiopulmonary bypass and may take up to 7 days to return to normal levels. In this group of patients, mechanical ventilation was provided for about four hours after surgery. (Turnbull KW et al: Can Anaesth Soc J 21:181, 1974)

lems. Obese patients should be urged to lose weight; heavy smokers should be instructed to stop smoking. Patients who have chronic bronchitis with profuse secretions are better operated on in the afternoon to allow vigorous physiotherapy and clearing of the overnight accumulations before surgery. Bedside pulmonary function tests such as forced vital capacity (FVC) and forced expiratory volume in one second (FEV1) are useful in defining the extent and reversibility of obstructive lung disease. Arterial blood gases (ABGs) are important in selected patients to determine the degree of intrapulmonary shunt (pulmonary edema or atelectasis) or the degree of CO_2 retention (chronic obstructive pulmonary disease; COPD). Patients with severe cardiac failure are admitted to the intensive care unit before surgery. Pulmonary artery catheters are placed so that hemodynamic manipulations with vasoactive drugs such as dopamine or nitroprusside may be used to improve cardiac function and reduce pulmonary extravascular water (PEVW) before operation.

Extensive atelectasis occurs when the lungs are deflated during cardiopulmonary bypass (CPB). Discrete areas may be easily visible to the naked eye. However, a graphic representation of the extent of FRC reduction is gained by noting how low the lungs sit in the thoracic cavity when ventilation is resumed after bypass. The provision of PEEP *during bypass* does not appear to prevent intrapulmonary shunting after bypass[94] and merely serves to irritate the surgeon. However, after bypass a series of sighs (Valsalva maneuvers) will visibly reexpand atelectasis, and as evidenced by the height at which the lungs sit at the end of a normal tidal volume, improve FRC. Unfortunately, to be effective in maintaining FRC, sighs must be repeated every 30 minutes; the impairment of venous return and hypotension they cause is dramatic. After the initial sighs, FRC is better maintained by the simple application of a PEEP valve (Boerhinger) in the expiratory limb of the circle. Because we uniformly use PEEP in the ICU, it seems logical to start in the operating room, unless there are contraindications to its use (see below).

Ventilatory settings in the operating room should conform to the same pattern found effective in the ICU (*i.e.*, relatively large tidal volumes with low ventilatory rates). Total minute ventilation requirements are frequently as low as 70 to 80 ml/kg/min because of decreased CO_2 production induced by hypothermia and anesthesia.

Because the left main bronchus is more difficult to enter, blind suctioning preferentially clears the right lung.[95] Repeated attempts at suctioning may so damage the mucosa around the carina as to physically dam up secretions distally. Atelectasis is much more common in the left lung for this reason. Some authors have recommended the use of flexible fiberoptic bronchoscopy in the ICU so that secretions may be selectively cleared; there may be a case for its use in the operating room if secretions have been profuse or obstructive.

Excessive fluid loading will obviously exacerbate postoperative pulmonary edema and atelectasis. However, restoration of intravascular volume and maintenance of adequate preload take precedence over the avoidance of edema because the latter can be supported by mechanical ventilation and later reversed by diuresis (Table 16-20).

Phase I: Restoration of Functional Residual Capacity

Admission to the ICU *Ventilator Set-up.* At Stanford, only two types of volume-triggered ventilator are presently used: the Bennet MA-1, for routine cases, and the Bourne Bear, for complicated ventilatory problems. Both are set up for intermittent mandatory ventilation (IMV) from admission, although this mode is not used until the commencement of weaning. Primary ventilatory settings in this section are based on the use of volume-triggered ventilators.

Examination of patient is a priority. It is important to quickly establish whether augmented sedation is required; agitation will interfere with proper ventilation. Check oxygenation by looking for good color and capillary perfusion; ensure satisfactory placement of the endotracheal tube by listening over the trachea for leak and over the periph-

Table 16-20. Prevention of Postoperative Atelectasis

PREOPERATIVE INTERVENTIONS
1. Encourage weight loss in obesity; curtail smoking
2. Morning physiotherapy to clear overnight secretions
3. Bedside FVC and FEVI; ABGs
4. Aggressive treatment of cardiac failure (ICU admission)

INTRAOPERATIVE INTERVENTIONS
1. Sighs after weaning off CPB
2. PEEP via circle system
3. Large V_T; slow f
4. Careful suctioning
5. Avoidance of excessive fluid loading

Table 16-21. Evaluation of Pulmonary Function on Admission to ICU: Checklist

1. Check that ventilation is adequate
   a. Chest movement
   b. Color, circulation
   c. Breath sounds
2. Check for complications
   a. Endotracheal tube
      Too high (cuff leak)
      Too low (endobronchial intubation)
      Obstruction
   b. Bronchospasm or air-trapping (Table 16-25)
   c. Pneumothorax
   d. Pleural effusion/hemothorax
3. Check chest tubes
   a. Air leak
   b. Bleeding
4. Check ventilator settings (Table 16-22)
5. Check chest film (Table 16-24)

Table 16-22. Ventilator Settings

F_IO_2	0.7
V_T	15 ml/kg
f	8/min
$\dot{V}_E$	90 ml/kg/min (34°C)
	120 ml/kg/min (37°C)
PEEP	5 cmH₂O

eral chest wall for bilateral equality of breath sounds. Bilateral wheeze and prolonged expiration confirm bronchospasm. A unilateral wheeze may be detected with endobronchial intubation or pneumothorax. Seek evidence of hemothorax or pneumothorax by careful percussion over the chest wall (Table 16-21).

Primary ventilator settings. Inspired oxygen fraction (F_IO_2) should be set at 0.7 or above to avoid hypoxemia. ABGs may be excellent immediately after bypass, but mild to marked

Contraindications to PEEP

1. Severe cardiovascular instability
2. Acute bronchospasm
3. Emphysema with air-trapping
4. Suspected pneumothorax
5. Suspected endobronchial intubation

deterioration should be anticipated by the time the patient enters the ICU. Pulmonary extravascular water (PEVW) increases with time after cardiopulmonary bypass, especially if high cardiac filling pressures are required to maintain adequate cardiac output. Ventilation may be suboptimal during transport from operating room to intensive care unit, and there is constant danger of malposition of the endotracheal tube during transfer. F_IO_2 should be lowered only after gas tensions have been measured in the ICU. In general, a combination of large tidal volumes and slow ventilator rates is best. Large tidal volumes (V_T) of 15 ml/kg or greater help reverse atelectasis. Slow rates (f) decrease the inspiration to expiration ratio (I:E ratio). A long expiratory time increases venous return and augments cardiac output; it facilitates full expiration and avoids air-trapping in obstructive lung disease. Slow rates allow slower inspiratory flow while maintaining an adequate I:E ratio. The slower inspiratory flow, the more laminar and less turbulent is the airstream. This decreases airway resistance, reduces airway trauma, and allows for better distribution of inspired gas to the small airways.

Minute ventilation ($\dot{V}_E$) should be adjusted to CO_2 production ($\dot{V}CO_2$) to maintain normal (uncorrected) pH: 7.35–7.45. $\dot{V}_E$ should be reduced below 120 ml/kg/min by 10% for every 1° below 37°C. For example, if a patient enters with a core temperature of 34°C, $\dot{V}_E$ is ideally set at 70% of 120, that is, 90 ml/kg/min. When V_T is set at 12 to 15 ml/kg, f of 8/minute or less avoids the adverse effects of hyperventilation, especially hypokalemic ventricular irritability.

Positive end expiratory pressure (PEEP) is routinely added to reverse atelectasis and shunting because this is not provided by large tidal volumes alone.[96, 97] A level of 5 cmH₂O provides adequate initial PEEP without interfering with venous return in the vast majority of cases. Contraindications to the institution of PEEP include cardiovascular instability, bronchospasm, emphysema, suspected pneumothorax, or suspected endobronchial intubation (Table 16-22).

Secondary Parameters. I:E ratio should be less than 1:2; if 1:1 or greater, impairment of venous return results. *Inspiratory flow rates* should be kept low, ideally around 30 l/min (500 ml/sec) to ensure laminar flow. *Peak inspiratory pressure* (PIP) should be less than 35 cmH2O. Apart from the complications mentioned below, high PIP may be caused by inadequate analgesia with agitation, chest wall rigidity with shivering, or excessively large tidal volumes. *The plateau pressure* (P_{plat}) is derived by use of an inspiratory hold (on the Bear ventilator) or occluding the expiratory limb at the end of inspiration (Bennett MA-1). P_{plat} is inversely proportional to the compliance of the lungs and chest wall. *Static compliance* (C_S) may be derived by dividing the tidal volume* by the difference between the plateau pressure and the baseline pressure (PEEP raises the baseline; Fig. 16-23). Normal C_S is 80 to 100 ml/cmH2O, although most patients after thoracotomy will have a C_S of about 60 ml/cmH2O. Marked decreases in static compliance may be found with pulmonary dysfunction caused by atelectasis, hemothorax, or edema.[98] However, changes in chest wall rigidity also affect C_S; as muscle relaxation wears off, these measurements become less useful as an index of pulmonary function. Increased *airway resistance* (R) is indicated by a difference between PIP and P_{plat} of greater than 3cmH2O; this may be very useful in determining the presence of air-trapping when overt bronchospasm is absent. Acute increases in R also occur with endobronchial intubation and pneumothorax because of reduction in airway volume (Table 16-23).

Check chest film. As soon as is convenient after admission, a chest film should be checked for possible complications. Those requiring immediate intervention include en-

---

* More accurately, volume lost by distension of ventilator tubing should be subtracted from the tidal volume in the MA-1. This is approximately 3 ml/cmH2O PIP.

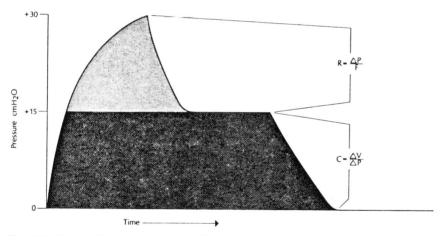

Fig. 16–23. Positive-pressure ventilation with end-inspiratory pause. The *lightly shaded area* represents the pressure change related to resistance phenomena. R = resistance; ΔP = pressure change; F = flow. The *darkly shaded area* represents the pressure change related to compliance factors. C = compliance; ΔV = change in volume. Static compliance (C) is calculated by dividing the inflationary pressure (ΔP) into the tidal volume (ΔV) when flow is stopped at the end of inspiration. Airway resistance (R) may be calculated by dividing inspiratory flow (F) into the difference between plateau and peak inspiratory pressures (ΔP). if F is constant, R may be estimated by simply examining the difference between the latter two pressures. (Shapiro BA, Harrison RA, Trout CA: Clinical Applications of Respiratory Care. 2nd edition, Year Book Press, Chicago, 1979)

Table 16-23. Secondary Parameters

I:E ratio	≤ 1:2
Peak inspiratory flow	~ 30 LPM (500 ml/sec)
PIP	< 35 cmH$_2$O
PIP − P$_{plat}$	≤ 3 cmH$_2$O
C$_S$	≥ 60 ml/cmH$_2$O

Table 16-24. Initial Management of Intrapulmonary Shunting*

Physical examination and chest film
  Complications requiring immediate intervention:
    Endobronchial intubation
    Pneumothorax
    Bleeding (hemothorax, hemomediastinum)
  Complications requiring ongoing therapy:
    Inadequate lung expansion (hypoventilation)
    Atelectasis
    Pulmonary edema
Maximize V$_T$ to ≥ 15 ml/kg if PIP < 25 cmH$_2$O
Trial of PEEP

*Significant Shunting = PaO$_2$ < 200 torr at F$_I$O$_2$ = 0.7

dobronchial intubation, high intubation, pneumothorax, or bleeding (hemomediastinum or hemothorax). The presence of inadequate expansion, atelectasis or pulmonary edema suggests that larger tidal volumes or PEEP will be useful in subsequent management.

Management of Intrapulmonary Shunting
Shunting. Formal calculation of the degree of intrapulmonary shunting is done through the alveolar air equation (Fig. 16-24). However, a useful guide is obtained by simply multiplying the F$_I$O$_2$ by 600. Ideally, if the F$_I$O$_2$ is 1.0, PaO$_2$ should be somewhere near 600 torr; if it is 0.7, somewhere near 420 torr. For clinical purposes, a PaO$_2$ of less than 200 torr at an F$_I$O$_2$ of 0.7 may be defined as significant shunting, requiring immediate attention.

The steps taken to address this problem are outlined in Table 16-24. Check the patient and chest film immediately to exclude bronchospasm, endobronchial intubation, or pneumothorax. If they are absent, hypoxemia is the result of decreased FRC. If PIP is low (*i.e.*, below 25 cmH$_2$O), immediate improvement in oxygenation is often achieved by increasing tidal volume to 15 ml/kg if it is

not already there, or to even higher levels as long as PIP does not exceed 30 to 35 cmH$_2$O. The latter maneuver is especially apt in tall, thin patients with large thoracic cages. If the tidal volume is already satisfactory, a trial of PEEP is performed, as outlined below. The ultimate goal of all these maneuvers is to maximize FRC while the patient is intubated because it will certainly decrease after extubation: *extubate from best FRC.*

Hyperinflation syndrome. If hypoxemia is caused by acute bronchospasm, attempts to correct it with PEEP will exacerbate air-trapping and result in progressive hyperinflation. In emphysema, areas of atelectasis and reduced FRC may indeed exist after surgery. However, PEEP is transmitted to the more compliant areas of the lung and further distends already distended alveoli, thereby increasing dead space (V$_D$). In emphysema, airway collapse may occur during expiration without obvious bronchospasm and other clues to air-trapping must be sought. On the other hand, it should be noted that in chronic bronchitis the basic pathology is excessive bronchial secretion caused by mucus cell hyperplasia, which accelerates atelectasis after surgery. In the absence of acute bronchospasm, these patients are helped by PEEP.

Progressive hyperinflation is reflected by a falling PaO$_2$ and rising PaCO$_2$ as PEEP is continued or increased, because of progressive increase in V$_D$. We have had one case in which the premonitory signs were not recognized. A low output state developed, with tachycardia, vasoconstriction, hypotension, and lactic acidosis. When complete cardiovascular collapse occurred, the patient was rushed back to the operating room because bleeding and cardiac tamponade were suspected as the cause. When the sternum was opened the lungs literally billowed out of the thoracic cage, with immediate and dramatic improvement in cardiovascular status (Table 16-25).

Management of the PEEP trial. Once the use of PEEP has been deemed appropriate, it is applied in a controlled manner. Most patients will already have a level of 5 cmH$_2$O. Increments are made by 2.5 cmH$_2$O at a time.

Because increasing PEEP decreases transmural cardiac filling pressures, the effect of each increment on cardiovascular status should be evaluated. In most patients, this may be judged simply by clinical observation of blood pressure and heart rate. In the unstable patient it is necessary to calculate oxygen delivery (cardiac output × arterial oxygen content) and mixed venous oxygen saturation (Sv_{O_2}) to ensure that PEEP does not adversely affect total oxygen transport and extraction. If cardiac output does fall, a fluid challenge or increased inotropic support can be given to restore it. In the early postoperative period, however, restoration of perfusion takes precedence over restoration of FRC, so that PEEP should be limited if it compromises stability or myocardial oxygen balance. Measurements of static compliance will improve after a PEEP increment if it reverses atelectasis and decreases lung stiffness, unless chest wall rigidity happens to be increasing. A widening of ($PIP - P_{plat}$) infers that PEEP is increasing airway resistance and dead space rather than decreasing shunting.

ABGs are drawn 20 minutes after a change in PEEP. Although theoretically any improvement should be immediate, we have often seen a favorable response after 1 or 2 hours. This may be the result of slow recruitment of collapsed alveoli, or it may merely be caused by the natural improvement that occurs as PEVW is slowly cleared after surgery. Not infrequently there appears to be a certain critical PEEP, after which there is a sudden, dramatic improvement in oxygenation. The goal of the PEEP trial is to reach a level that achieves a PaO_2 of 100 torr or more at an F_IO_2 of 0.4 or less, without hemodynamic instability. In the vast majority of cases, levels of 5 to 10 cmH_2O are sufficient for substantial reversal of intrapulmonary shunting; it is seldom necessary to go as high as 12.5 or 15 cmH_2O (Table 16-26).

Ventilatory Adjustments during Phase I (Rewarming). While rewarming is in progress, mechanical minute ventilation is adjusted to adapt to rising CO_2 production. Tidal volume should be increased to 15 ml/kg, if it is not

Table 16-25. Hyperinflation Syndrome: Evaluation of Air-Trapping

HIGH INDEX OF SUSPICION
Acute bronchospasm
Emphysema (barrel chest, "pink puffer")
Hyperinflation observed in OR
PHYSICAL EXAMINATION
(tracheal auscultation)
Audible wheeze
Prolonged expiratory time
Next breath before full expiration
VENTILATOR RESPONSE
Rising PIP
Widening PIP − P_{plat} (↑ R)
Slow return of inspired volume
ARTERIAL BLOOD GASES
Inappropriate hypoxemia
Inappropriate hypercarbia
Worsened by increase in PEEP
HEMODYNAMIC SEQUELAE
Low output syndrome
Cardiac tamponade

$$P_AO_2 = F_IO_2 (P_{ATM} - P_{H_2O}) - \frac{P_aCO_2}{R.Q.} \qquad (1)$$

$$AaDO_2 = P_AO_2 - P_aO_2 \qquad (2)$$

P_AO_2	Alveolar O_2 tension	P_{ATM}	Atmospheric pressure
PaO_2	Arterial O_2 tension	P_{H_2O}	Water vapor pressure
$PaCO_2$	Arterial CO_2 tension		(47 mmHg at 37°C)
F_IO_2	Inspired O_2 fraction	R.Q.	Respiratory quotient
			(0.85 is usually used)
$AaDO_2$	Alveolar-arterial O_2 difference.		

Fig. 16–24. The alveolar air equation in its simplest form. Normally at an F_IO_2 of 1.0, the $AaDO_2$ is <100 torr. Expect a 10% decrease with each reduction in F_IO_2 by 0.1. $AaDO_2$ of >300 torr at F_IO_2 1.0 represents severe shunting. PaO_2 may be used to derive Qs/Q_T, although this is not used during routine management. Studies are all done at ambient F_IO_2, because increasing the F_IO_2 increases shunting through absorption atelectasis.

Table 16-26. Utilization of PEEP

1. Increase PEEP in increments of 2.5 cmH_2O at a time
2. After each increment of PEEP,
   a. Observe cardiovascular status
   b. Critical patient: Calculate O_2 delivery
      $$(CO \times CaO_2)$$
      Measure Sv_{O_2}
   c. Calculate C_S
   d. Check ABGs after 20 minutes and estimate $AaDO_2$
3. If PEEP impairs O_2 delivery or Sv_{O_2}, consider risk versus benefit of fluid loading or inotropic support or both
4. Goal: Improve $AaDO_2$ such that $PaO_2 > 100$ torr at $FiO_2 < 0.4$ (seldom require > 10 cmH_2O PEEP)
5. At IMV rate $\leq 4/min$ PEEP may be increased with little impairment of venous return to optimize FRC before extubation.

already there, or above this to a PIP limit of 30 to 35 cmH_2O. Ventilator rate is increased once V_T is maximized. F_IO_2 is reduced as indicated to maintain a PaO_2 of between 75 and 85 torr.

Phase II: Ventilatory Weaning and Extubation

Debate continues as to the best time to extubate patients after cardiac surgery. With narcotic techniques, we feel there is nothing to be gained by premature extubation. Attempts at weaning during rewarming result in hypercapnia and acidosis. The ventilatory response to increasing $PaCO_2$ is depressed by narcosis and anesthesia; even if it were not, the increased work of breathing increases myocardial oxygen demand further. Reversal of narcosis and relaxants is hazardous (see below). IMV weaning is started when (1) rewarming has peaked and $\dot{V}CO_2$ stabilized, (2) muscle relaxation and narcosis have worn off, and (3) adequate spontaneous ventilation has returned. The latter is checked by direct verbal communication with the patient, ability to hand squeeze, and to take breaths off the ventilator. Once cardiovascular stability has been restored, FRC has been improved, and the patient is awake and comfortable, there is no advantage in continuing ventilatory support for its own sake. In most cases, IMV weaning is commenced 4 to 8 hours after return to the ICU.

Weaning Procedure *Wean F_IO_2.* Because high inspired oxygen concentrations predispose to oxygen toxicity and increase shunting by absorption atelectasis, they are weaned first. The goal is to achieve an F_IO_2 of between 0.4 and 0.3 as long as PaO_2 remains between 75 and 85 torr.

IMV rate. The IMV rate is reduced in decrements of 2/min, so long as the pH remains above 7.35. The rate of weaning depends entirely on the clinical condition of the patient; it may vary from 2 to 12 hours. If the PaO_2 falls as the IMV rate falls, it suggests that the FRC is still dependent on positive pressure support (*i.e.*, spontaneous ventilation is shallow). A means that enables weaning to be continued while FRC is maintained is to increase V_T to 20 ml/kg and PEEP by a further 2.5 or 5 cmH_2O, once the IMV rate is less than 4/min. The mean intra-thoracic pressure is less at slow ventilator rates and these maneuvers are usually well tolerated hemodynamically. At an IMV of 4/min, the patient is getting close to extubation. The head of the bed is elevated as much as possible to reduce pressure of abdominal contents on the diaphragm and also to allow the patient to re-establish contact with his or her environment. If CNS and neuromuscular status are assessed as adequate, most patients are weaned directly from an IMV of 4/min to 0/min. An IMV of 0/min with PEEP is known as *continuous positive airway pressure* (CPAP); without PEEP, it is called *T-tube mode*.

Wean PEEP. In the treatment of shunting, a high inspired oxygen concentration is symptomatic; PEEP is therapeutic. If PEEP improves oxygenation, wean F_IO_2, not PEEP. Optimal PEEP should be maintained throughout weaning of F_IO_2 and IMV rate so that extubation takes place at best FRC. Once CPAP has been achieved, high levels of PEEP should be weaned down to 7.5 or 5 cmH_2O. The requirement of an F_IO_2 greater than 0.6 to maintain adequate PaO_2 when PEEP is dropped suggests that extubation should be deferred because of significant residual shunting. Most patients do well when extubated off 5 to 7.5 cmH_2O PEEP, provided they have sufficient strength to breathe deeply and cough to maintain FRC once it is removed. The patient should be left on CPAP for at least 45 to 60 minutes before extubation to ensure that the patient does not become fatigued once off mechanical ventilation. This precaution will reveal a situation where normal ABGs are maintained at the cost of increased work of breathing.

Avoid CZAP. T-tube weaning (continuous zero airway pressure) is indicated for patients with air-trapping only. It is a low resistance circuit that bypasses the physiologic PEEP (about 2.5 cmH$_2$O) provided by the glottis and upper airway. Patients left on the T-tube for longer than 45 minutes can be expected to show gradual fall in FRC and PaO$_2$. It should not be used for longer than 1 hour without the restoration of some degree of IMV support. Ideally, it should be used only to assess readiness for extubation. In many patients, the presence of the endotracheal tube simply hampers their ability to breathe deeply and cough; ABGs usually improve *after* extubation (Table 16-27).

Indications for Extubation Lists of extubation criteria abound.[99-101] Readiness for extubation should be predicated on the achievement of three major goals; (1) reversal of the underlying pulmonary pathology; (2) ability to maintain homeostasis (*i.e.,* normal ABGs); and (3) adequate neuromuscular control.

Reversal of underlying pulmonary pathology. After cardiac surgery, the major pulmonary pathology is reduction in FRC. Adequate restoration of FRC is evident by a PaO$_2$ of 80 torr or above on an F$_I$O$_2$ of 0.4 or less, at levels of PEEP less than 7.5 cmH$_2$O.

If the pathology is excessive dead space caused by bronchospasm, this should be well controlled before extubation.

Maintenance of homeostasis. The patient should be able to maintain normal ABGs at a normal work rate. After 1 hour on CPAP or T-tube, pH should be greater than 7.35 with a respiratory rate of less than 28/min. This indicates maintenance of adequate tidal volume, without excessive dead space. However, normal ABGs do not reveal anything about the patient's ability to cough, breathe deeply, respond to stress, or maintain FRC.

Adequate neuromuscular control. In order to

ascertain the ability to maintain FRC after extubation an indication of ventilatory *reserve* must be obtained. The patient should be alert, cooperative, and eager to be extubated. Beware of the narcotized patient who is appropriate and strong when stimulated, but who slips back into stupor when left undisturbed. If there is any doubt, the patient should be left on CPAP for another 30 minutes and ABGs then repeated. Check the handgrip and thoracic excursion on voluntary deep breathing and sustained head raising (although this is painful after sternotomy—we don't insist). There are two quantitative tests of ventilatory reserve that may be helpful:

Forced Vital Capacity (FVC): Volume exhaled forcefully after maximal inspiration. This is an excellent indication of ability to respond to acute stress. Also, because it requires patient cooperation, it is guide to the potential success of breathing treatments after extubation. Normal range: 50–70 ml/kg; acceptable for extubation: > 15 ml/kg.

Table 16-27. Ventilatory Weaning

1. Wean Inspired O$_2$ Fraction
   a. Wean FiO$_2$ in decrements of 0.1 to achieve 0.35
2. Wean IMV Rate
   a. Wean IMV rate in decrements of 2/min (8 → 6 → 4)
   b. IMV rate weaned as long as pH > 7.35
   c. If PaO$_2$ falls as IMV rate falls (FRC ∝ V$_{Mech}$)
      Increase V$_T$ to 20 ml/kg if tolerated
      Increase PEEP
   d. Elevate head of bed when IMV rate 4/min
   e. Wean from IMV 4/min to CPAP after assessing CNS status
3. Wean PEEP
   a. If PEEP improves oxygenation, wean FiO$_2$, not PEEP
   b. Maintain optimal PEEP throughout IMV weaning to CPAP
      (extubate from best FRC)
   c. On CPAP, wean PEEP to 7.5 or 5 cmH$_2$O
   d. Evaluate for extubation after 1 hour on CPAP
4. Avoid CZAP!
   a. T-tube (continuous zero expiratory pressure) indicated in patients with air-trapping only
   b. In other patients lack of resistance → FRC ↓ → PaO$_2$ ↓
   c. Do not leave on T-tube alone longer than 1 hour
   d. Most patients do better extubated than on T-tube
      (except when used for airway protection)

Table 16-28. Indications for Extubation

1. Reversal of excessive shunting or dead space
   a. Shunt reduced, FRC restored as evidenced by good AaDO$_2$
      (PaO$_2$ > 80 torr at FiO$_2$ < 0.4)
   b. V$_D$ reduced: No acute bronchospasm or hypercapnia
2. Normal gas exchange on CPAP or T-tube for 1 hour
   a. pH > 7.35 at f < 28/min
   b. Maintenance of adequate V$_T$ and V̇$_E$ without excessive work
3. Ability to maintain FRC after extubation
   a. CNS status: Alert, cooperative, not narcotized
   b. Neuromuscular status
      Adequate hand grip, thoracic excursion
      FVC > 15 ml/kg (normal 50–70 ml/kg)
      MIF > −25 cmH$_2$O (normal −80 to −100 cmH$_2$O)

Maximum Inspiratory Force (MIF): Maximum negative pressure generated at airway when inspiration is artificially obstructed. This is a good indication of thoracic muscle strength. It is more objective than the FVC because it does not depend on patient motivation and may even be performed in the presence of coma. However, it provides little indication of subsequent voluntary activity. Normal range: −80 to −100 cmH$_2$O; acceptable for extubation: > −25 cmH$_2$O.

The FVC and MIF are most meaningful when used as serial rather than absolute measures. In most patients, clinical evaluation of muscle strength is sufficient; the FVC and MIF are helpful when the former is equivocal, especially after prolonged mechanical ventilation (Table 16-28).

Contraindications to Extubation The presence of residual neuromuscular paralysis or narcosis should contraindicate weaning. The side-effects of reversal agents justify the expedient of maintaining mechanical ventilatory support until spontaneous recovery is completed. Neostigmine or pyridostigmine, even if carefully used, may cause bradyarrhythmias, escape rhythms, excessive secretions, and bronchospasm. Atropine and other anticholinergic agents may provoke tachyarrhythmias; muscarinic blockade may be incomplete or short-lived. The use of nal-

oxone (Narcan) to reverse narcosis is particularly hazardous after cardiac surgery. The dramatic reversal of narcotic analgesia causes a sudden return of sympathetic tone which may precipitate pulmonary edema or myocardial ischemia. Although this can be avoided if naloxone is diluted and carefully titrated in 0.05 mg IV increments, its action is short-lived. The patient has to be monitored extremely closely for return of narcosis and the dose usually has to be repeated every 30 to 45 minutes.

Severe neurologic complications such as cerebral embolism or infarction obviously contraindicate extubation. Mechanical ventilation should be continued if it appears that the patient is unable to protect his or her airway, or if mental obtundation is such that spontaneous deep breathing, coughing, and compliance with respiratory therapy is unlikely.

If a severe degree of reversible shunting exists because of atelectasis or pulmonary edema, it is preferable to use mechanical ventilation with PEEP to improve FRC before extubation, even if this means continuing sedation. ABGs may be good and the chest film may look clear while positive pressure support and PEEP are provided, but after extubation there is a dramatic decrease in lung volumes and progressive deterioration in ABGs.

The sick mitral (*i.e.,* the elderly, debilitated patient with preexisting cardiac failure) is at particular risk of rebound pulmonary edema after extubation. PEVW, already extensive before surgery, is exacerbated during fluid loading. If the patient is still hemodynamically unstable, and is requiring fluid challenges to maintain a high filling pressure, respiratory failure is very likely to occur after extubation. Specific afterload reduction with intravenous hydralazine, with or without specific preload reduction with nitroglycerin, may be helpful in facilitating extubation in these patients. The patient who has had a complicated postoperative course (*e.g.,* bleeding requiring return to the operating room) will have received massive fluid replacement and also have large amounts of residual PEVW. The amount of weight gain after surgery is a reasonable indicator. In general, when weight gain is greater than 5 kg above preoperative weight, it is wise to defer extubation. Diuresis and fluid restriction are used until weight is near to the preoperative value. (Patients in controlled cardiac failure before operation may have been pruned to below their ideal weight.)

Patients with chronic atrial fibrillation often emerge in sinus rhythm when cardioversion is performed at the end of bypass. However, atrial fibrillation invariably recurs; if it does so shortly after extubation, it may so compromise cardiac output that pulmonary edema occurs. Atrial pacing commenced while sinus rhythm still exists can suppress the return of atrial fibrillation for 48 hours and ride out the danger period. Early reinstitution of digitalis therapy, within 12 hours of operation, may help defer its return or at least prevent a rapid ventricular response. If supraventricular irritability exists during weaning, it is wise to avoid extubation until the arrhythmia is controlled.

Ventricular arrhythmias provide a relative contraindication to extubation. Infusions of lidocaine or procainamide may cause mental obtundation even at therapeutic levels. Frequent cardioversion may be required. The patient who has already been extubated may get into a vicious cycle of hypoventilation, atelectasis, hypoxemia, and increased myocardial irritability.

In our experience, the presence of the IABP contraindicates extubation, although it does not preclude weaning down to low IMV rates. Usually the balloon has been placed because of myocardial dysfunction, so that higher filling pressures are required and PEVW is increased. The IABP prevents the patient from sitting up, and mobilization and proper respiratory therapy are markedly hampered. In addition, having the patient intubated facilitates general anesthesia should it be necessary when the IABP is removed. Sedation can be discontinued after balloon removal; extubation is usually achieved after 24 to 36 hours of slow weaning (Table 16-29).

Slow Ventilatory Weaning Even if extubation is not contemplated, as in the above situations, ventilatory weaning to low IMV rates has definite advantages: improved venous return, and respiratory muscle exercise and coordination. In the patient whose weaning is slow or difficult, there are certain principles that we have found helpful. Periods of ventilatory exercise are always followed by periods of rest to avoid the physical and psychological trauma of exhaustion, decompensation, sympathetic discharge, and delayed recovery time. Patients are rested at night (*e.g.*, from 8 PM to 6 AM) at IMV rates at which they are completely comfortable—usually in the 6 to 8/min range. During the day an exercise-rest pattern is alternated, such as 1 hour on CPAP and 1 hour on IMV 4/min. Gradually, exercise periods are lengthened at the expense of rest periods. In general, the longer the duration of previous mechanical support, the slower the weaning. Once CPAP is sustained for long periods, intermittent positive-pressure breathing (IPPB) treatments are instituted on a four hourly basis to interrupt the monotonous ventilatory pattern and prevent microatelectasis. The program of slow ventilatory weaning is an eclectic one, and has to be tailor-made to suit the individual needs of each patient. It is important to spend some time with the nursing staff and respiratory therapists to explain the rationale for delayed weaning because it may be quite different from the rapid weaning and extu-

Table 16-29. Contraindications to Extubation

1. Residual narcosis or muscle relaxation (avoid reversal agents)
2. Neurologic complications
3. Severe reversible intrapulmonary shunting
4. Unstable hemodynamic status
   a. Sick mitral → rebound pulmonary edema
   b. Excessive fluid loading: weight gain > 5 kg
   c. Persistent requirement for high filling pressures
5. Arrhythmias
   a. Return of atrial fibrillation in chronic fibrillators
   b. Ventricular arrhythmias requiring high-dose antiarrhythmic therapy or repeated cardioversion
6. IABP

bation that they have come to expect with the majority of postoperative patients.

Extubation Procedure The procedure at Stanford for extubation is fully outlined below. It is based on the recognition that the cuff is covered with a collection of mucus which may disperse into the distal trachea and bronchi when the cuff is deflated before extubation. Extubation with a suction catheter inside the tube to withdraw the plug is undesirable because the negative pressure decreases F_IO_2 and creates atelectasis just at the time when the patient can no longer be helped. Suctioning is always done ahead of time and is followed by bagging to overcome its detrimental effects. The patient is extubated with fully inflated lungs at the peak of a full voluntary inflation; the cuff is deflated at the last moment and, with that breath, the patient coughs out the mucus plug—often with devastating accuracy.

Extubation Procedure

1. Explain procedure fully to patient and sit upright as much as tolerated; have tissues and emesis basin ready.
2. Thorough endotracheal suctioning with reexpansion by bag and oxygen after each attempt; suction mouth.
3. Instruct patient to take deep breath and hold it.
4. While cords are open, rapidly deflate cuff and remove endotracheal tube.
5. Urge patient to cough with expiration from previous deep breath. Be prepared for large mucus plug (previously lying on cuff in trachea) which you catch with tissue in emesis basin.
6. Place aerosol oxygen mask with F_IO_2 0.1 higher than while intubated. Explain goals of postextubation respiratory therapy to patient.

Phase III: Postextubation Respiratory Therapy

Oxygen Therapy Because the precise oxygen concentration delivered by mask is uncertain, F_IO_2 is always raised by 0.1 above that through the endotracheal tube after extubation. Initially, an aerosol mask is used to pro-

vide humidification, but this can be quickly changed to nasal prongs, which at 4 to 6 l/min provide about 24 to 28 percent oxygen. The latter has the added advantage of being more comfortable and less likely to be removed by an agitated patient or solicitous nurse. In addition, they provide oxygen during eating and incentive spirometry. Continuous oxygen therapy should be provided for at least 24 hours after extubation because shunting increases. Inadvertent hypoxemia may contribute to the high incidence of supraventricular arrhythmias in the 2 to 4 days after operation. Patients with abnormal pulmonary function, especially with atelectasis, effusion or edema, should have oxygen provided for a longer time, especially when supine or asleep, when the FRC and PaO_2 are likely to decrease to lower levels.

ABGs should be checked 1 hour and again 6 hours after extubation, and more frequently if indicated.

We obtain daily chest films at 5 AM, before most patients are extubated. In fact, a chest film taken after extubation is much more meaningful because it will disclose atelectasis and effusions hidden by pressure support. In the sicker patient, it may be useful to obtain a chest film about 6 hours after extubation.

Respiratory Therapy and Mobilization The beneficial effects of incentive spirometry have been well documented.[102–104] We use the Triflo because it provides incentive for maximal voluntary inspirations cheaply and without the necessity for respiratory therapist intervention. However it must be realized that this device is a flowmeter rather than a spirometer; successive balls are raised with increasingly rapid inspiratory flow rates. In their zeal to achieve success, patients may be encouraged to hyperventilate themselves into a state of tetany or exhaustion. It must be made very clear that *sustained* elevation of one ball is more desirable than short-lived elevation of three balls, that the patient should breathe in slowly but strongly, and should rest completely between attempts. For best results, incentive spirometry should be performed for 5 minutes every hour while awake.

Aerosol treatments with a bronchodilator in suspension are indicated for active bronchospasm, patients with known COPD or a history of heavy cigarette smoking, or in the presence of diffuse rhonchi with secretions. In the latter case, the action of β-adrenergic agents in stimulating ciliary motility and the mucus cascade is utilized. Isoetharine (Bronkosol), 0.25 to 0.5 mg in 2 ml normal saline suspension, is used every 4 hours as indicated. Metoproterenol (Alupent) and terbutaline (Brethine) are alternative selective β₂-adrenergic agents. These agents are contraindicated in the presence of myocardial ischemia, sinus tachycardia, or supraventricular arrhythmias.

IPPB is reserved for patients who are too weak, tired, or otherwise unable to use incentive spirometry appropriately. It is not a panacea; in the mentally obtunded, who tend to air swallow to a large degree, we have seen ileus caused by gaseous distension of the entire gastrointestinal tract. The risks of regurgitation and aspiration are obvious. Many patients do not tolerate the sensation of IPPB. The rapid inspiratory flow causes sternal pain, splinting, decreases chest wall compliance, and reduces the effective tidal volume delivered. However, there are other patients in whom frequent IPPB treatments for the first 24 hours may well make the difference between recovery and reintubation. Common sense should prevail.

Mobilization is an essential component of the restoration of FRC. The more the patient can sit up, get out of bed, and walk, the more likely they are to overcome residual atelectasis and edema. Once the decision has been made to proceed with extubation and mobilization, as many catheters as possible which limit mobility, should be removed. This includes arterial lines, pulmonary artery catheters, urinary catheters, and chest tubes. In the vulnerable patient, there may be conflict between the need to closely monitor blood gases and filling pressures and the need for mobilization. Careful clinical consideration

has to be given to the right time to remove monitors.

Cough tubes (*i.e.,* the insertion of a 16- or 18-gauge catheter through the cricothyroid membrane for the instillation of saline to provoke cough), should be abandoned. They provide direct access for nosocomial infection below the glottis, and the cough provoked is not necessarily effective. Vigorous chest physiotherapy with drainage in the head-down position is poorly tolerated by most cardiac patients and may be dangerous, leaving the patient hypoxic, frightened, and exhausted. When CPT is performed it should be gentle and used appropriately. Unilateral severe atelectasis will frequently respond to positioning with the good lung down and gentle vibration or percussion therapy (Table 16-30).

Chest Tubes At Stanford, it is customary for the surgeons to place two mediastinal drains with or without a right pleural drain. These are usually removed after extubation (unless the latter is deferred more than 24 hours), once drainage has decreased to 20 ml/hr for 3 consecutive hours. However, if there is a suspicion of a pneumothorax (potential or otherwise) or of hemothorax, the tubes should be placed to underwater seal for 6 hours, a chest film taken to exclude the accumulation of air or fluid, and then removed. If there has been severe postoperative bleeding or hemomediastinum, the tubes are left another 24 hours. Occasionally, changes in position will result in a sudden efflux of blood; these are usually small pockets and not significant. Spontaneous gushes occur after 24 hours with clot lysis. If chest tubes are left in too long, they set up an irritative serosanguinous discharge.

Pleural effusions develop frequently in the postoperative period because of mobilization of interstitial and intraalveolar fluid by lymphatics. Often the effusion is inexplicably confined to one side. They almost invariably respond to diuresis and mobilization. Effusions are drained if they are obviously increasing the work of breathing, causing atelectasis, or suspected of being infected.

Table 16-30. Postextubation Respiratory Therapy

1. Oxygen therapy
   a. Check ABGs 1 hour and 6 hours after extubation, or prn
   b. Maintain on O_2 continuously for 24 hours
   c. Thereafter provide O_2 during sleep or supine position, as indicated
   d. Change to nasal prongs allows O_2 during eating and spirometry
   e. Check chest film 6 hours after extubation, if indicated, then daily
2. Respiratory therapy and mobilization
   a. Incentive spirometry q1h
   b. Aerosol treatments with bronchodilator q4h: Acute bronchospasm, heavy smoking, diffuse rhonchi
   c. IPPB treatments with bronchodilator q4h: Patient too weak or too tired to use spirometry or aerosol; severe, acute bronchospasm
   d. Gentle CPT and positioning for severe atelectasis
   e. Decannulation and mobilization (dangling, sitting, standing, walking) as soon as possible
   f. Contraindicated: Cough tubes, CPT in Trendelenberg
3. Hemodynamic interactions
   a. Augmented diuresis as indicated (furosemide, dopamine)
   b. Control of arrhythmias (potassium, digoxin, pacing)
   c. Inotropic support, afterload/preload reduction, as indicated
4. Decannulation procedure
   a. NG tube, urinary catheter removed at extubation
   b. Peripheral IV, arterial line removed 4–6 hours later if stable (pulmonary artery catheter removed when stable)
   c. Pleural tubes removed after extubation when drainage < 20 ml/hour for 3 consecutive hours (left atrial line removed before pleural tubes)
      (1) Suspected pneumo/hemothorax; Place tubes to underwater seal for 6 hours, check chest film, then remove
      (2) Postoperative bleeding: Leave tubes in place for 24 hours

Complications

Endotracheal Tube Position The dangers of endobronchial intubation have been covered already in this section. Suffice it to say that even careful clinical examination will not disclose endobronchial intubation in many cases. The roentgenograph is the ultimate arbiter.

In an effort to avoid this complication, many anesthesiologists cut the endotracheal tube (ET) too short. In the ICU, this will manifest as an urgent call for the attendant to replace the ET because of a cuff leak. Almost inevitably the cuff itself is fine; the leak exists because the cuff projects through the cords and prevents a complete seal. The more air injected into the balloon, the worse the apparent leak. In the extreme situation merely the tip of the tube projects through the cords, providing some lung inflation, while the entire balloon sits in the oropharynx. Because as much as 130 ml air can be inflated into the soft cuff, it may be some time before the true

cause of the leak is recognized, by which time dangerous hypoxemia or hypercarbia may occur.

Not infrequently, a tube that has been cut relatively short appears to be adequate in the operating room. However, after 24 hours, warming causes relative bending of the tube so that cuff leak first manifests on the second day.

The course is clear-cut. The first step in dealing with a cuff leak is to perform direct laryngoscopy and visualize the tube and cuff position. If the tube is long enough, the problem may be resolved by merely letting the cuff down and readvancing it through the cords under direct vision. If not, it will be necessary to replace the tube with one cut longer. A chest film is mandatory to confirm tube position after repositioning or replacement.

Non-Cardiac Pulmonary Edema This entity is usually defined as pulmonary edema secondary to a capillary leak syndrome, without elevated cardiac filling pressures, and with protein concentration in secretions virtually equivalent to that of serum. Because the combination of capillary leak and elevated filling pressures is so common after cardiopulmonary bypass, it may be inappropriate to define this as a separate entity unless it is fulminant. Cases labeled as delayed adult respiratory distress syndrome[105] may simply represent phase II fluid mobilization.

Putative causes of fulminant noncardiac pulmonary edema are summarized in Table 16-31. Anaphylactic drug and transfusion reactions may manifest predominantly as circulatory collapse rather than pulmonary edema. Protamine appears to be a frequent culprit. The drug is derived from salmon and not infrequently there is a history of allergy to fish. The postperfusion syndrome occurs unpredictably after prolonged cardiopulmonary bypass. Profound capillary leak with diffuse organ dysfunction, DIC, high cardiac output with low vascular resistance, fever, and leucocytosis are hallmarks of this condition.

Hemodynamic support with epinephrine infusion (1–4 μg/min), calcium chloride (1–2 g IV prn), and dopamine (3–8 μg/kg/min) is indicated. The patient is digitalized. Large amounts of saline, blood, or fresh frozen plasma may be required to replace the volume deficit; we avoid albumin because it leaks into the interstitial space and exacerbates pulmonary edema, although other authors report contrasting results.[106] A pharmacologic dose of methylprednisone, 30 mg/kg IV, is given, and repeated in 12 hours if the endotoxic shock-like state persists.[107] Ventilatory support with PEEP is provided as indicated by the degree of shunting. Vasodilator and diuretic therapy are of use only when the initial insult has dissipated, vascular tone returns, and interstitial fluid accumulation requires mobilization (see Table 16-31).

Pneumothorax Pneumothorax usually results from direct trauma to the lung at surgery. Management is by chest tube as discussed in the previous sections.

Pneumonia Acute pneumonia is relatively uncommon in the early postoperative period, unless secondary to aspiration pneumonitis complicating anesthesia, or occurring as a flare up of a preexisting infection. During initial rewarming, temperatures rise to above 38°C; this is a physiologic response and does not necessitate culturing for sepsis. On day one, temperature spikes may occur as a result of atelectasis, together with clinical signs of consolidation and productive cough. White counts are frequently elevated as an acute stress response.[108] Pneumonia is likely if the clinical signs persist for more than two days, if they are associated with obviously purulent sputum, a rising white cell count, and the presence of new infiltrates on chest film. Patients who require prolonged intubation with mechanical ventilation are at increased risk.

Etiologic diagnosis is best decided on the presence of intracellular organisms on a Gram stain of fresh sputum. Cultures are likely to grow out mixed organisms which are probably oral or endotracheal tube contaminants. In view of the high likelihood of hospital-borne nosocomial infection, antibiotic coverage should include staphylococcal

Table 16-31. Noncardiogenic Pulmonary Edema

ETIOLOGY
1. Anaphylactic shock
   a. Protamine sensitivity
   b. Leucoagglutinin, HL-A reactions
   c. Unknown antigens
2. Prolonged cardiopulmonary bypass
   Postperfusion syndrome
   (DIC, kinin, complement activation)
3. Endotoxic shock
   a. Valve replacement for active endocarditis
   b. Sepsis ab initio
4. Cardiac surgery after severe trauma
   Posttraumatic shock lung

MANAGEMENT
1. Hemodynamic support
   a. Epinephrine infusion 1–4 μg/min
   b. CaCl$_2$ 1–2 IV prn
   c. Dopamine 3–8 μg/kg/min
   d. Digoxin
2. Fluid support (saline, RBCs)
3. Methylprednisolone 30 mg/kg IV
4. Mechanical ventilation with PEEP
5. Coagulation factors (FFP, platelets):
   Given for bleeding only, not DIC

and Gram-negative organisms. Patients with prostheses should be vigorously treated because of the risk of endocarditis.

Pulmonary Embolism Although relatively uncommon, risk of embolism is increased by low cardiac output, arrhythmias and prolonged immobilization in the postoperative period. Coumadin therapy is routinely commenced on day 3 for all patients on most cardiac surgery services at Stanford, whatever the procedure. Differential diagnosis (myocardial infarction, tamponade) may be difficult, and pulmonary angiography is usually required for unequivocal confirmation. The risks and benefits of angiography, heparinization, or vascular procedures must be individualized according to the clinical situation.

SUMMARY

The primary purpose of intensive care is to integrate recovery from the acute stress of surgery with the restitution of cardiopulmonary independence. Early hemodynamic management is directed at restoration of intravascular volume to prevent cardiac and renal failure; later, interstitial fluid is mobilized to prevent pulmonary complications. Arrhythmias become the major problem after the first 48 hours. Pulmonary management is directed at restoration of functional residual capacity to prevent atelectasis and hypoxemia, followed by appropriate weaning from a mechanical ventilation. Respiratory therapy after extubation is equally important.

Complications should be promptly identified and treated. A rational and individualized approach to management permits low morbidity and mortality in association with these major surgical procedures.

Many aspects of the postoperative management of the patient undergoing cardiopulmonary bypass can be generalized to that of any acute cardiovascular insult. While the application of therapy depends on the nature of the insult, the physiologic principles remain the same.

REFERENCES

HEMODYNAMIC MANAGEMENT

Physiology

1. Lappas DG, Powell WMJ, Daggett WM: Cardiac dysfunction in the postoperative period: pathophysiology, diagnosis and treatment. Anesthesiology 47:117–137, 1977
2. Kouchoukos NO, Karp BB: Management of the postoperative cardiovascular surgical patient. Am Heart J 92:513–531, 1976
3. Berger RL, Weisel RD, Vito L et al: Cardiac output measurement by thermodilution during cardiac operations. Ann Thorac Surg 21:43–47, 1976
4. Utley JR, Michalsky GB, Bryant LR et al: Determinants of myocardial water content during cardiopulmonary bypass. J Thorac Cardiovasc Surg 68:8–16, 1974
5. Foglia RP, Steed DL, Follette DM et al: Iatrogenic myocardial edema with potassium cardioplegia. J Thorac Cardiovasc Surg 78:217–222, 1979
6. English TAH, Digerness S, Kirklin JW: Changes in colloid osmotic pressure shortly after open intracardiac operation. J Thorac Cardiovasc Surg 61:338–341, 1971
7. Gaasch WH, Quinones MA, Waisser E et al: Diastolic compliance of the left ventricle in man. Am J Cardiol 36:193–201, 1975
8. Levine HG, Gaatsch WH: Diastolic compliance of the left ventricle. Mod Concepts Cardiovasc Dis 47:95–102, ,1978
9. Estafanous FG, Tarazi RC, Viljoen JF et al: Systemic hypertension following myocardial revascularization. Am Heart J 85:731–738, 1976
10. Viljoen JF, Estafanous FG, Tarazi RG: Acute hypertension immediately after coronary artery surgery. J Thorac Cardiovasc Surg 71:548–550, 1976
11. Benzing G, Helmworth J, Stockert J et al: Human myocardial performance during surgical treatment of cardiac disease. J Thorac Cardiovascular Surg 59:800–809, 1970
12. Taylor KM, Morton IJ, Brown JJ et al: Hypertension and the renin angiotensin system following open-heart surgery. J Thorac Cardiovasc Surg 74:840–895, 1977
13. Kouchoukos NO, Karp RB: Management of the postoperative cardiovascular surgical patient. Am Heart J 92:513–531, 1976

14. Viljoen JF, Estafanous FG, Tarazi RG: Acute hypertension immediately after coronary artery surgery. J Thorac Cardiovasc Surg 71:548–550, 1976

15. Kissin I, Reves JG, Mardis M: Is the rate-pressure product a misleading question? Anesthesiology 52:373–374, 1980

16. Barash PG, Kopriva CJ: The rate-pressure product in clinical anesthesia: boon or bane? Anesth Analg (Cleve) 52:229–231, 1980

17. Hoffman JIE, Buckberg GD: The myocardial supply:demand ratio—a critical review. Am J Cardiol 41:327–332, 1978

18. Barnard RJ, MacAlpin R, Kattus AA et al: Ischemic response to sudden strenuous exercise in healthy men. Circulation 48:936–942, 1973

19. Oliveros RA, Boucher CA, Haycraft GL et al: Myocardial oxygen supply:demand ratio. A validation of peripherally vs. centrally determined values. Chest 75:693–696, 1979

20. Philips PA, Marty AT, Miyamoto AM: A clinical method for detecting subendocardial ischemia after cardiopulmonary bypass. J Thorac Cardiovasc Surg 69:30–39, 1975

21. Brazier J, Cooper N, Buckberg G: The adequacy of subendocardial oxygen delivery: interactions of determinants of flow, arterial oxygen content and myocardial oxygen need. Circulation 49:968–977, 1974

22. Oka Y, Frishman W, Becker RM et al: Clinical pharmacology of the new beta-adrenergic blocking drugs, part 10: beta-adrenoceptor blockade and coronary artery surgery. Am Heart J 99:255–269, 1980

23. Boudoulas H, Lewis RP, Kates RE, Dalamangas G: Hypersensitivity to adrenergic stimulation after propranolol withdrawal in normal subjects. Ann Intern Med 87:433–436, 1977

24. Taylor KM, Morton IJ, Brown JJ et al.: Hypertension and the renin angiotensin system following open-heart surgery. J Thorac Cardiovasc Surg 74:840–845, 1977

25. Nagaoka H, Katori M: Inhibition of kinin formation by a kallikrein inhibitor during extracorporeal circulation in open heart surgery. Circulation 52:325–332, 1975

26. Parker DJ, Cook S, Turner–Warwick M: Serum complement studies during and following cardiopulmonary bypass. In Junod AD, deHaller R (ed): Lung Metabolism, pp 481–491 New York, Academic Press, 1975

27. Chenoweth DE, Cooper SW, Hugli TE et al: Complement activation during cardiopulmonary bypass: evidence of generation of C3a and C5a anaphylatoxins. N Engl J Med 304:497–503, 1981

28. DeVries W, Kwan-Gett C, Kolff W: Consumptive coagulopathy, shock and the artificial heart. Trans Am Soc Artif Organs 16:29–36, 1970

29. Nordstrom S: Proteinase inhibitors in thoracic surgery. Acta Chir Scand Suppl 378:71–75, 1967

30. Davis FM, Parimelazhagan KN, Harris EA: Thermal balance during cardiopulmonary bypass with moderate hypothermia in man. Br J Anaesth 49:1127–1132, 1977

31. Henning RJ, Wiener F, Valdes S et al: Measurement of toe temperature for assessing the severity of acute circulatory failure. Surg Gynecol Obstet 149:1–7, 1979

32. Sladen RN: Unpublished data.

33. Noback CR, Tinker JH: Hypothermia after cardiopulmonary bypass in man: amelioration by nitroprusside-induced vasodilation during rewarming. Anesthesiology 53:277–280, 1980

Management

34. Coleman, RW: Paradoxical hypotension after volume expansion with plasma protein fraction. N Engl J Med 299:97–98, 1978

35. Benzing G, Helmsworth JA, Schrieber JT et al: Nitroprusside after open heart surgery. Circulation 54:467–471, 1976

36. Chiarello M, Gold HK, Leinback RC et al: Comparison between the effects of nitroprusside and nitroglycerin on ischemic injury during acute myocardial infarction. Circulation 54:766–763, 1976

37. Kaplan JA, Finlayson DC, Woodward S: Vasodilator therapy after cardiac surgery: a review of the efficacy and toxicity of nitroglycerin and nitroprusside. Can Anaesth Soc J 27:254–259, 1980

38. Stulz PM, Schneidegger D, Drop LJ et al: Ventricular pump performance during hypocalcemia. J Thorac Cardiovasc Surg 78:185–194, 1979

39. Miller RR, Awan NA, Joye JA et al: Combined dopamine and nitroprusside therapy in congestive heart failure—greater augmentation of cardiac performance by addition of inotropic stimulation to afterload reduction. Circulation 55:881–884, 1977

40. Stinson EB, Holloway, EL, Derby G et al:

Comparative hemodynamic responses to chlorpromazine, nitroprusside, nitroglycerin, and trimethaphan immediately after open heart operations. Circulation (Suppl I) 51, 52:26–33, 1975

41. Stinson EB, Holloway EL, Derby G et al: Control of myocardial performance early after open heart operations by vasodilator treatment. J Thorac Cardiovasc Surg 73:523–530, 1977

42. Sladen RN, Rosenthal MH: Specific afterload reduction with parenteral hydralazine following cardiac surgery. J Thorac Cardiovac Surg 78:195–202, 1979

43. Johnson LW, Dickst in RA, Fruehan CT et al: Prophylactic digitali..ation for coronary artery bypass surgery. Circulation 53:819–822, 1976

44. Tyras DH, Stothert JC, Kaiser GC et al: Supraventricular tachyarrhythmias after myocardial revascularization: a randomized trial of prophylactic digitalization. J Thorac Cardiovasc Surg 77:310–314, 1979

45. Oka Y, Frishman W, Becker RM et al: Clinical pharmacology of the new beta-adrenergic blocking drugs, part 10: beta-adrenoceptor blockade and coronary artery surgery. Am Heart J 99:255–269, 1980

46. Molu R, Smolinsky, A, Goor DA. Prevention of supraventricular tachyarrhythmias with low-dose propranolol after coronary bypass. J Thorac Cardiovasc Surg 81:840–845, 1981

47. Copeland JG, Stinson EB, Griepp R et al: Surgical treatment of chronic constrictive pericarditis using cardiopulmonary bypass. J Thorac Cardiovasc Surg 69:236–238, 1975

48. Ellison N: Diagnosis and management of bleeding disorders. Anesthesiology 47:171–180, 1977

49. Packam MA, Mustard JF: Pharmacology of platelet-affecting drugs. Circulation (Suppl V) 62:26–38, 1980

50. Tice DA, Worth MH: Recognition and treatment of postoperative bleeding associated with open heart surgery. Ann NY Acad Sci 146:745–753, 1968

51. Ellison N: Diagnosis and management of bleeding disorders. Anesthesiology 47:171–180, 1977

52. Gans H, Subramanian V, John S et al: Theoretical and practical (clinical) considerations concerning proteolytic enzymes and their inhibitors with particular reference to changes in the plasminogen-plasmin system observed during assisted circulation in man. Ann NY Acad Sci 146:721–734, 1968

53. Tsuji H, Reddington J, Kay J et al: The study of fibrinolytic and coagulation factors during open heart surg. Ann NY Acad Sci 146:763–773, 1968

54. Funk A, Gmur J, Herold R et al: Reptilase R, a new reagent in blood coagulation. Br J Haematol 21:43–52, 1971

55. Rossiter SJ, Miller DC, Raney AA et al: Hepatitis risk in cardiac surgery patients receiving factor IX concentrates. J Thorac Cardiovasc Surg 78:203–207, 1979

56. Weeks KR, Chatterjee K, Block S et al: Bedside hemodynamic monitoring: its value in the diagnosis of tamponade complicating cardiac surgery. J Thorac Cardiovasc Surg 71:250–252, 1976

57. Fraser DG, Ullyot DJ: Mediastinal tamponade after open heart surgery. J Thorac Cardiovasc Surg 66:629–631, 1973

58. Kaplan JA, Bland JW, Dunbar RW: The perioperative management of pericardial tamponade. South Med J 69:417–419, 1976

59. Weeks KR, Chatterjee K, Block S et al: Bedside hemodynamic monitoring: its value in the diagnosis of tamponade complicating cardiac surgery. J Thorac Cardiovasc Surg 71:250–252, 1976

60. Wechsler AS, Auerbach BJ, Graham TC et al: Distribution of intramyocardial blood flow during pericardial tamponade: correlation with microscopic anatomy and intrinsic myocardial contractility. J Thorac Cardiovasc Surg 68:847–856, 1974

61. Field J, Shiroff RA, Zelis RF et al: Limitations in the use of the pulmonary capillary wedge pressure: cardiac tamponade. Chest 70:451–453, 1976

62. Weeks KR, Chatterjee K, Block S et al: Bedside hemodynamic monitoring: its value in the diagnosis of tamponade complicating cardiac surgery. J Thorac Cardiovasc Surg 71:250–252, 1976

63. Culliford AT, Thomas S, Spencer FC: Fulminating noncardiogenic pulmonary edema: a newly recognized hazard during cardiac operations. J Thorac Cardiovasc Surg 80:868–875, 1980

64. Kaplan JA, Bland JW, Dunbar RW: The perioperative management of pericardial tamponade. South Med J 69:417–419, 1976

65. Kaplan JA, Bland JW, Dunbar RW: The perioperative management of pericardial tamponade. South Med J 69:417–419, 1976

66. Righetti A, Crawford MH, O'Rourke RA et al: Detection of perioperative myocardial

damage after coronary artery bypass graft surgery. Circulation 55:173–178, 1977

67. Fennell WH, Chua KG, Cohen L et al: Detection, prediction, and significance of perioperative myocardial infarction following aorto-coronary bypass. J Thorac Cardiovasc Surg 78:244–253, 1979

68. Flemma RJ, Singh HM, Tector AJ et al: Factors predictive of perioperative myocardial infarction during coronary operations. Ann Thorac Surg 21:215–220, 1976

69. Brewer DL, Bilbro RH, Bartel AG: Myocardial infarction as a complication of coronary bypass surgery. Circulation 47:58–64, 1973

70. Foglia RP, Steed DL, Follette DM et al: Iatrogenic myocardial edema with potassium cardioplegia. J Thorac Cardiovasc Surg 78:217–222, 1979

71. Fennell WH, Chua KG, Cohen L et al: Detection, prediction, and significance of perioperative myocardial infarction following aorto-coronary bypass. J Thorac Cardiovasc Surg 78:244–253, 1979

72. Flemma RJ, Singh HM, Tector AJ et al: Factors predictive of perioperative myocardial infarction during coronary operations. Ann Thorac Surg 21:215–220, 1976

73. Brewer DL, Bilbro RH, Bartel AG: Myocardial infarction as a complication of coronary bypass surgery. Circulation 47:58–64, 1973

74. Olson HG, Miller RR, Amsterdam EA et al: The propranolol withdrawal rebound phenomenon. Am J Cardiol 35:162, 1975

75. Alpert JS, Cohn LH: Medical/surgical treatment of acute myocardial infarction. In Cohn LH (ed): The Treatment of Acute Myocardial Ischemia: An Integrated Medical/Surgical Approach, pp 144–171. New York, Futura, 1979

76. Alpert JS, Cohn LH: Medical/surgical treatment of acute myocardial infarction. In Cohn LH (ed): The Treatment of Acute Myocardial Ischemia: An Integrated Medical/Surgical Approach, pp 144–171. New York, Futura, 1979

77. Righetti A, Crawford ME, O'Rourke RA et al: Detection of perioperative myocardial damage after coronary artery bypass graft surgery. Circulation 55:173–178, 1977

78. Righetti A, Crawford ME, O'Rourke RA et al: Detection of perioperative myocardial damage after coronary artery bypass graft surgery. Circulation 55:173–178, 1977

79. Righetti A, Crawford ME, O'Rourke RA et al: Detection of perioperative myocardial

damage after coronary artery bypass graft surgery. Circulation 55:173–178, 1977

80. Fennell WH, Chua KG, Cohen L et al: Detection, prediction, and significance of perioperative myocardial infarction following aorto-coronary bypass. J Thorac Cardiovasc Surg 78:244–253, 1979

81. Righetti A, Crawford ME, O'Rourke RA et al: Detection of perioperative myocardial damage after coronary artery bypass graft surgery. Circulation 55:173–178, 1977

82. Fennell WH, Chua KG, Cohen L et al: Detection, prediction, and significance of perioperative myocardial infarction following aorto-coronary bypass. J Thorac Cardiovasc Surg 78:244–253, 1979

83. Flemma RJ, Singh HM, Tector AJ et al: Factors predictive of perioperative myocardial infarction during coronary operations. Ann Thorac Surg 21:215–220, 1976

84. Brewer DL, Bilbro RH, Bartel AG: Myocardial infarction as a complication of coronary bypass surgery. Circulation 47:58–64, 1973

85. Righetti A, Crawford MH, O'Rourke RA et al: Detection of perioperative myocardial damage after coronary artery bypass graft surgery. Circulation 55:173–178, 1977

86. Righetti A, Crawford MH, O'Rourke RA et al: Detection of perioperative myocardial damage after coronary artery bypass graft surgery. Circulation 55:173–178, 1977

87. Fennell WH, Chua KG, Cohen L et al: Detection, prediction, and significance of perioperative myocardial infarction following aorto-coronary bypass. J Thorac Cardiovasc Surg 78:244–253, 1979

88. Brewer DL, Bilbro RH, Bartel AG: Myocardial infarction as a complication of coronary bypass surgery. Circulation 47:58–64, 1973

PULMONARY MANAGEMENT

Physiology

89. Downs JB, Mitchell LA: Pulmonary effects of ventilatory patterns following cardiopulmonary bypass. Crit Care Med 4:295, 1976

90. Wilson RS, Pontoppidan H: Acute respiratory failure: diagnostic and therapeutic criteria. Crit Care Med 2:293–304, 1974

91. Sladen RN, Jenkins LC: Intermittent mandatory ventilation and controlled mechanical ventilation without positive end-expiratory pressure following cardiopulmonary bypass. Can Anaesth Soc J 25:166–172, 1978

92. Turnbull KW, Miyagishima RT, Gerein AN: Pulmonary complications and cardiopulmonary bypass: a clinical study in adults. Can Anaesth Soc J 21:181–186, 1974
93. Craig DB: Postoperative recovery of pulmonary function. Anesth Analg (Cleve) 60:46–52, 1981

Management

94. Turnbull KW: Unpublished data.
95. Anthony JS, Sieniewicz DJ: Suctioning of the left bronchial tree in critically ill patients. Crit Care Med 5:161–162, 1977
96. Downs JB, Mitchell LA: Pulmonary effects of ventilatory patterns following cardiopulmonary bypass. Crit Care Med 4:295, 1976
97. Sladen RN, Jenkins LC: Intermittent mandatory ventilation and controlled mechanical ventilation without positive end-expiratory pressure following cardiopulmonary bypass. Canad Anaesth Soc J 25:166–172, 1978
98. Prakash O, Meij S, Bos E et al: Lung mechanics in patients undergoing mitral valve replacement—the value of monitoring of compliance and resistance. Crit Care Med 6:370–372, 1978
99. Prakash O, Jonson B, Meij S et al: Criteria for early extubation after intracardiac surgery in adults. Anesth Analg (Cleve) 56:703–708, 1977
100. Peters RM, Brimm E, Utley JR: Predicting the need for prolonged ventilatory support in adult cardiac patients. J Thorac Cardiovasc Surg 77:175–182, 1979
101. Hilberman M, Kamm B, Lamy M et al: An analysis of potential physiological predictors of respiratory adequacy following cardiac surgery. Proceedings of the Conference "Computers in Cardiology," October 2–4, 1974, National Institutes of Health, Bethesda, MD, IEEE, Cat. No. 74CH0879–7C, pp 171–175
102. Bartlett RH, Gazzaniga AB, Geraghty TR: Respiratory maneuvers to prevent postoperative pulmonary complications. JAMA 224:1017–1021, 1973
103. Dohi S, Gold MI: Comparison of two methods of postoperative respiratory care. Chest 73:592–595, 1978
104. Bartlett RH, Brennan ML, Gazzaniga AG et al: Studies on the pathogenesis and prevention of postoperative pulmonary complications. Surg Gynecol Obstet 137:925–933, 1973
105. Llamas R, Forthman HJ: Respiratory distress syndrome in the adult after cardiopulmonary bypass. JAMA 225:1183–1186, 1973
106. Culliford AT, Thomas S, Spencer FC: Fulminating noncardiogenic pulmonary edema: a newly recognized hazard during cardiac operations. J Thorac Cardiovasc Surg 80:868–875, 1980
107. Schumer W: Steroids in the treatment of clinical septic shock. Ann Surg 184:333–341, 1976
108. Pearl R, Sladen RN: Unpublished data.

17

Cardiac Transplantation

BRUCE A. REITZ
ROBERT E. FOWLES
ALLEN K. REAM

HISTORY

Widespread clinical interest in cardiac transplantation began in December 1967, but the procedure was based on laboratory investigation dating to the early part of the 20th century. The first attempts at transplantation of the heart were reported in 1905, with the experiments of Carrel and Guthrie, who developed techniques for blood vessel anastomoses.[1] In their experiments, canine hearts were transplanted heterotopically into the cervical region of the recipient by anastomosis of the donor heart aorta to the recipient carotid artery, and the pulmonary artery of the donor to the jugular vein of the recipient. With these early experiments, the problem of rejection by infiltration of the graft with host lymphocytes was recognized. Subsequent investigations in the 1930s were directed primarily toward modification and simplification of the surgical technique for heterotopic cardiac transplantation.[2]

The first experiments to use the donor heart to support the circulation were designed and carried out by Demikhov.[3, 4] Although the transplants he performed were heterotopic, they were intrathoracic and in parallel with the recipient heart so that the transplant could act as an auxiliary pump. In several instances, he was able to exclude the recipient's own heart from the circulation and thus successfully transfer the circulatory load to the donor organ.

Attempts at orthotopic transplantation of the canine heart were first reported by Goldberg in 1958.[5] The technique was cumbersome and maximum survival was only 117 minutes. The first fully successful orthotopic cardiac transplant was described by Lower and Shumway in 1960.[6] They removed both recipient and donor hearts at the midatrial level. By this technique, only a single continuous suture line was necessary in order to join the right and left atria appropriately. Myocardial preservation was provided by simple hypothermia, and reliable methods for cardiopulmonary bypass in the laboratory animals were also important in providing routine long-term survival.

These experiments also demonstrated that the host's immune response was elicited by the transplant. If not controlled, the response resulted in graft destruction within 5 to 10 days.[7] The first reliable indicator for the diagnosis of impending graft rejection was a decrease in QRS voltage as measured in a standard ECG.[8] Other indicators of rejection were the development of both atrial and ventricular arrhythmias, and the infiltration of lymphocytes as seen on cardiac biopsy.

Extension of survival after cardiac transplantation was first achieved with immunosuppressive drugs previously developed for treatment of cancer and successfully used to control rejection of renal transplants. The first investigator to show prolongation of cardiac allograft recipients was Reemtsma,[9] who treated recipients with methotrexate, and then azathioprine.[10] Further investigations of various immunosuppressive protocols led to development of therapy which closely resembles the present clinical regimen. This includes the use of prednisone, azathioprine, and antisera such as antithymocyte globulin (ATG) for control of the immune response. Using these drugs, a number of laboratory animals were maintained for extended periods of time with their circulation supported entirely by cardiac allografts.[11]

While this experimental work was being done, the first cardiac transplantation into a human patient took place at the University Hospital of the University of Mississippi in 1964.[12] This operation was performed by Hardy, and consisted of the implantation of a chimpanzee heart into a 68-year-old male who had recently suffered a severe myocardial infarction and was in cardiogenic shock. The transplant failed early, primarily because the chimpanzee heart was too small to effectively support the recipient's circulation.

On December 3, 1967, Barnard performed the first clinical cardiac transplant, in which the donor heart came from a patient who had suffered irreversible brain injury. The signs of congestive heart failure present preoperatively improved dramatically, and the recipient seemed to be doing well until he developed pneumonia and died on the 18th postoperative day.[13] Following the announcement of this procedure, a number of surgeons in various countries around the world attempted similar operations. Within the first year, 101 transplants had been performed.

The clinical cardiac transplant program at Stanford University Medical Center was initiated in January 1968 and has continued to be active since that time. Enthusiasm for the procedure in other centers waned because the initial survival rates were quite low. Figure 17-1 illustrates the number of clinical cardiac transplant procedures performed worldwide on a yearly basis since 1967; the decline of activity following the initial surge of enthusiasm is evident. The continued and steady activity of the Stanford program is also shown, as well as the gradual increase in activity during recent years at other centers.

WORLDWIDE CARDIAC TRANSPLANTS

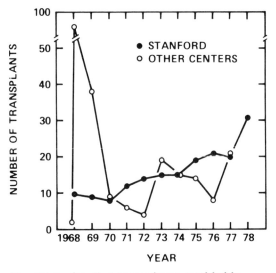

Fig. 17–1. Cardiac transplants worldwide, 1968–1978.

STANFORD CARDIAC TRANSPLANTATION

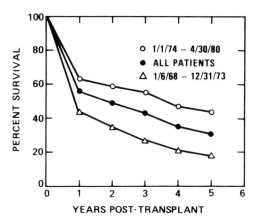

Fig. 17–2. Post-transplant survival; Stanford experience.

The experience that has been gained from the Stanford program forms the basis for this chapter. Presently 67 percent of transplant recipients at Stanford survive for one year or more (Fig. 17-2). Thereafter the attrition rate is approximately 5 percent per year. By contrast, less than 10 percent of untransplanted recipient candidates live more than 3 months after selection (Fig. 17-3). Nearly 90 percent of recipients living more than 3 months after transplantation have been able to return to their former occupations or other activities. In general, complications of chronic corticosteroid therapy have been responsible for the disability of the remaining 10 percent of surviving patients.

IMMUNOLOGY OF CARDIAC TRANSPLANTATION

The process of rejection remains a complex and substantial problem despite decades of research and clinical effort. The rapid progress already made in this field is mainly the result of powerful and nonspecific immunosuppressive agents. Rejection is a fundamental biologic process, as evidenced by the fact that even primitive organisms such as sea corals can effectively muster an immune re-

sponse against transplanted foreign tissue.[14] The following paragraphs briefly outline the basis by which an organism detects and rejects foreign tissue, and the lessons from immunologic research which are applied to modern cardiac transplantation.

The foundation of the rejection process is the immunologically distinct makeup of each individual. Allograft rejection results from the recipient's immune response against foreign donor antigens. These antigens are present on cell surfaces and can be classified into two main groups: *ABO* (blood groups) and *HL-A* (human leukocyte antigens).

Transplantation across the ABO barrier causes a decreased chance of graft survival. If anti-AB antibodies (isoagglutinins) are present in the host, rejection may be immediate.[15] This has been experimentally demonstrated in humans: when type O recipients were first sensitized by the injection of AB erythrocytes, later challenge with type AB skin grafts resulted in accelerated rejection;[16] whereas type O grafts were rejected in a normal (nonaccelerated) manner. Although some renal transplants done against an ABO barrier have been successful, this is probably because of the variable strength of these antigens. It is now common practice in renal and cardiac transplantation to require ABO compatibility between recipient and donor.[17]

STANFORD CARDIAC TRANSPLANTATION

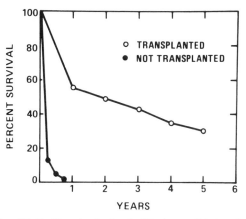

Fig. 17–3. Survival of admitted candidates for transplantation.

The other major transplant antigens are gene products of a single complex on human chromosome #6.[18] They are called human leukocyte antigens (HL-A) because they are identified in the laboratory on lymphocytes. These antigens are present on the surface of most tissue cells, including platelets. Currently, four loci on the HL-A chromosomal complex can be identified: A, B, C, and D. Each locus codes for one of many possible codominant alleles. Thus, each person has two alleles at each locus because of the presence of paired chromosomes. Because of the great diversity in possible alleles at each locus, it has been calculated that the chance of obtaining a perfect HL-A match between two unrelated persons is less than 1 in 20 million.

The effect of HL-A matching in organ transplantation has been variable. Early studies in renal transplant programs demonstrated better graft survival when donors were blood relatives of the recipients.[19-21] Experience in France and England indicated that cadaver kidney transplant survival was improved by HL-A matching,[22] but a series from San Francisco found no effect from HL-A matching.[23] In an early analysis of the Stanford heart transplant experience, the number of HL-A mismatches did not correlate with postoperative survival, severity or frequency of rejection, or with clinical status.[24] For this reason, cardiac transplantation is performed without insistence on HL-A compatibility between recipient and donor. The more dramatic improvement of HL-A-matched renal graft survival in northern Europe may be the result of the relative homogeneity of that population. Our understanding of all transplant antigens is incomplete, and thus simply identifying the HL-A A, B, C, and D loci may only be the beginning of immunologic fingerprinting.

The process of rejection is initiated with the detection of foreign tissue, or antigen. This recognition phase is part of the *afferent* arm of the immune response, and is primarily achieved by lymphocytes. A major advance in immunology has been the discovery that lymphocyte precursors differentiate into two main subsets according to function. *T* (thymus-derived) lymphocytes pass through the cortex of the thymus, where soluble substances induce them to differentiate into mature cells capable of mediating cellular immunity. Likewise, *B* (bone marrow-derived) lymphocytes differentiate into mature, immunoglobulin-secreting cells and are responsible for humoral immunity. Animal studies have shown that T lymphocytes are needed to recognize *allografts*.* Neonatally thymectomized rodents have impaired ability to reject grafts; this can be restored by thymic implants from genetically identical animals, underscoring the role of T lymphocytes in rejection. Lymphocyte recognition of allografts is demonstrated by studies in graft versus host (GVH) disease in animals. GVH results from an immune attack by lymphoid cells of the graft against antigens of the host. If mice are rendered immunologically incompetent by whole body irradiation and are then infused with incompatible lymphocytes, GVH occurs, thus indicating the ability of lymphocytes to recognize and attack the host.

Once foreign antigens are recognized, a complicated series of immune reactions begins, termed the *efferent* response. T lymphocytes proliferate after recognition of cellular antigen and produce various soluble substances which amplify, regulate, or recruit other cells into the immune response. For example, specific macrophage-arming factor (SMAF) can be transferred from antigen-sensitized T lymphocytes to macrophages, conferring upon the macrophages cytotoxic function specific for the involved antigen.[25] Another way in which T lymphocytes attack transplanted tissue is by direct cellular contact. This cell-mediated direct cytotoxicity is accomplished by effector T cells which specifically bind to and lyse foreign cells bearing the sensitizing HL-A A, B, and C antigens.[26, 27]

---

* The common terms are *autograft* (the donor is also the recipient); *allograft* or homograft—(the donor is of the same species as the recipient); and *heterograft* or xenograft (the donor is of a different species).

B lymphocytes also participate in graft destruction. Their role is limited to the production of antigen-specific immunoglobulins, but as such can be the most destructive component of the immune response. The types of immunoglobulins produced determine the nature of the immune response.[28] This includes triggering the complement cascade, opsonization, and antibody-dependent, cell-mediated cytotoxicity.[29] In the latter mechanism, the antigen-specific portion (F_{ab}) of the antibody adheres to the foreign cell, and the opposite (F_c) portion of the antibody attracts any cell which bears F_c receptors (polymorphonuclear leukocytes, monocytes, lymphocytes). These cells can then be transformed into cytotoxic effector (or "killer") cells. Such killer cells are found within rejecting allografts. Immune serum eluted from such a graft undergoing rejection, when injected into animals receiving new grafts, produces a mononuclear infiltrate histologically indistinguishable from that in a rejected allograft.[30]

Clearly, rejection manifests itself in several ways. *Hyperacute,* immediate, or accelerated rejection occurs in a recipient with preformed cytotoxic antibodies against donor antigens. This type of rejection occurs within minutes of transplantation, and presents immunologically as an antibody and complement-mediated vasculitis.[31] Most *acute* rejection episodes in cardiac transplants occur 5 to 30 days after operation, and appear as perivascular and interstitial mononuclear infiltration, with variable amounts of antibody deposition.[32] Animal studies indicate these mononuclear cells to be predominantly T-lymphocytes. Finally, *chronic* graft rejection as noted above appears insidiously, is related to endothelial injury, and results in vascular obliterative lesions.

Immunologic research has provided several lessons applicable to modern cardiac transplantation. First, blood group (ABO) and histocompatibility (HL-A) matching appear to be important for improving graft survival in general. Although HL-A mismatching doesn't preclude long-term survival and satisfactory cardiac graft function, this may

be because of incomplete typing methods, the strength of immunosuppressive agents, or the relative importance of certain HL-A antigens over others. For example, patients receiving cardiac grafts from donors incompatible with respect to specific HL-A antigens may be more prone to the development of chronic rejection and atherosclerosis. Evidence is accumulating to show that this is the case. Recipients of cardiac grafts mismatched at the HL-A-A2 locus have a significantly increased incidence of graft atherosclerosis 3 years after transplant ($p < 0.001$).

Second, the presence in the recipient's serum of antibody against donor antigens is known to decrease graft survival.[33–35] and may trigger hyperacute rejection.[36] Therefore, before transplantation a crossmatch is always performed between recipient serum and lymphocytes from the donor.

Third, various attempts at the induction of immunologic tolerance have shown promise. Immunodepressive factors in human serum can inhibit *in vitro* lymphocyte activity, and such factors have been administered to a cardiac transplant recipient successfully.[37]

Fourth, pretransplant screening of *in vitro* immunologic activity, such as lymphocyte stimulation studies, has occasionally discovered cardiac transplant patients with higher likelihoods of rejection.[38] These techniques are probably not yet sophisticated enough to accurately determine the prognosis for graft survival, and so are not routinely employed.

Fifth, the development of antihuman thymocyte globulin of rabbit origin (RATG) has proven to be a major advance in cardiac transplant immunosuppressive therapy. This preparation is superior to horse ATG in cardiac transplantation,[39] and is given by combined intramuscular and intravenous routes. Patients can be characterized according to their elimination of the globulin as detected in their serum. Those patients with slower elimination of globulin enjoy decreased frequency and severity of rejection episodes.[39, 40]

Sixth, frequent immunologic monitoring of postoperative patients within the first month after cardiac transplantation has been a valuable aid in detecting rejection. A rising level of circulating T-lymphocytes (as measured by sheep erythrocyte rosette formation) correlates very well with impending rejection,[40] and such a finding warrants endomyocardial biopsy and immunosuppressant augmentation.

PHYSIOLOGY OF THE TRANSPLANTED HEART

The early experiments by Lower and Shumway were the first to indicate that the transplanted heart devoid of innervation could adequately support normal activities. Their autotransplanted dogs survived for a number of years and were normally active.[41] Postoperative cardiac catheterization studies among human cardiac recipients demonstrate a return to normal hemodynamics in patients who previously exhibited the findings typical of end-stage myocardial disease.[42] Although resting hemodynamics are normal in most instances, a transplanted heart responds atypically to exercise and to certain cardioactive drugs, effects which are thought to be due primarily to the lack of direct neural control of the allograft.

The surgical technique utilized for cardiac transplantation results in the retaining of a small portion of the recipient's left and right atria, including the sinoatrial node tissue, which retains sympathetic and parasympathetic innervation. The donor heart also retains its own sinoatrial node which now no longer receives direct input from the autonomic nervous system. No electrical conduction occurs across the suture line. Partial reinnervation has been demonstrated in a few canine allografts; however, numerous studies in human cardiac recipients have failed to demonstrate reinnervation up to 8 years postoperatively. Occasionally one may observe synchronization of the donor and recipient atrium; in these cases the recipient atrium rate is controlled by the carotid baroreceptors. In the denervated heart, this control loop does not appear to be of practical significance.

Because both donor and recipient sinoatrial nodes are intact and functioning, P waves originating from both sources can be recorded electrocardiographically. This provides a model system for investigating the neural control of cardiac function. Such investigations have revealed that neurally mediated responses of the recipient sinoatrial node remain intact in the transplant recipient. Donor sinoatrial node activity is unaffected by neural activity. Thus, the administration of atropine causes an increase in recipient P wave rate with no change in donor heart rate. The same effect occurs in the response to the hypotension induced by inhalation of amyl nitrate. A decrease in recipient P wave activity also occurs after the rise in mean blood pressure produced by aramine infusion. The donor heart rate remains unchanged by these maneuvers, with the donor heart acting as a free-running pump.[43]

Despite the lack of neural control, the donor heart rate will vary depending upon circulating catecholamines, temperature, and mechanical factors. The heart transplant recipient responds to the stress of exercise in an abnormal fashion. Upon the initiation of exercise, the donor sinus node rate (donor heart rate) increases gradually, obtaining maximum levels toward the end of 10 minutes of steady effort. The deceleration phase following the termination of exercise is likewise gradual and prolonged. Detailed studies at Stanford have shown that the increase in heart rate follows closely the circulating level of catecholamines. These studies also show that the initial changes in myocardial contractile state follow preload augmentation from increased venous return secondary to muscular activity. Further increases in cardiac output occurring after several minutes of exercise are caused by increased ventricular inotropy and rate associated with a rise in plasma catecholamines. A normal progressive increase in systolic blood pressure is sustained as exercise progresses.

The adrenergic receptors remain intact and normally responsive to exogenously administered catecholamines. The denervated heart responds normally to isoproterenol, glucagon, norepinephrine, and propranolol.[43]

There does not seem to be a phenomenon of denervation hypersensitivity in the transplanted heart. Digoxin has been shown to have no immediate effect on heart rate or atrioventricular nodal conduction when administered acutely, but when administered chronically on an oral basis, digoxin causes a decrease in atrioventricular nodal conduction as in the normally innervated heart.[44]

RECIPIENT SELECTION

Cardiac transplantation is most likely to benefit those patients who have been carefully selected according to specific criteria. The procedure should be offered only to persons with advanced cardiac disease causing extreme disability or short life expectancy or both. All other modes of medical and surgical treatment must be exhausted.

Transplant candidates should be less than 55 years of age, free of active infection or any systemic disorder which would independently compromise survival or increase morbidity (such as severe peripheral vascular disease, irreversible renal or hepatic disease, or insulin-requiring diabetes mellitus). The candidate must be free of recent pulmonary infarction because this condition leads to disastrous lung infections after immunosuppression is begun. Chronically elevated left heart pressures in potential transplant candidates may cause increased pulmonary vascular resistance. This resistance must be less than 640 dyne-sec/cm^5 (8 Wood units), for the normal donor right ventricle cannot acutely augment its ability to work against excessive resistance.

In addition to fulfilling the above medical criteria, the cardiac transplant candidate must demonstrate psychosocial stability. This includes a supportive family environment and a history of compliance with prior treatment.

Of all patients intially proposed and screened for possible cardiac transplantation, approximately 20 percent are eventually accepted. Of those accepted for transplantation, about 80 percent receive the operation,

Table 17-1. Primary Diagnosis Leading to Cardiac Transplantation

CATEGORY	# PATIENTS
Coronary artery disease	90
Idiopathic cardiomyopathy	79
Valvular disease with ventricular dysfunction	9
Post-traumatic ventricular aneurysm	1
Congenital heart disease	1
Total	180

while the remainder die for lack of a suitable suitable donor.

Patients undergo cardiac transplantation for replacement of a poorly contractile, failing heart. The primary diagnoses leading to transplantation are categorized in Table 17-1. Coronary artery disease is the most frequent diagnosis, necessitating transplantation in 55 percent of recipients. Such recipients have left ventricular dysfunction not treatable by modern revascularization techniques. In recent years, idiopathic cardiomyopathy has become an increasingly more important category, accounting for 41 percent of the Stanford recipients.

DONOR SELECTION

It is clear that the donor heart functions better if there is no significant period of ischemia before removal. Whereas renal grafts had previously been removed following the cessation of the heartbeat, donor hearts removed in this manner are not satisfactory for transplantation. This consideration was primarily responsible for the development of guidelines and passage of laws which defined the concept of brain death. In 1967 the concept of brain death, though recognized widely on an informal basis within the medical community, remained undefined and guidelines for its formal recognition were undetermined. Subsequently, a number of organizations including the Harvard *ad hoc* Committee,[45] the neurological service at the University of Minnesota,[46] and the American Bar Association[47] have been responsible for the passage of laws in a number of states.

These state laws incorporate only minor differences in the criteria for the pronouncement of brain death. As an example, a California statute adopted in 1974 follows the American Bar Association recommendation. The pertinent portion of the law reads as follows.

> A person shall be pronounced dead if it is determined by a physician that the person has suffered a total and irreversible cessation of brain function. There shall be independent confirmation of the death by another physician. Nothing in this chapter shall prohibit a physician from using other usual and customary procedures for determining death as the exclusive basis for pronouncing a person dead.[48]

The requirements of cardiac transplantation, therefore, more than any other single event in recent medical history, stimulated recognition that death occurs with irreversible and total cessation of brain function, regardless of the status of the respiratory and circulatory subsystems that may be maintained by artificial means.

Potential cardiac donors have suffered neurologic catastrophes resulting in irreversible brain death. The pertinent characteristics of 183 cardiac donors evaluated at Stanford are shown in Table 17-2. The majority are male and the average age is 25. In one-half of the patients referred as donors, the family of the prospective donor first suggested the use of organs for transplantation, and in the remainder, the attending physician caring for the patient initiated the referral.

In preparation for cardiac transplanta-

tion, ABO blood group compatibility and approximate size match with a prospective cardiac recipient is first assured before transferring the donor to Stanford. After referral, tissue typing and crossmatching of donor cells with prospective recipient sera is performed. A positive crossmatch resulting in agglutination of donor cells with recipient serum is a contraindication to transplantation, but occurs only rarely. In a previous series of cardiac donors, the average time from hospital admission to certification of cerebral death was 61 hours, and the average time from certification of cerebral death to removal of the heart was 6.3 hours.[49]

Before use as a potential organ donor, the patient with neurologic death is evaluated as to cardiac status as thoroughly as possible. This involves history from the next-of-kin, physical examination, chest roentgenographic examination and electrocardiography. More definitive evaluation is performed if cardiac disease is suspected. This may include cardiac catheterization, coronary angiography, or echocardiography. At the present time, it is the practice at Stanford to perform routine coronary angiography for all male donors over the age of 35 years, and female donors over the age of 40 years. Among 37 potential donors thus evaluated, there were 10 patients who had significant coronary artery disease and three who had significant mitral regurgitation.[50]

The neurologically dead patient with increased intracranial pressure has an inherently unstable cardiovascular system. This requires meticulous attention to fluid balance as dictated by the arterial blood pressure and peripheral vascular resistance. Periods of hypotension before removing the heart are associated with poor postoperative graft function. Therefore, intensive care and vigorous supportive measures are necessary. The most important factors in avoiding hypotension are adequate volume administration and the use of vasopressor drugs. The administration of these agents is best regulated by continuous monitoring of the central venous and arterial pressure. Complicating this management is the development of diabetes

Table 17-2. Cause of Brain Death of Donors
for Cardiac Transplantation
(183 Donors)

ETIOLOGY	PERCENT
Cranial trauma: auto	34
Cranial trauma: motorcycle	19
Cerebrovascular accident	20
Gunshot wound	11
Falls	9
Anoxic brain death	3.5
Other	3.5
Total	100.0%

insipidus in the majority of neurologically dead patients, so that vasopressin must be administered to help control the marked diuresis resulting from the loss of pituitary function.[51] If the period following the development of cerebral death is prolonged, there is increasing difficulty with pulmonary function, and frequently cardiac donors will develop neurogenic pulmonary edema.[52] Thermoregulatory mechanisms are deranged and often body temperature must be maintained with warming blankets. After the donor has been declared neurologically dead, large doses of methylprednisolone are administered, as well as prophylactic antibiotics.

Recently, a method has been employed for the transport of donor hearts from distant hospitals.[53] This method for obtaining hearts is used when the family of the donor does not wish the body to be transported to Stanford, and in those instances where kidney removal is performed at the distant hospital. When hearts are removed at distant centers, close coordination is maintained between the heart retrieval team and the operating team performing the transplant. The operative procedure on the cardiac recipient is not initiated until the donor heart has been thoroughly evaluated and observed directly at the time of cardiectomy. When it has been determined that the heart is suitable, the recipient's operation commences, and continues during the period of transport of the heart back to Stanford. This requires close radio and telephone coordination of the activities of these two teams, as well as a method for rapid transportation of the graft.

The transported donor heart is first perfused through the aortic root with a hyperkalemic electrolyte solution (Table 17-3), and bathed in cold saline at 2 to 4°C. Hearts removed in this manner and protected by hypothermia have been successfully transplanted after 186 minutes of ischemia.[53] The longest transport has been 450 miles. Light and electron microscopic examination of ventricular biopsies obtained from distantly procured grafts have shown no significant structural damage. More than 40 hearts have been transported in this manner.

Table 17-3. Cardioplegia Solution for Donor Heart Preservation (Concentration Expressed per Liter)

Potassium	30 mEq
Sodium	25 mEq
Chloride	30 mEq
Bicarbonate	25 mEq
Dextrose	50 g
Mannitol	12.5 g
Osmolality	440 mOsm
pH (at 4°C)	8.1–8.4

In grafts which are removed on site, two adjacent operating rooms are employed. When this technique is used, the recipient heart is exposed through a median sternotomy and after systemic heparinization and placement of the patient on cardiopulmonary bypass, the heart is excised. When this has been accomplished, the donor heart is similarly excised and cooled by passing through a series of basins containing normal saline solution at 4°C. It is then brought into the recipient operating room where it is trimmed and sutured in place.

ANESTHETIC MANAGEMENT

DONOR

The donor is managed by the transplant team until the time of surgery. The anesthesiologist visits the patient before surgery to assure that physiologic status is adequate, and that any necessary preparations have not been overlooked. The donor is brought to an adjacent operating room when induction of the recipient has commenced.

Anesthesia is not required; the criteria for brain death assure that there is no potential discomfort. Muscle relaxants are usually not required, but often used in recognition of the exceptional case. Cardiorespiratory support is the major concern.

The donor is customarily maintained on 100 percent oxygen. Acute pulmonary injury is not a concern, and the risk of hypoxia is reduced. Minute ventilation and tidal volume must be maintained to assure adequate gas exchange. Despite the best efforts of the transplant team, volume and pressure status is never ideal. The almost certain presence of active diabetes insipidus, abnormal body temperature, and unstable autonomic behavior assures the necessity of constant monitoring. Vasopressors are sometimes essential, but most commonly can be discontinued when fluid volume is adequate. Donor evaluation should assure a normal myocardium, but occasionally, there will be evidence of modest compromise of contractility (such as in the patient dying in an auto accident, after suffering steering wheel impact to the chest). Modest inotropic stimulation may be required; the primary reason appears to be the failure of normal autonomic responses.

The time of the donor cardiectomy is determined by the recipient surgery. The chest is opened, and the heart and connecting vessels are exposed. The donor is heparinized, and the heart is removed when the recipient surgical team is ready for implantation. The ischemic time for this heart begins with donor cross-clamping, and ends when the recipient's aortic cross clamp is removed. If the kidneys will also be taken, regitine is administered as a bolus (15 mg), and removal performed after the blood pressure has decreased.

Because the patient has been declared legally dead before arriving in the operating room, no special measures are necessary after this time. The anesthesiologist should be sure that all records are complete and correct.

At Stanford, the major hazard is associated with inexperienced professional personnel. It is an instinctive diminution of concern for the welfare of the donor. This appears as a result of two considerations based on ethical grounds:

1. No additional effort can be expected to salvage the donor.
2. The surgery performed on the donor would be a shattering ethical violation if performed on a salvageable (legally living) patient.

This conflict is sometimes expressed as unusual anxiety on the part of otherwise competent professional personnel.

The remedies of this problem are direct and appropriate. Participants must be reminded that injury to the donor could assure the death of the recipient. No changes in procedure, from those appropriate for a patient with similar but possible nonlethal injuries, are warranted.

The person with overall anesthetic responsibility for the two procedures must be alert to this concern, and provide support or replacement if necessary. To the best of our knowledge, recipient injury associated with compromised donor care has not occurred, but we continue to observe instances of compromised individual behavior associated with this stress. Planning for backup must include both operating rooms.

RECIPIENT

Preoperative Activity

The selection procedure assures a relatively clear concept of patient status without detailed review of the record. The patient has end-stage heart disease, with unusually good noncardiac function. However, in addition to review for major considerations and the need of the usual anesthetic information (*e.g.*, status of teeth, airway), two special concerns must be addressed.

1. The patient is unusually anxious and requires reassurance. He has already participated in many hours of orientation, and does not require a detailed discussion of risks and outcomes. He needs to know that the anesthesiologist is alert, concerned, and aware of any special considerations.
2. Because of the organizational preoccupation with logistics, do not assume that any recent developments have been fully communicated. Evaluation must include a careful history of recent patient activities and any change in status. Specifics include current drugs (*e.g.*, what, dose, last given, any changes), pulmonary status (*e.g.*, orthopnea, supplementary oxygen), and

whether preoperative immunosuppressive agents have been administered.

The typical cardiovascular state is end-stage congestive failure, with evidence of hepatic congestion. Roentgenographic examination usually reveals cardiomegaly, with few or no pulmonary infiltrates. Catheterization documents a low cardiac output and ejection fraction, with elevated end-diastolic pressure. Pulmonary vascular resistance should not be more than moderately elevated.

Significant premedication is contraindicated; any agent used should treat anxiety or pain, not suppress consciousness.

Techniques

Transplant recipients begin immunosuppression before surgery, and will continue for the rest of their life. Because this regimen will be continued in a hospital environment for at least a month after surgery, their risk of infection is high. Strict adherence to aseptic technique is essential. The anesthesia circuit, monitors, and other equipment touching the patient should be previously gas sterilized. This includes all cleanable equipment. The intravascular lines are placed using a sterile prep and aseptic technique.

Monitoring is routine for cardiopulmonary bypass with the following exceptions. A Foley catheter is not placed; a suprapubic catheter is placed at the end of surgery. Two central venous lines are placed; one is used exclusively for drug administration and removed at the end of surgery. If possible, the right internal jugular vein is never entered, preserving it for postoperative cardiac biopsy.

A pulmonary artery catheter is not used because the catheter substantially increases the risk of patient infection and would be removed with the recipient heart.

Anesthetic Agents

Technique is more important than the selection of agents, but the same considerations affect both. Myocardial depression must al-ways be avoided. One should always plan for a complete failure to respond to inotropic agents. Abrupt changes in either preload or afterload can be lethal. Typically, large doses of inotropic agents are also lethal because oxygen consumption is increased in a heart which is incapable of significant hemodynamic response. Safety lies in minimal depression, and a slow rate of change of anesthetic level.

Techniques vary at Stanford, but a typical approach is pre-oxygenation, amnesia with low-dose ketamine (0.1 mg/kg intravenously every 5 minutes for three to five doses), paralysis (as pancuronium) with controlled ventilation, and the gradual infusion of a normal anesthetic dose of narcotic (such as 1.5 mg/kg of morphine) and amnesic agents over the first hour of anesthesia. The major errors to be avoided are overmedication during induction and undermedication during surgery. The patient with chronic low cardiac output has a small, fast circulating blood volume, providing abnormal sensitivity to induction doses, but equilibration ultimately requires normal cumulative drug doses.

The inhalation agents should normally be avoided because they carry no advantage, and some disadvantages. The usual drugs should be prepared in advance of induction (see Chap. 13).

Induction

Typically, the patient arrives when the room is prepared. Lines are placed in the operating room, with full facilities available. Induction commences immediately after line placement. With a distant donor, induction begins after direct inspection of the donor heart, by the team at the donor site. All stimulation is minimized; observers are excluded until the patient is asleep, laryngoscopy is double with anesthetic spray, and conversation is minimized.

Management

Prebypass management is typical of the severely compromised patient, with an important exception. If perfusion is less than ideal, appropriate therapy does not spare the heart. Subject only to the requirement that perfusion be maintained until bypass, the value of systemic perfusion outweighs any long-term insult to the heart (which will shortly be discarded). Thus a higher heart rate or modest hypertension is not of concern if there is no evidence of incipient failure. Conversely, evidence of a dilating heart is cause for response because failure can then be abrupt and immediate. Thus, inotropic agents are often appropriate after the induction, but must be used in moderation.

Concerns during the bypass period are routine for the anesthesiologist and discussed in Chapter 14. Anastomosis is accomplished by suturing the atria, aorta, and finally, the pulmonary artery, as shown in Figure 17-4. The cross-clamp may be removed as soon as the aorta is closed. Air maneuvers are absolutely essential because *every* chamber has been opened.

The distinctive aspects of post-bypass management rest on two considerations: the behavior of the denervated heart, and the severity of compromise of the recipient's heart. Defibrillation is often spontaneous because the donor heart is normal. However, isoproterenol is started as a drip before ending bypass, to assure adequate cardiac rate and output. Typically the drip is adjusted to provide a heart rate of 100 to 110 per minute. Pulmonary vascular resistance is never completely normal, and the combination of inotropy and vasodilation also appear to protect against right heart strain.

The lack of innervation increases the patient sensitivity to adequacy of preload, as discussed in Chapter 2. This must be controlled by a judicious combination of fluid administration and vasodilators, never with vasopressors.

It is customary to give methylprednisolone, 500 mg, immediately after the protamine, as part of the immunosuppressive protocol.

Frequently, hemostasis is more difficult to achieve in these patients, and appears related to suppression of clotting factors often exacerbated by preoperative coumadin therapy to reduce the incidence of pulmonary emboli. We commonly administer sufficient fresh frozen plasma to normalize the prothrombin time post-bypass.

IMMEDIATE POSTOPERATIVE CARE OF THE TRANSPLANT RECIPIENT

Postoperative monitoring is the same as for all open-heart patients including radial arterial pressure, internal jugular pressure, and continuous ECG. A total reverse-isolation environment is maintained during the patient's stay in the intensive care unit (ICU). Mechanical respiratory support is required for approximately 24 hours. Meticulous attention must be directed to maintaining sterility of all suction catheters and all tubing and equipment connected with the respirator. Because of the hazard of introducing contamination leading to pulmonary infection, extubation is accomplished as soon as possible.

Early postoperative complications are sim-

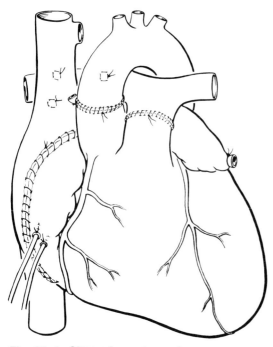

Fig. 17–4. Sites of anastomosis.

ilar to those observed in other severely ill patients undergoing open heart procedures. Mediastinal reexploration for bleeding has been performed in 13 patients (9%). Most patients exhibit a mild and reversible deterioration in renal and hepatic function as determined by blood chemistries. This is caused by secondary organ failure present before transplantation exacerbated by necessary surgical trauma. Postoperative thoracic drainage catheters and monitoring lines are removed as soon as possible commensurate with satisfactory condition of the patient. Patients are ambulatory within 2 days following surgery, and graded increases in physical activity are encouraged. Physical therapy begins within the first postoperative week.

Most recipients remain in the ICU under reverse-isolation precautions for approximately 4 weeks. Meticulous surveillance is necessary for the early detection and treatment of impending graft rejection, and also infectious complications arising from high-dose immunosuppression. Surveillance for impending graft rejection includes twice daily ECGs, in which the sum of leads I, II, III, V_1, and V_6 is serially tabulated and followed for a drop in voltage. Other measures of graft function include physical examination to look for the development of abnormal gallop rhythms, daily weight and urinary output changes, and fever. More sensitive indicators include the use of routine transvenous endomyocardial biopsy beginning at about the sixth postoperative day. Graft biopsies are obtained weekly for the subsequent 2-month period, and when indicated by a change in patient status. Other tests of immunologic reactivity are measured as well. This includes the number of circulating T and B cells, the number of circulating lymphocytes which undergo erythrocyte-rosette formation *in vitro*,[54] and the absolute level and clearance of circulating rabbit antithymocyte globulin which has been administered for the treatment of rejection.[55] The use of these tests and examinations for early detection and treatment of rejection are more fully explained in recent reviews.[56]

Equally as important as the detection and treatment of early rejection, is the early diagnosis and management of infectious complications. During the first three months postoperatively, when immunosuppressive drugs are at their highest level, the patient is at risk for opportunistic pathogens. Infections have been bacterial in origin in 61 percent of cases, viral in 17 percent, fungal in 12 percent, protozoal in 5 percent, and nocardia in an additional 5 percent. Despite the severity and gravity of such infections, rapid diagnosis and aggressive treatment have resulted in a successful outcome in the majority of cases. The majority of these infections involve the lungs, as evidenced by 193 episodes of pneumonitis in 92 patients. In addition to pneumonia, a number of patients have had empyema and cavitating pulmonary infections, especially those caused by aspergillus, nocardia, and various anaerobic organisms. In order to detect this complication in its early stages, close surveillance is mandatory in the early postoperative period. Daily chest films, physical examination, and routine sputum collections for bacterial and fungal cultures are taken. If a pulmonary infection is suspected, transtracheal aspiration is done with culture for aerobic, anaerobic, fungal, and mycobacterial organisms, as well as appropriate stains. If the specific diagnosis has not been obtained by this method, direct transthoracic needle aspiration of the lung under fluoroscopic control is performed. If the infection appears to be particularly severe, this may be the initial diagnostic maneuver because rapidly progressive infections can be lethal. Because of early experience with an inordinate number of complications and superinfections, transbronchial biopsy and open-lung biopsy are avoided.

Other sites of significant infection include the central nervous system and the urinary tract. Any new neurologic finding, change in personality, or persistent headache warrants diagnostic lumbar puncture and spinal fluid examination using Gram stain and India ink preparations, as well as cultures. Positive findings also warrant examination by computerized tomographic scanning.

Successful reversal of infectious episodes

Table 17-4. Primary Cause of Death in 97 Patients After 168 Cardiac Transplantations

	EARLY (0–3 MO)	LATE (> 3 MO)	TOTAL
Infection	31	20	51
Acute rejection	11	10	21
Graft atherosclerosis		13	13
Malignancy		4	4
Pulmonary hypertension	5		5
CVA	2		2
Suicide		1	1
Total	49	48	97

demands this type of aggressive diagnostic approach followed by specific and complete treatment programs. In the case of bacterial infections, two bactericidal antibiotics are usually employed concomitantly and are administered until complete resolution of the process has occurred. Fungal infections require treatment with amphotericin B, and nocardial infections are treated with sulfa derivatives combined with a brief course of an appropriate aminoglycoside. *Pneumocystis carinii* infections are treated with pentamidine isothionate or trimethorim-sulfamethoxasole combination or both. In several individuals with recurrent infection caused by a single organism, a program of continuous low-dose prophylactic antibiotic therapy has been used.

POST-TRANSPLANTATION COURSE AND MANAGEMENT

The first 3 months after cardiac transplantation are critical: rejection occurs with a mean frequency of one episode per 34 patient-days, and the required immunosuppressive regimen renders the graft recipient particularly vulnerable to infection.

In the late postoperative phase (more than 3 months after transplant), rejection frequency decreases markedly to one episode per 325 patient-days.[57] Currently, 85 percent of cardiac transplant recipients at Stanford are discharged from the hospital to be followed as outpatients. The postoperative return to normal cardiovascular hemodynamics is accompanied by similar improvement in exercise tolerance. At present, 91 percent of 74 one-year survivors enjoy rehabilitation to normal, Class I New York Heart Association activity status. Twenty-eight patients have survived more than 3 years, and the longest living Stanford recipient underwent transplantation 10 years ago.

Among 3-month survivors, infection is the most common primary cause of death, as indicated in Table 17-4. Potentially fatal infections occur in 75 percent of long-term recipients, at a mean rate of 1.3 infections per 1000 patient-days. As can be expected, this infection rate increases to 3.6 per 1000 patient-days during rejection, when immunosuppressive therapy is intensified.[58]

The late follow-up of heart transplant recipients requires an organized approach. Acute infection and graft rejection remain potential threats despite their decreased frequency in long-term survivors. New problems develop as a result of chronic immunosuppressive therapy. For these reasons, patients are seen regularly (at least every 4 to 6 weeks) in an outpatient setting. The ever-present possibility of infection, especially pulmonary, necessitates a pertinent history and physical exam, and usually a chest film. To help detect graft rejection, a 12-lead ECG is taken, using a standardized machine with precordial lead V_1 and V_6 placement guided by permanent, tattooed markers. Continuous azathioprine therapy requires monitoring of complete blood counts because of bone marrow suppression, and of liver function tests because of occasional hepatotoxicity.

One problem shared with renal transplantation is an increased risk of *de novo* malignancy.[59] The incidence of approximately 6 percent for both types of transplantation is much higher than would be expected in a normal population. Lymphomas are disproportionately common in post-transplant patients, with a 30 fold increase in risk over the general population; diffuse histiocytic lymphoma (reticulum cell sarcoma) is 300 times more common in transplant patients.[60, 61] At this writing, 11 malignancies have been discovered in 162 patients who have undergone cardiac transplantation at Stanford. Two patients had skin cancer, treated successfully; two deaths were caused by colon adenocarcinoma and acute myelogenous leukemia. The remaining seven malignancies were lymphomas (four diffuse histiocytic, three unclassified). The lymphoma patients have responded well to surgery or irradiation, underscoring the need for vigilant monitoring in the post-transplant period.[62]

Every 6 to 12 months, patients are admitted to the hospital for more extensive tests. Routine transvenous right ventricular endomyocardial biopsy is performed, and occasionally reveals unsuspected rejection. Roentgenographs of the hip joints are taken because of the increased incidence of femoral head aseptic necrosis associated with chronic corticosteroid administration. Ophthalmologic examination is performed to detect steroid-induced cataracts and cytomegalovirus retinitis. Finally, left ventriculography and coronary arteriography are performed to detect and monitor the development of graft atherosclerosis.

The phenomenon of accelerated graft atherosclerosis was recognized relatively early.[63] As more experience was accumulated with long-term recipients, it became more apparent that the transplanted heart was prone to develop coronary artery myointimal proliferation and atherosclerotic degeneration. This process probably results from continuing immune-mediated injury of the donor endothelium.[64] Eventually, occlusive coronary artery disease may develop, causing arrhythmias, sudden death, myocardial infarction, and ischemia-related left ventricular dysfunction with congestive heart failure. Graft ath-

erosclerosis is more frequent in hearts retrieved from older donors; accordingly, only donors younger than age 35 are now considered, except under unusual circumstances. A chronic program of weight control, serum lipid reduction, diet, and oral antiplatelet therapy (dipyridamole) has apparently reduced the incidence of graft coronary disease from nearly 100 percent at 3 years post-transplant to about 20 percent.[65] Nevertheless, the prevalence of this process increases with longer graft survival. Because of the diffuse nature of the graft atherosclerosis, coronary artery bypass surgery is not possible and retransplantation has therefore been electively performed in cases of significant coronary artery occlusion. This problem is an area of active research and current efforts are directed at further modes of antithrombotic-antiplatelet therapy as well as at identification of risk factors and ways of predicting or altering the chronic immune reactions felt to be responsible for accelerated graft atherosclerosis. Information gained from the heart transplant program may be helpful in the search for factors relating to atherosclerosis and coronary artery disease in the general population.

ANESTHESIA FOR POST-TRANSPLANT PROCEDURES

These patients may require surgery for complications arising from their post-transplant management. They are also exposed to all of the common indications for surgery associated with their age group. Thus, the procedure can be urgent, particularly in the first post-transplant year, such as with a bleeding gastric ulcer, acute abdomen, or heart block. Elective procedures may be secondary to transplant therapy, such as with hip replacement for aseptic necrosis, but should not be presumed related without investigation.[66] As shown in Table 17-5, the risk is high. The incidence of procedures is shown in Table 17-6.

The reader should also review the discussion of cardiac patients undergoing general

Table 17-5. Cardiac Transplant Recipients Requiring Reoperation

Total number of patients	42
Total number of surgical procedures	79
Age 12–55 (Mean 38.9)	
Sex Females	3
Males	39
Total survivors (49%)	19
Anesthetic complications	2

Table 17-6. Surgical Procedures

PROCEDURE	NUMBER
Cardiac retransplantation	10
Total hip replacement or open reduction	7
Craniotomy	3
Sternotomy	9
Thoractomy	1
Exploratory laparotomy	8
Major vascular surgery	4
Miscellaneous	37
	79

procedures (Chap. 21). The discussion in this chapter is confined to the concerns peculiar to this group, and is therefore incomplete.

ANESTHETIC CONSIDERATIONS

The major risks are associated with immunosuppressive therapy. The leading cause of injury is infection, and this concern must condition anesthetic technique. Aseptic technique is just as important as during the transplant procedure and must be observed. The most common lapse is contamination of intravenous equipment by airway equipment.

The major complications of immunosuppressive therapy are discussed under late course and management. Each must be considered, and therapy altered appropriately.

The second risk is a failure, at a reflexive level, to appreciate the behavior of the denervated heart. Of primary concern, for example, is the fact that even though the transplant patient may exhibit considerable cardiac reserve, reserve is mediated through changes in vascular resistance and compliance, and blood-borne catecholamines. Thus the response to any stress is abnormally slow, though ultimately effective. Though the pa-

tient may appear normal and vigorous, a crash induction with pentothal and succinylcholine is very dangerous. The anesthetist must examine each favored technique in this light, and omit those which are unsatisfactory. Similar obvious considerations, which habit obscures, include the special need to maintain preload if vasodilation occurs after the onset of anesthesia, and the possible failure to appreciate anesthetic lightness because of the relatively stable heart rate.

A wide choice of anesthetic agents can be used effectively. It is advisable to avoid agents and dosages which result in myocardial depression because the means of resuscitation are compromised. Ketamine can be very effective, but should never be used alone (immunosuppression is already a personality stress), and always in modest dosage (to avoid excessive changes in afterload). Drugs with a neural cardiac pathway (such as atropine) will have no effect on the heart. Drugs which exhibit ganglionic blocking (such as d-tubocurarine) should be ordinarily avoided, because of the consequent effect on afterload. Regional anesthesia is an acceptable alternative, but prophylactic ephedrine is recommended to avoid the larger decrease in blood pressure observed in association with the denervated heart.

Routine monitoring is appropriate; an ECG monitor should always be used. A suprapubic catheter is placed if urine output must be monitored. A pulmonary artery catheter is not appropriate. Remember the skin changes with chronic steroid therapy, and be gentle and sparing in the use of adhesives.

SUMMARY

Anesthetic management of the cardiac transplant patient has emerged as a clinical procedure. The Stanford statistics, with 50 percent 5-year survival, suggest the frequency of the procedure will continue to increase.

Intraoperative management of the recipient before transplantation is centered on the problem of end stage myocardial failure, with relatively good patient status aside from myocardial inadequacy and the associated side-effects. Post-bypass management substitutes the problem of management of a patient with a denervated heart, who retains the acute problems of organ dysfunction associated with chronic failure. The subsequent use of immunosuppressive techniques makes scrupulous aseptic technique essential.

These patients usually return to New York Heart Association Class I function and survive to return for other operative procedures associated with their age groups. Complications which influence anesthesia and are associated with their condition include sepsis and the risk of sepsis, an increased incidence of neoplasia, osteoporosis, steroid-induced cataracts and cytomegalovirus retinitis, and accelerated development of atheromatous coronary artery disease.

While the practice of cardiac transplantation was confined to a small number of centers during the first decade after the first human surgery was performed, it is now spreading to other institutions as the improved morbidity and mortality are appreciated, and the appropriate management techniques become better understood. It appears likely that more anesthesiologists will have the opportunity in the future to care for these patients, and in the process to more fully appreciate the physiologic behavior of the denervated heart.

REFERENCES

HISTORY

1. Carrel A and Guthrie CC: The transplantation of veins and organs. Am J Med 10:1101–1102, 1905
2. Mann FC, Priestly JR, Markowitz J et al: Transplantation of the intact mammalian heart. Arch Surg 26:219–224, 1933
3. Demikhov VP (assisted by Goryainov VM): Bull Eksp Biol Med 4, 1950
4. Demikhov VP: Experimental Transplantation of Vital Organs, Haigh B (trans): New York, Consultants Bureau, 1962
5. Goldberg M, Berman EF, Akman LC: Ho-

mologous transplantation of the canine heart. J Int Coll Surgeons 30:575–586, 1958
6. Lower RR and Shumway NE: Studies on orthotopic transplantation of the canine heart. Surg Forum 11:18–21, 1960
7. Lower RR, Dong E Jr, Shumway NE: Suppression of rejection crises in the cardiac homografts. Ann Thorac Surg 1:645–649, 1965
8. Lower RR, Dong E Jr, Glazener FS: Electrocardiograms of dogs with heart homografts. Circulation 33:455–460, 1966
9. Blumenstock DA, Hechtman HB, Collins JA et al: Prolonged survival of orthotopic homotransplants of the heart in animals treated with methotrexate. J Thorac Cardiovasc Surg 46:616–625, 1963
10. Reemtsma K, Williamson WE Jr, Iglesias F et al: Studies in homologous canine heart transplantation: prolongation of survival with a folic acid antagonist. Surgery 52:127–133, 1962
11. Kondo Y, Grogan JB, Cockrell JV et al: Comparison of the efficacy of immunosuppressive regimens on orthotopic heart allografts. J Thorac Cardiovasc Surg 67:612–620, 1974
12. Hardy JD, Chavez CM, Kurrus FD et al: Heart transplantation in man: developmental studies and report of a case. JAMA 188:1132–1140, 1964

IMMUNOLOGY OF CARDIAC TRANSPLANTATION

13. Barnard CN: A human cardiac transplant: an interim report of a successful operation performed at Goote Schuur Hospital. S Afr Med J 41:1257–1274, 1967
14. Hildemann WH, Raison RL, Hull CG et al: Tissue transplantation immunity in corals. In Proceedings of the Third International Symposium on Coral Reefs, 1977
15. Starzl TE, Marchioro TL, Holmes JH et al: Renal homografts in patients with major donor-recipient blood group incompatibility. Surgery 55:195–200, 1964
16. Dausset J, Rappaport FT: The role of blood group antigens in human histocompatibility. Ann NY Acad Sci 129:408–412, 1966
17. Ceppelini R, Curtoni ES, Mattiuz PL et al: Survival of test skin grafts in man: Effect of genetic relationship and of blood groups in compatibility. Ann NY Acad Sci 129:421–445, 1966

18. von Someren H, Westervold A, Hagemeier A et al: Human antigen and enzyme markers in man. Proc Natl Acad Sci USA 71:962, 1974

19. Hamburger J, Vaysse J, Crosner J et al: Renal homotransplantation in man after radiation of the recipient: experience with six cases since 1959. Am J Med 32:854–871, 1962

20. Starzl TE: Experience in Renal Transplantation. Philadelpha, WB Saunders, 1964

21. Hume DM, Lee HM, Williams GM et al: The comparative results of cadaver and related donor renal homografts in man, and the immunological implications of the outcome of second and paired transplants. Ann Surg 164:352–397, 1966

22. Amos DB: Genetic and antigenic aspects of human histocompatibility systems. Adv Immunol 10:251–297, 1969

23. Bach FH: The major histocompatibility complex in transplantation immunology. Transplant Proc 1:23–29, 1973

24. Stinson EB, Payne R, Griepp RB et al: Correlation of histocompatibility matching with graft rejection and survival after cardiac transplantation in man. Lancet 2:459–463, 1971

25. Evans R, Grant CK, Cox H et al: Thymus derived lymphocytes produce an immunologically specific macrophage arming factor. J Exp Med 136:1318–1322, 1972

26. Cerottini JC, Nordin AA, Brunner KT: Cellular and humoral response to transplantation antigens. J Exp Med 134:553–564, 1971

27. Brunner KT, Manuel J, Rudolf H et al: Studies of allograft immunity in mice. Immunology 18:501–515, 1970

28. Carpenter CB, D'Apice AJF, Abbas AK: The role of antibodies in the rejection and enhancement of organ allografts. Adv Immunol 22:1–65, 1976

29. Iwasaki Y, Talmage D, Starzl TE: Humoral antibodies in patients after renal homotransplantation. Transplantation 5:191–206, 1967

30. Spong F and Feldman JD: Transplantation antibody associated with first-set renal homografts. J Immunol 101:418–425, 1968

31. Caves PK, Dong E Jr, Morris RE et al: Hyperacute rejection of orthotopic cardiac allografts in dogs following solubilized antigen pretreatment. Transplantation 16:252–256, 1973

32. Bieber CP, Stinson EB, Shumway NE et al: Cardiac transplantation in man. VII. Cardiac allograft pathology. Circulation 41:753–772, 1970

33. Opelz G, Terasaki PI: Poor kidney transplant survival in recipients with frozen blood transfusions or no transfusions. Lancet 2:696–698, 1974

34. Terasaki PI, Kreisler M, Mickey MR: Presensitization and kidney transplant failures. Postgrad Med J 47:89–100, 1971

35. Van Hooff JP, Schippers HMA, Vandersteen GJ et al: Efficacy of HL-A matching in Eurotransplant. Lancet 2:1385–1388, 1972

36. Caves PK, Dong E Jr, Morris RE et al: Hyperacute rejection of orthotopic cardiac allografts in dogs following solubilized antigen pretreatment. Transplantation 16:252–256, 1973

37. Coulson AS, Zeitman VH, Stinson EB et al: Immunodepressive serum treatment of acute heart transplant rejection. Br Med J 1:749–750, 1976

38. Coulson AS, MacMillan F, Griepp RB et al: Lymphocyte tissue culture studies on human heart transplant recipients. II. Screening the lymphocyte reactivity of the recipients in vitro. Transplantation 18:409–416, 1974

39. Bieber CP, Griepp RB, Oyer PE et al: Use of rabbit antithymocyte globulin in cardiac transplantation. Relationship of serum clearance rates to clinical outcome. Transplantation 22:478–488, 1976

40. Bieber CP, Griepp RB, Oyer PE et al: Relationship of rabbit ATG serum clearance rate to circulating T-cell level, rejection onset, and survival in cardiac transplantation. Transplant Proc 9:1031–1036, 1977

PHYSIOLOGY OF THE TRANSPLANTED HEART

41. Dong E Jr, Hurley EJ, Lower RR et al: Performance of the heart two years after autotransplantation. Surgery 56:270–274, 1964

42. Stinson EB, Griepp RB, Schroeder JS et al: Hemodynamic observations one and two years after cardiac transplantation in man. Circulation 45:1183–1194, 1972

43. Cannom DS, Rider AK, Stinson EB et al: Electrophysiologic studies in the denervated transplanted human heart. II. Responses to norepinephrine, isoproterenol and propranolol. Am J Cardiol 36:859–866, 1975

44. Ricci DR, Orlick AE, Reitz BA et al: Depressant effect of digoxin on atrioventricular conduction in man. Circulation 57:898–903, 1978

DONOR SELECTION

45. Beecher HK, Adams RD, Barger C et al: A definition of irreversible coma. JAMA 205:337–340, 1968. (Report of the Ad Hoc Committee of the Harvard Medical School to examine the definition of brain death.)
46. Mohandas A, Chou SN: Brain death: a clinical and pathological study. J Neurosurg 35:211–218, 1971
47. De Mere M: Report on definition of death from Law and Medicine Committee, American Bar Association, adopted Feb 1975
48. California State Law, Assembly Bill 3560, Chap 3.7, Death—Section 7180
49. Griepp RB, Stinson EB, Clark DA et al: The cardiac donor. Surg Gynecol Obstet 133:792–798, 1971
50. Baumgartner WA, Reitz BA, Oyer PE et al: Cardiac homotransplantation. Curr Probl Surg 16(9):1–61, September 1979
51. Griepp RB, Stinson EB, Clark DA et al: The cardiac donor. Surg Gynecol Obstet 133:792–798, 1971
52. Ducker TB: Increased intracranial pressure and pulmonary edema. I. Clinical study of 11 patients. J Neurosurg 28:112–117, 1968
53. Watson DC, Reitz BA, Baumgartner W et al: Distant heart procurement for transplantation. Surgery 86:56–59, 1979

IMMEDIATE POST OPERATIVE CARE OF THE TRANSPLANT RECIPIENT

54. Bentwich Z, Douglas SD, Skultelsky E et al: Sheep red cell binding to human lymphocytes treated with neuramanidase; enhancement of T-cell binding and identification of a subpopulation of B cells. J Exp Med 137:1532–1537, 1973
55. Bieber CP, Griepp RB, Oyer PE et al: Relationship of rabbit ATG serum clearance rate to circulating T-cell level, rejection onset, and survival in cardiac transplantation. Transplant Proc 9:1031–1036, 1977
56. Baumgartner WA, Reitz BA, Oyer PE et al: Cardiac homotransplantation. Curr Probl Surg 16(9):1–61, September 1979

POST-TRANSPLANTATION COURSE AND MANAGEMENT

57. Rider AK, Copeland JG, Hunt SA et al: The status of cardiac transplantation. Circulation 52:531–539, 1975
58. Mason JW, Stinson EB, Hunt SA et al: Infections after cardiac transplantation: Relation to rejection therapy. Ann Intern Med 85:69–72, 1976
59. Krikorian JG, Anderson JL, Bieber CP et al: Malignant neoplasms following cardiac transplantation. JAMA 240:639–693, 1978
60. Hoover R and Fraumeni JF Jr: Risk of cancer in renal-transplant recipients. Lancet 2:55–57, 1973
61. Sheil AG: Cancer in renal allograft recipients in Australia and New Zealand. Transplant Proc 9:1133–1136, 1977
62. Anderson JL, Fowles RE, Bieber CP et al: Idiopathic cardiomyopathy, age and suppressor-cell dysfunction as risk determinants of lymphoma after cardiac transplantation. Lancet 2:1174–1177, 1978
63. Kosek J, Bieber CP, Lower RR: Heart graft arteriosclerosis. Transplant Proc 3:512–514, 1971
64. Griepp RB, Stinson EB, Bieber CP et al: Human heart transplantation: Current status. Ann Thorac Surg 22:171–175, 1976
65. Griepp RB, Stinson EB, Bieber CP et al: Control of graft arteriosclerosis in human heart transplant recipients. Surgery 81:262–269, 1977

ANESTHESIA FOR POST-TRANSPLANT PROCEDURES

66. Kanter SF, Samuels SI: Anesthesia for major operations on patients who have transplanted hearts. A review of 29 cases. Anesthesiology 46:65–68, 1977

Part V

PEDIATRIC CARDIAC SURGERY

Anatomy, Physiology, and Hemodynamics of Congenital Heart Disease

SUSAN PRINCE WATSON
DONALD C. WATSON, JR

INTRODUCTION

Congenital heart disease is one of the most frequent serious malformations occurring in infants and children.[1-7] Data collected from worldwide populations reveal an incidence of about 1 percent of live births.[8] Table 18-1 shows the incidence of various lesions in a large population of cardiac patients seen at the Hospital for Sick Children in Toronto, Canada. During the past 20 to 30 years, advances in diagnosis, operative technique, intraoperative monitoring, and postoperative care have enhanced the survival of these patients, especially in infancy.[9]

A successful outcome for the pediatric cardiac patient depends on adequate preoperative evaluation and preparation as well as a satisfactory operative result. Communication between the surgeons, pediatric cardiologists, and anesthesiologists will improve the optimal timing for operative intervention.

Pediatric patients and their parents should be told as completely and honestly as possible what to expect in the pre- and postoperative period. The use of hospital play, tours of the operating room and intensive care areas, and audiovisual aids can greatly assist in the parents' and patient's smooth adaptation to this new experience. The anesthesiologist's preoperative visit should include a detailed discussion with the child and his parents as well as a comprehensive medical evaluation (Table 18-2).

Medical complications of congenital heart disease should be treated as vigorously as possible before operation. Control of congestive heart failure with digitalis and diuretics and treatment of associated pulmonary infection is essential. Treatment of anemia may greatly improve oxygen delivery. Patients with extreme polycythemia (PCV > 70%) may have relief of symptoms by reduction of their packed cell volume.[10, 11]

Table 18-1. Incidence of Congenital Heart Defects Hospital for Sick Children, 1950–1973; 15,104 Cases

	PERCENT
Ventricular septal defect	28.3
Pulmonary stenosis	9.9
Patent ductus arteriosus	9.8
Tetralogy of Fallot	9.7
Aortic stenosis	7.1
Atrial septal defect	7.1
Coarctation of the aorta	5.1
Transposition of the great vessels	4.9
Endocardial cushion defect	3.4
Partial anomalous pulmonary venous drainage	1.4
Total anomalous pulmonary venous drainage	1.4
Vascular ring anomalies	1.2
Tricuspid atresia	1.2
Pulmonary atresia	0.7
Truncus arteriosus	0.7
Other	8.2

Table 18-2. Preoperative Evaluation of the Pediatric Cardiac Surgical Patient

History
  1. Exercise tolerance
  2. Drugs
  3. Disease complications
Physical findings
Laboratory data
  1. Blood count
  2. Electrolytes, calcium, glucose, BUN
  3. Clotting variables
  4. Urinalysis
Chest film findings
ECG
Echocardiogram
Cardiac catheterization data
  1. Oxygen saturations
  2. Shunt magnitude
  3. Variation from expected anatomy
Discussion with patient and family

HISTORY

The patient's general condition is helpful in assessing the severity of congenital heart disease. Poor appetite, decreased stamina, and poor growth suggest more serious disorders. In infancy the history is necessarily limited, but exercise tolerance can be evaluated through the infant's response to feeding; tachypnea is much more commonly seen than dyspnea. Abnormally frequent pulmonary infections suggest pulmonary vascular overload. Characteristics of congestive heart failure in infancy are outlined below.

In cyanotic patients, paroxysmal hyperpnea leading to cyanosis and obtundation suggest a more debilitating lesion. Squatting

**Characteristics of Congestive Heart
Failure in Infancy**

1. Grunting respirations
2. Nasal flaring
3. Tachypnea
4. Intercostal and Substernal Retractions
5. Tachycardia
6. Pallor
7. Hepatomegaly
8. Irritability
9. Difficulty feeding
10. Sweating
11. Failure to thrive

is also seen (as a response to increased oxygen demands with exercise) especially in those with tetralogy of Fallot. Other complications of cyanotic congenital heart disease are listed below.

Patients with pressure overload who have exertional chest pain or syncope or both are most severely affected. These symptoms with right-sided lesions are uncommon.[12]

PHYSICAL EXAMINATION

The general appearance of a child with congenital heart disease often reflects the magnitude of his problem. Weight gain is usually affected by chronic congestive heart failure; linear growth is less severely affected. Pallor may suggest anemia or vasoconstriction secondary to congestive heart failure. At sea level, cyanosis becomes visible at oxygen saturations of less than 95 percent if the hemoglobin is normal. Clubbing of the fingers and toes can be seen in cyanotic patients after 6 months of age.

Congenital heart disease is occasionally associated with other congenital anomalies. Chromosomal anomalies and environmental factors associated with congenital heart disease are shown on Table 18-3.[13, 14] In addition, patients with esophageal atresia, diaphragmatic hernia, omphalocoele, and imperforate anus also have an increased incidence of cardiac abnormalities.[15]

Examination of the chest should include inspection and palpation as well as auscultation. A precordial bulge is often seen with

severe, long-standing overactivity of either ventricle. A maximal impulse at the lower left sternal border indicates right ventricular predominance. Left-sided dominance is maximal at the apex.

A third heart sound is often present in children as a normal finding, but the presence of a fourth heart sound caused by atrial contraction is abnormal.

The intensity, location, transmission, timing, and quality of murmurs should be evaluated. Functional murmurs are generally short systolic murmurs, vibratory in quality, and varying with position or respiration. A venous hum may produce a loud, extra sound which disappears with the patient supine or with jugular venous compression.

The abdominal examination is important in evaluation of heart disease, especially in congestive heart failure. Infants normally have a liver edge palpable at 3 cm below the right costal margin. By 1 year of age, it may normally be felt at 2 cm, and by 4 to 5 years of age, it may be felt at 1 cm. The spleen is not normally palpable, and the presence of splenomegaly suggests infection rather than chronic congestive heart failure.[12]

LABORATORY DATA

Routine blood work should be evaluated. A complete blood count, urinalysis, electrolytes, BUN, glucose, and clotting studies should be available. Cyanotic patients with a hematocrit greater than 70 percent may benefit from phlebotomy to reduce the problems associated with hyperviscosity.[10, 11] Patients with chronic congestive heart failure

**Complications of Cyanotic Congenital
Heart Disease**

1. Cyanosis
2. Polycythemia
3. Clubbing
4. Squatting
5. Cyanotic spells
6. Paradoxical emboli
7. Cerebrovascular accidents
8. Brain abscess

Table 18-3. Syndromes With Cardiac Defects

LESION	INCIDENCE OF CONGENITAL HEART DISEASE (%)	CARDIAC DEFECT	OTHER ANOMALIES
Chromosomal Anomalies			
Trisomy 21 (Down's syndrome)	50	Endocardial cushion defect VSD, PDA, ASD	Characteristic facies, mental retardation, short neck, hypotonia, dysplasia of pelvis
Trisomy E (Edwards' syndrome)	95	VSD, PDA, ASD, bicuspid aortic value	Mental deficiency, low set ears, small mouth with narrow palate, micrognathia, rocker bottom feet, abnormal extremities, renal anomalies
Trisomy D (Patau syndrome)	90	VSD, PDA, ASD, dextrocardia	Microcephaly, microopthalmia, coloboma of iris, cleft lip/palate
4P (Wolf syndrome)	40	ASD, VSD	Mental motor retardation Cleft lip/palate, fishlike mouth
5P (Cri-du-chat syndrome)	30	Variable	Mental-motor retardation, microcephaly, epicanthal folds, hypotonia, cat-like cry
XO (Turner's syndrome)	30	Coarctation, AS	Ovarian dysgenesis, short stature Congenital lymphedema Broad chest, anomalous auricles Narrow maxilla, small mandible Short, webbed neck
Environmental Teratogens			
Rubella syndrome	50	PDA, peripheral PS, myocarditis, septal defects	Mental retardation, cataracts, deafness, glaucoma
Thalidomide	19	TOF, truncus	Extremity anomalies (amelia, phocomelia)
Fetal alcohol syndrome	40	VSD, ASD, TOF	Growth, mental retardation, microcephaly, maxillary hypoplasia, genital anomalies, dislocated hips
Fetal hydantoin syndrome	10	Variable	
Fetal trimethadione syndrome	50	VSD, TOF	Mental retardation, abnormal palate and teeth
Maternal lupus	?	Congenital heart block	

may show a high urine specific gravity with albuminuria and hematuria.

Patients should have normal potassium stores before operation, especially those on digitalis and diuretics. Both glucose and calcium levels may be low in stressed newborn or premature infants; preoperative and intraoperative replacement may be necessary. Hypoglycemia may be associated with neonatal polycythemia.

The chest film is essential to evaluate cardiac size, lung perfusion, and specific cardiac chamber enlargement. The contour of the cardiac silhouette may give some clues to specific lesions, as in transposition of the great vessels and tetralogy of Fallot. The trachea and esophagus, normally pushed to the right by the aorta descending on the left, will appear on the left with a right-sided aortic arch. The supracardiac area, normally occu-

pied by the thymus in a young infant, may appear narrowed in conditions producing stress in the newborn period. A very large, low-lying thymus may give the appearance of cardiomegaly. The pulmonary vascular pattern is variable in congenital heart disease. Increased pulmonary blood flow increases the caliber of arteries, well out into the peripheral lung fields. In pulmonary vascular obstruction, the proximal pulmonary vessels are large and the lung fields are relatively oligemic. When pulmonary blood flow is limited, the lung fields are highly penetrated with decreased hilar markings. Because respiratory infection commonly accompanies congestive heart failure, differentiation between these conditions may be difficult.[12] A summary of chest film findings in the lesions discussed is outlined on Table 18-4.

The ECG changes acutely during the first

Table 18-4. Chest Film Findings in Congenital Heart Disease

LESION	CHEST FILM FINDINGS
Aortic stenosis	Normal or enlarged left ventricle
	Normal pulmonary vascular markings
Coarctation of aorta	Normal or enlarged left ventricle, proximal aorta
	Rib notching after age 5–6 years
Endocardial cushion defect	Generalized cardiomegaly
	Increased pulmonary vascularity
Patent ductus arteriosus	Enlarged aorta, pulmonary artery
	Increased pulmonary vascular markings
Pulmonic stenosis	Normal or enlarged right ventricle, pulmonary artery
	Normal or decreased pulmonary vascular markings
Pulmonary atresia	Normal to increased heart size
	Decreased pulmonary vascularity
Secundum atrial septal defect	Normal or enlarged right atrium, right ventricle and pulmonary artery
	Increased pulmonary vascular markings
Tetralogy of Fallot	Boot-shaped heart; small main pulmonary artery
	Enlarged right ventricle
	Decreased pulmonary vascularity
Total anomalous pulmonary venous return	Normal to increased heart size
	Increased pulmonary vascularity
Transposition of the great vessels	Oval or "egg-shaped" heart
	Generalized cardiomegaly
	Increased pulmonary vascular markings
Tricuspid atresia	Normal to increased heart size
	Decreased pulmonary vascular markings
Truncus arteriosus	Wide mediastinum
	Generalized cardiomegaly
Ventricular septal defect	Normal to increased heart size
	Increased pulmonary vascularity

Table 18-5. ECG Findings in Congenital Heart Disease

LESION	ECG
Aortic stenosis	Normal → LVH
	LV strain if gradient > 50 mm (75%)
Coarctation of aorta	Normal → LVH
	RVH, S–T changes (infancy)
Endocardial cushion defect	Axis −60 to −140°
	BVH
Patent ductus arteriosus	Normal → LVH, LAE
	BVH (late)
Pulmonary atresia	Axis +30° to +100°
	Variable RV voltage
	Adult R/S progression
Pulmonic stenosis	Normal → RAD
	Normal → RVH
Secundum atrial septal defect	Axis +90° to +150°
	rsR′ In right chest leads
	Incomplete right bundle branch block
Tetralogy of Fallot	RAD − (+90° to +150°), RVH
Total anomalous pulmonary venous return	RAD
	RAE, RVH
Transportation of the great vessels	RAD, RVH, LVH
Tricuspid atresia	Biatrial enlargement
	LAD, LVH
Truncus arteriosus	Axis +90° to +150°
	1° or 2° heart block (10%)
	RVH or BVH

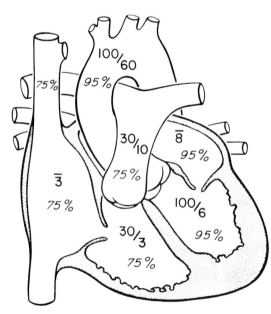

Fig. 18–1. Catheterization data in the normal pediatric heart with pressure (torr) and oxygen saturation (%).

few months of life, paralleling the physiologic events which occur in cardiorespiratory adaptation from intra- to extrauterine life. By 35 weeks' gestation, the right ventricle is predominant in size and cardiac output. At birth, this is seen as a right QRS axis of 125 to 135°, tall R waves in the right precordial leads, and R/S complex over the left precordium. By age 2 to 4 years, the R/S progression more clearly resembles that of the adult with left ventricular dominance. After 3 days of age, the T wave is usually upright in leads I, II, aVF, and V_6, and inverted in aVR, V_4R, and V_1. This T wave progression may persist through adolescence.

In children, the diagnosis of ventricular hypertrophy may be difficult because voltage criteria alone may not be adequate. The child's thin-walled chest brings the electrode closer to the heart, and this proximity increases the magnitude of the R and S waves. In premature infants, the ECG is variable. A tracing similar to that of a normal-term baby may be seen or generalized low voltage may be present. In other infants, left ventricular dominance similar to that of the older child may occur.[16]

A summary of ECG findings in the lesions discussed in this chapter is found in Table 18-5. Cardiac catheterization data in the normal heart are shown in Figure 18-1.

VALVULAR AND VASCULAR LESIONS

PATENT DUCTUS ARTERIOSUS

Isolated patent ductus arteriosis (PDA) accounts for about 10 percent of all types of congenital heart disease and occurs in 1 of 2000 full-term live births. It may be present in 45 percent of preterm infants less than 1750 grams. PDA is the most common cardiac anomaly after rubella exposure in the first trimester. Bacterial endocarditis at the ductus site represents a continued risk if closure is not performed.[17] Closure of the ductus by Gross in 1938 was the first cardiovascular procedure done.[18]

Embryology and Anatomy

By the sixth week of gestation, the aorta develops from the left fourth aortic arch to connect the left ventral and dorsal aorta. The pulmonary artery is formed from the left and right sixth aortic arch and a septation of the ventral aorta into the mature aorta and pulmonary artery. Normally intimal proliferation, in response to an increased arterial oxygen content, will cause the ductus arteriosus (previously the distal sixth arch) to close and form the ligamentum arteriosum. Failure of this constriction after birth causes a patent ductus arteriosus.

Physiology

In fetal life, because respiration is carried out in the placenta, oxygenated blood is carried through the umbilical veins to the inferior vena cava, through the right heart, and out the ductus arteriosus to the descending aorta and distal structures. After birth, respiration is transferred to the lungs. An increase in blood oxygen content causes the pulmonary arterioles to dilate, the pulmonary vascular resistance to decrease, and preferential blood flow through the lungs. The ductus arteriosus closes as a result of the increased local oxygen content and the decreased flow through it.

If the ductus arteriosus does not close, a large left-to-right shunt will occur as pulmonary vascular resistance falls. Initially, pulmonary flow will be much greater than systemic (Fig. 18-2A). As the shunt persists, pulmonary arteriolar reactive changes occur and increase the pulmonary vascular resistance. The magnitude of the left-to-right shunt will thus decrease. If the PDA is not appropriately treated, irreversible pulmonary vascular hypertensive changes often occur.

Clinical Features

Typically, patients are asymptomatic at birth with no murmur. A continuous machinery murmur will develop in early infancy. The pulmonary sound will increase and the pulse pressure will become larger than usual. As pulmonary vascular hypertension develops and the shunt magnitude decreases, the murmur will become systolic only and eventually disappear. A smaller group of neonates will fail to thrive and develop left ventricular congestive failure. These patients have a large PDA with an early high shunt ratio. In severe end-stage patients with right-to-left shunts, differential cyanosis may occur.

Laboratory Data

The ECG shows left ventricular hypertrophy early, biventricular hypertrophy at mid-course, and right ventricular hypertrophy late in the natural history of the disease. The chest film shows a large aorta, a large pulmonary artery, and increased pulmonary vascular markings. The left atrium and left ventricle are variable in size. An echocardiogram may show an enlarged left atrium. The right

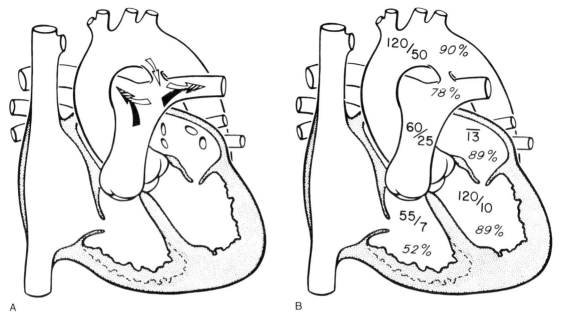

Fig. 18–2. A. Flow diagram of patent ductus arteriosus showing left-to-right shunting from the aorta to the pulmonary artery. *Dotted line* indicates normal right ventricular contour. *B.* Cardiac catheterization data on patent ductus arteriosus (PDA) with moderate pulmonary hypertension.

ventricular size and thickness will be increased with pulmonary vascular hypertension.

Cardiac catheterization can show the PDA by catheter passage from the right ventricle out the pulmonary artery into the descending aorta. An oxygen step-up is seen in the pulmonary artery early in the history of the disease (Fig. 18-2*B*). After the development of pulmonary vascular hypertension and right-to-left shunting, the oxygen tension will decrease between the proximal and descending aorta. On lateral aortic angiogram, the PDA will be seen to fill the pulmonary arteries.[19]

COARCTATION OF THE AORTA

Coarctation of the aorta comprises 5 to 8 percent of congenital heart disease. The male:female ratio is 2:1. It is the most common cardiovascular abnormality in Turner's syndrome. Associated lesions are common in infants presenting at less than 1 year of age including PDA (64 percent), bicuspid aortic valve (50 percent), ventricular septal defect (32 percent), and other left-sided lesions.[20]

Embryology and Anatomy

The aorta arises during the fifth to seventh weeks of gestation from the fourth left primitive arch. A coarctation is produced by narrowing of the aortic lumen because of an abnormality in the media of the vessel with cellular proliferation.

A coarctation may occur at any site along the aorta, but is most commonly seen just distal to the insertion of the liagmentum arteriosum. Coarctation can be divided into two groups: preductal, in which the upper body is supplied by the left ventricle and the lower body supplied by the right ventricle through the ductus arteriosus; and postductal coarctation, in which the left ventricle supplies the upper body and collaterals develop *in utero* through the intercostal and internal mammary arteries to supply the lower body (Fig. 18-3). Preductal coarctation is seen almost exclusively in infants, whereas post-ductal coarctation presents most commonly in older children and adults.

Physiology

Maintenance of blood flow to the lower body is accompanied by three mechanisms: increase in systolic blood pressure proximal to the coarctation; increase in arteriolar resistance with increased diastolic pressure; and development of collateral flow around the coarctation.[21]

After birth, the sudden increase in work load for the left ventricle may lead to congestive heart failure early in infancy, especially when other cardiac malformations are present.

Clinical Features

Fifty percent of all patients with coarctation of the aorta present at less than 1 year of age.[20] The preductal type is most commonly detected in the newborn period or early infancy with the sudden onset of congestive heart failure. Differential cyanosis in this type may be seen because the ductus arteriosus supplies the lower body wall with desaturated blood from the right ventricle. Diminished pulses are present in the lower body, although pulses may be decreased throughout if severe congestive heart failure is present. No bruit may be audible because collaterals are poorly developed.

Patients with postductal coarctation are acyanotic, with upper extremity hypertension and decreased lower extremity pulses. The systolic pressure of one arm may be 20 to 30 torr higher than the other. The patient may give a history of leg pain with exercise, easy fatigability, headache, or nosebleeds. A rough, midsystolic ejection murmur originating from the coaractation is audible over the left paravertebral area. Bruits from collateral flow through the intercostal and internal mammary arteries can be heard throughout the chest. A systolic murmur originating at a bicuspid aortic valve may be detected in the second right intercostal space.

Laboratory Data

The chest film in coarctation varies with the extent of the lesion, from a normal appearance to that of a dilated ascending aorta with an enlarged left ventricle. Rib notching is usually not evident until age 5 to 6 years. On a barium swallow, the aortic arch makes an E-shaped impression on the esophagus. This is produced by the proximal aortic segment, the coarctation, and the distal aortic segment with poststenotic dilatation.

The ECG varies from normal to a tracing with evidence of left ventricular hypertrophy. In infancy, right ventricular hypertrophy with or without left ventricular hypertrophy is common.

The echocardiogram is useful to evaluate left ventricular thickness and the nature of the aortic valve. A sector scan may help delineate the site of the coarctation. Cardiac catheterization may not be necessary in simple coarctation, if the classic clinical signs are present. Expected catheterization data are shown in Figure 18-4.

VASCULAR RINGS

Vascular rings are a group of anomalies of the aortic arch and great vessels which produce varying degrees of compression of the trachea or esophagus or both. They comprise

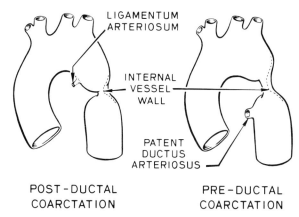

Fig. 18–3. Anatomy of postductal and preductal coarctation. *Dotted line* indicates internal vessel wall thickness.

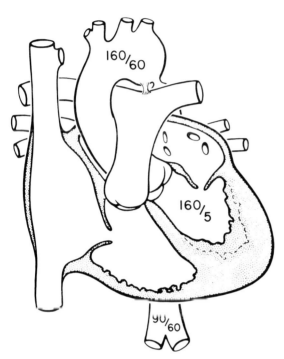

Fig. 18–4. Cardiac catheterization data in moderate postductal coarctation. *Dotted line* indicates normal left ventricular wall contour.

about 1 percent of congenital heart disease and are rarely associated with other cardiac anomalies.[22]

Embryology and Anatomy

Anomalous aortic arch structures result from abnormalities of the embryonic-paired aortic arch system. Abnormal regression of structures which normally remain patent or patency of structures which normally regress can occur. In double aortic arch, for example, there is failure of regression of the right fourth dorsal aortic segment.

The trachea and esophagus are normally located behind the great vessels. The anomalous vascular structures encircle and may entrap one or both of the trachea and esophagus. The most common types include double aortic arch, right aortic arch with left ligamentum arteriosum, anomalous right subclavian artery, anomalous left innominate artery, and anomalous left common carotid artery (Fig. 18-5).

Physiology

The degree of obstruction produced is variable, depending on the anatomic type. Double aortic arch leads to most severe symptoms in infancy as a result of pressure on the trachea and esophagus. In right aortic arch with

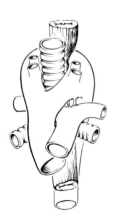

DOUBLE AORTIC ARCH

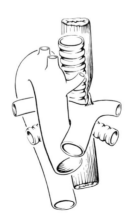

RIGHT AORTIC ARCH WITH
LEFT LIGAMENTUM ARTERIOSUM

Fig. 18–5. Sketch of the two most common, symptomatic types of vascular ring anomalies. Tracheal or esophageal compression or both can occur with both.

left ligamentum, symptoms and age of onset are more variable. The other anomalies seldom give significant symptoms.

Clinical Features

Patients who have significant obstruction usually present in infancy with severe respiratory distress, including retractions, wheezing, cyanosis, and pulmonary infection. Frequent vomiting caused by esophageal compression may lead to failure to thrive. The infant often lies with his head in hyperextension to minimize tracheal obstruction.

Laboratory Data

The chest film is usually normal, although hyperinflation caused by respiratory obstruction or narrowing of the trachea may be seen. The ECG is normal unless there are associated intracardiac anomalies. A barium swallow study should reveal the site of anomalous vessel. Preoperative angiocardiography often may not be necessary.[22]

PULMONIC STENOSIS

Pulmonic stenosis accounts for approximately 10 percent of patients with congenital heart disease.[23] Valvular involvement is most common, but supravalvular, infundibular, or peripheral arterial stenoses also occur. Congenital rubella, Williams syndrome, Noonan's syndrome, cutis laxa, and neurofibromatosis may have associated pulmonic stenosis.

Embryology and Anatomy

The pulmonary valve, infundibulum, and pulmonary arteries develop during the second and third months of gestation. The pulmonary valve is formed by enlargement and subsequent absorption of three tubercles within the pulmonary artery. Simultaneously, the primitive truncus arteriosus divides into the aorta and proximal pulmonary artery. The sixth aortic arch contributes to the distal pulmonary arteries as well as to the

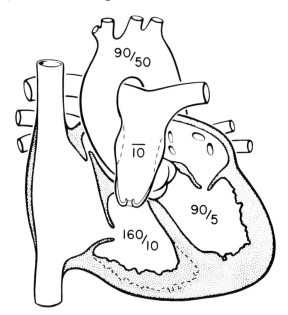

Fig. 18–6. Cardiac catheterization data in severe pulmonic valve stenosis. *Dotted lines* indicate normal right ventricular and pulmonary artery contours.

ductus arteriosus. The right ventricular infundibulum is formed from the bulbus cordis. Failure of normal development of the valve, infundibulum, or distal pulmonary arteries may give rise to obstruction. Most commonly, the valve is thickened with fusion of the leaflets at their commissures. Bicuspid valves may also occur. Poststenotic dilatation of the pulmonary artery is frequent, unless flow through the restricted orifice is extremely low. The right ventricle demonstrates compensatory hypertrophy with reduced cavity size (Fig. 18-6). Right atrial hypertrophy may also be seen in severe long-standing cases.

Physiology

Obstruction to right ventricular outflow leads to pressure overload in the right ventricle. When severe or long-standing disease is present, tricuspid regurgitation may occur, producing right atrial enlargement. If the foramen ovale is patent, right-to-left shunting may occur as right atrial pressure exceeds that in the left atrium. In severe cases, congestive heart failure and death are the ultimate outcome without surgical intervention.

With less severe obstruction, only moderate pressure increases are seen. Even with atrial or ventricular septal defects, shunting is predominantly left to right, and severe congestive heart failure is rare in childhood.

Clinical Features

Children with mild-to-moderate pulmonary stenosis usually appear healthy and are acyanotic. Exercise tolerance is generally good, although chest pain may accompany exercise in severe stenosis. Physical examination may reveal a systolic thrill in the second left intercostal space, a systolic ejection click, and a rough systolic ejection murmur whose intensity varies with the degree of obstruction. The first heart sound is normal, but the pulmonary component of the second sound may be diminished or delayed or both.

Laboratory Data

The ECG gives important information about the severity of obstruction. Right ventricular hypertrophy, shown by right axis deviation and large R-waves in the right precordial leads, parallels the gradient. The chest film shows a normal cardiac size with normal pulmonary vascular markings in mild-to-moderate stenosis. In severe stenosis, cardiomegaly with decreased pulmonary vascularity may be present. Poststenotic dilatation of the pulmonary artery is seen in valvular but not infundibular or supravalvular stenosis.

Cardiac catheterization will define the level and extent of obstruction as well as identify other lesions. A continuous pressure reading as the catheter is pulled back from the pulmonary artery into the right ventricle will define the degree and location of obstruction (Fig. 18-6). The right ventricular angiogram provides information about right ventricular cavity size, outflow tract anatomy, pulmo-

nary valve mobility, and distal pulmonary arterial anatomy.

AORTIC STENOSIS

Aortic stenosis accounts for 5 to 10 percent of congenital heart disease[24] and is associated with PDA, coarctation of the aorta, or both.[25] Eighty-three percent of patients have valvular involvement, 9 percent have subvalvular lesions, and 8 percent have supravalvular involvement.[26] The following discussion will focus on valvular disease. A bicuspid aortic valve is probably the most common congenital cardiac abnormality.

Embryology and Anatomy

Development of the aortic valve takes place during the sixth to ninth weeks of gestation. The valve appears as three tubercles within the aortic lumen. The tubercles grow toward the midline. Resorption of tissue at the aortic-tubercle junction creates the sinuses of the valve.

Aortic stenosis may occur with a unicuspid, bicuspid, tricuspid, or quadricuspid valve. The bicuspid valve occurs most commonly and is present in 1 percent of the population. The unicuspid valve is usually very abnormal with one commissure and an eccentric orifice. The bicuspid valve may have cusps of unequal size which open less completely than a normal valve. Prolapse of a larger cusp may lead to aortic insufficiency. An abnormal tricuspid valve may also have marked disparity in cusp size which causes fibrosis and obstruction later in life. A quadricuspid valve usually functions normally. If significant aortic obstruction is present, poststenotic dilatation of the aorta may occur.

Physiology

The increased work of maintaining adequate flow through the restricted orifice is assumed in the left ventricle by increased diastolic volume, increased systolic pressure, and prolonged systolic ejection time. As the left ventricle hypertrophies, oxygen consumption rises, but coronary blood flow does not increase proportionately. In severe cases, relatively coronary insufficiency may be present because of abnormalities of the coronary ostia, decreased diastolic filling time, and compression of the coronaries by the high left ventricular pressure.

Clinical Features

Children with aortic stenosis are often asymptomatic, but half may present before 1 year of age. Significant symptoms of angina or syncope occur in less than 10 percent of patients.[27] However, critical aortic stenosis may present in early infancy with left- and right-heart failure, tachypnea, tachycardia, and cyanosis.

Physical examination of these children shows normal general growth and appearance. A difference in blood pressure between the two arms may be seen, especially in supravalvular stenosis. Cardiac examination reveals a heaving cardiac impulse with a systolic thrill in the second right intercostal space or the suprasternal notch. An ejection click is often audible along the lower left sternal border in valvular stenosis. The second heart sound is narrowly split or single. A systolic ejection murmur, grade three or greater, is maximal in the second right intercostal space and transmits to the neck and back.

Laboratory Data

The chest film shows a variable degree of left ventricular hypertrophy with a prominent ascending aorta. The ECG is the most sensitive indicator of severity; 75 percent of patients with a gradient of greater than 50 torr show left ventricular strain.[28] Echocardiogram may detect the thickened, asymmetric valve and increased left ventricular wall thickness. Cardiac catheterization will delineate the location of obstruction, the magnitude of gradient, and the degree of left ventricular dysfunction (Fig. 18-7). A valve area of 0.5 cm^2/m^2 body surface area indicates severe obstruction.[29]

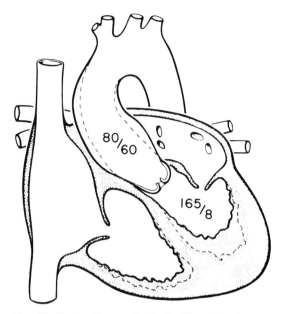

Fig. 18–7. Cardiac catheterization data in severe aortic valve stenosis. *Dotted lines* indicate normal left ventricular and right ventricular contours.

INTRACARDIAC LESIONS WITH LEFT-TO-RIGHT SHUNT

SECUNDUM ATRIAL SEPTAL DEFECT AND PATENT FORAMEN OVALE

Secundum atrial septal defect constitutes 7 percent of congenital heart defects and is commonly seen with other more complex congenital intracardiac defects and Holt Oram syndrome. The ratio of affected females to males is 2:1. Patients usually are asymptomatic and are diagnosed on routine physical examination or chest film.[30]

Embryology and Anatomy

In the fifth gestational week, the atrium is divided into two chambers by two closely approximated septa. A septum primum growing from the dorsal cephalic atrial wall moves toward and onto the endocardial cushions while a septum secundum grows from cephalad atrial wall at the right of the primum septum toward and onto the endo-

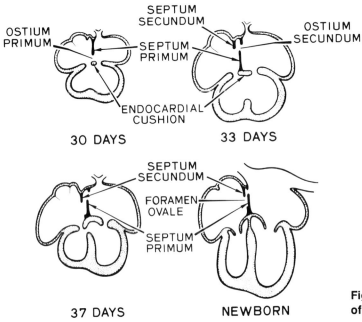

Fig. 18–8. Fetal development of the atrial septum.

Fig. 18–9. View of the atrial septum illustrating the location of various defects of the septum.

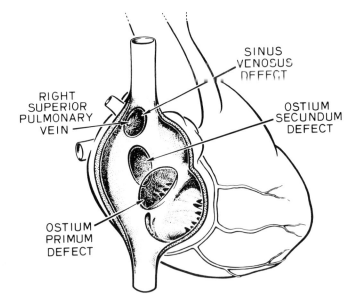

cardial cushions. The ultimate balance in the growth and resorption of the septa determine the nature of an atrial communication. Failure of the secundum system to grow sufficiently causes a secundum defect; failure of the primum and secundum septa to fuse causes a patent foramen ovale. Normal fetal development of the atrial septum is shown in Figure 18-8. The location of various types of atrial septal defects is shown in Figure 18-9.

Physiology

During fetal life, high pulmonary artery pressures are accompanied by a right atrial pressure which is greater than left atrial pressure, thus right-to-left shunting through the defect is created by pushing the primum atrial septum away from the secundum atrial septum. At birth, the lungs expand, pulmonary vascular resistance decreases, and pulmonary artery and right atrial pressures decrease. Left atrial pressures become greater than right atrial pressure and the primum atrial septum is pushed against the secundum atrial septum in a trap door manner to close the fossa ovalis. The secundum septal tissue may be insufficient to allow fossa ovalis closure. The secundum and primum septum may fail to fuse, leaving a patent fossa ovalis.

Clinical Features

Patients are usually asymptomatic but may be smaller in stature and weight than normal. The systolic ejection murmur of relative pulmonary stenosis is heard. A relative tricuspid stenotic diastolic rumble may be heard because the increased right atrial and right ventricular volume load. The second heart sound has a fixed split by a delay in pulmonary valvular closure as a consequence of right ventricular overload.

Laboratory Data

The chest film shows right ventricular enlargement and a prominent main pulmonary artery. Pulmonary arterial markings increase with the size of the left-to-right shunt. The ECG characteristically has an axis of 90 to 150°, a prolonged P-R interval, an rsR' in lead V_1, and incomplete right bundle branch block.[31] The echocardiogram shows an enlarged right ventricular dimension and paradoxical ventricular septal motion, especially with large defects. The cardiac catheterization should demonstrate an increased oxygen content in the right atrium, confirming the left-to-right shunt. Right-sided pressures may be normal, except in long-standing defects with pulmonary hypertensive disease (Fig. 18-10B). A contrast injection into the main pulmonary artery will demonstrate the shunt during the levophase.

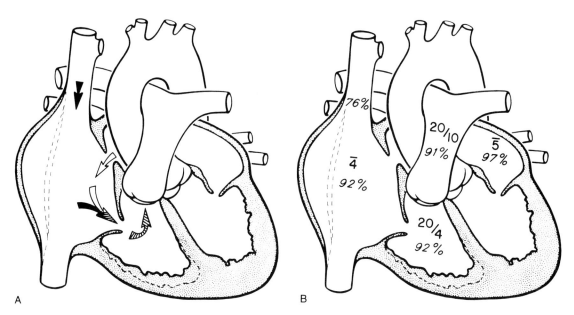

A

B

Fig. 18–10. *A.* Flow diagram diagram illustrating left-to-right shunting through the atrial septal defect. *Dotted lines* show normal right atrial and right ventricular contours. *B.* Cardiac cathetherization data in secundum atrial septal defect.

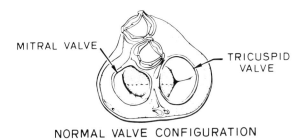

NORMAL VALVE CONFIGURATION

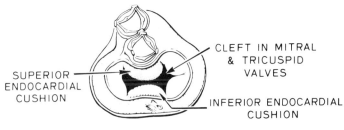

ENDOCARDIAL CUSHION DEFECT

Fig. 18–11. Sketch comparing normal valve configuration with that seen in complete endocardial cushion defect.

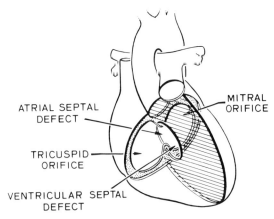

Fig. 18–12. Diagramatic view of endocardial cushion defect illustrating relative positions of atrioventricular (A-V) valves with ventricular and atrial septa.

ENDOCARDIAL CUSHION DEFECT

Endocardial cushion defects result in one of a complex spectrum of abnormalities involving the atrial septum, ventricular septum, and atrioventricular valves. It comprises 3 percent of congenital heart defects and is one of the most common cardiac lesions in Down's syndrome.[32]

Embryology and Anatomy

Normally, the heart is separated into four chambers by four to eight weeks' gestation. This is accomplished by atrial and ventricular septation, endocardial cushion proliferation, and proximal truncus arteriosus proliferation. The endocardial cushions form the primitive mitral and tricuspid tissue, and the truncus forms primitive aortic and pulmonary tissue. Failure of normal fusion of these elements will cause a partial, transitional, or complete endocardial cushion defect. The development of the mitral and tricuspid valves as well as the foundation for the ineferior atrial and superior ventricular septa may be affected (Fig. 18-11).

In the partial form, an atrial defect (ostium primum) near the mitral and tricuspid valves and a cleft mitral valve are found. The transitional form has the defects associated with the partial form with a more rudimentary mitral and tricuspid tissue. In the complete form, a primum atrial septal defect, cleft or primitive mitral or tricuspid valve (or both), and a ventricular septal defect are present (Fig. 18-12). Septal defects are occasionally present without abnormalities of the atrioventricular valves.

Endocardial cushion defects present with a spectrum of anatomic abnormalities, and any combination of the defects may be present. Only the complete form is discussed.

Physiology

A single connection between all four chambers of the heart makes possible both left-to-right and right-to-left shunts at any level. Shunt direction and size depend on the ratio of total pulmonic and systemic pressures.

Pulmonary arterial resistance is low and right ventricular compliance is high early in the disease, resulting in a large left-to-right shunt, (Fig. 18-13A). With prolonged exposure to high pulmonary artery pressures, pulmonary arteriolar hypertrophy initiates resistance increases. Further increases in pulmonary artery pressure cause right ventricular hypertrophy and a decrease in left-to-right shunting. In the late stages, shunting can reverse, becoming right-to-left and causing cyanosis.

Clinical Features

The balance between interchamber shunting and pulmonary vascular hypertension determines the clinical picture. Patients in the first 3 months of life have congestive heart failure and failure to thrive. Pulmonary infection associated with congestive heart failure is frequent. Cardiomegaly is easily palpated on physical examination. The murmur of an atrial septal defect, mitral regurgitation, tricuspid regurgitation, ventricular septal defect, or left-ventricular-to-right-atrial shunt or all of these may be present. As pulmonary vascular hypertensive disease progresses, the magnitude of the left-to-right shunt decreases, the second component of the second heart sound (pulmonic valve closure) increases in intensity, the heart size and right ventricular hypertrophy increase and interchamber shunting may not be audible. The more critically ill patients with an endocardial cushion defect have no murmur. Pulmonary vascular disease begins to develop in the first

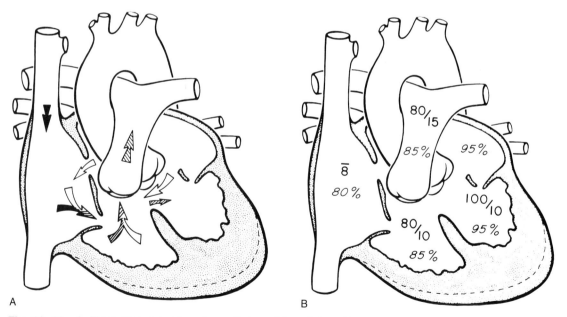

Fig. 18–13. *A.* **Flow diagram of endocardial cushion defect illustrating mixing at atrial and ventricular levels and biventricular hypertrophy.** *B.* Cardiac catheterization data in endocardial cushion defect.

year of life and may be irreversible by the age of 2 years.[33]

Laboratory Data

The ECG of patients with the complete form of endocardial cushion defect shows biventricular hypertrophy, left axis deviation, and a counterclockwise QRS loop. These findings help to distinguish this abnormality from other causes of pulmonary hypertension. The chest film shows cardiomegaly with increased pulmonary vascularity early in the course and pulmonary vascular pruning late in the course of this disease.

Cardiac catheterization is usually needed to confirm the diagnosis by catheter passage through the inferior vena cava into all four chambers. Pressures within the right ventricle will most commonly be systemic and the magnitude and direction of shunting will depend on the status of pulmonary vascular hypertensive disease (Fig. 18-13B). The angiogram shows mixture of dye in all four chambers regardless of which chamber is injected. Isolated chamber delineation is difficult. In the partial and transitional forms, an aortic outflow gooseneck deformity may be present because of abnormal mitral valve suspension and movement.[34]

VENTRICULAR SEPTAL DEFECT

Ventricular septal defect (VSD), presents an excellent opportunity to correlate anatomic abnormalities with physiologic sequelae. Twenty-eight percent of congenital heart disease patients have isolated ventricular septal defects.[35] Females are afflicted slightly more often than males. Ventricular septal defect is the most common heart defect in trisomy chromosomal syndromes.[36]

Embryology and Anatomy

By the eighth gestational week, the common ventricle is divided into two chambers by the fusion of the ventricular muscular septum (membranous extension), endocardial cushions, and bulbus cordis (proximal truncus arteriosus). The ventricular septum grows cephalad to join the right and left ridges of the bulbus cordis, the tricuspid valve orifice, and the endocardial cushions. The endocardial cushion also fuses with the muscular septum. A residual defect is closed by membranous tissue from the right truncoconal ridge. The endocardial cushion covers a defect between the inferior tricuspid valve annulus and the superior mitral valve annulus. A failure of any one of these developments will cause a ventricular septal defect. Defects are classified according to the size, location (sub-, inter-, or supracristal), and whether the muscular or membranous septum is involved. The location of various defects in the ventricular septum is shown in Figure 18-14A. The close proximity of the Bundle of His to the typical membranous defect is shown in Figure 18-14B.

Physiology

With lung expansion at birth, the pulmonary arterioles dilate and fetal arteriolar morphology regresses. As the pulmonary vascular resistance decreases, if a ventricular septal defect is present, a left-to-right shunt occurs with flow rates dependent upon the size of the ventricular septal defect (Fig. 18-15A). If the defect persists for a lengthy time, pulmonary arterioles respond by hypertrophy of the vessel musculature and intimal thickening. This increases the pulmonary vascular resistance and decreases the magnitude of the left-to-right shunt. Occasionally, an uncorrected ventricular septal defect shunt will reverse. Some patients have persistently high pulmonary vascular resistance throughout the newborn period and thus do not have a large left-to-right shunt. This high resistance eventually subsides and allows high shunt ratios.

Clinical Features

In the neonatal period, the pulmonary and systemic vascular resistances are similar, not allowing a large shunt and permitting normal early growth and development. Typically at

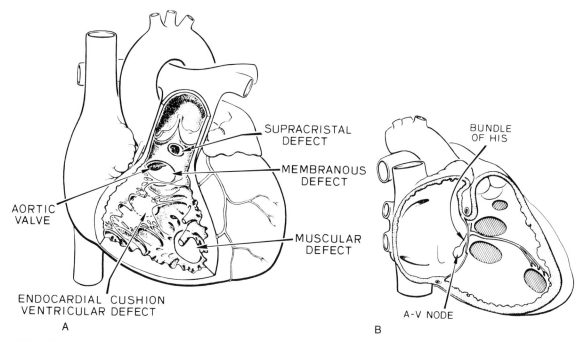

Fig. 18–14. *A.* **View of the ventricular septum showing the location of various types of ventricular septal defects.** *B.* View of the course of the bundle of His relative to ventricular defects.

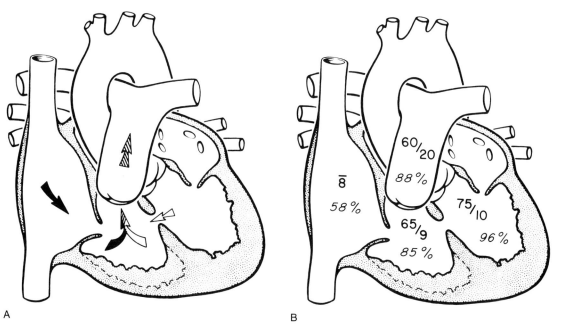

Fig. 18–15. *A.* **Flow diagram in ventricular septal defect (VSD) showing left-to-right shunt through the ventricular defect with enlarged pulmonary artery (PA) and hypertrophied right ventricle (RV).** *B.* Cardiac catheterization data in a large ventricular septal defect (VSD) with pulmonary hypertension.

about four weeks, the pulmonary vascular resistance decreases, as does the right ventricular pressure, and a shunt with its murmur develops and is first noticed. If this transition is rapid, congestive heart failure may ensue. Otherwise, cardiovascular compensation occurs and the patient remains asymptomatic. Approximately 25 percent of patients with small defects will spontaneously close the defect in the first 5 years of life.[35] Occasionally patients will develop right ventricular hypertrophy with infundibular or cristal hypertrophy leading to obstruction of the right ventricular outflow tract. The right ventricular outflow obstruction prevents blood from leaving the right ventricle and will decrease the amount of left-to-right shunting. Patients with defects that do not close or are not compensated for by right ventricular outflow obstruction may grow poorly and can remain in congestive heart failure. If allowed to persist, pulmonary vascular hypertrophic changes can occur with progression to Eisenmenger's reaction[37] and a right-to-left shunt.

Physical examination of the patient with the common membranous ventricular septal defect shows right ventricular hypertrophy, a systolic murmur of the ventricular septal defect shunt and relative pulmonary valve stenosis, a diastolic murmur of relative mitral valve stenosis, a presternal thrill, and a delayed pulmonary valve closing sound. If the defect is a small, muscular one, the shunting may be small late in systole secondary to muscular contraction. A decrescendo murmur will be heard.

Laboratory Data

The ECG will show right ventricular hypertrophy. The chest film will show right ventricular hypertrophy, pulmonary artery enlargement, increased pulmonary vascular markings, and left atrial and left ventricular enlargement. As the pulmonary vascular resistance increases, the right ventricle and right atrium will become large and the pulmonary vascular markings will become atten-

uated. Cardiac catheterization will show increased right ventricular and pulmonary artery pressures. An oxygen step-up will be present at the right ventricular outflow tract (Fig. 18-15B). If Eisenmenger's reaction develops,[37] right ventricular pressures become systemic, shunting decreases, and ultimately right-to-left shunting occurs with an oxygen step-down in the left ventricle. In the usual patient, a lateral angiocardiogram will show dye moving from the left ventricle to the right ventricle through the septal defect. Usually, an indication of the location and size of the defect is present on the angiocardiogram.

INTRACARDIAC LESIONS WITH RIGHT-TO-LEFT SHUNT

TETRALOGY OF FALLOT

Tetralogy of Fallot was one of the first complex congenital defects to be physiologically and anatomically corrected.[48] Approximately 10 percent of patients with congenital heart disease have this lesion, the most common type of cyanotic heart disease. The incidence increases with an advanced maternal age, particularly for mothers older than 35 years of age. Approximately 15 percent of these patients have an associated atrial septal defect while 25 percent have a right aortic arch.[39]

Embryology and Anatomy

Tetralogy of Fallot is a ventricular septal defect, aorta overriding the ventricular septal defect, right ventricular outflow obstruction, and secondary right ventricular hypertrophy. Normally at the fourth gestational week, the truncal artery is divided into the posterior aorta and anterior pulmonary artery by the truncoconal ridges spiraling caudad through a 180 degree rotation to join the bulbar ridges which fuse with the endocardial cushion and ventricular septum. The ventricular septal defect is in part formed by an absence of membranous septum. In tetralogy of Fallot, either abnormal truncal artery septation or abnormal development of the bulbus cordis distorts completion of the ventricular septum and leaves an abnormal amount of tissue in the right ventricular infundibulum. The overriding aorta and right ventricular hypertrophy are of secondary importance. Whether a patient is cyanotic or not depends upon the amount of right ventricular outflow obstruction and the degree of right-to-left shunting caused by this obstruction. Some may be so severely affected that a hypoplastic pulmonary valve or pulmonary artery may be present.

Physiology

An unobstructed right ventricular outflow tract with a ventricular septal defect will result in a large left-to-right shunt without cyanosis. In tetralogy of Fallot, there is right ventricular outflow obstruction, elevated right ventricular pressures to systemic levels, and thus right-to-left shunting with cyanosis. The distal pulmonary arteries are not exposed to high pressures and are thus protected from developing pulmonary vascular hypertensive disease. As right ventricular work persists, hypertrophy of the right ventricle and infundibulum increases, causing more right ventricular outflow obstruction and hence increased right-to-left shunting (Figure 18-16A). A restriction in the pulmonary blood flow usually stimulates the development of collateral bronchial and aortopulmonary communications.

Clinical Features

At birth, these patients are usually acyanotic. Cyanosis increases with time as a result of increasing infundibular stenosis. The fingers may become clubbed, squatting occurs, and

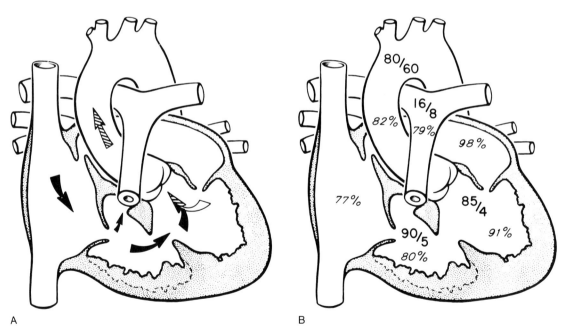

A   B

Fig. 18–16. *A.* Flow diagram in tetralogy of Fallot illustrating large right-to-left shunt through the ventricular septal defect (VSD), reduced pulmonary blood flow, and right ventricular hypertrophy. *B.* Cardiac catheterization data in tetralogy of Fallot.

hypercyanotic spells may ensue. Cyanosis, a result of hypoxia, may be accompanied by polycythemia and cause arterial thrombosis secondary to increased blood viscosity. The right-to-left shunt increases the risk of left-sided intravascular sepsis and a paradoxical embolus. A right ventricular lift, single S2, and systolic ejection murmur are usually present.

Laboratory Data

The ECG shows right axis deviation and right ventricular hypertrophy. The chest film has right ventricular hypertrophy, a boot-shaped heart, a small main pulmonary artery, and decreased pulmonary vasculature. An echocardiogram confirms these findings and may demonstrate septal overriding by the aorta and a ventricular septal defect. Cardiac catheterization shows right ventricular pressures equal to systemic, normal pulmonary artery pressures, and an oxygen step-down in the left ventricle (Fig. 18-16B). The angiocardiogram demonstrates a ventricular septal defect on a lateral view of the right ventricular injection with right-to-left shunting. Infundibular hypertrophy and stenosis should be seen. The pulmonary artery will be small, while the aorta is usually large.

TRICUSPID ATRESIA

Tricuspid atresia comprises 1 percent of all congenital heart disease.[40] Transposition of the great vessels occurs in 30 percent of cases, and extracardiac anomalies are seen in 20 percent of patients.[41]

Embryology and Anatomy

During the fifth gestational week, the anterior endocardial cushion, the posterior endocardial cushion, the posterior part of the ventricular septum, and the membranous ventricular septum fuse to form the tricuspid valve. A disruption in the balance between resorption and proliferation causes abnormal tricuspid valve formation. In tricuspid atre-

sia, no valvular tissue is found and no communication between the right atrium and ventricle is present.

There is considerable anatomic variation in tricuspid atresia, but absence of the right atrioventricular valve, a patent atrial septum, an enlarged mitral orifice and left ventricle, and rudimentary right ventricle are invariably present. The anatomic classification of tricuspid atresia depends on the relationship of the great vessels, the presence or absence of a ventricular septal defect, and the restrictive nature of the pulmonary outflow tract. The most common type includes normally related great vessels, a small ventricular septal defect, and pulmonary stenosis.

Physiology

All of the systemic venous blood is returned to the left atrium through an atrial septal defect, where complete mixing occurs with pulmonary venous blood (Fig. 18-17A). The relative flows of systemic and pulmonary venous blood determines the intensity of cyanosis. The amount of pulmonary blood flow is determined by the size of the ventricular septal defect, the degree of pulmonary outflow obstruction, and the position of the great vessels. A small, restrictive ventricular septal defect, intact ventricular septum, or pulmonic stenosis will severely restrict pulmonary flow. A patent ductus arteriosus or bronchial circulation will provide the main pulmonary flow. If a large ventricular septal defect or transposition of the great vessels is present, pulmonary blood flow is large, producing congestive heart failure and less intense cyanosis.

Clinical Features

The most common clinical presentation is that of an intensely cyanotic infant in the first 6 months of life without congestive heart failure. Hypoxic episodes are common. Clubbing is seen in older patients. The patient who is dependent on the patent ductus arteriosus for adequate pulmonary blood flow will rapidly deteriorate after it closes. Patients with unrestricted pulmonary blood flow may develop, early, severe left ventricular prominence, a single S_1 and S_2, and a variable murmur depending on the presence of associated lesions.

Laboratory Data

The chest film also varies with the anatomic situation. Most commonly, a normal heart size with decreased pulmonary vascularity is seen, but in cases with greatly increased pulmonary flow, cardiomegaly and pulmonary engorgement are present. The ECG shows left axis deviation, right atrial enlargement, and left ventricular enlargement. The echocardiogram should demonstrate an absent tricuspid valve, a small anterior ventricle, and large posterior ventricle. Cardiac catheterization will demonstrate no blood passing from the right atrium to the right ventricle (Fig. 18-17B). A balloon atrial septostomy may be beneficial in intensely cyanotic patients.

PULMONARY ATRESIA WITH INTACT VENTRICULAR SEPTUM

Pulmonary atresia represents the extreme form of valvular pulmonic stenosis and is seen in 1 percent of all congenital heart defects. The pulmonary valve is involved in 90 percent of cases. Without treatment, 50 percent of patients would die by age 1 month.[42]

Embryology and Anatomy

The pulmonary valve forms between the sixth and ninth weeks of gestation. Three tubercles enlarge within the pulmonary artery, initially growing toward the midline, and thinning out by resorption. Complete failure of absorption of this excess tissue will lead to pulmonary atresia.

The right ventricle is separated from the pulmonary artery by a diaphragm of tissue consisting of the fused pulmonary valve cusps. The right ventricular infundibulum and pulmonary trunk may rarely be in-

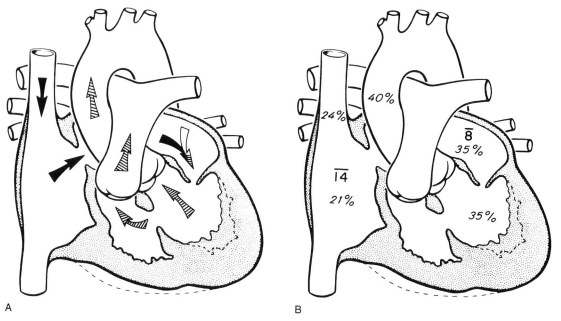

A

B

Fig. 18–17. *A.* **Flow diagram in tricuspid atresia illustrating obligatory right-to-left shunt at the atrial level with reduced right ventricular size.** *B.* Cardiac catheterization data in tricuspid atresia.

volved. The majority of cases also have a small right ventricle, but in 20 percent of cases it is normal or slightly dilated.[42]

Physiology

Blood passing through the tricuspid valve to the right ventricle is trapped and can only exit through an incompetent tricuspid valve or through sinusoids in the coronary circulation. Severe right ventricular pressure overload occurs if the tricuspid valve is competent. Most of the systemic venous return traverses the patent atrial septum to the left atrium. Pulmonary flow is solely dependent on the patent ductus arteriosus (Fig. 18-18A). Closure of the ductus at an early stage will lead to sudden, rapid deterioration.

Clinical Features

Cyanosis appears in the first few days of life and increases rapidly, except in the presence of a large patent ductus. Tachypnea and severe right heart failure are seen in cases with a large right ventricle and tricuspid regurgitation. A short systolic or continuous murmur may be heard as a result of patent ductus.

Laboratory Data

The chest film shows decreased pulmonary vascularity except in unusual cases with a large patent ductus. The heart size is variable, depending on the size of the right ventricle. The ECG also varies with right ventricular size. The usual patient with a small right ventricle will show a normal QRS axis and decreased right ventricular forces, thereby distinguishing pulmonary atresia from tetralogy of Fallot. Echocardiography may add information about the size of the right ventricle and tricuspid valves. The proximal pulmonary tree may be difficult to visualize. Car-

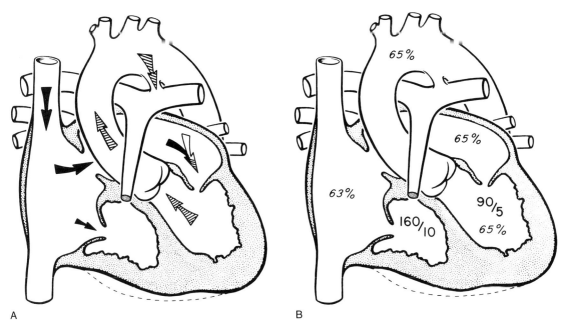

A   B

Fig. 18–18. *A.* Flow diagram in pulmonary atresia with intact ventricular septum showing obligatory right-to-left shunt at the atrial level and obligatory left-to-right shunt via the patent ductus arteriosus (PDA). *B.* Cardiac catheterization data in pulmonary atresia.

diac catheterization and angiography demonstrate no filling of the pulmonary artery or aorta from the right ventricle (Fig. 18-18B). The size of the proximal pulmonary arteries and ductus arteriosus can be evaluated with an aortic injection. Balloon atrial septostomy is performed in cases with a hypoplastic right ventricle to improve intracardiac mixing.

INTRACARDIAC LESIONS WITH BIDIRECTIONAL SHUNTS

TOTAL ANOMALOUS PULMONARY VENOUS RETURN

Total anomalous pulmonary venous return (TAPVR) is relatively rare, comprising about 1 percent of congenital heart disease. Other cardiovascular anomalies occur in 25 to 35 percent of patients.[43]

Embryology and Anatomy

Early in fetal life, the lung bud has vascular connections with the splanchnic plexus, which contributes to the four pulmonary veins. At three weeks' gestation, the common pulmonary vein appears as an evagination from the atrial wall and grows to join the splanchnic plexus. Subsequently, the common pulmonary vein is included in the atrial wall, leaving the four pulmonary venous channels draining into the left atrium. Failure of the common pulmonary vein to join the splanchnic plexus leads to development of anomalous channels which return pulmonary blood to the right side of the heart.

There are three primary sites of anomalous venous return (Fig. 18-19): supracardiac (47%), using a vertical connection to a persistent left superior vena cava and azygous vein or right superior vena cava; cardiac (30%),

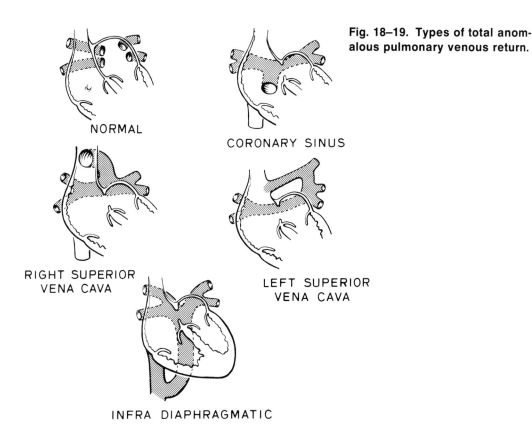

Fig. 18–19. Types of total anomalous pulmonary venous return.

NORMAL

CORONARY SINUS

RIGHT SUPERIOR VENA CAVA

LEFT SUPERIOR VENA CAVA

INFRA DIAPHRAGMATIC

including the right atrium and coronary sinus; and infradiaphragmatic (18%), using the portal vein or ductus venosus.[44] A secundum atrial septal defect or patent foramen ovale is almost always present.

Physiology

Total anomalous pulmonary venous return generally follows two patterns, depending on the degree of obstruction produced by the anomalous venous channels. If the veins are nonobstructed, few symptoms may appear, as the increased flow returning to the right atrium is returned to the lungs or to the left heart through the atrial defect (Fig. 18-20A). While congestive heart failure may appear in infancy, severe symptoms are uncommon until the fourth or fifth decade. Arterial oxygen saturation is usually decreased, but seldom clinically evident.

If pulmonary venous obstruction is present however, pulmonary vascular resistance increases, leading to increased pulmonary artery pressure with pulmonary edema and right ventricular pressure overload. With decreased pulmonary blood flow, cyanosis is more intense and congestive heart failure is severe.

Clinical Features

Total anomalous pulmonary venous return presents in three patterns. First, the infant with pulmonary venous obstruction has the most severe symptoms and presents with tachypnea, cyanosis, failure to thrive, and congestive heart failure. Without surgical treatment, the course rapidly deteriorates. Second, the infant with nonobstructed veins and an adequate atrial communication has a large pulmonary blood flow, but low pulmonary vascular resistance and may have congestive heart failure responding more easily to medical management. Third, the nonobstructed older child or adult who has normal pulmonary vascular resistance and an adequate atrial defect may have relatively few symptoms.

The physical examination shows a hyperactive precordium with left-sided prominence. The second heart sound has a fixed split. A soft ejection murmur is audible at the pulmonary area with a mid-diastolic rumble. A continuous murmur may be audible, from flow through the anomalous venous channels. Hepatomegaly may be prominent, especially if a subdiaphragmatic connection is present.

Laboratory Data

The chest film also assumes two patterns. With pulmonary venous obstruction, the heart size may be normal or increased. The lung fields are filled with fluffy opacification secondary to venous obstruction. If venous obstruction is absent, cardiomegaly and increased pulmonary blood flow are seen. The mediastinum and cardiac silhouette may have a "figure eight" contour as a result of the widened mediastinum of a supracardiac connection.

The ECG shows right axis deviation, right atrial enlargement, and right ventricular hypertrophy. Echocardiography demonstrates the large right ventricle and a small left atrium and left ventricle. Cardiac catheterization shows very similar oxygen saturations in the right atrium, pulmonary artery, and systemic artery (Fig. 18-20B). Angiocardiography should reveal the course of anomalous vein with a pulmonary artery injection.

TRUNCUS ARTERIOSUS

Truncus arteriosus represents approximately 1 percent of all congenital heart disease and is associated with right-sided aortic arch (30%), ventricular septal defect (100%), and patent foramen ovale (9%).[45]

Embryology and Anatomy

By the fourth gestational week, the common arterial trunk is divided into the posterolateral aorta and the anteriormedial pulmonary artery by the spiraling truncoconal ridges growing caudally to meet the bulbar ridges. Separation of the systemic and pulmonary cicuits is completed by the fusion of the bulbar ridges with the endocardial cushions and the membranous ventricular septum. Failure of maturation of the truncoconal ridges causes a persistent truncal artery and an inability of the ventricular septum to close. For this reason a ventricular septal defect is always present in trucus arteriosus.

Four basic types of truncus arteriosus have been classifed (Fig. 18-21).[46] In type I, the branch pulmonary arteries come off a common pulmonary artery trunk arising from the base of the aorta. Type II defects have two branch pulmonary arteries coming off a common artery posterior on the ascending aorta. In type III defects, the branch pulmonary arteries arise individually and laterally from the ascending aorta. Type IV defects have the pulmonary arteries arising from the descending aorta. The truncal valve is most commonly tricuspid, but will be quatricuspid in 24 percent of patients and bicuspid in 7 percent of patients.[47]

Physiology

All these patients have a common right and left ventricular outflow tract (Fig. 18-22A). Flow to the lungs can be increased, normal, or decreased, depending on the degree of pulmonary arterial obstruction. If the pulmonary artery is unobstructed, increased pulmonary artery blood flow causes abnormal left ventricular volume load and can cause congestive heart failure. If abnormally high pulmonary artery blood flow persists over a long period of time, pulmonary vascular resistance may increase and ultimately cause Eisenmenger's reaction with right-to-left shunting. Patients with low pulmonary blood flow have inadequate oxygenation and, therefore, develop cyanosis. The degree

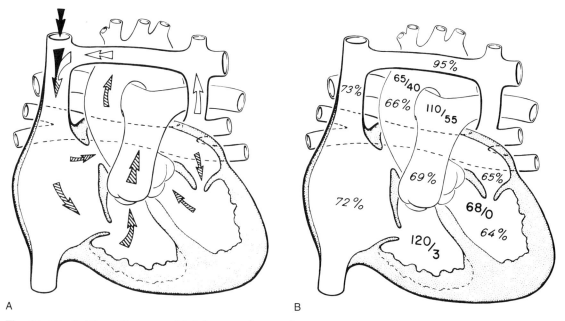

A
B

Fig. 18–20. *A.* **Flow diagram of total anomalous pulmonary venous return (TAPVR) (supradiaphragmatic) showing mixing of oxygenated blood at site of anomalous venous connection and obligatory right-to-left shunt at the atrial level.** *B.* Cardiac catheterization data in total anomalous pulmonary venous return (TAPVR) showing marked pulmonary hypertension and systemic desaturation.

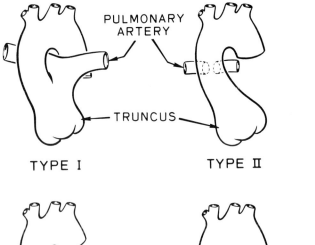

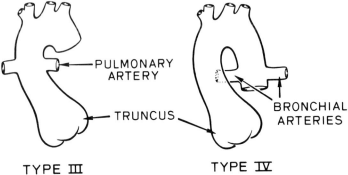

Fig. 18–21. Anatomic types of truncus arteriosus (Edwards classification).

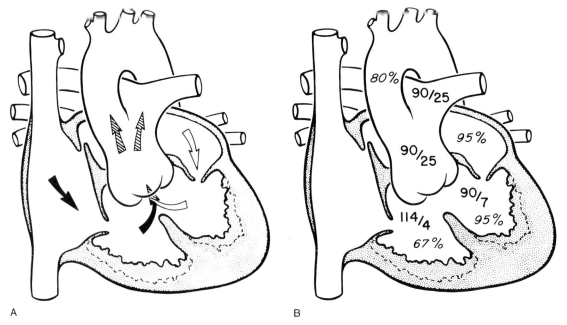

A   B

Fig. 18–22. **A. Flow diagram of truncus arteriosus showing systemic desaturation and biventricular hypertrophy.** B. Cardiac catheterization data in truncus arteriosus.

of cyanosis will depend upon the degree of pulmonary collateralization.

Clinical Features

Patients with truncus arteriosus usually present in the early weeks of life with congestive heart failure. Failure to thrive and dyspnea are prominent; cyanosis is variable. Cardiac examination reveals an increased heart size, right or biventricular hypertrophy, a systolic ejection murmur, an ejection click, and a single S2. A continuous murmur occasionally develops secondary to persistent flow from the systemic to the pulmonary circuit.

Laboratory Data

The chest film generally shows an increased size of the right atrium, right ventricle, pulmonary artery, and left ventricle. The pulmonary arteries arise superiorly and cause a widened mediastinum. The ECG shows biventricular hypertrophy. If no pulmonary artery is present or pulmonary stenosis is severe, cyanosis will be severe. The chest film in cyanotic patients will usually show a smaller than usual pulmonary artery shadow and a larger right ventricular shadow. The ECG shows a right ventricular hypertrophy in these cyanotic patients.

Cardiac catheterization discloses an oxygen decrease in the ascending aorta when compared to the left ventricular oxygen saturation. Pulmonary artery pressures can be systemic (Fig. 18-22B). The pulmonary artery may be difficult to enter. Angiocardiogram shows truncal anatomy and, in operable lesions, a satisfactory pulmonary artery and branch pulmonary artery size.

TRANSPOSITION OF THE GREAT VESSELS

Transposition of the great vessels occurs in 10 percent of infants presenting with congenital heart disease and is the most common cyanotic lesion evident at birth. Males are affected two to three times more frequently than females.[48] Commonly associated lesions include patent ductus arteriosus, atrial septal defect, ventricular septal defect, and pulmonic stenosis.[49] The incidence in infants of mothers with diabetes is 10 times that of the general population.[50]

Embryology and Anatomy

During the third to fourth weeks of gestation, the common truncus develops into the two great vessels by spiral growth distally of the truncoconal ridges. This spiral growth produces twisting of the great vessels into their normal orientation. Abnormal rotation of this truncal septation as well as abnormal partitioning of subvalvular conal tissue are thought to cause the transposed great vessel orientation.

In the most common form of transposition, the aorta arises from the anterior, anatomic right ventricle, and the pulmonary artery arises from the posterior, anatomic left ventricle (Fig. 18-23A). Therefore, the aorta lies anterior and to the right of the pulmonary artery which is posterior and to the left. Assuming no interchamber communications, the pulmonary and systemic circulations would operate in parallel, with desaturated venous blood being received by the right atrium and ventricle and then pumped to the aorta, while oxygenated blood returning to the left atrium and ventricle would exit to the pulmonary artery. One additional lesion which permits mixing must be present to allow life after birth. A ventricular septal defect (VSD) is seen in 40 percent of patients with transposition of the great vessels. Pulmonic stenosis occurs in 6 percent of patients with intact ventricular septum and in 31 percent of patients with a VSD.[49]

Physiology

Transposition of the great vessels presents a difficult physiologic circumstance because of the decreased oxygen supply to the tissues, the early development of congestive heart failure secondary to poor coronary oxygenation, pressure overload of one or both ventricles, and the early development of pulmonary vascular obstruction. The time of onset of symptoms is related to the extent and level of mixing of the parallel circulations. An atrial or ventricular septal defect producing good bidirectional shunting may delay the onset of cyanosis. Congestive heart failure would be the main problem. However, if a PDA is the only communication between circuits, PDA closure in the first few days of life may lead to sudden, rapid deterioration.

Clinical Features

Simple transposition with an intact ventricular septum is usually seen in the first days of life with severe cyanosis and congestive heart failure. If a ventricular septal defect is present, the resultant mixing delays the appearance of congestive heart failure until 2 to 6 weeks of age, with less intense cyanosis. Transposition with a VSD and pulmonic stenosis has very early cyanosis, but congestive heart failure is less severe.

The physical examination varies with the spectrum of cardiac anomalies. Most infants are well-developed and of normal birth weight. Associated extracardiac anomalies are rare. Differential cyanosis may be present if the large patent ductus is shunting from the pulmonic to the distal systemic circulation. Clubbing is uncommon until 5 to 6 months of age.

Cardiac murmurs may be absent, especially in the first few days of life. Patients with an intact ventricular septum develop a soft systolic ejection murmur at the upper left sternal border from flow across the left ventricular outflow. Patients with a VSD develop a lower pansystolic murmur with a diastolic rumble and loud sound of pulmonic closure.

Laboratory Data

The chest film early in the neonatal period may be surprisingly normal if the usual drop in pulmonary vascular resistance has not oc-

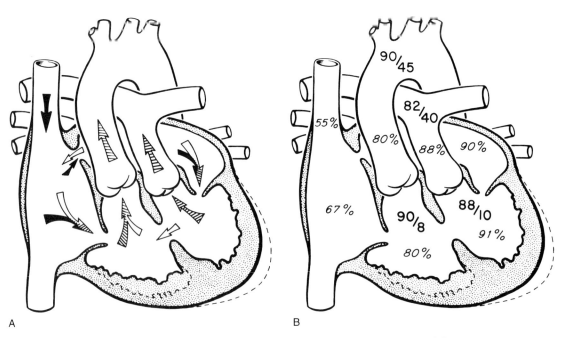

A   B

Fig. 18–23. *A.* **Flow diagram in simple transposition of the great vessels (TOGV) showing shunting at the atrial and ventricular levels and right ventricular hypertrophy.** *B.* Cardiac catheterization data in simple TOGV.

curred. After 2 to 3 days with the onset of congestive heart failure and increasing cyanosis, the heart size increases and pulmonary arterial congestion appears. The characteristic oval or egg-shaped cardiac silhouette with narrow superior mediastinum is caused by an enlarged right atrium, anterior-posterior relationship of the great vessels, and shrinking of the normally prominent thymus. The ECG may appear normal during the first days of life, but right axis deviation and right ventricular hypertrophy soon become evident. Left ventricular hypertrophy may be seen if pulmonic stenosis or a ventricular septal defect place an extra load on the left ventricle. The echocardiogram should detect abnormal position of the great vessels and may suggest the presence of a ventricular septal defect or pulmonic obstruction. Cardiac catheterization (Fig. 18-23B) is essential and may provide lifesaving palliation by balloon atrial septostomy in patients with intact ventricular septum.[51]

GENERAL OPERATIVE CONSIDERATIONS

The determinants of the type of operation to be performed upon a patient with congenital heart disease depends upon age, size, symptoms, anatomic status, and physiologic status of the patient. These factors need to be acknowledged during consideration of timing of an operation and type of operation to be performed.

The types of operation can be categorized broadly as *anatomic, physiologic,* or *palliative.* In the anatomic repair, the morphology of the correction exactly duplicates or approximates normal cardiac anatomy and physiology. The best example is ligation of a PDA. Other examples include coarctation repair, secundum atrial septal defect closure, simple ostium primum atrial septal defect closure, VSD closure, milder forms of aortic valvular stenosis, tetralogy of Fallot, double outlet

right ventricle, transposition of the great vessels associated with a large VSD close to the aorta, and truncus arteriosus in which the aortic valve is normal. In many of these repairs, prosthetic material is necessary which improves sequence of blood flow through the cardiac chambers but does not allow a perfect anatomic reconstruction. The right ventricle provides pulmonary blood flow, and the left ventricle provides sytemic blood flow.

In a physiologic correction, the systemic venous drainage is directed toward the morphologic systemic (left) ventricle rather than the morphologic pulmonary (right) ventricle. A good example is that of a transposition of the great vessels without a VSD. After physiologic repair, namely the Mustard[52] or Senning[53] intra-atrial baffle, systemic venous return is directed to the left atrium, left ventricle, then out of the pulmonary artery to the lungs. The pulmonary venous drainage is shunted to the right atrium, right ventricle, aorta, and hence to the systemic periphery. The right ventricle is performing systemic work while the left ventricle is performing a relatively smaller amount of work delivering pulmonary blood flow. The remote long-term sequelae of this hemodynamic circuit have not clearly been established.

The third, and least corrective type of operation performed is the palliative procedure, including systemic-to-pulmonary shunts, pulmonary artery banding, and intraatrial baffling with pulmonary vascular hypertension. In the very small cyanotic child with too little pulmonary blood flow and anatomy that does not allow the physiologic or anatomic repair, systemic-to-pulmonary shunts are usually indicated. The shunt can be created at the atrial level by balloon septostomy (Rashkind procedure)[51] or operative atrial septectomy (Blalock–Hanlon procedure).[54] Most situations, however, require systemic-to-pulmonary shunting between the aorta or its branches and the main pulmonary artery or its branches. The subclavian artery can be brought down and anastomosed to the corresponding pulmonary artery in an end-to-side manner (Blalock–Taussig shunt).[55] The ascending aorta can also be approximated with the underlying pulmonary artery (Waterston shunt).[56] If none of these are possible, the descending thoracic aorta can be approximated to an adjacent pulmonary artery (Potts shunt).[57] Patients who have these palliative procedures may then grow large enough to be corrected in an anatomic or physiologic manner. Often the final corrections are limited by the absence or diminutive nature of the main pulmonary arteries or ventricles.

Patients with increased pulmonary blood flow, often seen with VSDs and normal pulmonary vascular resistance, can be palliated by use of a pulmonary artery band. Occasionally more complex lesions with very elevated pulmonary blood flow will also require pulmonary artery banding. Recently, several centers have shown the efficacy of correcting these lesions in a single stage rather than performing two procedures, namely the palliative and subsequent anatomic repair. In simple defects, the overall mortality and morbidity are decreased by a single-staged anatomic repair in spite of small patient size.

Finally, in patients with a severe long-standing congenital abnormality who have developed pulmonary arteriolar hypertension, an operative procedure may be done to improve the patient's symptoms in spite of a well-documented low probability of long-term survival. The best example is that of transposition of the great vessels with a VSD in which abnormally high pulmonary vascular resistance has already occurred. A Mustard or Senning baffle can be used in an effort to decrease the amount of unfavorable shunting. The ventricular septum is not closed in order to allow decompression of the pulmonary ventricle and to avoid severe congestive heart failure.

Every attempt is made by the surgeon, pediatrician, and anesthetist to design a therapeutic regimen which will allow the best outcome for the patient. The details of this decision making vary among localities, surgeons, pediatricians, and anesthetists. A high degree of skill is required on all participants' parts in order to achieve an optimal outcome.

GLOSSARY*

aortic stenosis. Narrowing of the aortic outflow; may be subvalvular, valvular, or supravalvular

atrial septal defect. Abnormal opening in the atrial septum

Baffes procedure. Prosthetic shunt from inferior vena cava to anatomic left atrium through proximal right pulmonary veins and distal right pulmonary venous anastomosis to anatomic right atrium

Blalock–Hanlon procedure. Operative atrial septectomy

Blalock–Taussig shunt. Subclavian artery to pulmonary artery anastomosis

Brock procedure. Right transventricular infundibulectomy without cardiopulmonary bypass

coarctation of the aorta. Localized narrowing of the aortic lumen, usually at the ligamentum arteriosum

Eisenmenger's reaction. Pulmonary vascular obstructive changes

endocardial cushion defect. Defect which may involve atrial septum, ventricular septum, tricuspid, or mitral valve

Fontan procedure. System venous return directed to right ventricle, proximal pulmonary artery, or distal pulmonary artery using prosthetic conducts or direct vascular connection, primarily used for tricuspid or pulmonary atresia or both

Glenn procedure. Superior vena cava to right pulmonary artery anastomosis, end to end

Mustard procedure. Intraatrial baffling to redirect systemic venous blood to the anatomic left atrium, left ventricle, and out the pulmonary artery and to direct pulmonary venous blood to the anatomic right atrium, right ventricle, out the aorta uses either precordium or prosthetic material

---

* Aortic stenosis (AS); atrial septal defect (ASD); electrocardiogram (ECG); left ventricle (LV); patent ductus arteriosus (PDA); patent foramen ovale (PFO); pulmonary artery (PA); pulmonic stenosis (PS); right ventricle (RV); tetralogy of Fallot (TOF); total anomalous pulmonary venous return (TAPVR); transposition of the great vessels (TOGV); ventricular septal defect (VSD).

patent ductus arteriosus (PDA). Persistent communication between the aorta and the pulmonary artery distal to the left subclavian artery.

patent foramen ovale. Opening in the atrial septum at the site of the foramen secundum

Potts shunt. Descending aorta to pulmonary artery anastamosis

pulmonary atresia with intact ventricular septum. Separation of the right ventricle from the pulmonary artery by a diaphragm of tissue

pulmonic stenosis. Narrowing of the pulmonary outflow tract; may involve muscular infundibulum, valve, or peripheral pulmonary artery

Rashkind procedure. Balloon atrial septostomy performed at cardiac catheterization to improve intraatrial mixing of venous and oxygenated blood

Rastelli procedure. Left ventricular blood flow directed out aorta using ventricular septal defect patch, proximal PA oversewn, and a valved conduit placed between RV and distal PA. Used primarily in transposition of the great vessels with a large ventricular septal defect and tetralogy of Fallot, or double outlet right ventricles with severe pulmonary stenosis.

Senning procedure. Intra- and extraatrial baffling using atrial wall and a prosthesis to direct blood flow as in a Mustard procedure.

tetralogy of Fallot. Ventricular septal defect, pulmonic stenosis, overriding aorta, and right ventricular hypertrophy

total anomalous pulmonary venous return. Return of pulmonary venous blood through anomalous channels to the right atrium

transposition of the great vessels. Abnormal great vessel anatomy with aorta arising from the anatomic right ventricle and pulmonary artery arising from the anatomic left ventricle.

tricuspid atresia. Absent tricuspid valve, with patent atrial septum, enlarged mitral orifice, and rudimentary right ventricle

truncus arteriosus. Persistent fetal common arterial trunk supplying the systemic and pulmonary circulations

vascular ring. Anomaly of the aorta or its branches or both, leading to compression of the trachea or esophagus or both

ventricular septal defect. Abnormal communication between the left and right ventricle through the ventricular septum

Waterston shunt. Ascending aorta to pulmonary artery anastomosis

REFERENCES

GENERAL READING

1. Nadas AS, Fyler DC: Pediatric Cardiology, Philadelphia, WB Saunders, 1972 (Coarctation: p 453; Vascular rings: p 496–502; aortic stenosis: 476, 478; tricuspid atresia p 588; TAPVR: pp 640–641)
2. Moss AJ, Adams FH, and Emmanouilides GC (eds): Heart Disease in Infants, Children and Adolescents, ed 2. Baltimore, Williams and Wilkins, 1977
3. Keith JD, Rowe RD, Vlad P (eds): Heart Disease in Infancy and Childhood, pp 4–6. New York, Macmillan, 1978
4. Netter FH: The CIBA Collection of Medical Illustrations, vol 5, The Heart. Summit, NJ, CIBA, 1969
5. Fink BW: Congenital Heart Disease. Chicago, Year Book Medical Publishers, 1975
6. Morgan BC (ed): Symposium on Pediatric Cardiology. Pediatr Clin North Am 25:4, 1978
7. Langman J: Medical Embryology, ed 2. Baltimore, Waverly Press, 1969

INTRODUCTION

8. Keith JD, Rowe RD, Vlad P (eds): Heart Disease in Infancy and Childhood, p 4. New York, Macmillan, 1978
9. Keith JD, Rowe RD, Vlad P (eds): Heart Disease in Infancy and Childhood, pp 5–6. New York, Macmillan, 1978
10. Kontas SB, Bodenbender JG, Haenen J et al: Hyperviscosity in congenital heart disease. J Pediatr 76:214, 1970
11. Epert H, Gilchrist GS, Stanton R et al: Hemostatis in cyanotic congenital heart disease. J Pediatr 76:221, 1970
12. Gunteroth WG: Initial evaluation of the child for heart disease. Pediatr Clin North Am 25:657–675, 1978
13. Noonan JA: Association of congenital heart disease with syndromes or other defects. Pediatr Clin North Am 25:809, 1978
14. Smith DW: Recognizable Patterns of Human Malformation, ed 2, Major Problems in Clinical Pediatrics, vol 7. Philadelphia, WB Saunders, 1976
15. Greenwood RC et al: Extracardiac abnormali-

ties in infants with congenital heart disease. Pediatrics 55:485, 1975

16. Gunteroth WG: Pediatric Electrocardiography. Philadelphia, WB Saunders, 1965

VALVULAR AND VASCULAR LESIONS

Patent Ductus Arteriosus

17. Heymann MA: The ductus arteriosus. In Moss AJ, Adams FH, Emmanouilides GC (eds): Heart Disease in Infants, Children and Adolescents, 2 ed. Baltimore, Williams and Wilkins, 1977

18. Gross RE, Hubbard JP: Surgical ligation of a patent ductus arteriosus: report of first successful case. JAMA 112:729, 1939

19. Rowe RD: Patent ductus arteriosus. In Keith JD, Rowe RD, Vlad P (eds): Heart Disease in Infancy and Childhood, ed 3, pp 418–451. New York, Macmillan, 1978

Coarctation of the Aorta

20. Keith JD: Coarctation of the aorta. In Keith JD, Rowe RD, Vlad P (eds): Heart Disease in Infancy and Childhood, ed 3, pp 736–760. New York, Macmillan, 1978

21. Nadas AS, Fyler DC: Pediatric Cardiology, p 453. Philadelphia, WB Saunders, 1972

Vascular Rings

22. Nadas AS, Fyler DC: Pediatric Cardiology, pp 496–502. Philadelphia, WB Saunders, 1972

Pulmonic Stenosis

23. Rowe RD: Pulmonary stenosis with normal aortic root. In Keith JD, Rowe RD, Vlad P (eds): Heart Disease in Infancy and Childhood, pp 761–788. New York, Macmillan, 1978

Aortic Stenosis

24. Stevenson JG: Acyanotic lesions with normal pulmonary blood flow. Pediatr Clin North Am 25:736, 1978

25. Friedman WF, Kirkpatrick SE: Congenital aortic stenosis. In Moss AJ, Adams FH, Emmanouilides GC (eds): Heart Disease in Infants, Children and Adolescents ed 2, p 178. Baltimore, Williams and Wilkins, 1977

26. Olley PM, Bloom KR, Rowe RD: Aortic stenosis: valvular, subaortic and supravalvular. In Keith JD, Rowe RD, Vlad P (eds): Heart Disease in Infancy and Childhood ed 3, p 698. New York, Macmillan, 1978

27. Nadas AS, Fyler DC: Pediatric Cardiology, p 476. Philadelphia, WB Saunders, 1972

28. Nadas AS, Fyler DC: Pediatric Cardiology, p 478. Philadelphia, WB Saunders, 1972

29. Friedman WF, Pappelbaum SJ: Indications for hemodynamic evaluation and surgery in congenital aortic stenosis. Pediatr Clin North Am 18:1207, 1971

INTRACARDIAC LESIONS WITH A LEFT-TO-RIGHT SHUNT

Secundum Atrial Septal Defect

30. Feldt RH, Weidman WH: Defects of the atrial septal defect and endocardial cushion. In Moss AJ, Adams FH, Emmanouilides GC (eds): Heart Disease in Infants, Children and Adolescents. 2nd ed, p 129. Baltimore, Williams & Wilkins, 1977

31. Keith JD: Atrial septal defect. In Keith JD, Rowe RD, Vlad P (eds): Heart Disease in Infancy and Childhood, 3rd ed, p 387. New York, Macmillan, 1978

Endocardial Cushion Defect

32. Rowe RD, Uchida IA: Cardiac malformation in mongolism. Am J Med 31:726, 1961

33. Feldt RH, Weidman WH: Defects of the atrial septal defect and endocardial cushion. In Moss AJ, Adams FH, Emmanouilides GC (eds): Heart Disease in Infants, Children and Adolescents. 2nd ed, p 138. Baltimore, Williams & Wilkins, 1977

34. Baron MG et al: Endocardial cushion defects: specific diagnosis by angiocardiography. Am J Cardiol 13:162, 1964

Ventricular Septal Defect

35. Keith JD: Ventricular septal defect. In Keith JD, Rowe RD, Vlad P (eds): Heart Disease in Infancy and Childhood, 3rd ed, pp 320–379. New York, Macmillan, 1978

36. Nora JJ, Fraser FLC: Medical Genetics, pp 334–338. Philadelphia, Lea and Febiger, 1974

37. Abott M-E: Congenital heart disease. In Nel-

son's Loose-Leaf Medicine, vol 5, p 207. New York, Thomas Nelson & Sons, 1932

INTRACARDIAC LESIONS WITH RIGHT-TO-LEFT SHUNT

Tetralogy of Fallot

38. Lillehei CW et al: Direct vision intracardiac surgical correction of the tetralogy of Fallot, pentalogy of Fallot and pulmonary atresia defects. Report of first ten cases. Ann Surg 142:418, 1955
39. Guntheroth WG, Kawabari I: Tetrad of Fallot. In Moss AJ, Adams FH, Emmanouilides GC (eds): Heart Disease in Infants, Children and Adolescents, ed 2, pp 276–279. Baltimore, Williams and Wilkins, 1977

Tricuspid Atresia

40. Nadas AS, Fyler DC: Pediatric Cardiology, p 558. Philadelphia, WB Saunders, 1972
41. Rosenthal A: Tricuspid atresia. In Moss AJ, Adams FH, Emmanouilides GC (eds): Heart Disease in Infants, Children and Adolescents, ed 2, pp 290–291. Baltimore, Williams and Wilkins, 1977

Pulmonary Atresia with Intact Ventricular Septum

42. Emmanouilides GC: Obstructive lesions of the right ventricle and the pulmonary arterial tree. In Moss AJ, Adams FH, Emmanouilides GC (eds): Heart Disease in Infants, Children and Adolescents; ed 2, pp 226–232. Baltimore, Williams and Wilkins, 1977

INTRACARDIAC LESIONS WITH BIDIRECTIONAL SHUNTS

Total Anomalous Pulmonary Venous Return

43. Nadas AS, Fyler DC: Pediatric Cardiology, pp 640–641. Philadelphia, WB Saunders, 1972
44. Rowe RD: Anomalies of venous return. In Keith JD, Rowe RD, Vlad P (eds): Heart Disease in Infancy and Childhood, ed 3, p 565. New York, Macmillan, 1978

Truncus Arteriosus

45. Mair DD, Ritter DG: Truncus arteriosus. In Moss AJ, Adams FH, Emmanouilides GC (eds): Heart Disease in Infants, Children and Adolescents, ed 2, pp 417–418. Baltimore, Williams and Wilkins, 1977
46. Collett RW, Edwards RE: Persistent truncus arteriosus: a classification according to anatomic types. Surg Clin North Am 29:1245–1270, 1949
47. Kidd BSL: Persistent truncus arteriosus. In Keith JD, Rowe RD, Vlad P (eds): Heart Disease in Infancy and Childhood, ed 3, p 457. New York, Macmillan, 1978

Transposition of the Great Vessels

48. Paul MH: D-Transposition of the great arteries. In Moss AJ, Adams FH, Emmanouilides GC (eds): Heart Disease in Infants, Children and Adolescents, ed 2, p 301. Baltimore, Williams and Wilkins, 1977
49. Kidd BSL: Complete transposition of the great arteries. In Keith JD, Rowe RD, Vlad P: Heart Disease in Infancy and Childhood, ed 3, pp 592–593. New York, Macmillan, 1978
50. Rowland TW, Hubbell JP Jr, Nadas AS: Congenital heart disease in infants of diabetic mothers. J Pediatr 83:815, 1973
51. Rashkind WJ, Miller WW: Creation of an atrial septal defect without thoracotomy. JAMA 196:991, 1966

OPERATIVE CONSIDERATIONS

52. Mustard WT: Successful two-stage correction of transposition of the great vessels. Surgery 55:469, 1964
53. Senning A: Correction of the transposition of the great arteries. Ann Surg 182:287, 1975
54. Blalock A, Hanlon CR: The surgical treatment of complete transposition of the aorta and the pulmonary artery. Surg Gynecol Obstet 90:1, 1950
55. Blalock A, Taussig HB: The surgical treatment of malformations of the heart. JAMA 128:189, 1945
56. Waterston DH: Treatment of Fallot's tetralogy in children under 1 year of age. Rozhl Chir 41:181, 1962
57. Potts WJ, Smith S, Gibson S: Anastomosis of the aorta to a pulmonary artery. JAMA 132:627, 1946

19

Anesthetic Management of the Pediatric Patient

ALVIN HACKEL

HISTORICAL NOTES

The development of methods to diagnose and correct surgically congenital cardiac lesions represents one of the most exciting chapters in recent medical history. Anesthesia operating room and intensive care techniques which allow the surgeon to correct the malformed heart followed the development of anesthesia for thoracic surgery, beginning in the 1930s, and intensive care techniques, beginning in the 1950s in response to epidemic poliomyelitis.[1]

In 1937, Graybiel attempted ligation of a patent ductus arteriosus, in a patient with subacute bacterial endocarditis. The patient survived the operation but then died after acute gastric dilation.[2] In 1938, Gross and Hubbard reported the successful ligation of a ductus arteriosus.[3] Tubbs and Keele reported a similar case in 1940.[4] In 1944, the close collaboration of two medical pioneers at the Johns Hopkins University School of Medicine, Helen Taussig, a pediatric cardiologist, and Alfred Blalock, a cardiac surgeon, culminated in the first attempt at a palliative cardiac operative procedure. An artificial aortic-pulmonary artery anastomosis, the Blalock–Taussig shunt, was created surgically.[5] This procedure was used initially for patients with tetralogy of Fallot. Successful repair of coarctation of the aorta was reported in 1944 and 1945 by Blalock, Crafoord, and Gross.[6-8] These reports heralded the beginning of a new era in cardiac surgery. Potts and Waterston created operations for surgical anastomosis between the aorta and a pulmonary artery, pallative procedures for cyanotic congenital heart disease.[9, 10] Brock devised a surgical technique for treating pulmonic stenosis by valvotomy through the pulmonary artery without bypass.[11] Blalock and Hanlon reported a technique for surgical creation of an atrial septostomy for increased intracardiac mixing in patients with transposition of the great vessels.[12]

The realization that surgical procedures were being developed for complete physiologic correction of congenital cardiac defects stimulated development of pediatric cardiac catheterization and angiography. A major contribution was the pioneering work of Rudolph in studying newborn infants with suspected congenital heart disease.[13, 14]

Following the early success of palliative procedures, more aggressive techniques were developed. Lillehei successfully performed cardiac surgery in children using a cross-circulation technique.[15] Drew, Lewis, and Swan demonstrated the efficacy of deep hypothermia for cardiac surgery.[16-18] Gibbon performed the first successful open-heart procedure with the assistance of cardiopulmonary bypass in 1953 on an 18-year-old girl with a large atrial septal defect.[19] Subsequently, a steady stream of surgical triumphs utilizing new innovative surgical techniques transformed the outlook for infants and children with congenital heart disease from despair to optimism.[20-32]

Anesthesiologists have responded to the challenge to develop methods for operating room anesthesia and intensive care that allow the surgeons to work successfully on severely ill patients.[33-44] The least difficult has been the selection of anesthetic agents and techniques. The most difficult has been the creation of an appropriate operating room environment with emphasis on temperature control, maintenance of an appropriate acid-base balance, regulation of fluid and electrolyte balance, regulation of ventilation and oxygenation, and intensive care monitoring.[45]

PEDIATRIC CARDIAC ANESTHESIA: SPECIAL CONCERNS

Pediatric patients undergoing cardiac anesthesia differ from adult cardiac patients in physiology, anatomy, and the disease entities involved. Of particular interest is the variation of cardiac output, heart rate, and blood pressure with age. The higher metabolic rate leads to an increased cardiac index and heart rate in the neonate and child. Cardiac output

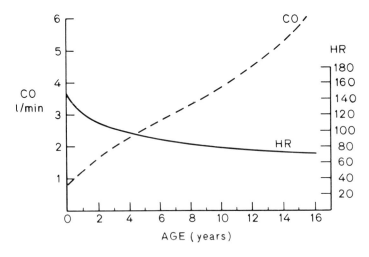

Fig. 19–1. The effect of age on cardiac output and heart rate. (Modified from Rudolph AM: Congenital Diseases of the Heart p 27. Chicago, Year Book Medical Publishers, 1974)

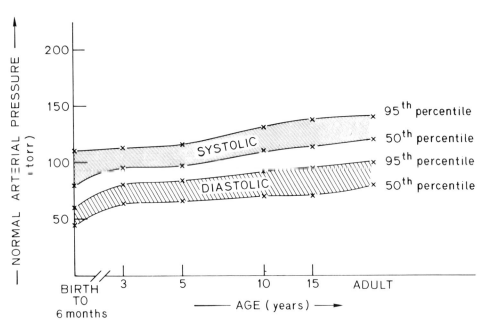

Fig. 19–2. Arterial pressure norms versus age. (Modified from Rudolph AM: p 1485. New York, Appleton–Century Crofts, 1977)

increases and heart rate descreases with age (Fig. 19-1). Arterial pressure, on the other hand, increases with age (Fig. 19-2). The blood volume as a fraction of body mass varies in the first 2 years, gradually decreasing from 8.5 to 10 percent of body weight at birth to 7 percent at 2 years of age. Hemoglobin and hematocrit changes with age are shown in Table 19-1. The red cell mass:blood volume ratio changes as fetal hemoglobin is replaced by adult hemoglobin in the first 6 months of life. This process of replacement also leads to a significant shift in hemoglobin saturation versus pO_2 (Fig. 19-3).

Temperature regulation is a major concern in the pediatric patient. Because hypothermia is part of the surgical armamentarium, the rate of cooling and warming must be controlled.[46–51] But the newborn infant has little ability to control body temperature. This difficulty is accentuated in the presence of a decreased cardiac output or hypovolemia leading to peripheral vasoconstriction. Hypothermia interacts with metabolic acidosis and pulmonary blood flow to increase pulmonary vascular resistance.[52] It should be avoided except when used to decrease tissue oxygen consumption.

Pediatric patients differ from adults in their psychological reactions to hospitalization, anesthesia, and surgery. Greater preparation is required for successful surgery and postoperative intensive care. Pediatric cardiac patients (and their parents) suffer from the chronic anxiety of a prolonged debilitating and restricting illness associated with a shortened life expectancy.[53, 54] It is logical that special attention should be given to their psychological needs. Although the studies are not definitive, some suggest anxiety may contribute to a poor prognosis in these patients.[55]

The cardiovascular abnormalities requiring surgery usually differ from those of adults. Whereas adult cardiovascular surgery is mainly the treatment of coronary artery disease and left-sided valvular abnormalities, pediatric cardiac surgery is usually concerned with the treatment of congenital, rheumatic, and endocardial heart disease. In recent years, the rheumatic and endocardial lesions have decreased in frequency, leaving the congenital lesions as the most common concern.

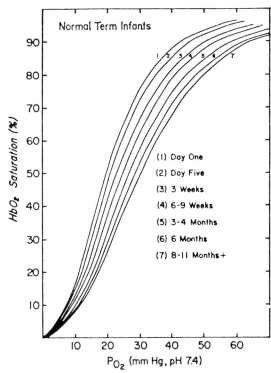

Fig. 19–3. Hemoglobin saturation versus arterial PO₂. Oxygen equilibrium curves of blood from term infants at different postnatal ages; each curve represents the mean value of the infants studied in each age group. (Delivoria et al: Pediatr Res 5:235, 1971)

Table 19-1. Normal Blood Values of Infants and Children

AGE	HEMOGLOBIN (g/dl)	HEMATOCRIT PRCV/100 ml (means)
Birth (cord values)	13.6–19.6	56.6
1 day	21.2	56.1
1 week	19.6	52.7
4 weeks	15.6	44.6
2 months	13.3	38.9
6 months	12.3	36.2
1 year	11.6	35.2
2 years	11.7	35.5
4 years	12.6	37.1
8 years	12.9	38.9
10–12 years	13.0	39.0

(Smith CH: Blood Diseases of Infancy and Childhood, ed 3, p 16. St. Louis, CV Mosby 1972)

These lesions are intra- and extracardiac shunts, valvular abnormalities, and inappropriate connections between the great arteries and veins and the heart. The physiologic problems involve arterial oxygen content, cardiac output, and pulmonary blood flow.

All of these differences affect the selection of the most appropriate environment for administration of anesthesia.

PREOPERATIVE PREPARATION OF PATIENT AND FAMILY

Preparation of the pediatric patient for cardiac anesthesia begins with a detailed review of the patient's history and diagnostic evaluation. By the time the anesthesiologist evaluates the patient, every other preoperative facet of the child's care should be documented, and available for review. Cardiac surgery is a team effort that must be carefully planned, with the plan understood by all of the team members. The best format for review is a weekly conference attended by all team members. The anesthesiologist supplements this information with that obtained from the chart at the time of the preoperative visit.

PHYSIOLOGIC EVALUATION

The preoperative evaluation begins with a determination of the patient's general state of health. Cardiac surgery is a major insult to patients with severely abnormal cardiovascular physiology. Postoperative infection, particularly with foci in the heart and lungs, is a feared complication frequently leading to death.[56] Unless the surgery is an emergency, the presence of infection is an indication for delay. Postponing surgery can be a source of patient stress because the patient and family are on a psychological time-table pointing to a specific surgical date. In addition, the commitment of medical and nursery personnel, postoperative intensive care bed, blood for the surgical procedure, and special operating room equipment is such that changing a surgical date or even the time of the surgery is disruptive. But it is better to be disruptive than to incur an avoidable major complication.

The preoperative evaluation must include a cardiac history stressing growth and development with possible failure to thrive, exercise response, evidence of congestive heart failure, cyanotic episodes, pneumonia, and asthma. The response to hospitalization for previous surgery or cardiac catheterization should be considered. Diet and drugs prescribed should be evaluated. Of particular importance in this respect are digitalis preparations, propanolol, and diuretics.

Evaluation of the cardiovascular and pulmonary status depends on the type of congenital cardiac pathology present, its effect on the patient as a whole, and specifically its effect on the cardiac and pulmonary systems. In order to determine the effect of anesthesia on the patient, one needs a summation of the effects of the anatomic variations on the cardiovascular physiology. The disease may involve a single anatomical shunt (*e.g.*, an atrial or ventricular septal defect) or a complex of abnormalities (*e.g.*, transposition of the great vessels with pulmonic stenosis and a ventricular septal defect).

Congestive heart failure with an increase in pulmonary vascular congestion may be caused by a left-to-right shunt which increases pulmonary blood flow, or obstruction to flow of blood returning from the lungs to the heart because of lesions of the left heart. For a more complete discussion of the pathology of congenital heart disease, the reader is referred to the previous chapter.

The basic questions are (1) is a cyanotic (right-to-left) shunt or a noncyanotic (left-to-right) shunt present? (2) what is the pulmonary blood flow and the pulmonary vascular resistance? (3) can the pulmonary vascular resistance be decreased by altering pulmonary blood flow? (4) will changing systemic or pulmonary vascular resistance or both affect the balance of systemic and pulmonary blood flow (the degree of shunting) or the cardiac output or both significantly? and (5) has congestive heart failure, if present, been controlled by medical therapy?

PSYCHOLOGIC EVALUATION

Psychological preparation of the patient and family should begin long before the anesthesiologist meets the family. Children scheduled for cardiac surgery live in an environment of chronic stress. The anesthesiologist enters the picture at a late stage when preoperative anxiety is greatest. A good portion of this anxiety relates to the work of the anesthesiologist: "will I (or, my child) live through the operation and wake up at the end?"

Because of this chronic state of stress, the preoperative visit by the anesthesiologist with the child's parents cannot be completely effective in allaying anxiety, but with care and confidence, reassurance can be provided. This reassurance may have a direct effect on the ease of induction and anesthesia. Present a careful but simple, non-threatening explanation of the role of the anesthesiologist and principles of the anesthetic technique to be used. Explain the events of the day of surgery to the family and, in general terms, the type of anesthesia planned and the concepts to be applied in postoperative care. The child and family may not remember all of the details but they will remember the general tone of the discussion and can be instilled with confidence by the manner in which the presentation is made. Simplicity is helpful. Upon completion of the evaluation of the patient, an anesthetic plan is made and discussed with the family and patient, if he is able to understand.

PREOPERATIVE FEEDING AND FLUID ADMINISTRATION

The decision to withhold oral feedings preoperatively is made on the same basis as for other pediatric patients undergoing surgery. For infants receiving oral feedings every 3 to 4 hours, the last feeding is withheld and the previous feeding is restricted to clear liquids. For children eating three meals a day, there should be a 6-hour *NPO* period.

If the environmental temperature is above normal, if there is a delay in the beginning of surgery, or if the patient has polycythemia, it may be necessary to administer intravenous fluids.

With patients in congestive heart failure, fluid restriction must be managed carefully. These patients may be dehydrated as a result of their preoperative medical preparation. Further dehydration will enhance hypovolemia and further decrease peripheral perfusion increasing the risk of patient injury.

THE NEONATE: SPECIAL CONSIDERATIONS

Infants requiring cardiac surgery require unusual attention. These patients have surgery at an early age because of failure of medical therapy or the concern that irreversible changes will occur to the pulmonary vasculature as a result of abnormally increased pulmonary blood flow. Included in this group are patients with extracardiac and intracardiac lesions. Medical therapy may be directed at treatment of congestive heart failure secondary to left-sided obstructive lesions such as coarctation of the aorta, of right-sided obstructive lesions such as pulmonary stenosis, or of complex lesions which include cyanotic or non-cyanotic shunts such as transposition of the great vessels or total anomalous pulmonary venous return. In recent years, as mortality from cardiac surgery has dropped dramatically, less urgent problems associated with failure to thrive or retardation of growth and development have also been surgically corrected in the first year of life. Included in this last group are patients with ventricular septal defects and tetralogy of Fallot.

A persistent patent ductus arteriosus frequently occurs in premature infants with the respiratory distress syndrome (RDS).[57] Hypoxia and elevated pulmonary vascular resistance are associated with the patent ductus arteriosus. The increased pulmonary vascular resistance causes a right-to-left shunt through the ductus arteriosus, if it is greater than the systemic vascular resistance, a frequent finding in RDS. With treatment, the pulmonary vascular resistance gradually falls to a level below the systemic vascular resistance. The result is closure of the ductus arteriosus or reversal of the shunt (to left-to-right). Cardiac failure may ensue. If medical therapy, including the use of indomethacin, is unsuccessful, ligation is usually recommended.[58, 59] Prompt improvement of pulmonary compliance may not follow the ligation, particularly if chronic pulmonary changes have already occurred.[60]

Particular attention must be paid to the FIO_2 required to maintain the arterial pO_2 in the normal range. An inspired oxygen concentration which leads to an arterial pO_2 of greater than 100 torr for even a short period of time is believed by some authors to predispose these patients to retrolental fibroplasia.[61] Hyperoxia should be avoided during transport as well as during anesthesia.

The infant must be evaluated with reference to blood volume, the ability to place arterial and venous catheters, temperature control, fluid and electrolyte balance, pulmonary compliance, and neurologic status. He may require endotracheal intubation and assisted ventilation in preparation for surgery.

Assessment of blood volume is difficult in the neonate. There is no accurate quantitative means of determining an infant's blood volume on a repetitive basis in a clinical setting. The best methods available are indirect and measure other parameters which blood volume affects. Included in this group are the hematocrit and hemoglobin, central venous pressure, arterial pressure, urine output, and peripheral and pulmonary perfusion. These variables do not give an absolute indication of blood volume, but when considered with the cardiovascular abnormalities present in a given patient, an approximation can be obtained to compare with normal values. It is rarely necessary to change blood volume in these patients before surgery. The exceptions are patients with very low or very high red blood cell volumes. The blood volume may decrease during cardiac catheterization or intensive care because of the operative loss or frequent withdrawal of blood for tests. These changes in blood volume can be minimized with diligent attention to sample volumes.

If the volume is significant, it should be replaced.

PHARMACOLOGIC CONSIDERATIONS

PREOPERATIVE MEDICATION

The anesthetic goal in the immediate preoperative period is to achieve a relaxed non-threatening psychological state. This goal may be difficult to achieve. As noted, the chronic anxiety of the patient can only be partially alleviated by the preoperative visit. Leaving parents and entering the operating room setting increases patient anxiety. The anesthesiologist must choose between the psychic advantages of further sedation or tranquilization, and the cardiac and respiratory side effects of these drugs. Whenever possible, a drug and a dosage should be selected which will minimize respiratory depression, changes in cardiac output or vascular resistance or both, and contribute to tranquilization of the patient. The final determinant is the preference of the anesthesiologist (based on experience), the anesthesia to be used for the induction and maintenance phases of the procedure, and the severity of illness.

Preoperative medication is recommended in all but the most unusual circumstances for patients weighing more than 10 kg or who are more than 1 year of age. Patients weighing less than 10 kg or less than 1 year of age are not usually given preoperative medication (other than atropine). The uncertainty of the response is too great. Because of concern about hypoventilation secondary to the sedative and respiratory depressant effects of premedicant drugs, administration of these drugs should be timed so that the child is in the operating room suite, and under the surveillance of the anesthesia team, *before* the time of maximum drug effect. If a narcotic will be used during the procedure, it should also be used as premedication, so that the dose-response relationship can be evaluated before induction.

Table 19-2. Suggested Premedication for Infants and Children

1. Less than 1 year old or less than 10 kg or both
   a. Atropine intramuscular: 0.02 mg/kg
2. 1 year and older or more than 10 kg or both
   a. Demerol: 1–2 mg/kg intramuscularly, maximum 50 mg
   b. Phenergan (promethazine): 0.51–1 mg/kg intramuscularly, maximum 25 mg
   c. Atropine: 0.02 mg/kg intramuscularly, maximum 0.5 mg

The method of administration and the ability to combine the selected premedication with other drugs is an important factor in selection. Prophylactic antibiotics are often given in the immediate preoperative period. If these drugs are given intramuscularly, one injection for antiobiotics and one injection for premedication is necessary. If the premedication drugs are a combination, than an additional injection may be necessary. Such is the case with the barbiturates and atropine.

Several drug combinations have been recommended.[62] The drug dose should be regulated according to the cardiovascular status of the patient. The critically ill patient requires no premedication. The active child in relatively good health with a stable cardiovascular system needs the upper level of the dose range. My choice is meperidine (1–2 mg/kg) and atropine (0.02 mg/kg), with or without promethazine (0.5–1 mg/kg) (Table 19-2). This choice is based mainly on the work of Eger[63] as well as my own experience during the last 20 years. Meperidine appears to have a limited effect on systemic vascular resistance. It produces sedation and tranquilization, and is a good choice as an agent for maintenance of anesthesia. Meperidine in this dose range is more predictable in its sedative effect than morphine in a dose of 0.1 mg/kg. Promethazine can be added for additional tranquilization if the child is hyperactive. Atropine or glycopyrrolate is given for the antisialic effect. Barbiturates are not used, despite the recommendation of other authors.[64] They cannot be given in the same syringe with atropine. In addition, despite the sedative effect, the patient may awaken just before induction and be disoriented, confused, and anxious.

ANESTHESIA FOR INDUCTION

The induction of anesthesia is often the most physiologically traumatic phase of pediatric anesthesia. Maintenance of the physiologic status quo and/or an increase in systemic oxygenation or both are the anesthesiologists's goals for this phase. Conversely, a decrease in pulmonary blood flow, an increase in right-to-left shunting, or a decrease in the left-sided cardiac output must be avoided. Children with borderline oxygenation and perfusion will have chronic metabolic acidosis, increased systemic vascular resistance, and minimal cardiac reserve. The appropriate induction technique depends on whether or not a shunt is present, the adequacy of pulmonary blood flow, and cardiac output.

The child with cyanotic congenital heart disease has at least partially compensated for his abnormal physiologic state. Severe instability can occur during the induction phase, when physiologic parameters are changed, including vascular resistance, ventilation, intrathoracic pressure, and myocardial contractility. These patients *must* be handled with the utmost diligence and care. *Introduction or enhancement of hypoxia may set up an irreversible downhill cycle of hypoxia, acidosis, and decreased cardiac output.* In particular, decreased cardiac output may reverse a left-to-right shunt or enhance a right-to-left shunt through a disproportionate decrease in systemic pressure, further increasing tissue hypoxia. A rapid induction for its own sake is completely inappropriate.

The most commonly used anesthetic agents for pediatric cardiac anesthesia are halothane, morphine, meperidine, nitrous oxide, and ketamine.

Halothane is a pleasant induction agent but decreases systemic vascular resistance and myocardial contractility. For these reasons, it is a particularly hazardous agent to use with patients with cyanotic congenital heart disease, with acyanotic congenital heart disease with a potentially reversible intracardiac shunt, or with any patient with low cardiac output or impaired contractility. Unfortunately, once a toxic level of an inhalation anesthetic has been administered, excretion through the lungs may be very slow.[65] Halothane, or enflurane, may be appropriate in the patient with good cardiac output and a small VSD or ASD. Enflurane, an inhalation agent recently introduced for general anesthetic use, is similar to halothane in use for cardiac anesthesia. The induction time is prolonged, but arrhythmias are less common. Respiratory depression is more severe. Hepatic toxicity has not proven to be a concern.

Morphine sulfate is used frequently in adults.[66] A factor in its favor is the relatively small effect on myocardial contractility. An undesirable factor in pediatric patients with congenital heart disease is the early reduction in systemic vascular resistance with rapid administration. This reduction, although improving tissue perfusion, may increase right-to-left intracardiac or extracardiac shunting when these abnormal anatomic pathways exist. In addition, morphine is most effective when administered intravenously, a less reliable avenue during induction in the pediatric age group.

Meperidine also has a relatively small effect on myocardial contractility. In the pediatric age group, systemic vascular resistance does not appear to be significantly affected in the usual anesthetic dose range,[67] although this lack of effect has not been well substantiated. Unfortunately, it is most effective when used intravenously and is therefore not suitable as an induction agent unless an intravenous route is available before induction.

Fentanyl has recently achieved popularity as a cardiac anesthetic agent, primarily because of its relatively minimal effect on cardiovascular function.[68] Its use in pediatric cardiac anesthesia closely follows the pattern of meperidine, except for a shorter duration of action.

Nitrous oxide is used frequently as a second anesthetic agent in pediatric anesthesia during induction for general surgery. It is more hazardous in the induction phase of pediatric cardiac anesthesia because of the sudden episodes of hypoxia which can occur in patients with cyanotic or potentially cyanotic heart disease. When shunts and the possibility of air embolism coexist, nitrous oxide increases patient risk. For these reasons, nitrous oxide is not recommended for use with this group of patients. However, it is quite useful in patients who have good contractility and no shunting.

Ketamine, a dissociative anesthetic agent, is also used in cardiac anesthesia.[69–71] In my opinion, it is the current drug of choice for induction of pediatric patients with cyanotic or potentially cyanotic (as with shunt reversal) congenital heart disease. It has little effect on myocardial contractility and is protective of increased right-to-left shunting in cyanotic congenital heart disease, as a result of its tendency to increase systemic vascular resistance.[72, 74] In adults, it enhances sympathetic activity and can increase contractility, cardiac output, blood pressure, and heart rate. It increases myocardial oxygen consumption and pulmonary artery pressure, and may increase systemic vascular resistance.[75, 76] However, its use as an anesthetic agent for pediatric cardiac catheterization and surgery preceded many of the studies of its effect on cardiac physiology. The clinical results have been good, but not carefully documented with physiologic studies.

An intramuscular dose of 10 mg/kg is effective in pediatric patients for 30 to 45 minutes. Its main disadvantage is the postoperative psychological dysfunction that can occur. This effect is obliterated by using sedative or analgesic drugs after induction and in the immediate postoperative period, and by using it only as an induction agent. In order to decrease preoperative anxiety, ketamine should be administered in a quiet section of the operating room suite, before bringing the patient into the operating room.

ANESTHESIA FOR MAINTENANCE

The choice of maintenance anesthesia follows the same philosophy as that for induction, except that intravenous agents are always acceptable. The decision depends on the pathophysiology and plan for postoperative care. In a patient with an acyanotic (left-to-right) shunt (*e.g.*, a simple atrial septal defect with normal pulmonary vascular resistance), inhalation agents such as halothane and enflurane are acceptable. If a cyanotic (right-to-left) shunt is present or potentially present (*e.g.*, transposition of the great vessels or a ventricular septal defect with pulmonary stenosis), then agents which decrease systemic vascular resistance more than pulmonary vascular resistance must be avoided. For this second group, a narcotic such as meperidine or fentanyl is the drug of choice. Additional anesthetic agents are not usually necessary if a dose of meperidine of 1 to 2 mg/kg each 45 minutes is used. Halothane or enflurane can be used for this purpose, but the dose must be carefully titrated.

Postoperative care plans should be reviewed before beginning anesthesia. The most important decision is the time of endotracheal extubation. If extubation will occur before transport, management of maintenance anesthesia is directed to produce an awake patient at that time. But, except for the most minor procedures, which do not require cardiopulmonary bypass, early extubation is not indicated. We recommend never extubating a pediatric cardiac patient in the operating room (see the following chapter for futher discussion).

In the immediate post-bypass period, cardiovascular instability is secondary to the complex relationships between myocardial contractility, cardiac output, vascular resistance, hypothermia, hypovolemia, anesthetic and other drug effects, ventilation, and oxygenation. The patient must be stable for a period before extubation. The ventilatory and oxygenation requirements must be manageable without endotracheal intubation before the endotracheal tube is removed. The anesthetic plan, therefore, is prepared with ex- tubation in the postoperative intensive care unit in mind.

MUSCLE RELAXANTS

The most desirable muscle relaxant has minimal cardiovascular effects with a reasonably long (45 minutes to 1 hour) duration of action, so that complete relaxation can be maintained without frequent redosing. It need not be easily reversible as these patients routinely receive ventilatory support in the immediate postoperative period.

While the concept is simple, the choice is more difficult (see Chap. 10). Succinylcholine, by mimicking acetylcholine at muscarinic and nicotinic receptors, can produce bradycardia. This effect can be blocked by atropine and, clinically at least, appears to either be blocked or weakened by ketamine. Bradycardia must be avoided in neonatal cardiac patients whose cardiac output is rate-dependent because of a nearly fixed stroke volume. With this concept in mind, succinylcholine can be used during induction, provided steps are taken to avoid bradycardia. Its routine use is uncommon.

Until recently, d-tubocurarine was the neuromuscular relaxant agent of choice, despite the associate histamine release and hypotension. Pancuronium bromide is now the preferred muscle relaxant for pediatric cases.[77-79] If given slowly, its only significant physiologic side effect, tachycardia, is minimized. The initial dose is 0.08 to 0.1 mg/kg, intravenously. An added dose of 25 to 50 percent more pancuronium may be required to achieve complete paralysis. Further doses are administered as needed at 30 to 60 minute intervals, depending on the duration of paralysis in the individual patient. Approximately 25 percent of the initial dose is required to maintain muscle relaxation. It is wise to give a prebypass dose equal to the initial dose to avoid inadequate relaxation during bypass. A larger dose may be necessary for adequate relaxation because of dilution caused by the priming volume of the bypass circuit.

CARDIOVASCULAR DRUGS

Cardiotonic drugs should be prepared in the appropriate dosage/ml before the beginning of the case and be immediately available to the anesthesiologist during every phase of the anesthesia (see Table 19-3). If the induction and maintenance of anesthesia are handled properly, these drugs will not be needed during the bypass period, except in the most critically ill patient.

The drugs are delivered most effectively by a quantitative method of infusion independent of the central venous pressure or other drugs being administered through the same line. The drug chosen is prepared in a volume of solution such that it can be delivered at a rate of 2 to 10 microdrops/min (60 microdrops/ml). As an example, if the desired dose is 5 µg/kg-min in a 10 kg child and the concentration of dopamine in the infusion fluid is 800 µg/ml, the infusion rate is 4 microdrops/min. The desired dose in µg/kg-min multiplied by body weight in kilograms, divided by the concentration in micrograms/ml, multiplied by 60 microdrops/ml gives the desired drip rate.

The vasoactive drugs can be divided into those with primary inotropic and chronotropic effects. The most popular pediatric inotropic agents are dopamine and isoproterenol. Dopamine is the present drug of choice.[80] Its recommended dose range is 1 to 10 µg/kg/min. At that dose level, in addition to its adrenergic action, dopamine selectively reduces the renal and mesenteric vascular resistance. It may be contraindicated in patients with a fixed increased pulmonary vascular resistance, or when a possible increase in heart rate must be avoided.

Table 19-3. Cardiovascular Drugs*

NAME	IV DOSE RANGE
Calcium chloride	20 mg/kg/dose
Dopamine	1–10 µg/kg/min
Epinephrine hydrochloride	0.1–1.0 µg/kg/min
Isoproterenol	1–12 µg/kg/min
Sodium nitroprusside	1–12 µg/kg/min

*See also chapters 11 and 12.

Isoproterenol has both chronotropic and inotropic effects and, thus, may be of value in the neonate with decreased cardiac output and a slow heart rate. Infants have relatively fixed stroke volumes and increase or decrease their cardiac outputs by changing heart rate. The appropriate starting dose range for isoproterenol is 0.1 µg/kg/min.[81]

MONITORING TECHNIQUES

Careful evaluation of the patient's clinical condition is mandatory. The tentative decisions as to monitoring techniques are made during the preoperative visit. Monitoring begins when the patient enters the operating room area, and continues through each phase of the anesthesia/surgical procedure. It ends for the operating room anesthesiologist after the patient has arrived in the postoperative intensive care unit. Whenever possible, direct but noninvasive monitoring is preferred to avoid unnecessary delays in obtaining significant information, reduce the incidence of artifacts, and reduce the risk to the patient. The anesthesiologist's eyes, ears, hands, and brain remain the primary source of information. The most likely causes of anesthetic catastrophies are simple problems buried in a complex environment.[82]

CARDIOVASCULAR CONSIDERATIONS

The intent of pediatric cardiovascular monitoring is to ensure optimal tissue perfusion of all organs through careful observation and appropriate regulation of the systems involved. The simplest techniques are the precordial stethoscope, digital palpation of the peripheral pulse, visual evaluation of skin color and tissue perfusion, and visual evaluation of cardiac function when the thoracic cavity is open. Slightly more complex techniques include cuff and Doppler blood pressure measurement, the ECG, and finger pulse plethysmography. The most complex techniques used routinely in clinical situations are on-line monitoring of arterial and central venous pressures. Most of these techniques are appropriate in every pediatric cardiac surgery procedure. The intent is to utilize the best tools available to acquire needed information for patient management.

INSERTION OF VASCULAR LINES

One of the greatest challenges of pediatric anesthesia is the insertion of a catheter into a small vascular channel, perhaps not even palpable or visible through the skin.

Peripheral venous catheterization is accomplished after the patient is asleep unless the patient is either a neonate, critically ill, or older than 6 to 8 years of age. With the use of a tourniquet, the dorsa of the hands and feet are examined and the most easily cannulated vein chosen. If a suitable vein is not found at one of those sites, the saphenous vein may be palpable at the ankle, or an external jugular vein may be visible in the neck.

There are several different techniques for inserting a cannula into the peripheral vein of an infant or child. The one chosen will depend on the personal experience of the anesthesiologist. The general considerations are summarized below.

The insertion of an arterial catheter is also a challenge, but is associated with a high success rate with proper technique.[83-87] If the catheter cannot be placed within a reasonable period of time by a percutaneous method, it should be placed by surgical cutdown. The radial artery is usually best.

The chosen extremity should be immobilized before attempting cannulation. Palpate the artery with one hand and insert the catheter with the other at a 45° angle into and through the artery (Fig. 19-4a). With the stylus of the catheter at least partially removed, withdraw the catheter slowly (Fig. 19-4b). When a pulsating stream of blood is encountered, advance the catheter slowly. Multiple attempts may be needed to hit the artery with the catheter and then the catheter may not advance satisfactorily. If a hematoma develops, discontinue the attempt. If either of the above problems occur, perform surgical cutdown of the artery or percutaneous cannu-

General Rules for Peripheral Venous Catheterization

1. It is *essential* that the intravenous set-up not have any *air bubbles*. Search for bubbles several times.
2. Place the hand on a splint or armboard before inserting the catheter.
3. Do not try to put the largest possible catheter into a vein. The success rate will be higher if you do not. Size 20–22 French catheters are usually adequate.
4. Avoid forcing the catheter forward in the vein. Forcing it against resistance leads to infiltration. The catheter can be secured when barely in the vein. A muscle relaxant can be given and the anesthesiologist can progress to the next phase without undue delay.
5. If the catheter passes through a vein, an attempt to reinsert the catheter by pulling it back first will fail. Look for another vein.

lation of another artery. Use size 22 French catheters for infants and Size 20–22 French catheters for patients 1 year of age or older.

To perform the cutdown, make a transverse incision over the artery. Expose the artery by blunt dissection using a curved hemostat, avoiding traumatization of the artery because spasm will occur. Any attached veins are separated from the artery. Two nylon sutures are gently looped around the artery to enhance exposure. Introduce the catheter into the artery, remove the inner needle, and advance the catheter. After connecting the catheter to a monitoring line, the wound is closed and covered with a sterile dressing. With this technique, ligation of the distal portion of the artery is contraindicated. Occlusion for control of bleeding is no more necessary than with the percutaneous technique.

As with the peripheral venous catheter, the catheter *must* be free of gas bubbles. A heparinized saline solution (1 unit heparin/ml) is used to flush the line, preferably with a continuous technique. Flushing should be kept to a minimum to avoid arterial spasm. An infusion rate of 2 ml/hour is recommended. Blood withdrawn as the wash sample should not be inserted into the artery, because microemboli may be thus injected. The catheter, the arterial line, and their interconnections *must* be secured firmly with tape to avoid

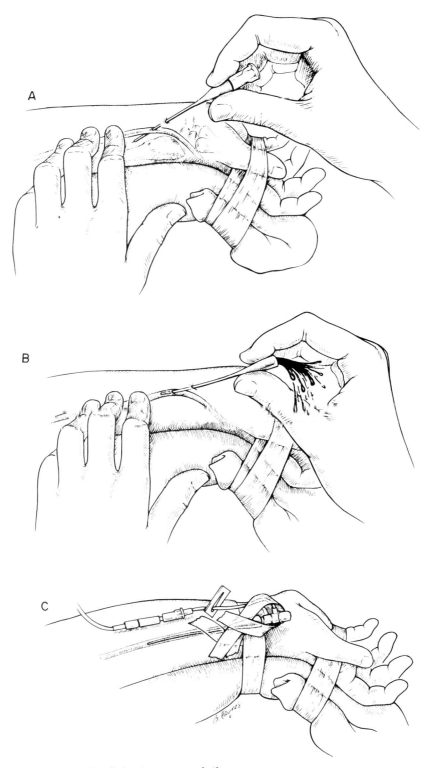

Fig. 19–4. Radial artery cannulation.

accidental disconnection. The splint should be left attached to avoid arterial spasm caused by movement of the catheter in the artery (Fig. 19-4c). With these precautions, the catheter will usually remain patent for at least 3 to 4 days and may continue to function for 2 weeks.

The insertion of the central venous catheter is accomplished by cannulation of an external or internal jugular vein.[88-90] If an external jugular vein is visible, it should be tried first because the chance of a complication is presumed to be less than with an internal jugular vein. The right side is preferred because passage of a catheter into the superior vena cava is more direct. The patient is placed in the Trendelenberg position and the right shoulder pulled caudally. A thin-walled arterial needle is then passed into the vein. A J-wire aimed to the left is passed through the arterial needle and guided into the superior vena cava. The accompanying cannula is then passed over the wire and the cannula secured in place with a skin suture. If cannulation of an external jugular vein is not possible, an attempt to pass a catheter into an internal jugular vein should be made.

For insertion of an internal jugular vein catheter, the patient is placed in the Trendelenberg position with the head turned 45° to the opposite side. The borders of the triangle, the sternocleidomastoid muscle divisions and the clavicle, are defined and the common carotid artery palpated. The internal jugular vein lies just lateral and dorsal to the internal carotid artery, and is usually visible and distinguishable from the artery by its pulsations. Insert the needle in the upper one-third of the triangle just lateral to the artery at a 45° angle. Anticipate entry into the vein in the mid-one-third of the triangle. *The vein is superficial.* If the needle is inserted past the mid-one-third of the triangle and blood has not returned into the syringe, you have missed the vein or gone through it. Withdraw slowly, with mild negative pressure. If you have passed through it, you will observe good blood return. If so, carefully keep the needle position and pass the wire. If it does not go easily, do not force the wire (Fig. 19-5).

The complications which may be encountered with an internal jugular vein catheterization include carotid artery puncture, pneumothorax, and Horner's syndrome.[91] If the carotid artery is entered, the needle should be withdrawn and the vascular puncture site (not the cutaneous puncture site) compressed for 5 minutes. An internal jugular vein catheterization may be attempted on the other side. If a pneumothorax occurs, it may have to be treated immediately if clinical symptoms occur. Horner's syndrome may last weeks, but usually is temporary.

DURING INDUCTION

The anesthetic technique determines how monitoring begins. With intramuscular ketamine, even the simplest monitoring equipment may be applied after the patient is asleep. As previously stated, ketamine in modest doses does not depress cardiac output or cause bradycardia. Modest hypertension does not significantly alter the intraoperative management of the patient. On the other hand, because inhalation anesthetic drugs cause vasodilation and bradycardia and reduce myocardial contractility, application of ECG leads and a blood pressure cuff is mandatory before induction with these agents.

When the patient is anesthetized, a precordial stethoscope, electrocardiographic leads, and a cuff or Doppler blood pressure instrument should be used. It is essential that the blood pressure cuff be the appropriate size for the infant or child to avoid obtaining artifactually high blood pressures. The cuff bladder width must be approximately equal to one-half the circumference of the arm.

A direct arterial pressure monitor is of great value in assessing myocardial contractility, stroke volume, and vascular volume and tone. It is used routinely in pediatric cardiac anesthesia. The arterial line is placed after induction, usually by a second anesthesiologist.

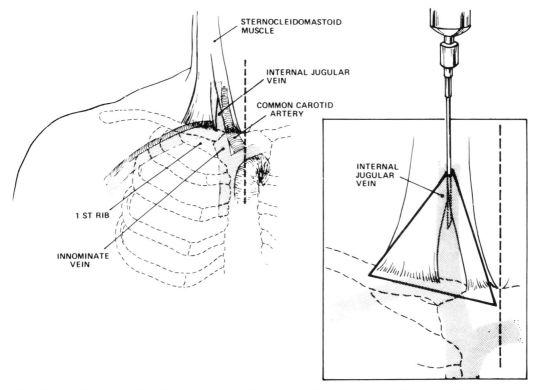

STERNOCLEIDOMASTOID
MUSCLE

INTERNAL JUGULAR
VEIN

COMMON CAROTID
ARTERY

INTERNAL
JUGULAR
VEIN

1 ST RIB

INNOMINATE
VEIN

Fig. 19–5. Diagram of the landmarks used to locate the internal jugular vein. The internal jugular vein lies just behind the sternocleidomastoid muscle within the center of the triangle (*inset*). The common carotid artery is in a posterior (deeper) and medial position in relation to the internal jugular vein. (Prince SR, Sullivan RL, Hackel A: Percutaneous catheterization of the internal jugular vein in infants and children. Anesthesiology 44(2):170–174, 1976)

The central venous (pressure) catheter measures right atrial pressure and is of particular value in the immediate post-bypass and postoperative periods because it provides an indication of the right-sided cardiac volume. The CVP catheter is inserted into the right external or internal jugular vein after endotracheal intubation is accomplished. If right internal jugular vein placement is difficult or unsuccessful, the catheter can be placed in the left internal jugular vein, or under direct vision by the cardiac surgeon. In my opinion, turning to a cutdown or subclavian approach is not acceptable. The hazards outweigh the contribution to monitoring.

Pulmonary artery (Swan–Ganz) catheters are of controversial value in congenital car-

diac surgery. They may pass through the lesion to be corrected, may not pass because of the congenital cardiac abnormalities, or may cause an increased hazard by diminishing an already partially obstructed valve or channel. Their main valve is in patients with nonreactive pulmonary hypertension for monitoring of the pulmonary pressure, cardiac output, and pulmonary vascular resistance during the postoperative period, as in patients with impaired cardiac output.

OXYGENATION/VENTILATION

Patients with cyanotic congenital heart disease frequently have chronic hypoxia and a low systemic cardiac output. These both cause metabolic acidosis. Because of the sensitive relationship between catecholamine excretion, pulmonary and systemic vascular resistance, and acid-base balance, ventilation must be carefully controlled.

The optimal method for monitoring oxygenation in these patients is a continual noninvasive technique, such as cutaneous oxygen tension or transcutaneous hemoglobin saturation. These techniques are difficult in these patients. In the absence of such a technique, the primary technique is direct observation of the color of the blood in the operative site. Remember that if the temperature is less than 23°C, hypoxic blood may be cherry red, an event which could occur during bypass.

Arterial blood gases should be monitored as frequently as possible without compromising other necessary activities. The minimum number of blood gas determinations depends on the ventilatory stability of the patient. There is no fixed rule. Certainly they should be obtained after induction, shortly after beginning and ending bypass, and before transfer to the ICU.

TEMPERATURE

Temperature monitoring is important as an indicator of metabolic requirements and the degree of peripheral vasoconstriction. There is no one true measurement of the body's core temperature during cooling and warming because thermal gradients develop (see Chap. 26). The rectal temperature changes more slowly and thus is not representative of cardiac or cerebral temperatures.[92] Esophageal temperature is more representative of the cardiac and cerebral temperatures but differs from peripheral temperatures. It is affected by pericardial cooling with iced saline solution during bypass. The auditory canal or nasopharyngeal temperature is most representative of the cerebral temperature. Auditory canal measurement may cause traumatic injury to the ear, especially if actually applied to the tympanic membrane (which is unnecessary). A combination of rectal and nasopharyngeal temperature provides the most information with least risk. This com-

bination is particularly valuable during the late bypass and immediate post-bypass periods during rewarming.

The airway temperature should be monitored when using a heated humidified anesthesia circuit, and maintained between 32 and 35°C, to ensure adequate humidification and to avoid accumulation of mucous secretions in the endotracheal tube.

AIRWAY MANAGEMENT

GENERAL

The anesthesia system chosen depends on the pediatric anesthesia circuit(s) usually used in a given hospital. The criteria for selection are no different than for other pediatric patients. The system chosen should be familiar to the anesthesiologist because it is the lifeline for the child during all but the bypass portion of the procedure. Pediatric anesthesia centers tend to choose a specific anesthesia ventilatory system for all procedures. This decision is largely arbitrary, but better patient care results, by reducing errors.

Humidification of the pediatric anesthesia circuit is necessary to avoid excessive heat loss (warming inspired gas requires only a fraction of the heat of humidification), to prevent postoperative dysfunction, and to avoid dried secretions in the endotracheal tube.[93] Warmed humidified exhaled gas mixing with cooler inhaled gas causes condensation of secretions within the endotracheal tube. These secretions cause an already narrow conduit to become even narrower with increased turbulence and airway resistance. The degree of humidification in an anesthesia circuit cannot be measured readily in the operating room. For this reason, every attempt should be made to deliver 100 percent humidity at an airway temperature which is just below body temperature. This is best accomplished with a heated blow-over humidifier in a nonrebreathing circuit such as the Bain circuit.[94] Significant amounts of water must be vaporized; 100 percent humidity at 20°C is less than 50 percent at 37°C.[95] In the younger child, the airway temperature must be maintained at 32 to 35°C with gas humidified to greater than 90 percent. A margin of thermal safety is created by not heating the gas to 37°C. A circle system with low flow may provide adequate humidification in the older child.

CONTROLLED VENTILATION

Close attention to oxygenation and ventilation is obviously of great importance in these patients. The already cyanotic patient does not tolerate hypoxia. Hyperventilation decreases systemic vascular resistance with a secondary decrease in pulmonary blood flow. Hypoventilation causes a decrease in arterial pH with an increase in pulmonary vascular resistance (and a decrease in pulmonary blood flow). In addition, the relationships between intrathoracic pressure and intratracheal pressure are altered with assisted ventilation. Profound changes in the venous return to the heart may result from increased intrathoracic pressure. For example, with cyanotic heart disease and decreased pulmonary blood flow but normal or above normal pulmonary compliance, a continuous distending pressure greater than 3 cmH$_2$O, an end-inspiratory pressure greater than 20 cmH$_2$O, or a prolonged inspiratory time is likely to obstruct venous blood return to the heart and decrease cardiac output.

The anesthesiologist is faced with a different set of problems if the pulmonary vascular pressures are increased as a result of a left-sided obstructive lesion or a large left-to-right shunt. In that case, pulmonary compliance is less than normal. Increased end-inspiratory and continuous distending pressure will be necessary to achieve a normal functional residual capacity and adequate ventilation. The increased end-inspiratory pressure, if not excessive, does not cause increased intrathoracic pressure. The ventilation technique must therefore be customized to the needs of the patient.

The ventilation and oxygenation variables of importance include the inspiratory and expiratory times, the end-inspiratory and end-expiratory pressures, the inspiratory and expiratory flow rates, and the inspired oxygen concentration. These variables are the same as those for assisted ventilation for any patient undergoing surgery and anesthesia. But because of the interaction of the cardiovascular and pulmonary systems in these patients with congenital heart disease, the fine tuning is more critical.

Perhaps the most important rule is to begin assisted ventilation with a manual technique and determine the ease of ventilation directly with the use of the experienced hand sensor. Pulmonary compliance can be easily determined by squeezing the anesthesia bag, watching the chest (and addominal/diaphragmatic) expansion, monitoring the ventilation system pressure with an in-line pressure gauge, and noting the patient's blood pressure and heart rate. A rational basis for setting of the above-mentioned variables can then be made and the mechanical ventilator set to deliver the prescribed variables. For an infant or a small child with normal pulmonary compliance, inspiratory and expiratory times of 1 and 2 seconds, end-inspiratory and end-expiratory pressures of 20 and 3 cmH$_2$O, and inspiratory and expiratory flow rates of 80 ml/sec are typical. For optimal expansion of the lungs during inspiration, the flow versus time relationship should create a sine wave pattern. For further discussion see the following chapter.

FLUID MANAGEMENT

GENERAL CONCEPTS

The management of intraoperative fluid therapy is difficult at best. The predicted maintenance fluid volume required is a small quantity; drugs must be given and flushed through intravenous lines, of which there are usually two, and the patency of the intra-arterial catheter must be maintained by continuous or intermittent fluid infusion. In order to quantify the volumes given, the intravenous apparatus should have pediatric-sized volumetric chambers. There is no excuse (other than laziness) for not using one of the readily available quantified pediatric intravenous setups. For patients weighing less than 10 kg, the use of infusion pumps are recommended. The sites of drug administration into the intravenous lines should be as close as possible to the catheters to avoid unnecessarily large flush volumes and delayed onset of drug effect. Whenever possible, the peripheral intravenous site should be in an upper extremity, positioned so that the catheter is readily visible to the anesthesiologist during the procedure.

Infants and children undergoing cardiac surgery may be relatively dehydrated secondary to fluid restriction as part of the management of cardiac failure. When it exists, this state of relative dehydration does not *have to be corrected* before the initiation of bypass unless there is clinical evidence of hypovolemia. Partial correction of intravascular volume can be performed under anesthesia provided correction does not adversely alter existing intracardiac shunts, pulmonary blood flow, or cardiac output.

Patients who exhibit polycythemia should have intravenous fluids delivered at an infusion rate which will keep them hydrated, so that the polycythemia is not accentuated. Enhancement of polycythemia increases the viscosity of the blood and increases the likelihood of a thrombotic complication.

The composition of the intravenous fluid (*i.e.*, whether it is a maintenance or a replacement solution) is not of great importance for the older pediatric patient. A maintenance solution such as 5 percent dextrose/0.225 percent normal saline is recommended. If the patient is an infant, a parenteral solution of 10 percent dextrose should be given.

The infusion rate depends on the volume state of the patient. If there is no contraindication to the usual hourly rate of maintenance solution, 4 ml/kg should be given. If the child weighs less than 10 kg, an additional 2 ml/kg should be given. If the child weighs between 10 and 20 kg, an additional 1 ml/kg should be added. Fastidious attention to fluid volume and rate is required to avoid inadvertent administration of excessive volumes of parenteral fluids. The volume of fluid used to administer drugs and flush intravenous and intraarterial lines must be quantified, and included in the calculation of the total volume administered.

THE PREBYPASS PERIOD

The relative size of a patient's blood volume compared to his body weight decreases with age, reaching the adult level at 2 years of age. The hemoglobin and hematocrit also change with age (see Table 19-1).

Congestive heart failure, left-to-right, and right-to-left shunts affect blood volume. Because of the complexity of the pathology in congenital heart disease, each case must be evaluated individually. For this reason, the normal value for blood volume may not apply to these patients. If the patient is prepared and stable preoperatively, one may assume that the blood volume with which the patient comes to the operating room is appropriate for the vascular volume at that time. However, anesthetic agents usually increase vascular volume, requiring volume infusion for stability (see Chap. 2).

If there is a significant blood loss before bypass, with a decrease in the blood pressure or a decrease in the cardiac output, a vascular replacement solution must be given. Whole blood is usually the appropriate choice. An exception is in patients with polycythemia. They should receive nonblood volume expanders (crystalloid solutions).

INTRAOPERATIVE CONSIDERATIONS

PREBYPASS

In the 10- to 15-minute period before cardiopulmonary bypass, preparations should be completed for management during bypass. The following matters must be considered. During bypass, the circulating blood volumes of the patient and bypass equipment are combined. Anesthetic and muscle relaxant drugs administered during this period, if given in the usual dosage, are diluted, decreasing their effects. The body temperature is lowered, changing the effects of administered drugs. It is wise to administer anesthetic drugs and muscle relaxants at the beginning of the bypass period, immediately before (within 1–2 minutes) to the initiation of bypass to minimize acute effects during the onset of bypass (see Chap. 14). The anesthetic drug(s) selected should have minimal effects on myocardial contractility and vascular resistance in their usual dosage, and should be given just before going on bypass. Careful observation of the patient is required while going on bypass and immediately thereafter to determine whether the dose administration has been correct. Diaphragmatic respiratory movements are a good indication of too light anesthesia, inadequate muscle relaxation, or excessive P_{CO_2} in the bypass circuit. Remember that movement at this stage rarely increases patient risk or compromises the surgical result, and is often a sign of the need to alter physiologic (*not* anesthetic) management.

Utilization of the ACT test for adequate anticoagulation during bypass has become popular in the past few years.[96] The control ACT value is obtained from the CVP line. If a CVP line is not available as may be the case with pediatric patients, the control value cannot be measured accurately unless the surgeon provides a sample. The heparin is given into the right atrium to reduce the possibility of local sequestration (see Chaps. 13, 14, and 24). The dose should give an ACT five times control. Typically 300–400 units/kg are required (3–4 mg/kg).

In order to accomplish drainage of the blood returning to the right atrium through the inferior and superior venae cavae, to the bypass system, a cannula is placed in each of the cavae through an incision made in the right atrial wall. The cannulae must be inserted with care to avoid obstruction to flow to the heart before and during bypass. If there is obstruction to flow before bypass, the decreased venous return will reduce cardiac output. This drop is readily detected by monitoring the heart rate and arterial pressure. A fall in cardiac output may also occur

as a result of patient exsanguination to fill the vena caval and aortic cannulae. It is surprising how infrequently a fall in cardiac output from this cause occurs. As much as 50 ml of the patient's blood may be used to fill the cannulae.

If there is adequate venous return to the heart around the cannulae before bypass and the cardiac output is decreased, additional vascular volume or placing the patient in the Trendelenberg position may be of help. The most efficient maneuver is to connect the cannulae to the bypass system and go immediately on bypass. If the onset of bypass is delayed, this volume should be replaced, *even if* the patient appears stable.

BYPASS

During bypass, the anesthesiologist must monitor bypass perfusion and its impact on the patient, as well as the surgery. The reader is referred to Chapter 14 for a general discussion. Here we emphasize differences associated with the pediatric patient. Venous drainage into the bypass system should provide continuous flow without obstruction or interruption. Before fibrillating or opening the heart, tapes placed around the vena cavae cannulae may be tightened, forcing all of the vena caval blood into the venous cannulae. If vena caval blood flow is obstructed, the interference with emptying of the venous system will cause secondary changes in perfusion because of a decrease in output and an increase in venous pressure. The anesthesiologist should monitor perfusion of the superior circulation by direct observation of the patient's cranial skin color and suffusion.

The presence of air in the venous cannulae may cause an air lock with diminution or cessation of venous drainage from one or both cannulae. This decrease in venous return will be noted by a decrease in the venous reservoir volume by the perfusionist, but the anesthesiologist can note it first by direct observation of the cannulae.

Assisted ventilation must be continued until total cardiopulmonary bypass is accomplished and there is evidence that oxygenation is adequate. It is wise to continue ventilation until the heart is opened or fibrillated, the umbilical tapes are tightened around the venous cannulae restricting venous return to the heart, or the cardiac surgeon requests a quieter operating field. In any case, assisted ventilation should not be discontinued until it is deemed safe to do so.

Oxygenation of the patient by the bypass machine, particularly in the first 5 minutes, must be monitored closely. There are two ways to do this. First, the color of the blood in the venous and arterial bypass system lines is checked. The differences in the color of the blood in the two lines gives a gross indication of the degree of oxygenation in the oxygenator. The color of the blood in the surgical field will also indicate if adequate oxygenation is occurring unless the patient is very cold. An arterial blood sample should be obtained from the radial artery line after 5 minutes to verify the patient's oxygenation and ventilation status.

Diaphragmatic movement may occur with the initiation of bypass. This movement usually indicates either inadequate anesthesia and muscle relaxation or inadequate ventilation by the bypass system. A sudden rise in the Pa_{CO_2} with the initiation of cardiopulmonary bypass will cause diaphragmatic movement in the presence of otherwise satisfactory muscle relaxation. Inadequate perfusion will also cause acidosis with the same symptom. The mixture of gases being used for bypass ventilation should be checked and changed accordingly. Flow through the venous and arterial bypass catheters should be checked for obstruction. If these are in order, supplementary doses of the anesthetic agent and muscle relaxant should be given and an arterial blood gas sample obtained.

The correct mean arterial pressure during bypass is a source of controversy. Which is the more important variable for adequate perfusion: pressure or flow? In pediatric patients, a flow of 75 ml/kg will provide a bypass perfusion which is in the adequate range. With that flow, one would expect to have a mean arterial pressure during bypass within the expected normal range for the given patient. Unfortunately, physiologic factors other than cardiac output intervene to cause a fall in the mean arterial pressure, particularly in the first phase of bypass. With the initiation of bypass, the mean arterial pressure falls because of the lowered viscosity of the perfusate and peripheral vasodilation. After 10 to 15 minutes, mixing is nearly complete, vasoconstriction begins, and the mean arterial pressure rises. The anesthesiologist should be aware of these expected changes in arterial pressure, monitor them carefully, and respond to exceptions.

There are other causes for a blood pressure decrease with initiation of bypass. An undetected extracardiac left-to-right shunt, either a patent ductus arteriosus or over-developed bronchial collateral circulation, may be the cause. If such an event occurs, blood return to the left side of the heart will increase, causing cardiac dilation, or, if the heart is open, increasing the volume of blood in the surgical field.

Apportioning of the blood between the patient and the bypass machine may be unbalanced. In pediatric patients, this balance is difficult to maintain because of the small blood volume of the patient and the difference between the size of the patient's blood volume and the priming volume of the bypass machine. An imbalance can cause a significant change in the mean arterial pressure.

Obstruction of venous return by kinking of a cannula or an air lock can cause a series of events which will decrease the bypass system output with a resultant decrease in arterial pressure.

And finally, a surgical event may cause sudden blood loss necessitating blood transfusion or a change in the volume of the bypass system.

If a thorough check of the above causes for arterial hypotension is negative, then the anesthesiologist can watch and wait for the mean arterial pressure to gradually increase from its initially low level to a normal level. It is our practice not to attempt to raise a low mean arterial pressure by the use of vasopressors, if the flow and volume are adequate in these patients. Subsequent neurologic evaluation on a clinical basis, although not studied in a scientific manner, has not indicated any resultant problems, and there is no convincing evidence that vasopressor therapy reduces the incidence of renal failure (see Chap. 14).

As with adult bypass patients, serum potassium, hematocrit, platelets, and arterial blood gases should be monitored during bypass.

As noted previously, the patient's temperature should be monitored from several sites. The nasopharyngeal or tympanic membrane temperature will indicate the temperature of the blood circulating to the brain and to the heart if it is perfused. Rectal temperature, even though a core measurement, will give a better indication of peripheral perfusion. During bypass with temperature changes caused by heating or cooling of the blood by the bypass system, the esophageal or nasopharyngeal temperatures will react faster than the rectal temperature.

POST-BYPASS

Immediate Post-bypass Period

The reader is referred to the chapter on adult post-bypass management for a general discussion. We concentrate here on pediatric considerations special to pediatric patients.

The transition time between bypass support and non-bypass support is one of the high-risk periods of the procedure. Many factors interact. The success of the surgeon's efforts to correct the abnormal pathophysiology is tested and the effects of cardiopulmonary bypass on the heart and general body perfusion must be reversed. Bypass should be discontinued as soon as possible to minimize damage to the blood and to improve perfusion by use of the patient's own pump. The core and peripheral body temperatures are usually less than normal (32 to 35°C) at the end of bypass. Because of the low cardiac temperature, myocardial contractility is decreased. The surgical procedure, particularly if a ventriculotomy has been peformed, decreases contractility of the heart.

Air may have entered the coronary artery system and the conduction system may be affected in the surgical repair. Thus, arrhythmias or heart block is likely. Pulmonary hypertension, if persisting after surgical correction, places an added workload on the right heart. The degree of right-sided failure will depend, therefore, on the type of surgical repair and the ability of the heart in its new post-bypass configuration to pump against the existing pulmonary vascular resistance.

Controlled ventilation is reinstituted in the bypass period when the heart is closed and beating, and blood is passing through the pulmonary vascular system. Controlled ventilation during the partial bypass period enhances oxygenation and ventilation, increases the rate of rewarming if the gases are heated and humidified, and assists in the removal of air from the pulmonary and coronary vascular circuits. Manual ventilation is desired rather than mechanical ventilation initially, as the hand is a more flexible and sensitive ventilating instrument. With the use of manual ventilation, the anesthesiologist can readily discern the compliance of the lungs, important information during this transition period. In addition, controlled ventilation can be changed more rapidly with a manual technique, to assist the surgeons as they prepare the heart and its adjacent structures for the post-bypass period. After ending bypass, the ventilatory parameters should be adjusted as noted in the previous discussion for the prebypass period. Oxygenation and ventilation should be monitored with arterial blood gases, and the end tidal CO_2, if a device for that purpose is available.

Supplementation of cardiac action by an inotropic agent (dopamine, isoproterenol, or calcium chloride or all of these) may be needed. Dopamine is administered at a continuous rate of 5 to 10 μg/kg/min if cardiac contractility is decreased. The dopamine infusion should be prepared beforehand and be ready for use through the CVP line before discontinuing bypass. Calcium chloride may be administered in repeated doses of 20 mg/kg to enhance cardiac action. Prophylactic use of calcium chloride to enhance myocardial contractility is controversial.[97–100] The ionized calcium level is decreased during bypass, and administration of calcium chloride will increase myocardial contractility and blood pressure. It will also increase systemic vascular resistance and myocardial oxygen consumption. Administration of this drug may be counterproductive if the main goal is to increase cardiac output. Administration of calcium chloride through a peripheral vein may lead to a severe local tissue reaction and should be avoided.

Heart block may be temporary or permanent. In the presence of hypothermia, temporary heart block cannot be differentiated from permanent heart block. If it persists more than a few minutes, direct electrical pacing of the heart is necessary. A heart rate consistent with the optimal cardiac output for the age and body size of the individual patient is used.

The most important intravenous agent to be administered in the post-bypass period is blood. During this period, the patient should be warming and vasodilating. On the average, one-half of the patient's normal blood volume is administered in the first 4 hours of the post-bypass period. The volume administered is determined by monitoring the mean arterial pressure, the central venous pressure, and the size of the heart (by direct vision). The mean arterial pressure should be kept within the normal range for the patient. The central venous pressure can serve as a guide to whether the patient is full or empty. The anticipated range will depend on the degree of right-sided failure and/or pulmonary hypertension present at the end of the bypass period. *The use of a balance calculation alone is inadequate and can lead to lethal errors.* With left-sided failure, a pulmonary artery catheter would be helpful as a monitoring aid. Unfortunately, because of the complex pathologic anatomy usually encountered in those patients in whom it would be most useful, such catheters are infrequently inserted during surgery.

The post-bypass blood administration setup should be prepared before discontinuing bypass, and *tested* for the ability to ad-

minister large quantifiable volumes of *warm* blood rapidly. The blood will usually be administered through a peripheral vein, so that the central venous pressure catheter can be used for pressure measurements and administration of drugs.

Whole blood obtained less than 48 hours before surgery is requested for postoperative transfusion, so that red cell fragility and microemboli are minimized and coagulation factors are present. Fresh whole blood, less than 2 hours old is ideal.

The control of coagulation mechanisms post-bypass is a three-part effort. Protamine is administered IV in a dose sufficient to restore the ACT to control values, or the lowest obtainable value. This usually requires a protamine dose of approximately 1.2 mg for each 1 mg of heparin received by the patient; however, individual variability is the rule. Residual heparin effect may be double-checked with a thrombin time; a normal thrombin time signifies no heparin effect. An abnormal thrombin time signifies either heparin effect, presence of fibrin split products, or a low or abnormal fibrinogen (Fig. 19-6).

Once the inhibitor heparin has been treated with protamine, an evaluation of coagulation factor levels is continued. A normal ACT or aPTT signifies reasonable factor levels and function. An abnormal ACT, aPTT, or PT, in the presence of a normal thrombin time (no heparin effect), signifies the need for factor administration by fresh frozen plasma administered at 10 ml/kg. Rarely, Factor IX concentrate (Proplex, Konyne) may be required for administration of Factors II, VII, IX, and X in the small patient who cannot receive sufficient intravascular volume factor replacement with fresh frozen plasma (see Chapters 15, 24, and a separate textbook[101] for further details).

Platelets are administered if platelets are deficient in number (platelet count < 80,000/mm³) or deficient in function (bleeding time > 8 minutes). One platelet pack unit is administered for each 10 kg of patient body weight, and the above two tests repeated. Because of platelet storage deficits, the function of administered platelets may not be optimal

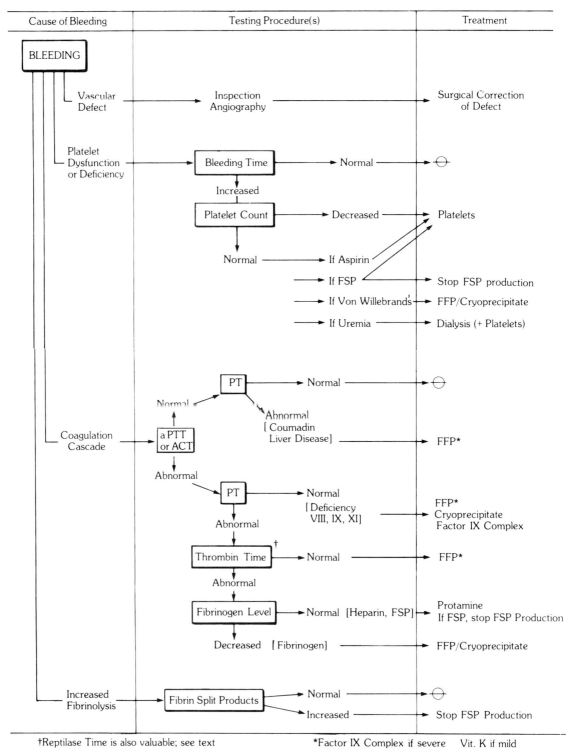

Fig. 19–6. Summary: Analysis and treatment of postbypass bleeding. (From Fischbach DP, Fogdall RP: Coagulation: The Essentials. Baltimore, Williams & Wilkins, 1981)

for several hours. (The reader is referred to the above three sources for further details.)

REMAINING POST-BYPASS PERIOD

During the remainder of the surgery, the emphasis is on life support in the sicker patients. Supplementation of anesthesia or muscle relaxation is not usually required. The healthier patient may require supplementation.

Cardiovascular function should be monitored to optimize cardiac contractility and body perfusion. Cardiac contractility, as viewed directly in the operative field and noted in the arterial pressure recording, is correlated with the central venous pressure, the heart rate, and the core temperatures, and the measurements of pulmonary function and peripheral perfusion. Vasodilating drugs may be helpful in enhancing the normalizing of vascular resistance and intravascular volume. However, vasodilation occurs with rewarming postbypass provided cardiac output is adequate. Because of the small intravascular volumes and the difficulty in maintaining optimal cardiovascular status, rapid changes in vascular resistance should be avoided.

TRANSPORT AND THE POSTOPERATIVE PERIOD

The patient should arrive in the postoperative intensive care unit with as many of the routine procedures required for the postoperative period accomplished as possible. Procedures, at the end of the surgical period before leaving the operating room, include changing the endotracheal tube from oral to nasotracheal and inserting a nasogastric tube.

The oral endotracheal tube can be changed to a nasal tube to facilitate postoperative care. The pediatric patient is more comfortable with a nasotracheal tube. If the anticipated postoperative intubation period is greater than 12 hours or the time cannot be predicted, nasal intubation may be appropriate. If the anticipated postoperative intubation is less than 6 hours, nasal intubation is not recommended. I prefer not to perform nasal intubation at the beginning of the procedure because nasal bleeding before, and particularly during, bypass may occur. Postoperative nasal intubation is avoided if the patient is in a precarious physiologic state or is an infant. Infants tolerate oral intubation better than older pediatric patients and are more sensitive to direct nasal mucosa pressure causing subsequent cosmetic deformities.[102]

The patient must be stable before transport. Cardiovascular stability and hemostasis are usually accomplished in the early postbypass period and maintained for the remainder of the case. If at the end of the operation cardiovascular stability and hemostasis have not been achieved, further time should be spent in the operating room. The patient is moved with less than optimal monitoring and control over the infusion of blood and drugs. The patient transit time between the operating room and intensive care unit should be no longer than 5 to 10 minutes. Adequate monitoring and life support for these patients cannot be sustained easily for longer periods of time.

If the patient is hypovolemic, the movement from the operating table to an intensive care bed will cause a decrease in cardiac output and hypotension. A change in ventilation may cause arrhythmias. Replacement of serum potassium deficits should be completed before the initiation of transport, as the potassium administration rate may change without the anesthesiologist noticing during transport with deleterious results. Active bleeding, either surgical or nonsurgical, will be accentuated during this period.

Specific attention should be directed to using a blood pressure monitoring technique which allows continous monitoring of blood pressure during transport. The technique may allow the use of a transducer or a simple sphygmomanometer connected to the arterial cannula. The smaller the patient, the lower the mean arterial pressure, and the narrower the pulse pressure. In neonates, the transducer technique is recommended.

Monitoring of body temperature is not critical during short transports of older pediatric patients. These patients will continue to re-warm during this period. Neonatal transport is different. These patients, because of their inability to maintain their body temperature, may become hypothermic. This tendency is accentuated by the presence of peripheral vasoconstriction, decreased neurologic tone, and increased muscle relaxation. The postoperative cardiac infant must be transported in a warm, carefully monitored environment.

Our approach to postoperative transport of the newborn infants involves the same techniques as those used for transport, either inter- or intra-hospital, of critically ill neonates at any time.[103] They are transported in portable battery-powered transport incubators which provide a neutral thermal environment while allowing open-type intensive care. A life support module allows ventilation and oxygenation to be controlled and drug or fluid infusion or both to be precise. A monitoring module provides electronic measurement of inspired oxygen concentration, core and skin temperatures, arterial pressure, and ECG and heart rate.[104]

The importance of a careful transition between the operating room setting and the postoperative intensive care unit cannot be stressed too strongly. There must be an appreciation and understanding by the medical and nursing personnel in both areas of each others' roles and the absolute need to communicate meaningful information. The operating room personnel who have spent considerable time monitoring and controlling the cardiovascular physiology of the anesthetized patient have the responsibility to pass on all the information available concerning the patient, and to offer a prediction of the postoperative course. The intensive care unit personnel have the responsibility to listen.

REFERENCES

HISTORICAL NOTES

1. Hilberman M: The evolution of intensive care units. Crit Care Med 3:159–165, 1975

2. Strieder JW et al: Attempt to obliterate a patent ductus arteriosus in a patient with subacute bacterial endocarditis. Am Heart J 15:621–624, 1938

3. Gross RE, Hubbard JP: Surgical ligation of patent ductus arteriosus. JAMA 112:729–731, 1938

4. Tubbs OS, Keele KD: Combined ligation of ductus arteriosus and sulphapyridine therapy in case of influenzal endarteritis. St. Bartholomew's Hospital Journal War Bulletin 1:175–177, 1940

5. Blalock A, Trussig H: Surgical treatment of malformations of the heart in which there is pulmonary atresia. JAMA 128:189–202, 1945

6. Blalock A, Park EA: Surgical treatment of experimental coarctation (atresia) of the aorta. Ann Surg 119:445–456, 1944

7. Crafoord C, Nylin G: Congenital coarctation of the aorta and its surgical treatment. J Thorac Surg 14:347–362, 1945

8. Gross RE, Hufnagel CA: Coarctation of the aorta. N Engl J Med 233:287–293, 1945

9. Potts WJ, Smith S, Gibson S: Anastomosis of the aorta to a pulmonary artery. Certain types in congenital heart disease. JAMA 132:627–631, 1946

10. Waterston DJ: The treatment of Fallot's Tetralogy in infants under the age of one year. Kozhledy v Chirurgii 41:181, 1962

11. Brock RC: Pulmonary valvotomy for the relief of congenital pulmonary stenosis. Br Med J 1:1121–1128, 1948

12. Blalock A, Hanlon CR: The surgical treatment of complete transposition of the aorta and pulmonary artery. Surg Gynecol Obstet 90:1–15, 1950

13. Rudolph AM, Caylor GG: Cardiac catheterization in infants and children. Pediatr Clin North Am 5:907:943, 1958

14. Rudolph AM: Cooperative study on cardiac catheterization: complication occurring in infants and children. Circulation (Suppl III)37:59–66, 1968

15. Lillehei CW et al: Direct vision intracardiac surgery by means of controlled cross circulation or continuous arterial reservoir perfusion for correction of ventricular septal defects, atrioventricular communis, isolated infundibular pulmonic stenosis, and Tetralogy of Fallot. Cardiovascular Surgery, In Lam CR (ed): Henry Ford Hospital International Symposium on Cardiovascular Surgery, Philadelphia, WB Saunders, 1955

16. Drew CE, Keen G, Benazon DB et al: Profound hypothermia. Lancet 1:745–750, 1959
17. Lewis FJ, Taufic M: Closure of atrial septal defects with the aid of hypothermia. Surgery 33:52–59, 1953
18. Swan H: Clinical hypothermia: A lady with a past and some promise for the future. Surgery 73:736–758, 1973
19. Gibbon JH: Application of a mechanical heart and lung apparatus to cardiac surgery. Minn Med 37:171–180, 1954
20. Senning A: Surgical correction of transposition of the great vessels. Surgery 45:966–980, 1959
21. Gerbode F, Johnston JB, Robinson S et al: Endocardial cushion defects: diagnosis and technique of surgical repair. Surg 49:69–76, 1961
22. Shumway NE, Lower RR, Hurley EJ et al: Total surgical correction of Fallot's anomaly. Am J Surg 106:267–272, 1963
23. Mustard WT: Successful two stage correction of transposition of the great vessels. Surgery 55:469–472, 1964
24. Rastelli GC, Ongley PA, Kirklin JW et al: Surgical repair of persistent common atrioventricular canal. J Thorac Cardiovasc Surgery 55:299–308, 1968
25. Starck J, Hucin B, Aberdeen E et al: Cardiac surgery in the first year of life: experience with 1049 patients. Surgery 69:483–497, 1971
26. Barratt–Boyes BG, Neutze JM, Seelye ER et al: Complete correction of cardiovascular malformations in the first year of life. Prog Cardiovasc Dis 15:229–253, 1972
27. Kirklin JW: Advances in Cardiovascular Surgery. New York, Grune & Stratton, 1973
28. Castaneda AR, Lamberti J, Sade RM et al: Open heart surgery during the first three months of life. J Thorac Cardiovasc Surg 68:719–731, 1974
29. Subramanian S: Early correction of congenital cardiac defects using profound hypothermia and circulatory arrest. Ann Coll Surg Engl 54:176–187, 1974
30. Shumway NE, Griepp RB, Stinson EB: Surgical management of transposition of the great arteries. Am J Surg 130:233–236, 1975
31. Sorland SL, Tjonneland S, Hall KV: Transposition of great arteries: Early results of Mustard's operation in pediatric patients. Br Heart J 38:584–588, 1976
32. Coto EO, Norwood WI, Lang P et al: Modified Senning operation for treatment of transposition of the great arteries. J Thorac Cardiovasc Surg 78:721–729, 1979
33. Harmel MH, Lamont A: Anesthesia in the surgical treatment of congenital pulmonic stenosis. Anesthesiology 7:477–498, 1946
34. Adelman MH: Anesthesia in surgery of patent ductus arteriosus. Anesthesiology 9:42–47, 1948
35. McQuiston WO: Anesthetic problems in cardiac surgery in children. Anesthesiology 10:590–600, 1949
36. Harris AJ: Management of anesthesia for congenital heart operations in children. Anesthesiology 11:328–332, 1950
37. Bailey P, Gerbode F, Garlington L: An anesthetic technique for cardiac surgery which utilizes 100% oxygen as the only inhalant. Arch Surg 76:437–440, 1958
38. Adams AK, Parkhouse J: Anesthesia for cardiac catheterization in children. Br J Anaesth 32:69–75, 1960
39. Strong MJ, Keats AS, Cooley DA: Anesthesia for cardiovascular surgery in infancy. Anesthesiology 27:257–265, 1966
40. Moffit EA, Tarhan S, Lundborg RO: Anesthesia for cardiac surgery: Principles and Practice. Anesthesiology 29:1181–1205, 1968
41. Okamura H: Inhalation anesthesia for simple deep hypothermia induced by surface cooling. Med J Osaka Univ 20:29–79, 1969
42. Vaughan RW, Stephen CR: Ketamine for corrective cardiac surgery in children. South Med J 66:1226–1230, 1973
43. Steward DJ, Sloan IA, Johnston AE: Anesthetic management of infants undergoing correction of congenital heart defects. Can Anaesth Soc 21:15–22, 1974
44. Laver MB, Bland JHL: Anesthetic Management of the pediatric patient during open-heart surgery. Int Anesthesiol Clin 13:149–182, 1975
45. Rackow H, Salanitre E: Modern concepts in pediatric anesthesiology. Anesthesiology 30:208–234, 1969

PEDIATRIC CARDIAC ANESTHESIA: SPECIAL CONCERNS

46. Bruck K: Temperature regulation in the newborn infant. Biol Neonate 3:65–119, 1961
47. Adamsons K, Gandy GM, James LS: The influence of thermal factors upon oxygen consumption of the newborn human infant. J Pediatr 66:495–508, 1965

48. Stern L, Lees MH, Leduc J: Environmental temperature, oxygen consumption, and catecholamine excretion in newborn infants. Pediatrics 36:367–373, 1965

49. Silverman WA, Sinclair JC: Temperature regulation of the newborn infant. N Engl J Med 274:92–94, 146–148, 1966

50. Stephen CR, Dent SJ, Hall KD et al: Body temperature regulation during anesthesia in infants and children. JAMA 174:1579–1585, 1969

51. Scopes JW: Metabolic rate and temperature control in the human body. Br Med Bull 22:88–91, 1960

52. Rudolph AM, Yuan S: Response of the pulmonary vasculature to hypoxia and H^+ ion concentration changes. J Clin Invest 45:399–411, 1966

53. Smith RM: Children, hospitals and parents. Anesthesiology 25:461–465, 1963

54. Jackson K: Psychological preparation as a method of reducing the emotional trauma of anesthesia in children. Anesthesiology 12:293–300, 1951

55. Barnes CM, Kenny FM, Call T et al: Measurement in management of anxiety in children for open-heart surgery. Pediatrics 49:250–259, 1972

PREOPERATIVE PREPARATION OF PATIENT AND FAMILY

Physiologic Evaluation

56. Lord JW, Imparato AM, Hackel A et al: Endocarditis complicating open-heart surgery. Circulation 23:489–497, 1961

The Neonate: Special Considerations

57. Siassi B, Emmanouilides G, Cleveland R et al: Patent ductus arteriousus complicating prolonged assisted ventilation in respiratory distress syndrome. J Pediatr 74:11–19, 1969

58. Friedman W, Hirschklav MJ, Printz MP et al: Pharmacologic closure of patent ductus arteriosus in the premature infant. N Engl J Med 295:526–529, 1976

59. Heymann MA, Rudolph AM, Silvermann NH et al: Closure of the ductus arteriosus by inhibition of prostaglandin synthesis. N Engl J Med 295:530–533, 1976

60. Edmunds LH: Surgical management of the ductus arteriosus. Report of the 75th Ross Conference on Pediatric Research, p 86–88. Columbus, OH, Ross Labs, 1978

61. Betts EK, Downes JJ, Schaffer DB et al: Retrolental fibroplasia and oxygen administration during general anesthesia. Anesthesiology 47:518–500, 1977

PHARMACOLOGIC CONSIDERATIONS

Preoperative Medication

62. Smith RM: Anesthesia for infants and children, 4th ed, pp 101–102. St. Louis, CV Mosby, 1980

63. Eger EI, Kraft ID, Keasling HH: A comparison of atropine or scopolamine plus pentobarbital, meperidine, or morphine as pediatric preanesthetic medication. Anesthesiology 22:962–969, 1961

64. Smith RM: Anesthesia for infants and children. 4th ed, pp 101–102. St. Louis, CV Mosby, 1980

Anesthesia for Induction

65. Eger EI: Recovery from anesthesia. In Anesthetic Uptake and Action, pp 229–230. Baltimore, Williams & Wilkins, 1974

66. Lowenstein E, Hallowell P, Levine FH et al: Cardiovascular response to large doses of intravenous morphine in man. N Engl J Med 281:1389–1393, 1969

67. Bailey P, Gerbode F, Garlington L: An anesthetic technique for cardiac surgery which utilizes 100% oxygen as the only inhalant. Arch Surg 76:437–440, 1958

68. Stanley TH, Webster LR: Anesthetic requirements and cardiovascular effects of fentanyl-oxygen and fentanyl-diazepam-oxygen anesthesia in man. Anesth Analg (Cleve) 57:411–416, 1978

69. Vaughan RW, Stephen CR: Ketamine for corrective cardiac surgery in children. South Med J 66:1226–1230, 1973

70. Levin RM, Seleny FL, Streczyn MV: Ketamine-Pancuronium-Narcotic technique for cardiovascular surgery in infants—a comparative study. Anesth Analg (Cleve) 54:800–805, 1975

71. Radnay PA, Arai SH, Nagashima H: Ketamine-gallamine anesthesia for great-vessel operations in infants. Anesth Analg (Cleve) 53:365–369, 1974

72. Dowdy EG: Studies of the mechanism of car-

diovascular response to CI–5. Anesthesiology 29:931–943, 1968

73. Tweed WA, Minuck M et al: Circulatory responses to ketamine anesthesia. Anaesthesia 37:613–619, 1972

74. Taber DL, Wilson RD, Priano II: The effects of beta-adrenergic blockade on the cardiopulmonary response to ketamine. Anesth Analg (Cleve) 49:604–613, 1970

75. Demaster RJ, Fogdall RP: The effects of ketamine on the pulmonary and systemic circulations in patients with coronary artery disease (abstr). Annual meeting of the Am Soc Anesthesiology, Scientific Papers:721–722, 1977

76. Gassner S, Cohen M, Aygen M, Levy E et al: The effect of ketamine on pulmonary artery pressure. Anaesthesia 29:141–146, 1974

Muscle Relaxants

77. Bennett EJ, Daughety MJ, Bowyer DE et al: Pancuronium bromide: Experiences in 100 pediatric patients. Anesth Analg (Cleve) 50:798–807, 1971

78. Nightingale DA, Burh GH: A clinical comparison between tubocurarine and pancuronium in children. Br J Anaesth 45:63–70, 1973

79. Goudsouzian NG, Ryan JF, Savarese JJ: The neuromuscular effects of pancuronium in infants and children. Anesthesiology 41:95–98, 1974

Cardiovascular Drugs

80. Driscoll DJ, Gillette PC, Duff DF et al: The hemodynamic effect of dopamine in children. J Thorac Cardiovasc Surg 78:765–768, 1979

81. Levin DL, Morriss FC, Moore GC: A practical guide to pediatric intensive care, p 61. St. Louis, CV Mosby, 1979

MONITORING TECHNIQUES

82. Hackel A, Bland JW, Schwartz AJ: Monitoring the pediatric patient. American Society of Anesthesiologists Annual Refresher Course Lectures, No. 220, 1980

Insertion of Vascular Lines

83. McClish A, Benazura A: Prolonged percutaneous radial artery cannulation in infants and children. Annual meeting of the Am Soc Anesthesiology:143, 1971

84. Todres SD, Rogers MC, Shannon DC: Percutaneous catheterization of the radial artery in the critically ill neonate. J Pediatr 87:273–275, 1975

85. Spoerel WE, Deimling P, Aitken R: Direct arterial pressure monitoring from the dorsalis pedia artery. Can Anaesth Soc J 22:91–99, 1975

86. Adams JM, Rudolph AJ: The use of indwelling radial artery catheters in neonates. Pediatrics 55:261–265, 1975

87. Galvis AG, Donahue JS, White JJ: An improved technique for prolonged arterial catheterization in infants and children. Crit Care Med 4:166–169, 1976

88. English ICW, Frew RM, Pigott JF et al: Percutaneous catheterization of the internal jugular vein. Anaesthesia 24:521–531, 1969

89. Prince SR, Sullivan RL, Hackel A: Percutaneous catheterization of the internal jugular vein in infants and children. Anesthesiology 44:170–174, 1976

90. Cote CJ et al: Two approaches to cannulation of a child's internal jugular vein. Anesthesiology 50:371–373, 1979

91. Prince SR, Sullivan RL, Hackel A: Percutaneous catheterization of the internal jugular vein in infants and children. Anesthesiology 44:170–174, 1976

Temperature

92. Molnar GW, Read RC: Studies during open-heart surgery on the special characteristics of rectal temperature. J App Physiol 36:333–336, 1974

AIRWAY MANAGEMENT

General

93. Graff TD: Humidification: Indications and hazards in respiratory therapy. Anesth Analg (Cleve) 54:444–448, 1975

94. Bain JA, Spoerel WE: Flow requirements for a modified mapleson D system during controlled ventilation. Can Anaesthsiol Soc J 20:629–636, 1973

95. MacIntosh R, Mushin WW, Epstein HG: Physics for the anaesthetist, 3rd ed, pp 399–401. Philadelphia, FA Davis, 1963

INTRAOPERATIVE CONSIDERATIONS

Prebypass

96. Hattersley PG: Activated coagulation time of whole blood. JAMA 196:436–440, 1966

POSTBYPASS

97. Drop LS, Laver MB: Low plasma ionized calcium and response to calcium therapy in critically ill man. Anesthesiology 43:300–306, 1975
98. Stanley TH, Isern-Amaral J, Lieu W et al: Peripheral vascular versus direct cardiac effects of calcium. Anesthesiology 45:46–58, 1976
99. Hempelman G, Prepenbroch S, Frerk CHR et al: The effect of calcium gluconate and calcium chloride on cardiac and circulatory parameters. Anaesthetist 27:516–522, 1978

100. Stulz PM, Scheidegger D, Drop LJ et al: Ventricular pump performance during hypocalcemia. J Thorac Cardiovasc Surg 78:185–194, 1979
101. Fischbach DP, Fogdall RP: *Coagulation: The Essentials,* Baltimore, Williams & Wilkins, 1981

TRANSPORT AND THE POSTOPERATIVE PERIOD

102. Baxter RJ, Johnson D. Goetzman BW et al: Cosmetic nasal deformities complicating prolonged nasotracheal intubation in critically ill newborn infants. Pediatrics 55:884–887, 1975
103. Hackel A: A medical transport for the neonate. Anesthesiology 43:258–267, 1975
104. Hackel A: The infant environment and monitoring during air transport. Proceedings of the Mead Johnson Conference on Air Transport, Denver, Colorado, 1978.

20

Care of the Pediatric Patient Following Cardiovascular Surgery

JAMES C. LOOMIS

INTRODUCTION

In the past two decades, the variety of congenital heart lesions amenable to corrective or palliative surgery and the rate of postoperative survival have substantially increased.[1-7] Many factors contributed to these improvements. The immediate postoperative care of the cardiac surgical patient in a specialized intensive care unit is an important step in the overall sequence of surgical management.[8-10] When the surgical procedure produces adequate anatomic correction or palliation, and when intraoperative monitoring and support are optimal, the patient generally does well postoperatively. A high standard of postoperative care speeds recovery and prevents complications. With less favorable anatomic results, intensive care may provide the margin necessary for survival.

REQUIREMENTS

The purpose of an intensive care unit (ICU) is to provide the necessary personnel and equipment in an environment which ensures effective use of these scarce resources. Success depends primarily on the involvement of medical and nursing personnel with interest, training and experience in the care of critically ill infants and children.

The basic requirements for intensive care of infants and children following cardiovascular surgery are listed in Table 20–1.[11-12]

TRANSITION BETWEEN OPERATING ROOM AND ICU

Sudden physiologic changes may occur immediately following surgery, while the patient is being transferred from the operating room to the ICU. Vital functions must be monitored closely, and an anesthesiologist and surgeon should accompany the patient. The minimal acceptable monitoring during transport includes a precordial stethoscope and a means of continually measuring blood pressure, generally a manometer or transducer connected to an arterial catheter. The ECG should be monitored in any patient who has, or is likely to have, an arrhythmia. Fluid, colloid or blood, and resuscitation drugs should accompany the patient. Unless extubated in the operating room, the patient is ventilated with oxygen using either a Mapleson nonrebreathing system, a self-inflating resuscitation bag, or a portable ventilator. Infants should be moved in a transport isolette to maintain body temperature. A source of gas with adjustable oxygen content should be provided for ventilation of premature infants.

A means of accurately infusing drugs, such as a battery-powered portable infusion pump, is desirable for those patients who require inotropic or vasodilator drugs which must be precisely controlled.

The ICU should be notified far enough in advance of the patient's arrival so that preparations can be made. All monitoring systems should be assembled, calibrated, and ready for use. Respiratory support equipment should be in position, checked, and ready for final adjustment.

Those transferring the patient should verify that the appropriate monitors are attached and functioning, that the cardiovascular function is stable, that required drug infusions are appropriate and that ventilation is adequate. The anesthesiologist and surgeon should transmit to the intensive care nurses and to other physicians involved in postoperative care all relevant information regarding the patient's history, anatomic lesion, surgical repair, anesthetic management, other drugs given and anticipated problems. The physician to be called, in case of an emergency or significant change in condition, must be identified.

POSTOPERATIVE MONITORING

MONITORING SYSTEMS EMPLOYED

The most important monitoring technique in the cardiac surgical patient is continuous surveillance by experienced nurses and physicians. The choice of other techniques depends on the patient, the lesion, and the

Table 20-1. Resource Requirements for Pediatric Intensive Care Following Cardiovascular Surgery

NURSING

Numbers

1. 1:1 Nurse-patient ratio immediately postsurgery or during major cardiovascular or respiratory support
2. At least 1:2 nurse-patient ratio for remainder of intensive care stay

Qualifications

1. Training and experience in both pediatric and cardiac surgical nursing
2. Participation in continuing education program

PHYSICIANS

Primary

24-hour immediate availability of physician capable of managing problems or complications (surgeon, intensivist, cardiologist, or other specialist–according to local arrangement)

Consultants

Cardiology, anesthesiology, radiology, clinical pathology, pediatric subspecialties (infectious disease, nephrology, neurology)

PHYSICAL FACILITY

1. Adequate space: 120–150 ft²/bed
2. Environmental control: Temperature, lighting, noise
3. Adequate utilities: Electricity, water, oxygen, air, suction
4. Isolation facilities
5. Traffic control
6. Provision for family visitation and consultation
7. Adequate storage space for equipment and supplies

MONITORING SERVICES AND EQUIPMENT

1. Continuous ECG monitors
2. 2 to 4 pressure channels per patient
3. 24-hour clinical laboratory facilities, including microtechniques
4. Radiology technicians and portable roentgenographic equipment
5. Cardiac output determinations
6. Echocardiography

SUPPORT SERVICES

1. Respiratory therapy: Setup, adjustment and maintenance of ventilators; respiratory therapy and chest physical therapy treatments
2. Biomedical engineering: Maintenance of electronic monitoring equipment
3. Pharmacy: Provision of drugs and special solutions
4. Social services
5. Clerical and logistical services

preferences of the personnel involved (Table 20–2).[13, 14]

ARTERIAL CATHETERS

Meticulous technique is required to use intravascular catheters effectively in infants and small children. Patency of arterial lines is maintained with a continuous infusion of dilute heparinized saline solution.[15, 16] Dressing changes, inspection, and cleaning of insertion sites should be carried out daily. Careful aseptic technique in drawing blood

Table 20-2. Monitoring of Pediatric Patients After Cardiovascular Surgery

IMMEDIATE POSTOPERATIVE PERIOD

All patients
1. Continuous ECG with high and low rate alarms
2. Continuous display of arterial blood pressure with high and low pressure alarms
3. Temperature: Continuous or every hour
4. Intake and output every hour
5. Neurologic status: Simple rating system
6. Arterial blood gases: Every 1 to 4 hours, and with any changes in ventilator settings or clinical condition
7. Blood chemistries (electrolytes, glucose, BUN, calcium, osmolality) and hematologic studies (hematocrit, platelets, PT, PTT) every 4–24 hours (frequency determined by patient condition)
8. Body weight 1–2 times/day
9. Chest film on admission and daily while in ICU

As indicated
1. Central venous pressure monitoring
2. Pulmonary artery catheter for measurement of PAP, PCWP, thermodilution cardiac output, mixed venous blood sampling, derived indices
3. Left atrial catheter
4. Dye dilution cardiac output determinations
5. Echocardiography
6. Transcutaneous PO_2 or O_2 saturation monitors
7. 12-lead ECG for diagnosis of arrhythmias

REMAINDER OF POSTOPERATIVE INTENSIVE CARE
Continuation of the above modalities depends on the patient and his condition; those continued throughout the ICU stay usually include
1. ECG, heart rate, and rhythm
2. Blood pressure (intraarterial or noninvasive measurement)
3. CVP
4. Temperature
5. Intake and output
6. Daily weights
7. Hematocrit, blood chemistries every 4–24 hours
8. Chest radiographs daily
Additional studies or monitoring devices may be indicated by the patient's condition or complications

samples reduces the risk of infection. Avoidance of arterial catheter movement or excessive negative pressure helps to prevent vascular spasm and occlusion.

The incidence of distal vascular complications following peripheral arterial cannulation is low in children.[17] Vasospastic, thrombotic, or embolic complications are probably more common with aortic catheterization through the umbilical artery in neonates. The incidence of complications reported varies with the methods of detection, but clinically significant problems which may include lower extremity, renal, or mesenteric arterial occlusion occur in 3 to 5 percent of patients with umbilical catheters.[18]

The most common vascular complication with prolonged peripheral arterial cannulation seems to be ischemia of the skin secondary to small vessel occlusion.[19] Blanching or discloration of the skin is an indication to remove the catheter to prevent necrosis and sloughing. This complication seems to be most common in patients with low cardiac output or polycythemia.

A more serious complication of peripheral arterial lines is the retrograde flushing of air or clot into the systemic circulation. Cerebral vascular occlusion with hemiplegia has been associated with temporal artery lines.[20] Adequate heparinization, careful exclusion of air or particulate matter from lines, and limitation of the flush volume to 0.1 to 0.2 ml at one time reduce the risk of emboli. Attempts to clear an occluded arterial catheter by vigorous flushing are hazardous.

Despite the potential problems with arterial catheters, long-term arterial cannulation is often helpful, especially in monitoring arterial blood gases (ABGs) in infants with respiratory impairment. Repeated arterial punctures are difficult and time-consuming in these patients. Arterialized capillary heelstick samples are often used as a substitute for arterial blood but are less accurate, particularly for determining PaO_2.[21] In addition, the crying and agitation caused by arterial or heel puncture may significantly change the arterial blood gases from the previous quiet state. Continuous noninvasive monitoring methods such as transcutaneous oxygen electrodes[22] or oximeters[23] may replace invasive blood gas monitoring but, for the present, frequent sampling by an indwelling arterial catheter seems to be the best alternative.

CENTRAL VENOUS CATHETERS

Although specific practices vary from center to center, central venous or atrial catheters are commonly used for monitoring cardiac filling pressures (Table 20–3).[24–27] The risks of inserting and using these catheters in children with congenital heart disease may be substantial, especially with left atrial lines.[28] Any air or particulate matter inadvertently injected into the left atrium may embolize to the systemic circulation, including the coronary or cerebral arteries. The patient with a persistent right-to-left or bidirectional shunt poses a similar risk of paradoxical embolization to the systemic circulation from any venous line. The removal of transthoracic atrial catheters is associated with a small but significant risk of bleeding.

PULMONARY ARTERY CATHETERS

The balloon-tipped, flow-directed pulmonary artery catheter (Swan–Ganz catheter) can provide useful information in a number of situations.[29–31] The frequency of its use in patients with congenital heart disease varies from center to center. Insertion is more difficult in infants and children, even with the smaller size 4 or 5 French catheters. Fluoroscopic control is often needed for accurate placement. Many congenital heart lesions, such as those with right-to-left shunts or right ventricular outflow obstruction, make flow-directed placement of the catheter difficult or impossible. If a pulmonary artery catheter or thermodilution flow probe is to be inserted in a patient with such a lesion, it must usually be placed by the surgeon at operation, either guiding it through the open heart or passing it directly through the wall of the right ventricle or pulmonary outflow tract into the pulmonary artery. Some contend that the risks of pulmonary artery cath-

Table 20-3. Indications for Central Vein or Atrial Cannulation in Pediatric Patients

CENTRAL VENOUS OR RIGHT ATRIAL CATHETER
1. Monitoring of central venous (right atrial) pressure
2. Reliable large-bore venous line (volume replacement, exchange transfusion)
3. Central site for fluid or drug administration
   a. Hypertonic solutions (*e.g.*, hyperalimentation)
   b. Irritating drugs (*e.g.*, calcium chloride)
   c. Vasoactive drugs (inotropes, vasodilators)
4. Site for venous blood sampling without repeated venipuncture
5. Site for indicator injection for cardiac output determinations

LEFT ATRIAL CATHETER
1. Monitoring left heart filling pressure

Indications for Pulmonary Artery Catheterization in Pediatric Patients

1. Monitoring of pulmonary capillary wedge pressure (approximating left heart filling pressure) when right atrial pressure differs significantly from left atrial pressure (*e.g.*, cardiac failure involving predominantly one ventricle
2. Monitoring of pulmonary artery pressure
3. Treatment of increased pulmonary vascular resistance by direct infusion of vasodilator into pulmonary artery
4. Cardiac output determination by thermodilution technique
5. Mixed venous blood sampling

eterization, such as pulmonary embolization or infarction and arrhythmias or valvular damage, are greater in children because of the greater catheter size in relation to the heart and vasculature. However, this has not been well documented.

The risks associated with these monitoring devices are mentioned, not to condemn their use in the pediatric patient, but to emphasize that any invasive monitor should be used with specific indications, not from habit.

ECHOCARDIOGRAPHY

In recent years, improvements in noninvasive techniques, especially echocardiography, have made it possible to evaluate many aspects of cardiac structure and function without resorting to invasive catherization techniques. Though certainly not replacing invasive monitoring methods as yet, echocardiography may provide valuable information about cardiac chamber size, valve function, contractility or residual defects in the postoperative patient.[32, 33]

CARDIOVASCULAR MANAGEMENT

CARDIAC OUTPUT ASSESSMENT

A primary goal in postoperative management is to maintain adequate circulation while the heart recovers from the stress of surgery, cardiopulmonary bypass, and anesthesia. In most patients, the adequacy of circulation can be estimated by relatively simple clinical examinations. If cardiac output is adequate, the blood pressure should be in the normal range. Peripheral pulses should be full and easily palpated. The skin of the extremities should be warm and well perfused, as demonstrated by rapid refill of capillaries following pressure to the skin or nailbed. If blood flow to the kidneys is adequate, urine output should exceed 0.5 to 1 ml/kg/hr, although urine flow may be spuriously increased by the inclusion of mannitol in the bypass pump prime or the use of diuretics postoperatively. Oliguria always suggests diminished renal perfusion.

Inadequate organ perfusion results in a conversion from aerobic to anaerobic metabolism, reflected in the development of metabolic acidosis. Acidosis is a sign of inadequate tissue perfusion until proven otherwise. In the patient who has recovered from the effects of anesthetic drugs, mental status is another sensitive indicator of circulatory adequacy. The alert and oriented patient has adequate cerebral perfusion. Inadequate cerebral blood flow must always be considered in the patient who is somnolent, disoriented, or combative. Agitation should always suggest the possibility of hypoxia or low cardiac output in the child.

When these signs are equivocal or indicate that cardiac output is insufficient, quantitative measurement may be necessary to evaluate circulatory function. Most available methods of measuring cardiac output in children require invasive procedures (Table 20–4).[34] The thermodilution technique is probably the most widely used at present, and provides reasonably good correlation with other techniques (Fig. 20–1).[35–37]

In children with shunt lesions, the systemic and pulmonary blood flow rates are not equal. Therefore, a simple measurement of cardiac output does not adequately describe the functional state of the circulation; one must know both the systemic and pulmonary flow rates. This is not possible with simple thermal or dye dilution cardiac output methods. The techniques of measuring sys-

Table 20-4. Cardiac Output Measurement in Pediatric Patients

COMMONLY USED

Thermodilution
1. Requires quadrilumen pulmonary artery catheter or pulmonary artery thermistor plus central venous line
2. Requires repeated injections of saline or D5W; volume of injectate may become a problem in small, fluid-restricted infants
3. Requires careful technique for accuracy

Dye Dilution (Cardiogreen)
1. Requires central venous or atrial line for injection and an arterial line for sampling
2. Requires removal of significant quantity of blood for each determination (5–20 ml); number of determinations limited in infants or small children.

UNCOMMONLY USED

Fick
1. Requires pulmonary artery catheter for mixed venous blood sampling
2. Requires arterial blood sampling
3. Requires measurement (difficult) or estimation (? accuracy) of oxygen consumption

Arterial Pulse Wave Analysis
1. Requires presence of arterial line (preferably central aortic) for pulse wave
2. Requires computer system for analysis
3. Questionable accuracy in infants and children

Noninvasive Methods
1. Echocardiography: Unproven accuracy
2. Impedance plethysmography: Unproven accuracy

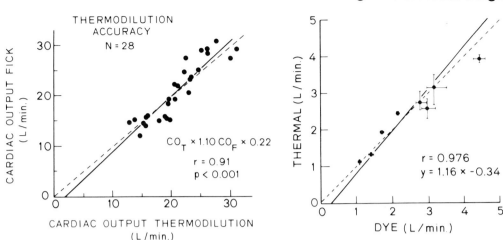

Fig. 20–1. Comparison of thermodilution cardiac output measurement in children with Fick and dye dilution techniques. (Freed MD, Keane JF: Cardiac output measured by thermodilution in infants and children. J Pediatr 92:39–42, 1978; Colgan FJ, Stewart S: An assessment of cardiac output by thermodilution in infants and children following cardiac surgery. Crit Care Med 5:220–225, 1977)

temic and pulmonary blood flow are described in Chapter 4.

Following surgical procedures, plotting a dye-dilution curve may be helpful in determining if a significant residual right-to-left or left-to-right shunt is present (Fig. 20–2).[38]

On a weight basis, cardiac output in normal infants and children is significantly greater than in adults (Fig. 20–3). Normal cardiac output is linearly related to body surface area and approximates 4.5 1/min/m² (Fig. 20–4). A cardiac index of less than 2.0 1/min/m² is inadequate for maintaining perfusion.[39,40] When the cardiac output is low, a number of potential causes must be considered (Table 20–5).

DETERMINANTS OF CARDIAC OUTPUT

Anatomic Structure

The usual congenital heart lesions consist of abnormal connection of cardiac chambers and major vessels, malfunction of one-way valves, or the presence of abnormal obstruction to blood flow. Surgical repair involves anatomic correction of these structural abnormalities (*e.g.*, closure of an abnormal connection or relief of an obstruction). When total correction cannot be achieved, a palliative procedure may be performed in an attempt to improve cardiovascular function until growth or improved general condition allows anatomic correction. For those lesions which cannot be corrected by present techniques, a palliative procedure may allow prolonged survival, perhaps with the development of a corrective operation in the future.

The success of an operative procedure depends upon how closely the function of the repaired heart approximates the normal. This is the single most important factor in determining cardiovascular function postoperatively and the chance of survival.

Excitation and Conduction

A second factor is the integrity of the conduction system. Optimal cardiac function depends on cardiac pacemaker tissue firing at an appropriate rate, and on conduction of the pacemaker impulses to the remainder of the myocardium in a normal sequence. Arrhythmias may result when the normal pacemaker is depressed or when an abnormal pace-

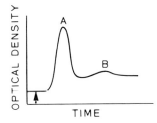

Fig. 20–2. Detection of residual shunts with dye dilution curve. Normal. Injection of indicator dye (indocyanine green) into central venous catheter at arrow. *A* represents initial passage of dye through systemic circulation. *B* represents recirculation.

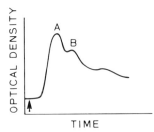

Left-to-right shunt. Injection at arrow. *A* represents initial passage of dye. *B* represents early recirculation peak from dye short-circuiting back through pulmonary circulation.

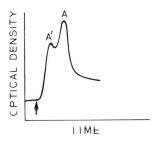

Right-to-left shunt. Injection at arrow. *A'* represents an early peak caused by appearance of dye in the peripheral artery, having entered the left heart directly from the right without passing through the lungs.

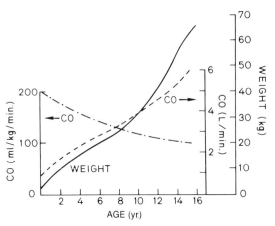

Fig. 20–3. Change in cardiac output, cardiac output relative to weight, and weight, with age. (Rudolph AM: Congenital Diseases of the Heart. Chicago, Year Book Medical Publishers, 1974)

maker focus is unusually irritable. The frequency of myocardial excitation may be too fast or too slow, or abnormal conduction pathways may produce asynchronous myocardial contraction. Factors which may cause postoperative arrhythmias in children include hypoxia, hypercarbia, acidosis, electrolyte abnormalities (especially potassium), inadequate coronary perfusion, surgical injury to the conduction system, irritation of the myocardium by intracardiac catheters, and toxicity of drugs such as digitalis.[41, 42] A search should be made for one of these factors before resorting to nonspecific drug therapy, except when critical depression of cardiac output necessitates urgent treatment.

Bradycardia may result from an abnormally slow supraventricular pacemaker or from a block of atrioventricular conduction. Bradycardia is poorly tolerated in the infant because cardiac output is more rate dependent than in the adult. Hypoxia and severe hypotension are the most frequent causes of profound sinus bradycardia in the infant or young child. Atrioventricular block usually results from surgical trauma to the conduction system, or from digitalis toxicity.[43, 44]

If the heart rate is so slow that cardiac output is impaired and the specific etiology cannot be corrected, then the rate may be increased by the use of drugs or an artificial pacemaker. Atropine increases the frequency of SA node discharge and atrioventricular conduction. Isoproterenol may be used to temporarily increase the rate of discharge of the sinus node in sinus bradycardia, or the ventricular rate in atrioventricular block.

During open-heart procedures, most surgeons place temporary epicardial pacing wires from the right ventricle or atrium through the chest wall to allow artificial pacing. This is especially important for operations which include dissection or suturing in the vicinity of the A-V node or Bundle of His. If wires have not been placed at operation, a

Table 20-5. Factors Determining Cardiac Output and Adequacy of Circulation in Congenital Heart Disease

FUNCTIONAL ANATOMIC STRUCTURE
Anatomy of congenital lesion
Adequacy of surgical correction or palliation
ELECTRICAL ACTIVITY
Site, frequency, and regularity of pacemaker activity
Conduction of electrical impulse to myocardium
Abnormal electrical activity—dysrhythmias
PRELOAD
Adequacy of cardiac filling
AFTERLOAD
Vascular resistance
MYOCARDIAL CONTRACTILITY

temporary transvenous pacemaker wire may be inserted, although this is difficult in the small child. External pacing electrodes or a transthoracic lead may also be used in an emergency.[45] If complete A-V block persists, a permanent pacemaker may be required.[46]

With complete A-V block and a slow ventricular rate, pacing with a ventricular epicardial lead at a faster rate improves cardiac output.[47] Even with normal A-V conduction, treatment of bradycardia by pacing usually increases cardiac output.

Pacing with a ventricular lead sacrifices the effect of atrial contraction. If cardiac output is too low with ventricular pacing, a sequential atrioventricular pacemaker may produce another 10 to 30 percent increase in output.[48] The sequential pacemaker delivers an impulse first to the atrium and then, after a period approximating the normal PR interval, to the ventricle.[49] This requires the placement of both atrial and ventricular leads at the time of surgery.

Tachycardia is extremely common after cardiac surgery, and is generally well tolerated in children unless extreme. In the normal infant, cardiac output increases along with increasing heart rate up to about a frequency of at least 180 to 200/min before being limited by time for diastolic filling. Sinus tachycardia most frequently results from pain or agitation. It may reflect other treatable conditions

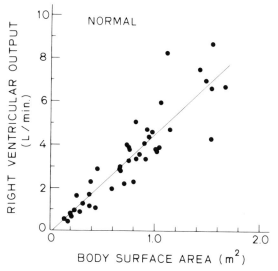

Fig. 20–4. Relation of cardiac output to body surface area. (Moss AJ, Adams FH, Emmanouilides GC: Heart Disease in Infants, Children and Adolescents, p 129. Baltimore, Williams & Wilkins Co 1977)

Table 20-6. Energy Selection for Electrical Cardioversion

ARRHYTHMIAS	INITIAL SHOCK (WATT-SEC)		
	Infant	Child	Adult
Atrial flutter	5	10	10
PAT	10	25	50
Atrial fibrillation	25	50	100
Ventricular tachycardia	5	10	25
Ventricular fibrillation	2–4/kg	2–4/kg	2–4/kg

(Modified from Sade RM, Cosgrove DM, Casteneda AR: Infant and Child Care in Heart Surgery, p 115. Chicago, Year Book Publishers, 1977; Gutgesell HP, Tacker WA, Geddes LA et al: Energy dose for ventricular defibrillation of children. Pediatrics 58:898–901, 1976)

such as fever, hypovolemia, or hypoventilation.

Pathologically fast heart rates may result from a rapidly discharging irritable focus in the atrium, conduction system or ventricle, corresponding to atrial, junctional or ventricular tachycardia. If the cardiac output is severely compromised by a tachyarrhythmia, producing hypotension and signs of poor perfusion, the preferred treatment is immediate electrical cardioversion. A synchronized DC defibrillator is best, with the energy level adjusted to the patient's size and the type of arrhythmia (Table 20-6).[50, 51]

If the hemodynamic status is stable, an effort should be made to determine the type of tachyarrhythmia present.

Supraventricular tachyarrhythmias include atrial flutter or fibrillation with rapid ventricular response, paroxysmal atrial tachycardia and junctional tachycardia. In these types, carotid massage may decrease the rate or convert the heart to a normal rhythm. Slowing of the rate with carotid massage may allow more accurate diagnosis of the arrhythmia by the detection of P waves, flutter waves or fibrillation. When conversion of a supraventricular tachycardia does not occur with carotid massage, digitalis may slow conduction and ventricular response rate. Propranolol (0.01–0.1 mg/kg) may be added if digitalis is ineffective.

Ventricular tachycardia is characterized by abnormal QRS complexes with absent or dissociated P waves. It may be difficult to distinguish ventricular tachycardia from supraventricular tachyarrhythmia with aberrant conduction and abnormal QRS morphology.

Ventricular tachycardia must be treated immediately because this rhythm often grossly impairs cardiac output and may quickly degenerate into ventricular fibrillation. The initial treatment is a bolus of lidocaine (1 mg/kg). If conversion is not immediate, electroshock is indicated.

Ventricular fibrillation inevitably stops effective cardiac contraction. Immediate cardiopulmonary resuscitation and electrical cardioversion are essential.

A summary of the relative efficacy of the most-commonly used pediatric antiarrhythmic drugs is given in Table 20-7.[52, 53]

Preload

Ejection of an adequate stroke volume depends upon the degree of diastolic filling of the ventricle. Under most conditions, stroke volume increases with increased preload until maximum acceptable distention is reached (see Chap. 2).

The most important factor in maintaining adequate preload is the replacement of blood and fluids lost during and after surgery. Assessment of intravascular volume requires accurate measurement of losses, which is difficult during cardiac surgery in children, and monitoring of intracardiac filling pressures. Monitoring of central venous or right atrial pressure is usually adequate, but in some circumstances monitoring of both right and left atrial pressures may be necessary for optimal management.[54, 55] The amount of blood actually administered post-operatively to maintain adequate filling pressure is usually greater than the measured loss, the difference being accounted for by vasodilation with rewarming. Continued blood loss of greater than 10 ml/kg/hour is generally an indication for reexploration of the chest as well as blood replacement and correction of any coagulation disorders.

With good ventricular function, cardiac output should be adequate with right and left atrial pressures of 5 to 12 torr. When the heart functions less efficiently because of impaired contractility or loss of ventricular compliance or both, improved cardiac output can usually be gained by increasing the left-sided filling pressure up to a maximum of 12 to 15 torr.[56] Pulmonary edema generally begins to appear when the left atrial pressure is increased above 18 to 20 torr. It may develop at even lower pressures if the pulmonary capillaries are damaged or plasma colloid osmotic pressure is low. Right atrial pressure may occasionally have to be elevated to 20 to 25 torr to achieve adequate output in the presence of right-heart failure. Markedly elevated right-sided pressure may result in peripheral edema and hepatomegaly, but is less ominous than elevated left-sided pressure.

In general, it is best to give volume supplements in small increments, observing the effect on filling pressure and adequacy of circulation. Choice of the specific fluid or blood component will depend on the character of

losses being replaced, the patient's hematocrit and the possible need for supplementing coagulation factors (see *Blood Components and Coagulation*).

A number of mechanical factors may interfere with filling of the heart even though conventionally measured atrial pressures are normal or elevated. An infrequent but dreaded complication is cardiac tamponade from postoperative bleeding which accumulates in the mediastinum and is not drained because of occluded chest tubes. The blood in the mediastinum restricts cardiac filling and reduces stroke volume. The blood pressure and cardiac output are decreased despite elevated filling pressure. Heart sounds are often muffled and the mediastinum appears widened on the chest film. The treatment is prompt volume replacement to maintain circulation, reopening of the chest, evacuation of accumulated blood, and control of persistent bleeding. If cardiac tamponade is detected early, the patient can usually be taken to the operating room for reexploration of the chest. If severe cardiovascular depression has occurred and does not respond to volume replacement, the chest may have to be opened immediately in the ICU as a lifesaving measure.[57]

Cardiac function may also be impaired by a tension pneumothorax. This interferes with

Table 20-7. Clinical Effectiveness of Antiarrhythmic Drugs*

ARRHYTHMIA	QUINIDINE	PROCAINAMIDE	PROPRANOLOL	DIPHENYLHYDANTOIN	LIDOCAINE
Atrial premature extrasystole	4	4	2	2	2
Paroxysmal atrial tachycardia†	3	3	3	2	2
Atrial flutter	2	2	2	1	1
Atrial fibrillation	4	4	2	1	1
Junctional extrasystoles	3	3	1	1	2
Junctional tachycardia	3	3	1	1	1
Ventricular premature extrasystole	4	4	2	4	4
Ventricular tachycardia	4	4	2	4	4
Digitalis-induced atrial arrhythmia	2	2	3	4	4
Digitalis-induced ventricular arrhythmia	2	2	3	4	4

*4 = Highly effective; 3 = moderate effect; 2 = fairly effective; 1 = poorly effective
†Digitalis, drug of choice
(Moss AJ, Adams FH, Emmanouilides GC: Heart Disease in Infants, Children and Adolescents, p 692. Baltimore, Williams and Williams, 1977)

venous return because of increased intrathoracic pressure or deviation of the mediastinum with compression and kinking of the great vessels (see below).

Excessive airway pressure, either as peak inflating pressure (PIP) or positive end expiratory pressure (PEEP), may interfere with venous return and decrease cardiac output.[58] High airway pressure increases measured filling pressures while the diastolic volume or true preload is decreased. Cardiac output can usually be increased despite elevated intrathoracic pressure by intravascular volume loading.[59] One method of estimating true preload in the presence of high levels of PEEP is the calculation of transmyocardial filling pressure by subtracting intrathoracic pressure (measured from an esophageal balloon or intrapleural catheter) from the pulmonary capillary wedge or left atrial pressure.[60]

Afterload

Another prominent factor influencing cardiac output is the pressure against which the heart must pump blood, the so called *afterload*. A marked increase in the resistance to flow of either the systemic or pulmonary vascular bed may increase the work load of the respective ventricle to the point that it cannot maintain normal cardiac output. As the ventricle fails, it may become overdistended and poorly contractile, further impairing its function.

When the ventricle is functioning marginally or beginning to fail, decreasing the afterload or vascular resistance may improve cardiac output by allowing more efficient ejection of blood and reducing end systolic volume.[61, 62]

Eliminating physiologic factors which tend to increase systemic vascular resistance (*e.g.,* hypothermia, acidosis, hypoxia or pain) may decrease left ventricular afterload. A further reduction may be produced by vasodilator drugs (Table 20–8).[63–72] Most of these drugs affect capacitance vessels as well as resistance vessels. When the heart is overdistended and failing, venodilation and decrease in preload may be helpful. However, if function on the Starling curve has already been optimized, preload should be held constant by volume infusion. Therefore, cardiac filling pressure must be carefully monitored when using a vasodilator drug, and appropriate supplementation of intravascular volume given if preload decreases (see Chap. 2).

When vasodilation with controlled preload does not adequately increase cardiac output, adding an inotrope along with the vasodilator may further improve cardiac function.

Aortic balloon counterpulsation has not been widely applied in pediatric patients, primarily because of technical problems of patient size. In larger children, balloon counterpulsation should be considered for indications similar to those in adults.

Pulmonary hypertension, often with in-

Table 20-8. Systemic Vasodilator Drugs

| MECHANISM OF ACTION | Drug | EFFECT ON | | Toxicity or Adverse effects |
		Arterial Resistance	Capillary and Venous Capacitance	
Vascular smooth muscle relaxants	Sodium*[63] nitroprusside	+ + +	+ + +	Cyanide toxicity in high dose
	Nitroglycerin[64]	+	+ + +	
	Hydralazine*[65]	+ + +	+	Lupus-like syndrome
	Diazoxide[66, 67]	+ + +	−	Hyperglycemia, salt and water retention
Alpha blockers	Prazosin[68, 69]	+ + +	+ +	
	Chlorpromazine*[70]	+ +	+	Sedation; rare extrapyramidal side effects; rare hepatotoxicity
Ganglionic blockers	Phentolamine*[71]	+ + +	+	Flushing, tachycardia
	Trimethaphan*[72]	+ +	+ +	Tachyphylaxis, ileus, urinary retention

*Most commonly used

creased pulmonary vascular resistance, is a frequent complicating factor in patients with congenital heart disease, particularly those with large left-to-right shunts.[73, 74] A significant increase in pulmonary vascular resistance in patients undergoing repair of lesions such as VSD, ASD, PDA, or truncus arteriosus increases the perioperative mortality rate and risk of complications.[75, 76] This is most commonly caused by right ventricular failure secondary to the increased afterload. Part of the increased pulmonary vascular resistance may be reactive or potentially reversible.

In such patients, physiologic factors which increase pulmonary vascular resistance must be carefully avoided. These include hypoxia, hypercarbia, acidosis, excessive airway pressure, and marked sympathetic stimulation. The use of alpha-adrenergic drugs such as norepinephrine, phenylephrine or high doses of dopamine may cause pulmonary vasoconstriction.[77-79] In the newborn infant, hyperventilation to produce a moderate degree of hypocarbia seems to reduce the pulmonary vasoconstriction of persistent fetal circulation.[80]

A wide variety of vasodilating drugs have been tried in an attempt to reduce pulmonary vascular resistance as listed below.[81-100] There is insufficient information at present to indicate that any one is superior. Most of these drugs have vasodilating effects on systemic as well as pulmonary vessels, complicating their use.

Contractility

The ability of the myocardium to pump effectively is another important factor determining postoperative cardiovascular function. In congenital or acquired heart disease, the function of myocardial tissue may be impaired by a myopathy, fibrosis, inflammation or the changes of chronic congestive heart failure. The surgical procedure may involve an incision through the ventricular wall or excision of hypertrophic muscle from the right or left ventricular outflow tracts. Injury to the myocardium itself or to its blood supply interferes with contractility.

Pulmonary Vasodilators

Sodium nitroprusside* [81-83]
Tolazoline* [84-88]
Phentolamine* [89,90]
Hydralazine[91]
Diazoxide[92, 93]
Isoproterenol[94, 95]
Prostaglandins[96-98]
  (PGE, prostacyclin)
Acetyl choline[99, 100]

* Most commonly used

During cardiopulmonary bypass, especially when cross-clamping of the aorta is required, the myocardium may suffer from periods of inadequate perfusion and oxygen supply. A number of methods have been used to protect the myocardium and preserve its functional integrity. These are discussed in Chapter 26. Myocardial function may also be impaired by embolization of air into the coronary arteries, interfering with perfusion.

The contractility of the heart depends on the adequacy of myocardial blood flow and oxygen delivery. There is rarely an anatomic impairment to coronary flow in the pediatric patient unless a coronary artery has anomalous origin[101] or is injured surgically. Myocardial oxygen delivery, therefore, depends on the maintenance of adequate arterial perfusion pressure, oxygenation, and oxygen-carrying capacity of the blood.

Myocardial performance is also temperature dependent, with hypothermia tending to decrease cardiac output. Hypothermia also decreases oxygen consumption proportionally, and for practical purposes, does not grossly impair cardiovascular function unless the body temperature is below 30°C.

When myocardial contractility is impaired to such a degree that cardiac output and tissue perfusion are inadequate despite optimal preload and afterload adjustment, an attempt may be made to increase cardiac output by the use of inotropic drugs.[102, 103] In the immediate postoperative period, it is generally desirable to use short-acting, titratable drugs because the situation may change acutely.

Table 20-9. Catecholamine Infusion in Children

DRUG	CARDIAC OUTPUT	HEART RATE	PERIPHERAL RESISTANCE
Dopamine	↑ ↑ ↑	————dose dependent————	
Isoproternol	↑ ↑ ↑	↑	sl. ↓ or —
Dobutamine	↑ ↑	— or sl. ↑	sl. ↓ or —
Epinephrine	↑ ↑	↑	dose dependent, generally ↑
Norepinephrine	↑ or —	— or ↓	↑

Table 20-10. Dose-response Relationship of Dopamine*

	DOSE		EFFECT
Low dose	1–5	μg/kg/min	β and δ predominate—renal and splanchnic vasodilation; ↑ cardiac output
Medium dose	5–15	μg/kg/min	Mixed α, β, and δ effects— ↑ cardiac output, preservation of renal and splanchnic blood flow, variable increase in systemic vascular resistance
High dose	> 15	μg/kg/min	α effects predominate—vasoconstriction, including renal and splanchnic vessels

*Dose response may vary in infants, who may require a higher dose for an equivalent effect.[112, 113]

When the serum-ionized calcium level is low, as is often the case following cardiopulmonary bypass or massive blood transfusion,[104] administration of calcium has a positive inotropic action on the heart.[105] The effect is transient, lasting approximately 10 to 15 minutes, but may be quite useful when a rapid increase in myocardial contractility is desired. When the ionized calcium concentration is normal or high, administration of calcium may increase systemic vascular resistance and blood pressure without increasing cardiac output.[106]

For a more prolonged, titratable inotropic effect an infusion of a catecholamine is generally chosen (Table 20–9). At present, dopamine is probably the most frequently used inotrope in the postoperative period.[107–110] The cardiovascular effects of this drug vary considerably with the dose infused (Table 20–10). Dopamine has been used extensively in infants and children,[111] but the dose-response relationships have not been investigated fully. Older children seem to respond in a manner quite similar to adults. The myocardium of some newborn animals has been shown to be less sensitive to the effects of dopamine than that of older animals.[112] A study in infants after cardiac surgery suggests that higher doses may be required in

these patients than in adults to increase cardiac output.[113] The potential increase in pulmonary vascular resistance produced by high doses of dopamine may also be a problem in the patient with severe pulmonary hypertension or the newborn who is prone to pulmonary hypertension.[114]

Isoproterenol also may be a useful inotrope in infants and small children because these younger patients tolerate and may benefit from the increase in heart rate it produces. Impairment of coronary artery integrity is rarely a problem in children, so there is less concern for increased myocardial oxygen consumption and potential intramyocardial steal. The increased cardiac output produced by isoproterenol may not be optimally distributed, however, because blood flow may be increased primarily in the skin and muscle rather than in the kidney and other viscera.[115]

Because of the possible insensitivity of the newborn myocardium to dopamine and the potential increase in pulmonary vascular resistance which dopamine may produce, some authorities recommend the use of isoproterenol as the preferred inotrope in the neonate.[116, 117] We usually select dopamine as our initial inotrope, however.

Dobutamine has not been used extensively in children.[118] Its main advantage is purported to be a lesser tendency to increase heart rate or potentiate arrhythmias.[119, 120] Therefore, its selection over isoproterenol may be indicated if tachycardia or dysrhythmias are a problem. In a study of children after cardiac surgery, however, dobutamine appeared to increase cardiac output primarily by increasing heart rate rather than enhancing contractility.[121]

Epinephrine, with both alpha- and beta-adrenergic activity, may be useful when both inotropic and vasopressor effects are needed. In an emergency when arterial pressure is so low that coronary blood flow is impaired, a bolus or short-term infusion of epinephrine may produce the simultaneous increase in blood pressure and cardiac contractility needed to reverse an otherwise self-perpetuating cycle of hypotension and decreasing cardiac output. A low-dose epinephrine infusion may sustain blood pressure over a prolonged period, but the prominent vasoconstrictor effects with higher doses are usually undesirable.

Catecholamines with predominant vasopressor effects such as norepinephrine and phenylephrine are rarely used alone. An increased systemic resistance impairs cardiac output and interferes with optimal distribution of blood flow.

Combining an inotrope and a vasodilator seems to be particularly effective following cardiac surgery. A simultaneous increase in contractility and decrease in afterload may allow even the seriously-compromised myo-cardium to maintain adequate cardiac output during recovery.[122] We commonly use a combination of sodium nitroprusside and dopamine. Other catecholamines with a prominent component of alpha activity may also be more effectively used in combination with a vasodilator, such as nitroprusside or phentolamine.

Continued inotropic support may be needed during a prolonged period of myocardial recovery. This is likely to be the case when the patient is in congestive heart failure preoperatively, when complete surgical correction of the lesion is not possible, or when there is a large ventriculotomy or other major myocardial injury. When extended inotropic support is needed, digitalization or resumption of the preoperative digitalis regimen is indicated. Digoxin is the most commonly-used digitalis preparation in children. Guidelines for its use are given in Table 20-11.[123 – 126]

RESPIRATORY MANAGEMENT

Better respiratory care is a key element in improved survival following cardiovascular surgery.[127] The most important contributions are a greater understanding of respiratory physiology and pathophysiology, the development of specific maneuvers for treating respiratory impairment in the perioperative period, and advances in the technical aspects of

Table 20-11. Use of Digoxin in Pediatric Patients

AGE	TOTAL DIGITALIZING DOSE (μg/kg)		MAINTENANCE DOSE (μg/kg)	
	Parenteral	Oral	Parenteral	Oral
Premature	20–30	30–40	5–8	8–10
Term newborn	30–35	40–50	8–10	10–12
1 mo–2 yr	40–45	50–60	10–12	12–15
2–5 years	30–35	30–50	8–10	10–12
> 5 years	20–30	30–40	6–8	8–10

1. For rapid digitalization, give 1/2 total digitalizing dose (TDD) initially, then 1/4 TDD in 4–8 hr and another 1/4 TDD in 8–16 hr, monitoring for signs of toxicity.
2. Individual sensitivity to digitalis preparations varies considerably; dosage must be adjusted to the patient's response.[123]
3. Accumulation of digoxin or increased sensitivity is likely with renal or hepatic insufficiency, myocarditis, potassium depletion, simultaneous use of quinidine or in the immediate postoperative period.[124]
4. Serum digoxin levels vary more widely in effectively digitalized infants and children (0.9–3.7 ng/ml) than in adults (0.9–1.7 ng/ml). Toxicity is generally indicated by a serum digoxin level greater than 4–5 ng/ml in infants, greater than 3 ng/ml in young children, and greater than 2 ng/ml in older children and adults.[125]
5. Signs of digitalis intoxication may be nonspecific in children and include lethargy, poor feeding, nausea, vomiting, ECG changes, or dysrhythmias.[126]

Table 20-12. Evaluation of Respiratory Function

PHYSICAL EXAMINATION

Color
Respiratory frequency
Signs of respiratory effort or distress: nasal flaring, grunting, retractions, gasping
Chest expansion: depth of respiration, symmetry, I:E ratio
Auscultation
1. Breath sounds: intensity, quality, symmetry
2. Abnormal sounds: stridor, wheezes, rales, rhonchi

RADIOLOGIC EXAMINATION

Chest radiographs
1. Lung expansion and aeration
2. Abnormal densities, masses, or fluid collections
3. Pulmonary vasculature
4. Tube and catheter position
Chest fluoroscopy: diaphragm and chest wall motion

BLOOD GAS ANALYSIS: ARTERIAL OR ARTERIALIZED CAPILLARY SAMPLES

PaO_2, $PaCO_2$, pH
Derived measurements: $AaDO_2$, shunt fraction

NONINVASIVE MEASUREMENTS

End-tidal CO_2
Transcutaneous PO_2
O_2 saturation

PULMONARY FUNCTION TESTING

Simple spirometry: tidal volume, vital capacity
Maximum negative inspiratory pressure (inspiratory force)
Compliance estimates

respiratory care including maintenance of artificial airways, mechanical ventilation, and support of oxygenation.

ASSESSMENT OF RESPIRATORY FUNCTION

Evaluation of respiratory function in the postoperative period entails of a combination of physical, laboratory, and radiographic examinations (Table 20–12).

ANATOMIC AND PHYSIOLOGIC DIFFERENCES IN CHILDREN

The general approach to postoperative respiratory management in the pediatric patient is quite similar to that in the adult (Chapter 16).[128] However, a number of structural (Table 20–13) and functional (Table 20–14) differences between adults and children must be considered.[129–131] The smaller the patient, the more significant these differences become.

CHANGES IN RESPIRATORY FUNCTION AFTER SURGERY

Following a cardiovascular surgical procedure, many changes occur which may adversely affect pulmonary function. A thoracic incision with resulting postoperative pain causes splinting of the chest wall, reduced compliance, and interference with deep breathing and coughing. Decreased lung volume, retention of secretions, small airway closure, atelectasis, and increased intrapulmonary shunting may result. Failure to suction the trachea adequately during surgery or prolonged use of dry anesthetic gases may also result in the retention of thick secretions. Accumulation of blood or serous effusions in the pleural spaces or mediastinum postoperatively may compress the lung and restrict ventilation.

The effects of anesthetic drugs may persist for some time after surgery and adversely affect respiration. Most intravenous and inhalational anesthetic agents are respiratory depressants. They may reduce minute ventilation by decreasing tidal volume or frequency, or may reduce the respiratory drive from hypercarbia. Anesthetic agents and neuromuscular blocking drugs may also abolish normal periodic sighing or deep breathing and may interfere with the ability to maintain and protect the airway.

Some anesthetic agents, vasodilators, and inotropes may alter normal compensatory hypoxic pulmonary vasoconstriction and increase ventilation-perfusion mismatching.[132, 133]

Following intraoperative hypothermia, rewarming to normal body temperature may be delayed considerably beyond the termination of the operation. The body's own efforts to regain normal temperature by nonshivering thermogenesis in the newborn, or

Table 20-13. Structural Differences in Respiratory System of Pediatric Patients

	ANATOMIC CHARACTERISTIC	IMPORTANCE
All pediatric patients	Narrow larynx and trachea	Increased susceptibility to upper airway obstruction from mucosal edema, granulation tissue, and so on
	Short tracheal length	Position of endotracheal tube critical to prevent accidental dislodgement or endobronchial intubation
	Smaller terminal airways and alveoli	Increased tendency to small airway obstruction and alveolar collapse
Infants	Greater dependence on diaphragm for respiratory work	Significant respiratory impairment from interference with movement of diaphragm (phrenic nerve palsy, abdominal distention)
Newborn	Greater elasticity of chest wall	Tendency to retraction of thoracic cage with inspiration; inefficient ventilatory effort
	Increased thickness of muscular layer of wall of pulmonary arterioles; smaller lumina	Increased pulmonary vascular resistance
Premature	Immature central control of respiration	Periodic breathing; apneic episodes
	Surfactant deficiency	Increased surface tension and tendency to atelectasis; respiratory distress syndrome

Table 20-14. Comparisons of Pulmonary Function between Infants and Adults: Normal Values

	INFANT	ADULT
Body weight (kg)	3	70
Oxygen consumption (ml/kg/min)	6	3.5
CO_2 production (ml/kg/min)	6	3
Tidal volume (ml/kg)	6–7	6–7
Respiratory frequency (breaths/min)	30–40	10–15
Minute ventilation (ml/kg/min)	200–250	75–105
Dead space (ml/kg)	2–3.5	~2
Functional residual capacity (ml/kg)	~30	~34
Lung compliance (ml/cmH$_2$O)	4–6	200
Specific compliance (ml/cmH$_2$O/ml)	0.04–0.05	0.07
Airway resistance (cmH$_2$O/1/sec)	18–25	2–3
Arterial blood gases		
PaO$_2$ (torr)	55–85	85–100
PaCO$_2$	35–45	37–44
pH	7.32–7.38	7.37–7.43
Base excess (mEq/l)	−1 to −5	−2 to +2

(Compiled from: Motoyama EK, Cook CD: Respiratory Physiology. In Smith RM (ed): Anesthesia for Infants and Children, ed 4, pp 38–86. St. Louis, CV Mosby 1980;
Doershuk CF, Fisher BJ, Matthews LW et al: Pulmonary Physiology of the Young Child. In Scarpelli E, Auld P (eds): Pulmonary Physiology of the Fetus, Newborn and Child, p 174. Lea & Febiger, Philadelphia, 1975;
Polgar G, Weng TR: Functional development of the respiratory system. Am Rev Resp Dis 120:625–695, 1979)

by shivering in the older child, markedly increase the metabolic rate.[134] Oxygen consumption, carbon dioxide production, minute ventilation, work of breathing, and cardiac output are proportionally increased. This may occur at a time when the cardiorespiratory system is least able to support increased demands.

The functions of the circulatory and respiratory systems are interrelated in a complex manner. Low cardiac output causes an increased functional deadspace and may significantly alter the degree of intrapulmonary shunting or ventilation-perfusion mismatching.[135] When cardiac output is low, oxygen extraction by the tissues is greater, increasing the effect of venous admixture on arterial oxygen tension. To compensate for the metabolic acidosis produced by inadequate tissue perfusion the respiratory system must increase ventilation and carbon dioxide elimination.

Increased left atrial and pulmonary capillary pressure secondary to left ventricular failure may cause increased interstitial lung water, decreased compliance, and increased work of breathing.[136] Even in the absence of overt congestive failure, the infusion of blood, colloid, or crystalloid to increase cardiac filling pressures and improve cardiac output may cause similar changes. With overt pulmonary edema, fluid is extravasated into the alveoli, causing a further decrease in compliance and increase in intrapulmonary shunting.

The excessive pulmonary blood flow in left-to-right shunt lesions leads to ventilation-perfusion imbalance and increases bronchial secretions, potentiating atelectasis and infection. With right-to-left shunt lesions, pulmonary blood flow is diminished, functional dead space increases, and a greater minute ventilation is required to maintain normocarbia.[137, 138]

The effects of cardiopulmonary bypass on postoperative lung function are controversial. Most evidence indicates that a short, well-managed perfusion alone does not have a significant adverse effect on pulmonary function.[139] However, prolonged cardiopulmonary bypass, especially if followed by a low cardiac output state or massive transfusion, may result in pulmonary capillary endothelial damage with increased intrapulmonary shunting and potential for pulmonary edema (see Chap. 14).

PRE- AND INTRAOPERATIVE FACTORS IN RESPIRATORY CARE

Optimal postoperative respiratory care begins in the preoperative period. Certain categories of patients have an increased risk of postoperative respiratory complications or are likely to need prolonged respiratory support.

In some of these children, simple preoperative testing of pulmonary function (e.g., arterial blood gases, basic spirometry) may help with the prediction of postoperative problems and formulation of a treatment plan. Preoperative counseling with the patient and parents should include discussion of the risk of respiratory complications and the possibility of prolonged respiratory support. A program of chest physical therapy begun preoperatively, when the child is alert and free from pain, is more likely to result in cooperation postoperatively. In the patient with preoperative infection or increased secretions, physical therapy may help to expel

---

Patients in Whom Prolonged Respiratory Support May be Anticipated or in Whom Respiratory Complications are Likely

1. Preexisting respiratory disease: respiratory distress syndrome, bronchopulmonary dysplasia, pneumonia, cystic fibrosis
2. Severe congestive heart failure
3. Pulmonary hypertension or pulmonary venous obstruction
4. Severe cyanotic lesions
5. Severe growth retardation (failure to thrive); malnutrition
6. Lesions for which prolonged cardiopulmonary bypass is anticipated or less than optimal hemodynamic results are expected.

secretions, clear the airways, and reduce atelectasis.[140] When the surgical procedure is elective, the presence of a significant respiratory infection is generally cause for delaying the operation.

During the procedure, careful, atraumatic placement of an appropriately sized endotracheal tube, humidification of inspired gases and suctioning of secretions help to prevent postoperative respiratory complications. The potential benefits of constant distending pressure or periodic inflation of the lungs during cardiopulmonary bypass are unproved.[141]

EARLY EXTUBATION VERSUS POSTOPERATIVE RESPIRATORY SUPPORT

The necessity for and optimal duration of elective postoperative endotracheal intubation and mechanical ventilation is also a matter of controversy.[142–144] For patients in good condition preoperatively who have uncomplicated nonbypass (closed) procedures or even simple bypass procedures, the endotracheal tube can usually be removed shortly after the procedure. The patient must be awake enough to maintain a patent airway and to ensure adequate ventilation and oxygenation. The endotracheal tube may be removed in the operating room or soon after arrival in the ICU. We usually prefer the latter because a patent airway and adequate ventilation are assured during transfer. Figure 20–5 presents a flow chart for determining the time for postoperative extubation.

AIRWAY MANAGEMENT

When prolonged support of ventilation is anticipated, a nasotracheal tube is generally inserted in the operating room; an orotracheal tube is usually left in place when early extubation is anticipated. Many prefer the use of oral tubes in newborn infants, even when mechanical ventilation is prolonged.

If an artificial airway is to remain in place for an extended period, the selection of an appropriate type and size of tube is necessary to minimize the incidence of airway complications. Endotracheal tubes should be of minimally reactive, implant-tested, plastic material.[145] Uncuffed tubes are generally used for children of less than 8 to 10 years of age. For older children, low-pressure cuffed tubes similar to those used in adults are recommended. The endotracheal tube should fit easily into the trachea. With an uncuffed tube, a small air leak should be present when airway pressures of 20 to 30 cm H_2O are generated. Proper fixation of the tube with waterproof tape applied to the benzoin-prepared skin is important not only to prevent accidental dislodgement of the tube, but also to prevent trauma to the airway by back-and-forth movement.

The indications for tracheostomy in pediatric patients following cardiac surgery have undergone revision in recent years.[146, 147] While in the past some surgeons performed elective tracheostomy at the time of surgery when postoperative mechanical ventilation was planned, it is now considered safe to maintain endotracheal tubes in place for 7 to 10 days (or longer). Because of the reported high incidence of tracheostomy complications in small infants, many neonatalogists advocate the use of endotracheal tubes in these patients for even 30 days or more if necessary. The relative risks of tracheostomy versus prolonged endotracheal intubation in various age groups with current methods and materials remain incompletely defined.

SUPPORT OF RESPIRATORY FUNCTION

The purpose of postoperative respiratory support is to maintain adequate oxygenation and ventilation during recovery. Respiratory causes of inadequate oxygenation of arterial blood include grossly inadequate ventilation, intrapulmonary shunting, and ventilation-perfusion mismatching. Regardless of the etiology, hypoxia may rapidly produce impairment of cellular function followed by structural damage and cell death. Prevention of hypoxic injury is the first priority in respiratory management.

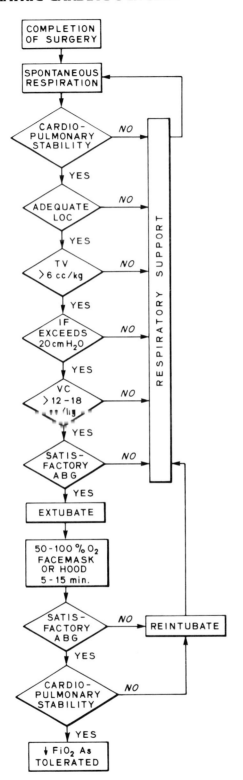

Fig. 20–5. Flow chart used in postoperative decision-making for early extubation. LOC = level of consciousness; TV = tidal volume; IF = inspiratory force; VC = vital capacity. (Modified from Barash PG, Lescovich F, Katz JD et al: Early extubation following pediatric cardiothoracic operations. Ann Thorac Surg 29:230, 1980)

Oxygenation

The most immediately effective maneuver for treating hypoxia in most situations is the administration of an increased inspired oxygen concentration, accompanied by assisted or controlled ventilation. High inspired oxygen concentrations may produce toxic effects to the lung[148-150] or, in the newborn, to the retina.[151, 152] However, concerns about such toxicity should not lead to failure to administer sufficient oxygen because the adverse effects of hypoxia are more rapid and devastating than those of hyperoxia.

In the lung, hyperoxia over a period of hours or days causes decreased compliance, alveolar collapse, increased intrapulmonary shunting, pulmonary edema, intraalveolar exudate, and hyaline membrane formation. An inspired oxygen tension less than 40 to 50 percent appears to be slower to produce pulmonary injury. But in any given patient it is impossible to determine exactly what concentration and duration of supplemental oxygen is safe. Therefore, it is prudent to give only the concentration required for adequate arterial oxygen tension. Arterial oxygen desaturation, as seen in cyanotic congenital heart disease, does not seem to provide protection against pulmonary oxygen toxicity.[153]

Excessive arterial oxygen tension in the premature infant may produce changes in the retinal vasculature which lead to retrolental fibroplasia (RLF) and impaired vision or blindness.[154] This toxic effect appears to be related to arterial rather than inspired oxygen tension. The risk of RLF is highest in the smallest, most immature babies. In tiny premature infants, RLF may occur despite attempts to carefully control blood oxygen tension.[155] RLF has also been reported in immature infants who have never received supplemental oxygen. Any newborn infant should be considered to be at risk of developing RLF until it has reached a gestational age of 44 weeks.[156] Efforts should be made to avoid excessive arterial hyperoxia in infants younger than this. Absolutely safe limits have not been determined for infants of any specific size or gestational age, but the presently accepted standard is that the PaO_2 for term infants to be maintained in the range of 60 to 80 torr and for premature infants, 50 to 70 torr.[157]

When severe intrapulmonary pathology exists, even 100 percent inspired oxygen may not produce adequate arterial oxygenation. In this situation, the addition of constant distending pressure to the lung may reduce intrapulmonary shunting. Constant distending pressure may also reduce the need for prolonged, elevated inspired oxygen concentrations.[158] The mechanism by which positive pressure throughout the respiratory cycle improves arterial oxygenation is not entirely clear, but the primary beneficial effects are probably an increase in functional residual capacity and a decrease in atelectasis and small airway closure.[159]

Although often of benefit, the application of constant distending pressure to the airway may produce detrimental effects as well. The transmission of positive pressure through the lung to the intrathoracic vasculature may decrease venous return, effective intracardiac filling pressure and cardiac output.[160, 161] The proportion of airway pressure transmitted to the vasculature varies with lung compliance (*i.e.*, the stiffer the lung the less transmission of pressure).[162] Elevated intrapulmonary pressure also increases the risk of lung injury, pneumothorax, pneumomediastinum, and interstitial emphysema.[163, 164] The benefits and risks of using constant distending airway pressure in infants and children after cardiac surgery have been debated extensively.[165-169]

Constant distending pressure may be applied to the airway either with spontaneous ventilation (continuous positive airway pressure or CPAP)[170] or in conjunction with mechanical support of ventilation (PEEP).[171] CPAP is generally applied through an endotracheal tube, although modest levels of constant distending pressure may also be applied to infants with nasal prongs,[172] a face mask or a negative-pressure chamber surrounding the chest.[173, 174] When positive-pressure breathing with PEEP is employed for more than very short periods, an endotracheal tube or tracheostomy is virtually always required.

Ventilation

Inadequate ventilation may result from impaired central control of respiration, upper or lower airway obstruction, or inability to do the work of breathing. Hypoventilation of any cause will result in increased carbon dioxide tension in arterial blood and, if severe, hypoxemia as well. The magnitude of arterial pH change with CO_2 retention decreases with time as the kidney compensates for respiratory acidosis by bicarbonate retention.

Hypercarbia and respiratory acidosis may produce sympathetic stimulation with tachycardia and hypertension, an increased susceptibility to cardiac arrhythmias, increased pulmonary vascular resistance and, if severe, depression of cardiac and cerebral function.[175, 176]

Treatment of inadequate ventilation requires a patent airway and a secondary source of work, either manual or mechanical, to produce gas exchange. In the simplest, short-term situation, this consists of manual ventilation with a bag and mask. For longer periods, a mechanical ventilator is employed. A ventilator may be used to assume all work of breathing (controlled ventilation), or the patient may breathe spontaneously with the ventilator supplying part of the work by periodic inflations (intermittent mandatory ventilation or IMV).[177, 178] The IMV principle has been widely used in managing infants with respiratory distress syndrome,[179] and has also been successfully applied with older children. It is the preferred method of ventilatory support in most pediatric centers, and has particular advantage for gradual weaning from ventilatory support.[180]

With IMV, periodic ventilation may be supplied in a regular sequence, or may be synchronized with the patient's spontaneous ventilations by periodically allowing the patient to trigger ventilator breaths by the generation of negative airway pressure (synchronized IMV).

Either controlled ventilation, regular or synchronized IMV may be employed along with PEEP to increase FRC and improve oxygenation.

A wide variety of mechanical ventilators are available for use in infants and children (Table 20–15). They all generate a flow of gas in a controlled manner. Some are pediatric adaptions of adult ventilators; others are specifically designed for use in children. Their effectiveness in pediatric patients, especially small infants, varies considerably.

At present, the two most frequently used types of pediatric ventilators are the volume-limited devices and the pressure- or time-limited constant flow generators.[181] A volume-limited ventilator terminates inspiratory flow when a preselcted volume of gas has been delivered. The gas flow may be generated by a piston, bellows, or valve mechanism. Such ventilators are preferred in adults and older children because a relatively constant tidal volume is delivered despite changes in compliance. With any volume ventilator, part of the preset tidal volume is expended in compression of gas within the ventilator, humidifier and delivery tubing, and also in expansion of the delivery tubing itself. This amount of gas or *compression volume* is a reflection of

Table 20-15. Ventilators for Pediatric Use

PEDIATRIC ADAPTION OF ADULT VENTILATORS
MA1
Bourns Bear
Emerson
Engstrom
Veriflow CV 2000
Seimens Servo

SPECIFICALLY DESIGNED PEDIATRIC VENTILATORS

Volume
Bourns LS 104–150

Time/pressure cycled flow generators
BabyBird
Bourns BP 200
Healthdyne
Veriflow CV 200
Sechrist

the *internal compliance* of the ventilator, and does not contribute to effective ventilation of the patient.[182] When exhaled tidal volume is measured as the gas exists from the ventilator circuit, as is common practice in adults, this compression volume will be included in the measured tidal volume. To avoid this error, one must measure exhaled tidal volume at the endotracheal tube (which is possible but difficult to do reliably with presently available equipment), or subtract the calculated compression volume from the exhaled tidal volume of the ventilator. To measure the internal compliance of the ventilator, a known tidal volume is delivered with the circuit occluded at the patient connector and the peak pressure generated is observed. The set tidal volume divided by the peak pressure yields the internal compliance. This factor, in ml/cmH_2O, is multiplied by the PIP (cmH_2O) observed when delivering the approximate desired tidal volume to the patient, giving an estimate of the compression volume of the system. This compression volume must be subtracted from the set tidal volume to determine the effective tidal volume. For the usual adult ventilators and circuits, this internal compliance varies from approximately 3 to 10 ml/cmH_2O. Therefore, when smaller children or infants are ventilated with these devices, the compression volume generated with normal inflating pressures (15–25 cmH_2O) may equal or exceed the delivered tidal volume. When the lung compliance is low, this effect will be magnified. Also, changes in compliance, by affecting the compression volume, will markedly alter the delivered tidal volume, defeating the original intention. Another complicating factor in the use of volume ventilators is the leak of gas around an uncuffed endotracheal tube.

Volume ventilators are adapted for use in infants in one of two ways. The internal compliance of the ventilator may be reduced to an absolute minimum by the use of small internal gas volumes in the ventilator and humidifier, and the use of short, small diameter, non-compliant delivery tubing. With some specifically designed infant volume ventilators, such as the Bourns LS 104, the internal compliance may be reduced to as little as 0.25 ml/cm H_2O, producing a much smaller and more manageable compression volume.[183] The other approach is to use an adapted adult ventilator which is set with a machine tidal volume approximating desired patient tidal volume plus compression volume.[184, 185] Adjustments are made based on the observed PIP, chest expansion and ABG measurements. This approach works reasonably well with children weighing more than about 10 kg. Below this size, a pressure-limited, constant-flow generator or a specifically designed infant volume ventilator is more effective.

Another problem encountered with some adult volume ventilators is the relatively high lower limit of inspiratory flow rate which requires a very short inspiratory time with small tidal volumes. Virtually all the available volume ventilators have been designed or adapted for the use of an IMV or synchronized IMV mode with adjustable PEEP levels.

For ventilatory management of infants with respiratory distress syndrome, many neonatologists prefer a time-cycled, pressure- or time-limited, constant-flow generator. We have found this type of ventilator quite useful in infants following cardiac surgery. It is most commonly operated in an IMV mode, delivering a relatively high, constant flow of gas from which the patient may inspire at any time with the continuous flow preventing significant rebreathing. At specifically set intervals, the outflow of gas from the system is occluded for a period of time, resulting in pressurization of the system and gas flow into the lungs. The peak pressure generated is limited to a preset level in most cases, although inspiratory flow may also be time limited. When time limited, this ventilator will actually function as a volume ventilator, subject to the previously described inaccuracies caused by compression volume and leaks. In the majority of situations, these ventilators are used in the pressure-limited mode. This approach automatically compensates for volume loss from small leaks around the endotracheal tube, but the delivered tidal volume varies with compliance. Therefore, the peak inflating pressure may have to be periodically adjusted on the basis of observed chest expansion and ABG measurements. The inspiratory flow rate and inspiratory-to-expiratory time ratio are easily adjustable. When inspiration is time cycled but pressure limited, a variable period of *inspiratory hold* may be produced during which the airway pressure is held at the peak level. In some circumstances, this may improve intrapulmonary gas distribution. PEEP is easily produced in this type of ventilator by a variable threshold or flow resistor in the expiratory limb of the circuit.

When rapid respiratory rates are employed, the expiratory time may be too short for complete exhalation of gas from the lung. If there is inadequate time for airway pressure to return to zero before the next inspiration begins, inadvertent PEEP, gas trapping, and overdistention of the lung may occur. Some ventilators attempt to compensate for this problem by adding a negative-pressure or expiratory-assist phase to the cycle (e.g., the "Baby Bird").

For the larger child (> 10-15 kg), we use a volume-cycled ventilator, setting the initial patient tidal volume (corrected for compression volume) at about 10 to 12 ml/kg and the cycling frequency at about two-thirds to three-fourths normal for age (Table 20-16). If compliance and resistance are not grossly abnormal, this produces adequate chest expansion with a peak inflating pressure of 15 to 30 cmH$_2$O. The inspiratory flow rate is generally set so as to produce an I:E ratio of approximately 1:2. The initial FiO$_2$ is selected on the basis of ABG measurements during

surgery or by predicting the efficiency of gas exchange postoperatively, tending to err on the high side of oxygen concentration. Unless there is a specific contraindication, we employ low end expiratory pressure (2–5 cmH$_2$O) following thoracic surgery to maintain FRC above closing volume and help prevent atelectasis. If the chest film shows poor lung expansion and areas of segmental or lobar atelectasis, or if oxygenation is inadequate because of intrapulmonary shunting from atelectasis, small airway closure or pulmonary edema, then higher levels of PEEP may be employed. In each situation, one must weigh the relative risks of hypoxia or oxygen toxicity versus potential barotrauma or circulatory compromise from PEEP. If inadequate pulmonary perfusion is a problem, high levels of PEEP are usually avoided to prevent further impairment of pulmonary circulation by high intrathoracic pressure.

With infants or children smaller than 10 kg, we generally use a time-cycled, pressure-limited, constant flow generator with an initial flow rate of 4 to 8 1/min, PIP of 15 to 25 cmH$_2$O, I:E ratio of 1:1.5 to 1:2, and a frequency of 15 to 30/min. Low levels of end expiratory pressure are also commonly used. Adjustments are made in a similar manner as for the volume ventilator except that tidal volume is adjusted by varying the peak inflating pressure, and inspiratory flow rate by varying the total gas flow.

Adjustments in ventilator settings are made on the basis of arterial blood gas results. The PaCO$_2$ is altered by changing the tidal volume or ventilator frequency, and the PaO$_2$ by adjusting the FiO$_2$ and the end expiratory pressure levels. Changes in ventilatory pattern, such as a larger tidal volume and lower frequency, a slow inspiratory flow rate or a period of hold at PIP may also improve distribution of ventilation and oxygenation in some situations. As a general rule, we try to maintain a low normal PaCO$_2$, a normal pH, and a PaO$_2$ of greater than 80 to 100 torr except in neonates. An obvious exception to this would be the child with a persistent intracardiac right-to-left shunt le-

Table 20-16. Normal Respiratory Rate

AGE	FREQUENCY (BREATHS/MIN)
Newborn	30–40
1 month–1 year	25–35
1–2 years	22–30
2–4 years	20–28
4–6 years	18–24
6–10 years	16–22
10–16 years	14–20
> 16 years	12–18

sion in whom a PaO_2 of 30 to 40 torr may be accepted, so long as tissue oxygenation is adequate, as evidenced by a stable blood pH.

The arterial gas tensions also depend on cardiovascular function and metabolic rate (oxygen consumption and CO_2 production). Low cardiac output or increased metabolic rate (fever, shivering) magnify the effect or an intrapulmonary shunt because venous oxygen content is decreased, increasing the effect of venous admixture on arterial oxygen tension.[186, 187] Increased carbon dioxide production is reflected in increased $PaCO_2$ if ventilation remains unchanged. Therefore, it is usually necessary to increase minute ventilation as the body temperature increases after hypothermia. Arterial carbon dioxide tension can usually be normalized even when cardiac output is low by increasing alveolar ventilation, unless pulmonary blood flow is extremely small. When cardiac output is very low, augmentation with volume expansion or inotropic support may be more effective in improving oxygenation than any ventilator adjustment.

Other Supportive Measures

In addition to mechanical support of ventilation, a number of other factors are important in maintaining optimal respiratory function and in preventing complications.

The effects of anesthetics, relaxants, and sedatives may impair the ability to breathe deeply, sigh, and cough. An artificial airway interferes with the patient's normal ability to warm and humidify inspired air. All of these functions must be supplied artificially. Inspired gases should be warmed to near body temperature (generally 32–34°C) and humidified in order to prevent thickening of secretions and the adverse effects of drying on the airway mucosa. This is particularly important in infants where the small size of airways and endotracheal tubes make them particularly susceptible to obstruction from secretions.

Many humidifier systems are available as part of ventilators or for attachment to them. These vary considerably in efficiency and safety. The ultrasonic-type humidifier has been virtually abandoned for pediatric ventilators because inappropriate use may produce overhydration and hyponatremia.[188] With most other humidifiers, the inspired gas is drawn over or through heated water. If the gas temperature at the patient's airway is 32 or 34°C, then the water content at saturation will be 35 to 38 mg/l, which appears adequate to minimize airway mucosal damage.[189,190] Unless the delivery tubing is warmed or insulated, the gas must be heated to a greater temperature in the humidifier to compensate for cooling in the delivery tubing.[191] The temperature near the airway must be monitored and the humidifier temperature regulated to prevent inadequate humidity or dangerous overheating. Excessive temperature of inspired gas may result in increased body temperature with increased demand for oxygen and cardiac output, or even thermal injury to the airway.[192]

When humidified gas cools in the delivery tubing, water condenses. This is bothersome because of noise, and may be dangerous if large amounts of water are allowed to run into endotracheal tube. Therefore, water traps must be included in the circuit or the tubing emptied very frequently. A controlled heating element in the delivery tubing would minimize these problems, but is an available feature of few ventilators at present.

The lungs of an intubated patient should be vigorously inflated at frequent intervals in order to help prevent atelectasis. This may be done by incorporating a sigh mechanism into a volume ventilator, but is more commonly done by manually inflating the lungs in conjunction with suctioning and chest physical therapy. The concentration of inspired oxygen should be increased during manual inflation before suctioning because alveolar oxygen concentration decreases rapidly during this procedure. The frequency and vigor of suctioning will, of course, depend on the amount of secretions, but suctioning should be carried out at least every hour initially. The duration of actual suctioning after manual inflation should be limited to 10 to 15 seconds before repeat inflation of the lungs. Smooth, sterile, end-hole plastic catheters should be used with sterile technique and without excessive negative pressure to avoid trauma to the airway mucosa.

The removal of secretions, especially when viscid, may be facilitated by frequent change of position, vibration, and percussion of the chest. A physical therapy session of 10 to 20 minutes every 2 to 6 hours may be helpful in preventing or treating atelectasis.[193]

In those patients for whom a period of mechanical support of ventilation is anticipated, the effects of narcotics or muscle relaxants are not reversed pharmacologically at the completion of surgery. When prolonged respiratory support is required and agitation interferes with effective ventilation, supplemental doses of a narcotic, sedative, or muscle relaxant may be needed. Before resorting to large doses of these drugs, however, one should assure that agitation is not caused by hypoxia, inadequate ventilation, or low cardiac output. Children generally require no more than usual analgesic doses of narcotics (morphine 0.05–0.1 mg/kg, meperidine 0.5–1 mg/kg) to make them comfortable as long as they are adequately ventilated and oxygenated. In the older child in whom excessive anxiety also seems to be a problem, small supplemental doses of a sedative such as diazepam (0.05 mg/kg) may also be helpful.

It is rare that muscle relaxants are needed because of agitation and restlessness, and they should not be used alone without sedation in the conscious patient. The most common use for muscle relaxants in the postoperative period is to prevent shivering and increased oxygen consumption during the initial rewarming period or when cardiac output is marginal. The circulatory effects of the various muscle relaxant drugs should be considered when selecting one for use in a particular situation. Pancuronium may at times cause tachycardia and hypertension,[194] while D-tubocurarine may cause transient hypoten-

sion because of histamine release and vasodilatation.[195] Metocurine appears to have the fewest cardiovascular side effects[196, 197] and has been shown to be safe in infants and children.[198]

Bronchospasm and increased airway resistance may occasionally complicate respiratory management in the cardiac patient. When wheezing and a prolonged expiratory phase are apparent, inhaled bronchodilators may be helpful, but there is no indication for their routine use in all patients. The more specific $beta_2$-agonist drugs such as isoetharine (Bronkosol) or terbutaline appear to be as effective as isoproterenol as bronchodilators with less $beta_1$ side effects such as tachycardia.[199] The beta agonists may block compensatory hypoxic vasoconstriction in the lung and increase ventilation-perfusion mismatching and shunting.[200, 201] Isoetharine (Bronkosol) is generally administered as a 1:4 or 1:8 dilution with normal saline by an in-line nebulizer. In the patient with a history of asthma, the use of intravenous theophylline[202] or corticosteroids[203] may also be indicated if severe bronchospasm occurs.

Poor gas exchange because of increased lung water or pulmonary edema may be improved by fluid restriction or the use of potent diuretics such as furosemide (Lasix) along with measures to improve cardiac performance.[204] Maintaining colloid osmotic pressure in the normal range may also help to prevent or treat pulmonary edema, although experimental evidence for this is lacking.[205]

Weaning from Respiratory Support

In most children following open-heart procedures, mechanical support of ventilation is continued for 12 to 48 hours, although practice varies from center to center. The use of IMV has greatly simplified weaning from respiratory support.[206] Once the patient has recovered sufficiently to begin spontaneous ventilation, the IMV rate is gradually decreased, usually in increments of 2 to 4 breaths/min. As long as the patient breathes comfortably and carbon dioxide retention does not occur, the weaning process is continued until the IMV rate is zero and the patient is breathing without mechanical support. Because the appropriate $PaCO_2$ level depends on the metabolic state and serum bicarbonate concentration, the arterial pH must also be considered. When metabolic alkalosis is present, increased $PaCO_2$ levels may be acceptable as long as the pH remains greater than 7.35. If CO_2 retention and acidemia occur, the IMV rate is increased back to that which produced adequate ventilation and further weaning attempted later.

During weaning of IMV rate, PEEP is generally maintained to prevent atelectasis and improve compliance by increasing FRC. The FiO_2 can usually be decreased gradually from initial levels of 40 to 70 percent as the patient recovers. When the FiO_2 is decreased to 40 percent or less, the end expiratory pressure is then decreased in increments of 1 to 2 cmH_2O.

When the patient is able to comfortably maintain adequate ABG measurements with spontaneous ventilation on a CPAP of 2 to 4 cmH_2O[207] and 40 percent oxygen or less, removal of the endotracheal tube is considered. Other criteria which must be met before extubation include

1. Stable cardiovascular function: normal blood pressure, adequate cardiac output, no significant arrhythmias
2. Adequate hemostasis, absence of significant bleeding from chest tubes
3. Normal temperature and oxygen demand
4. Normal metabolic state: electrolytes, glucose
5. Adequate neurologic status: patient awake enough to maintain the airway, clear secretions, cough and deep breathe; complete reversal of muscle relaxants

Simple bedside measurements, such as vital capacity or maximum inspiratory force, may be helpful predictors in older children, but are less useful in infants.[208]

When the child is ready for extubation, a few simple preparations should be made.

The stomach should be empty and if a nasogastric tube is in place, this should be suctioned. The airway, mouth, and nasopharynx should also be cleared of secretions. A source for humidified supplemental oxygen, such as a hood, mask, or nasal prongs should be ready. Also a bag and mask, laryngoscope and endotracheal tubes should be at hand in case support of ventilation or reintubation is required. The endotracheal tube is then removed while applying positive pressure. The pharynx is again suctioned and the child placed in an oxygen concentration approximately 10 percent higher than before extubation. The adequacy of ventilation and oxygenation is determined by examination and confirmed by ABG measurement in 15 to 30 minutes.

Edema of the larynx and subglottic trachea in infants and small children may occasionally produce signs of obstruction or postextubation croup. The incidence is highest in the 6-month to 3-year age groups, especially when prolonged intubation is required. This problem can be reduced by atraumatic intubation, minimal movement of the tube within the airway, and the use of minimally reactive, properly fitting tubes.

When stridor occurs after extubation, an aerosolized vasoconstrictor such as epinephrine seems to help transiently reduce edema and obstruction.[209] Racemic epinephrine (2.25%) is given as a 1:8 to 1:4 dilution in 2 ml with normal saline, aerosolized over 10 to 15 minutes in a hand-held nebulizer with a face mask or mouth piece. The heart rate and blood pressure should be carefully monitored during and after treatment to detect tachycardia and hypertension.

High-dose corticosteroids have been advocated for treatment or even prevention of postextubation croup.[210] Although the efficacy of steroids is unproven, we administer dexamethasone 0.2 to 0.5 mg/kg as a single dose when postextubation stridor is anticipated because of traumatic insertion of an endotracheal tube or prolonged duration of intubation; it is also used in patients with severe stridor not responding to a vasoconstrictor aerosol. In rare instances, drug therapy may not relieve severe stridor. If hypoxia, hypercarbia, or markedly increased work of breathing ensue, reinsertion of an endotracheal tube may be required (usually with a smaller diameter tube than before).

Chest physical therapy is continued after extubation. Suctioning of the pharynx may help to clear secretions and stimulate cough, but excessive or traumatic suctioning may cause airway edema and agitation. Intermittent positive-pressure breathing by mask or mouthpiece continues to be used in some centers, though its benefits are questionable.[211] When positive-pressure inflation of the lungs is indicated in an infant or child after extubation, this is best accomplished manually with a bag and mask.

Supplemental oxygen is gradually withdrawn as indicated by physical signs and ABG measurements. Chest roentgenographs are repeated daily during the intensive care stay, looking for signs of atelectasis, lobar collapse, or infection.

RESPIRATORY COMPLICATIONS

Respiratory complications are among the most frequent following cardiovascular surgery. Airway complications include accidental extubation, occlusion of the endotracheal tube with clot or secretions, and trauma to the airway. Accidental extubation can be almost entirely prevented by proper tube position and fixation along with restraint and sedation of the patient as necessary. Nevertheless, equipment and personnel for emergency reintubation must be kept immediately available, and all nurses should be trained in the technique of bag and mask ventilation. Endotracheal tube obstruction should be suspected whenever ventilation is inadequate, when resistance and peak airway pressure increase, or when the patient develops respiratory distress, cyanosis, and retractions. The failure to hear breath sounds with attempted manual inflation of the lungs and the inability to pass a suction catheter through the endotracheal tube confirm the presence of an obstruction and indicate immediate removal and replacement of the tube.

In addition to transient edema following extubation, more prolonged and serious sequelae of artificial airways may occur.[212] These include erosion of tracheal mucosa, granuloma formation, fibrotic bands, or circumferential subglottic stenosis.[213, 214] The occurrence of these lesions is minimized by careful attention to equipment and techniques and by avoiding prolonged endotracheal intubation whenever possible.

The most common complications involving the lung are atelectasis, infection and barotrauma. Atelectasis is minimized by maintaining FRC with end expiratory pressure, periodic hyperinflation, and chest physical therapy. Infection generally results from preexisting conditions, airway trauma, contaminated equipment, or breaks in aseptic technique. Barotrauma can be minimized by limiting the PIP and end expiratory pressure to the minimum levels necessary to maintain oxygenation and prevent atelectasis.[115, 116] Whenever sudden deterioration in respiratory or cardiovascular status occurs, pneumothorax or pneumomediastinum should be suspected. Tension penumothroax is usually characterized by decreased breath sound on the involved side and asymmetric chest expansion. Wheezing, increased PIP, deviation of the cardiac apex, cyanosis, and hypotension are commonly seen as well. When the cardiovascular status is reasonably stable, the suspicion of a pneumothorax should be confirmed by a chest film, but when hypotension, bradycardia, or severe cyanosis accompany suggestive physical signs, immediate syringe and needle aspiration or chest tube placement should proceed without waiting for film confirmation. In the premature infant, in whom barotrauma is particularly common, a suspected pneumothorax can usually be confirmed immediately by transilluminating the chest with a specifically designed fiberoptic light source.[217] The presence of a large pneumothorax is detected by increased lucency of the chest on the involved side.

Pneumomediastinum and pneumopericardium, unusual in older children, are more commonly seen in newborns, especially those with severe respiratory distress syndrome or meconium aspiration.[218, 219] Signs of pneumopericardium are similar to those of cardiac tamponade from other causes, and include decreased intensity of heart sounds, hypotension, venous distention, and increased central venous pressure. The diagnosis is confirmed by roentgenograph if time permits. Emergency treatment consists of needle aspiration of air, usually followed by placement of a pericardial drainage tube. Gas may occasionally track from the mediastinum into the peritoneal cavity and cause marked abdominal distention requiring drainage.

In the neonate with respiratory disease, prolonged mechanical ventilation or oxygen therapy may result in the syndrome of bronchopulmonary dysplasia, characterized by fibrotic changes in the lung with multiple small areas of hyperinflation and atelectasis.[220] The etiology of this syndrome is unclear. Suggested causes are oxygen toxicity, barotrauma, and specific nutritional deficiencies.

Mechanical ventilation and surgical stress may stimulate ADH secretion with fluid retention.[221] Careful fluid balance, at times supplemented by diuretics, is required to prevent this complication.

Respiratory support depends on the use of complicated equipment with the risk of malfunctions, such as power-source failure, accidental disconnection from the endotracheal tube, gas leaks in the ventilator or tubing, kinking of tubing, malfunction of valves, overheating of humidifiers, and malfunction of controls, pressure gauges or alarms. These problems can be minimized by selection of reliable equipment, conscientious preventative maintenance, and proper use of alarms and monitoring equipment. The most important factor is the continual presence of personnel familiar with the equipment and capable of substituting manual ventilation immediately if any malfunction is suspected.

TEMPERATURE CONTROL

In the pediatric patient, control of body temperature within the normal range requires close monitoring and the ability to regulate the thermal environment. This is particularly true in the newborn or premature infant in whom heat loss occurs rapidly because of the large ratio of body surface area to mass and also thinner layers of insulating tissue. When the infant is subjected to cold stress, it attempts to maintain body temperature by increased heat production from the metabolism of free fatty acids released from brown fat stores.[222, 223] This may be effective in maintaining body temperature, but at the expense of a marked increase in metabolic rate and oxygen consumption. This places a great stress on the cardiorespiratory system, perhaps exceeding the ability of the infant to compensate. The infant may then develop metabolic acidosis, respiratory failure, and apnea.[224]

To avoid this situation, the infant should be maintained in a neutral thermal environment, regulated by monitoring ambient or skin temperature.[225] At present, the thermal environment of the infant is most commonly maintained by the use of an Isolette incubator, or a servocontrolled radiant overhead warming unit.[226] The latter offers greater access to the infant and facilitates nursing care in the critically ill patient.

In the older child, the primary intrinsic mechanism to reverse hypothermia is shivering. This vigorous muscle activity increases oxygen consumption. In the hypothermic patient after cardiopulmonary bypass, it is often desirable to avoid this increased oxygen demand. If the patient is kept paralyzed to prevent shivering and external heat is supplied from a warming mattress or radiant source, the thermal stress on the cardiovascular system is reduced. Overheating must be avoided because increased body temperature also increases oxygen consumption.

During hypothermia, systemic vasoconstriction occurs, increasing peripheral vascular resistance. With rewarming, volume

Table 20-17. Renal Function in Children with Congenital Heart Disease*

STRUCTURAL AND FUNCTIONAL CHANGES
Observed in *some* patients; varies with lesion
1. Decreased total glomerular mass
2. Increased size of individual glomeruli
3. Hyalinization or sclerosis of glomeruli
4. Reduced renal plasma flow
5. Increased filtration fraction
6. Decreased PAH clearance
7. Shift of blood flow from cortical to medullary nephrons
8. Decreased ability to clear sodium load

CONTRIBUTING FACTORS
1. Anomalies of GU tract
2. Reduced renal blood flow with congestive heart failure
3. Chronic hypoxia with cyanotic lesions
4. Malnutrition and growth retardation
5. Extreme polycythemia
6. Diuretics or salt restriction
7. Bacterial endocarditis

(*Compiled from Gruskin AB: The kidney in congenital heart disease—an overview. Adv. Pediatr 24:133–189, 1977)

infusion is required to compensate for vasodilation.

RENAL FUNCTION, FLUIDS, AND ELECTROLYTES

CHANGES IN RENAL FUNCTION WITH HEART DISEASE AND SURGERY

In patients with congenital heart disease, the ability of the kidney to maintain normal fluid and electrolyte balance may be altered by a number of factors (Table 20-17).[227]

Renal function, as measured by glomerular filtration rate postoperatively, is generally not adversely affected by uncomplicated extracorporeal circulation and cardiovascular surgery.[228] However, the stress of anesthesia and major surgery may produce changes in the regulation of fluid balance, probably by release of ADH and aldosterone. Cardiopulmonary bypass also tends to increase extracellular fluid and total body water.[229–231] Careful monitoring is necessary to accurately assess intravascular volume status, fluid and electrolyte balance, and renal function (Table 20-18).

FLUID AND ELECTROLYTE THERAPY

Water

The usual postsurgical approach is to maintain sufficient intravascular volume and cardiac output to assure adequate renal perfusion and urine output, while avoiding the accumulation of excessive water and sodium. This is especially important in the patient with congestive heart failure. The ideal postoperative fluid and electrolyte intake remains controversial.[232–234] For patients who have undergone cardiopulmonary bypass, our approach is to give about 50 percent of the normal maintenance water requirement on the first postoperative day and to increase to full maintenance over 2 to 4 days. Normal maintenance fluid requirements are given in Table 20-19. Patients undergoing procedures without cardiopulmonary bypass are given 80 to 100 percent of maintenance volumes throughout the postoperative period unless congestive heart failure or other complications indicate the need for fluid restriction. Adequate fluid administration is particularly important in the cyanotic polycythemic pa-

Table 20-18. Evaluation of Fluid Balance in Children

BODY WEIGHT

PHYSICAL EXAMINATION
1. Signs of edema: Puffy eyelids or hands and feet
2. Signs of dehydration: Decreased skin turgor, dry mucous membranes, sunken eyes or fontanelle
3. Signs of circulatory adequacy: Peripheral pulses, perfusion
4. Signs of intravascular volume overload: Rales, gallop rhythm, hepatomegaly, tachypnea

INTAKE AND OUTPUT MEASUREMENT

INTRAVASCULAR PRESSURE MEASUREMENTS
1. Arterial blood pressure
2. Central venous pressure (RAP)
3. Pulmonary capillary wedge pressure (LAP)

URINE MEASUREMENTS
1. Volume
2. Specific gravity
3. Osmolality
4. Electrolytes

BLOOD MEASUREMENTS
5. Electrolytes
6. Hematocrit
7. Osmolality

Table 20-19. Maintenance Fluid Requirements*

BODY WEIGHT	FLUID VOLUME/DAY	OR	FLUID VOLUME/HOUR
1st 10 kg	100 ml/kg/24 hr		4 ml/kg/hr
Next 10 kg	50 ml/kg/24 hr		2 ml/kg/hr
Each kg > 20	25 ml/kg/24 hr		1 ml/kg/hr
Example:	25 kg patient would receive		
	1000 + 500 + 125 = 1625 ml/day		
	or approximately		
	40 + 20 + 5 = 65 ml/hour		

*These are basal requirements for the normal individual. Actual fluid volume administered will vary with the situation (e.g., less following CPB or with congestive heart failure; more with greater than normal losses or dehydration). Calculation of fluid requirements on the basis of body surface area or caloric expenditure may be more theoretically accurate but adds little in actual practice.

tient because of possible thrombotic complications secondary to dehydration.

When losses exceed those normally expected, fluid administration rates must be altered.[235, 236] Gastrointestinal losses from diarrhea, vomiting, or nasogastric drainage must be added to the maintenance volume. Fever also increases insensible water loss by 10 to 12 percent for each degree Centigrade increase in body temperature. Nursing an infant under a radiant warmer will also increase insensible water loss by 10 to 20 ml/kg/day in the term neonate, and even more in the small, premature infant.[237, 238] On the other hand, mechanical ventilation with adequate humidification of inspired gases reduces insensible loss, decreasing fluid requirements about 10 to 15 percent.[239]

Sodium

The daily intake of sodium is generally restricted to about 1 to 2 mEq/kg or less in the immediate postoperative period. For the larger child, 5 percent glucose with 0.2 percent saline is a reasonable choice as a maintenance solution. For the small infant, a solution with a higher glucose concentration is given. Calculation of sodium intake must include the sodium content of drugs and flush solutions as well as intravenous fluids. The minimal infusion rate for maintaining patency of an arterial line with heparinized normal saline (2–3 ml/hr) may provide most or all of the daily sodium needs for the small infant.

Electrolyte abnormalities are common in the postoperative cardiac surgery patient. There is a tendency to retain water in excess of sodium, producing a dilutional hyponatremia, probably as a result of ADH stimulation.[240] Total body sodium is usually increased to a lesser extent than total body water and may be decreased. Dilutional hyponatremia may be accompanied by edema, increased body weight, decreased urine output, and increased urine osmolality coincident with decreased serum osmolality. Management should consist of adequate sodium administration, fluid restriction and, if necessary, the use of diuretic such as furosemide or ethracrynic acid.[241]

Severe hyponatremia (< 120mEq/l) may produce neurologic abnormalities including disorientation, agitation, cerebral edema, seizures, or coma. When life-threatening complications of hyponatremia exist, the serum sodium may be increased by the use of hypertonic saline solution along with fluid restriction and diuresis. Increasing the serum sodium by about 5 mEq/l over 15 to 30 minutes is usually sufficient to reverse acute symptoms. More rapid sodium administration is particularly hazardous. In the presence of an already expanded extracellular volume in the postcardiac surgery patient prone to congestive heart failure, fluid restriction is the preferred treatment.

Potassium

Maintenance of normal serum potassium concentration is important in the postoperative patient because abnormal levels, either high or low, may potentiate cardiac arrhythmias.[242] There are many causes of low serum potassium in the perioperative period. Preoperative chronic diuretic therapy may deplete total body potassium.[243] Extracorporeal circulation tends to diminish serum potassium.[244, 245] If a potassium-poor priming solution is used, dilution may contribute to hypokalemia. Acid-base status also affects the serum potassium concentration; respiratory or metabolic alkalosis tends to shift potassium into cells. The postoperative use of potent diuretics such as furosemide to treat fluid retention may enormously increase potassium loss in the urine.[246]

Potassium should be added to intravenous fluids soon after operation, provided that renal function is adequate and serum potassium levels are not increased.[247] Usual potassium maintenance consists of 1 to 3 mEq/kg/day or 10 to 40 mEq/1 of intravenous fluids. These are approximations; actual potassium requirements may vary considerably and must be determined on the basis of frequent serum potassium measurements. Prevention of hypokalemia is particularly important in the patient treated with digitalis preparations to avoid toxicity.

Hypokalemia may be treated by increasing the potassium concentration in maintenance fluids or by repeated infusions of small amounts of potassium. It is not possible to accurately estimate total body potassium deficit on the basis of serum potassium measurement because the extracellular component is only a small fraction of total body potassium. To treat acute severe hypokalemia, it is generally safe to infuse 0.2 to 0.5 mEq/kg of potassium over 30 to 60 minutes. If intracellular potassium is markedly depleted, this dose may have to be repeated several times. During the administration of supplemental potassium the electrocardiogram should be monitored continually for the high peaked T waves of hyperkalemia. Extreme care must be exercised when infusing concentrated potassium solutions, especially into central venous catheters, because very high blood concentrations delivered to the myocardium may produce serious arrhythmias or cardiac arrest.

Hyperkalemia may result from excessive potassium administration, renal failure or acute acidemia. When blood is drawn from infants by heel stick, laboratory serum potassium measurements often exceed the true value. Venous or arterial blood samples should be used when accurate potassium measurement is required.

Hyperkalemia will generally produce typical electrocardiographic changes including high-peaked T waves, depressed S-T segments, and prolonged QRS complexes. Extreme increases in serum potassium may cause bradycardia, conduction abnormalities, ventricular fibrillation, or asystole.

The mode of treatment for hyperkalemia depends on the urgency of the situation.[248] When acute, life-threatening arrhythmias occur, the depressant effects of potassium may be partially opposed by the infusion of calcium chloride 10 to 20 mg/kg or calcium gluconate 30 to 60 mg/kg. This infusion should be slowed if significant bradycardia results. Extracellular potassium may be rapidly reduced by administration of sodium bicarbonate 1 to 2 mEq/kg or glucose 1 to 2 gm/kg along with insulin 1 unit per 4 g of glucose. None of the above removes potassium from the patient. Although the effect on serum potassium concentration is slower, total body potassium may be reduced by Kayexalate enemas, 1 to 2 g/kg in 10 percent sorbitol. Removal of potassium by Kayexalate results in absorption of significant amounts of sodium which may be a problem in the patient with renal failure and congestive heart failure. In this situation dialysis is the most effective treatment.

Calcium

Following cardiovascular surgery, calcium homeostasis may be significantly altered. The calcium content of the blood is comprised of three factors: free ionized calcium, protein-bound calcium, and anion-complexed calcium. The total amount of calcium in the blood is small compared with the amount in bone, with which it is in equilibrium. The blood calcium concentration is normally maintained within close limits by the activity of parathormone and calcitonin, which regulate the rates of mobilization and deposition of bone calcium, and also affect the rates of absorption and excretion of calcium.

During cardiac surgery, total serum calcium usually decreases with the onset of cardiopulmonary bypass, primarily because of dilution and decreased serum protein concentration.[249] The change in serum calcium will, of course, be affected by the amount of calcium added to the pump priming solution; if an adequate amount is added, the ionized calcium concentration generally remains in the normal range. Total or ionized calcium levels may also be altered by changes in acid-base status or by citrate complexing during the transfusion of CPD blood.

An adequate ionized calcium concentration is necessary for normal excitation, conduction, and contractile function of the myocardium. Acute reduction of ionized calcium, as occurs with rapid infusion of citrated blood, produces a negative inotropic response,[250] while rapid infusion of calcium generally increases contractility and cardiac output.[251] Calcium chloride or gluconate is often used for inotropic support, but the effect of a single dose is brief because calcium rapidly reequilibrates with bone stores.

In the newborn infant, hypocalcemia is especially common. It is most frequent in premature infants, infants of diabetic mothers, and infants with birth asphyxia or other severe stress such as hypoxia or sepsis.[252] Even the smallest infants have large stores of calcium in bone, but the homeostatic mechanisms responsible for mobilization of calcium in response to hypocalcemia may not function normally for several days after birth. Parathyroid activity is insufficient for about 2 days in the term infant and longer in the premature.[253] The blood calcitonin level may be transiently increased in the neonate.[254] Severe hypocalcemia may cause seizures or tetany in the newborn, as well as adversely affecting cardiovascular function.

For these reasons, it is important to moni-

tor serum calcium in children, especially newborn infants, and to correct hypocalcemia when detected. Methods for measuring total serum calcium are widely available. With these methods, however, the total serum calcium must be correlated with the serum protein concentration (McClean–Hastings nomogram) to make some estimate of ionized calcium.[255] A calcium-specific electrode is now available (Orion Research Corporation) to directly measure the physiologically active ionized fraction.[256] If this method proves to be reliable in large scale clinical use, it will be quite helpful in managing the postoperative patient in whom rapid changes may occur.

Treatment of hypocalcemia in indicated when symptomatic or when the ionized calcium is less than about 3 to 3.5 mg/dl, usually corresponding to a total calcium of 7.5 to 8.0 mg/dl. The rapidity of treatment of hypocalcemia depends on the urgency of the clinical situation.[257] Asymptomatic hypocalcemia in the newborn may be treated by the addition of 20 to 30 mg/kg of elemental calcium to the maintenance intravenous solution. Several calcium preparations are available for intravenous use. Calcium chloride is supplied as a 10 percent solution which contains 27.2 mg or 1.36 mEq/ml of calcium per milliliter. Calcium gluconate, which is somewhat less irritating when infused through a peripheral vein, is also supplied as a 10 percent solution containing 9 mg or 0.45 mEq/ml. Calcium gluceptate has less tendency to precipitate when administered with sodium bicarbonate, and is supplied as a 23 percent solution containing 18 mg or 0.9 mEq/ml.

The usual intravenous dose given as a slow injection for inotropic effect or rapid treatment of symptomatic hypocalcemia is 10 to 20 mg/kg (0.1–0.2 ml/kg) of calcium chloride or 30 to 60 mg/kg (0.3–0.6 ml/kg) of calcium gluconate. For emergency treatment of hypocalcemic seizures, this dose may be repeated up to three to four times at 3- to 5-minute intervals if necessary to control seizure activity. Calcium should always be injected slowly, especially into central lines, continually monitoring the ECG for QT prolongation, bradycardia, or other arrhythmias. Calcium toxicity is more likely in the presence of hypokalemia or digitalis intoxication. Subcutaneous injection of calcium salts, especially chloride, with an infiltrated intravenous infusion may cause skin necrosis and sloughing.

If symptomatic hypocalcemia persists or recurs, the daily dose of calcium in the intravenous fluids may be increased to as much as 50 to 60 mg elemental calcium/kg/day. In some circumstances, magnesium deficiency may cause hypocalcemia which is unresponsive to usual therapy.[258, 259]

RENAL FAILURE

Etiology

The kidney may be subjected to a number of potentially harmful effects in the perioperative period (Table 20-20). Chesney and coworkers observed postoperative acute renal

Table 20-20. Contributing Factors in Acute Renal Failure after Cardiac Surgery

DECREASED RENAL PERFUSION
1. Hypovolemia
2. Low cardiac output states (cardiogenic shock)
3. Septicemia
4. Disseminated intravascular coagulation
5. Prolonged use of vasoconstrictor drugs (epinephrine, norepinephrine)
6. Prolonged cardiopulmonary bypass
7. Prolonged aortic cross-clamping (coarctation repair)

NEPHROTOXINS
1. Aminoglycoside antibiotics (gentamicin, kanamycin)
2. (?) Cephalosporins
3. (?) Other antibiotics (methicillin, sulfonamides, tetracyclines)
4. Hemoglobin, myoglobin
   a. Transfusion reaction
   b. Prolonged CPB
   c. Hemolysis from prosthetic material or valve
   d. Massive tissue trauma or necrosis
5. Angiography dye administered shortly before surgery

PREEXISTING RENAL DISEASE
1. GU tract anomalies
2. Glomerulonephritis
3. Chronic pyelonephritis

failure in 8 percent of infants undergoing cardiac surgery; 65 percent of these patients died.[260] The risk of renal failure in older children following cardiac surgery is less than in infants.[261]

Most frequently, acute renal failure follows a prolonged period of inadequate cardiac output and renal hypoperfusion.[262-263] Glomerular filtration rate and urine output decrease. Both water and sodium excretion are reduced, presumably to increase plasma volume. The clearance of protein catabolites is decreased as well. This initial state of *prerenal* or *functional* oligura and azotemia is rapidly reversible if cardiac output and renal perfusion are restored to normal.

If renal hypoperfusion persists for a prolonged period, however, parenchymal changes occur in the kidney which are not immediately reversible. Preglomerular vascular constriction becomes severe and persistent, especially in the cortical region, reducing renal blood flow to 25 to 50 percent of normal.[264] Functional, and often structural, changes occur in the renal tubules as well, hence the descriptive, but not always applicable, term *acute tubular necrosis.*[265] These changes in renal structure and function may persist for days or weeks despite return of cardiac output to normal, and are better termed *vasomotor nephropathy* or simply *acute renal failure.*

Diagnosis

Persistent oliguria after surgery (2 or more consecutive hours during which the urine output is less than 0.5 ml/kg/hr in the infant, 0.4 ml/kg/hr in the young child, or 0.3 ml/kg/hr in the older child) may be a sign of inadequate renal perfusion or impaired renal function. Complete anuria is unusual in postoperative renal failure, and is more commonly caused by an obstruction of urinary drainage, such as an occluded or kinked catheter, than by renal parenchymal injury.

Restoration of normal urine output with improved cardiovascular function is the best indication that oliguria is the result of func-

Table 20-21. Differential Diagnosis of Oliguria

	PRERENAL (FUNC-TIONAL) OLIGURIA	ACUTE RENAL FAILURE (VASOMOTOR NEPHROPATHY)
Urine Sodium*	< 30 (Usually < 10)	30–90 (Usually 40–60)
Urine/plasma ratios:*		
Osmolality	> 1.15	< 1.15
Urea nitrogen	>20	<10 (usually 2–5)
Creatinine	>40	<15 (usually 3–8)
Renal Failure Index)* (urinary sodium conc. ÷ urine: plasma creatinine ratio)	< 1–2**	> 5
Urine sediment	Usually normal (may have some hemoglobin, protein, or cells immediately after CPB or with congestive failure)	Proteinuria, hematuria, granular or tubular casts, occasional RBC casts

*May not be accurate for several hours after administration of mannitol or diuretics
**May be higher in premature infants

tional or prerenal causes. If oliguria persists in spite of adequate blood volume and cardiac output, then acute renal failure or vasomotor nephropathy is more likely. Further evidence in differentiating a renal parenchymal from prerenal etiology of oliguria may be gained by examining urine and serum chemistries, and the urine sediment (Table 20-21). The absolute serum level of urea nitrogen or creatinine is rarely of diagnostic value when oliguria is initially observed. Azotemia may occur with either prerenal or true renal failure.

When oliguria does not respond to restoration of intravascular volume and cardiac output, many authorities recommend administration of an osmotic diuretic such as mannitol or a loop diuretic such as furosemide.[266–268] These drugs are used in an attempt to restore urine output and prevent acute renal failure, or at least to convert it from the oliguric to nonoliguric form. Diuretics have not been proven conclusively to be of benefit in this situation, and their use remains controversial.[269, 270]

The apparent benefit of mannitol in some studies may be the result of its effect as a plasma volume expander,[271] an effect which may be duplicated by other more physiologic volume expanders such as blood, plasma, or saline. It has been proposed, but not proven, that mannitol has a renal vasodilator effect which might partially reverse the vasoconstriction of early vasomotor nephropathy.[272, 273] The use of mannitol may be dangerous in a patient with an expanded intravascular volume (e.g., congestive heart failure) and acute renal failure. Infusion of a large dose of mannitol without a subsequent diuresis may produce a marked increase in serum osmolality and expansion of intravascular volume with ensuing acute congestive heart failure and pulmonary edema.[274]

The use of furosemide in patients with impending acute renal failure is more widely accepted, but its efficiency in preventing or ameliorating renal failure is far from certain.[275] After adequate intravascular volume is established, an initial dose of 1 to 2 mg/kg may be given intravenously. If a diuresis is not produced, the dose is often increased up to a maximum of 10 mg/kg, although this dose may be excessive. Failure to produce a diuresis in response to this dose of furosemide confirms the diagnosis of renal failure.

A more insidious form of renal dysfunction without oliguria may also be seen in the postoperative period.[276] In this situation, urine output may be normal or greater, while BUN and creatinine increase progressively. Evidence of tubular dysfunction is present, and the patient has a diminished capacity to concentrate the urine.

Treatment

Even though the overall mortality rate from postoperative renal failure is high, most patients who die have associated circulatory failure. For the patient in whom adequate circulation is restored, recovery from acute renal failure is reasonably likely with meticulous care.

Gross impairment of renal function produces a number of physiologic effects (Table 20-22). The primary threats to the patient in acute renal failure are fluid overload, congestive heart failure, hyperkalemia, acidosis, and infection.

Initial treatment of renal failure should include elimination or careful restriction of potassium intake and limitation of fluid administration to insensible loss (approximately 300 ml/m^2/day) plus urine output and other losses (*e.g.*, nasogastric drainage or diarrhea).[277] Sodium intake should also be limited to replacement of losses. Hyponatremia usually indicates excess body water rather than diminished total body sodium. Adequacy of fluid and electrolyte management should be assessed by twice daily weights and frequent electrolyte determinations. Except when treating preexisting fluid overload, weight loss in excess of 1 percent per day associated with a rising serum sodium and osmolality is an indication of too vigorous fluid restriction. On the other hand, rapid weight gain and signs of vascular congestion are an indication for further restriction or removal of excess fluid by dialysis.

Hyperkalemia may be an acute and life-threatening complication of renal failure. Emergency treatment is described above. When potassium remains above 6.5 despite this regimen, immediate dialysis is indicated.

Metabolic acidosis develops in the patient with renal failure as a result of inability to excrete endogenously-produced acid. This acidosis may be treated by the infusion of sodium bicarbonate, but the ability to do so is often grossly limited by the amount of sodium which bicarbonate therapy entails. Intractable acidosis requires dialysis.

If renal failure is prolonged and signs of uremia develop (BUN > 150–200 mg/dl) dialysis may also be required. The rate of increase in BUN is determined more by the catabolic state of the patient than the state of renal dysfunction. Daily increases of 15 to 20 mg/dl may be seen in the surgical patient. Serum creatinine is less influenced by the catabolic state and gives a more accurate index of renal function.

Maintenance of adequate nutrition during acute renal failure is difficult. The infusion of hypertonic glucose and essential amino acid solutions (renal failure fluid) may help maintain nutrition and decrease tissue catabolism.

Peritoneal dialysis is simpler than hemodialysis in children and seems to be preferred

Table 20-22. Results of Renal Insufficiency

EARLY
1. Impaired water and electrolyte homeostasis
2. Impaired excretion of protein catabolites
3. Impaired acid-base homeostasis
4. Diminished drug excretion
5. Hypertension

LATE
1. Impaired erythropoesis
2. Altered blood coagulation
3. Susceptibility to infection
4. Impaired neurologic function
5. Abnormal bone formation

for acute management in most centers.[278, 279] For this procedure, a flexible, multihole catheter is inserted into the abdominal cavity using local anesthesia. The peritoneal dialysis solution is then infused into the abdomen and allowed to equilibrate with the plasma across the peritoneal membranes for a specified period, the *dwell time.* Initially about 20 ml/kg are infused and, if tolerated, the volume may be increased to as much as 40 ml/kg for each run. The dwell time may vary from 10 to 30 minutes.

The composition of the dialysate depends on the purpose of dialysis. In general, the dialysate consists of an electrolye solution containing sodium, chloride, calcium, magnesium, and acetate in either 1.5 percent or 4.25 percent dextrose. For treatment of hyperkalemia, a 1.5 percent dextrose solution with no added potassium is used. For removal of excess fluid, a 4.25 percent Dextrose solution, which has a higher osmotic gradient, might be employed. Successful dialysis requires appropriate selection or modification of dialysis solutions, careful measurement of the volumes of dialysate infused and removed, frequent determination of serum chemistries, monitoring of cardiovascular status, and observation for complications.

Dialysis may produce a number of problems.[280] The patient in renal failure is at high risk for infection, and the presence of a catheter into the abdomen surrounded by an excellent culture medium invites peritonitis or sepsis. Therefore frequent culture of the dialysate and observation for signs of infection are essential.

The use of hypertonic glucose solutions in the peritoneal cavity may result in the absorption of large amounts of glucose, especially in the infant who may develop extreme hyperglycemia and hyperosmolality. Even the 1.5 percent glucose solution is hyperosmotic relative to plasma, and prolonged dialysis may result in a net removal of water from the body, producing dehydration and hyperosmolality if adequate fluid replacement is not maintained.

The infusion of large quantities of dialysate into the peritoneal cavity may distend the abdomen so much that diaphragmatic movement is restricted and respiration impaired. If respiratory difficulty is detected by clinical examination or ABG changes, the volume of dialysate may have to be reduced or ventilation supported. Impaired respiration is particularly likely when the dialysate is not completely drained after each infusion, allowing an increasingly positive dialysis balance. In this case, the catheter may have to be repositioned or replaced.

When a patient survives acute renal failure, the duration of oliguria may vary from 3 days to 3 weeks, usually lasting 10 to 12 days.[281] The urine output typically increases over several days, often reaching levels considerably greater than normal (the so-called *polyuric phase*) before full recovery. The serum level of creatinine and urea nitrogen may not begin to plateau and decrease until several days after the urine output increases. Continued careful attention to fluid, electrolyte, and acid-base balance is necessary during this period until the kidney's ability to maintain homeostasis returns.

In the patient with renal failure, the dosage of drugs excreted or metabolized by the kidney must be adjusted to avoid drug accumulation and potential toxicity. This may be done either by decreasing the amount of individual doses or by increasing the interval between doses. Plasma drug levels should be measured whenever possible to further regulate dosages.[282]

BLOOD COMPONENTS AND COAGULATION

CHANGES WITH CONGENITAL HEART DISEASE

Congenital heart disease and cardiovascular surgery may produce a number of hematological changes. The child with chronic hypoxia usually develops polycythemia, presumably as an attempt to increase oxygen-carrying capacity and total tissue oxygen delivery. Extreme polycythemia increases viscosity, increases the risk of thrombotic complications, and may produce a state of low-grade intravascular coagulation with consumption of clotting factors and abnormalities of platelet function.[282-285] This may increase the risk of bleeding problems during and after surgery.[286] Preoperative erythrophoresis (removal of blood and replacement with 5% albumin or plasma) to produce a final hematocrit of 55 to 60 percent may help to correct these problems.[287, 288]

CHANGES WITH CPB AND SURGERY

Cardiovascular surgical procedures are often accompanied by significant blood loss. Blood given to replace losses is changed in several ways during collection and storage.[289] The blood is diluted with an anticoagulant and has a lower hematocrit. When a large volume of citrated blood is given, the anticoagulant may produce cardiovascular effects by binding calcium. If the blood is anticoagulated with heparin, systemic anticoagulation may result. Platelets, soluble-clotting factors, and 2,3 diphosphoglycerate (DPG) are depleted in stored blood. With time, red cell metabolism causes a decreased blood pH; red cells also release increasing amounts of potassium during storage.

Cardiopulmonary bypass requires systemic anticoagulation with heparin and subsequent reversal with protamine. Incomplete reversal or gross overdosage with protamine may result in coagulation problems postoperatively.[290, 291] The concentration of platelets is reduced during bypass by dilution with the pump-prime volume (which is larger relative to blood volume in the pediatric patient); by adherence to surfaces of the oxygenator, filters, and tubing; by mechanical trauma to platelets; and by formation of platelet aggregates which are cleared from the circulation.[292, 293] Similarly, levels of soluble coagulation factors are reduced by dilution and by denaturation.[294] Massive transfusion may further dilute coagulation factors.[295]

MANAGEMENT OF POSTOPERATIVE COAGULATION PROBLEMS

Continued bleeding in the postoperative period may result from inadequate surgical hemostasis, from incomplete reversal of heparin, from dilution or inactivation of platelets and soluble clotting factors, or from DIC.[296] Evaluation of abnormal coagulation should include an activated clotting time (ACT), prothrombin time (PT), partial thromboplastin time (PTT), and platelet count. Incomplete heparin reversal will be manifest by a prolonged ACT and PTT, and is treated by slow infusion of 0.25 to 0.5 mg/kg of protamine. Deficiency of soluble clotting factors, such as that evidenced by prolongation of PT and PTT, may be treated by administration of fresh frozen plasma 10 to 20 ml/kg, factor concentrates, or fresh whole blood. Thrombocytopenia (platelet count $< 100,000/mm^3$) associated with abnormal bleeding may be treated with infusion of platelet concentrates. Administration of 0.2 units of platelets per kilogram body weight should transiently increase the platelet count by about 100,000/mm^3. (See also Chaps. 15, 16 and 24.)

HEMOLYSIS

Prolonged cardiopulmonary bypass damages red cells which are lysed and cleared from the circulation.[297] Hemolysis may also occur secondary to sepsis, transfusion or drug reactions, or erythrocyte damage by prosthetic valves or other synthetic materials. In the newborn infant, transplacental transfer of maternal antibodies to the infant's red cell antigens (Rh or ABO) may produce hemolytic disease of the newborn. Hemolytic reactions, regardless of etiology, are manifest by a decreasing hematocrit, reticulocytosis, and jaundice.

Massive hemolysis should be treated by correction of the etiologic factors if possible. It is also essential to maintain an adequate hematocrit by infusion of red cells, and to prevent complications, primarily renal impairment caused by the release of hemoglobin and red cell stroma. In the newborn infant, jaundice caused by hemolysis may be more profound because of immaturity of the liver enzyme systems for conjugation and elimination of bilirubin.[298] The newborn, especially the premature infant, is at risk for central nervous system damage from high bilirubin levels (kernicterus), presumably because of immaturity and increased permeability of the blood-brain barrier.[299] An increasing serum indirect (unconjugated) bilirubin concentration, approaching 18 to 20 mg/dl in the term infant or 12 to 15 mg/dl in the premature infant, is an indication of the need for immediate exchange transfusion. An incremental exchange transfusion with two times the patient's blood volume should decrease the serum bilirubin level, remove some tissue bilirubin, and replace a large portion of the sensitized red cells subject to further rapid hemolysis.

ANEMIA

The optimal postoperative hematocrit (*i.e.,* the appropriate balance between oxygen-carrying capacity and viscosity) is uncertain. It is generally recommended that normal values be approximated—a hematocrit of 40 to 50 percent in the newborn, and 30 to 40 percent in the older pediatric patient.

Anemia in the postoperative period is corrected with whole blood or packed red cells. The former may be chosen if whole blood losses are being replaced and intravascular volume needs to be increased as well as red cell volume. When intravascular volume is normal or increased, slow infusion of packed red cells is preferred to whole blood to correct anemia. Further volume overload may be prevented by concomitant use of diuretic such as furosemide, or a partial exchange transfusion may be done, replacing aliquots of the patient's blood with packed red cells.

DISSEMINATED INTRAVASCULAR COAGULATION

Infection or low cardiac output states with inadequate tissue perfusion are the most frequent causes of postoperative disseminated intravascular coagulation (DIC), with consumption of platelets and soluble clotting factors.[300, 301] This condition is diagnosed by abnormal bleeding accompanied by the presence of fibrin-split products, thrombocytopenia, prolonged prothrombin and partial thromboplastin times, and decreased fibrinogen. DIC is most appropriately treated by reversing the etiologic factors such as infection or shock, and by replacing platelets or coagulation factors as necessary to control bleeding.[302] Heparinization is indicated only if DIC produces gross vascular occlusion with evidence of ischemia or infarction.[303]

NEUROLOGIC COMPLICATIONS

ETIOLOGY AND CLASSIFICATION

Central nervous system complications are uncommon following surgery for congenital heart disease.[304, 305] When neurologic impairment does occur, it is usually in a high-risk patient with poor cardiovascular results or multisystem failure. In rare situations, however, devastating neurologic impairment may occur despite excellent anatomic correction and adequate cardiovascular function. The neurologic disorders seen most commonly after cardiovascular surgery are listed in Table 20-23.

MANAGEMENT

Treatment of neurologic disorders is directed primarily at reversing the etiologic cause (*e.g.,* improving cerebral oxygenation or correcting metabolic disorders). A diffuse insult, such as hypoxia, multiple microemboli, or severe hyponatremia, may produce cerebral edema and increased intracranial pressure. Therapy designed to decrease such edema and pressure may be useful in preventing further damage from ischemia or herniation.[306, 307] Moderate fluid restriction, avoidance of increases in venous pressure by coughing and straining, hyperventilation to an arterial carbon dioxide tension ($PaCO_2$) of 25 to 30 torr, and the use of muscle relaxants

Table 20-23. Postoperative Neurologic Complications

NEUROLOGIC LESION	ETIOLOGY	SITUATION OR POTENTIATING FACTORS
1. Diffuse cerebral impairment (coma, stupor)	Hypoxia	Cyanotic lesion Respiratory complications
	Cerebral hypoperfusion	Cardiac arrest Low cardiac output states Inadequate perfusion during CPB (low pressure and flow; obstruction of venous return)
	Inadequate cerebral protection during profound hypothermia	Insufficient or uneven cooling
	Diffuse microemboli	Improper perfusion techniques
	Metabolic abnormalities	Hypoglycemia Hyponatremia Renal or hepatic failure
2. Focal cerebral lesions	Air or particulate emboli	Air in arterial line during CPB or in left side of heart following repair Paradoxical emboli from venous system with right-to-left or bidirectional shunt Inadequate heparinization during CPB
	Cerebral vascular thrombosis	Extreme polycythemia Anemia in hypoxic infants
	Brain abscess	Cyanotic lesions
3. Intracranial hemorrhage (may produce focal or diffuse impairment)	Premature infant	Birth asphyxia Hypoxia, hypercarbia, acidosis (?) Rapid osmotic changes (sodium bicarbonate)
	Coagulation disorders	Cyanotic lesions with polycythemia Prolonged CPB Massive transfusion Hepatic insufficiency
	Coarctation repair	Extreme hypertension Cerebral vascular malformations
4. Seizures	Any of above lesions 1–3	See above
	Metabolic derangements in the newborn	Hypoglycemia Hypocalcemia
	Preexisting seizure disorder	Especially likely if previous anticonvulsants not restarted postoperatively
	CNS infection	Meningitis, encephalitis
5. Paraplegia	Inadequate spinal cord perfusion during aortic cross-clamping	Coarctation repair
6. Phrenic nerve injury	Cutting, crushing, stretching nerve; electrocautery	Subclavian-to-aorta shunts, PDA ligation, pericardial dissection during repeat operations
7. Recurrent laryngeal nerve injury	Cutting, crushing, stretching nerve; electrocautery	PDA, coarctation repair
8. Horner's syndrome	Sympathetic nerve injury	Subclavian-to-aortic shunts
9. Peripheral nerve injury	Improper positioning during surgery	Brachial plexus Ulnar nerve Peroneal nerve
	Injury during attempted vascular cannulation	Median nerve Ulnar nerve

may all help decrease intracranial pressure. Corticosteroids, such as dexamethasone, have not been proven useful in such situations, but are often employed. When markedly increased intracranial pressure is suspected, its presence should be confirmed by monitoring the pressure.[308] Life-threatening increases in ICP (> 25–30 torr) may be treated by more extreme hyperventilation ($PaCO_2 < 25$–30), osmotic diuretics (mannitol or glycerol), or barbiturates. It has been postulated that treatment with barbiturates shortly after a hypoxic or ischemic insult to the brain, such as cardiopulmonary arrest, may prevent or ameliorate the degree of neurologic injury.[309] Such therapeutic benefit has not as yet been proven in clinical trials. Because barbiturate therapy poses some risks, it cannot be recommended in this situation until benefit is proven.

The occurrence of frequent or persistent seizure activity (status epilepticus) requires prompt treatment.[310] Adequacy of the airway and ventilation must be immediately assured because seizure activity or its treatment may interfere with respiration. Maintenance of adequate oxygenation and ventilation must be the prime initial consideration in treating a seizure. If a rapidly reversible cause of seizures such as hypoxia or hypoglycemia cannot be established, then nonspecific suppression of seizure activity with anticonvulsants is employed. The initial drug of choice for seizures is generally phenobarbital. A dose of 5 to 10 mg/kg may be infused slowly, carefully monitoring respiration and cardiovascular status. Following a loading dose of about 10 mg/kg, a maintenance dose of about 5 mg/kg/day may be continued. If phenobarbital alone does not control the seizure, dilantin 5 to 8 mg/kg or diazepam 0.1 mg/kg may also be infused slowly, again with careful monitoring. Maintenance doses of anticonvulsants should generally be regulated by monitoring serum drug concentrations.

In the newborn infant, metabolic causes of seizures are especially frequent, and after serum is obtained for chemical determinations, sequential empiric treatment with glucose (1/2 to 1 g/kg), calcium gluconate (100–200 mg/kg slowly), or magnesium sulfate (1–2 ml/kg of 3% solution slowly) may be attempted.[311, 312] Cessation of seizure activity following one of these drugs may be coincident or nonspecific, and etiology should not be attributed to such a deficiency unless it is confirmed by laboratory determinations.

INFECTIONS

CAUSES OF INCREASED RISK

The child with congenital heart disease has an increased risk of serious infections for a number of reasons. Chronic congestive heart failure, hypoxia, malnutrition, and failure to thrive may decrease resistance to infection. Structural abnormalities in the cardiovascular system predispose to endocarditis, probably because of damage to the vascular intima by abnormally turbulent blood flow.[313] Surgery adds increased risk because of tissue trauma, further depression of host resistance to infection, and the possible introduction of organisms.

PROPHYLACTIC ANTIBIOTICS

Because of the high risk and potentially serious nature of infections following cardiac surgery, prophylactic antibiotics are generally administered before and after the surgical procedure.[314, 315] Antibiotic coverage should include staphylococci and, in infants or debilitated patients, gram-negative organisms as well. A loading dose is given before the surgical procedure, and therapy continued 24 to 48 hours postoperatively. A longer duration of treatment may be employed for the high-risk patient or one in whom a prosthetic valve is inserted.[316]

COMMON INFECTIONS

Frequent sites of infection after surgery include the respiratory tract, urinary tract, surgical wound, or intravascular catheter sites.

Generalized septicemia may result from extension from any of these sites or from primary introduction of organisms into the blood stream. Following cardiac surgery, septicemia commonly results in seeding of organisms onto the heart valves and endocardium, or onto prosthetic valves or other materials. The newborn infant is particularly prone to septicemia.

Systemic signs of infection usually include fever and leukocytosis. Inflammation or purulent discharge may also appear at the site of infection. Less specific changes with septicemia include deteriorating cardiovascular status (septic shock), impaired respiratory function (shock lung), or impaired neurologic function. Signs of infection are particularly nonspecific in the newborn infant who may exhibit lethargy, poor feeding, hypothermia, jaundice, hypoglycemia, or seizures rather than the previously mentioned signs.[317]

Because of the potentially devastating results of infections in the cardiac surgery patient, treatment is often indicated on the basis of clinical signs without waiting for confirmation of infection by culture. However, cultures of all likely sites of infection should be obtained before starting or changing antibiotic therapy. Such cultures should always include the blood, tracheal aspirate, urine, and any suspicious wound or catheter sites. In the infant or any older patient with central nervous system signs, a lumbar puncture for cerebrospinal fluid culture, Gram stain, and cell count should also be included. The choice of antibiotics before isolation and identification of a specific organism must be based on Gram stains of potentially infected material and the likelihood of various organisms in the particular clinical situation and environment.

Bacterial endocarditis may produce destruction of heart valves, septic shock or septic emboli to the brain, heart, lung or kidney.[318-320] Optimal treatment of endocarditis requires identification of the infecting organism by multiple blood cultures. An appropriate antibiotic or combination and the dosage should be selected on the basis of the sensitivity of the isolated organism, and the minimum inhibitory concentrations or serum killing levels.[321] A prolonged period of parenteral therapy (6 to 8 weeks' duration) is generally required. When prosthetic material is infected, it may have to be removed and replaced in order to eradicate the infection.[322-323]

Wound infections following cardiac surgery may result in dehiscence, sternal osteochondritis, or mediastinitis. Reddening, swelling, or purulent discharge from a wound should be treated by limited opening of the wound, drainage of any purulent collections, culture, irrigation or packing of the wound with antibiotic or antiseptic solution, and systemic antibiotics.[324, 325]

Respiratory infections should be treated by the use of systemic antibiotics appropriate for the organisms isolated from tracheal aspirates and by physical measures to remove secretions and reverse atelectasis.

Urinary tract infections are most often caused by contamination from an indwelling bladder catheter. Treatment consists of removal of the contaminated catheter and the use of an appropriate antibiotic. If prolonged bladder drainage is required, irrigation of the catheter with an antibiotic solution may help to prevent or control infection. Suprapubic drainage of the bladder may be less likely to potentiate infection than urethral catheterization.

FEVER AND FEBRILE SYNDROMES

Fever occurs quite commonly in patients following cardiovascular surgery, so much so that a low-grade fever on the first few days after surgery may be considered normal. The etiology of this temperature elevation is not clear, but may be caused by the presence of blood in the pericardial or pleural spaces, reaction to damaged cells or proteins produced by cardiopulmonary bypass, or the presence of atelectasis. Fever that exceeds 39°C, persists for more than 3 or 4 days, or is accompanied by other systemic signs should be cause for concern and further evaluation.

Causes for fever other than infection include drug reactions, minor blood reactions, malfunction of warming devices or heated humidifiers, or the postpericardotomy or postperfusion syndromes.

Fever alone may be detrimental because of the resulting increased oxygen consumption, increased demands on the cardiorespiratory system, and the potential for febrile seizures in young children. Acetaminophen (5–10 mg/kg) is generally preferred to aspirin for treatment of fever because the latter may cause platelet dysfunction and impaired hemostasis. Cooling by a thermal mattress or sponging with cool water may also be useful, but is of little use if shivering is permitted.

A relatively common cause of persistent postoperative fever is the so-called *postpericardotomy syndrome.*[326] The etiology is unclear but an autoimmune, antigen-antibody reaction, possibly triggered by a viral infection, is suspected.[327] Symptoms, which include fever, leukocytosis, and pericardial and/or pleural effusions, may appear anytime during the first few months after surgery and may persist from several days to weeks. This syndrome rarely causes serious problems other than concern over the fever and possibility of infection. Some patients may be troubled by chest pain, malaise, or respiratory impairment from large pleural effusions. These occasionally need drainage. Cardiac tamponade from pericardial effusion, although rare, is a serious problem which may require pericardiocentesis. Treatment of the postpericardotomy is usually symptomatic with aspirin and rest. Corticosteroids may be even more effective if troublesome symptoms persist.

The *postperfusion syndrome* begins with fever, leukocytosis (primarily atypical lymphocytes), and splenomegaly 2 weeks to 2 months postoperatively.[328, 329] Viral infections such as cytomeglovirus or Epstein-Barr virus transmitted by blood products apparently produce this syndrome at least in the majority of cases.[330] This condition is self-limited and symptomatic treatment with aspirin is usually sufficient.

GASTROINTESTINAL FUNCTION AND NUTRITION

In uncomplicated cardiovascular surgery, the gastrointestinal system is generally not greatly affected. As with any other major surgical procedure, a transient ileus may result and it is common practice to avoid oral feedings and maintain gastric drainage through a nasogastric tube. This prevents gastric distention which may interfere with respiration and also helps to avoid nausea and vomiting.

GASTROINTESTINAL COMPLICATIONS

In unusual situations, gastrointestinal complications may occur. Gastrointestinal bleeding from an ulcer or as a result of a generalized coagulopathy is occasionally seen. Bowel infarction or perforation may result from embolic phenomena or a low-cardiac output state.[331, 332] This is particularly likely in the premature infant in whom the syndrome of necrotizing enterocolitis may occur.[333] This condition is manifest by abdominal distention, bloody stools, vomiting, and usually thrombocytopenia. Abdominal roentgenographs may show the characteristic picture of pneumotosis intestinalis or gas within the wall of the bowel. Intestinal perforation, peritonitis, and shock are common complications. The etiology of this condition has not been established, but it most likely results from invasion of fecal organisms into the bowel wall in a patient with inadequate mesenteric perfusion. When necrotizing enterocolitis is suspected, initial treatment includes the discontinuing of oral feedings, nasogastric drainage, systemic antibiotics, and monitoring for signs of bowel infarction or perforation.[334] Large volume transfusions with fresh frozen plasma or blood may be required to support the circulation. The use of antibiotics, orally or by nasogastric tube, to prevent or treat this lesion is controversial. Signs of perforation or peritonitis require laparotomy and appropriate surgical treatment.

Following repair of coarctation of the aorta, a form of mesenteric arteritis may occur. This begins with abdominal pain, vomiting, and ileus, and may proceed to bowel infarction or perforation in some patients.[325, 326]

Prolonged ileus may be seen following any cardiac operation when overall recovery is delayed, most commonly because of marginal cardiovascular functions or congestive heart failure with ascites and edema of the bowel. Other factors which may interfere with normal gastrointestinal function include pain, narcotic drugs, hypokalemia, or drugs which affect smooth muscle function such as sodium nitroprusside. An extreme form of venous congestion and edema of the bowel may result when the inferior vena cava is obstructed, most commonly due to an obstructing atrial baffle following the Mustard procedure for transposition of the great arteries.[337] A syndrome of chronic diarrhea and protein-losing enteropathy has been reported in this situation.[338]

NUTRITION

Maintenance of adequate nutrition is not a major problem for most pediatric patients undergoing elective cardiac surgery. When the child has preexisting failure to thrive or chronic malnutrition, when the postoperative recovery is long and complicated, or when the patient is a small infant, nutrition may play a more important role. Aggressive measures may be necessary to provide adequate nutritional substrate to meet the demands of the surgical stress and wound healing in these patients.

In the well-nourished child, adequate supplies of energy substrate are available from glycogen and other stores, plus the small amounts of glucose infused intravenously, to maintain blood glucose levels in the normal range. In the stressed newborn or cachectic, chronically ill older infant, minimal energy stores may be present and hypoglycemia is a frequent problem.[339] Low blood glucose levels (< 30–40 mg/dl) may produce impaired consciousness, seizures, impaired cardiac performance, and even permanent brain damage. It is important, therefore, to monitor blood glucose concentrations by laboratory determinations or by Dextrostix and to supply extra glucose as needed. In the infant weighing less than 10 kg, we routinely provide intravenous fluids as a 10 percent glucose solution. Occasionally it is necessary to increase the concentration to 15 or 20 percent glucose. When symptomatic hypoglycemia is detected, the blood glucose level should be rapidly increased by injection of about 1 ml/kg of 50 percent glucose solution, followed by an increase in the glucose concentration in maintenance fluids and frequent monitoring of glucose levels.

When normal enteral nutrition cannot be established within 3 to 5 days after surgery, intravenous nutrition with concentrated glucose, amino acids, vitamins, and trace elements. (hyperalimentation) should be considered.[340, 341] This technique requires a central venous line and carries the risks of infection or metabolic abnormalities such as hyperglycemia and hyperosmolality.[342, 343] Estimated daily requirements for total intravenous nutrition in infants are listed in Table 20-24. The solution infused through a central venous line contains 20 to 25 percent glucose and crystalline amino acids. A similar solu-

Table 20-24. Estimated Daily Needs for TPN*
Metabolic Maintenance, Growth, and Tissue Repair of Infants

Proteins	1.5–4.0 g/kg
Calories	120–200/kg
Water	120–180 ml/kg
Sodium	3–8 mEq/kg
Potassium	2–4 mEq/kg
Chloride	2–4 mEq/kg
Calcium	1 mEq/kg
Phosphorus	1 mEq/kg
Magnesium	1 mEq/kg
Vitamins	
A	2,000 IU
B$_1$	0.5–5 mg
B$_2$	0.5–2 mg
B$_6$	0.5–2 mg
B$_{12}$	1 µg
C	75–100 mg
D	300–400 IU
E	1 IU
K	1–1.5 mg
Folic acid	0.35–0.5 mg
Niacin	10–30 mg

*TPN = total parenteral nutrition.
Mize CE, Hartwig R: In Levin DL, Morris FC, Moore GC (eds): A Practical Guide to Pediatric Intensive Care, p 459. St. Louis, CV Mosby, 1979

tion with a lower glucose concentration (10–12.5%) may be given through peripheral veins and may help to minimize protein catabolism. However, administration of adequate calories for maintenance and growth is difficult with this peripheral solution without a very high fluid intake. The addition of a parenteral lipid solution (Intralipid) allows a greater caloric intake with less volume, especially important in the cardiac patient requiring fluid restriction.[344]

PSYCHOLOGIC FACTORS

Major surgery is a significant psychologic and emotional stress for a child.[345, 346] The long-term effects of such a stress are uncertain, but a number of things can be done to reduce psychologic trauma throughout the perioperative period.

Preoperative preparation should include a tour of the intensive care area for the child and parents, and a full explanation of the expected postoperative course and procedures. The child, regardless of age, should be told what is going to happen within his ability to understand, including the fact that he will have some pain and discomfort. To do otherwise violates the child's trust. He should be assured that someone will always be with him to take care of his needs and help relieve the pain.

Younger children are probably more stressed by separation from their parents than any other factor and every effort should be made to avoid unnecessary separation. The traditional practice of excluding parents from the ICU except for short visitation periods for the convenience of physicians and nurses should be replaced with a philosophy which gives high priority to allowing the parents at the child's bedside as soon and as much as possible. Allowing familiar objects from home and otherwise providing a child-oriented environment also helps to reduce the stress of unfamiliar and often threatening surroundings.

Continued communication with the patient and parents as to progress and plans is an important aspect of postoperative care which is often neglected by physicians preoccupied with technical aspects of intensive care, despite repeated admonitions to do otherwise. In many hospitals, a special team of social workers, nurses, or other professionals is organized to support the patient and family and to improve communications. These personnel may be responsible for preoperative teaching, emotional and logistical help during hospitalization, discharge planning, and arrangements for follow up. The physician's responsibility to the patient and parents is not diminished by the existence of such a support group. However, the presence of such personnel with the time and skills for communication and emotional support makes the experience of surgery easier for the patient and his family. It is especially helpful to have such a person with whom the parents are familiar and comfortable when the postoperative course is complicated and setbacks occur.

SUMMARY

Provision of optimal postoperative intensive care requires more than adherence to a routine management protocol. A tremendous variety of anatomic lesions occur in infants and children.[347–349] It is essential that the medical and nursing staff caring for the pediatric heart patient understand the anatomy of the cardiac lesion and the surgical procedure performed to correct it, as well as the physiologic alterations and potential complications that may occur (see Chap. 18 and Table 20–25).[350–445] By applying this knowledge along with skilled nursing care and appropriate monitoring techniques, the intensive care team can provide an environment where adverse physiologic changes are detected early so that appropriate interventions can be made to correct them before irreversible harm occurs. In this environment, the patient has the best chance for survival and recovery.

**Table 20-25. Problems and Complications Associated with Specific
Surgical Procedures and Lesions**

SURGICAL PROCEDURE OR LESION	PROBLEMS-COMPLICATIONS
1. Pulmonary artery banding[350, 351]	Inadequate banding → persistent CHF Excessively tight band, right-to-left shunt, cyanosis
2. Systemic to pulmonary anastomosis[352, 353]	Shunt occlusion (thrombosis, kinking)
a. Waterston;[354–357] Potts[358]	Shunt too large → excessive pulmonary blood flow, CHF, pulmonary hypertension[359]
b. Blalock–Taussig[360–364]	Phrenic nerve injury[365] Vascular insufficiency to arm secondary to ligation of the subclavian artery[366, 367] Chylothorax[368]
c. Glenn[369]	Superior vena cava syndrome Persistent cyanosis, insufficient pulmonary blood flow
3. Atrial balloon septostomy[370] (Rashkind procedure)	Insufficient atrial mixing
4. Patent ductus arteriosus[371–373]	Phrenic nerve injury Recurrent laryngeal nerve injury Persistent CHF (usually secondary to unsuspected associated lesion) Persistent respiratory insufficiency (infants) Recanalization of ductus
5. Coarctation of the aorta[374–376] a. Infants, emergency	Persistent congestive heart failure or low output state (usually with associated lesions or endocardial fibroelastosis) Restenosis at site of anastomosis[377] Renal failure (cross-clamping of aorta; low output states)
b. Older children, elective[378, 379]	Persistent hypertension[380, 381] Postcoarctectomy syndrome; mesenteric arteritis, abdominal pain, vomiting; rarely bowel infarction or perforation[382] Paraplegia[383] Cerebral hemorrhage secondary to hypertension, cerebral aneurysm[384] Valve dysfunction (associated bicuspid aortic valve or parachute mitral value)[385, 386]
6. Pulmonic stenosis[387, 388]	Persistent stenosis Pulmonic regurgitation Right ventricular failure
7. Aortic stenosis[389–391] a. Valvotomy	Persistent stenosis Aortic regurgitation Left ventricular failure; low output state
b. Valve replacement[392–393]	Systemic emboli Hemolysis
8. Ventricular septal defect[394–396]	Persistent VSD (multiple defects; patch leak)[397] Pulmonary hypertension[398] Right heart failure Complete atrioventricular block[399–401] Ventricular arrhythmias[402] Aortic regurgitation (supracristal defects)[403]

Table 20-25. Continued

SURGICAL PROCEDURE OR LESION	PROBLEMS-COMPLICATIONS
9. Atrial septal defect a. Secundum[404]	Persistent ASD (multiple defects; patch leak) Atrial arrhythmias[405] Pulmonary hypertension[406] Congestive heart failure[407] Mitral valve prolapse[408]
b. Primum[409, 410]	Pulmonary hypertension[411] Mitral or tricuspid valve dysfunction or both Atrioventricular block Congestive heart failure
10. Atrioventricular canal[412–416]	Pulmonary hypertension[417] Atrioventricular block Mitral or tricuspid valve dysfunction or both Congestive heart failure
11. Total anomalous pulmonary venous return[418, 419]	Low output state; congestive heart failure[420] Persistent pulmonary venous obstruction (pulmonary hypertension and/or pulmonary edema)
12. Truncus arteriosus[421, 422]	Congestive heart failure Pulmonary hypertension Regurgitant truncal valve Conduit obstruction (kinking, calcific stenosis)
13. Tetralogy of Fallot[423, 424]	Persistent right ventricular outflow obstruction[425] Pulmonic regurgitation Right heart failure[426] Atrioventricular block[427] Ventricular arrhythmias[428] Persistent VSD Outflow tract aneurysm[429, 430] Thrombotic or hemorrhagic complications secondary to polycythemia
14. Tricuspid atresia (Fontan procedure)[431–433]	Systemic venous hypertension (right heart failure): hepatomegaly, ascites, pleural effusions, edema Atrial arrhythmias Respiratory insufficiency
15. Pulmonary atresia[434–436]	See Tetralogy of Fallot Conduit obstruction
16. Transposition of the great arteries (Mustard procedure)[437–439]	Atrial arrhythmias[440] Atrial baffle obstruction:[441] Superior vena cava syndrome Inferior vena cava syndrome Pulmonary venous obstruction[442] Baffle leak Inadequate atrial size (insufficient ventricular filling) Congestive heat failure[443] Pulmonary vascular disease[444, 445]

Appendix. Commonly Used Drugs in Pediatric Intensive Care*

DRUG	ROUTE	DOSE FREQUENCY
Acetaminophen	PO, PR	5–10 mg/kg q4hrs
Acetazolamide	PO, IM, IV	5–30 mg/kg/day (1–3 doses)
Amikacin	IV, IM	Newborn 15 mg/kg/day (2 doses)
		Child 22.5 mg/kg/day (3 doses)
Aminophylline	IV	4–5 mg/kg q6h or
		5–6 mg/kg loading dose
		and ~ 1.0 mg/kg/hour continuous infusion
Amoxicillin	PO	100 mg/kg/day (3–4 doses)
Ampicillin	IV, IM, PO	100–400 mg/kg/day (4–6 doses)
Atropine	IV, IM	0.01–0.02 mg/kg/dose (maximum 0.4 mg)
Calcium chloride	IV	10–20 mg/kg/dose
Calcium gluconate	IV	30–60 mg/kg/dose
Calcium gluceptate	IV	20–40 mg/kg/dose
Carbenicillin	IV	Newborn 200–400 mg/kg/day (4 doses)
		Child 300–600 mg/kg/day (6 doses)
Cefalothin	IV	50–300 mg/kg/day (4–6 doses)
Cephamandole	IV, IM	Newborn 50–130 mg/kg/day (3–4 doses)
		Child 100–300 mg/kg/day (q4h)
Cefazolin	IV, IM	Newborn *Do not use*
		Child 25–100 mg/kg/day (4 doses)
Chloral hydrate	PO, PR	10–40 mg/kg/dose
Chloramphenicol	IV	Premature (avoid if possible)
		25 mg/kg/day (1–2 doses)
		Term infant 50 mg/kg/day (1–2 doses)
		(↓ if jaundiced)
		Child 100 mg/kg/day (4 doses)
Chlorothiazide	PO, IV	20–40 mg/kg/day (2–4 doses)
Chlorpromazine	IV	0.1–0.5 mg/kg/dose
	IM, PO	0.5 mg/kg/dose
Cimetidine	IV, PO	5 mg/kg q6h
Clindamycin	IV	Infants < 1 mo: *Do not use*
		Child 25–40 mg/kg/day (3–4 doses)
Cloxacillin	PO	50–100 mg/kg/day (4 doses)
Codeine	IM, PO	0.5–1.0 mg/kg/q4–6h
Dexamethasone	IV, PO	0.1–1.0 mg/kg/dose
Diazepam	IV	0.05–0.1 mg/kg/dose
	PO	0.1–0.3 mg/kg/dose
Diazoxide	IV	2–10 mg/kg rapid bolus
Dicloxacillin	PO, IM	50–100 mg/kg/day (4 doses)
Digoxin	IV, IM, PO	see Table 20-11
Diphenhydramine	IV	0.2–0.5 mg/kg/dose
	PO	0.5–1.5 mg/kg/dose
Dobutamine	IV	0–20 μg/kg/min constant infusion
Dopamine	IV	0–20 μg/kg/min constant infusion
		(see table 20-10)
Droperidol	IV, IM	0.05–0.1 mg/kg
Edrophonium	IV	0.1–0.2 mg/kg slowly
Epinephrine	IV, IC	5–10 μg/kg bolus
	IV	0.1–1.0 μg/kg/min constant infusion
Ethacrynic acid	IV, IM	0.5–1.0 mg/kg/dose
Furosemide	IV	0.5–1.0 mg/kg/dose
	PO	1–4 mg/kg/day (1–2 doses)
Gentamicin	IV, IM	Premature (< 3 days old) 6 mg/kg/day
		Newborn 7.5 mg/kg/day
		Child 5.0–7.5 mg/kg/day (3 doses)
		> 10 years 5 mg/kg day
Glucagon	IV	40–100 μg/kg/hr constant infusion
Glucose	IV	0.5–2 ml of 50% solution
		(0.25–1.0 g)
Glycopyrrolate	IV, IM	0.005–0.01 mg/kg/dose
Heparin	IV	CPB 200–300 units/kg
		Therapeutic anticoagulation 50–100 units/kg q4h or 10–25 units/kg-hour
Hydralazine	IV, IM	0.2–0.5 mg/kg q4–6h slowly IV
	PO	initial 0.75 mg/kg/day (3–4 doses); max ~ 3.5 mg/kg/day
Hydrocortisone	IV	shock 50–75 mg/kg/dose
Hydroxyzine	IM	0.5–1.5 mg/kg/dose
Isoproterenol	IV	0.1–3.0 μg/kg/min constant infusion
Kanamycin	IM	Premature or newborn < 7 days
		15 mg/kg/day (2 doses)
		Infant > 7 days 30 mg/kg/ (3 doses)
		Child 30 mg/kg/day (3 doses)

DRUG	ROUTE	DOSE FREQUENCY
Kayexalate (Sodium polystyrene sulfonate)	PR	1–2 g/kg/dose in 10% sorbitol
Lidocaine	IV	0.5–1.0 mg/kg/dose bolus 20–50 μg/kg/min constant infusion
Magnesium sulfate	IV	Neonatal seizures (1% solution) 50–100 mg/kg/dose very slowly
	IM	50% sol. 0.2 ml/kg/dose 8–12 h
Mannitol	IV	0.25–2.0 g/kg q4–6h
Meperidine	IV	0.25–1.0 mg/kg/ql–4h
Methicillin	IV	Premature, term < 4 days 100–200 mg/kg/day (3–4 doses) Term newborn > 7 days 150–200 mg/kg/day (4 doses) Child 200–300 mg/kg/day (6 doses)
Methyldopa	IV	10–40 mg/kg/day (4 doses)
	PO	10–50 mg/kg/day (3 doses)
Methylprednisolone	IV	shock 30 mg/kg/dose
Metocurine	IV	0.15–0.25 mg/kg q1–2h
Morphine	IV	0.05–0.1 mg/kg q2–4h
	IM	0.1–0.2 mg/kg q4–6h avoid in newborn
Nafcillin	IV	Child 150–300 mg/kg/day (6 doses)
Naloxone	IV	0.005–0.01 mg/kg/dose
Nitroprusside	IV	0.5–10 μg/kg/min constant infusion
Norepinephrine	IV	0.1–1.0 μg/kg/min constant infuson
Oxacillin	IV	200–300 mg/kg/day (3 doses)
	PO	50–100 mg/kg/day (4 doses)
Pancuronium	IV	0.05–0.1 mg/kg q1–2h
Paraldehyde	PR	0.1–0.3 ml/kg/dose
Penicillin G	IV	Newborn < 7 days 100,000–200,000 units/kg/day (4–6 doses) Newborn < 7 days 200,000–400,000 units kg/day (6 doses) Child 200,000–400,000 units/kg/day (6 doses)
Pentobarbital	PO, IM, IV	2–4 mg/kg/dose
Phenobarbital	IV, PO	loading dose 10 mg/kg slowly IV maintenance 5–6 mg/kg/day (2–3 doses)
Phentolamine	IV	0.1 mg/kg/dose 1–7 μg/kg/min constant infusion
Phenytoin (diphenylhydantoin)	IV, PO	seizures: loading dose 10–15 mg/kg slowly IV maintenance 5 mg/kg/day (1–2 doses) arrhythmias: 1–5 mg/kg JV slowly
Procainamide	IV	3–6 mg/kg loading dose over 5–10 min 20–80 μg/kg/min continuous infusion
	PO	30–50 mg/kg/day (4–6 doses)
Promethazine	IV	0.25–0.5 mg/kg/dose
	IM, PO	0.5–1.0 mg/kg/dose
Propranolol	IV	0.01–0.1 mg/kg slowly (maximum 1 mg)
	PO	0.5–2 mg/kg/day (3 doses)
Prostaglandin E$_1$	IV	0.05–0.1 μg/kg/min constant infusion
Protamine	IV	1–1.5 mg/100 units heparin to be reversed Supplemental Doses 0.25–0.5 mg/kg
Quinidine gluconate	IV, IM	2–10 mg/kg q3–6h (*very slowly* if IV)
Quinidine sulfate	PO	initial 3–6 mg/kg q3h maximum 12 mg/kg/dose
Sodium bicarbonate	IV	1–2 mEq/kg/dose
Spironolactone	PO	1.5–3.0 mg/kg/day (2–4 doses)
Succinylcholine	IV, IM	1–2 mg/kg/dose
Thiopental sodium	IV	1–4 mg/kg/dose
Ticarcillin	IV, IM	Premature, newborn < 7 days 200 mg/kg/day (4 doses) Term newborn > 7 days 200–300 mg/kg/day (4–6 doses) Child 300–600 mg/kg/day (6 doses)
Tobramycin	IV, IM	Newborn < 7 days 4–5 mg/kg/day (2 doses) Infant > 7 days 6–7.5 mg/kg/day (3 doses) Child 7.5–9.0 mg/kg/day (3 doses)
Tolazoline HCl	IV	1 mg/kg/dose 2 mg/kg/hr constant infusion
Trimethaphan	IV	0.5 mg/ml solution—titrate to response
d-Tubocurarine	IV	0.3–0.5 mg/kg/dose q1–2h
Vitamin K	IM, IV	1–5 mg
Warfarin	PO, IM	loading dose ~ 0.5 mg/kg regulate subsequent dose and frequency by prothrombin time

*The best single reference is Benitz WE, Tatro DS. The Pediatric Drug Handbook. Chicago. Yearbook Medical Publishers. 1981

REFERENCES

GENERAL REFERENCES

1. Sade RM, Castaneda AR: Recent advances in cardiac surgery in the young infant. Surg Clin North Am 56:451–465, 1976
2. Hallman GL, Cooley DH: Surgical Treatment of Congenital Heart Disease, ed 2. Philadelphia, Lea and Febiger, 1975
3. Stark J, DeLeval M, Macartney F et al: Open heart surgery in the first year of live. Current state and future trends. Adv Cardiol 27:243–253, 1980
4. Manners JM, Monro JL, Edwards JC: Corrective cardiac surgery in infants. Anaesthesia 35:1149–1156, 1980
5. Rowe RD: Evaluation of late results of surgical treatment of congenital heart disease. Can Med Assoc J 113:853–863, 1975
6. Macartney FJ, Taylor JFN, Graham GR et al: The fate of survivors of cardiac surgery in infancy. Circulation 62:80–91, 1980
7. Mansfield PB, Hall DG, Rittenhouse EA et al: Cardiac surgery under age two years. J Thorac Cardiovasc Surg 77:816–825, 1979
8. Sade RM, Cosgrove DM, Castaneda AR (eds): Infant and Child Care in Heart Surgery. Chicago, Year Book Medical Publishers, 1977
9. Aberdeen E: The care of infants and children after heart operations. In Ravitch MM et al (eds): Pediatric Surgery, pp 598–611. Chicago, Yearbook Medical Publishers 1979
10. Radney PA: Anesthetic considerations for pediatric cardiac surgery. Int Anesthesiol Clin 18:1–231, 1980

Requirements

11. Levin DL, Morriss FC, Moore GG (eds): A Practical Guide to Pediatric Intensive Care. St. Louis, CV Mosby, 1979
12. Engle MA, Adams FH, Betson C et al: Resources for the optimal acute care of patients with congenital heart disease. Circulation 43:A123–133, 1971

POSTOPERATIVE MONITORING

13. Piepenbrock S, Hempelman G: Intraoperative and postoperative monitoring of cardiocirculatory function in pediatric and adult cardiosurgical patients. Int Anesthesiol Clin 14(3):49–62, 1976
14. Baker RJ: Monitoring in critically ill patients. Surg Clin North Amer 57(6):1139–1158, 1977

Arterial Catheters

15. Galvis AG, Donahoo JS, White JJ: An improved technique for prolonged arterial catheterization in infants and children. Crit Care Med 4:166–169, 1976
16. Adams JM, Rudolph AJ: The use of indwelling radial artery catheters in neonates. Pediatrics 55:261–265, 1975
17. Miyasaka K, Edmonds JF, Conn AW: Complications of radial artery lines in the paediatric patient. Can Anaesth Soc J 23:9–14, 1976
18. Goetzman BW, Stadalnik RC, Bogren HG et al: Thrombotic complications of umbilical artery catheters: a clinical and radiographic study. Pediatrics 56:374–379, 1975
19. Miyasaka K, Edmonds JF, Conn AW: Complications of radial artery lines in the paediatric patient. Can Anaesth Soc J 23:9–14, 1976
20. Prian AW, Wright GB, Rumack CM et al: Apparent cerebral embolization after temporal artery catheterization. J Pediatr 93:115–118, 1978
21. Sadove MS, Thomason, RD, Jobgen E: Capillary versus arterial blood gases. Anesth Analg (Cleve) 52:724–727, 1973
22. Huch R, Huch A, Albani M et al: Transcutaneous PO_2 monitoring in routine management of infants and children with cardiorespiratory problems. Pediatrics 57:681–690, 1976
23. Sarnquist FH, Todd C, Whitcher C: Accuracy of a new non-invasive oxygen saturation monitor. Anesthesiology 53:S163, 1980

Central Venous Catheters

24. Prince SR, Sullivan RL, Hackel A: Percutaneous catheterization of the internal jugular vein in infants and children. Anesthesiology 44:170–174, 1976
25. Coté CJ, Jobes DR, Schwartz AJ et al: Two approaches to cannulation of the child's internal jugular vein. Anesthesiology 50:371–373, 1979
26. Kaplan S, Benzing G: Ventricular function in the immediate postoperative period. In Kidd BSL, Rowe RD (eds): The Child with Congenital Heart Disease after Surgery pp 265–

275. Mount Kisco, NY, Futura Publishing Co, 1976

27. Aberdeen E: The care of infants and children after heart operations. Ravitch MM et al (eds): Pediatric Surgery, pp 598–611. Chicago, Yearbook Medical Publishers, 1979
28. Mills LJ: Left atrial catheters. In Levin DL, Morriss FC, Moore GC (eds): A Practical Guide to Pediatric Intensive Care, p 361. St Louis, CV Mosby, 1979

Pulmonary Artery Catheters

29. Swan HJC, Ganz W, Forrester J et al: Catheterization of the heart in man with the use of a flow directed balloon-tipped catheter. N Engl J Med 283:447–451, 1970
30. Mills LJ: Pulmonary artery catheters. In Levin DL, Morriss FC, Moore GC (eds): A Practical Guide to Pediatric Intensive Care, pp 351–356. St Louis, CV Mosby, 1979
31. Pollack MM, Reed TP, Holbrook PR et al: Bedside pulmonary artery catheterization in pediatrics. J Pediatr 96:274–276, 1980

Echocardiography

32. Goldberg SJ, Allen HD, Sahn DJ: Pediatric and Adolescent Echocardiography, ed 2. Chicago, Year Book Medical Publishers, 1980
33. Williams RG, Tucker CR: Echocardiography Diagnosis of Congenital Heart Disease. Boston, Little, Brown, & Co, 1977

CARDIOVASCULAR MANAGEMENT

Cardiac Output Assessment

34. Fixer DE: Measurement of cardiac output. In Levin DL, Morriss FC, Moore GC (eds): A Practical Guide to Pediatric Intensive Care, pp 362–365. St Louis, CV Mosby, 1979
35. Freed MD, Keane JF: Cardiac output measured by thermodilution in infants and children. J Pediatr 92:39–42, 1978
36. Wyse SD, Pfitzner J, Rees A et al: Measurement of cardiac output by thermal dilution in infants and children. Thorax 30:262–265, 1975
37. Callaghan ML, Weintraub WH, Coran AH: Assessment of thermodilution cardiac output in small subjects. J Pediatr Surg 11:629–634, 1976
38. Jarmakani JM: Cardiac catheterization. In Moss AJ, Adams FH, Emmanouilides GC

(eds): Heart Disease Infants, Children and Adolescents, ed 2, pp 113–118. Baltimore, Williams & Wilkins, 1977
39. Parr GVS, Blackstone EH, Kirklin JW: Cardiac performance and mortality early after intracardiac surgery in infants and young children. Circulation 51:867–874, 1975
40. Truccone NJ, Spotnitz HM, Gersony WM et al: Cardiac output in infants and children after open heart surgery. Circulation 50(Suppl III):73, 1974

Determinants of Cardiac Output

41. Roberts NK, Yabek S: Arrhythmias Following Atrial and Ventricular Surgery. In Roberts NK, Gelband H (eds): Cardiac Arrhythmias in the Neonate, Infant and Child, pp 405–436. New York, Appleton-Century-Crofts, 1977
42. Angelini P, Feldman MI, Lufschanowski R, et al: Cardiac arrhythmias during and after heart surgery: diagnosis and management. Prog Cardiovasc Dis 16:469–495, 1974
43. Hofschire PJ, Nicoloff DM, Moller JH: Postoperative complete heart block in 64 children treated with and without cardiac pacing. Am J Cardiol 39:559–562, 1977
44. Squarcia U, Merideth J, McGoon DC et al: Prognosis of transient atrioventricular conduction disturbances complicating open heart surgery for congenital heart defects. Am J Cardiol 28:648–652, 1971
45. Zoll PM: Resuscitation of the heart in ventricular standstill by external electric stimulation. N Engl J Med 247:768–771, 1952
46. Gamble WJ, Owens JP: Pacemaker Therapy for Conduction Defects in the Pediatric Population. In Roberts NK, Gelband H (eds): Cardiac Arrhythmias in the Neonate, Infant and Child, pp 469–525. New York, Appleton–Century Crofts, 1977
47. Litwak RS, Kuhn LA, Gadboys HL et al: Support of myocardial performance after open cardiac operations by rate augmentation. J Thorac Cardiovasc Surg 56:484–496, 1968
48. Samet P, Castillo C, Bernstein WH: Hemodynamic sequelae of atrial, ventricular and sequential atrioventricular pacing in cardiac patients. Am Heart J 72:725–729, 1966
49. Hartzler GO, Maloney JD, Curtis JJ et al: Hemodynamic benefits of atrioventricular sequential pacing after cardiac surgery. Am J Cardiol 40:232–236, 1977

50. Sade RM, Cosgrove DM, Casteneda AR: Infant and child care in heart surgery, p 115. Chicago, Year Book Medical Publishers, 1977

51. Gutgesell HP, Tacker WA, Geddes LA et al: Energy dose for ventricular defibrillation of children. Pediatrics 58:898–901, 1976

52. Gelband H, Myerburg RJ, Bassett AL: Management of Cardiac Arrhythmias. In Roberts NK, Gelband H (eds): Cardiac Arrhythmias in the Neonate, Infant and Child, pp 437–468. New York, Appleton–Century Crofts, 1977

53. Gelband H, Rosen MR: Pharmacologic basis for the treatment of cardiac arrhythmias. Pediatrics 55:59–67, 1975

54. Aberdeen E: The care of infants and children after heart operations. In Ravitch MM et al (eds): Pediatric Surgery, Chicago, Yearbook Medical Publishers, 1979

55. Kouchoukos NT, Sheppard LC, Kirklin JW: Effect of alterations in arterial pressure on cardiac performance early after open intracardiac operations. J Thorac Cardiovasc Surg 64:563–572, 1972

56. Kaplan S, Benzing G: Ventricular function in the immediate postoperative period. In Kidd BSL, Rowe RD (eds): The Child with Congenital Heart Disease after Surgery, pp 265–275. Mt. Kisco, Futura Publishing, 1976

57. Thomas TV: Emergency evacuation of acute pericardial tamponade. Ann Thorac Surg 10:566–570, 1970

58. Sturgeon CL, Douglas ME, Downs JB et al: PEEP and CPAP: Cardiopulmonary effects during spontaneous ventilation. Anesth Analg (Cleve) 56:633–641, 1977

59. Qvist J, Pontoppidan H, Wilson RS et al: Hemodynamic responses to mechanical ventilation with PEEP: the effect of hypervolemia. Anesthesiology 42:45–55, 1975

60. Douglas ME, Downs JB: Cardiopulmonary effects of intermittent mandatory ventilation. Int Anesthesiol Clin 18(2):97–121, 1980

61. Appelbaum A, Blackstone EH, Kouchoukos NT et al: Afterload reduction and cardiac output in infants early after intracardiac surgery. Am J Cardiol 39:445–451, 1977

62. Benzing A: Nitroprusside after open heart surgery. Circulation 54:467–471, 1976

63. Miletick DJ, Ivankovich AD: Sodium nitroprusside and cardiovascular hemodynamics. Int Anesthesiol Clin 16:31–49, 1978

64. Stetson, JB: Intravenous nitroglycerin: a review. Int Anesthesiol Clin 16:261–298, 1978

65. Albrecht RF, Toyooka ET, Polk SL et al: Hydralazine therapy for hypertension during anesthetic and postanesthetic periods. Int Anesthesiol Clin 16:299–312, 1978

66. Koch–Weser J: Diazoxide. N Engl J Med 294:1271–1274, 1976

67. Paulissian R: Diazoxide. Int Anesthesiol Clin 16:201–237, 1978

68. Awan NA, Miller RR, Mason DT: Comparison of effects of nitroprusside and prazosin on left ventricular function and the peripheral circulation in chronic refractory congestive heart failure. Circulation 57:152–159, 1978

69. Lowenstein J, Steele JM: Prazosin. Am Heart J 95:262–265, 1978

70. Stinson EB, Holloway EL, Derby G et al: Comparative hemodynamic responses to chlorpromazine, nitroprusside, nitroglycerine and trimethaphan immediately after open heart operations. Circulation 52 (Suppl 1):26–32, 1975

71. Gould L, Reddy CV: Phentolamine. Am Heart J 92:397–402, 1976

72. Miletich DJ, Ivankovich AD: Cardiovascular effects of ganglionic blocking drugs. Int Anesthesiol Clin 16:151–170, 1978

73. Heath D, Edward JE: The pathology of hypertensive pulmonary vascular disease. A description of six grades of structural changes in the pulmonary arteries with special reference to congenital cardiac septal defects. Circulation 18:533–547, 1958

74. Vogel JHK, Grover RJ, Blount SG: Progressive pulmonary hypertension in ventricular septal defect. Clin Res 11:100, 1963

75. Cartwill TB, DuShane JW, McGoon DC et al: Results of repair of ventricular septal defect. J Thorac Cardiovasc Surg 52:486–501, 1966

76. Kouchoukos NT, Blackstone EH, Kirklin JW: Surgical implications of pulmonary hypertension in congenital heart disease. Adv Cardiol 22:225–231, 1978

77. Rudolph AM, Yuan S: Response of the pulmonary vasculature to hypoxia and H^+ ion concentration changes. J Clin Invest 45:399–411, 1966

78. Kliegman R, Fanaroff AA: Caution in the use of dopamine in the neonate. J Pediatr 93:540–541, 1978

79. Mentzer R, Alegre CA, Nolan SP: The effect of dopamine and isoproterenol on the pulmonary circulation. J Thorac Cardiovasc Surg 71:807–814, 1976

80. Peckham GJ, Fox WW: Physiologic factors affecting pulmonary artery pressure in infants with persistent pulmonary hypertension. J Pediatr 93:1005–1010, 1978

81. Faraci PA, Rheinlander HF, Clevaland RJ: Use of nitroprusside for control of pulmonary hypertension in repair of ventricular septal defect. Ann Thorac Surg 29:70–73, 1980

82. Knapp E, Gmeiner R: Reduction of pulmonary hypertension by nitroprusside. Int J Clin Pharmacol Biopharm 15:75–80, 1977

83. Pace JB: Pulmonary vascular response to sodium nitroprusside in anesthetized dogs. Anesth Analg (Cleve) 57:551–557, 1978

84. Goetzman BW, Sunshine P, Johnson JD et al: Neonatal hypoxia and pulmonary vasospasm: response to tolazoline. J Pediatr 89:617–621, 1976

85. Levin DL, Gregory GA: The effect of tolazoline on right-to-left shunting via a patient ductus arteriosus in meconium aspiration syndrome. Crit Care Med 4:304–307, 1976

86. Grover RF, Reeves JT, Blount SG: Tolazoline hydrochloride (Priscoline): an effective pulmonary vasodilator. Am Heart J 61:5–15, 1961

87. Rudolph AM, Paul MH, Sommer LS et al: Effects of tolazoline hydrochloride (Priscoline) on circulatory dynamics of patients with pulmonary hypertension. Am Heart J 55:424–432, 1958

88. Wheller J, George BL, Mulder DG et al: Diagnosis and management of postoperative pulmonary hypertensive crisis. Circulation 60:1640–1644, 1979

89. Taylor SH, MacKenzie GJ, George M et al: Effects of adrenergic blockade on the pulmonary circulation in man. Br Heart J 27:627–639, 1965

90. Ruskin JN, Hutter AM: Primary pulmonary hypertension treated with oral phentolamine. Ann Intern Med 90:772–774, 1979

91. Rubin LJ, Peter RH: Oral hydralazine therapy for primary pulmonary hypertension. N Engl J Med 302:69–73, 1980

92. Wang SWS, Pohl JEF, Rowlands DJ et al: Diazoxide in treatment of primary pulmonary hypertension. Br Heart J 40:572–574, 1978

93. Klinke WP, Gilbert JAL: Diazoxide in primary pulmonary hypertension. N Engl J Med 302:91–92, 1980

94. Shettigar UR, Hultgren HN, Specter M, et al: Primary pulmonary hypertension: favorable effect of isoproterenol. N Engl J Med 295:1414–1415, 1976

95. Daoud FS, Reeves JT, Kelly DB: Isoproterenol as a potential pulmonary vasodilator in primary pulmonary hypertension. Am J Cardiol 42:817–822, 1978

96. Watkins WD, Peterson MB, Crone RK: Prostacyclin and prostaglandin E_1 for severe idiopathic pulmonary artery hypertension. Lancet 1:1083, 1980

97. Szczeklik J, Dubiel JS, Mysik M et al: Effects of prostaglandin E_1 on pulmonary circulation in patients with pulmonary hypertension. Br Heart J 40:1397–1401, 1978

98. Kadowitz PJ, Joiner PD, Hyman AL, et al: Influence of prostaglandins E_1 and F_{2a} on pulmonary vascular resistance, isolated lobar vessels and cyclic nucleotide levels. J Pharmacol Exp Ther 192:677–687, 1975

99. Crittenden IH, Adams FH, Latta H: Preoperative evaluation of the pulmonary vascular bed in patients with pulmonary hypertension associated with left to right shunts. I. Effect of acetylcholine: preliminary report. Pediatrics 24:448–454, 1959

100. Sarnet P, Bernstein WH, Widrich J: Intracardiac infusion of acetylcholine in primary pulmonary hypertension. Am Heart J 60:433–439, 1960

101. Askenazi J, Nadas AS: Anomalous left coronary artery originating from the pulmonary artery: report on 15 cases. Circulation 51:976–987, 1975

102. Lappas DG, Powell WMJ, Daggett WM: Cardiac dysfunction in the perioperative period: pathophysiology, diagnosis and treatment. Anesthesiology 47:117–137, 1977

103. Driscoll DJ, Pinsky WW, Entman ML: How to use inotropic drugs in children. Drug Therapy (HOSP), pp 39–51, November 1979

104. Yoshioka K, Tsuchioka H, Abe T et al: Changes in ionized and total calcium concentrations in serum and urine during open heart surgery. Biochem Med 20:135–143, 1978

105. Drop LJ, Laver MB: Low plasma ionized calcium and response to calcium therapy in critically ill man. Anesthesiology 43:300–306, 1975

106. Drop LJ, Scheidegger D: Plasma ionized calcium concentration. Important determinant of the hemodynamic response to calcium infusion. J Thorac Cardiovasc Surg 79:425–431, 1980

107. Rosenblum R, Frieden J: Intravenous dopamine in the treatment of myocardial dys-

function after open heart surgery. Am Heart J 83:743–748, 1972

108. Truccone JN, Farooki Z, Green E et al: Cardiocirculatory effects of dopamine in infants and children with low cardiac output after open heart surgery. Program for Scientific Sessions, American Academy of Pediatrics, Section on Cardiology, 1977

109. Holloway EL, Stinson EB, Derby GC et al: Action of drugs in patients early after cardiac surgery. I. Comparison of isoproterenol and dopamine. Am J Cardiol 35:656–659, 1975

110. Stephenson LW, Blackstone EH, Kouchoukos NT: Dopamine vs. epinephrine in patients following cardiac surgery: a randomized study. Surg Forum 27:272–275, 1976

111. Driscoll DJ, Gillette PC, McNamara DC: The use of dopamine in children. J Pediatr 92:309–314, 1978

112. Driscoll DJ, Gillette PC, Ezrailson EG et al: Inotropic response of the neonatal canine myocardium to dopamine. Pediatr Res 12:42–45, 1978

113. Lang P, Williams RG, Norwood WI et al: Hemodynamic effects of dopamine in infants after cardiac surgery. Circulation 58(Suppl 2):149, 1978

114. Driscoll DJ, Gillette PC, Duff DF et al: The hemodynamic effect of dopamine in children. J Thorac Cardiovasc Surg 78:765–768, 1979

115. Driscoll DJ, Gillette PC, Lewis RM et al: Comparative hemodynamic effects of isoproterenol, dopamine and dobutamine in the newborn dog. Pediatr Res 13:1006–1009, 1979

116. Driscoll DJ, Pinsky WW, Entman ML: How to use inotropic drugs in children. Drug Therapy (HOSP) pp 39–51, November 1979

117. Kliegman R, Fanaroff AA: Caution in the use of dopamine in the neonate. J Pediatr 93:540–541, 1978

118. Driscoll DJ, Gillette PC, Duff DF et al: Hemodynamic effects of dobutamine in children. Am J Cardiol 43:581–585, 1979

119. Loeb HS, Bredakis J, Gunnar RM: Superiority of dobutamine over dopamine for augmentation of cardiac output in patients with chronic low output cardiac failure. Circulation 55:375–381, 1977

120. Kersting F, Foliath F, Moulds R et al: A comparison of cardiovascular effects of dobutamine and isoprenaline after open heart surgery. Br Heart J 38:622–626, 1976

121. Bohn DJ, Poirier CS, Edmonds JF, et al: The hemodynamic effects of dobutamine after cardiopulmonary bypass in children. Crit Care Med 8:367–371, 1980

122. Stephenson LW, Edmunds LH, Raphaely R et al: Effects of nitroprusside and dopamine on pulmonary vasculature after cardiac surgery. Circulation 58(Suppl 2):149, 1978

123. Soyka LF: Clinical pharmacology of digoxin. Pediatr Clin North Am 19:241–256, 1972

124. Singh, S: Clinical pharmacology of digitalis glycosides: a developmental viewpoint. Pediatr Ann 5:81–97, 1976

125. Hayes CJ, Butler VP, Gersony WM: Serum digoxin studies in infants and children. Pediatrics 52:561–568, 1973

126. Krasula R, Yanagi R, Hastreiter HR et al: Digoxin intoxication in infants and children: correlation with serum level. J Pediatr 84:265–269, 1974

RESPIRATORY MANAGEMENT

127. Downes JJ, Nicodemus HF, Pierce WS: Acute respiratory failure in infants following cardiovascular surgery. J Thorac Cardiovasc Surg 59:21–37, 1970

Anatomic and Physiologic Differences in Children

128. Edmunds LH, Downes JJ: Assisted ventilation in infants. In Sabiston DC, Spencer FC (eds): Gibbons Surgery of the Chest, pp 224–238. Philadelphia, WB Saunders, 1975

129. Motoyama EK, Cook CD: Respiratory Physiology. In Smith RM: Anesthesia for Infants and Children, ed 4. pp 38–86. St Louis, CV Mosby, 1980

130. Doershuk CF, Fisher BJ, Matthews LW et al: Pulmonary physiology of the young child. In Scarpelli E, Auld P (eds): Pulmonary Physiology of the Fetus, Newborn and Child, pp 166–182. Philadelphia, Lea & Febiger, 1975

131. Polgar G, Weng TR: Functional development of the respiratory system. Am Rev Respir Dis 120:625–695, 1979

Changes in Respiratory Function After Surgery

132. Mathers J, Benumof JL, Wahrenbrock EA: General anesthetics and regional hypoxic pulmonary vasoconstriction. Anesthesiology 46:111–114, 1977

133. Fordham RMM, Resnekov L: Arterial hypoxemia. A side effect of intravenous isoprenaline used after cardiac surgery. Thorax 23:19–23, 1968

134. Stern L, Lees MH, Leduc J: Environmental temperature, oxygen consumption and catecholamine excretion in newborn infants. Pediatrics 36:367–373, 1965

135. Smith G, Cheney FW, Winter PM: The effect of change in cardiac output on intrapulmonary shunting. Br J Anaesth 46:337–342, 1974

136. Lees MH, Way RC, Ross BB: Ventilation and respiratory gas transfer of infants with increased pulmonary blood flow, Pediatrics 40:259–271, 1967

137. Bancalari E, Jesse MJ, Gelband H et al: Lung mechanics in congenital heart disease with increased and decreased pulmonary blood flow. J Pediatr 90:192–195, 1977

138. Lees MH, Burnell RH, Morgan CL et al: Ventilation-perfusion relationships in children with heart disease and diminished pulmonary blood flow. Pediatrics 42:778–785, 1968

139. Laver MB, Hallowell P, Goldblatt A: Pulmonary dysfunction secondary to heart disease. Anesthesiology 33:161–192, 1970

Pre- and Intraoperative Factors in Respiratory Care

140. Howell S, Hill JD: Chest physical therapy procedures in open heart surgery. Phys Ther 58:1205–1214, 1978

141. Stanley TH, Liu WS, Gentry S: Effects of ventilatory techniques during cardiopulmonary bypass on post-bypass and postoperative pulmonary compliance and shunt. Anesthesiology 46:391–395, 1977

Early Extubation Versus Postoperative Respiratory Support

142. Laver MD, Bland JHL: Anesthetic management of the pediatric patient during open heart surgery. Int Anesthesiol Clin 13:149–182, 1975

143. Tarhan S, White RD, Moffitt EA: Anesthesia and postoperative care for cardiac operations. Ann Thorac Surg 23:173–193, 1977

144. Barash PG, Lescovich F, Katz JD et al: Early extubation following pediatric cardiothoracic operation: a viable alternative. Ann Thorac Surg 29:228–233, 1980

Airway Management

145. Aberdeen E, Downes JS: Artificial airways in children. Surg Clin North Am 54:1155–1170, 1974

146. Aberdeen E, Downes JS: Artificial airways in children. Surg Clin North Am 54:1155–1170, 1974

147. Filston HC, Johnson DG, Crumrine RS: Infant tracheostomy. Am J Dis Child 132:1172–1176, 1978

Support of Respiratory Function

148. Winter PM, Smith G: The toxicity of oxygen. Anesthesiology 37:210–241, 1972

149. Deneke SM, Fanburg BL: Normobaric oxygen toxicity of the lung. N Engl J Med 303:76–86, 1980

150. Wolfe WG, Ebert PA, Sabiston DC: Effect of high oxygen tension on mucociliary function. Surgery 72:246–252, 1972

151. Kinsey VE, Arnold HJ, Kalina RE et al: PaO_2 levels and retrolental fibroplasia: A report of the cooperative study. Pediatrics 60:655–668, 1977

152. James SL, Lanman JT (eds): History of oxygen therapy and retrolental fibroplasia. Pediatrics (suppl)57:591–642, 1976

153. Miller WW, Waldhausen JA, Rashkind WJ: Comparison of oxygen poisoning of the lung in cyanotic and acyanotic dogs. N Engl J Med 282:943–947, 1970

154. James SL, Lanman LT (eds): History of oxygen therapy and retrolental fibroplasia. Pediatrics (suppl)57:591–642, 1976

155. Adamkin DH, Shott RS, Cook LN et al: Non-hyperoxic retrolental fibroplasia. Pediatrics 60:828–830, 1977

156. Betts EK, Downes JJ, Schaffer DB et al: Retrolental fibroplasia and oxygen administration during general anesthesia. Anesthesiology 47:518–520, 1977

157. Kinsey VE, Arnold HJ, Kalina RE et al: PaO_2 levels and retrolental fibroplasia: a report of the cooperative study. Pediatrics 60:655–668, 1977

158. Ashbaugh DG, Petty TL: Positive end-expiratory pressure: physiology, indications and contraindications. J Thorac Cardiovasc Surg 65:165–170, 1973

159. Abboud N, Rehder K, Rodarte JF et al: Lung volumes and closing capacity with continu-

ous positive airway pressure. Anesthesiology 42:138–142, 1975

160. Powers SR, Mannal R, Neclerio M et al: Physiologic consequences of positive end-expiratory pressure (PEEP) ventilation. Ann Surg 178:265–272, 1973

161. Suter PM, Fairley HB, Isenburg MD: Optimum end-expiratory airway pressure in patients with acute pulmonary failure. N Engl J Med 292:284–289, 1975

162. Pollack MM, Fields AI, Holbrook PR: Cardiopulmonary parameters during high PEEP in children. Crit Care Med 8:372–376, 1980

163. Kumar A, Pontoppidan H, Falke KJ et al: Pulmonary barotrauma during mechanical ventilation. Crit Care Med 1:181, 1973

164. Pollack MM, Fields AI, Holbrook PR: Pneumothorax and pneumomediastinum during pediatric mechanical ventilation. Crit Care Med 7:536–539, 1979

165. Stewart S, Edmunds LH, Kirklin JW et al: Spontaneous breathing with continuous positive airway pressure after open intracardiac operations in infants. J Thorac Cardiovasc Surg 65:37–44, 1973

166. Gregory GA, Edmunds LH, Kitterman JA et al: Continuous positive airway pressure and pulmonary and circulatory function after cardiac surgery in infants less than three months of age. Anesthesiology 43:426–431, 1975

167. Hatch DJ, Taylor BW, Glover WJ et al: Continuous positive airway pressure after open heart operations in infancy. Lancet 2:469–471, 1973

168. Crew AD, Varkonyi PI, Gardner LG et al: Continuous positive airway pressure breathing in the postoperative management of the cardiac infant. Thorax 29:437–445, 1974

169. Colgan FJ, Stewart S: PEEP and CPAP following open-heart surgery in infants and children. Anesthesiology 50:336–341, 1979

170. Gregory GA, Kitterman JA, Phibbs RH et al: Treatment of the idiopathic respiratory-distress syndrome with continuous positive airway pressure. N Engl J Med 284:1333–1340, 1971

171. Falke KJ, Pontoppidan H, Kumar A et al: Ventilation with end-expiratory pressure in acute lung disease. J Clin Invest 51:2315–2323, 1972

172. Kattwinkel J, Fleming D, Cha CC et al: A device for administration of continuous positive airway pressure by the nasal route. Pediatrics 52:131–134, 1973

173. Fanaroff AA, Cha CC, Sosa R et al: Controlled trial of continuous negative external pressure in the treatment of severe respiratory distress syndrome. J Pediatr 82:921–928, 1973

174. Chernick V: Continuous negative chest wall pressure therapy for hyaline membrane disease. Pediatr Clin North Am 20:407–417, 1973

175. Cullen DJ, Eger EI: Cardiovascular effects of carbon dioxide in man. Anesthesiology 41:345–349, 1974

176. Rasmussen JP, Dauchot PJ, DePalma RG et al: Cardiac function and hypercarbia. Arch Surg 113:1196–1200, 1978

177. Downs JB, Klein EF, Desautels D et al: Intermittent mandatory ventilation: a new approach to weaning from mechanical ventilators. Chest 64:331–335, 1973

178. Kirby RR, Graybar GB: Intermittent mandatory ventilation. Int Anesthesiol Clin 18:1–196, 1981

179. Kirby RR; Intermittent mandatory ventilation in the neonate. Crit Care Med 5:18–22, 1977

180. Downs JB, Klein EF, Desautels D et al: Intermittent mandatory ventilation: a new approach to weaning from mechanical ventilation. Chest 64:331, 1973

181. Kirby RR: Design of mechanical ventilators In Thibeault DW, Gregory GA (eds): Neonatal Pulmonary Care, pp 154–167. Menlo Park, Cal, Addison–Wesley Publishing Co, 1979

182. Haddad C, Richards CC: Mechanical ventilation of infants: Significance and elimination of ventilator compression volume. Anesthesiology 29:365–370, 1968

183. Binda RE, Fischer CG, Cook DR: Advantages of infant ventilators over adapted adult ventilators in pediatrics. Anesth Analg (Cleve) 55:769–772, 1976

184. Robbins LS, Crocker D, Smith RM: Tidal volume losses of volume-limited ventilators. Anesth Analg (Cleve) 46:428–431, 1967

185. Haddad C, Richards CC: Mechanical ventilation of infants: Significance and elimination of ventilator compression volume. Anesthesiology 29:365–370, 1968

186. Kelman GR, Nunn JF, Prys–Roberts C et al: The influence of cardiac output in arterial oxygenation: a theoretical study. Br J Anaesth 39:450–458, 1967

187. Smith G, Cheney FW, Winter PM: The effect of change in cardiac output on intra-pulmonary shunting. Br J Anaesth 46:337–342, 1974

188. Shakoor MA, Sabean J, Wilson KM et al: High-density water environment by ultrasonic humidification: pulmonary and systemic effects. Anesth Analg (Cleve) 47:638–646, 1968

189. Dick W: Aspects of humidification: requirement and techniques. Int Anesthesiol Clin 12:217–239, 1974

190. Walker JEC, Wells RE, Merrill EW: Heat and water exchange in the respiratory tract. Am J Med 30:259–267, 1961

191. Nelson D, McDonald J: Heated humidification temperature control and "rainout" in neonatal ventilation. Respiratory Therapy 7:41, 1977

192. Klein EF, Graves SA: "Hot Pot" tracheitis. Chest 65:225–226, 1974

193. Rowe MI, Weinberger M, Poole CA: An experimental study of the vibrator in postoperative tracheobronchial clearance. J Pediatr Surg 8:735–738, 1973

194. Kelman GR, Kennedy BR: Cardiovascular effects of pancuronium in anesthetized man. Br J Anaesth 43:335–338, 1971

195. Stoelting RK: The hemodynamic effects of pancuronium and d-tubo curarine in anesthetized patients. Anesthesiology 36:612–615, 1972

196. Antonio RP, Philbin DM, Savarese JJ: Comparative hemodynamic effects of D-tubocurarine and metocurine in the dog. Anesthesiology 51:S281, 1979

197. Savarese JJ, Ali HH, Antonio RP: The clinical pharmacology of metocurine. Anesthesiology 47:277–284, 1977

198. Goudsousian NG, Liu LMP, Savarese JJ: Metocurine in infants and children: neuromuscular and clinical effects. Anesthesiology 49:266–269, 1979

199. Seigel S, Rachelefsky GS, Katz RM et al: Pharmacologic management of pediatric allergic disorders. Current Prob Pediatr 9:1–76, 1979

200. Knudson RJ, Constantine HP: An effect of isoproterenol on ventilation perfusion in asthmatic versus normal subjects. J Appl Physiol 22:402–406, 1967

201. Fordham RMM, Resnekov L: Arterial hypoxemia. A side effect of intravenous isoprenaline used after cardiac surgery. Thorax 23:19–23, 1968

202. Weinberger M: Theophylline for treatment of asthma. J Pediatr 92:1–7, 1978

203. Pierson WE, Bierman CW, Kelly VC: A double-blind trial of corticosteroid therapy in status asthmatics. Pediatrics 54:282–288, 1974

204. Moylan FMB, O'Connel KC, Todres ID et al: Edema of the pulmonary interstitium in infants and children. Pediatrics 55:783–787, 1975

205. Virgilio RW, Smith DE, Rice CL et al: The effect of colloid osmotic pressure and pulmonary capillary wedge pressure on intrapulmonary shunt. Surg Forum 27:168, 1976

206. Downs JB, Klein EF, Desautels D et al: Intermittent mandatory ventilation: a new approach to weaning from mechanical ventilation. Chest 64:331, 1973

207. Berman LS, Fox WW, Raphaely RC et al: Optimum levels of CPAP for tracheal extubation of newborn infants. J Pediatr 89:109–112, 1976

208. Shimada Y, Yoshiya I, Tanaka K et al: Crying vital capacity and maximal inspiratory pressure as clinical indicators of readiness for weaning of infants less than a year of age. Anesthesiology 51:456–459, 1979

209. Jordan WS, Graves CL, Elwyn RA: New therapy for post-intubation laryngeal edema and tracheitis in children. JAMA 212:585–598, 1970

210. Goddard JF, Phillips OC, Marcy JH: Betamethasone for prophylaxis of postintubation inflammation: a double-blind study. Anesth Analg (Cleve) 46:348–353, 1967

211. Iverson LIG, Ecker RR, Fox HE et al: A comparative study of IPPB, the incentive spirometer, and blow bottles: the prevention of atelectasis following cardiac surgery. Ann Thorac Surg 25:197–200, 1978

Respiratory Complications

212. Battersby EF, Hatch DJ, Towey RM: The effects of prolonged naso-tracheal intubation in children. A study in infants and young children after cardiopulmonary bypass. Anaesthesia 32:154–157, 1977

213. Striker TW, Stool S, Downes JJ: Prolonged nasotracheal intubation in infants and children. Arch Otolaryngol 85:210–215, 1967

214. Allen TH, Steven IM: Prolonged nasotracheal intubation in infants and children. Br J Anaesth 44:835–840, 1972

215. Kumar A, Pontoppidan H, Falke KJ et al: Pulmonary barotrauma during mechanical ventilation. Crit Care Med 1:181, 1973

216. Pollack MM, Fields AI, Holbrook PR: Pneumothorax and pneumomediastinum during pediatric mechanical ventilation. Crit Care Med 7:536–539, 1979
217. Wyman ML, Kuhns LR: Accuracy of transillumination in the recognition of pneumothorax and pneumomediastinum in the neonate. Clin Pediatr 16:323–324, 1977
218. Brans YW, Pitts M, Carsady G: Neonatal pneumopericardium. Am J Dis Child 130:393–396, 1976
219. Reppert SM, Ment LR, Todres ID: The treatment pneumopericardium in the newborn infant. J Pediatr 90:115–117, 1977
220. Workshop on bronchopulmonary dysplasia. J Pediatr (5):815–920, 1979
221. Sladen A, Laver MB, Pontoppidan H: Pulmonary complications and water retention in prolonged mechanical ventilation. N Engl J Med 279:448:453, 1968

TEMPERATURE CONTROL

222. Stern L, Lees MH, Leduc J: Environmental temperature, oxygen consumption and catecholamine excretion in newborn infants. Pediatrics 36:367–373, 1965
223. Adamson K, Gandy GM, James LS: The influence of thermal factors upon oxygen consumption of the newborn human infant. J Pediatr 66:495–508, 1965
224. Perlstein PH, Edwards NK, Sutherland JM: Apnea in premature infants and incubator air temperature changes. N Engl J Med 282:461–466, 1970
225. Hey EN, Katz G: The optimum thermal environment for naked babies. Arch Dis Child 45:328–334, 1970
226. Agate FJ, Silverman WA: The control of body temperature in the small newborn infant by low-energy infra-red radiation. Pediatrics 31:725–733, 1963

RENAL FUNCTION, FLUIDS, AND ELECTROLYTES

Changes in Renal Function with Heart Disease and Surgery

227. Gruskin AB: The kidney in congenital heart disease—an overview. Adv Pediatr 24:133–189, 1977
228. Bourgeois BFD, Donath A, Paunier L et al: Effects of cardiac surgery on renal function in children. J Thorac Cardiovasc Surg 283–286, 1979
229. Beall AC, Johnson PC, Shirkey AL et al: Effects of temporary cardiopulmonary bypass on extracellular fluid volume and total body water in man. Circulation 29(Suppl 1):59–62, 1964
230. Breckenridge IM, Digerness SB, Kirklin JW: Increased extracellular fluid after open intracardiac operation. Surg Gynecol Obstet 131:53–56, 1970
231. Cohn LH, Angell WW, Shumway NE: Body fluid shifts after cardiopulmonary bypass. I. Effects of congestive heart failure and hemodilution. J Thorac Cardiovasc Surg 62:423–430, 1971

Fluid and Electrolyte Therapy

232. Aberdeen E: The care of infants and children after heart operations. In Ravitch MM et al (eds): Pediatric Surgery, pp 598–611. Chicago, Yearbook Med Pub, 1979
233. Sade RM, Cosgrove DM, Castaneda AR (eds): Infant and Child Care in Heart Surgery. Chicago, Year Book Medical Publishers, 1977
234. Joseph M: Rapid calculation of children's fluid requirement after cardiac surgery. Br Med J 1:306, 1978
235. Heird W, Winters RW: Fluid therapy for the pediatric surgical patient. In Winters RW (ed): The Body Fluids in Pediatrics, pp 595–611. Boston, Little, Brown & Company, 1973
236. Kaplan SA: Fluid and electrolyte therapy; maintenance, abnormal states, methods of administration. Pediatr Clin North Am 16:581–591, 1969
237. Yeh TF, Vidyasagar D, Pildes RS: Critical care problems of the newborn: insensible water loss in small premature infants. Crit Care Med 3:238–241, 1975
238. Williams PR, Oh W: Effects of radiant warmer or insensible water loss in newborn infants. Am J Dis Child 128:511–514, 1974
239. Walker JEC, Wells RE, Merrill EW: Heat and water exchange in the respiratory tract. Am J Med 30:259–267, 1961
240. Pacifico AD, Digerness S, Kirklin JW: Sodium-excreting ability before and after intracardiac surgery. Circulation 41,42(Suppl II):142–146, 1970

241. Engle MA, Lewy JE, Lewy PR et al: The use of furosemide in the treatment of edema in infants and children. Pediatrics 62:811–818, 1978

242. Fisch C: Relation to electrolyte disturbances to cardiac arrhythmias. Circulation 47:408–419, 1973

243. Walker WG, Cooke, CR: Diuretics and electrolyte abnormalities in congestive heart failure. III. Electrolyte disturbance in congestive heart failure. Mod Concepts Cardiovasc Dis 34:17–22, 1965

244. Kirsch MM, Morales J, Kahn DR et al: Effect of extracorporeal circulation on total body potassium. Arch Surg 101:500–502, 1970

245. Babka R, Pifarre R: Potassium replacement during cardio-pulmonary bypass. J Thorac Cardiovasc Surg 73:212–215, 1977

246. Nuutinen LS: The effect of furosemide on potassium balance in open heart surgery. Ann Chir Gynecol 65:277–281, 1976

247. Breckenridge IM, Deverall PB, Kirklin JW et al: Potassium intake and balance after open intracardiac operations. J Thorac Cardiovasc Surg 63:305–311, 1972

248. Hogg RJ: Acute Renal Failure. In Levin DC, Morriss FC, Moore GC (eds): A Practical Guide to Pediatric Intensive Care, pp 70 77. St. Louis, CV Mosby, 1979

249. Yoshioka K, Tsuchioka H, Abe T et al: Changes in ionized and total calcium concentrations in serum and urine during open heart surgery. Biochem Med 20:135–143, 1978

250. Bunker JP, Stetson JB, Coe RC et al: Citric acid intoxication. JAMA 157:1361–1367, 1955

251. Stanley TH, Isern–Amaral J, Liu WS et al: Peripheral vascular versus direct cardiac effects of calcium. Anesthesiology 45:46–58, 1976

252. Tsang RC, Donovan EF, Steichen JJ: Calcium physiology and pathology in the neonate. Pediatr Clin North Am 23:611–626, 1976

253. Root, AW, Harrison HE: Recent advances in calcium metabolism. J Pediatr 88:177–199, 1976

254. Dirksen H, Anast CS: Interrelationship of serum immunoreactive calcitonin and serum calcium in newborn infants (abstr). Pediatr Res 10:408, 1976

255. McLean FC, Hastings AB: The state of calcium in the fluids of the body. I. The conditions affecting the ionization of calcium. J Biol Chem 108:285–322, 1935

256. Sorell M, Rosen JF: Ionized calcium: serum levels during symptomatic hypocalcemia. J Pediatr 87:67–70, 1975

257. Mizrahi A, London RD, Gribetz D: Neonatal hypocalcemia: its causes and treatment. N Engl J Med 278:1163–1165, 1968

258. Snodgrass GJ, Stimmler L, Went J et al: Interrelations of plasma calcium, inorganic phosphate, magnesium and protein over the first week of life. Arch Dis Child 48:279–285, 1973

259. Cockburn F, Brown JK, Belton NR et al: Neonatal convulsions associated with primary disturbance of calcium, phosphorus, and magnesium metabolism. Arch Dis Child 48:99–108, 1973

Renal Failure

260. Chesney RW, Kaplan BS, Freedom RM et al: Acute renal failure: an important complication of cardiac surgery in infants. J Pediatr 87:381–388, 1975

261. Krian A: Incidence, prevention and treatment of acute renal failure following cardiopulmonary bypass. Int Anesthesiol Clin 14:87–101, 1976

262. Levinsky NG, Alexander F.A: Acute renal failure. In Brenner BM, Rector FC (eds): The Kidney, pp 806–837. Philadelphia, WB Saunders, 1976

263. Conger JD, Schrier RW: Pathogenesis and diagnosis of acute renal failure. In Strauss J (ed): Pediatric Nephology. Volume 4. Renal Failure, pp 3–28. New York, Garland STPM Press, 1978

264. Hollenberg NK, Epstein M, Rosen SM et al: Acute oliguric renal failure in man: evidence for preferential renal cortical ischemia. Medicine 47:455–474, 1968

265. Oliver J, MacDowell M, Tracy A: The pathogenesis of acute renal failure associated with traumatic and toxic injury: renal ischemia. Nephrotoxic damage and the ischemuric episode. J Clin Invest 30:1307–1351, 1951

266. Barry KG: Post-traumatic renal shutdown in humans: its prevention and treatment by the intravenous infusion of mannitol. Milit Med 128:224–230, 1963

267. Barry KG, Malloy JP: Oliguric renal failure: evaluation and therapy by the intravenous infusion of mannitol. JAMA 179:510–513, 1962

268. Cantarovich R, Locatelli A, Fernandez JC et

al: Furosemide in high doses in the treatment of acute renal failure. Postgrad Med J 47:13–17, 1971

269. Epstein M, Schneider NS, Befeler B: Effect of intrarenal furosemide on renal function and intrarenal hemodynamics in acute renal failure. Am J Med 58:510–516, 1975

270. Harrington JT, Cohen JJ: Acute oliguria. N Engl J Med 292:89–91, 1975

271. Barry KG, Berman AR: Mannitol infusion. III. The acute effect of the intravenous infusion of mannitol on blood and plasma volumes. N Engl J Med 264:1085–1088, 1961

272. Stahl WM: Effect of mannitol on the kidney. Changes in intrarenal hemodynamics. N Engl J Med 272:381–386, 1965

273. Morris CR, Allexander EA, Burns FJ et al: Restoration and maintenance of glomerular filtration by mannitol during hypoperfusion of the kidney. J Clin Invest 51:1555–1564, 1972

274. Barry KG, Berman AR: Mannitol infusion III: the acute effect of the intravenous infusion of mannitol on blood and plasma volumes. N Engl J Med 264:1085–1088, 1961

275. Muth RG: Furosemide in acute renal failure. In Friedman EA, Eliahou HE (eds): Proceedings of Acute Renal Failure, pp 245–263. Washington, DC, DHEW Publication No. (NIH) 74-608, 1973

276. Anderson RJ, Linas SL, Berns AS et al: Non-oliguric acute renal failure. N Engl J Med 296:1134, 1977

277. Kjellstrand CM, Lynch RE, Mauer SM et al: Acute renal failure in children: conservative and dialysis management. In Strauss J (ed): Pediatric Nephrology, vol 4, Renal Failure, pp 89–110. New York, Garland STPM Press, 1978

278. Hogg RJ, Stein P: Acute peritoneal dialysis. In Levin DL, Morriss FC, Moore GC (eds): A Practical Guide to Pediatric Intensive Care, pp 446–456. St Louis, CV Mosby, 1979

279. Day RE, White RHR: Peritoneal dialysis in children. Arch Dis Child 52:56–61, 1977

280. Vaamonde CA, Michael UF, Metzger RA et al: Complications of acute peritoneal dialysis. J Chronic Dis 28:637–659, 1975

281. Oken DE: Clinical aspects of acute renal failure. In Edelman CM (ed): Pediatric Kidney Disease, pp 1108–1119. Boston, Little, Brown & Co, 1978

282. Bennett WM, Singer I, Coggins CJ: A guide to drug therapy in renal failure. JAMA 230:1544–1553, 1974

BLOOD COMPONENTS AND COAGULATION

Change with Congenital Heart Disease

283. Ekert H, Sheers M: Pre- and post-operative studes of fibrinolysis and prothrombin in cyanotic congenital heart disease. Haemostasis 3:158–166, 1974

284. Ekert H, Sheers M: Pre- and post-operative platelet function in cyanotic congenital heart disease. J Thorac Cardiovasc Surg 67:184–190, 1974

285. Wedermyer AL, Edson JR, Krurt W: Coagulation in cyanotic congenital heart disease. Am J Dis Child 124:650–652, 1972

286. Wedermyer AL, Castaneda AR, Edson JR et al: Serial coagulation studies in patients undergoing Mustard procedure. Ann Thorac Surg 15:120–127, 1973

287. Maurer HM, McCue CM, Robertson LW et al: Correction of platelet dysfunction and bleeding in cyanotic congenital heart disease by simple red cell volume reduction. Am J Cardiol 35:831–835, 1975

Changes in CPB and Surgery

288. Wedermyer AL, Lewis JH: Improvement in hemostasis following phlebotomy in cyanotic patients with heart disease. J Pediatr 83:46–50, 1973

289. Collins JA: Problems associated with massive transfusion of stored blood. Surgery 75:274–295, 1974

290. Coon WW: Some recent developments in the pharmacology of heparin. J Clin Pharmacol 19:333–349, 1979

291. Ellison N, Ominsky AJ, Wollman H: Is protamine a clinically important anticoagulant? Anesthesiology 35:621–629, 1971

292. Harding SA, Shakoor MA, Grindon AJ: Platelet support for cardiopulmonary bypass surgery. J Thorac Cardiovasc Surg 70:350–353, 1975

293. deLeval MR, Hill JD, Mielke CH et al: Blood platelets and extracorporeal circulation. J Thorac Cardiovasc Surg 69:144–151, 1975

294. Bachmann F, McKenna R, Cole ER et al: The hemostatic mechanisms after open heart surgery. I. Studies on plasma coagulation factors and fibrinolysis in 512 patients after extracorporeal circulation. J Thorac Cardiovasc Surg 70:76–85, 1975

295. Collins JA: Problems associated with massive

transfusion of stored blood. Surgery 75:274–295, 1974

Management of Postoperative Coagulation Problem

296. Ellison N: Diagnosis and treatment of bleeding disorders. Anesthesiology 47:171–180, 1977

Hemolysis

297. Andersen MN, Kuchiba K: Blood trauma produced by pump oxygenators. J Thorac Cardiovasc Surg 57:238–244, 1969
298. Poland RL, Ostrea EM: Neonatal hyperbilirubinemia. In Klaus MH, Fanaroff AA (eds): Care of the High Risk Neonate, pp 243–266. Philadelphia, WB Saunders, 1979
299. Odell GB: The distribution and toxicity of bilirubin. Pediatrics 46:16–24, 1970

Disseminated Intravascular Coagulation

300. Inglis TC, Breeze GR, Stuart J et al: Excess intravascular coagulation complicating low cardiac output. J Clin Pathol 28:1–7, 1975
301. Boyd AD, Engelman RM, Beaudet RL et al: Disseminated intravascular coagulation following extracorporeal circulation. J Thorac Cardiovasc Surg 64:685–693, 1972
302. Hathaway WE: Disseminated intravascular coagulation. In Smith CA (ed): The Critically Ill Child: Diagnosis and Management, pp 307–318 Philadelphia, WB Saunders, 1977
303. Buchanan GR, Moore GC: Disseminated intravascular coagulation. In Levin DL, Morriss FC, Moore GC (eds): A Practical Guide to Pediatric Intensive Care, pp 91–95. St. Louis, CV Mosby, 1979

NEUROLOGIC COMPLICATIONS

Etiology and Classification

304. Leading Article: Brain damage after open heart surgery. Lancet 2:399–400, 1975
305. Aguilar MJ, Gerbode F, Hill JD: Neuropathologic complications of cardiac surgery. J Thorac Cardiovasc Surg 61:676–685, 1971

Management

306. Mickell JJ, Reigel DH, Cooke DR et al: Intracranial pressure: monitoring and normaliza-tion therapy in children. Pediatrics 59:606–613, 1977
307. Morriss FC: Increased intracranial pressure. In Levin DL, Morriss FC, Moore GC (eds): A Practical Guide to Pediatric Intensive Care, pp 39–44. St. Louis, CV Mosby, 1979
308. Bruce DA, Berman WA, Schut L: Cerebrospinal fluid pressure monitoring in children: physiology, pathology and clinical usefulness. Adv Pediatr 24:233–290, 1977
309. Safar P (ed): Brain resuscitation. Crit Care Med 6:199–291, 1978
310. Dodson WE, Prensky AL, DeVivo DC et al: Management of seizure disorders: selected aspects. Part I. J Pediatr 89:527–540, 1976
311. Freeman JM: Neonatal seizures—diagnosis and management. J Pediatr 77:701–708, 1970
312. Volpe JJ: Neonatal seizures. Clin Perinatol 4:43–63, 1977

INFECTIONS

Causes of Increased Risk

313. Angrist AA, Oka M: Pathogenesis of bacterial endocarditis. JAMA 183:249–252, 1963

Prophylactic Antibiotics

314. Myerowitz PD, Caswell K, Lindsay WG et al: Antibiotic prophylaxis for open heart surgery. J Thorac Cardiovasc Surg 73:625–629, 1977
315. AHA Committee Report: Prevention of bacterial endocarditis. Circulation 56:139A–143A, 1977
316. Amoury RA: Infection following cardiopulmonary bypass. In Norman JC (ed): Cardiac Surgery, ed 2, pp 555–598. New York, Appleton–Century Crofts, 1972

Common Infections

317. Gotoff SP, Behrman RE: Neonatal septicemia. J Pediatr 76:142–153, 1970
318. Blumenthal S, Griffiths SP, Morgan BC: Bacterial endocarditis in children with heart disease. Pediatrics 26:993–1017, 1960
319. Weinstein L, Schlesinger JJ: Pathoanatomic, pathophysiolgic and clinical correlation in endocarditis. N Engl J Med 291:832–837, 1974
320. Johnson DH, Rosenthal A, Nadas AS: A forty-year review of bacterial endocarditis in infancy and childhood. Circulation 51:581–588, 1975

321. Blumenthal S: Infective endocarditis. In Gellis SS, Kagan BM (eds): Current Pediatric Therapy, pp 528–531. Philadelphia, WB Saunders, 1980

322. Richardson JV, Karp RB, Kirklin JW et al: Treatment of infective endocarditis: a 10 year comparative analysis. Circulation 58:589–597, 1978

323. Amoury RA, Bowman FO, Walm JR: Endocarditis associated with intracardiac prosthesis. Diagnosis, management and prophylaxis. J Thorac Cardiovasc Surg 51:36–48, 1966

324. Culliford AT, Cunningham JN, Zeff RH et al: Sternal and costochondral infections following open heart surgery. J Thorac Cardiovasc Surg 72:714–726, 1976

325. Barois A, Grosbuis S, Simon N et al: Treatment of mediastinitis in children after cardiac surgery. Intensive Care Med 4:35–39, 1978

Fever and Febrile Syndrome

326. Engle MA, Zabriskie JB, Senterfit LB, Ebert PA: Postpericardiotomy syndrome: a new look at an old condition. Mod Concepts Cardiovasc Dis 44:59–64, 1975

327. Engle MA, Zabriskie JB, Senterfit LB et al: Viral illness and the postpericardiotomy syndrome. A prospective study in children. Circulation 62:1151–1158, 1980

328. Wheeler EO, Turner JD, Scannell JG: Fever, splenomegaly and atypical lymphocytes. A syndrome observed after cardiac surgery utilizing a pump oxygenator. N Engl J Med 266:454–456, 1962

329. Kreel T, Zaroff LI, Canter JW et al: A syndrome following total body perfusion. Surg Gynecol Obstet 111:317–321, 1960

330. Paloheimo JA, vonEssen R, Klemola E et al: Subclinical cytomegalovirus infections and cytomegalovirus mononucleosis after open heart surgery. Am J Cardiol 22:624–630, 1968

GASTROINTESTINAL FUNCTION AND NUTRITION

Gastrointestinal Complications

331. Silane MF, Symchych PS: Necrotizing enterocolitis after cardiac surgery. A local ischemic lesion? Am J Surg 133:373–376, 1977

332. Kleinman PK, Winchester P, Brill PW: Necrotizing enterocolitis after open heart surgery employing hypothermia and cardiopulmonary bypass. AJR 127:757–760, 1976

333. Ross Conference on Pediatric Research: Necrotizing enterocolitis in the newborn infant. Columbus, OH, Ross Laboratories, 1975

334. Burrington JD: Necrotizing enterocolitis in the newborn infant. Clin Perinatol 5:29–44, 1978

335. Ho EC, Moss AJ: The syndrome of "mesenteric arteritis" following surgical repair of aortic coarctation. Report of nine cases and review of the literature. Pediatrics 49:40–45, 1972

336. Perez-Alvarez JJ, Oudkerk S: Necrotizing arteriolitis of the abdominal organs as a postoperative complication following correction of coarctation of the aorta. Surgery 37:833–837, 1955

337. Moodie DS, Feldt RH, Wallace RB: Transient protein-losing enteropathy secondary to elevated caval pressures and caval obstruction after the Mustard procedure. J Thorac Cardiovasc Surg 72:379–383, 1976

338. Krueger SK, Burney DW, Ferlic RM: Protein-losing enteropathy complicating the Mustard procedure. Surgery 81:305–306, 1977

Nutrition

339. Pagliara AS, Karl IE, Haymond M et al: Hypoglycemia in infancy and childhood. J Pediatr 82:365–379, 1973

340. Abel RM: Malnutrition in cardiac patients: results of a prospective, randomized evaluation of early postoperative total parenteral nutrition. Acta Chir Scand (Suppl)466:77–77A, 1976

341. Blackburn GL, Maini BS, Pierce EC: Nutrition in the critically ill patient. Anesthesiology 47:181–194, 1977

342. Heird WC, Winters RW: Total parenteral nutrition. The state of the art. J Pediatr 86:2–16, 1975

343. Winters RW: Total parenteral nutrition in pediatrics: the Borden Award address. Pediatrics 56:17–23, 1975

344. Bryan H, Shennan A, Griffin E et al: Intralipid—its rational use in parenteral nutrition of the newborn. Pediatrics 58:787–790, 1976

PSYCHOLOGIC FACTORS

345. Visintainer MA, Wolfer JA: Psychological preparation for surgical pediatric patients: the effects on children's and parents' stress responses and adjustment. Pediatrics 56:187–202, 1975

346. Gabriel HP, Danilowicz D: Postoperative responses in "prepared" child after cardiac surgery. Br Heart J 40:1046–1051, 1978

SUMMARY

347. Moss AJ, Adams FH, Emmanouilides GC (eds): Heart Disease in Infants, Children and Adolescents, ed 2. Baltimore, Williams & Wilkins, 1977
348. Keith JD, Rowe RD, Vlad P (eds): Heart Disease in Infancy and Childhood, ed 3. New York, Macmillan, 1978
349. Rudolph AM: Congenital Diseases of the Heart. Chicago, Year Book Medical Publishers, 1974

SPECIFIC SURGICAL PROCEDURES

350. Hunt CE, Formanek G, Levine MA et al: Banding of pulmonary artery: results in 111 children. Circulation 43:395–406, 1971
351. Dooley KJ, Parisi–Buckley L, Fyler DC et al: Results of pulmonary arterial banding in infancy. Survey of 5 years experience in the New England Regional Infant Cardiac Program. Am J Cardiol 36:484–488, 1975
352. Neches WH, Naifeh JG, Park SC et al: Systemic-pulmonary artery anastamoses in infancy. J Thorac Cardiovasc Surg 70:921–927, 1975
535. Ebert PA: Past, present and future of palliative shunts. Adv Cardiol 26:127–128, 1979
354. Idriss FS, Cavallo CA, Nikaidoh H et al: Ascending aorta-right pulmonary artery shunt. J Thorac Cardiovasc Surg 71:49–57, 1976
355. Greenwood RD, Nadas AS, Rosenthal A et al: Ascending aorta-pulmonary artery anastomosis for cyanotic congenital heart disease. Am Heart J 94:14–20, 1977
356. Vetter VL, Rashkind WJ, Waldhausen JA: Ascending aorta-right pulmonary artery anastomosis. Long-term results in 137 patients with cyanotic congenital heart disease. J Thorac Cardiovasc Surg 76:115–125, 1978
357. Stewart S, Harris P, Manning J: Current results with construction and interruption of the Waterson anastomosis. Ann Thorac Surg 25:431–437, 1978
358. Daniel FJ, Clarke CP, Richardson JP et al: An evaluation of Potts aortopulmonary shunt for palliation of cyanotic heart disease. Thorax 31:394–397, 1976
359. Newfield EA, Waldman JD, Paul MH et al: Pulmonary vascular disease after systemic-pulmonary arterial shunt operations. Am J Cardiol 39:715–720, 1977
360. Laks H, Marco JD, William VL: The Blalock–Taussig shunt in the first six months of life. J Thorac Cardiovasc Surg 70:687–691, 1975
361. Chopra PS, Levy JM, Dacumos GC et al: The Blalock–Taussig operation: the procedure of choice in the hypoxic infant with Tetralogy of Fallot. Ann Thorac Surg 22:235–238, 1976
362. Tyson KR, Larrien AJ, Kirchmer JT: The Blalock–Taussig shunt in the first two years of life: a safe and effective procedure. Ann Thorac Surg 26:38–41, 1978
363. Laks H, Fagan L, Barner HB et al: The Blalock–Taussig shunt in the neonate. Ann Thorac Surg 25:220–224, 1978
364. Edmunds LH, Stephenson LW, Gadzik JP: The Blalock–Taussig anastomosis in infants younger than 1 week of age. Circulation 62:597–603, 1980
365. Mickell JJ, Oh KS, Siewers RD et al: Clinical implications of postoperative unilateral phrenic nerve paralysis. J Thorac Cardiovasc Surg 76:297–304, 1978
366. Currarino G, Engle MA: The effects of ligation of the subclavian artery on the bones and soft tissues of the arm. J Pediatr 67:808–811, 1965
367. Mearns AJ, Deverall PB, Kester RC: Revascularization of an arm for incipient gangrene after Blalock-Taussig anastomosis. Br J Surg 65:467–468, 1978
368. Hargus EP, Carson SD, McGrath RL et al: Chylothorax and chylopericardial tamponade following Blalock–Taussig anastomosis. J Thorac Cardiovasc Surg 75:642–645, 1978
369. Laks H, Mudd JG, Standeven JW et al: Long-term effect of the superior vena cava-pulmonary artery anastomosis on pulmonary blood flow. J Thorac Cardiovasc Surg 74:253–260, 1977
370. Hurwitz RA, Girod DA: Percutaneous balloon atrial septostomy in infants with transposition of the great arteries. Am Heart J 91:618–622, 1976
371. Trusler GA, Arayangkoon P, Mustard WT: Operative closure of isolated patient ductus arteriosus in the first two years of life. Can Med Assoc J 99:879–881, 1968
372. Horsley BL, Lerberg DB, Allen AC et al: Respiratory distress from patient ductus arteriosus in the premature newborn. Ann Surg 177:806–809, 1973
373. Nelson RJ, Thibeault DW, Emmanouilides GC et al: Improving the results of ligation of

patent ductus arteriosus in small preterm infants. J Thorac Cardiovasc Surg 71:169–178, 1976

374. Fishman NH, Bronstein MH, Berman W et al: Surgical management of severe aortic coarctation and interrupted aortic arch in neonates. J Thorac Cardiovasc Surg 71:34–48, 1976

375. MacManus Q, Starr A, Lambert LE et al: Correction of aortic coarctation in neonates: mortality and late results. Ann Thorac Surg 24:544–549, 1977

376. Herrmann VM, Laks H, Fagan L et al: Repair of aortic coarctation in the first year of life. Ann Thorac Surg 25:57–63, 1978

377. Hartmann AF, Goldring D, Hernandez A et al: Recurrent coarctation of the aorta after successful repair in infancy. Am J Cardiol 25:405–410, 1970

378. Pennington DG, Liberthson RR, Jacobs M et al: Critical review of experience with surgical repair of coarctation of the aorta. J Thorac Cardiovasc Surg 77:217–229, 1979

379. Liberthson RR, Pennington DG, Jacobs ML et al: Coarctation of the aorta: review of 234 patients and clarification of management problems. Am J Cardiol 43:835–840, 1979

380. Sealy WC, Harris JS, Young WG et al: Paradoxical hypertension following resection of coarctation of the aorta. Surgery 42:135–147, 1957

381. Will RJ, Walker OM, Traugott RC et al: Sodium nitroprusside and propranolol therapy for management of postcoarctectomy hypertension. J Thorac Cardiovasc Surg 75:722–724, 1978

382. Ho ECK, Moss AJ: The syndrome of mesenteric arteritis following surgical repair of aortic coarctation. Pediatrics 49:40–45, 1972

383. Brewer LA, Fosburg RG, Mulder GA et al: Spinal cord complications following surgery for coarctation of the aorta: a study of 69 cases. J Thorac Cardiovasc Surg 64:368–381, 1972

384. Shearer WT, Rutman JY, Weinberg WA et al: Coarctation of the aorta and cerebrovascular accident: a proposal for early corrective surgery. J Pediatr 77:1004–1009, 1970

385. Simon AB, Zloto AE: Coarctation of the aorta. Longitudinal assessment of operated patients. Circulation 50:456–464, 1974

386. Rosenquist GC: Congenital mitral valve disease associated with coarctation of the aorta. Circulation 49:985–993, 1974

387. Danielson GK, Exarhos ND, Weidman WH et al: Pulmonic stenosis with intact ventricular septum. Surgical considerations and results of operation. J Thorac Cardiovasc Surg 61:228–234, 1971

388. Reid JM, Coleman EN, Stevenson JG et al: Long-term results of surgical treatment for pulmonary valve stenosis. Arch Dis Child 51:79–81, 1976

389. Keane JF, Bernhard WF, Nadas AS: Aortic stenosis surgery in infancy. Circulation 52:1138–1143, 1975

390. Chiariello L, Agosti J, Vlad P et al: Congenital aortic stenosis. Experience with 43 patients. J Thorac Cardiovasc Surg 72:182–193, 1976

391. Fisher RD, Matson DT, Morrow AG: Results of operative treatment in congenital aortic stenosis. J Thorac Cardiol Surg 59:218–224, 1970

392. Chen S, Laks H, Fajan L et al: Valve replacement in children. Circulation 56(Suppl 2):117, 1977

393. Mathews RA, Parks SC, Neches WH et al: Valve replacement in children and adolescents. J Thorac Cardiovasc Surg 73:872–876, 1977

394. McNicholas KW, Bowman FO, Hayes CJ et al: Surgical management of ventricular septal defects in infants. J Thorac Cardiovasc Surg 75:346–353, 1978

395. Rein JG, Freed MD, Norwood WI et al: Early and late results of closure of ventricular septal defect in infancy. Ann Thorac Surg 24:19–27, 1977

396. Hoffman JI: Indications for and results of surgery in ventricular septal defects. Adv Cardiol 17:40–50, 1976

397. Theye RA, Kirklin JW: Physiologic studies following surgical correction of ventricular septal defect. Circulation 27:530–540, 1963

398. Suzuki Y, Ishizawa E, Tanaka S et al: Surgical treatment of large ventricular septal defect with pulmonary hypertension in the first 24 months of life. Ann Thorac Surg 22:228–234, 1976

399. Lauer RM, Ongley PA, DuShane JW et al: Heart block after repair of ventricular septal defect in children. Circulation 22:526–534, 1960

400. Lev M, Fell EH, Arcilla R et al: Surgical injury to the conduction system in ventricular septal defect. Am J Cardiol 14:464–476, 1969

401. Hobbins SM, Izukawa T, Radford DJ et al: Conduction disturbances after surgical

correction of ventricular septal defect by the atrial approach. Br Heart J 41:289–293, 1979

402. Angelini P, Feldman MI, Lufschanowski R et al: Cardiac arrhythmias during and after heart surgery: diagnosis and management. Prog Cardiovasc Dis 16:469–495, 1974

403. Nadas AS, Thilenius OG, LaFarge CG et al: Ventricular septal defect with aortic regurgitation: medical and pathological aspects. Circulation 29:862–873, 1964

404. DaCosta JC, Rebocho MJ, Real MT et al: Results following closure of ostium secundum atrial septal defects. J Cardiovasc Surg (Torino) 19:567–570, 1978

405. Sealy WC, Farmer JC, Young WG et al: Atrial dysrhythmia and atrial secundum defects. J Thorac Cardiovasc Surg 57:245–250, 1969

406. Zaver AG, Nadas AS: Atrial septal defect-secundum type. Circulation 32(Suppl III):24–32, 1965

407. Beyer J: Atrial septal defect: acute left heart failure after surgical closure. Ann Thorac Surg 25:36–43, 1978

408. Leachman RD, Cokkinos DV, Cooley DA: Association of ostium secundum atrial septal defects with mitral valve prolapse. Am J Cardiol 38:167–169, 1976

409. Ward RE, Anderson RM, Goldberg SJ et al: Septum primum defect repair. Ann Thorac Surg 24:291–293, 1977

410. Losay J, Rosenthal A, Castaneda AR et al: Repair of atrial septal defect primum. Results, course and prognosis. J Thorac Cardiovasc Surg 75:248–254, 1978

411. Somerville J: Ostium primum defect: factors causing deterioration in the natural history. Br Heart J 27:413–419, 1965

412. Rastelli GC, Weidman WH, Kirklin JW: Surgical repair of the partial form of persistent atrioventricular canal, with special reference to the problem of mitral valve imcompetence. Circulation 31 (Supp 1):31–35, 1965

413. McCabe JC, Engle MA, Gay WA et al: Surgical treatment of endocardial cushion defects. Am J Cardiol 39:72–77, 1977

414. Mair DD, McGoon DC: Surgical correction of atrioventricular canal during the first year of life. Am J Cardiol 40:66–69, 1977

415. Kahn DR, Levy J, France NE et al: Recent results after repair of atrioventricular canal. J Thorac Cardiovasc Surg 73:413–415, 1977

416. Berger TJ, Kirklin JW, Blackstone EH et al: Primary repair of complete atrioventricular canal in patients less than 2 years old. Am J Cardiol 41:906–913, 1978

417. Newfeld EA, Sher M, Paul MH et al: Pulmonary vascular disease in complete atrioventricular canal defect. Am J Cardiol 39:721–726, 1977

418. Clarke DR, Paton BC, Stewart JR: Surgical treatment of total anomalous pulmonary venous drainage. Adv Cardiol 26:129–137, 1979

419. Whight CM, Barratt-Boyes BG, Calder L et al: Total anomalous pulmonary venous connection. Long-term results following repair in infancy. J Thorac Cardiovasc Surg 75:52–63, 1978

420. Mathew R, Thilenius OG, Replogle RF et al: Cardiac function in total anomalous pulmonary venous return before and after surgery. Circulation 55:361–370, 1977

421. Sullivan H, Sulayman R, Replogle RF et al: Surgical correction of truncus arteriosus in infancy. Am J Cardiol 38:113–116, 1976

422. Appelbaum A, Bargeron LM, Pacifico AD et al: Surgical treatment of truncus arteriosus, with emphasis on infants and small children. J Thorac Cardiovasc Surg 71:436–440, 1976

423. Chiariello L, Meyer J, Wukasch DC et al: Intracardiac repair of Tetralogy of Fallot. Five year review of 403 patients. J Thorac Cardiovasc Surg 70:529–535, 1975

424. Castaneda AR, Freed MD, Williams RG et al: Repair of Tetralogy of Fallot in infancy. Early and late results. J Thorac Cardiovasc Surg 74:372–381, 1977

425. Joransen JA, Lucas RV, Moller JH: Postoperative hemodynamics in Tetralogy of Fallot. A study of 132 children. Br Heart J 41:33–39, 1979

426. Rocchini AP, Rosenthal A, Freed M et al: Chronic congestive heart failure after repair of Tetralogy of Fallot. Circulation 56:305–310, 1977

427. Sondheimer HM, Izukawa T, Olley PM et al: Conduction disturbances after total correction of Tetralogy of Fallot. Am Heart J 92:278–282, 1976

428. James FW, Kaplan S, Chou TC: Unexpected cardiac arrest in patients after surgical correction of Tetralogy of Fallot. Circulation 52:691–695, 1975

429. Rosenthal A, Gross RE, Pasternac A: Aneurysms of right ventricular outflow patches. J Thorac Cardiovasc Surg 63:735–740, 1972

430. Seybold-Epting W, Chiariello L, Hallman GL et al: Aneurysm of pericardial right ventric-

ular outflow tract patches. Ann Thorac Surg 24:237–240, 1977

431. Williams WG, Rubis L, Fowler RS et al: Tricuspid atresia: results of treatment in 160 children. Am J Cardiol 38:235–240, 1976

432. Scrratto M, Miller RA, Tatoules C et al: Hemodynamic evaluation of Fontan operation in tricuspid atresia. Circulation 54 (Suppl 3):99–101, 1976

433. Gale AW, Danielson GK, McGoon DC et al: Fontan procedure for tricuspid atresia. Circulation 62:91–96, 1980

434. Moore CH, Martelli V, Ross DN et al: Reconstruction of right ventricular outflow tract with a valved conduit in 75 cases of congenital heart disease. J Thorac Cardiovasc Surg 71:11–19, 1976

435. Rocchini AP, Rosenthal A, Keane JF et al: Hemodynamics after surgical repair with right ventricle to pulmonary artery conduit. Circulation 54:951–956, 1976

436. Norwood WI, Freed MD, Rocchini AP et al: Experience with valved conduits for repair of congenital cardiac lesions. Ann Thorac Surg 24:223–232, 1977

437. Stark J: Operation results for transposition of the great arteries. Adv Cardiol 17:20–31, 1976

438. Sorland SJ, Tjonneland S, Hall KV et al: Transposition of great arteries. Early results of Mustard's operation in pediatric patients. Br Heart J 38:584–588, 1976

439. Shumway NE, Griepp RB, Stinson EB: Surgical management of transposition of the great arteries. Am J Surg 130:233–236, 1975

440. Lewis AB, Lindesmith GG, Takahashi M et al: Cardiac rhythm following the Mustard procedure for transposition of the great vessels. J Thorac Cardiovasc Surg 73:919–926, 1977

441. Stark J, Silove ED, Taylor JFN et al: Obstruction to systemic venous return following the Mustard operation for transposition of the great arteries. J Thorac Cardiovasc Surg 68:742–749, 1974

442. Berman MA, Barash PS, Hellenbrand WE et al: Late development of severe pulmonary venous obstruction following the Mustard operation. Circulation 56 (Suppl 2):91–94, 1977

443. Graham TP, Atwood GF, Boucek RJ et al: Abnormalities of right ventricular function following Mustard's operation for transposition of the great arteries. Circulation 52:678–684, 1975

444. Newfeld EA, Paul MH, Muster AJ et al: Pulmonary vascular disease in transposition of the great vessels and intact ventricular septum. Circulation 59:525–530, 1979

445. Borman W, Whitman V, Pierce WG et al: The development of pulmonary vascular obstructive disease after successful Mustard operation in early infancy. Circulation 58:181–185, 1978

Part VI

ANESTHESIA FOR NONCARDIAC SURGERY

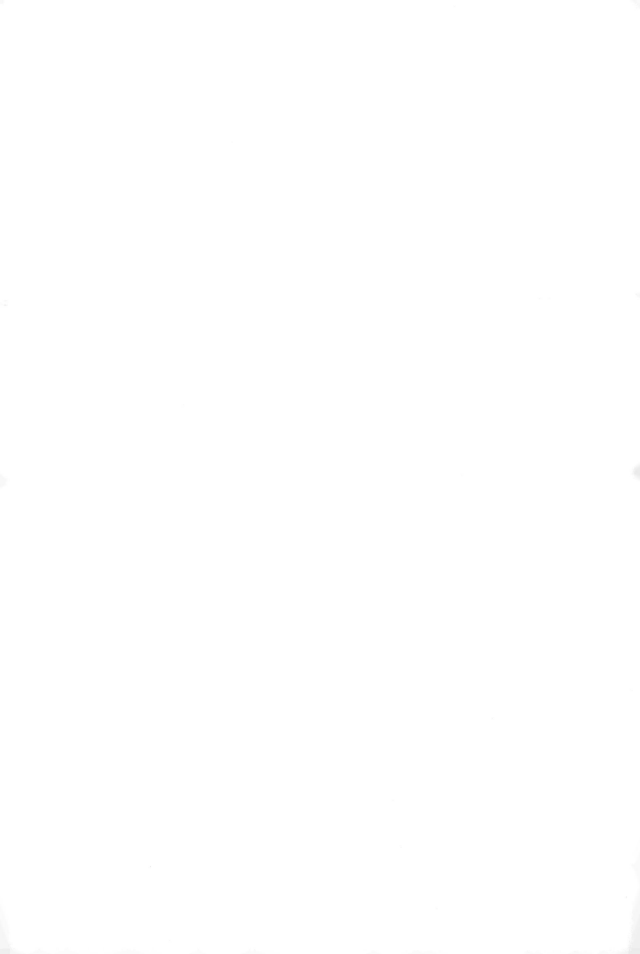

21

General Surgery and Anesthesia in the Adult Patient with Cardiovascular Disease

THEODORE H. STANLEY

The aim of any anesthetic technique is to assure a state in which a diagnostic or therapeutic procedure or surgical operation can be performed with as little physiologic and psychological trauma to the patient as possible. In this respect, anesthesia for general surgery in patients with cardiovascular disease is not different from anesthesia for patients without cardiovascular disease. However, significant impairment of respiratory, renal, cardiovascular, and other organ system function is frequent in patients with cardiovascular pathology and, in general, they can tolerate less alteration in cardiovascular dynamics and in other organ functions than patients without cardiovascular disease.[1, 2] It is undoubtedly because of this that the risk for patients with cardiovascular disease is higher than that of similar patients without cardiovascular disease undergoing the same operative procedures.[3, 4] The object of this chapter is to examine some of the influences of anesthesia and perianesthetic care on patients with cardiovascular disease and to delineate a rational approach to the management of these patients. The chapter is divided into three sections: preoperative considerations, anesthesia, and postoperative considerations.

PREOPERATIVE CONSIDERATIONS

PREOPERATIVE EVALUATION AND PREPARATION

Preoperative evaluation and preparation of the patient with cardiovascular disease should be designed to answer the following questions. Is the patient in the best possible physiologic and psychological condition? What can be done to ensure that the patient is in the best possible condition? What specific cardiovascular pathology exists and how does this further endanger the patient? Specific inquiries in the history, physical examination and laboratory studies should be designed to clarify and quantify, as much as possible, the extent of functional impairment

of the heart and peripheral vascular system (including cerebral and renal vascular systems); the pulmonary conducting and gas exchange systems; renal function; cellular metabolism; intravenous, interstitial, and cellular volume status; hepatic metabolic and excretory capabilities; and the extent of neurologic impairment. Attention to detail cannot be overemphasized because, in these patients, any minor oversight can lead to a major complication. The temptation to operate on a patient whose condition can be improved by appropriate medical management, but will take additional time, should be strongly resisted (except in life-endangering emergency situations). In this respect the following points are important.

Cardiovascular System

Congestive Heart Failure. A carefully performed experiment comparing the dangers (*i.e.*, increased morbidity and mortality) of anesthetizing patients in congestive heart failure with the dangers to similar patients adequately prepared so that they are not in congestive heart failure has never been reported. However, Goldman and coworkers did show that the presence of congestive heart failure is one of the factors that leads to an increase in postoperative complications.[5] Other factors include a recent (less than 6 months previously) myocardial infarction, frequent (more than 5/min) premature ventricular contractions, age greater than 70 years, and significant valvular aortic stenosis.

The hazard of anesthesia in patients with congestive heart failure is magnified because of the increased probability of hypoxia, reduced cardiac output, overt pulmonary edema, hypotension, and malignant arrhythmias. These patients have greatly reduced myocardial reserve and cardiac output.[6] Their congested lungs and the presence of pleural effusions foster severe ventilation/perfusion defects with increased pulmonary shunting and dead space ventilation.[7] On the other hand, their decreased cardiac output can promote rapid changes in depth of anesthesia and concomitant alterations in cardiovascular dynamics and critical organ perfusion during anesthetic induction, or following even small changes in inspired concentrations of inhalation agents or minimal doses of intravenous compounds.

Patients in early congestive heart failure present signs and symptoms which are subtle and often missed in a cursory history and physical examination.[8] Occasional coughing, especially at night, as well as insomnia (perhaps caused by early respiratory distress), nocturia, unexplained fatigue, irritability (perhaps secondary to reduced cerebral blood flow) abdominal discomfort (particularly right upper-quadrant pain), and evidence of increased sympathetic activity (such as sweating) are early symptoms of congestive heart failure which can be easily overlooked.

While it is beyond the scope of this discussion to elaborate on the details of medical treatment for congestive heart failure, therapy should include bed rest, a low-salt diet, vigorous diuresis, adequate digitalization, potassium supplementation, and appropriate pharmacologic therapy for or conversion of serious arrhythmias. Therapy for congestive heart failure in the preoperative period should be vigorous. This does not mean "a dose of digitalis, a little diuretic, and some potassium today and operation tomorrow." Indeed, adquate therapy for congestive heart failure can rarely be accomplished in a few hours. For this reason, attempts to treat patients in congestive heart failure overnight so that they can be ready for morning surgery should be discouraged regardless of operating room expediency.

Some clinicians are of the opinion that diuretics used in the management of patients with congestive heart failure should be discontinued 24 to 48 hours before surgery, especially prior to intra-abdominal vascular operations, to ensure an adequate intravascular volume during anesthesia and operation.[9] Others do not recommend this therapy, reasoning that if a relative or absolute hypovolemia exists upon induction of anesthesia, intravenous crystalloids or colloids or both can be rapidly administered at that time.[10] The author's opinion is closer to the latter belief.

The rationale supporting this position is that hypovolemia can be more easily and rapidly treated than overt congestive heart failure (which can develop in some patients in the short span of one or two days without diuretics).

Myocardial Ischemia or Infarction. Demonstration of myocardial ischemia or a previous myocardial infarction is extremely important in the preoperative assessment of patients before vascular surgery because of the significantly increased risks of infarction, other postoperative complications, and death that accompany anesthesia with these conditions.[11] While an old myocardial infarction (greater than 6 months old) and stable angina were not associated with an increased incidence of perioperative complications, in the study by Goldman and coworkers, patients with unstable angina and a myocardial infarction within 6 months were found to be a greater risk.[12] Optimal preoperative preparation and careful anesthetic and postanesthetic management have, in recent years, reduced the risk of perioperative reinfarction following initial infarction (even within the crucial first 6-month period), from approximately 40 percent to less than 10 percent.[13] Nonetheless these patients are more likely to sustain malignant arrhythmias, congestive heart failure, reinfarction, and death than are patients without cardiac ischemic disease.[14-16]

Every effort must be made throughout the preoperative period to recognize and treat early evidence of myocardial ischemia. Medications that patients bring to the hospital to relieve ischemia should be maintained throughout the preoperative period. Perhaps the patients with cardiac ischemia pathology most difficult to identify are those who (because of their sedentary ways, early phase of the disease, or for unknown reasons) are symptomless and thus unaware of the serious progression of their disease. Even a standard ECG accomplished under resting conditions may not assist in diagnosis of the pathology. Recent data obtained by Roberts[17] and others suggest that ECGs during stress testing are more likely to demonstrate myocardial ischemia and therefore help clinicians choose ideal anesthetic techniques in these patients.[18] Unfortunately, ECGs during stress testing are more time consuming and costly.

Because the incidences of reinfarction and death decrease as the time between infarction and operation increases,[19, 20] it is absolutely necessary to postpone elective operations considered early after myocardial infarction. Tarhan and associates[21] showed that patients operated on within 3 months of myocardial infarction have a reinfarction rate of 37 percent. This rate decreases to 16 percent in patients operated on 3 to 6 months after infarction, and remains at 4 to 5 percent when patients are operated on 6 months or more after infarction. From the above it appears clear that operative procedures during the first 3-month period following infarction (when most of the healing of the infarcted tissue is taking place) are probably dangerous and should only be attempted when there is no other alternative. Elective surgery during the third- to sixth-month period after infarction should only be undertaken when delay would be more dangerous than waiting. Increased recognition of the risk factors associated with patients having coronary artery disease, as well as modern monitoring techniques and new anesthetic adjuvants (vasodilators and beta-adrenergic blockers) may eventually make the above restrictions to operation in patients with ischemic cardiac disease less rigid. However, until evidence to the contrary is presented, all available data indicate that elective operations should be postponed until at least 6 months after myocardial infarction.

Hypertension. As many as 30 percent of all American adults and approximately 50 percent of patients with cardiovascular disease have elevated blood pressure, the etiology of which is unknown.[22-24] Because life expectancy is inversely related to the magnitude and duration of hypertension, most patients with known hypertension are taking antihypertensive medications when admitted to the hospital. However, it has been demonstrated that approximately 40 percent of patients with aortic occlusive or aneurysmal disease and more than 50 percent of patients with carotid artery disease have hypertension upon hospital admission whether taking antihypertensives or not.[25, 26] These figures demonstrate the high incidence of inadequate antihypertensive therapy in this population and underline the importance of frequent blood pressure measurements in the preoperative period.

For years there was concern that patients who were receiving hypertensive medications would become hypotensive during anesthesia.[27, 28] A number of studies in the late 1950s and early 1960s evaluating the advantages and disadvantages of continuing antihypertensive therapy with reserpine and other rawolfia alkaloids produced conflicting results and conclusions.[29-33] However, by 1965 it became apparent that reserpine should not be discontinued before anesthesia.[34] This position was solidified by the studies of Prys–Roberts and coworkers, who evaluated the cardiovascular responses of patients who were not hypertensive, patients who were untreated or inadequately treated, and patients who had their hypertension well controlled with a wide variety of antihypertensive drugs.[35, 36] It was found that while cardiac output was reduced to a similar degree by anesthesia in all three groups, untreated patients had a more marked fall in systemic vascular resistance and a much greater reduction in mean arterial blood pressure than in the patients in the other two groups. In addition, the untreated hypertensives experienced a 70-percent incidence of severe dysrhythmias and electrocardiographic evidence of ischemia, while severe dysrhythmias only occurred in 20 percent of the treated hypertensive patients and in none of the normals. The untreated hypertensive patients also experienced severe hypertensive response during endotracheal intubation and during the awakened period. However, these responses were not significantly different from those of patients having their hypertension well treated before operation. It appears clear from these studies that the cardiovascular responses to anesthesia are more dependent on the preanesthesia arterial blood pressure than on whether the elevation in blood pressure is treated. Patients who are hypertensive regardless of treatment behave similarly to untreated hypertensives and, as a result, suffer the same type and number of cardiovascular complications. Therefore, it is important that patients coming to operation have their hypertension treated and well controlled before induction of anesthesia.

Because hypertension is so common in patients with cardiovascular disease and is associated with significant increases in coronary artery occlusion, stroke, uremia, and congestive heart failure,[37] it is imperative that scrupulous attention be focused upon careful evaluation of cardiac and renal function as well as cerebral and peripheral vascular integrity before operation.

Patients with diastolic hypertension usually have a reduced plasma volume.[38] Most antihypertensive compounds, with the exceptions of the thiazides and propranolol, increase plasma volume towards normal.[39, 40] Reductions in plasma volume in inadequately treated or uncontrolled hypertensive patients undoubtedly contribute to the cardiovascular instability experienced by these patients during anesthesia. Ideally, intravascular volume should be controlled before induction of anesthesia by adequate preoperative and antihypertensive medication. If that is not possible, appropriate volume expansion with intravenous fluids should occur before anesthetic induction.

There are many drugs available to treat hypertension. Selection of the drug to use depends upon the etiology of the hypertension, magnitude of blood pressure elevation, response of the patient, bias of the primary physician, and other associated clinical and practical considerations. Antihypertensive drugs have different mechanisms of action but can be classified as diuretics, central or peripheral sympathetic blockers or both, depletors, modifiers or false transmitters, central nervous system depressants, direct-acting vasodilators, and compounds which influence renin, angiotension, aldosterone or some of the other hormonal systems involved in blood pressure regulation. Many of these drugs alter total body or serum electrolyte concentrations or both, which can lead to serious arrhythmias and myocardial contractility problems during anesthesia. For this reason, careful evaluation and treatment of abnormal electrolyte concentrations, particularly potassium and sodium, must be accomplished before anesthesia.

Electrolyte Abnormalities. Many patients with cardiovascular disease, as mentioned above, take diuretics and digitalis for congestive heart failure or hypertension or both and develop hypokalemia because of urinary loss of potassium and inadequate potassium replacement.[41-43] Hypokalemia can also follow acute respiratory or chronic metabolic disease. In both of the above conditions the K^+ ion migrates into cells in exchange for the H^+ ion. Gastrointestinal disorders, hyperaldosteronism, and chronic steroid therapy may result in both hyponatremia and hypokalemia. Uremia can lead to hyperkalemia. All of these conditions are dangerous because electrolyte abnormalities increase the risk of arrhythmias during anesthesia. In addition, severe hyponatremia ($Na^+ < 125$ meq/1) is associated with impaired myocardial contractility.[44, 45]

Cellular and interstitial fluid concentrations of electrolytes are as important as plasma concentrations because they help determine the cellular: plasma ratio of these ions. The latter is important because it determines the resting membrane potential of a cell (K^+) and the height or magnitude of a depolarization (Na^+). Electrolyte defects of a chronic nature are often much different in their physiologic implications than acute defects. For example, acute plasma hypokalemia (hypokalemia without total body potassium loss) is often observed under anesthesia during conditions of hypocapnia and is usually well tolerated.[46, 47] On the other hand, chronic hypokalemia, as occurs following long-term diuretic therapy without proper K ion replacement, is associated with a significant loss of total body K^+ and a high incidence of arrhythias followings small changes in K^+ during anesthesia.[48]

How should the busy clinician deal with electrolyte abnormalities in the patient with cardiovascular disease before anesthesia? First, it is clear that plasma K^+ alone is not a reliable indicator of total body K^+. However, reviewing the history, ECG, and objective measurements of K^+ loss in the urine, makes it possible to determine whether hypokalemia is acute or chronic. Rapid intravenous repletion of potassium is not only ineffective in treating chronic hypokalemia (most of the potassium is excreted in the urine) but actually may be more dangerous in terms of arrhythmia production during subsequent anesthesia than no K^+ supplementation.[49] This is true because the rapid increase in plasma K^+ to normal levels can unbalance the intracellular: extracellular K^+ ratio, producing a condition not unlike that which occurs with acute hyperkalemia. The author's guidelines to this condition are listed below.

Chronic hyperkalemia implies increased intracellular and extracellular potassium. The most common condition producing this effect is chronic renal failure. The fact that patients in chronic renal failure often tolerate plasma K^+ concentrations > 6 meq/l without cardiovascular symptoms supports the belief that the intravenous cellular–extracellular K^+ ratio across the cell membrane is more crucial than the absolute plasma K^+ value in terms of preventing or producing cardiac arrhythmias. Preoperative treatment of hyperkalemia in patients with cardiovascular disease should follow the schema outlined below.

Arrhythmias. Patients with cardiovascular disease often have cardiac arrhythmias preoperatively.[50, 51] The most frequent causes for arrhythmias preoperatively are cardiac disease with direct or indirect involvement of the myocardial conducting system, drug-induced changes in the cardiac conducting system, electrolyte, pH, blood gas, or hormonal abnormalities, and hypertension.[52] It is important in evaluating a patient with heart disease to determine the probable cause of his arrhythmia and to treat the treatable arrhythmias before anesthetic induction. The reason for this is that arrhythmias which may be benign in frequency or type before anesthesia may not remain so during anesthesia. Premedicants, anesthetics, muscle relaxants, and the variety of other drugs used during anesthesia promote arrhythmias. While it would appear rational to assume that patients having arrhythmias inadequately treated or not treated at all should have a higher morbidity and mortality than patients having adequate treatment for arrhythmias before anesthesia and operation, there is little hard data available to support this concept. Goldman and coworkers did find that patients with frequent premature ventricular contractions, as previously mentioned, have a higher incidence of postoperative complications.[53] However, patients with bundle-branch blocks and nonspecific S-T and T wave abnormalities (conditions which may or may not be treatable) did not have an increased anesthetic risk.

Atrial premature beats are usually harmless and caused by excessive sympathetic stimulation.[54] However, they can precede the development of atrial tachycardia or atrial fibrillation in patients with organic heart disease. Atrial fibrillation and atrial flutter may or may not require treatment. Conversion to sinus rhythm, while desirable in most patients, is not always possible and does carry a risk of embolization of atrial thrombi. Consultation with the patient's internist or car-

---

Implications of Preoperative Hypokalemia

1. When chronic hypokalemia is suspected and serum K^+ is less than 3.0 meq/l and total body K^+ is estimated at 20% or greater, avoid all but emergency operations.
2. Replace potassium orally, if possible, over 3 to 4 days with twice daily plasma potassium determinations.
3. When plasma potassium returns to normal the patient is ready for operation.
4. When oral replacement is not feasible follow the guidelines for intravenous potassium replacement.

diologist can be of great benefit in this kind of a situation.

Isolated ventricular premature contractions (VPCs) are also common in patients with cardiovascular disease and are usually of little consequence.[55, 56] However, when VPCs become frequent or assume a bigeminal pattern, they are serious and demand that a cause and treatment be found before induction of anesthesia.

Current Pharmacologic Therapies. Patients with heart disease coming to operation are almost always taking a variety of medications for their cardiovascular problems, as well as other pathology. These compounds can interact with each other and thereby alter the effectiveness of the intended therapy as well as significantly influence the anesthetic requirements and cardiovascular actions of the administered anesthetics[57-61] While there are a variety of noncardiac drugs that these patients may take which must be considered in the preoperative evaluation, this discussion will consider only digitalis preparations, propranolol, clonidine, and nitroglycerin.

The questions that most frequently confront anesthesiologists caring for patients taking the above medications are the following. Which drugs should be decreased or stopped? How long before induction should the last dose be given? Are the blood levels of the drug in question optimal considering the increased stresses of the operation? Are there indications for prophylactic administration of any of these medications in patients with cardiac disease who are not presently receiving these medications?

Prophylactic preoperative administration of digitalis in patients with evidence of some but not serious cardiac dysfunction is controversial.[62-67] Routine digitalization of all elderly patients and younger patients with clinical or historical evidence of heart disease before major surgery has been advocated by some clinicians.[68-70] Their belief is that preoperative digitalization avoids the development of unexpected acute heart failure or serious arrhythmias or both intraoperatively or in the early postoperative period. Others be-

---

Guidelines for Typical Intravenous Potassium Replacement

1. Give up to but no more than 20 meq/l/hr of K^+ intravenously.
2. Give no more than 240 meq of K^+ each 24 hours.
3. Continuously monitor the electrocardiogram for T wave and QRS alteration as well as rate and rhythm disturbances.
4. Frequently (every 4 hours) measure plasma electrolyte concentrations.
5. Allow at least 13 hours for minimal to moderate depletion of K^+ (< 20% total body loss or plasma K^+ = 2.8 − 3.2 meq/l) and at least 24–48 hours of therapy for greater losses or a plasma K^+ of < 2.5 meq/l.

Guidelines for Treatment of Preoperative Hyperkalemia

1. Hemodialysis or peritoneal dialysis are the treatments of choice, if possible.
2. Continous electrocardiographic monitoring is always desirable but especially so in nondialysis treatments.
3. Cation exchange resins by mouth or rectum (20–50 g/day) when the condition is not emergent or rapidly progressing and the patient can take and tolerate the medications
4. Slow intravenous calcium (for emergency treatment) until the arrhythmia reverts to a normal electrocardiographic complex
5. Slow intravenous $NaHCO_3$ when hyperkalemia is accompanied by acidosis
6. Insulin and glucose intravenously (for emergency treatment)

---

lieve that because overt intraoperative and postoperative heart failure is a rare complication of noncardiac operations (even in patients with preoperative signs of early failure) digitalis should never be administered prophylactically.[71-73] They argue that because the therapeutic margin of safety with digitalis preparations is so narrow and the effective dose so variable, it is equally easy to administer a noneffective, effective, or toxic amounts of the drug in attempting to produce adequate digitalization. Furthermore, there may be a higher incidence of arrhythmias and even a higher mortality in digitalized patients.[74]

In order to resolve these conflicts, the author tries to determine whether a patient, regardless of his age, type of operation, and previous cardiac history, shows any signs or symptoms of cardiac failure. If he does and if, in my clinical judgment, he might benefit from positive inotropic support, he is digitalized slowly over a 1- to 3-day period. If he does not, or if I do not think additional positive inotropic support will produce an advantage, prophylactic digitalization is not considered. Management of patients who are already taking digitalis is conducted in a similar fashion. That is, if additional doses of digitalis are indicated, they are given, with careful monitoring of clinical and electrocardiographic signs and symptoms that will indicate toxicity and maintenance of normal serum electrolytes.

Propranolol, a beta-adrenergic blocking compound, decreases myocardial inotropy and chronotropy, diminishes the velocity of mechanical cardiac systole, and reduces systemic arterial blood pressure.[75, 76] These effects are also produced by the most potent inhalation anesthetic agents and by various combinations of nitrous oxide and narcotics or other supplements. Faced with the problem of adding the depressant cardiac effects of propranolol to the cardiovascular depressant effects of most modern anesthetic techniques, the anesthesiologist must decide if he should discontinue or reduce the dosage of propranolol preoperatively and, if so, when. When propranolol was first introduced, Viljoen and coworkers experienced severe problems in reestablishing normal circulatory dynamics after cardiopulmonary bypass in patients receiving large doses of propranolol.[77] They suggested that propranolol be discontinued for at least 2 weeks before anesthesia to permit full return of cardiac reserve. A number of other cardiac centers acted in a similar fashion and it was the practice in those centers that all patients taking propranolol (for whatever reason) had the compound discontinued for 1 day to a few weeks before operation. It soon became clear that this might not always be beneficial. A high incidence of angina, arrhythmias, and even myocardial infarction after preoperative discontinuation of propranolol was reported.[78–80] Presently, most clinicians favor continuation of propranolol up to or at least until a few hours before surgery. What data are available suggest that maintaining patients on propranolol is safer than letting the pathology, which is being controlled by the beta-blocker, surface.[81] Treatment for excessive beta blockage is rarely required. However, when necessary, atropine, calcium, alpha-adrenergic stimulating drugs, epinephrine, isoproterenol, careful digitalization, glucagon, and pharmacologic doses of steroids have all been effectively used.[82–85] The author has adopted the general policy of neither reducing nor terminating any dosage of propranolol when the drug is used to treat angina, myocardial ischemia or infarction, or severe arrhythmias. Patients having extremely high doses of propranolol (>1000 mg/day) to control hypertension do have these doses of the drugs reduced, but only approximately 8 hours before the operation.

Clonidine is one of a number of new orally administered antihypertensive compounds. It usually stimulates both peripheral alpha-adrenergic receptors and the central adrenergic apparatus and thereby produces transient increases in arterial blood pressure.[86–89] This is rapidly followed by an inhibition of sympathetic outflow from the brain and a reduction in arterial blood pressure.[90, 91] Problems with clonidine include severe hypertension and, on occasion, tachycardia, and occur when the compound is suddenly withdrawn, such as during the perioperative period in patients undergoing operation.[92] Prevention of hypertension can be achieved by early reinstitution of clonidine therapy (the same day) or employment of other intravenous antihypertensive compounds.

Oral nitroglycerin has long been used in the treatment of angina and other symptoms of myocardial ischemia. Recently, intravenous nitroglycerin has gained popularity in the acute treatment of hypertension and as a preload and afterload reducer intraoperatively and in the perioperative period.[93–96] Nitroglycerin increases blood flow to the ventricular endocardium, the tissues most at risk.[97] At present, there is no reason why nitroglycerin, regardless of dosage or frequency of administration, should be decreased or terminated in patients coming to operation. Indeed, this author feels that nitroglycerin, when routinely taken by a patient, should always accompany that patient (perhaps attached to the chart) to the operating room so that it can be instantly available for use in case of angina.

Specific Cardiac Lesions. Knowledge of the specific pathology and secondary derangements produced by that abnormality is critically important in anesthetizing patients with cardiovascular disease undergoing any kind of operative procedure. Patients with long standing mitral valve stenosis, for example, usually have interstitial pulmonary fibrosis and pulmonary hypertension.[98, 99] Their pulmonary shunt fraction is frequently elevated, necessitating the administration of higher than usual inspired concentrations of oxygen.[100] Besides digitalis, these patients are usually receiving one or more diuretics and as a result are often hypovolemic and in a state of electrolyte imbalance. This must be corrected before anesthetic induction.

Premedication is not easy in patients with long-standing mitral stenosis because belladonna drugs and other compounds that increase heart rate can result in significant decreases in left ventricular filling pressure and sudden cardiovascular collapse. Analgesics, hypnotic compounds, and anesthetics, which have only minimal central nervous system depressant effects in other patients, often produce marked depressioin in patients with mitral stenosis.[101] This may be related to the decreased cardiac output or the reduced effective circulating blood volume or both that these patients have. However, the exact mechanism has not been defined.

Patients with mitral stenosis also have more postoperative problems than other patients.[102–104] They require mechanical postoperative respiratory support more frequently and for longer periods of time. In addition, modest degrees of arterial oxygen desaturation can cause severe increases in pulmonary artery blood pressure and even sudden cardiovascular collapse in these patients.

Patients with ischemic cardiac disease undergoing vascular operations also have particular problems of great concern. While these patients often have a normal cardiac output and little or no pulmonary parenchymal disease, they frequently have systemic hypertension and sometimes pulmonary hypertension as well.[105–107] Like the patient with mitral valvular stenosis, tachycardia is also a problem for patients with ischemic disease, but for a different reason. Tachycardia, and for that matter, hypertension, increases in myocardial contractility, and increases in preload and afterload are not well tolerated because they all increase myocardial oxygen demands.[108, 109] Patients with ischemic cardiac disease suffer from an unbalanced myocardial oxygen demand: oxygen supply ratio. A change such as tachycardia, which alters the balance so that demand exceeds availability of oxygen, will produce additional ischemia in a heart that is close to or already ischemic. This may result in angina (if the patient is still conscious), impaired myocardial function, arrhythmias, and infarction. Therefore, patients with ischemic cardiac disease about to undergo surgery require heavy premedication to prevent anxiety-induced increases in heart rate and blood pressure. They also need deep, or at least adequate levels of anesthesia,[110] especially during endotracheal intubation and the start of the operation, when surgical stimulation is most likely to result in hypertension and tachycardia. However, some patients with ischemic cardiac disease have such a compromised myocardium and cardiac output that they cannot tolerate deep levels of anesthesia. These patients need alternative forms of pharmacologic therapy, such as peripheral arterial vasodilation or beta-adrenergic blockade. Occasionally, these therapies may be necessary even before or during anesthetic induction.

Patients with aortic valvular stenosis and high pressure gradients coming to cardiovascular surgery do not tolerate sudden changes in systemic arterial blood pressure or cardiac output.[111–113] Sudden increases in pressure, as can occur after intubation in a poorly anesthetized patient, markedly impair ventricular emptying and coronary artery blood flow. This could cause acute left ventricular failure and circulatory collapse. Similar results occur with sudden hypotension in this patient population. In patients with aortic insufficiency, sudden hypotension associated with a decrease in cardiac output can also cause circulatory failure. Therefore, drugs that decrease heart rate must be used with caution.

Patients with hypertrophic subaortic stenosis are a unique group. In these individuals increased myocardial contractility, such as might occur from sympathetic stimulation or administration of dopamine or digoxin, can cause constriction of the infundibulum or the outflow tract of the left ventricle with resultant impaired ventricular ejection.[114–116] Therefore, overtly or accidentally increased inotropism must be studiously avoided.

Patients with combined aortic and cerebrovascular disease, both requiring operation, present the dilemma of which operation should be performed first. Because arterial hypotension is not uncommon during major aortic vascular operations and is a serious risk in the presence of cerebral vascular disease,[117] it would appear rational to perform the carotid surgery before the aortic operation.

Myocardial Function. Preoperative myocardial function can be assessed clinically by history, physical examination, and simple laboratory examinations such as chest film (size of heart and chambers, evidence of cardiac failure), ECG, and circulation time. More time-consuming, sophisticated, and often invasive techniques measure indices reflecting myocardial contractility, left-ventricular filling pressure, left-ventricular work, left-ventricular ejection fraction and a plethora of other variables. Work in our laboratories and operating rooms of the University of Utah College of Medicine has demonstrated preoperative resting and stress or exercise-in-

duced cardiac output to be a very valuable additional variable which not only reflects myocardial function but perhaps anesthetic requirements as well in patients with cardiac disease.[118]

Patients who have a reasonably normal cardiac output and, more importantly, who experience an appropriate increase in output upon exercise, invariably have good left ventricular function. They also tend to have normal or close to normal MAC values when subjected to any anesthetic technique.[119] On the other hand, patients who do not experience appropriate increases in cardiac output with exercise or who experience evidence of left ventricular failure or inadequate systemic perfusion with exercise, usually have diminished myocardial function.[120, 121] Still worse in terms of overall myocardial function are those patients with inadequate cardiac output at rest. Not only do they have little, if any, cardiac reserve, but they also poorly tolerate the usual concentrations or dosage of whatever anesthetic is used.[122] They require little anesthetic depression for complete anesthesia and typify the kind of patients who need a light anesthetic technique that stimulates and supports the cardiovascular system. Unfortunately, some of these patients cannot tolerate too much stimulation (*i.e.,* anesthetic techniques that allow tachycardia to occur). The safety margin between too light and too deep anesthesia can be very small in these patients and therein lies the difficulty in providing them with the best anesthetic.

The Lungs

Chronic Obstructive Pulmonary Disease. Patients with cardiovascular pathology frequently have pulmonary disease as well.[123] Although it has not been carefully evaluated, the most common pulmonary pathology encountered in this population is probably chronic obstructive pulmonary disease.[124, 125] While it would appear obvious that preoperative pulmonary function in these patients should be evaluated and optimized by the use of appropriate breathing exercises, postural drainage, bronchodilators, and antibiotics, it has not been conclusively demonstrated that this kind of therapy significantly decreases postoperative morbidity or mortality in patients with cardiovascular disease. However, a recent study by Gracey and co-workers has suggested that patients undergoing extensive surgery of the upper abdomen have a lower incidence of pulmonary complications after preoperative pulmonary preparation than patients who are not subjected to such preparation.[126] In addition, it is beneficial to evaluate pulmonary function in this group of patients if for nothing else but to have a baseline for comparison in the postoperative period. An abnormally low Pa_{O_2} or high Pa_{CO_2} in the postoperative period has much more diagnostic meaning when compared to a known preoperative value than when these values are unknown.

An irritating and potentially serious problem in patients with obstructive pulmonary disease is bronchorrhea. These secretions are especially prevalent in patients with a long history of smoking. Frequently even the most meticulous and dedicated postoperative tracheal toilet cannot eliminate secretions that accumulate in the smaller airways. Small airway secretions not only interfere with adequate ventilation-perfusion matching and decrease PaO_2, but also provide an ideal culture medium for any bacteria that are introduced during intubation, tracheobronchial suctioning or contamination from a breathing circuit or ventilator. It is not surprising therefore that there is a threefold increase in the incident of postoperative pulmonary complications in the smoker as compared to the nonsmoker after major operative procedures.[127] What is less clear is at what time smoking should be stopped preoperatively or whether it should be stopped at all. There are some who believe that the irritating effects of cigarette smoke on the morning of surgery actually help mobilize small airway secretions.[128] Whether this is true or not has not been demonstrated.

Obesity. Cardiovascular disease occurs more frequently in the obese patient and is more severe.[129] The obese patient is also much more likely to develop a postoperative pulmonary complication, particularly atelectasis,

than the nonobese patients.[130–132] This is especially true following intraabdominal operations and even more so in patients subjected to xyphoid-to-pubis incisions.[133, 134] The most important cause of atelectasis in the obese patient during and following abdominal operation is diaphragmatic compression.[135, 136] Whether the use of positive end expiratory pressure (PEEP) or continuous positive airway pressure (CPAP) during operation or in the early postoperative period is of any advantage to these patients (in terms of reducing the incident of postoperative atelectasis) is unclear.[137]

Pulmonary Hypertension. The markedly obese patients as well as those with significant pulmonary obstructive disease or severe ischemic cardiac disease can have pulmonary hypertension.[138–140] In some cases, pulmonary hypertension is severe enough to result in right ventricular failure. Significant left-to-right shunts, arterial hypoxemia, and ventricular arrhythmias are associated with pulmonary hypertension and right ventricular failure.

It is difficult to diagnose pulmonary hypertension and early right ventricular failure.[141] The chest film might be quite normal. Although these patients almost always have marked exercise limitations, are frequently hypoxemic and are prone to pulmonary infections, these are not specific signs of pulmonary hypertension and often go unnoticed. The best method of diagnosing pulmonary hypertension is by pulmonary artery catheterization.[142] Consistent increases of pulmonary artery blood pressure and further increases with moderate exercise are cardinal signs of pulmonary artery hypertension. Proper management of these patients preoperatively consists of water and salt restriction, digitalization, appropriate diuretics, weight loss if obesity is present, and, if possible, correction of pulmonary lesions.

The Kidneys

Analysis of preoperative renal function is important in all patients with cardiovascular disease, but especially in those about to undergo major operations in whom significant blood loss or volume translocations are possible. In patients with impaired renal function, hypotension from blood loss can quickly result in acute tubular necrosis and renal failure.[143, 144] A usual preoperative renal function evaluation in these patients includes a complete urine analysis, blood urea nitrogen and creatinine, and blood electrolyte determinations including sodium, potassium, chloride, bicarbonate, calcium, and phosphorus. In patients with known renal impairment or those likely to sustain renal damage during operation or postoperatively (because of the nature of their pathology and the kind of operation to be performed), it is desirable to obtain more specific tests including those evaluating glomerular function (creatinine or inulin clearances) and renal blood flow (para-aminohippurate clearance), as well as osmolar, free water, and sodium clearances.

PREMEDICATION

Anxiety and excitement in the immediate preoperative period often cause increases in heart rate, arterial blood pressure, peripheral vascular resistance, and myocardial contractility, all of which may predispose to myocardial ischemia in patients with coronary artery disease and which may impair ventricular filling or ejection in patients with valvular heart disease. Therefore, it is important in patients with cardiovascular disease to sedate before operation. Perhaps more importantly, all possible emotional and psychological influences should be used during the preoperative visit to allay anxiety. On the other hand, it is also important to be frank with the patient in describing the discomfort which may be associated with insertion of arterial, venous, or pulmonary artery cannulae before induction of anesthesia. He should also be informed that he might not be able to speak in the early postoperative period because of an endotracheal tube in his trachea, and that he might find himself in the stressful environment of the intensive care unit. A supportive and frank preoperative

visit not only relieves anxiety, but it also enables smoother induction of anesthesia.

In choosing preoperative medication, the objective should be maximum sedation and minimum depression of respiration and circulation. Many drug combinations are effective in achieving these ends. A favorite of this author's is morphine (0.1 mg/kg), diazepam (0.1 mg/kg), and atropine (0.05 mg/10 kg).

In patients with severe myocardial disease and little or no myocardial reserve, premedicants should be reduced or entirely eliminated because of the increased risk of impaired consciousness and respiratory depression. It is unknown why these patients have an increased susceptibility to depressants. The author believes it is related to a reduced cardiac output or circulating blood volume,[145] but this has yet to be confirmed.

There are some who feel that the preoperative use of belladonna compounds is not indicated in patients with cardiac disease.[146] They state that besides the risk of tachycardia, these compounds produce severe dry mouths, which result in unnecessary patient discomfort. They prefer administering atropine or scopolamine in small amounts just before or after anesthetic induction or completely omitting these compounds unless they are clinically indicated. Others have adopted a less radical approach and still use the belladonnas intramuscularly for premedication 1 hour before surgery in cardiac patients.[147] More recently, glycopyrrolate has become popular and, in some centers, replaced the belladonnas because it appears to produce less dry mouth, causes little, if any, tachycardia, and precipitates little, if any, postoperative excitement or agitation,[148] the latter because it possesses a quarternary carbon and therefore does not penetrate the central nervous system.

MONITORING DURING OPERATION

Extensive intra- and postoperative monitoring of all patients with cardiovascular disease is an accepted standard.[149–153] The minimum monitoring which we consider adequate includes continuous measurement of the ECG, esophageal temperature and heart sounds (including heart rate), and indirect, intermittent measurements of arterial blood pressure. When blood loss or volume translocation is more than a remote possibility, hemodynamic instability is likely, when less than adequate oxygenation or ventilation is a possibility, direct arterial and central venous blood pressures and frequent determinations of arterial blood gases, pH, body color, and urine output are also mandatory. In addition to the above, cardiac output, pulmonary artery and left atrial, or pulmonary artery occlusion or wedge pressures are particularly useful in managing patients with cardiac disease in operations in which dramatic increases and decreases of cardiac output and arterial pressure often occur or in which cardiac reserve is minimal.

The pulmonary artery catheter, one of the most important monitoring tools developed in the last 10 years, has revolutionized cardiovascular monitoring in patients with cardiac disease.[154] Besides providing pulmonary artery and right arterial pressures, this instrument has enabled monitoring of left ventricular filling pressure (by pulmonary artery wedge pressure) and thus left ventricular function, as well as cardiac output determinations (by the thermodilution technique) on a moment-to-moment basis. In addition, measurement of pulmonary artery or mixed venous oxygen tension is an extremely sensitive index of the adequacy of cardiac output for total body metabolic needs. Thus it is now possible, with the pulmonary artery catheter, to assess the total body metabolic requirement to perfusion ratio. Experiments in our laboratories and others suggest that total body or even better specific organ metabolic/ perfusion rates are far superior in assessing the adequacy of circulation and prediction of its early degeneration than standard blood pressure, blood gas, pH, or even cardiac output monitoring.[155] Recent work suggests that routine continuous monitoring of muscle gas tensions, particularly muscle P_{O_2} will predict early circulatory derangement minutes to hours before standard techniques will show

similar changes.[156] Unfortunately, there is not yet commercially available a reliable device that gives consistently reproducible values and is resistant to the rigors (*i.e.*, will not easily break) of the clinic environment.

ANESTHESIA

INDUCTION

The ideal anesthetic induction technique would provide a rapid, excitement-free passage from awareness to adequate maintenance levels of anesthesia with significant muscle relaxation but without any, or at least minimal, alterations in all cardiovascular variables.[157] Neither sympathetic nor parasympathetic stimulation nor depression would be observed. Unfortunately, an ideal anesthetic induction agent is not currently available.[158] However, ideal inductions should be constantly strived for with what agents are available.

In the author's opinion, speed of induction is the least important of all of the above criteria for the ideal induction for patients with cardiovascular disease. The most important criteria are stability or circulatory dynamics and absence of excitement. In considering the technique of choice, it is extremely important to recall the specific pathology of the patient involved. A rapid induction with a sleep dose of thiopental followed by paralysis with succinylcholine and endotracheal intubation is obviously not the technique of choice for the patient with associated coronary artery disease and angina or an expanding aortic aneurysm because it will often produce, because of inadequate analgesia, tachycardia and hypertension during or shortly after introduction of the endotracheal tube in the trachea.[159] Rather, one should slowly introduce anesthesia with either an intravenous or inhalation agent and only when the patient is adequately anesthetized, and therefore not likely to become hypertensive or significantly increase his heart rate, should he be intubated. A smooth, safe induction and intubation without cough, rather than a speedy one (with stimulation or depression of cardiovascular dynamics) is the better one.

It should be realized that patients with low cardiac output may have a slow circulation time and experience a delay in onset of action with intravenous agents. On the other hand, inhalation agents will rapidly come to equilibrium with alveolar gas in patients and produce onset of deep levels of anesthesia much faster than normal.[160] Patients with significant pulmonary pathology (chronic bronchitis) frequently have marked ventilation/perfusion abnormalities. As a result, induction with an inhalation agent may be longer and, if not skilfully managed, more stormy and dangerous in these patients.[161]

Patients with a cardiac or prepulmonary right-to-left shunt will also experience a slow induction time with inhalation agents but often a speedier one with intravenous compounds. Increased right-to-left shunt and secondary hypoxemia is a danger in patients with a right-to-left ventricular shunt who experience a significant reduction in systemic vascular resistance with induction of anesthesia. Many inhalation and intravenous anesthetics reduce systemic vascular resistance.[162, 163] Some also increase venous compliance and pooling.[164] The latter compounds would be dangerous to use in patients with cardiac tamponade or shock secondary to blood loss (*i.e.,* an expanding aneurysm), who depend on an increased venous pressure for adequate ventricular filling.[165]

The same principles that apply to anesthetic induction agents also apply to the muscle relaxants that are used during this period. When tachycardia and hypertension are not desirable, a large bolus dose of pancuronium or gallamine should be avoided. On the other hand, when induction produces hypotension or bradycardia or both, pancuronium is the muscle relaxant of choice. When the onset or speed of action of a muscle relaxant employed during induction is of no consequence, slow administration of adequate amounts of d-tubocurarine, metocurine, or pancuronium can be used. When rapid paralysis is thought desirable, succinylcholine

should be used in large amounts (1.5 mg/kg). The use of barely adequate doses of succinylcholine (0.5–0.75 mg/kg) should be condemned, for such techniques risk the possibility of less than optimal relaxation and, perhaps even more dangerous, occasionally necessitate the use of a second dose of succinylcholine with its associated high incidence of arrhythmias.[166] Succinylcholine usually is preceded by a small dose of a nondepolarizing muscle relaxant (pancuronium 1 mg, d-tubocurarine 3 mg, or gallamine 20 mg) to reduce or prevent muscle fasciculations or increases of intraocular, intra-abdominal, or intragastric pressure.[167–169] This practice is mandatory in the patient with a full stomach. Succinylcholine is omitted if there is an open-eye injury.

MAINTENANCE

Many patients with cardiac disease also have peripheral vascular disease and therefore have marginal blood flows to some or all major organ systems. This mandates that anesthesia be conducted so that cardiovascular dynamics are minimally altered. The goal is to produce and maintain optimal cardiovascular dynamics at all times. In order to accomplish this goal, it may be necessary, on occasion, to use compounds which produce profound neuromuscular blockade or agents that result in significant and prolonged respiratory or central nervous system depression and necessitate reversal or antagonism for immediate recovery of all depressed organ systems at the end of operation. Sometimes reversal may produce dangerous alterations in circulatory dynamics (*i.e.,* following reversal of a high dose opiate technique in a patient having a long abdominal vascular operation who also has coronary artery disease).[170] In these situations, reversal should not be undertaken. At all times, maintenance of optimal circulatory dynamics is the primary goal both during and following anesthesia. In addition to providing myocardial and cardiovascular stability, the anesthesiologist anesthetizing patients with vascular and cardiac disease must be concerned with avoiding agents or techniques which stimulate atrial or ventricular irritability and, particularly in patients with ischemic disease, techniques that result in excessive stimulation or increased myocardial work requirements and oxygen consumption. In patients with cerebral vascular disease, attention must be paid to maintaining normotension and normocarbia.

As discussed in the previous section on anesthetic induction, the specific pathology of the patient coupled with the operation to be performed and operative position will often indicate which anesthetic technique will be best. Patients with chronic fibrotic pulmonary changes and a high preoperative pulmonary shunt undergoing extensive upper abdominal vascular surgery or a thoracotomy in the lateral position cannot be safely anesthetized with a nitrous oxide-narcotic technique that allows an inspired oxygen concentration of only 30 percent because of the dangers of potential hypoxemia. Rather, they require an anesthetic regimen that will employ a high inspired concentration of oxygen, sometimes 70 percent or more. In this situation, it might be easier to use a halogenated anesthetic plus oxygen rather than nitrous oxide plus a narcotic. On the other hand, if prolonged postoperative ventilation is desirable, an opiate (morphine or fentanyl) oxygen technique might be most desirable.

It has been suggested by some authors that patients with ischemic myocardial disease will benefit from anesthetic techniques that produce moderate myocardial depression.[171,172] For example, moderate halothane-induced myocardial depression improves the myocardial oxygen supply/demand ratio and is, therefore, a good anesthetic to use in patients with coronary artery disease.[173] On the basis of this and other work, it has been suggested that the old dictum, "avoid hypotension and hypoxia," should be changed to "produce moderate hypotension and normoxia and avoid hypertension" in patients with coronary artery disease.[174] Considering this, it is important in choosing an anesthetic technique for patients with coronary artery disease undergoing noncardiac surgery that

cardiovascular dynamics, particularly myocardial contractility, preload and afterload, and heart rate not be stimulated but rather be unchanged or moderately depressed. The key is to preserve myocardial blood flow and decrease heart rate (the most important determinant of myocardial oxygen consumption) and the other factors which influence myocardial energy needs.

Patients who are hypovolemic, in severe congestive heart failure, shock, or who have significant valvular disease often require stimulation and support of the heart and circulatory system to maintain adequate amounts of myocardial, cerebral, and total body blood flow. Indeed, preoperative urine and plasma epinephrine and norepinephrine are usually increased in these patients.[175] Light levels of anesthesia with low concentrations of halothane or enflurane with or without nitrous oxide or with agents that maintain or increase circulatory levels of epinephrine and norepinephrine (morphine, fentanyl, and perhaps, on some occasions, ketamine)[176,177] are most desirable in these patients.

In considering the properties of the specific general anesthetic techniques available to modern anesthesiologists having to anesthetize patients with cardiovascular disease the old dictim, "it is not so important what you have but rather what you do with what you have," is quite appropriate. In the author's opinion, the skill of the anesthesiologist plus his knowledge of the specific cardiac and other organ systems pathology involved and the physiologic ideals to be strived for are far more important in choosing whether an inhalation technique, a balanced nitrous oxide-narcotic technique, a pure narcotic or ketamine technique, or one of a variety of mixtures of the above is optimal for any patient. In other words, the ideal anesthetic state can probably be achieved in many, if not most, patients with cardiovascular disease by a number of different routes. It is true that certain techniques might be easier than others. For example, trying to maintain normotension and normocarbia and at the same time avoiding a marked increase in intracranial pressure and intracerebral steal is difficult to do with deep halothane anesthesia in a spontaneously breathing patient.

PARTICULAR SURGICAL PROCEDURES

Transurethral Prostatic Resection

Transurethral prostatic resection presents problems peculiar to this procedure because of the difficulty of estimating blood loss and the necessity of irrigating the surgical field continuously with a nonelectrolyte solution.[178, 179] The combination of unknown blood loss, intravascular absorption of water, and extravasation of water into tissues outside the bladder or the prostatic capsule produces a dilutional hyponatremia and anemia and can lead to rapid multiple organ system failure and death if not detected early.

The key to successful treatment of this problem is early recognition. While it is well known that overload and hyponatremia are directly related to time and volume of irrigation, occurrence of the problem is variable in individual patients. With early symptoms, patient anxiety, confusion, and abdominal pain (in patients anesthetized with regional anesthesia), and signs, slowing pulse rate, and increase in blood pressure, the surgeon should be warned so that he will bring the procedure to an end as soon as possible.[180–182] Confirmation of the diagnosis and quantification of the defect(s) should be made by measurements of serum osmolarity and electrolytes (particularly Na^+ and K^+) and blood hemoglobin concentration. In addition, measurements of central venous and pulmonary capillary wedge pressures will quantitate the magnitude of overload volume or degree of myocardial compromise or both and indicate whether myocardial support is necessary. Arterial blood gases, particularly Pa_{O_2}, can be used to document pulmonary dysfunction.

In treating these patients, it is imperative that serum electrolytes and osmolarity be measured frequently. In patients with a normal serum osmolarity and low plasma sodium it has been found by some that usually no treatment is necessary. In contrast, for the patient who experiences changes in both serum osmolarity and plasma sodium, heart failure is likely, and active measures must be taken quickly to avoid or treat it. Diuretics and 5 percent saline with half-hour to hourly repeated measurements of plasma electrolytes and serum osmolarity are the treatment of choice. While treatment should be vigorous, it also must be accomplished with some caution because the cardiac reserve of these patients is usually limited at best. In addition, other factors such as hemorrhage, different kinds and depths of anesthesia, hypotension, and hypertension, to name a few, will alter the speed with which therapy can be administered safely.

Ophthalmic Surgery

Operations on the eye are frequently performed on the very young and very old. Because ocular operations are usually elective, there should be little difficulty in ensuring that these patients are optimally prepared. While there are some data that show that the incidence of ocular problems after operation (vitreous loss, iris prolapse, and wound dihiscence) is similar irrespective of whether local or general anesthesia is used,[183] the same is not true with regard to morbidity and mortality in patients with cardiac disease. Backer, Tinker, and Robertson showed that the remyocardial infarction and mortality rate were significantly higher in patients subjected to general anesthesia for ophthalmologic surgery than to local anesthesia.[184] This, however, does not mean that serious complications cannot occur with local anesthetic techniques. Disadvantages of retrobulbar block include retrobulbar hemorrhage, optic nerve injury, stimulation of the oculocardiac reflex with resultant severe bradycardia and inadvertent tachycardia, and hypertension secondary to system absorption of vasopressors used in and around the eye.

Some clinicians are of the opinion that patients undergoing ocular operations under local anesthesia do not need the same type of cardiovascular monitoring as do patients undergoing similar operations with general anesthesia. The result is that these patients often have no monitoring at all. Unfortunately, older patients with ophthalmic disease frequently have significant ischemic cardiac disease and, because of this, are quite anxious. Absence of an ECG, heart rate monitor, and arterial blood pressure recordings in these patients may allow them to develop dangerous levels of undetected hypertension and tachycardia and with these changes, myocardial ischemia. Such alterations may occur frequently in anxious patients, as well as those subjected to retrobulbar or ocular injections of vasopressors; they demand immediate diagnosis and treatment. Diagnosis and treatment can only be made early if adequate, continuous monitoring of those cardiovascular variables is available and utilized throughout the operative and postoperative periods.

POSTOPERATIVE CONSIDERATIONS

The same principles that applied during induction and maintenance of anesthesia apply during termination of anesthesia and the recovery period (*i.e.,* anesthesia should be discontinued in a fashion that least disturbs cardiovascular dynamics, myocardial oxygen requirements, oxygen delivery, and so on). In this respect, the postanesthetic recovery period is of no less importance than the period of induction or maintenance of anesthesia. Reversal of anesthetic and neuromuscular blocking compounds, if done at all, should be done cautiously during this period. Because of the potential cardiovascular dangers of pharmacologic reversal, the author does not routinely antagonize narcotic or neuromuscular compounds in patients previously in shock or after prolonged abdominal or thoracic surgery, especially when large fluid shifts or massive blood replacement has occurred. Instead, patients are mechanically

ventilated until they can sustain a normal Pa_{CO_2} while breathing unassisted for an hour, draw a negative pressure of at least 25 cm H_2O against an occluded airway, and possess a tidal volume of at least 5 ml/kg and a vital capacity of at least 12 to 15 ml/kg. Then, the pharynx is suctioned and the patient extubated. Often lidocaine (50 mg) is injected down the endotracheal tube or administered intravenously to prevent coughing upon extubation. Less concern is necessary in patients with reasonable cardiovascular, pulmonary, hepatic, and renal function. In these patients, reversal of residual neuromuscular blockade and narcotic action is usually done in the operating or recovery rooms. Because of the length of the incision, extensiveness of the dissection, duration of the procedure, anesthetics sometimes used (high doses of narcotics), presence of significant preoperative pulmonary disease, intraoperative requirements for large amounts of intravenous fluids and blood, and the possibility of hypothermia, early endotracheal extubation after prolonged abdominal, thoracic, and sometimes urogenital surgery is often not desirable. In addition, postoperative hemorrhage and respiratory and renal insufficiency are not uncommon in these patients. For these reasons, careful evaluation of cardiovascular and respiratory dynamics and renal function should continue for at least some hours after operation before endotracheal intubation is even contemplated after major abdominal or thoracic surgery. In some of these patients (particularly those with aortic disease), hypertension may develop postoperatively.[185, 186] The mechanism producing it is not entirely clear. If small doses of intravenous narcotics or sedatives cannot effectively treat postoperative hypertension, a vasodilator may be required. However, it is important that intravascular volume be normal to avoid decreases in cardiac output during vasodilator therapy.

Patients usually have shorter and less complicated postoperative courses after less invasive, shorter operations. However, hypertension and hypotension are significant complications of radical neck and carotid artery procedures.[187-190] Hypertension with systolic arterial pressures above 200 torr has been described in more than 33 percent of patients in one series.[191] The mechanism is thought to be denervation of the carotid sinus during mobilization of the carotid bifurcation with resultant loss of tonic baroreceptor stimulation. Treatment is similar to hypertension after aortic operations.

Patients with cardiovascular disease can experience all of the problems and complications that normal patients do in the postoperative period. Some of these are listed below. Unfortunately, because their cardiovascular reserve is often significantly less than that of normal patients, the risk of sustaining permanent damage for any one of those complications is significantly greater in patients with cardiovascular disease. For this reason, it is mandatory that administration of the increased concentrations of oxygen; careful monitoring of electrolytes; evaluation of arterial blood gases; and recognition of hypovolemia, impaired renal function, cardiac arrhythmias or altered cardiac output, arterial blood pressure, heart rate, and so on be more compulsively carried out in these patients than in those without cardiovascular disease.

Common Postoperative Complications of Patients With Cardiovascular Disease Undergoing General Surgery

1. Atelectasis
2. Pneumonia
3. Hypoxia
4. Hypercarbia
5. Cardiac arrhythmias
6. Reduced cardiac output
7. Hypotension
8. Hypertension
9. Hypovolemia
10. Congestive heart failure
11. Persistent neuromuscular blockade
12. Renarcotization following antagonists
13. Prolonged CNS depression
14. Urinary retention
15. Decreased urine flow rate
16. Thromboembolism
17. Myocardial ischemia
18. Myocardial infarction
19. Gastric distention
20. Hemorrhage

SUMMARY

Ideal anesthetic management consists of adequate preanesthetic preparation, provision of a state in which a diagnostic or therapeutic procedure or surgical operation can be performed with as little physiologic and psychologic trauma as possible, and, finally, a speedy and event-free postoperative course. Anesthesia for general surgery in patients with cardiovascular disease is not, in this respect, different from anesthesia for patients without cardiovascular disease. However, significant impairment of respiratory, renal, and other organ systems functions is frequent in patients with cardiovascular pathology, who also tolerate less alteration in cardiovascular dynamics. For this reason, it is imperative that preoperative evaluation be more complete in these patients than patients without cardiovascular disease. It is necessary that signs of congestive heart failure, myocardial ischemia or infarction or both, hypertension, electrolyte abnormalities, and cardiac arrhythmias be compulsively looked for and aggressively treated before these patients are brought to the operating room. In addition, knowledge of the specific associated lesions (cardiac and otherwise), drugs being used to treat these derangements, and the adequacy of the current therapies for derangements must be obtained before induction of anesthesia.

Premedication is important in patients with cardiovascular disease and should be carefully administered to enable a smooth and event-free induction. Speed of anesthetic induction is not usually important; rather, a smooth change from consciousness to unconsciousness without alterations in cardiovascular dynamics and arterial blood gases is the better course.

Monitoring is obviously important in patients with cardiovascular disease undergoing general surgery and should not be neglected even in patients subjected to regional or local anesthetic techniques. As a general rule, it is difficult not to monitor too many things (*i.e.*, the more monitoring the better).

Maintenance and recovery from anesthesia

should be as event-free as induction. To this end, it may be better not to antagonize muscle relaxants or narcotic compounds in some patients with very unstable cardiovascular dynamics or those requiring long abdominal or thoracic procedures where much blood has been lost, third space fluid translocations have occurred, or when hypothermia is present. Even in those patients in whom these events have not occurred, antagonism of these compounds can produce dangerous alterations in cardiovascular dynamics and therefore should be done carefully and slowly.

REFERENCES

GENERAL REFERENCES

1. Föex P: Preoperative assessment of patients with cardiac disease. Br J Anaesth 50:15–22, 1978
2. Goldman L, Caldera DL, Nussbaum R et al: Multifactorial index of cardiac risk in noncardiac surgical procedures. N Engl J Med 297:845–850, 1977
3. Goldman L, Caldera DL, Nussbaum R et al: Multifactorial index of cardiac risk in noncardiac surgical procedures. N Engl J Med 297:845–850, 1977
4. Nachlan MM, Abrams SJ, Goldberg MM: The influence of arteriosclerotic heart disease on surgical risk. Am J Surg 101:447–455, 1961

PREOPERATIVE CONSIDERATIONS

Congestive Heart Failure

5. Goldman L, Caldera DL, Nussbaum R et al: Multifactorial index of cardiac risk in noncardiac surgical procedures. N Engl J Med 297:845–850, 1977
6. Goldman L, Caldera DL, Nussbaum R et al: Multifactorial index of cardiac risk in noncardiac surgical procedures. N Engl J Med 297:845–850, 1977
7. Hudson REB: Cardiovascular Pathology, pp 1004-1023. London, Edward Arnold Ltd, 1965
8. Hudson REB: Cardiovascular Pathology, pp 1004-1023. London, Edward Arnold Ltd, 1965
9. Davison JK: Anesthesia for peripheral vascular disease. Int Anesthesiol Clin 17: 129–141, 1979
10. Sabawala PB, Strong MJ, Keats AS: Surgery of the aorta and its branches. Anesthesiology 33:229–259, 1970

Myocardial Ischema or Infarction

11. Goldman L, Caldera DL, Nussbaum R et al: Multifactorial index of cardiac risk in noncardiac surgical procedures. N Engl J Med 297:845–850, 1977
12. Goldman L, Caldera DL, Nussbaum R et al: Multifactorial index of cardiac risk in noncardiac surgical procedures. N Engl J Med 297:845–850, 1977
13. Kaplan JA: Unpublished data.
14. Föex P: Preoperative assessment of patients with cardiac disease. Br J Anaesth 50:15–22, 1978
15. Goldman L, Caldera DL, Nussbaum R et al: Multifactorial index of cardiac risk in noncardiac surgical procedures. N Engl J Med 297:845–850, 1977
16. Nachlan MM, Abrams SJ, Goldberg MM: The influence of arteriosclerotic heart disease on surgical risk. Am J Surg 101:447–455, 1961
17. Roberts et al: Personal communication.
18. Froelicher VF, Thomas MM, Pillow C et al: Epidemiologic study for asymptomatic men screened by maximal treadmill testing for latent coronary artery disease. Am J Cardiol 34:770–776, 1974
19. Topkins MJ, Artusio JF: Myocardial infarction and surgery. Anaesth Analg (Cleve) 43:716–720, 1964
20. Tarhan S, Moffet EA, Taylor WF et al: Myocardial infarction after general anesthesia. JAMA 220:1451–1454, 1972
21. Tarhan S, Moffet EA, Taylor WF et al: Myocardial infarction after general anesthesia. JAMA 220:1451–1454, 1972

Hypertension

22. Föex P: Preoperative assessment of patients with cardiac disease. Br J Anaesth 50:15–22, 1978
23. Nachlan MM, Abrams SJ, Goldberg MM: The influence of arteriosclerotic heart disease on surgical risk. Am J Surg 101:447–455, 1961
24. Stamler J, Stamler R, Pullman TN: The Epidemiology of Hypertension. Edition, New York, Grune and Stratton, 1967

25. De Bakey ME. Crawford ES, Cooley DA et al: Cerebral arterial insufficiency: one to 11 year results following arterial reconstructive operation. Ann Surg 161:921–945, 1965

26. Dunn E, Prager RL, Fry W et al: The effect of abdominal aortic cross-clamping on myocardial function. J Surg Res 22:463–468, 1977

27. Cookley CS, Alpert S, Boling JS: Circulatory responses during anesthesia of patients on rauwolfia therapy. JAMA 161:1143–1144, 1956

28. Munson WM, Jenicek JA: Effects of anesthetic agents on patients receiving reserpine therapy. Anesthesiology 23:741–746, 1963

29. Cookley CS, Alpert S, Boling JS: Circulatory responses during anesthesia of patients on rauwolfa therapy. JAMA 161:1143–1144, 1956

30. Munson WM, Jenicek JA: Effects of anesthetic agents on patients receiving reserpine therapy. Anesthesiology 23:741–746, 1963

31. Alper MH, Flacke W, Kroyer O: Pharmacology of reserpine and its implications for anesthesia. Anesthesiology 24:524–542, 1963

32. Morrow DH, Morrow AG: The response to anesthesia for non-hypertensive patients pretreated with reserpine. Br J Anaesth 35:313–316, 1963

33. Hamelberg W. Current concepts on antihypertensive drugs and steroids. Anaesth Analg (Cleve) 43:104–107, 1964

34. Papper EM: Selection and management of anesthesia in those suffering from disorders and disease of the heart. Cana Anaesth Soc J 12:245–254, 1965

35. Prys–Roberts C, Meloche R, Föex P: Studies of Anesthesia in relationship to hypertension. I. Cardiovascular responses of treated and untreated patients. Br J Anaesth 43:122–137, 1971

36. Prys–Roberts C, Greene LT, Meloche R et al: Studies of anaesthesia in relation to hypertension. II. Haemodynamic consequences of induction and endotracheal intubation. Br J Anaesth 43:531–547, 1971

37. Perera GA: Hypertensive vascular disease: description and natural history. J Chron Dis 1:33–42, 1955

38. Tarazi RC, Dustan HP, Frolich ED et al: Plasma volume and chronic hypertension. Relationship to arterial pressure levels in different hypertensive diseases. Arch Intern Med 123:835–842, 1970

39. Dustan HP, Tarazi RC, Bravo EL: Dependence of arterial pressure on intravascular volume in treated hypertensive patients. N Engl J Med 286:861–866, 1972

40. Tarazi RC, Frolich ED, Dustan HP: Plasma volume changes with long-term beta-adrenergic blockade. Am Heart J 82:770–776, 1971

Electrolyte Abnormalities

41. Goldman L, Caldera DL, Nussbaum R et al: Multifactorial index of cardiac risk in noncardiac surgical procedures. N Engl J Med 297:845–850, 1977

42. Tarazi RC, Dustan HP, Frolich ED et al: Plasma volume and chronic hypertension. Relationship to arterial pressure levels in different hypertensive

43. Katz RL, Bigger JT: Cardiac arrhythmias during anesthesia and operation. Anesthesiology 33:193–213, 1970

44. Katz RL, Bigger JT: Cardiac arrhythmias during anesthesia and operation. Anesthesiology 33:193–213, 1970

45. Trautwein W: Generation and conduction of impulses in the heart as affected by drugs. Pharmacol Rev 15:277–307, 1963

46. Wong KC, Wetstone D, Martin WE, et al: Hypokalemia during anesthesia: The effects of D-tubocurarine, gallamine, succinylcholine, thiopental and halothane with or without respiratory alkalosis. Anesth Analg (Cleve) 52:522–528, 1973

47. Wright BD, De Giovanni AJ: Respiratory alkalosis, hypokalemia and repeated ventricular fibrillation associated with mechanical ventilation. Anesth Analg (Cleve) 48:467–473, 1969

48. Scribner BH, Burnell JM: Interpretation of the serum potassium concentration. Metabolism 5:469–479, 1956

49. Wong KC, Kawamura R, Hodges MR et al: Acute intravenous administration of potassium chloride to furosemide pretreated dogs. Cana Anaesth Soc J 24:203–211, 1977

Arrhythmias

50. Föex P: Preoperative assessment of patients with cardiac disease. Br J Anaesth 50:15–22, 1978

51. Katz RL, Bigger JT: Cardiac arrhythmias during anesthesia and operation. Anesthesiology 33:193–213, 1970

52. Katz RL, Bigger JT: Cardiac arrhythmias during anesthesia and operation. Anesthesiology 33:193–213, 1970

53. Goldman L, Caldera DL, Nussbaum R et al: Multifactorial index of cardiac risk in noncardiac surgical procedures. N Engl J Med 297:845–850, 1977

54. Föex P: Preoperative assessment of patients with cardiac disease. Br J Anaesth 50:15–22, 1978

55. Föex P: Preoperative assessment of patients with cardiac disease. Br J Anaesth 50:15–22, 1978

56. Goldman L, Caldera DL, Nussbaum R et al: Multifactorial index of cardiac risk in noncardiac surgical procedures. N Engl J Med 297:845–850, 1977

Current Pharmacologic Therapy

57. Goldman L, Caldera DL, Nussbaum R et al: Multifactorial index of cardiac risk in noncardiac surgical procedures. N Engl J Med 297:845–850, 1977

58. Sabawala PB, Strong MJ, Keats AS: Surgery of the aorta and its branches. Anesthesiology 33:229–259, 1970

59. Morrow DH, Morrow AG: The response to anesthesia of non-hypertensive patients pretreated with reserpine. Br J Anaesth 35:313–316, 1963

60. Hamelberg W: Current concepts on antihypertensive drugs and steroids. Anaesth Analg (Cleve) 43:104–107, 1964

61. Papper EM: Selection and management of anesthesia in those suffering from disorders and disease of the heart. Cana Anaesth Soc J 12:245–254, 1965

62. Deutsch S, Dalen JE: Indications for prophylactic digitalization. Anesthesiology 30:648–656, 1969

63. Wheat MW, Burford TR: Digitalis in surgery: extension of classical indications. J Thorac Cardiovasc Surg 41:162–168, 1961

64. Burman S: The prophylactic use of digitalis before thoracotomy. Ann Thorac Surg 14:358–368, 1972

65. Strong MJ, Keats AS: Digitalis and heart disease. Anesthesiology 31:583–584, 1969

66. Selzer A, Colin KE: Some thoughts concerning the prophylactic use of digitalis. Am J Cardiol 26:214–216, 1970

67. Juler GL, Stemmer EA, Connolly JE: Complications of prophylactic digitalization in thoracic surgical patients. J Thorac Cardiovasc Surg 58:352–360, 1969

68. Deutsch S, Dalen JE: indications for prophylactic digitalization. Anesthesiology 30:648–656, 1969

69. Wheat MW, Burford TR: Digitalis in surgery: extension of classical indications. J Thorac Cardiovasc Surg 41:162–168, 1961

70. Burman S: The prophylactic use of digitalis before thoracotomy. Ann Thorac Surg 14:358–368, 1972

71. Strong MJ, Keats AS: Digitalis and heart disease. Anesthesiology 31:583–584, 1969

72. Selzer A, Colin KE: Some thoughts concerning the prophylactic use of digitalis. Am J Cardiol 26:214–216, 1970

73. Juler GL, Stemmer EA, Connolly JE: Complications of prophylactic digitalization in thoracic surgical patients. J Thorac Cardiovasc Surg 58:352–360, 1969

74. Strong MJ, Keats AS; Digitalis and heart disease. Anesthesiology 31:583–584, 1969

75. Shand DG: Propranolol. N Engl J Med 293:280–285, 1975

76. Viljoen JF, Estafanous FG, Kellner GA: Propranolol and cardiac surgery. J Thorac Cardiovasc Surg 64:826–830, 1972

77. Viljoen JF, Estafanous FG, Kellner GA: Propranolol and cardiac surgery. J Thorac Cardiovasc Surg 64:826–830, 1972

78. Shand DG: Propranolol. N Engl J Med 293:280–285, 1975

79. Viljoen JF, Estafanous FG, Kellner GA: Propranolol and cardiac surgery. J Thorac Cardiovasc Surg 64:826–830, 1972

80. Alderman EL, Coltart DJ, Wetlock GE et al: Coronary artery symptoms after sudden propranolol withdrawal. Ann Intern Med 81:625–627, 1974

81. Kaplan JA, Dunbar RW, Blard JW et al: Propranolol and cardiac surgery: A problem for the anesthesiologist? Anesth Analg (Cleve) 54:571–577, 1975

82. Shand DG: Propranolol. N Engl J Med 293:280–285, 1975

83. Viljoen JF, Estafanous FG, Kellner GA: Propranolol and cardiac surgery. J Thorac Cardiovasc Surg 64:826–830, 1972

84. Alderman EL, Coltart DJ, Wetlock GE et al: Coronary artery symptoms after sudden propranolol withdrawal. Ann Intern Med 81:625–627, 1974

85. Kaplan JA, Dunbar RW, Blard JW et al: Pro-

pranolol and cardiac surgery: A problem for the anesthesiologist? Anesth Analg (Cleve) 54:571–577, 1975

86. Constantine JW, McShane: Analysis of the cardiovascular effects of 2-(2,6-dichlorophenylamine)-imidazoline hydrochloride (Catapres). Eur J Pharmacol 4:109–123, 1968

87. Starke K, Hontell H: Involvement of a- receptors in clonidine-induced inhibition of transmitter release from central monamine neurons. Neuropharmacology 12:1073–1080, 1973

88. McRaven D, Kroltz F, Kioschos JM et al: The effect of clonidine on hemodynamics in hypertensive patients. Am Heart J 81:482–489, 1971

89. Mroczek W, Davidor M, Finnerty F: Intravenous clonidine in hypertensive patients. Clin Pharmacol Ther 14:847–851, 1973

90. Bucher TJ, Buckingham RE, Fanch L et al: Studies on the central hypertensive effects of clonidine. J Pharm Pharmacol 25:139–143, 1973

91. Schmitt H and Schmitt H: Localization of the hypotensive effect of 2-(2,6-dichlorophenylamino)-2imidazoline hydrochloride (ST-155, Catapresan). Eur J Pharmacol 6:8–12, 1969

92. Hansson L, Hunyor SN: Blood pressure overshoot due to acute clonidine (Catapres) withdrawal: studies on arterial and urinary catecholamines and suggestions for management. Clin Sci Mol Med 45:181–184, 1973

93. Kaplan JA, Dunbar JW, Jones EL: Nitroglycerin infusion during coronary artery surgery. Anesthesiology 45:14–21, 1976

94. Miller RR, Vismara LA, William DO et al: Pharmacological mechanism for left ventricular unloading in clinical congestive heart failure. Circ Res 39:127–133, 1976

95. Epstein SE, Kent KM, Goldstein RE et al: Reduction of ischemic injury by nitroglycerin during acute myocardial infarction. N Engl J Med 292:29–35, 1975

96. Fahmy NR: Nitroglycerin as a hypotensive drug during general anesthesia. Anesthesiology 49:17–20, 1978

97. Chiarello M, Gold HK, Leinbach RC et al: Comparison between the effects of nitroprusside and nitroglycerin on ischemic injury during acute myocardial infarction. Circulation 54:766–773, 1976

98. Hutchins GM, Ostrow PT: The pathogenesis of the two forms of hypertensive pulmonary vascular disease. Am Heart J 92:797–803, 1976

99. Laver MB, Hallowell P, Goldblatt A: Pulmonary dysfuction secondary to heart disease: Aspects relevant to anesthesia and surgery. Anesthesiology 33:161–192, 1970

100. Laver MB, Hallowell P, Goldblatt A: Pulmonary dysfuction secondary to heart disease: Aspects relevant to anesthesia and surgery. Anesthesiology 33:161–192, 1970

101. Stanley TH, Isern-Amaral J, Lathrop GD: Urine norepinephrine excretion in patients undergoing mitral or aortic valve replacement with morphine anesthesia. Anaesth Analg (Cleve) 54:509–516, 1975

102. Bedford RF, Wollman H: Postoperative respiratory effects of morphine and halothane anesthesia: a study in patients undergoing cardiac surgery. Anesthesiology 43:1–9, 1975

103. Stanley TH, Lathrop GD: Excretion of urinary morphine during and after valvular and coronary artery surgery with morphine anesthesia. Anesthesiology 46:166–169, 1977

104. Chambers DA: Acquired valvular heart disease. in Kaplan JA (ed): Cardiac Anesthesia. New York, Grune and Stratton, 1979

105. Kaplan JA, Dunbar JW, Jones EL: Nitroglycerin infusion during coronary artery surgery. Anesthesiology 45:14–21, 1976

106. Stanley TH, Lathrop GD: Excretion of urinary morphine during and after valvular and coronary artery surgery with morphine anesthesia. Anesthesiology 46:166–169, 1977

107. Gracey DR, Divertie MB, Didier ER: Preoperative pulmonary function of patients with chronic obstructive pulmonary disease; a prospective study. Chest 76:123–129, 1975

108. Kaplan JA, Dunbar JW, Jones EL: Nitroglycerin infusion during coronary artery surgery. Anesthesiology 45:14–21, 1976

109. Epstein SE, Kent KM, Goldstein RE et al: Reduction of ischemic injuray by nitroglycerin during acute myocardial infarction. N Engl J Med 292:29–35, 1975

110. Stanley TH, Lathrop GD: Excretion of urinary morphine during and after valvular and coronary artery surgery with morphine anesthesia. Anesthesiology 46:166–169, 1977

111. Chambers DA: Acquired valvular heart disease. In Kaplan JA (ed): Cardiac Anesthesia. New York, Grune and Stratton, 1979

112. Gracey DR, Divertie MB, Didier ER: Preoperative pulmonary function of patients with chronic obstructive pulmonary disease; a prospective study. Chest 76:123–129, 1975

113. Carroll RM, Laravuso RB, Schauble JF: Left

ventricular function during aortic surgery. Arch Surg 111:740–745, 1976

114. Chambers DA: Acquired valvular heart disease. In Kaplan JA (ed): Cardiac Anesthesia. New York, Grune and Stratton, 1979

115. Gracey DR, Divertie MB, Didier ER: Preoperative pulmonary function of patients with chronic obstructive pulmonary disease; a prospective study. Chest 76:123–129, 1975

116. Carroll RM, Laravuso RB, Schauble JF: Left ventricular function during aortic surgery. Arch Surg 111:740–745, 1976

117. De Bakey ME. Crawford ES, Cooley DA et al: Cerebral arterial insufficiency: one to 11 year results following arterial reconstructive operation. Ann Surg 161:921–945, 1965

Myocardial Function

118. Roberts L, Stanley TH: Unpublished data.
119. Stanley TH: Unpublished data.
120. Stanley TH, Isern-Amaral J, Lathrop GD: Urine norepinephrine excretion in patients undergoing mitral or aortic valve replacement with morphine anesthesia. Anaesth Analg (Cleve) 54:509–516, 1975
121. Stanley TH, Lathrop GD: Excretion of urinary morphine during and after valvular and coronary artery surgery with morphine anesthesia. Anesthesiology 46:166–169, 1977
122. Davison JK: Anesthesia for peripheral vascular disease. Int Anesthesiol Clin 17:129–141, 1979

Chronic Obstructive Pulmonary Disease

123. Sabawala PB, Strong MJ, Keats AS: Surgery of the aorta and its branches. Anesthesiology 33:229–259, 1970
124. Davison JK: Anesthesia for peripheral vascular disease. Int Anesthesiol Clin 17:129–141, 1979
125. Sabawala PB, Strong MJ, Keats AS: Surgery of the aorta and its branches. Anesthesiology 33:229–259, 1970
126. Gracey DR, Divertie MB, Didier ER: Preoperative pulmonary function of patients with chronic obstructive pulmonary disease; a prospective study. Chest 76:123–129, 1975
127. Gaensler EA, Weisel AD: The risks in abdominal and thoracic surgery. Postgrad Med 53:183–192, 1973
128. Dannemiller FJ: Personal communication

Obesity

129. Wilens SL: Bearing of the general nutritional state of atherosclerosis. Arch Intern Med 79:129–136, 1947
130. Bedford RF, Wollman H: Postoperative respiratory effects of morphine and halothane anesthesia: a study in patients undergoing cardiac surgery. Anesthesiology 43:1–9, 1975
131. Fisher A, Waterhouse TD, Adams APL: Obesity: its relation to anesthesia. Anaesthesia 30:633–647, 1975
132. Vaughan RW, Wise L: Choice of abdominal operative incision in the obese patient: a study of blood gas measurements. Ann Surg 181:829–835, 1975
133. Fisher A, Waterhouse TD, Adams APL: Obesity: its relation to anesthesia. Anaesthesia 30:633–647, 1975
134. Vaughan RW, Wise L: Choice of abdominal operative incision in the obese patient: a study of blood gas measurements. Ann Surg 181:829–835, 1975
135. Fisher A, Waterhouse TD, Adams APL: Obesity: its relation to anesthesia. Anaesthesia 30:633–647, 1875
136. Holley HS, Milic–Enuli J, Becklake MR et al: Regional distribution of pulmonary ventilation and perfusion in obesity. J Clin Invest 46:475–481, 1967
137. Patton CM, Dannemiller FJ, Broennle AM: CPPB during surgical anesthesia: Effect on oxygenation. Anesth Analg (Cleve) 53:309–316, 1974

Pulmonary Hypertension

138. Fisher A, Waterhouse TD, Adams APL: Obesity: its relation to anesthesia. Anaesthesia 30:633–647, 1975
139. Vaughan RW, Wise L: Choice of abdominal operative incision in the obese patient: a study using blood gas measurements. Ann Surg 181:829–835, 1975
140. Wogenvoort CA, Heath DH, Edwards JE: The Pathology of the Pulmonary Vasculature. Springfield, Ill, Charles C Thomas, 1964
141. Laver MB, Hallowell P, Goldblatt A: Pulmonary dysfuction secondary to heart disease: Aspects relevant to anesthesia and surgery. Anesthesiology 33:161–192, 1970
142. Laver MB, Hallowell P, Goldblatt A: Pulmonary dysfuction secondary to heart disease:

Aspects relevant to anesthesia and surgery. Anesthesiology 33:161–192, 1970

The Kidneys

143. Davison JK: Anesthesia for peripheral vascular disease. Int Anesthesiol Clin 17:129–141, 1979
144. Sabawala PB, Strong MJ, Keats AS: Surgery of the aorta and its branches.

Premedication

145. Stanley TH, Lathrop GD: Excretion of urinary morphine during and after valvular and coronary artery surgery with morphine anesthesia. Anesthesiology 46:166–169, 1977
146. Falick YS, Smiler BG: Is anticholinergic premedication necessary? Anesthesiology 43:472–473, 1975
147. Chambers DA: Acquired valvular heart disease. In Kaplan JA (ed): Cardiac Anesthesia. New York, Grune and Stratton, 1979
148. Baraka A, Yared JP, Karam AM et al: Glycopyrrolate-Neostigmine and atropine-neostigmine mixtures affect postanesthetic arousal times differently. Anesth Analg (Cleve) 59:431–434, 1980

Monitoring During Operation

149. Föex P: Preoperative assessment of patients with cardiac disease. Br J Anaesth 50:15–22, 1978
150. Goldman L, Caldera DL, Nussbaum R et al: multifactorial index of cardiac risk in noncardiac surgical procedures. N Engl J Med 297:845–850, 1977
151. Nachlan MM, Abrams SJ, Goldberg MM: The influence of arteriosclerotic
152. Davison JK: Anesthesia for peripheral vascular disease. Int Anesthesiol Clin 17:129–141, 1979
153. Sabawala PB, Strong MJ, Keats AS: Surgery of the aorta and its branches. Anesthesiology 33:229–259, 1970
154. Buchbinder N, Ganz W: Hemodynamic monitoring. Invasive techniques. Anesthesiology 45:146–155, 1976
155. Stanley TH, Isern–Amaral J: Periodic mixed venous oxygen tension analysis as a measure of the adequacy of perfusion during and after cardiopulmonary bypass. Can Anaesth Soc J 21:454–460, 1974

156. Stanley TH: Arterial pressure and deltoid muscle oxygen tensions during cardiopulmonary bypass in man. Can Anaesth Soc J 26:277–281, 1979

ANESTHESIA

Induction

157. Stanley TH: Narcotics as complete anesthetics. In Aldrete JA, Stanley TH (eds): An International Symposium on Intravenous Anesthesia, pp 43-58. Chicago, Grune and Stratton, 1980
158. Stanley TH: Narcotics as complete anesthetics. In Aldrete JA, Stanley TH (eds): An International Symposium on Intravenous Anesthesia, pp 43-58. Chicago, Grune and Stratton, 1980
159. Stoelting RK: Circulatory changes during direct laryngoscopy and tracheal intubation. Influence of duration of laryngoscopy with and without prior lidocaine. Anesthesiology 47:381–384, 1977
160. Eger EL II: Anesthetic Uptake and Action. Baltimore, Williams & Wilkins, 1974
161. Eger EL II: Anesthetic Uptake and Action. Baltimore, Williams & Wilkins, 1974
162. Smith NT, Calverly RK, Prys–Roberts C et al: Impact of nitrous oxide on the circulation during enflurane anesthesia in man. Anesthesiology 48:345–349, 1978
163. Whitman JG, Russell WJ: The acute cardiovascular changes and adrenergic blockade by droperidol in man. Br J Anaesth 43:581–591, 1971
164. Stanley TH, Gray NH: The effect of high dose morphine on blood and fluid requirements of open heart operations. Anesthesiology 38:536–541, 1973
165. Stanley TH, Wideauer H: Anesthesia for cardiac tamponade. Anesth Analg (Cleve) 52:110–114, 1973
166. Lupprian KG, Churchill–Davidson HC: Effect of suxamethonium on cardiac rhythm. Br Med J 2:1774–1777, 1960
167. Miller RD, Way WL, Hickey RL: Inhibition of succinylcholine increased intraocular pressure by nondepolarizing muscle relaxants. Anesthesiology 29:123–126, 1968
168. Miller RD, Way WL: Inhibition of succinylcholine induced increased intragastric pressure by nondepolarizing muscle relaxants

and lidocaine. Anesthesiology 34:185–188, 1972

169. La Cour D: Rise in intragastric pressure caused by suxamethonium fasciculations. Acta Anesthesiol Scand 13:255–261, 1969

Maintenance

170. Desmonds JM, Bohm G, Couderc E: Hemodynamic responses to low doses of naloxone after narcotic-nitrous oxide anesthesia. Anesthesiology 49:12–16, 1978
171. Hamilton WK: Do let the blood pressure drop and do use myocardial depressants. Anesthesiology 45:273–274, 1976
172. Bland JHL, Lowenstein E: Halothane-induced decreased in experimental myocardial ischemia in the non-failing canine heart. Anesthesiology 45:287–293, 1976
173. Bland JHL, Lowenstein E: Halothane-induced decreased in experimental myocardial ischemia in the non-failing canine heart. Anesthesiology 45:287–293, 1976
174. Hamilton WK: Do let the blood pressure drop and do use myocardial depressants. Anesthesiology 45:273–274, 1976
175. Stanley TH, Isern-Amaral J, Lathrop GD: Urine norepinephrine excretion in patients undergoing mitral or aortic valve replacement with morphine anesthesia. Anaesth Analg (Cleve) 54:509–516, 1975
176. Stanley TH, Isern-Amaral J, Lathrop GD: Urine norepinephrine excretion in patients undergoing mitral or aortic valve replacement with morphine anesthesia. Anaesth Analg (Cleve) 54:509–516, 1975
177. Liu WS, Bidwai AV, Lunn JK et al: Urine catecholamine excretion after large doses of fentanyl, diazepam and pancuronium. Can Anaesth Soc J 24:371–379, 1977

Transurethral Prostatic Resection

178. Desmonds J: Complications of transurethral prostatic surgery. Can Anaesth Soc J 17:25–36, 1970
179. Aashein GM: Hyponatremia during transurethral surgery. Can Anaesth Soc J 20:274–280, 1973

180. Desmonds J: Complications of transurethral prostatic surgery. Can Anaesth Soc J 17:25–36, 1970
181. Aashien GM: Hyponatremia during transurethral surgery. Can Anaesth Soc J 20: 274–280, 1973
182. Hastings K, Wright D: Severe postoperative hyponatremia without symptoms of water intoxication. Surg Gynecol Obstet, 115:553–556, 1962

Opthalmic Surgery

183. Lynch S, Wolf GL, Berline I: General anesthesia for cataract surgery: a comparative review of 2217 consecutive cases. Anesth Analg (Cleve) 53:909–913, 1974
184. Backer CL, Tinker JH, Robertson DM: Myocardial infarction following local anesthesia. Anesthesiology 51:561, 1979

POSTOPERATIVE CONSIDERATIONS

185. Davison JK: Anesthesia for peripheral vascular disease. Int Anesthesiol Clin 17:129–141, 1979
186. Sabawala PB, Strong MJ, Keats AS: Surgery of the aorta and its branches. Anesthesiology 33:229–259, 1970
187. Davison JK: Anesthesia for peripheral vascular disease. Int Anesthesiol Clin 17:129–141, 1979
188. Sabawala PB, Strong MJ, Keats AS; Surgery of the aorta and its branches. Anesthesiology 33:229–259, 1970
189. Boutrous AR, Ruess R, Olsen L et al: Comparison of hemodynamic, pulmonary and renal effects of use of three types of fluid after major surgical procedures on the abdominal aorta. Crit Care Med 7:9–13, 1979
190. Wade JG, Larson CP, Jr, Hickey RH et al: Effect of carotid endarterectomy on carotid chemoreceptor and baroreceptor function. Surg Forum 19:144–145, 1968
191. Sabawala PB, Strong MJ, Keats AS: Surgery of the aorta and its branches. Anesthesiology 33:229–259, 1970

22

Surgery on the Aorta and Peripheral Arteries

RONALD A. DRITZ

INTRODUCTION

In the past 25 years, rapid advances have occurred in detection and treatment of vascular disease. Surgical intervention is now possible in many patients with occlusive or aneurysmal diseases of the aorta and its main branches. Thromboendarterectomy, first reported in the early 1950s by Wylie[1] and Barker and Cannon,[2] is now a routine operation in most community hospitals. Replacement of aneurysmal segments of arteries with tubular protheses has gained increasing application with improvements in both surgical and anesthetic techniques.

The anesthetic management of the patient undergoing surgery on the aorta may be one of the most challenging undertakings faced by an anesthesiologist. Yet the challenge is worth the effort involved; operative intervention can decrease mortality in some cases from 95 to 25 percent. This chapter will focus on the perioperative management for surgery for two types of aortic lesions, aortic aneurysm (both thoracic and abdominal) and acute aortic dissection, as well as aortic arch replacement and major extremity vascular surgery.

PATHOPHYSIOLOGY OF AORTIC LESIONS

There has long been confusion concerning the two major aortic lesions: aortic aneurysm and acute aortic dissection. They are two distinct lesions with different etiologies. While some principles of anesthetic management are similar, important differences exist.

Acute dissection of the thoracic aorta is a surgical emergency of the first magnitude. Without prompt, intensive intervention, mortality in the first 48 hours after the onset of symptoms is 1 percent per hour! Until the early 1970s an acute aortic dissection was referred to as a dissecting aortic *aneurysm*. This misnomer probably resulted from the appearance on the patient's chest film, which showed the characteristic increase in aortic size of an aortic aneurysm. However, in this instance, the picture resulted not from aneurysmal ballooning of the aortic lumen, but from penetration of blood into the aortic wall—a dissecting *hematoma*. Throughout this chapter, such a dissecting hematoma will be referred to as an *aortic dissection*, while true aneurysmal dilation of the aortic lumen will be referred to as an *aortic aneurysm*. (Fig. 22–1) To add to the confusion, approximately 1 percent of aortic aneurysms can dissect, resulting in a true dissecting aortic aneurysm.

ETIOLOGY OF AORTIC LESIONS

AORTIC ANEURYSM

Numerous autopsy series show that syphilis was the major cause of aortic aneurysm during the first five decades of this century.[3-5]

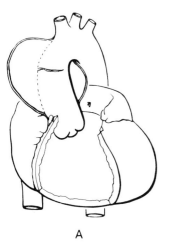 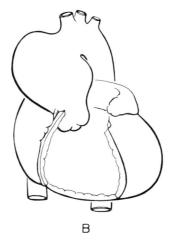

A   B

Fig. 22-1. Aortic dissection and aortic aneurysm. The pathologic process differs between an acute aortic dissecton (*A*), where a medial hematoma results from intimal rupture, and an aortic aneurysm (*B*), resulting from distention of the aortic wall. The ascending aorta may appear similar on chest film.

Effective antibiotic treatment decreased the incidence of syphilitic aortic disease. However, the incidence of atherosclerotic aneurysms increased to keep the overall rate of aortic aneurysm at 1 to 3 percent in most postmortem series.[3-5] Consistent with this change in principle etiology, the location of aortic aneurysms has changed from primarily thoracic (syphilitic) to abdominal (atherosclerotic).[3]

Atherosclerosis is a systemic disease of the large and medium-sized arteries causing intimal deposition of plaques rich in lipid and cholesterol. In the adult, intimal disease is generally most severe in the abdominal aorta. Chronologically over the population at large, coronary artery lesions lag behind those of the aorta by about a decade, and lesions in the cerebral arteries appear even later.[6]

Several factors predispose to the premature and augmented onset of atherosclerosis. Of most concern to the anesthesiologist are hypertension (defined here as a blood pressure of 150/90 torr or greater), diabetes mellitus, obesity, and cigarette smoking. Forty to fifty percent of patients presenting for various forms of arterial surgery are hyperten-sive.[7, 8] Hypertension not only augments the development of atherosclerosis, but, by increasing arterial wall tension, predisposes to aneurysm formation.

Sixteen percent of the patients in the Joint Study of Extracranial Arterial Occlusion were diabetic.[7] Several studies show a positive correlation between cigarette smoking and coronary artery disease in populations with high serum cholesterol levels.[9, 10] No such relationship has been found in Chile, where serum cholesterol levels are lower.[10] The Framingham Study has demonstrated augmented peripheral vascular disease among cigarette smokers.[11] Obesity alone has never been shown to be a risk factor in the development of atherosclerosis. It probably operates through its strong association with diabetes mellitus, hypertension, and lipid disturbances.[12]

AORTIC DISSECTION

Almost 50 years ago, Erdheim's careful pathologic accounts of two cases of aortic rupture localized the medial layer of the aorta as the site of pathology in aortic dissection.[13, 14] The

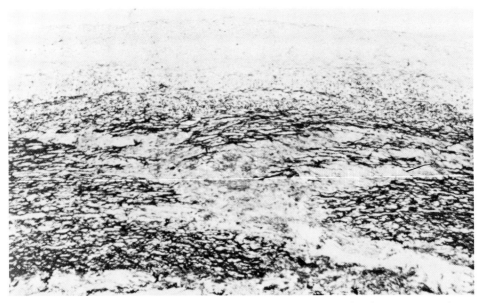

Fig. 22-2. Idiopathic medial necrosis. The large defect in the laminar pattern of the aortic wall is highlighted by the elastic tissue stain (Robbins SL: Pathology, 3rd ed. WB Saunders, 1967)

media is the strong central layer which provides the chief support for the aortic wall. It consists of an interwoven network of elastic tissue and muscle cells. Lesions of the media can be categorized by noting whether degeneration of the elastic tissue or muscle cells predominates.[15]

Muscle cells are metabolically active. In the inner media, they derive their metabolic requirements by diffusion through the intima. The outer media is supplied by the vasa vasorum. Intimal thickening or sclerosis of the vasa vasorum (both of which may be aggravated by long-standing hypertension) place these cells in jeopardy and may predispose to aortic dissection.[15] Although some series show muscle cell lesions to be more frequent than elastic tissue lesions in aortic dissection,[16] these lesions occur just as frequently in the absence of aortic dissection, causing some to be reluctant to ascribe to them etiologic significance.

As opposed to muscle cell lesions which are found mainly in older patients, elastic tissue lesions are encountered in a population usually under the age of 40.[16] These lesions, classically found in Marfan's syndrome, are thought to be hereditary and consist of interruption of laminae of the media with microscopic voids which become filled with ground substance.[16] The result is the lesion Erdheim originally described (Fig. 22–2). Rarely, aortic dissections arise from inflammatory disease of the vessel wall or advanced atherosclerosis.

PATIENT PRESENTATION AND ASSOCIATED DISEASES

ATHEROSCLEROTIC THORACIC AORTIC ANEURYSM

Atherosclerotic aortic aneurysms can involve any portion of the aorta. Regardless of the location, the symptoms experienced by the patient are surprisingly mild for such a potentially catastrophic lesion.

Patients with aneurysms of the ascending aorta are frequently asymptomatic. Though expanding saccular aneurysms can cause symptoms because of compression of the superior vena cava or the trachea, the diagnosis is often made when a widened mediastinum is noted on a chest film performed for other purposes. The first symptom is often congestive heart failure caused by aortic valvular insufficiency as the aneurysm stretches the aortic annulus. Repair of ascending aortic aneurysm is often combined with aortic valve replacement. It does not offer routinely special considerations and this will not be discussed further.

Aneurysms of the aortic arch are rare and almost always are caused by atherosclerosis. Again, symptoms are mild and usually the result of compression of adjacent structures by the expanding mass. Diagnosis is suspected by the characteristic findings on chest film and confirmed by aortography.

An aneurysm of the descending thoracic aorta usually is found as an asymptomatic mass on a chest film. As the aneurysm expands, it can cause compression of the left lung or left main stem bronchus. Compression of the bronchus can lead to dyspnea or atelectasis. Continued pressure can lead to bronchial erosion and hemoptysis. Occasionally, the left recurrent laryngeal nerve can become involved at the point where it encircles the ligamentum arteriosum leading to paralysis of the vocal cord and hoarseness.

Widespread atherosclerotic processes are common among all patients with aortic disease. Coronary artery disease, cerebrovascular disease, and hypertensive renal disease may complicate perioperative management (Table 22–1) making careful preoperative assessment imperative.[17]

ACUTE DISSECTION OF THE THORACIC AORTA

Acute dissection of the thoracic aorta is a catastrophic illness. From an initial point of penetration through the intimal layer of the aortic wall, a dissecting hematoma can propagate both proximally and distally through a weakened medial layer. Death can result from rupture or from organ ischemia as the hematoma interrupts blood flow to the aorta's major branches. The highly emergent

Table 22-1. Incidences of Other Manifestations of Arterial Disease in Patients Treated Primarily for Localized Disease

	NUMBER OF PATIENTS	OTHER MANIFESTATIONS				
		Hypertension (%)*	Heart Disease (%)†	Cerebrovascular Disease (%)	Other Occlusive vascular Disease (%)	Other Aneurysms (%)
Carotid or vertebral occlusive disease	804	52	19	100	52	
Occlusive disease of vessels arising from the aortic arch	67	35	37		58	6
Peripheral aneurysms	107	40	54	10		55
Abdominal aneurysms	1449	39	29	7	30	9
Aortoiliac occlusive disease	134	40	42			
Renovascular occlusive disease	432	100			26	13
Thoracoabdominal aneurysms	42	45	38			
Thoracic and arch aneurysms	51	43	57	8	16	
Nondissecting thoracic aneurysms	107	47		10	11	10

*Pressures greater than 150 torr systolic or 90 torr diastolic
†ECG Abnormality, angina, or congestive heart failure
(Sabawala PB, Strong MJ, Keats AS: Surgery of the aorta and its branches. Anesthesiology 33:229, 1970)

nature of the disease is striking, with a 20 percent mortality in the first 6 hours after the onset of symptoms.[18] If untreated, or with only supportive therapy, 3-month mortality is 90 percent.[19]

The sudden onset of severe, unremitting, tearing or ripping chest pain is the most frequent presenting symptom. The most common complications are rupture (usually a fatal event), aortic valvular insufficiency (the result of stretching of the aortic annulus by the dissecting hematoma), and major vessel obstruction with symptoms of coronary, cerebral, spinal, gastrointestinal, or renal vascular insufficiency depending on the vessel(s) involved.

The section on thoracic aortic surgery concentrates on management of patients with acute aortic dissection. Management of chronic (aneurysmal) disease of the thoracic aorta is similar though less emergent. Differences in management are noted.

ANESTHESIA FOR THORACIC AORTIC SURGERY

PREOPERATIVE ASSESSMENT AND MANAGEMENT

Despite early surgical intervention, mortality from acute aortic dissection remained disappointingly high in early series, ranging from 60 to 100 percent.[20-22] In view of these discouraging results, Wheat and coworkers devised a preoperative pharmacologic regimen designed to slow or stop the progress of the dissecting hematoma, and decrease the hazard of acute aortic rupture.[22]

Wheat chose agents which rapidly decreased systemic blood pressure and diminished propulsive forces within the aorta. He believed that the ejection of blood from the left ventricle generated an impulse against the aortic wall that was the major factor responsible for propagation of dissection and aortic rupture. Thus, by choosing agents which decrease the velocity of left ventricular contraction (approximated by the derived value, $dp/dt_{max.}$) short-term survival could be enhanced. To support this contention, he cited the following evidence:

1. The aorta is remarkably resistant to static pressure increases.[23]
2. Static pressure provides no pressure gradients as driving forces to induce shear stresses or other stresses on aortic tissue.[24]
3. In experimental models, tygon-tubing aortas with rubber cement intimas dissect only when the flow is pulsatile and do not dissect when flow is laminar or nonturbulent. Experiments with dog aortas show the same relationship to pulsatile flow as do the artificial aortas.[25]

4. Protection from aortic rupture in a susceptible strain of turkeys can be accomplished with propranolol, a beta-adrenergic blocking agent,[26] or reserpine, a catecholamine depleting agent,[27] at a dose that does not affect mean aortic pressure, but does alter the quality of pulsatile blood flow.

To attain these twin goals on controlled systemic hypotension and reduction of dp/dt_{max}, Wheat administered trimethaphan, reserpine, and guanethidine. His aim was to convert all acute dissections into subacute or chronic dissections.

Early results from groups employing this protocol—adding propranolol, methyldopa, and diuretics when needed—demonstrated an impressive 1-year survival of 84 percent *without surgery.*[28, 29] However, as experience accumulated, it became evident that blanket adoption of Wheat's method could not assure this high 1-year survival.

Trimethaphan proved a less than ideal hypotensive agent, despite its associated ability to lower dp/dt_{max} because of the problems of taxyphylaxis and occasional respiratory arrest. The association of reserpine with central nervous system depression and duodenal ulcers made it an unattractive agent.

Nitroprusside has become the hypotensive agent of choice because of its effectiveness in lowering blood pressure and ease of control. Some have argued against the use of nitroprusside because it increases dp/dt_{max} in dog experiments.[30] Others have refuted these arguments[31] and recent data show that nitroprusside does not change the maximum acceleration of aortic blood flow in humans given the drug after cardiac surgery.[32]

Propranolol has replaced reserpine because it can reduce effectively dp/dt_{max} through beta-adrenergic blockage, without central nervous system depression or duodenal ulceration.

Once short-term survival with medical therapy had stabilized at 65 to 70 percent, late complications, primarily saccular aneurysms and progressive aortic valvular insufficiency began to emerge.[33] Certain patients seemed more prone to develop these complications, especially those with dissections involving the ascending aorta. These patients should be offered early surgery.

On the basis of widespread experience, a consensus has emerged concerning major principles of management of acute aortic dissections.[34–38] During the first 4 hours following admission, the patient should be stabilized using the Wheat protocol with antihypertensive and negative inotropic medications and *then* taken to aortography. *At the same time,* the operating room should be prepared for surgery.

Based on the results of aortography, the lesion can be classified as type A or B (Fig. 22–3). This information, coupled with the patient's in-hospital course and response to emergency therapy, dictate whether immediate surgery, further stabilization with later surgery, or no surgery will be required.

AORTOGRAPHY

Once the patient has been stabilized aortography should begin (Table 22–2). The patient should be accompanied during transport to the radiologic facility by a cardiac surgeon,

Table 22-2. Emergency Preoperative Stabilization of Acute Thoracic Aortic Dissection (in sequence)

Monitoring*
Two large-bore intravenous catheters
Wheat protocol
    Sodium nitroprusside: to systolic BP 110–100
    Propranolol: to heart rate 60–70
Laboratory analysis sent
    CBC
    Electrolytes
    BUN/Creatinine
    Clotting studies
        PT/PTT/Bleeding time/Platelet count
Type and crossmatch
    10 units whole blood
12 lead ECG
If stable: Transfer for aortography
If unstable: Transfer to operating room

*1. Electrocardiogram
 2. Intraarterial catheter—left radial artery, if possible. (Most aortic dissections arise in the ascending aorta, which may involve the right subclavian artery. Once the ECG and intraarterial catheter are operational, the Wheat protocol should be initiated *without delay.*)
 3. Urinary catheter
 4. Central venous pressure catheter or pulmonary artery catheter
 5. Cerebral function—talking with patient; pupils

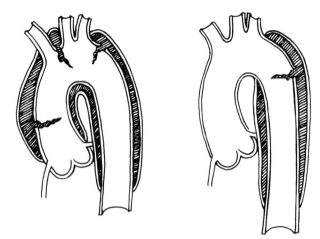

Fig. 22-3. Classification of aortic dissection. Classification is based upon the presence or absence of involvement of the ascending aorta. The primary intimal tear in type A dissections can be in the ascending aorta, the transverse aortic arch, or the descending aorta. Ten percent (8/82) of the type A and 23% (10/43) of the type B dissections originated in the aortic arch.

LESIONS	THERAPY
Type A	Immediate Surgery
Type B Complicated*	Immediate Surgery
Type B Uncomplicated	Continue Wheat protocol
	Later elective surgery

* Type B dissection with *any* of the following:
  Failure to control hypertension
  Continued pain
  Expanding aortic diameter
  Development of neurologic deficit
  Evidence of compromise of major subdiaphragmatic aortic branch
    vessel
  Development of aortic valvular insufficiency
  (Miller DC et al: Operative treatment of aortic dissection. J Thorac
  Cardiovasc Surg 78:365, 1979)

an anesthesiologist, and a nurse trained in intensive care. Such a patient should always have at least one physician and nurse present at all times in this critical preoperative period.

In the radiology department, the anesthesiologist should have the necessary equipment available for endotracheal intubation or resuscitation or both, should the need arise. The patient should receive supplemental oxygen during this period through a facemask at the rate of 4 to 6 l/min. A sample of arterial blood should be sent for determination of acid-base status, and sodium bicarbonate given to correct metabolic acidosis.

Overzealous use of pain medications or sedatives during this period is a dangerous practice. The persistance of pain despite the adequate decrease of arterial blood pressure and depression of left ventricular contractile state is a sign of failure of medical therapy and continuing aortic dissection. Depression of mental status is an ominous clinical finding which may indicate involvement in the dissection of one of the major extracranial cerebral vessels. Both these valuable and important signs (pain and mental status) are masked by overmedication with narcotics or sedatives. Small doses of a mild hypnotic agent such as diazepam should provide adequate relief of patient anxiety.

INTRAOPERATIVE AND ANESTHETIC MANAGEMENT

Once the necessary preoperative evaluation and, if needed, resuscitation, has been performed, the operating room properly prepared, and cannulae placed for adequate monitoring and vascular access, anesthesia may begin.

While there is never a time during the management of such an anesthetic when one's attention can wander, there are certain critical periods when particular care and attention must prevail. During these times, failure to recognize warning signs can lead to major complications and can significantly increase postoperative morbidity and mortality. These periods are the following:

1. Induction and endotracheal intubation
2. Application of the aortic cross-clamp
3. Release of the aortic cross-clamp
4. Transfer of the patient from the operating room to the intensive care unit

In discussing the intraoperative anesthetic care, these periods will receive special emphasis.

Induction of Anesthesia and Endotracheal Intubation

Laryngoscopy and endotracheal intubation produce responses, probably mediated by the sympathetic nervous system, which result in increases in blood pressure and heart rate.[39] Among patients with preexisting arterial hypertension, the increases are greater than in nonhypertensive subjects. This heightened response is unaltered by prior treatment with antihypertensive medications,[40] including all medications except those drugs containing β-adrenergic blocking properties. However, when treated hypertensive patients receive β-adrenergic blocking drugs before induction and intubation, the response is significantly attenuated.[41] Topical laryngeal anesthesia[42] or intravenous

---

Intraoperative Monitoring for Aortic Surgery

ECG
Intraarterial catheter*
Arterial blood gases
Urinary catheter
Central venous or pulmonary artery catheter
Temperature probe

*During surgery on the ascending aorta, the arterial catheter should be placed in the left radial artery; during surgery on the descending thoracic aorta the arterial catheter should be placed in the right radial artery because the left subclavian artery may be compromised during aortic cross-clamping. Additionally, an arterial catheter should be placed in a dorsalis pedis artery (opposite side from femoral-femoral bypass, if used) to measure distal perfusion pressure during cross-clamping.

Indications for Pulmonary Artery Catheterization for Aortic Surgery

A history of, or evidence of, congestive heart failure
History of acute myocardial infarction within 6 months of admission
Cor pulmonale
Hypovolemic shock
Oliguria
Contemplated resection of descending thoracic aorta with femoral-femoral bypass.

---

lidocaine[43] also attenuate the response, but to a lesser degree.

Table 22–3 shows the high incidence of ECG abnormalities among non β-blocked hypertensive patients and the significant diminution of this finding with β blockade. Other complications occurring during induction and intubation among hypertensive patients include congestive heart failure[44] and rupture of a previously unrecognized cerebral aneurysm.[44]

Most patients with acute thoracic aortic dissection who require surgery, arrive in the operating room within hours of the onset of symptoms. The need for a smooth and rapid *but controlled* (not "crash") induction, with cricoid pressure to protect against gastric regurgitation and pulmonary aspiration of stomach contents is well documented.[45]

These patients are doubly at risk from the pressor response to laryngoscopy and intubation. Besides the possibility of inducing

Table 22-3. Effect of Prior β Blockade on Response of Treated Hypertensive Patients to Induction* and Endotracheal Intubation

GROUP	INCREASE IN HEART RATE	INCREASE IN MEAN ARTERIAL PRESSURE	INCIDENCE OF ECG ABNORMALITY†
I	< 5 beats/min	+ 24 torr ⎫	
			4%
II	< 5 beats/min	+ 14 torr ⎭	
III	20 beats/min	+ 60 torr	38%

β BLOCKADE

    Group I: Preinduction, practolol 0.4 mg/kg intravenously and atropine 1.2 mg intravenously

    Group II: Practolol 1.5 mg/kg/6hr orally for 48 hr before surgery

    Group III: None

*Pentothal, succinylcholine, then N_2O: O_2 and Halothane 1%.

†ECG abnormality defined as ST segment depression or elevation indicative of myocardial ischemia or appearance of ventricular extrasystoles (singly, in bigeminy, or runs of ventricular tachycardia)

(Prys–Roberts C, Foëx P, Biro GP: Studies in anaesthesia in relation to hypertension. V. Adrenergic β-receptor blockade. Br J Anaesth 45:671, 1973)

myocardial ischemia, sympathetically mediated increases in blood pressure and heart rate can lead to further propagation of the dissecting hematoma or aortic rupture or both. Fortunately, most of these patients will have received β-adrenergic blocking medication as part of their therapy before surgery. Nonetheless, extreme care and caution must be taken and prompt intervention with further doses of propranolol or sodium nitroprusside or both initiated if needed.

In patients presenting for elective resection of thoacic aortic aneurysms who have been placed on NPO status overnight, a more leisurely induction can be used. Sympathetically mediated reflexes can still cause aortic rupture and should be avoided or promptly treated.

The choice of anesthetic agent(s) must be made based on known effects of the available agents on the various organ systems and the physical status of the patient presenting for a given operation. For instance, a pure narcotic and oxygen technique might be the anesthetic of choice in hypovolemic shock but not be recommended for elective thoracic aneurysm resection where high-velocity left ventricular contractility could result in aneurysmal rupture. The converse would apply to an enflurane, nitrous oxide, and oxygen technique with its attendant myocardial depression.

PRECROSS-CLAMPING MANAGEMENT

During initial surgical dissection, a stable level of anesthesia should be maintained. Fluid management will depend on initial cardiovascular parameters and the fluid loss attendant with surgical dissection. Arterial blood gas values should be checked and therapy given as indicated. In patients in whom a period of cardiopulmonary bypass will be necessary in order to resect the lesion an initial determination of activated clotting time (ACT) should be made.

One-lung Ventilation and Anesthesia. Surgical resection of dissection originating in, or aneurysms of, the descending thoracic aorta is approached through a left thoracotomy. For several reasons, tracheal intubation in such a patient using a double-lumen (or right endobronchial) tube is of advantage. First, surgical exposure, especially during the difficult period of initial aortic mobilization, is considerably enhanced by the ability to collapse the adjacent left lung. Secondly, initial surgical dissection can cause bleeding into the bronchi of the left (up) lung because the aorta is often adherent to the adjacent lung tissue. The double-lumen tube protects the right (down) lung, which might otherwise be flooded by this blood traversing the carina.

If femoral-femoral bypass is used (see Fig. 22–4D), the patient is in the unique position

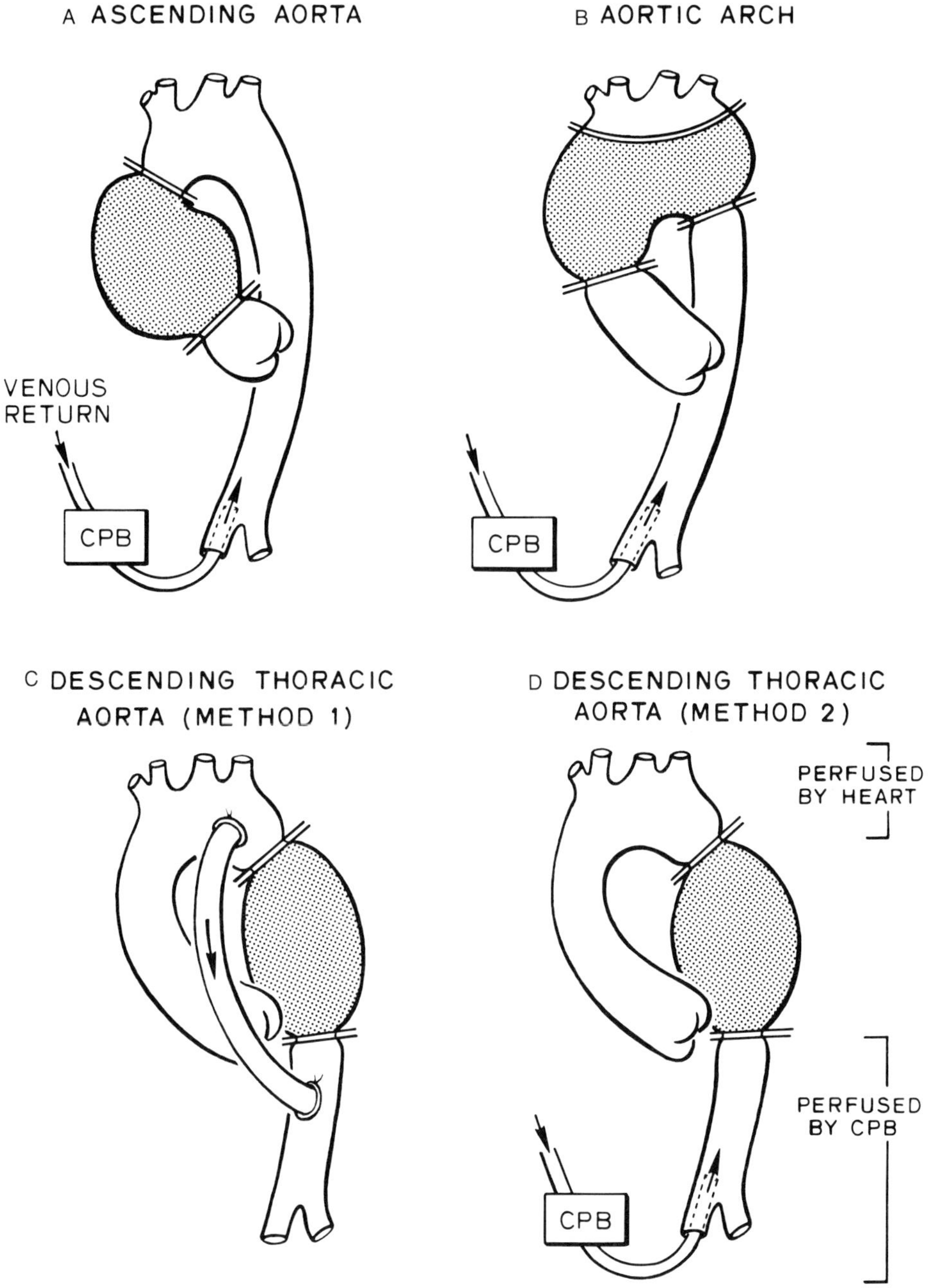

A ASCENDING AORTA

B AORTIC ARCH

VENOUS
RETURN

CPB

CPB

C DESCENDING THORACIC
AORTA (METHOD 1)

D DESCENDING THORACIC
AORTA (METHOD 2)

PERFUSED
BY HEART

PERFUSED
BY CPB

CPB

Fig. 22-4. Methods of bypass during aortic surgery. *A.* Complete cardiopulmonary bypass; cardioplegia for myocardial preservation. *B.* Cardiopulmonary bypass for cooling prior to cross clamping, *then,* cessation of bypass with profound hypothermia during cross clamping. *C.* TDMAC-heparin shunt. *D.* Partial femoral-femoral bypass.

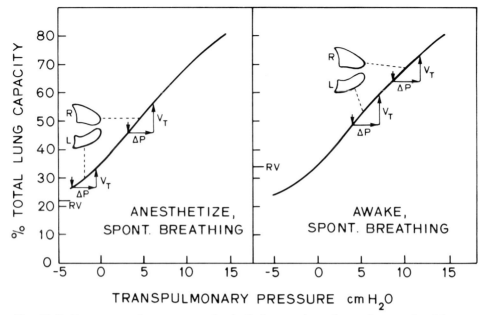

Fig. 22-5. Pressure-volume curves for both lungs of awake and normal subjects in left lateral position. *Left Panel.* Mean relative dependent lung volume 27% and mean relative nondependent lung volume 45% of TLC in anesthetized and spontaneously breathing subjects. Let transpulmonary pressure during inspiration increase uniformly by 3 cm H_2O; lung volume change of nondependent lung then will be greater than that of the dependent lung (longer upward arrow). *Right Panel.* Mean relative dependent lung volume 49% and nondependent lung volume 61% of TLC in awake and spontaneously breathing subjects. If transpulmonary pressure is again increased uniformly by 3 cm H_2O, volume change of dependent lung will be greater than that of nondependent lung (*longer upward arrow*). (Rehder K, Sessler AD: Anesthesiology 38:320–327, 1973)

of being on bypass and thus fully heparinized, but still ventilated actively to maintain proper oxygenation to those body areas proximal to the aortic cross-clamp. If the left lung were being ventilated during this period, considerable retraction would have to be placed on it to allow adequate surgical access. This, in a fully heparinized patient, could again initiate bleeding capable of severely compromising function in the right lung.

At Stanford University, a Robert–Shaw right endobronchial tube is usually employed for this purpose. Obviously the same care and attention to the cardiovascular responses of intubation must be taken when using a double lumen tube in such a patient.

In the normal awake human lying in the lateral position, the dependent lung receives both the majority of pulmonary blood flow (because of the effect of gravity) and pulmonary ventilation. Figure 22–5 illustrates that during spontaneous awake breathing, the dependent lung is on a steeper portion of the pulmonary pressure-volume curve and thus receives a greater volume of gas for a given change in transpulmonary pressure. When anesthesia is induced but spontaneous breathing is maintained, this relationship changes because of a decrease in lung volumes. Anesthesia causes a relaxation of the diaphragm, allowing abdominal contents to exert a greater pressure from below.[46] The result is some small airway collapse at the bases of both lungs and a shift in their position on the pressure-volume curve. Again referring to Figure 22–5, the *nondependent* lung is now in a steeper portion of the curve and thus will receive a greater portion of an inspired breath. Because the distribution of pulmonary blood flow is unchanged, this causes a relative ventilation-perfusion abnormality. The imbalance persists when muscle paralysis and positive pressure ventilation are instituted.

When an endobronchial tube is used and ventilation of the up lung is terminated, all blood flowing through that lung is shunted (unventilated) and thereby contributes to a venous admixture, which can result in significant hypoxemia. Fortunately, hypoxic vasoconstriction of the pulmonary vasculature in this unventilated lung helps redirect some of this blood flow to the dependent lung. A special note of caution is important here. Patients undergoing descending thoracic aortic surgery with one-lung ventilation may require infusions of sodium nitroprusside (SNP) or other hypotensive agents to control hypertension in the proximal circulation once the cross-clamp is placed. SNP has been shown to overcome the hypoxic pulmonary vasoconstriction induced by one-lung ventilation in dogs.[47] Thus venous admixture may worsen. In an attempt ot offset this admixture, the blood flowing through the dependent, ventilated lung should be saturated maximally with oxygen.

When one lung is collapsed, the ventilated lung may or may not tolerate the full tidal volume used before collapse. Tidal volume may need to be reduced slightly, but no change is preferred. Pa_{CO_2} should be controlled to normal levels by ventilatory rate changes as needed.

Five minutes after institution of one-lung anesthesia, a sample of arterial blood should be sent for blood gas analysis. If hypoxemia is present despite high inspired oxygen concentration, periods of ventilation of the up (left) lung may be necessary. If this is not possible, temporary clamping of the left pulmonary artery may eliminate or reduce the shunt.

The collapsed lung should be reexpanded fully before closing the chest. Despite this maneuver, atelectasis may result in the lung and a period of ventilation with positive end expiratory pressure (PEEP) may be required immediately post-operatively.

Placement of the Aortic Cross-clamp and Perfusion

Once the section of diseased aorta has been freed and mobilized, arterial cross-clamps will be placed proximal and distal to the lesion. Before placement of the cross-clamps, the anesthesiologist should make certain that a sample of unheparinized blood has been drawn from the patient by the surgeon to preclot the prosthetic graft, and then that the patient has been adequately anticoagulated with intravenous heparin. An ACT approximately four times the control value is desired[48] (see Chaps. 13 and 24).

Placement of an aortic cross clamp causes an increase in left ventricular afterload. If the ascending aorta or aortic arch is cross-clamped, the heart is fibrillated and cardiopulmonary bypass used (Figs. 22–4A and 4B). However in the case of descending aortic cross-clamping, the circulation is divided. Proximal structures are still perfused by the heart (Figs. 22–4C and 4D). Structures distal to the cross-clamp, especially the kidneys and lower spinal cord, must also receive blood flow (Fig. 22–6). At Stanford University, two methods have been used to avoid left ventricular dilation and to provide distal blood flow during cross-clamping of the descending aorta.

Femoral-femoral bypass. This form of bypass is employed in the majority of patients undergoing descending thoracic aortic surgery at Stanford University. The venous cannula is placed in the femoral vein and threaded well up into the inferior vena cava to insure adequate venous drainage. Venous blood is passed through an oxygenator and transfused through the arterial cannula into the femoral artery (see Fig. 22–4D). Advantages of this technique include a means of distal perfusion that is independent of cardiac output and a direct means of altering venous return to the proximal circulation so the problem of proximal hypertension and

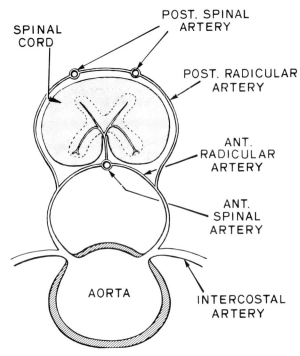

Fig. 22-6. Anterior spinal artery anatomy. If blood flow to the lower spinal cord is interrupted by cross-clamping for too great a time period, permanent damage can result. The anterior spinal artery supplies arterial blood to 75% of the cross-sectional area of the cord, while the two posterior spinal arteries only supply 25% of the cord. In thoracic and lumbar regions, these arteries are supplied from the aorta by the anterior and posterior radicular arteries. The major anterior radicular artery responsible for the lower 2/3 of the spinal cord originates between T_{11} and L_3. If blood flow through this artery is terminated by cross-clamping, the anterior 75% of the lower 2/3 of the cord may be damaged as collateral flow from the posterior spinal arteries is not sufficient to overcome the deficit.

left ventricular dilation can be avoided. Alteration of venous drainage into the pump is used to maintain left ventricular preload within desired limits. Obviously some form of adjustable clamping device is required on the venous line to perform this task. Some perfusionists prefer a second roller pump, interposed in the venous line to control venous flow. This may offer tighter control over venous drainage. The routine use of a pul-

monary artery (Swan–Ganz) catheter has enabled the anesthesiologist and perfusionist to control tightly left ventricular preload without large changes in proximal blood pressure. Previously, changes in proximal blood pressure occurred because preload could not be controlled as well.

TDMAC-heparin shunt (see Fig. 22–4C). This is a flexible polyvinyl tube bonded with triiodododecylmethylammonium-heparin. Clotting is retarded in blood flowing through it, and systemic heparinization is not used. The shunt is inserted proximally in the ascending aorta, apex of the left ventricle, or, if neither is available, the left subclavian artery, and distally into the aorta or femoral artery.

Though use of the shunt appears simple and convenient, there are several potential problems. First, the shunt can obscure the operative field and attempts to reposition it can cause kinking with loss of distal perfusion pressure.[49] Second, if the shunt is placed in the left subclavian artery, it has been suggested that there is an increased likelihood of spinal cord ischemia.[50] In the upper thoracic area, the anterior spinal artery is supplied by the vertebral arteries. Placing the shunt in the left subclavian artery can initiate a subclavian steal which reverses blood flow in the vertebral artery with a resultant decrease of blood flow to the anterior spinal artery. To date there is no study which substantiates this hypothesis.

Finally, one should not be lulled into thinking that, with a shunt in place, the hemodynamics are returned to their precross-clamping state. Careful hemodynamic monitoring has revealed a significant decrease in cardiac index and left ventricular stroke work in patients during use of TDMAC-heparin shunts.[49] Associated with the decrease in cardiac index was a decrease in urinary output, although no overt renal failure resulted among the eight patients studied. The findings suggest a depression in cardiac performance possibly caused by the increased impedance the heart must face when the relatively noncompliant shunt is substituted for the aorta during cross-clamping.[51]

Some physicians use no bypass during descending aortic cross-clamping, feeling that distal organs can withstand short periods of anoxia without permanent damage. Their results would tend to confirm this contention,[52] though others do not report a similar experience.[53] What is not discussed, however, is the second major problem induced by descending aortic cross-clamping: that of increased ventricular afterload and left-heart failure. Many physicians feel that the syndrome can be anticipated if proximal hypertension is noted when the cross-clamp is placed, and then the patient treated with hypotensive agents.[52] Others feel that left heart dilation can be better avoided through the use of some form of bypass with diversion of excess blood volume, either into a pump oxygenator[53] or through a shunt.[54]

Volume Management Before Unclamping

Just as the placement of the cross-clamp decreased the arterial space and vascular compliance, unclamping will have the opposite effect. To prepare for this sudden return to normal vascular size and compliance, the anesthesiologist should begin transfusion to high-normal cardiac filling pressures as the final vascular anastomosis is performed. If hypotensive agents have been necessary to treat hypertension or evidence of myocardial ischemia during cross-clamping, careful drug infusion tapering should begin. Adequate amounts of blood and blood products should be available if further transfusion is necessary once the cross-clamp is removed.

In surgery on the ascending aorta, where total cardiopulmonary bypass is used, unclamping and cessation of bypass are managed jointly by surgeon, anesthesiologist, and perfusionist. Rapid transfusion from the pump reservoir provides initial volume support, augmented later by IV blood infusion by the anesthesiologist. Unclamping, in surgery on the descending thoracic aorta when a TDMAC-heparin shunt is in place, involves simultaneous cross-clamping of the shunt. Unclamping when femoral-femoral partial bypass has been used requires the perfusionist to decrease venous drainage into the pump by 100 to 200 ml/min just before unclamping, thus enhancing the patient's venous volume.

Metabolic Stabilization

Much has been made of the sudden release of lactic acid into the circulation with unclamping. Lactic acid accumulates in the unperfused areas distal to the cross-clamp. This has been given as a possible explanation for "declamping shock" (see below). The importance of the phenomenon has been overstated. The body's natural buffering mechanisms should be adequate to handle the hypoxic metabolites under most circumstances. However, a sample of arterial blood should be sent shortly after unclamping and metabolic acidosis corrected with bicarbonate, if necessary.

For many years, the phenomenon of declamping shock was widely discussed but poorly understood. Certain patients with descending aortic lesions would appear stable during the operation until the cross-clamp was removed. At this point, the blood pressure would decrease suddenly to very low levels. Attempts at resuscitation were unsuccessful. Various theories were advanced to explain the phenomenon. Causative factors were thought to be the sudden increase in the vascular space, sudden liberation of an acid load into the circulation, and inadequate vascular volume loading before unclamping. With the recent emphasis on control of left ventricular dilation during cross-clamping, this syndrome occurs less frequently. One possible explanation is that previously during cross-clamping some patients suffered severe left ventricular dilation and ischemia; when the cross-clamp was removed without adequate prior volume loading, the blood pressure decreased, further aggravating myocardial ischemia. Myocardial damage was then too great and resuscitation proved futile. When left ventricular dilation is avoided and volume loading is initiated before cross-clamp removal, this problem should not occur.

Anesthetic Management After Unclamping

After the immediate hemodynamic problems of unclamping or discontinuance of bypass have occurred, further stabilization of physiologic variables should be undertaken.

Respiratory. A sample of arterial blood should be sent for determination of pH and blood gas tensions. The results should act as a guide to further intraoperative respiratory and bicarbonate management. In the case where one-lung anesthesia has been used, reinstitution of bilateral ventilation may require alteration of tidal volume and respiratory rate.

Coagulation Management After Aortic Unclamping (in Sequence)

Reverse heparin with protamine
Check ACT; give additional protamine as indicated to return ACT to control
Perform coagulation tests (laboratory)
  1. Thrombin time
  2. Activated PTT (aPTT)
  3. Prothrombin time
  4. Platelet count
Treat according to results of clotting studies[48] (Table 22–4)

Management of Patient Transfer From Operating Room to Intensive Care Unit (in sequence)*

  1. Taper inhalational anesthetic agents slowly to 0% in 100% oxygen.
  2. Supplement anesthesia with intravenous narcotic agents as needed.
  3. Adjust all cardiovascular medication infusions.
  4. Check all equipment for transport.
  5. Gently transfer patient to gurney or ICU bed.
  6. Stabilize on gurney or bed before leaving OR (CV, respiratory, position, etc.).
  7. Maintain arterial blood pressure monitoring and ECG monitoring during transfer.
  8. Transport with sufficient assistance.
  9. Provide adequate report of intraoperative events to ICU nursing staff.
 10. Check all ICU equipment, drugs, responses.
 11. Leave patient only if stable.

*See also Chap. 15 on postbypass management and operating room to ICU transport.

Hemodynamic. With unclamping and initial perfusion of the graft, bleeding may occur, especially along the fresh suture lines. Blood loss can be significant especially if complicated by derangements in the clotting system.

Coagulation. Management of the coagulation system is outlined above[48] and in Table 22–4 (see also Chaps. 15 and 24).

Renal. This is also the time to recheck urine output, most especially in cases where suprarenal aortic cross-clamping has been required. Oliguria should be managed as described later in the section on *Management of Renal Function during Major Vascular Surgery.*

During closure of the incision, the anesthesiologist should begin preparing the patient for the move from operating room to intensive care unit (see above). If an endobronchial tube or double-lumen tube has been used during surgery, it should be replaced by a standard low-pressure endotracheal tube before patient transfer.

ANESTHESIA FOR AORTIC ARCH REPLACEMENT

Acute dissection or aneurysm involving the aortic arch is fortunately relatively rare. Acute dissection in which the intimal tear was found in the aortic arch occurred in 34 of 236 patients reported by Shennan.[55] The decreased prevalence of syphilitic aortitis has made the aortic arch a rare location for aneurysmal dilation. Takayasu's aortitis, a progressive obliterative intimal disease of the aortic arch and neck vessels characterized by giant cell formation and most prevalent among young women, is a third cause of aortic arch pathology.

Attempts to treat any of these disorders medically (nonsurgically) have met with dismal results. Yet surgical replacement of the aortic arch could not, until recently, offer more hope for survival. Even in the most experienced centers, mortality approached 50 percent.[56] Recently, a technique involving the use of profound hypothermia and a period of total circulatory arrest has been employed

Table 22-4. Treatment of Coagulation Abnormalities During Aortic Surgery

ABNORMALITY	ETIOLOGY	ABNORMAL TEST	THERAPY
Residual Heparin	Inadequate reversal with protamine sulfate	↑ ACT	Protamine sulfate
Thrombocytopenia	Massive transfusion Prolonged CPB	↓ Platelet count ↑ Bleeding time	Platelet transfusion
Qualitative platelet defect	Drugs (aspirin and the like) Fibrin split products (FSP)	↑ Bleeding time	Platelet transfusion Remove FSP
DIC (rare)	Prolonged hypotension Circulatory stasis Inadequate heparinization	↓ Platelet count ↑ PTT ↓ Fibrinogen level ↑ FSP	Treat cause Replace consumed components Optimize circulation
Fibrinolysis (rare)	CPB	↑ PTT ↓ Fibrinogen level ↑ Bleeding time	ε-aminocaproic acid (consult a hematologist)?

Abbreviations: ACT—activated clotting time; CPB—cardiopulmonary bypass; PTT—partial thromboplastin time; DIC—disseminated intravascular coagulation; FSP—fibrin split products.
(See also Chap. 24 and Fischbach DP, Fogdall RP: Coagulation: The Essentials. Baltimore, Williams & Wilkins, 1981)

in such patients at Stanford University. Initial results are encouraging with mortality well below that reported using other techniques.[57] The technique is complex and should not be attempted unless previous experience with both aortic vascular surgery and profound hypothermia is extensive. What follows is a brief description of the technique and some of the problems encountered. For a more thorough discussion of hypothermia and its effects on the cardiovascular system, see Chap. 26.

The patient is anesthetized and intubated. Initial cooling to a core body temperature of 30 to 31°C is accomplished externally by total immersion in an ice bath. The patient is dried and moved onto the operating table where surgical incision is made and the patient is placed on total cardiopulmonary bypass (see Fig. 22–4B). During this period, core temperature continues to drift downward and is usually in the vicinity of 26 to 28°C when cannulation is complete. Further cooling to a core temperature of 12 to 16°C is accomplished on bypass. Once adequate cooling is completed, bypass is temporarily discontinued (total circulatory arrest) and the aortic arch replaced with a prosthetic graft. The button of aorta containing the origin of the neck

vessels is preserved in the surgical dissection and an anastomosis is made into the graft. This saves valuable time, allowing one anastomosis to take the place of three. Total arrest times average 45 minutes and cross-clamp times are approximately 75 minutes.

Some of the problems encountered when body temperature is lowered to these levels are listed below:

1. *Blood viscosity.* As body temperature is lowered, blood viscosity increases. Hemodilution to a hematocrit of 14–18 must precede cooling or considerable red cell sludging and organ damage will occur.
2. *Cardiac rhythm disturbances.* As body temperature decreases into the low 30s and high 20s (°C), arrhythmias become an important management problem. Ventricular fibrillation usually occurs around 26°C;[58, 59] thus care must be taken lest this occur before cannulation is complete.
3. *Coagulation disturbances.* Profound hypothermia affects both platelets and circulating clotting factors. Platelet counts decrease with body temperature and, though normal counts return with rewarming,[60] platelet function may be abnormal. Circulating clotting factors are

also adversely effected. To treat this bleeding abnormality, the phlebotomized blood collected during hemodilution, fresh frozen plasma, and platelet concentrates are infused once rewarming is complete.

ANESTHESIA FOR ABDOMINAL AORTIC SURGERY

PATIENT PRESENTATION

The patient with an aneurysm of the abdominal aorta is often unaware of the problem until it is discovered by a physician at routine physical examination. Occasionally low back pain may be the presenting symptom and must be differentiated from similar pain of orthopedic or neurologic origin. The patient also may present with impending aneurysmal leak or rupture. Aneurysmal pain or back pain produced by gentle pressure on the aneurysm are the most consistent signs of active or impending leak.[61] The most common presentations for aneurysmal rupture are (in descending order of frequency): back pain, cardiovascular collapse, and abdominal pain.[61] Aneurysmal size appears to be the only finding which correlates with likelihood of rupture. Aneurysms with 4 cm diameter have a 25 percent risk of rupture.[62] Once rupture has occurred, perioperative mortality increases from less than 5 percent[63, 64] to greater than 40 percent.[65, 66] Therefore all

Table 22-5. Mainstays of Initial Anesthetic Management in Ruptured Abdominal Aortic Aneurysm

VOLUME RESUSCITATION
Blood and blood products or crystalloid if blood not available
Temporizing, short-term use of dopamine or G-suit or both

RESPIRATORY MANAGEMENT
Oxygen by mask

METABOLIC STABILIZATION
Frequent arterial blood gases
Vigorous correction of lactic acidosis

ASSESSMENT OF RENAL FUNCTION
See Fig. 22 8 and text

aneurysms of 4 cm diameter or greater should be resected electively once discovered. The high prevalence of coronary artery disease, hypertension, diabetes mellitus, and other peripheral vascular disease in these patients may complicate anesthetic management (see Table 22–1).

ANESTHETIC MANAGEMENT WHERE DIFFERENT FROM ROUTINE

Intraoperative monitoring procedures have been shown above. Awake intubation may be indicated in patients with aneurysmal rupture associated with hypotension, while a slow anesthetic induction and intubation, which minimizes stress on the cardiovascular system, is appropriate in elective patients. Anesthetic agents of choice are those which provide cardiovascular stability, as dictated by patient pathophysiology. This usually is a narcotic technique supplemented with potent inhalation agents. The principles of intraoperative resuscitation in patients with ruptured abdominal aortic aneurysm are outlined in Table 22–5. After preclotting of the aortic graft and then heparin administration into the patient, the aortic cross-clamp is placed (usually below the origin of the renal arteries). Increases in afterload may be associated with myocardial ischemia, especially in patients with history of angina pectoris.[67] Vasodilating agents given during this period will return afterload to normal levels. Prior to cross-clamp removal, volume loading is mandatory to avoid hypotension with unclamping. In cases where a Y-shaped graft is used, with distal anastomosis into the iliac or femoral arteries, the clamp will be removed in stages. Once the proximal and first distal anastomoses are complete, one leg will be reperfused and the cross-clamp moved to the unattached limb of the graft to be removed when the final anastomosis is complete. Acid-base status should be rechecked after unclamping. Protamine sulfate may be necessary to counteract residual heparin. Most patients will require a period of mechanical ventilation postoperatively, because of preoperative pulmonary dysfunction (from smoking) or intraabdominal interference with pulmonary function.

ANESTHESIA FOR EXTREMITY VASCULAR SURGERY

In the past 10 years, numerous procedures have been developed to augment blood flow in vessels distal to the aorta. Before this, the only surgical intervention that could be offered in an attempt to salvage an ischemic limb was a sympathectomy. Now procedures which bypass the obstruction (femoral-popliteal venous graft), divert blood flow into the area from other vessels (axillary-femoral or femoral-femoral bypass), and which enhance the diameter of the affected vessel lumen (femoral profundoplasty) can be offered.

Patients in surgery for these procedures come from a population similar to that of patients with aortic lesions. The strong association with hypertension, heart disease, diabetes mellitus, and other vascular occlusive disease has been discussed earlier in this chapter. Indeed, in some cases, patients who may have been candidates for major aortic surgery are instead subjected to one of these lesser procedures because their other associated problems make them a poor operative risk. Thus, the anesthesiologist must be prepared to manage a patient whose physical status is poor and whose anesthetic risk is high.

Regional anesthetic techniques have been advocated for these patients as a means of augmenting blood flow into the ischemic area.[68] Sympathetic blockade has been shown to increase skin and muscle blood flow and decrease peripheral vascular resistance in ischemic limbs.[69] Whether this temporary blockade in any way enhances the clinical outcome of the procedure is not known. Continuous regional anesthesia with placement of catheters in either the extradural or subarachnoid space may not be indicated in patients who will receive some form of systemic heparinization during surgery.[70] Indeed, some have argued against the use of spinal anesthesia on this ground.[71] The extent and duration of anticoagulation is variable and unpredictable, creating the possibility of peri- or subdural hemorrhage with subsequent spinal cord compression. Thus general anesthesia may be the anesthesia of choice for many of these patients. Because adequate operating conditions will not require thorough muscle relaxation, a light inhalational technique with spontaneous respiration has proven a popular choice for some practitioners. As always, the patient's general status is the determining factor in choosing which anesthetic technique to employ.

For selected procedures which do not require extensive dissection in very high-risk patients, infiltration with a local anesthetic combined with mild intravenous sedation may offer adequate operating conditions with the least alteration in physiologic parameters. Certainly careful prior consultation with the surgeons is necessary. In some cases, the anesthetic risks may argue for a less invasive procedure in a very high-risk patient (*e.g.*, axillary-femoral graft rather than aortofemoral graft). It is important that the anesthesiologist not hesitate to express feelings regarding the patient's ability to withstand surgery when alternative surgical procedures may be possible.

RELATED TOPICS OF SPECIAL CONCERN
AUTOTRANSFUSION

Several devices are available presently to reinfuse blood removed from the operative field. Some, adapted from cardiopulmonary bypass units, incorporate roller pumps and a blood reservoir. Blood aspirated through suction tips from the surgical field is stored in the reservoir, filtered, and reinfused without further treatment into the patient's intravenous catheters. The technique decreases the need for homologous blood transfusion with its attendant risk of hepatitis and isoimmunization. Disadvantages include the need

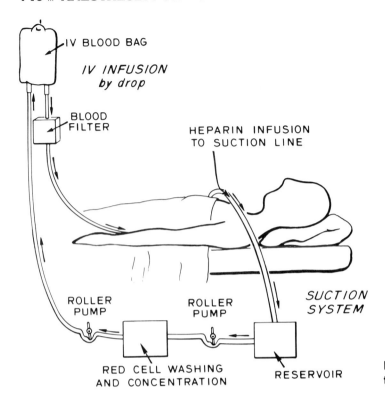

Fig. 22-7. An idealized auto-transfusion system.

for systemic heparinization to levels normally required only for cardiopulmonary bypass, destruction of some red cells with postoperative hemoglobinemia,[72] some degree of thrombocytopenia because of platelet destruction,[73] and the risk of air embolism. Because the equipment is cumbersome, complex, and hazardous, the technique has never gained widespread enthusiasm.

A new device has appeared recently which overcomes some of the drawbacks of the older unit. It has the capability to wash the collected aspirate, discard the supernatant and return only washed red cells for reinfusion, overcoming the problem of hemoglobinemia. Because heparin is added directly to the aspiration *tubing* and discarded in the washing process, the need for systemic heparinization is avoided. The device is expensive but many hospitals already use similar systems for plasmaphoresis. Whether it will gain popularity in the operating room remains to be seen. An idealized autotransfusion system is shown in Fig. 22–7.

G-SUIT

The G-suit is a wrap-around vinyl bag which is applied to the patient up to the level of the epigastrium. Originally described by Crile in 1903, it was largely forgotten in clinical medicine until the late 1950s when a series of case reports of its efficacy in resuscitation of vital signs in patients with uncontrollable abdominal hemorrhage revived interest in it.[74] The principle also was applied successfully in the modern aviation antigravity suit, first introduced during World War II to combat retinal ischemia induced by centrifugal forces generated in certain aerial maneuvers. Most of the early clinical reports concerned patients suffering from intraabdominal hemorrhage in whom all available means to control bleeding had failed, including surgical exploration and massive infusion of blood products. When the G-suit was applied and inflated to only 20 to 30 torr, blood pressure which had been 40 torr or less in some cases returned to near normal levels and stayed there for prolonged periods. Its major role is that of a time-buyer (*e.g.*, leaking abdominal aortic aneurysm) when delays in getting the patient to the operating room occur or when transfer to another hospital is necessary.

A variety of explanations have been forwarded to explain how 20 to 30 torr external counterpressure can tamponade bleeding from a vessel whose internal hydrostatic mean pressure may reach 80 to 90 torr, a seeming contradiction in the laws of physics. Experiments in dogs suggest two mechanisms are involved: tamponade and clot formation with sealing of the bleeding point.[75] A 5-cm laceration was made in the aortas of dogs and intraperitoneal and arterial pressure measured. In control dogs without G-suits, blood pressure decreased rapidly and all dogs expired within 15 minutes. In the dogs with G-suits, blood pressure decreased rapidly to the level of intraperitoneal pressure, now raised by the external pressure of the G-suit and remained at that level for approximately 10 minutes. Blood pressure then gradually increased to approximately 60 percent of control levels during the next 20 minutes, and stabilized. A last group of animals was placed in G-suits, and each animal completely heparinized. In these dogs, blood pressure decreased to the level of intraperitoneal pressure, stabilized briefly, and then continued to decrease. All of these animals expired in an average of 90 minutes. These data suggest strongly that the mechanism of blood pressure resuscitation when the G-suit is applied, is initially tamponade of bleeding at a level equal to intraperitoneal pressure, and that the cessation of active bleeding at this level allows clot formation and temporary sealing of the leak site.

Because the G-suit is inflated to a pressure which is above venous pressure, the suit will shunt venous blood from the lower portion of the body towards the heart, an internal autotransfusion. Structures cephalad to the compressed region, including heart, lungs, and brain, will enjoy increased blood flow. For structures within the compressed region, most notably the kidneys, this is not the case. In intact (nonhemorrhaging) dogs subjected to 40 torr external counterpressure, blood flow in the compressed region decreased.[76]

MANAGEMENT OF RENAL FUNCTION DURING MAJOR VASCULAR SURGERY

When acute renal failure (ARF) complicates the in-hospital course of a patient undergoing major vascular surgery, mortality ranges from 57 to 95 percent.[77–81] In patients spared this complication, in-hospital mortality is less than 10 percent.[77, 82] Hence, the early recognition of impending ARF and intervention to maintain renal function is critical in such a patient's care. Many of these patients have suffered acute hemorrhage and require emergency surgery. Thus, it is often the anesthesiologist in the operating room who must recognize the condition and initiate treatment.

Despite intensive research, the precise pathophysiologic mechanisms responsible for the production of ARF in a patient with previously adequate renal function remain unclear. At present, evidence suggests that ARF results from a combination of vasomotor alterations in the microvasculature of the kidney and tubular and capillary cell damage.

A marked increase in renal cortical vascular resistance, apparently in the afferent arteriole, with a decrease in renal cortical blood flow has been demonstrated in both animals and humans suffering from ARF.[83, 84] The renin-angiotensin system has been shown to play a major role in this vascular response. Both the angiotensin II competitive receptor antagonist P113 and the angiotensin I converting enzyme antagonist SQ20881 (captopril) block the decreased renal blood flow and increase renal vascular resistance associated with glycerol-induced ARF in the rat.[85] However, a parallel improvement in renal excretory function does not occur.[85] Attempts to reverse the vascular abnormality in established ARF in humans with adrenergic blocking agents failed to reestablish renal function.[86]

The decrease in cortical blood flow and resultant ischemia has been shown to result in swelling of cells lining renal capillaries and tubules.[87] This cell swelling has been implicated as the cause of persistent blockage of precapillary arterioles, resistant to the use of vasodilating agents, the so-called *no reflow phenomenon.*

Factors Affecting Renal Function During Aortic Surgery

Anesthetic agents. While it is certainly beyond the scope of this chapter to undertake a thorough discussion of the effect of anesthetic agents on the kidney, certain concepts do pertain to aortic surgery. Anesthetic agents can depress renal function in three general ways. First, by the direct nephrotoxic effect of the agent or its metabolites on the kidney, as in the case of methoxyflurane's,[88] and to a lesser extent enflurane's,[89] inorganic fluoride metabolite. Second, through the liberation of catecholamines, as with cyclopropane and diethyl ether, which severely diminish renal cortical blood flow.[90] And lastly, through the depressant effect of some anesthetic agents on cardiac output with resulting diminution of total renal blood flow, as with halothane.[91]

Aortic cross-clamping. Cross-clamping of the aorta below the renal arteries has been associated with a decrease in urine flow.[92] Experiments in dogs show this to be associated with a decrease in both renal plasma flow and glomerular filtration rate.[93] In early studies of patients undergoing abdominal aortic aneurysmectomy, there was a high incidence of acute renal failure. However, as clinical experience has accumulated and anesthetic techniques improved, the incidence of ARF in elective aneurysm resection has decreased to well below 10 percent in most large series.[94, 95] Thus, the decrease in urine output during infrarenal cross-clamping should be classified as a reversible functional acute renal impairment, the etiology of which is not presently known. Some have suggested prophylactic pre-cross-clamp volume loading in these patients, using hypertonic solutions such as mannitol[92] or dextrose.[94] Though the oliguria associated with infrarenal aortic cross-clamping is avoided by these measures, there is no evidence in humans, either prospective or retrospective, to show that the incidence of postoperative ARF is affected.

When a cross-clamp is placed across the aorta above the origin of the renal arteries, renal blood flow obviously decreases to zero. Thus, the question becomes, how long a period of anoxia can the kidneys withstand without permanent damage? And second, what can be done to minimize the insult incurred during this period? Among a group of 17 patients undergoing elective replacement of portions of the descending thoracic aorta without shunting or bypass during cross-clamping, there was no incidence of renal failure postoperatively. Aortic cross-clamp times ranged from 6.5 to 34 minutes. No particular maneuvers were undertaken to protect the kidneys either before or during cross-clamping.[96] Many surgeons and anesthesiologists feel that mannitol given before suprarenal aortic cross-clamping may help the kidneys better withstand ischemia. There is some evidence in rats subjected to 60 to 180 minutes of renal artery cross-clamping that treatment with mannitol helps preserve renal cortical blood flow in the postischemic period.[87] This work is controversial and studies in humans are inconclusive.[92] Furosemide appears to be of *no* value in preventing renal failure in humans.[97]

Cardiopulmonary Bypass. Bypass techniques, whether total or partial, alter renal hemodynamics by several methods. Renal perfusion pressure decreases and pulsatile flow ceases. For a thorough discussion of the effects of bypass on renal function see the chapter on renal function (Chap. 25).

Oliguria During Major Vascular Surgery

A period of hypotension is the strongest predisposing factor in the development of ARF in patients undergoing vascular surgery. The incidence of ARF among hypotensive patients is eight- to tenfold greater than in patients without hypotension. Thus, the anesthesiologist should be particularly attentive

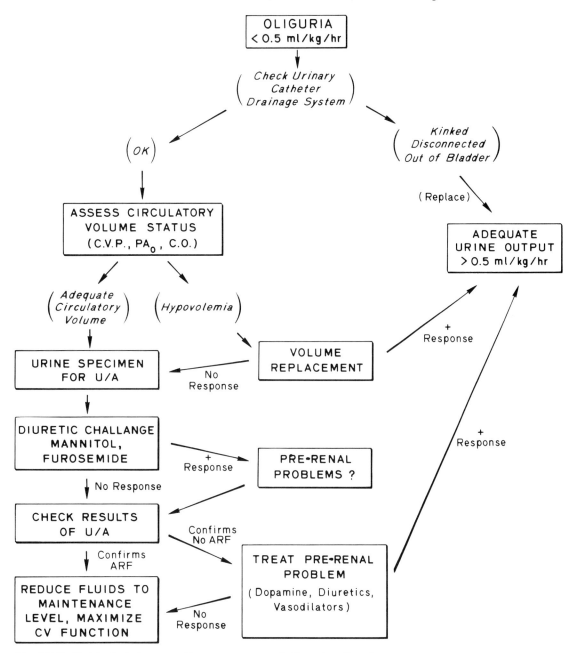

Fig. 22-8. Guide to intraoperative management of acute oliguria.

to renal function when managing such a patient.

If urine output decreases to less than 0.5 ml/kg/hr, the anesthesiologist should initiate intensive investigation of possible impending ARF (Fig. 22–8). Malfunction of the urinary catheter system should be ruled out. The pa-

tient's volume status should be reassessed and augmented if necessary. If these maneuvers fail to elicit an increase in urine flow, a sample of the last hour's urine should be sent for a urinalysis, including microscopic examination for casts and determinations of urine sodium, urea, and osmolality. A sam-

Table 22-6. Nephrotoxins of Concern During Aortic Surgery

PIGMENT
  Myoglobin
  Hemoglobin

MISMATCHED TRANSFUSION

ANESTHETIC AGENTS
  Methoxyflurane
  Enflurane*

ANTIBIOTICS
  Coly-Mycin
  Polymyxin
  Gentamycin
  Kanamycin
  Tobramycin
  Amphotericin B

---

*If enflurane is being used and an oliguric state develops it should be discontinued.

ple of blood also should be sent for concomitant determination of serum osmolality. *After a urine sample is collected,* a diuretic challenge may be helpful. Urine collected after diuretics have been given is of no value in distinguishing between prerenal azotemia and ARF. The best available knowledge suggests that diuretics are not therapeutic in established ARF.[97, 90] If a patient responds to a diuretic challenge, it is strong evidence that renal impairment has not progressed to ARF. It also calls for further assessment of volume status, first because the positive response suggests that hypovolemia may indeed be the cause of the oliguria, and secondly because the diuresis alone may aggravate hypovolemia. A note of caution should be sounded concerning the rapid infusion of large doses of furosemide-deafness, sometimes permanent, may result from too rapid infusion of large doses. Therefore, doses greater than 100 mg should be given by a continuous infusion at the rate of 100 to 150 mg/hr.

If the patient does not respond to the diuretic challenge, a presumptive diagnosis of ARF can be made. The urinalysis should now be available to confirm. Urine sodium will be increased because the ARF kidney loses the ability to conserve sodium. Urine urea will be decreased and urine and blood will show isoosmolality because of loss of renal tubular concentrating ability. Such a urinalysis is diagnostic of ARF. Once the diagnosis of ARF

is made, all potential nephrotoxins should be avoided (Table 22–6).

Until recently, once the diagnosis of ARF was made, fluid replacement was restricted to maintenance levels. Vigorous volume-loading to maintain pulmonary artery occluded pressure in the range of 16 to 18 torr may convert a significant number of these patients from oliguric to nonoliguric ARF. This seems not only to decrease the need for dialysis but also may enhance ultimate survival.[99]

SUMMARY

Surgery on the aorta and major branches is becoming more common. Anesthesia for major cardiovascular procedures, often performed on the critically ill patient, is challenging. Complications are not uncommon, but can be minimized. A combination of a thorough understanding of the pathophysiology and of the various disease processes, pharmacology of available therapeutic agents, appropriate monitoring, and skilled attention to detail, all should provide optimal results. The patient with major vascular disease or injury is not routine, and cannot be treated as routine for optimal survival. The anesthesiologist, surgeon, and critical care specialists all have a coordinated role in the successful management of this patient.

REFERENCES

INTRODUCTION

1. Wylie E, Kerr E, Davies O: Experimental and clinical experiences with use of fascia lata applied as a graft about major arteries after thromboendarectomy and aneurysmorrhaphy. Surg Gynecol Obstet 93:257, 1951
2. Barker WF, Cannon JA: An evaluation of endarterectomy. Arch Surg 66:488, 1953

ETIOLOGY OF AORTIC LESIONS

3. Maniglia R, Gregory JE: Increasing incidence of arteriosclerotic aortic aneurysms. Analysis of 6,000 autopsies. Arch Pathol Lab Med 54:298, 1952

4. Blakemore AH, Voorhees AB: Aneurysm of aorta: review of 365 cases. Angiology 5:209, 1954

5. Parkhurst GF, Decker JP: Bacterial aortitis and mycotic aneurysm of aorta. Am J Pathol 31:821, 1955

6. McGill JC Jr (ed): Geographic Pathology of Atherosclerosis, pp 523, 645. Baltimore, Williams & Wilkins, 1969

7. Bauer RD, Meyer JS, Fields WS et al: Joint study of extracranial arterial occlusion (III). JAMA 208:509, 1969

8. Gore I, Hirst AE, Jr: Arteriosclerotic aneurysms of the abdominal aorta: a review. Prog Cardiovasc Dis 16:113, 1973

9. Auerbach O, Hammond EC, Garfinkel L: Smoking in relation to atherosclerosis of the coronary arteries. N Engl J Med 273:775, 1965

10. Viel B, Donoso S, Salcedo D: Coronary atherosclerosis in persons dying violently. Arch Intern Med 122:97, 1968

11. Kannel WB, Dawler TR, Slanner JJ et al: Epidemiological aspects of intermittent claudication: the Framingham Study. Circulation 31–32 (Suppl II):121, 1967

12. Thomas CS, Cohen BH: The familial occurrence of hypertension and coronary artery disease with observations concerning obesity and diabetes. Ann Intern Med 42:A55, 1970

13. Erdheim J: Medionecrosis aortae idiopathica. Virchows Archiv [Pathol Anat] 273:454, 1929

14. Erdheim J: Medionecrosis aortae idiopathica cystica. Virchows Archiv [Pathol Anat] 276:187, 1930

15. Hirst AE, Gore I: Is cystic medionecrosis the cause of dissecting aortic aneurysm? Circulation 53:915–916, 1976

16. Gore I, Seiwert VJ: Dissection aneurysm of the aorta. Pathologic aspects. An analysis of 85 fatal cases. Arch Pathol Lab Med 53:121, 1952

17. Cutler BS, Wheeler HB, Paraskos JA et al: Assessment of operative risk with electrocardiographic exercise testing in patients with peripheral vascular disease. Am J Surg 137:484, 1979

PATIENT PRESENTATION AND ASSOCIATED DISEASES

18. Anagnostopoulos CE, Prabhaker MJS, Kittle CF: Aortic dissections and dissecting aneurysms. Am J Cardiol 30:263, 1972

19. Hirst AE, Jr, Johns VJ, Kime SW: Dissecting aneurysm of the aorta. A review of 505 cases. Medicine 37:217, 1958

ANESTHESIA FOR THORACIC AORTIC SURGERY

20. Warren WD, Beckwith J, Muller WH Jr: Problems in surgical management of acute dissecting aneurysm of aorta. Ann Surg 144:530, 1956

21. Hume DM, Porter RR: Acute dissecting aortic aneurysms. Surgery 53:122, 1963

22. Wheat MW, Jr, Palmer RF, Bartley TD et al: Treatment of dissecting aneurysm of the aorta without surgery. J Thorac Cardiovasc Surg 50:364–373, 1965

23. Hirst AE, Jr, Johns VJ Jr: Experimental dissection of media of aorta by pressure: its relation to spontaneous dissecting aneurysm. Circ Res 10:897, 1962

24. Wheat MW, Jr, Palmer RF: Dissecting aneurysms of the aorta: present status of drug vs. surgical therapy. Prog Cardiovasc Dis 11:198–210, 1968

25. Prokop EK, Palmer RD, Wheat MW, Jr: Hydrodynamic forces in dissecting aneurysms. Circ Res 27:121–127, 1970

26. Simpson CF, Kling JM, Palmer RD: Beta-aminoproprionitril induced dissecting aneurysm of turkey: Treatment with propranolol. Toxicol Appl Pharmacol 16:143–153, 1970

27. Ringer RK (ed): Influence of reserpine and early growth, blood pressure and dissecting aneurysms in turkeys. Conference on the Use of Serpasil in Animal and Poultry Production. May 7, 1959, Rutgers University, New Brunswick, NJ, CIBA, Summit, NJ, pp 21–28.

28. Harris PD, Bowman FO, Jr, Malm MR: The management of acute dissections of the thoracic aorta. Am Heart J 78:419, 1969

29. Wheat MW, Jr, Harris PD, Malm MR et al: Acute dissecting aneurysm of the aorta. J Thorac Cardiovasc Surg 58:344, 1969

30. Palmer RF, Lasseter KC: Nitroprusside and aortic dissecting aneurysm. Correspondence, N Engl J Med 294:1403–1404, 1976

31. Cohn JN: Letter to the Editor. Nitroprusside and dissecting aneurysm of aorta (continued). N Engl J Med 295:567, 1976

32. Pool–Wilson PA, Lewis G, Angerpourter T et al: Haemodynamic effects of salbutamol and nitroprusside after cardiac surgery. Br Heart J 39:721, 1977

33. McFarland J, Willerson JT, Dinsmore RE et al: The medical tratment of dissecting aortic aneurysms. N Engl J Med 286:115–119, 1972

34. Wolfe WG, Moran JF: The evolution of medical and surgical management of acute aortic dissection. Circulation 56:503–505, 1977

35. Anagnostopoulos CE, Athanasuleas CL, Garrick TR et al: Acute Aortic Dissections. Baltimore, University Park Press, 1975

36. Wheat MW, Jr: Treatment of dissecting aneurysms of the aorta. Ann Thorac Surg 12:582, 1971

37. Appelbaum A, Karp RB, Kirklin JW: Ascending vs. descending aortic dissections. Ann Surg 183:296, 1976

38. Kidd JN, Reul GJ, Jr, Cooley DA, et al: Surgical treatment of aneurysms of the ascending aorta. Circulation 54 (Suppl II-111):118–122, 1976

39. King BD, Harris LC, Greifenstein FE et al: Reflex circulatory responses to direct laryngoscopy and tracheal intubation performed under general anesthesia. Anaesthesia 12:556, 1951

40. Prys–Roberts C, Greene LT, Medoche R: Studies in anesthesia in relation to hypertension: II. Hemodynamic consequences of induction and endotracheal intubation. Br J Anaesth 43:531, 1971

41. Prys–Roberts C, Foëx P, Biro GP: Studies in anaesthesia in relation to hypertension. V. Adrenergic β-receptor blockade. Br J Anaesth 45:671, 1973

42. Foëx P, Prys–Roberts C: Anaesthesia and the hypertensive patient. Br J Anaesth 46:575, 1974

43. Denlinger JK, Messner JT, D'Orazio DJ et al: Effect of intravenous lidocaine on the circulatory response to tracheal intubation. Anesthesiology Review 3:13, 1976

44. Fox EJ, Sklar GS, Hill CH et al: Complications related to the pressor response to endotracheal intubation. Anesthesiology 47:524, 1977

45. Sellick DA: Cricoid pressure to control regurgitation of stomach contents during induction of anesthesia. Lancet 2:404, 1961

46. Froese AB, Bryan AC: Effects of anesthesia and paralysis on diaphragmatic mechanics in man. Anesthesiology 41:242, 1974

47. Hill AB, Sykes MK, Reyes A: A hypoxic pulmonary vasoconstrictor response in dogs during and after infusion of sodium nitroprusside. Anesthesiology 50:484, 1979

48. Fischbach DP, Fogdall RP: Coagulation: The Essentials. Baltimore, Williams & Wilkins, 1981

49. Kopman EA, Ferguson TB: Intraoperative monitoring of femoral artery pressure during replacement of aneurysm or descending thoracic aorta. Anesth Analg (Cleve) 561:603, 1977

50. Sabawala PB, Strong MJ, Keats AS: Surgery on the aorta and its branches. Anesthesiology 33:229, 1970

51. Chaux A, Bussell JA, Matloff JM et al: Hemodynamic effects of the TDMAC-heparin shunt during descending thoracic aortic surgery. J Thorac Cardiovasc Surg (in press)

52. Crawford ES, Fenstermacher M, Richardson W et al: Reappraisal of adjuncts to avoid ischemia in the treatment of thoracic aortic aneurysms. Surgery 67:182, 1970

53. Hug HR, Taber RE: Bypass flow requirements during thoracic aneurysmectomy with particular attention to prevention of the left heart failure. J Thorac Cardiovasc Surg 57:203, 1969

54. Connors JP, Ferguson TB, Roper CL et al: The use of the TDMAC-heparin shunt in replacement of the descending thoracic aorta. Ann Surg 181:735, 1975

ANESTHESIA FOR AORTIC ARCH REPLACEMENT

55. Shennan T: Dissecting aneurysms. Medical Research Council Special Report Serial 193, p 138. London, HMSO 1934

56. DeBakey ME, Henly WS, Cooley DA et al: Aneurysms of the aortic arch. Factors influencing operative risk. Surg Clin North Am 42:1543, 1962

57. Griepp RB, Stinson EB, Hollingsworth JF et al: Prosthetic replacement of the aortic arch. J Thorac Cardiovasc Surg 70:1051, 1975

58. Boyan CP: Cold or warmed blood for massive transfusion. Ann Surg 160,282, 1964

59. Swan H: Clinical hypothermia: a lady with a past and some promise for the future. Surgery 73:736, 1973

60. Waddell WG, Fairley HB, Bigelow WG: Improved management of clinical hypothermia based upon related biochemical studies. Ann Surg 146:542, 1957

ANESTHESIA FOR ABDOMINAL AORTIC SURGERY

61. Darling RC: Ruptured arteriosclerotic abdominal aortic aneurysms. A pathologic and clinical study. Am J Surg 119:397, 1970

62. Darling RC, Messina CR, Brewster DC et al: Autopsy study of unoperated abdominal aortic aneurysms: the case for early resection. Circulation 56:II:161, 1977

63. Brewster DC, Buth J, Darling RC et al: Com-

bined aortic and renal artery reconstruction. Am J Surg 131:457, 1976

64. Volpetti G, Barker CF, Berkowitz H et al: A 22 year review of elective resection of abdominal aortic aneurysms. Surg Gynecol Obstet 142:321, 1976

65. van Heeckeren DW: Ruptured abdominal aortic aneurysms. Am J Surg 119:402, 1970

66. Couch NP, Lane FC, Crane C: Management and mortality in resection of abdominal aortic aneurysms. A study of 114 cases. Am J Surg 119:408, 1970

67. Attia RR, Murphy JD, Snider MT et al: Myocardial ischemia due to infrarenal aortic cross-clamping during aortic surgery in patients with severe coronary artery disease. Circulation 53:961, 964, 1976

ANESTHESIA FOR EXTREMITY VASCULAR SURGERY

68. Sabawala PB, Strong MJ, Keats AS: Surgery on the aorta and its branches. Anesthesiology 33:229, 1970

69. Folser R, Mack RM, Cantrell JR: Alterations in femoral blood flow and resistance following sympathetic blockade. Ann Surg 162:873, 1965

70. Bromage PR: Epidural anesthesia: indications, contraindications and complications. American Society of Anesthesiologists. Annual Refresher Course Lectures, 1977

71. Bromage PR: Personal communication.

RELATED TOPICS OF SPECIAL CONCERN

Autotransfusion

72. Brener BJ, Raines JK, Darling RC: Intraoperative autotransfusion in abdominal aortic resections. Arch Surg 107:78–84, 1973

73. Raines JK, Buth J, Brewster DC et al: Intraoperative autotransfusion: Equipment, protocols and guidelines. J Trauma 16:616–623, 1976

G-Suit

74. Crile GW: Blood Pressure in Surgery: an Experimental and Clinical Research, p 228. Philadelphia, JB Lippincott Co, 1903

75. Ludewig RM, Wangensteen SL: Aortic bleeding and the effect of external counterpressure. Surg Gynecol Obstet 128:252, 1969

76. Wangensteen SL, Ludewig RM, Eddy DM: Effects of external counterpressure on the intact circulation. Surg Gynecol Obstet 127:253, 1968

Management of Renal Function during Major Vascular Surgery

77. Couch NP, Lane FC, Crane C: Management and mortality in resection of abdominal aortic aneurysms: a study of 114 cases. Am J Surg 119:408, 1970

78. Luft FC, Hamburger RJ, Dyer JK et al: Acute renal failure following operation for aortic aneurysm. Surg Gynecol Obstet 141:374, 1975

79. Tilney NL, Bailey GL, Morgan AD: Sequential system failure after rupture of abdominal aortic aneurysms. Ann Surg 178:117, 1972

80. Chawla CK, Najafi H, Ing TS et al: Acute renal failure complicating ruptured abdominal aortic aneurysm. Arch Surg 110:521, 1975

81. van Heeckeren DW: Ruptured abdominal aortic aneurysms. Am J Surg 119:402, 1970

82. Thompson JE, Hollier LH, Patman RD et al: Surgical management of abdominal aortic aneurysms. Ann Surg 181:654, 1975

83. Chedru M, Baethke R, Oken D: Renal cortical blood flow and glomerular filtration in myohemoglobinuric acute renal failure. Kidney Int 1:232, 1972

84. Hollenberg NK, Epstein M, Rosen SM et al: Acute oliguric renal failure in man: evidence for preferential renal cortical ischemia. Medicine 47:455, 1968

85. Ishikawa I, Hollenberg NK: Pharmacologic interruption of the renin-angiotensin system in myohemoglobinuric acute renal failure. Kidney Int 10:S-183, 1976

86. Reubi FC, Vorburger C, Tuckman J: Renal distribution volumes of indocyanine green (^{51}Cr) EDTA, and ^{24}Na in man during acute renal failure after shock. Implications for the pathogenesis of anuria. J Clin Invest 52:233, 1973

87. Flores J, Dibona DR, Beck CH et al: The role of cell swelling in ischemic renal damage and the protective effect of hypertonic solute. J Clin Invest 51:118, 1972

88. Mazze RI, Trudell JR, Cousins MJ: Methoxyflurane metabolism and renal dysfunction: Clinical correlation in man. Anesthesiology 35:247, 1971

89. Eichhorn JH, Hedley–Whyte J, Steinman TI et al: Renal failure following enflurane anesthesia. Anesthesiology 45:557, 1976

90. Larson CP Jr, Mazze RI, Cooperman LH et al: Effects of anesthetics on cerebral, renal, and splanchnic circulations. Anesthesiology 41:167, 1974

91. Deutsch S, Goldberg M, Stephen GW et al: Effects of halothane anesthesia on renal function in normal man. Anesthesiology 27:793, 1966

92. Barry KG, Coehn A, Knochel JP et al: Mannitol infusion II: The prevention of acute renal failure during resection of an aneurysm of the abdominal aorta. NEJM 264:967, 1961

93. Gagnon JA, Bolt DA, Clarke RW et al: Effect of lower aortic occlusion on renal function in dogs. Surgery 47:240, 1960

94. Thompson JE, Hollier LH, Patman RD et al: Surgical management of abdominal aortic aneurysms. Ann Surg 181:654, 1975

95. Stokes J, Butcher HR: Abdominal aortic aneurysms. Factors influencing operative mortality and criteria of operability. Arch Surg 107:297, 1973

96. Crawford ES, Fenstermacher JM, Richardson W et al: Reappraisal of adjuncts to avoid ischemia in the treatment of thoracic aortic aneurysms. Surgery 67:182, 1970

97. Lucas CE, Zito JG, Carter KM et al: Questionable value of furosemide in preventing renal failure. Surgery 82:314, 1977

98. Cantarovich F, Galli C, Benedetti L et al: High-dose furosemide in established acute renal failure. Br Med J 4:449, 1973

99. Shin B, Mackenzie CF, McAslan TC et al: Postoperative renal failure in trauma patients. Anesthesiology 51:218, 1979

23

Extracranial Carotid Artery Surgery

RONALD A. DRITZ

INTRODUCTION

Cerebral vascular disease accounts for approximately 10 percent of the total deaths within the United States.[1] Since the introduction of carotid endarterectomy in 1954, cerebrovascular insufficiency caused by lesions arising in the extracranial arterial system has been amenable to surgical intervention.[2] Symptomatic lesions usually are located at the junction of the internal and external carotid arteries and produce symptoms of cerebral ischemia either by reduction of flow because of arterial stenosis or by embolization of platelet thrombi from an ulcerative plaque (Fig. 23–1).

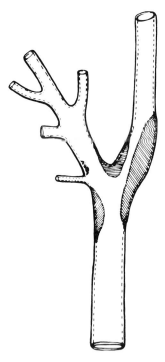

Fig. 23-1. Location of carotid lesions. The typical location of an atherosclerotic plaque at the bifurication of the common carotid artery, which may lead to reduction of cerebral blood flow or embolization. Major manifestations are an asymptomatic bruit, transient ischemic attacks (TIAs), or stroke (CVA). (Thompson JE, Talkington CM: Ann Surg 184:1, 1976)

PHYSIOLOGY OF THE CEREBRAL CIRCULATION

A thorough, working knowledge of the physiology of cerebral blood flow and the effect of anesthetic drugs on those parameters is the foundation of modern anesthetic care of patients with cerebrovascular occlusive disease.

The brain can withstand relatively large decreases in the cross-sectional area of the carotid artery without symptoms of cerebral ischemia.[3] Cerebral blood flow is substantially maintained, even in the presence of a complete unilateral carotid occlusion because of two main mechanisms:[4] a rich collateral vascular network and the ability of the local cerebral vasculature to vasodilate.

COLLATERAL FLOW

Collateral flow within the cerebral arterial system can compensate for decreased carotid blood flow. The major collateral conduits are the following:

1. Circle of Willis. This is by far the most important source of collateral blood flow in carotid arterial disease. Normally there is no crossover flow within the circle of Willis, but in the presence of decreased flow in the carotid system, crossover flow through the communicating arteries occurs to divert blood towards the jeopardized region (Fig. 23–2). Fifty percent of the population has no posterior communicating artery in the circle of Willis,[5] severely restricting the ability to compensate for decreases in carotid blood flow, and thereby enhancing the likelihood of stroke.
2. Vertebral arteries. The vertebrals act as collateral vessels through their contribution of blood flow through the circle of Willis.
3. External to internal carotid artery through superficial temporal and ophthalmic arteries. It is measurement of the extent to which this collateral pathway is partici-

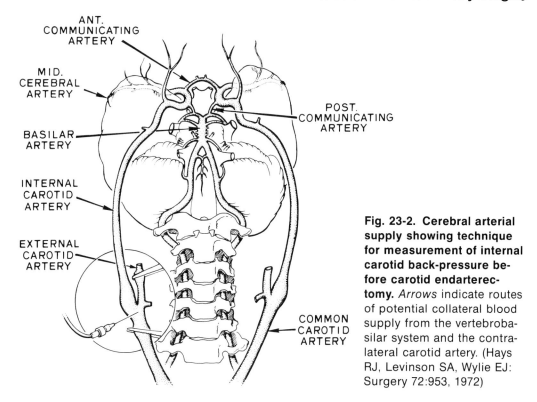

ANT.
COMMUNICATING
ARTERY

MID.
CEREBRAL
ARTERY

POST.
COMMUNICATING
ARTERY

BASILAR
ARTERY

INTERNAL
CAROTID
ARTERY

EXTERNAL
CAROTID
ARTERY

COMMON
CAROTID
ARTERY

Fig. 23-2. Cerebral arterial supply showing technique for measurement of internal carotid back-pressure before carotid endarterectomy. *Arrows* indicate routes of potential collateral blood supply from the vertebrobasilar system and the contralateral carotid artery. (Hays RJ, Levinson SA, Wylie EJ: Surgery 72:953, 1972)

pating that forms the basis of the Doppler ophthalmic test.

4. External carotid to vertebral artery through the occipital artery.

VARIABLES AFFECTING LOCAL CEREBRAL BLOOD FLOW

Metabolic Factors

Although global blood flow to the brain is maintained relatively constant at about 50 ml/100 g of brain tissue, regional blood flow is subject to considerable alteration. Changes in regional cerebral blood flow are coupled to the level of metabolic activity in the area of brain.[6] In areas of increased metabolic activity, regional cerebral blood flow (rCBF) is augmented. Because the venous oxygen content *increases* at sites with enhanced metabolic activity, some mechanism other than hypoxia may be responsible for the coupling of metabolic activity to flow. Changes in H^+ and K^+

concentration in the extracellular fluid surrounding the brain arterioles are possible mediators.[7]

Arterial Carbon Dioxide Tension (PaCO$_2$)

Changes in $PaCO_2$ strongly affect cerebral blood flow (CBF). Within a relatively wide range of $PaCO_2$ (20–60 torr), CBF changes linearly, at a rate of 1 ml/100 g for each 1 torr change in $PaCO_2$.[8] Carbon dioxide affects arteriolar smooth muscle tone by altering cerebrospinal fluid pH (Fig. 23–3).[9]

Arterial Oxygen Tension (PaO$_2$)

CBF is insensitive to changes in oxygen tension until arterial PO_2 falls below 50 torr. At this level, hypoxic metabolism in brain tissue results in lactic acidosis. This would then result in a decrease of periarteriolar pH and vasodilatation (see Fig. 23–3).[7]

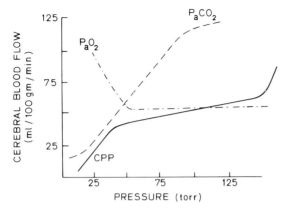

Fig. 23-3. Cerebral blood flow changes as a result of alterations in PaCO$_2$ (---), PaO$_2$ (–·–) and cerebral perfusion pressure (CPP) (—). CPP equals mean arterial blood pressure minus central venous or intracranial pressure. In patients with chronic hypertension, the autoregulation (CPP) curve is shifted to the right. (Modified from Shapiro HM: ASA Refresher Course Lectures, Number 11, 1976)

Cerebral Perfusion Pressure (CPP)*

CBF is kept constant over a wide range of CPPs by a direct vascular response of the brain arterioles known as *autoregulation*. This response is not mediated by the autonomic nervous system but instead appears to be a direct response of the arteriolar smooth muscle cells to the distending transmural pressure.[7] If CPP decreases, arterioles vasodilate, but if CPP increases, arterioles vasoconstrict, thus maintaining CBF relatively constant. In normal human, maximal vasodilation is achieved at a CPP of approximately 55 torr. Below this level, no further vasodilatation is possible and CBF decreases in a pressure-dependent fashion (see Fig. 23–3). There is an *upper limit* of autoregulation at a CPP of about 130 torr. Above this level, the pressure head will break through the vasoconstrictor response and may result in multifocal ruptures of the blood-brain barrier with edema for-

mation. This is the pathogenesis of hypertensive encephalopathy seen in malignant hypertension.[10]

In patients with *chronic* hypertension, the vessel walls adapt through hypertrophy and the autoregulation curve is shifted to the right.[7] These patients will thereby be better able to withstand high CPP. More importantly however, they will withstand low CPP *less* well with symptoms of cerebral ischemia developing at higher CPPs than normotensive persons. Thus the hypertensive patient is at *increased risk of cerebral ischemia* should blood pressure decrease.

Cerebral Ischemia and the Luxury Perfusion Syndrome

In patients with cerebral ischemia, a situation in which perfusion is inadequate to supply the metabolic demands of brain cells, there is an intense local production of lactic acid. This is a potent stimulus to local arteriolar vasodilation. Called the *luxury perfusion syndrome*,[11] this response causes shunting of blood into the ischemic area inducing a relative hyperemia.

Factors affecting vascular tone in areas of the brain *not* suffering ischemia may govern the extent of the increased perfusion in the ischemic region. If relative vasodilatation is induced in areas of nonischemic brain by hypercarbia, more blood will be shunted into this region and away from the acidic brain tissue where further vasodilatation is not possible, the so called *intracerebral steal*.[12] Conversely, stimuli inducing a vasoconstrictor response in normal brain (*i.e.*, hypocarbia) may shunt blood *into* the ischemic zone, the inverse intracerebral steal or *Robin Hood syndrome*, though clinical evidence for this phenomenon is incomplete.[13]

EFFECT OF ANESTHETIC AGENTS ON CEREBRAL BLOOD FLOW

Anesthetic agents can affect CBF through their ability to alter vascular tone of intracranial vessels. These effects can be direct (*i.e.*, alteration of perivascular hydrogen ion

---

*CPP equals mean arterial pressure (MAP) minus central venous (CVP) or intracranial pressure (ICP), whichever is *higher*. In cases where CVP and ICP are normal, the CPP is approximated by MAP. When CVP or ICP is high it will oppose the flow of arterial blood to the brain.

concentration) or indirect (*i.e.*, alteration in brain metabolic rate and compensatory reduction in flow). Specific information concerning the mechanism of action of a drug or combination of drugs in the clinical setting is not always available.

Volatile anesthetic agents cause a dose-related cerebrovascular dilatation manifested by a progressive loss of autoregulation (Fig. 23–4). As the inspired concentration of a volatile anesthetic agent is increased, cerebral blood flow progressively increases even though cerebral perfusion pressure is kept constant.[14] With high concentrations of volatile anesthetics, cerebral vasculature is maximally vasodilated making cerebral blood flow totally pressure dependent, a situation analogous to extreme hypercapnia. Two potential disadvantages could result under these conditions which would potentiate cerebral ischemia. First, cerebral vasodilatation would act as an intracranial steal, as previously discussed. Secondly, at high cerebral perfusion pressures, cerebral edema formation in injured areas would be enhanced.[15]

Intravenous agents affect CBF as sumarized in Table 23–1. Of particular importance is ketamine, which through its cerebral vasodilatory action could potentiate ischemia by intracranial steal, and thiopental, which as a potent vasoconstrictor can shunt blood towards ischemic regions. Thiopental will also reduce cerebral edema which can accompany acute ischemia. Because it is also a potent depressor of cerebral metabolic rate, it may also be beneficial by prolonging the brain's ability to withstand an ischemic insult (see section below on treatment of cerebral ischemia).

EFFECT OF VASOACTIVE AGENTS ON CEREBRAL BLOOD FLOW

The effect on vasoactive agents is summarized in Table 23–2. Both norepinephrine and metaraminol are mild cerebral vasoconstrictors in normotensive humans. Thus, if these drugs are used to treat intraoperative hypo-

tension, blood pressure must be raised to slightly supranormal levels to maintain normal CBF.[13] Mephentermine is a potentially poor choice for systemic blood pressure support in patients with potential cerebral ischemia because it increases cerebral oxygen consumption (CMR_{O_2}) without a compensatory increase in CBF (see Table 23–2). Angi-

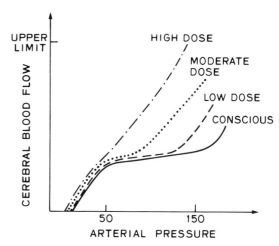

Fig. 23-4. Cerebral blood flow autoregulation. Schematic representation of the effect of a progressively increased dose of a typical anesthetic agent on CBF autoregulation. Both the upper and lower thresholds are shifted to the right. (Shapiro HM: ASA Refresher Course Lectures number 11, 1976)

Table 23-1. Effect of Anesthetic Agents on Cerebral Blood Flow and Metabolism

DRUG	CBF	CMR_{O_2}
Inhalational		
Volatile	+ + +	+ + +
Nitrous Oxide	0 +	±
Intravenous		
Ketamine	+ + +	+ +
Fentanyl	– –	–
Droperidol	– –	– –
Diazepam	– –	–
Thiopental	– – –	– – –

+ increase, – decrease; suspected relative potency for effect indicated, although direct comparative data in humans are not complete
(Shapiro HM: ASA Refresher Course Lectures, no. 11, 1976)

Table 23-2. Effect of Vasoactive Agents on CBF and Cerebral Oxygen Consumption (CMR$_{O_2}$)*

	CBF	CMR$_{O_2}$
Epinephrine	0 (+)†	0 (+)†
Norepinephrine	(mild)	0
Metaraminol	− (mild)	0
Mephentermine	0	+
Angiotensin	0	0
Phenylephrine	0	0

*At doses which do not affect systemic arterial pressure
†At higher doses (36.9 g/min)
(Modified from Smith AL: Anesthesiology 36:378, 1972)

otensin and phenylephrine would appear the most attractive agents to treat hypotension.

Sodium nitroprusside is a direct-acting, potent, cerebral vasodilator. Cerebral autoregulation is blunted in a dose-dependent fashion in the same manner as discussed with volatile anesthetic agents.[16]

PATIENT PRESENTATION

Carotid thromboendarterectomy can be considered in patients with any of three findings.

TRANSIENT CEREBRAL ISCHEMIC ATTACKS (TIAs)

TIAs are defined as "nonconvulsive, reversible focal neurologic deficits lasting minutes to several hours and presumably related to cerebral ischemia."[17]

Risk of a completed stroke within 1 year of the onset of TIAs is 4 to 10 percent.[17] In a group of 82 patients with TIAs followed for 40 months, 42 (51%) developed strokes, of which 12 died, 4 were totally disabled, 7 were left with moderate disability, and 19 made a complete recovery.[18]

TIAs involving the areas perfused by the carotid artery present in two ways:

1. Transient monocular blindness (TMB; amaurosis fugax). This is the onset of a gray or black shade obscuring the vision of one eye for 1 to 30 minutes. Of 32 patients with TMB, 19 (60%) had tight (≤ ?

mm) stenosis of the internal carotid artery at angiography.[19]
2. Transient hemispheric attacks (THAs). Symptoms of THAs can include any or all of the following: speech disturbances, numbness or weakness of the face, arm, hand, fingers or leg. Of 52 patients with THAs, 23 (44%) had a tight carotid lesion.[19]

TMB and THAs appear not to occur at the same time although both can occur at different times in the same patient. Of ten patients who had both TMB and THAs, at different times, eight (80%) had tight carotid stenosis.[19]

Patients with TIAs should have angiography of the carotid and cerebral arterial system. Those with tight stenosis or evidence of ulceration of an atheroma should have carotid endarterectomy.[17]

CEREBRAL VASCULAR ACCIDENTS (CVA): STROKE

Stroke is usually defined as a fixed focal neurologic deficit. "It has become quite evident that carotid endarterectomy is inappropriate in the treatment for an acute stroke or for relief of a fixed or evolving neurologic deficit."[20]

ASYMPTOMATIC BRUITS

The appropriate treatment of patients presenting with asymptomatic carotid bruits is an extremely controversial subject. As with most such areas of heated medical debate, differences arise because of lack of sufficient data for any one view. Based on the best available studies,[20, 21] it seems clear that this is a group of patients who are at increased risk of developing a stroke, though to what extent is not clear.[21, 22] A carefully done study has shown that in *male* patients suffering *TIAs*, the incidence of TIAs, stroke, and death was reduced by a regimen of 325 mg aspirin taken four times a day. No such benefit was found among female patients, and the stroke rate among treated male patients was still greater than among patients subjected to carotid endarterectomy.[23] This study has formed the basis for medical therapy among patients with TIAs who have either no carotid lesion or one not accessible to surgery. Furthermore, it also forms the basis for conservative *medical therapy* of patients with *asymptomatic* carotid bruits.

At present there is no prospective randomized study of best medical versus best surgical therapy among patients with asymptomatic carotid bruits. Treatment therefore ranges from "do nothing" to carotid endarterectomy. Until the appropriate studies are undertaken the confused situation will continue.

ANESTHETIC PLANNING

Once the decision is reached to undertake carotid endarterectomy, proper anesthetic management can reduce mortality and morbidity.[24] Emphasis in preoperative evaluation of these patients should center on the following areas:

Check the blood pressure in *both* arms. All patients having this type of surgery require meticulous care in blood pressure management, care that can only be provided with an intraarterial line in place. The atherosclerotic process often extends into the subclavian or innominate arteries, therefore blood pressure may be lower in one arm. Use of this arm for blood pressure determination can lead to improper management and complications. Allen's test should be done on the radial artery chosen before cannulation.

A thorough history concerning heart disease and evaluation of the ECG are a must. These patients have a high incidence of hemodynamically significant coronary artery disease.[24] Perioperative *mortality* caused by coronary artery disease is around 1 percent in a large series.[25] Fifty-two percent of all patients who died in the follow-up period died of cardiac disease.[25] Hypertension is found among almost half of these patients.[25, 26] Antihypertensive medications should be continued until the morning of surgery.[27]

EVALUATION OF THE CAROTID LESION

Never palpate the neck! Emboli can be dislodged and strokes induced!

During the operation the patient will be positioned with his head turned to the contralateral side with the neck in moderate hyperextension. This position can cause flow reduction in the vertebral arteries, and may thereby decrease an important source of collateral blood flow. Part of the preoperative evaluation should be to have the patient lie in the operative position for a minute while checking for any symptoms of cerebral ischemia.

Check the carotid arteriogram; it is important to evaluate collateral blood flow. Is there contralateral carotid occlusion? Is the circle of Willis patent? These findings may have important implications during carotid cross-clamping because in such patients collateral blood flow may be especially poor.[28]

PREOPERATIVE MEDICATION

Premedication should be light. A mild sedative-hypnotic drug or no premedication at all, when combined with a careful and thoughtful preoperative visit, should present a calm patient in the operating room. Heavy doses of premedication (including scopolamine) can mask or confuse symptoms of cerebral ischemia in the preinduction period. All anticoagulants should be discontinued and clotting studies shown to be normal before surgery.

OPERATIVE MANAGEMENT

Armed with this information, one would think that a certain uniformity might exist in anesthetic technique. Yet there appear to be almost as many different anesthetic techniques as there are anesthesiologists.[29] From among this seeming chaos there does appear consensus on certain points. Rather than attempt to devise the perfect anesthetic in these pages, I will try to correlate available data and present the major trends in the anesthetic approach to carotid endarterectomy as practiced in major centers where this surgery is undertaken on a large scale.

MONITORING

Careful monitoring of arterial blood pressure and the ECG is a must. Intraarterial catheter placement for monitoring of systemic blood pressure is now routine practice. Mild induced hypertension is increasingly used to protect the brain during initial dissection and carotid cross-clamping (see below).

This patient group is particularly at risk for intraoperative myocardial ischemia. V_5 lead or MCL monitoring are more sensitive in detection of left ventricular ischemia than standard limb leads and should be employed.

ANESTHETIC INDUCTION

On arrival in the operating room, a brief neurologic examination should be performed. After placement of intravenous and intraarterial catheters under local anesthesia, general anesthesia is induced with thiopental, the trachea intubated after neuromuscular blockade, and ventilation controlled. Anesthesia is maintained with 65 percent nitrous oxide and 35 percent oxygen, supplemented with light levels of an inhalational agent (0.5 MAC) or intravenous narcotic. Arterial PCO$_2$ is usually maintained between 35 and 40 torr and checked by means of blood gas determination. After initial surgical dissection and exposure of the carotid artery, an intravenous dose of heparin is administered and a cross-clamp placed on the artery proximal to the lesion.

ASSESSMENT OF CEREBRAL BLOOD FLOW

The area of brain normally perfused by the artery must now rely totally on collateral circulation for metabolic needs. Some method *must* be employed to assess whether collateral flow is sufficient to proceed with the operation. Several alternatives have been suggested.

Regional anesthesia and the conscious patient

Before other means became available routinely to judge regional cerebral perfusion, the procedure was performed under regional anesthesia with the patient awake. The patient's own level of consciousness served as a measure of adequacy of perfusion. Though some surgeons still use this technique routinely, most centers have abandoned the practice. The major disadvantages are the following.

1. A shunt may need to be placed quickly and under stress in a patient exhibiting seizure activity.
2. Airway management under surgical drapes in a patient having a transient (hopefully) ischemic attack or seizure is woefully inadequate.
3. Some measures which might offer protection against cerebral ischemia (see below), such as alterations in PaCO$_2$, use of barbiturates, or inhalational anesthetics, cannot be employed.

Measurement of regional cerebral blood flow by scintillation counting

This technique involves intracarotid injection of radioactive ^{133}Xe and detection of radioactivity by multiple external scintillation counters located adjacent to the affected cerebral hemisphere.[30] [32] rCBF is calculated from the radioactive decay curve. Normal CBF is approximately 50 ml/100 g brain/min, though CBF is nonuniform and can vary widely between different areas of the brain.[29] The question is, what is the lower limit of safety? Generalization is difficult because alteration of physiologic parameters (PaCO$_2$, PaO$_2$, body temperature) alter the ischemic threshold. "Our present knowledge about the critical lower level of CBF may [be] thus summarized: in the normothermic, normocapnic or slightly hypocapnic halothane-N$_2$O anesthetized patient, the critical level is 18 ml/100 g·min."[33]

The apparatus is expensive and cumber-

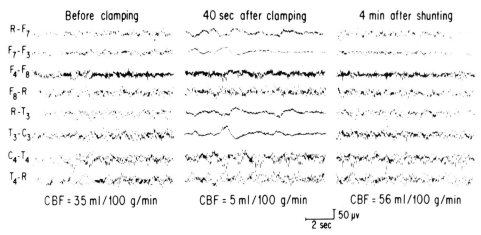

Before clamping	40 sec after clamping	4 min after shunting
$R-F_7$		
F_7-F_3		
F_4-F_8		
F_8-R		
$R-T_3$		
T_3-C_3		
C_4-T_4		
T_4-R		
CBF = 35 ml/100 g/min	CBF = 5 ml/100 g/min	CBF = 56 ml/100 g/min

50 μv
2 sec

Fig. 23-5. Electroencephalographic alterations with cerebral ischemia. *Left.* EEG recording before left carotid artery clamping (77-year-old woman) shows lower amplitude fast activity over left hemisphere. *Middle.* EEG recording 40 seconds after clamping shows major EEG changes on left side when the blood flow was reduced to 5 ml/100 g/min. *Right.* EEG recording, 4 minutes after internal shunting, has returned to baseline levels (R = midline electrode 4 cm below inion). (Sundt TM Jr, Sharbrough SW, Anderson RE et al: J Neurosurg 41:315, 1974)

some and therefore not suited for any but the most active centers undertaking this type of surgery. Its chief benefit is to provide data to correlate with other more easily employed methods.

Electroencephalographic monitoring (EEG)

Continuous monitoring of 8 or 16 lead EEG has been employed as the most reliable method of detecting ongoing cerebral ischemia.[34] Patients who show EEG changes consistent with cerebral ischemia usually have them reversed by placement of a shunt (Fig. 23–5). In one study, *no* patient with *reversible* EEG changes woke up with a new, fixed neurologic deficit, while one patient whose changes did not reverse had a new, fixed neurologic deficit.[35] EEG changes that mimic ischemia can be induced by changes in level of anesthesia or hypocapnia. This has been the basis of criticism for the technique[36] and the proviso that anesthetic level and $PaCO_2$ be maintained constant to make EEG interpretation more accurate.[35]

Because the equipment is cumbersome, and interpretation and running the machine require extra people in the operating room, it has not gained wide acceptance. Recently an EEG filter processor (EFP), a small, relatively inexpensive, and easy-to-operate piece of equipment has been introduced in an attempt to overcome the EEGs drawbacks. Initial results have proven promising,[37] but further experience will have to be gained before widespread use can be recommended.

Collateral cerebral blood pressure: stump pressure.

Measurement of the distal internal carotid artery blood pressure immediately after cross-clamping has been touted as an easy and reliable means of assessing cerebral perfusion (see Fig. 23–2).[38, 39] There has been considerable debate as to the lower limit of stump pressure, that is, the stump pressure below which regional cerebral ischemia can be expected to occur. Various proponents have advocated stump pressures of 25,[38] 50,[33, 39] and 60[36, 40] torr as the level below which a shunt should be placed. A recent study has shed some light on the topic in correlating measurement of regional CBF using the ^{133}Xe injection method (see above) with internal carotid artery stump pressure *and* type of anesthetic agent.[40] Figure 23–6 summarizes the data. First, there is tremendous scatter in the results. But what of the question of the safe lower limit for stump pressure? Seven patients who had stump pressures *greater* than 50 torr, had rCBF *less* than 18 ml/100 g brain/min (considered the level of cerebral ischemia). Four of the seven patients had EEG changes consistent with regional cerebral ischemia. When a stump pressure of 60 torr was used as the lower limit, three patients still had rCBF below 18 ml/100 g brain/min, but *none* of these patients had an EEG consistent with ischemia. Indeed no patient in the study (90 patients) with a stump pressure of 60 torr or greater had EEG evidence of ischemia.[40] Of the three anesthetic agents used, none was shown to be clearly safer with regard to cerebral ischemia. Based on these data, one could conclude that stump pressure greater than 60 torr ensured safety. This should not lull one into a sense of complete security. Patients have been reported with stump pressure as great as 90 torr associated with an EEG pattern demonstrating changes consistent with ischemia.[41]

Jugular Venous Oxygen Saturation

Some investigators postulated that cerebral ischemia could be detected by a decrease in mixed venous oxygen saturation aspirated from the jugular bulb. This has proven *not* to be the case. In five awake patients in whom loss of consciousness occurred after test clamping of the internal carotid artery, internal jugular venous oxygen saturation did not change.[42] Venous mixing is too great to detect *focal* areas of increased oxygen extraction which occur with regional cerebral ischemia. This method is unreliable and is not recommended.

As experience accumulates, it is clear that this operation should be performed with an operative mortality of less than 1 percent and a perioperative stroke incidence of less than 3 percent. It is therefore necessary to detect intraoperative cerebral ischemia with considerable sensitivity. The easiest method to estimate cerebral perfusion is the internal carotid artery stump pressure. When stump pressure is greater than 60 torr, signs consistent with cerebral ischemia on EEG analysis are rare, regardless of anesthetic agent used. A stump pressure of less than 60 torr may indicate cerebral ischemia, and some method to augment cerebral blood flow should be employed.

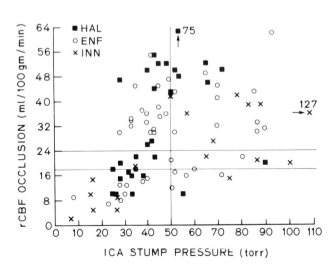

Fig. 23-6. Scattergram of occlusion regional cerebral blood flows (*rCBF*) plotted against internal carotid artery (*ICA*) stump presures. The *vertical line* represents a stump pressure of 50 torr (considered the critical level). The *two horizontal lines* represent the critical flow level (*rCBF* ≤ 18 ml/100 g/min) and the marginal zone (*rCBF* 18–24 ml/100 g/min). Regression lines for each anesthetic agent were calculated. Expressed for halothane, $rCBF_{occl} = 0.51$ (stump pressure) + 9.94; $r = 0.43$. Expressed for enflurane, $rCBF_{occl} = 0.26$ (stump pressure) + 16.51; $r = 0.39$. Expressed for Innovar, $rCBF_{occl} = 0.27$ (stump pressure) + 0.93; $r = 0.68$. (McKay RD: Anesthesiology: 45:393, 1976)

Some patients appear to be at particular risk of cerebral ischemia and additionally have particularly poor correlation between stump pressure and EEG ischemic changes. These patients appear to lack at least one communicating branch in the circle of Willis as visualized on preoperative angiography.[41] These patients should have some other method available to assess rCBF (^{133}Xe washout or EEG) or have shunts placed regardless of stump pressure.

TREATMENT OF CEREBRAL ISCHEMIA

Once cerebral ischemia is detected, treatment must involve either increasing cerebral blood flow to the ischemic area or decreasing cerebral oxygen consumption.

Methods Which Increase Cerebral Blood Flow (CBF)

Temporary Shunt Placement. Placement of a temporary in-lying shunt which bypasses both the carotid occlusion and the cross-clamp would seem a sound maneuver to avoid cerebral ischemia, and indeed some surgeons routinely shunt every patient. Others, however, argue against its routine use[43] because it interferes with the performance of the endarterectomy, particularly at the distal portion of the arteriotomy and can give rise to emboli (air, thrombus, or atherosclerotic material). Mortality or incidence of postoperative neurologic deficit gives no clear indication whether shunting or no shunting is preferable. Most surgeons employ a middle ground, using some method to assess cerebral perfusion, and then place a shunt if it seems indicated.

Induced Hypertension. Pharmacologic elevation of the systemic blood pressure has been advocated as a means of increasing blood flow to ischemic areas of the brain. Presumably, these areas would have lost autoregulatory ability in the arterioles and increased pressure would result in increased flow. Studies using both stump pressure or ^{133}Xe washout or both have tended to substantiate this impression.[44, 45] In instances in which stump pressure or rCBF was extremely low (<40 torr or <20 ml/100 g/min, respectively), induced hypertension was ineffective in raising these parameters to acceptable levels.[44] However, when stump pressure was only slightly depressed (41 to 50 torr), hypertension could increase stump pressure to acceptable levels and the operation could proceed without a shunt and without postoperative deficit.[39] Many anesthesiologists routinely increase arterial pressure by 15 to 20 percent during cross-clamping.[36, 47]

Induced Hypocapnia. A moderate level of hypocapnia ($PaCO_2 = 25$–35 torr) has been invoked in an attempt to shunt blood flow towards ischemic areas within the brain.[45]

The response to alteration of $PaCO_2$ in a given patient appears difficult to predict[29] and although stump pressure may increase in response to induced hypocapnia,[45] it is not clear whether this change indicates increased perfusion. The present consensus appears to be in favor of normocapnia or mild hypocapnia (30–35 torr) during operation and use of other means to enhance perfusion, if necessary.[29, 47]

Methods Which Decrease Cerebral Oxygen Consumption

Hypothermia. Hypothermia has long been thought of as a means of protecting living tissue against ischemia. Indeed, it was the method used to protect the brain during the first surgical attempt to reconstruct a carotid artery.[48] Despite the known ability of hypothermia to slow accumulation of anoxic metabolites in brain tissue,[29] enthusiasm for the technique was short-lived because of its complexity and because clinical outcome was no better than with other methods.[49] (See Chap. 26.)

General anesthesia. Some have argued that general anesthetics alone may serve to protect against cerebral ischemia in humans[50] and possibly protect the brain during hypotension.[29] Evidence for this speculation is incomplete and is certainly not the sole basis for choosing the technique.[47]

Barbiturates. Considerable interest has recently been focused on the use of barbiturates to protect against various forms of cerebral hypoxia.[51] Evidence showing protection against the effects of focal cerebral ischemia in animals forms the basis of enthusiasm for possible application in carotid endarterectomy. To summarize the animal data, animals (primates, dogs, cats) subjected to focal cerebral ischemia induced by cerebral artery ligation appeared to withstand the insult with smaller cerebral infarctions and less accumulation of ischemic metabolites when anesthetized with barbiturates than when anesthetized with other agents.[52, 53]

Total dose of barbiturates used in these studies was large (40 mg/kg) and clinical data to substantiate these findings in humans are unavailable. Because a thiopental loading dose may be relatively innocuous and because the animal data are so intriguing, some have recommended a 10 to 15 mg/kg dose during initial surgical dissection in carotid endarterectomy.[36] Clinical efficacy will have to await adequate human studies. Investigational drugs such as etomidate *may* provide cerebral protection; again, efficacy has yet to be proven.

If cerebral ischemia is suspected and the surgeon is strongly against the use of a shunt, induced hypertension is the next best alternative while maintaining careful surveillance for signs of *myocardial* ischemia. If this fails (*i.e.,* stump pressure still < 60 torr, EEG changes not reversed), hypocapnia to a $PaCO_2$ of 25 torr can be tried. Many would also argue for a 4 to 5 mg/kg infusion of thiopental.

CONCLUSION OF SURGERY

Once thromboendarterectomy is completed, the arterial incision is closed and the carotid cross-clamp removed. Protamine sulfate may be given intravenously at this time to reverse any residual heparin effect. Some surgeons prefer not to administer protamine sulfate if possible hoping to avoid sudden clot formation in the newly sutured vessel.

As the wound is being closed, the level of anesthesia should be lightened. Careful neurologic evaluation is critical in the early postoperative period and is hampered by residual anesthesia.

It is very important that neuromuscular blockade be antagonized and the patient's trachea be extubated at the conclusion of the procedure if at all possible. Neurologic assessment is more difficult in the intubated patient. The patient cannot respond verbally to questions and may have some degree of residual neuromuscular blockade, making neurologic testing uninterpretable. In the patient with severe pulmonary disease, a period of postoperative mechanical ventilation may be unavoidable.

POSTOPERATIVE CONCERNS

NEUROLOGIC

As just stressed, early reliable neurologic assessment of the patient in the recovery room is very important. A new neurologic deficit referable to the cerebral hemisphere at risk may signal the presence of an intimal flap, partially occluding carotid blood flow, or platelet aggregation in the arterial lumen. In either case, emergency carotid angiography and reexploration may reverse the cerebral ischemia and avoid a permanent deficit.

CARDIOVASCULAR

Patients undergoing carotid thromboendarterectomy are at risk for myocardial ischemia unless proven otherwise. Care to avoid insults which provoke myocardial ischemia must be continued in the recovery room. Electrocardiographic and intraarterial blood pressure monitoring should be continued.

An occasional patient may exhibit a syndrome of severe arterial hypotension in the early postoperative period requiring pharmacologic blood pressure support for several days. This is thought to occur when a plaque has formed over the carotid sinus. The carotid sinus is thus shielded from normal arterial distending pressures. When the operation is performed and the plaque removed, the carotid sinus is suddenly exposed to normal blood pressure, which it interprets as hypertension and begins firing at a rapid rate, thus eliciting profound vasodilation. Both norepinephrine and phenylephrine infusions have been successfully used to counteract the syndrome for the 2 or 3 days required for the carotid sinus to reset.

RESPIRATORY

The Upper Airway

The trachea is directly adjacent to the operative field. Bleeding from the arterial suture line can form a hematoma that can externally compress the upper airway. This complication can be recognized more easily if a *small* dressing is placed over the incision. A large compressive dressing will not hinder the hematoma formation but only hide it. In some patients, a hematoma may compress the trachea without external signs. Frequent checks of the dressing, neck, and upper airway are essential.

Carotid Body Function

In patients who have undergone bilateral carotid endarterectomy or unilateral endarterectomy with a contralateral carotid artery occlusion, there is a strong likelihood of bilateral carotid body denervation. This results in permanent loss of hypoxic ventilatory drive and 15 percent blunting of the respiratory response to CO_2. Resting $PaCO_2$ increases about 6 torr.[54] Four of seven patients studied by Wade and coworkers also had loss of the circulatory response to hypoxia.[54] Blood pressure increased in response to hypoxia preoperatively and decreased postoperatively. This is extremely important in patients with severe chronic respiratory disease, CO_2 retention, and hypoxic ventilatory drive.

Patients at risk for bilateral carotid body denervation should be warned to take supplemental oxygen if they go to high altitudes or contemplate airplane travel.

COMBINED CORONARY AND CAROTID ARTERIAL DISEASE

Because of the widespread nature of the atherosclerotic process, it is not surprising that patients will present with significant disease in both the coronary and carotid arteries. Of 874 consecutive candidates for coronary artery surgery, 49 (5.6%) had extracranial carotid lesions.[55] The best surgical approach to these patients is the subject of considerable debate. Bernhard[56] presented a group of such patients in which mortality was 33 percent when carotid surgery preceded coronary artery surgery. These patients died in the postoperative period before coronary artery bypass could be undertaken. When both procedures were done at the same sitting there was no mortality and no permanent neurologic deficit among 16 patients.[56] These results are cited by those favoring the simultaneous approach.[57, 58] Others did not find the same high mortality when the procedures were staged (carotid then coronary). Of 59 patients, operative mortality was 1.7 percent. Simultaneous surgery was reserved only for patients where both lesions were considered critical. Among this high-risk group, mortality was 4.4 percent.[59]

Patients with bilateral carotid disease appear to tolerate cardiopulmonary bypass poorly.[55] Of six patients with bilateral carotid disease in whom there was contralateral carotid artery occlusion and who underwent unilateral carotid endarterectomy and coronary artery bypass as the same sitting, five (83%) suffered neurologic deficit referable to the unoperated cerebral hemisphere.

At present, there is no clear choice in staged versus combined procedures. With skilled anesthetic management and postoperative care, patients can undergo staged procedures (carotid then coronary) with acceptable morbidity and mortality and *maybe* have a decreased incidence of neurologic deficit attendant with the combined procedure. Patients with bilateral carotid disease should probably have *staged* procedures.

ANESTHETIC CONCERNS

Anesthesia performed upon these patients is a challenge. While there is nothing unique in the management of these patients as opposed to those with isolated coronary or carotid artery disease, both lesions must be treated. Hypotension can be disastrous to *both* heart and brain. Hypertension may damage the heart.

Criteria for adequate cerebral perfusion during carotid artery cross-clamping remain the same. Some surgeons favor institution of cardiopulmonary bypass before carotid endarterectomy when combined surgery (carotid then coronary) is contemplated, with hypothermia to provide added protection against cerebral ischemia.[58]

If these patients can undergo surgery without morbidity and mortality, they appear to enjoy the possibility of increased life expectancy.[55] Such a result is not only gratifying to all involved but indeed the point of the entire undertaking.

REFERENCES

INTRODUCTION

1. Cerebral vascular disease and strokes. US Public Health Service Publication #513, 1969
2. Eastcott HHG, Pickering GW, Rob CG: Reconstruction of internal carotid artery in a patient with intermittent attacks of hemiplegia. Lancet 2:994, 1954

PHYSIOLOGY OF THE CEREBRAL CIRCULATION

3. Brice JG, Dowsett DJ, Lowe RD: Haemodynamic effect of carotid artery stenosis. Br Med J 2:1363, 1964

4. Symon L: A comparative study of middle cerebral artery pressure in dogs and macaques. J Physiol (Lond) 191:449, 1967
5. Alpers BJ, Berry RG, Paddison RM: Anatomical studies of the circle of Willis in normal brain. Archives of Neurology and Psychology 81:25, 1959
6. Olesen J: Contralateral focal increase of cerebral blood flow in man during arm work. Brain 94:635, 1971
7. Lassen NA, Christensen MS: Physiology of cerebral blood flow. Br J Anaesth 48:719, 1976
8. Kety SS, Schmidt CF: The effects of altered tensions of carbon dioxide and oxygen on cerebral blood flow and cerebral oxygen consumption of normal young men. J Clin Invest 27:487, 1948
9. Severinghaus JW, Chiodi H, Eger EI et al: Cerebral blood flow in man at high altitude: role of cerebrospinal fluid pH in normalization of flow in chronic hypocapnia. Circ Res 19:274, 1966
10. Lassen NA, Agnoli A: Upper limit of autoregulation of cerebral blood flow: on the pathogenesis of hypertensive encephalopathy. Scand J Clin Lab Invest 30:110, 1972
11. Lassen NA: The luxury perfusion syndrome and its possible relation to acute metabolic acidosis localized within the brain. Lancet 2:1113, 1966
12. Symon L: Regional cerebrovascular responses to acute ischaemia in normocapnia and hypercapnia. J Neurol Neurosurg Psychiatry 83:756, 1970
13. Smith AL, Wollman H: Cerebral blood flow and metabolism: effects of anesthetic drugs and techniques. Anesthesiology 36:378, 1972
14. Murphy FL, Kennell EM, Johnstone RE et al: The effects of enflurane, isoflurane and halothane on cerebral blood flow and metabolism in man. Abstracts of Scientific Papers, pp 62–63. Annual Meeting of the American Society of Anesthesiologists, 1974
15. Shapiro HM: Physiologic and pharmacologic regulation of cerebral blood flow. Annual Refresher Course Lectures, No. 11. Annual Meeting of the American Society of Anesthesiologists, 1976
16. Shapiro HM: Physiologic and pharmacologic regulation of cerebral blood flow. Annual Refresher Course Lectures, No. 11. Annual Meeting of the American Society of Anesthesiologists, 1976

PATIENT PRESENTATION

17. Duncan GW, Pessin MS, Mohr JP et al: Transient cerebral ischemic attacks. Adv Intern Med 21:1, 1976
18. Acheson J, Hutchinson EC: Observations on the natural history of transient cerebral ischemia. Lancet 2:871, 1964
19. Pessin MS, Duncan GW, Mohr JP et al: Clinical and angiographic features of carotid transient ischemic attacks. N Engl J Med 296:358, 1977
20. Machleder HI: Strokes, transient ischemic attacks and asymptomatic bruits. (Medical Progress) West J Med 130:205, 1979
21. Thompson JE, Patman RD: Endarterectomy for asymptomatic carotid bruits. Surgical Digest 7:9, 1972
22. Samples JR, Wiederhold WC: Treatment of asymptomatic carotid bruit. West J Med 127:130, 1977
23. Bennett HJM: A randomized trail of aspirin and sulfinpyrazone in threatened stroke. The Canadian Cooperative Study Group. N Engl J Med 299:53, 1978

ANESTHETIC PLANNING

24. Sabawala PB, Strong MJ, Keats AS: Surgery of the aorta and its branches. Anesthesiology 33:229, 1970
25. Thompson JE, Austin DJ, Patman RD: Carotid endarterectomy for cerebrovascular insufficiency: long-term results in 592 patients followed up to thirteen years. Ann Surg 172:663, 1970
26. Bauer RB, Meyer JS, Fields WS et al: Joint study of extracranial arterial occlusion (III). JAMA 208:509, 1969
27. Edwards WT: Letter to the Editor: Preanesthetic management of the hypertensive patient. N Engl J Med 301:158, 1979
28. Matsumoto GH, Baker JD, Watson CW et al: EEG surveillance as a means of extending operability in high risk carotid endarterectomy. Stroke 7:554, 1976

OPERATIVE MANAGEMENT

29. Smith AL, Wollman H: Cerebral blood flow and metabolism: effects of anesthetic drugs and techniques. Anesthesiology 36:378, 1972
30. Murphy FL, Kennell EM, Johnstone RE et al: The effects of enflurane, isoflurane and halothane on cerebral blood flow and metabolism in man. Abstracts of Scientific Papers, pp 62–63. Annual Meeting of the American Society of Anesthesiologists 1974
31. Shapiro HM: Physiologic and pharmacologic regulation of cerebral blood flow. Annual Refresher Course Lectures, No. 11. Annual Meeting of the American Society of Anesthesiologists, 1976
32. Duncan GW, Pessin MS, Mohr JP et al: Transient cerebral ischemic attacks. Adv Intern Med 21:1, 1976
33. Boysen G, Engell HC, Pistolese GR et al: Editorial: On the critical lower level of cerebral blood flow in man with particular reference to carotid surgery. Circulation 69:1023, 1974
34. Baker JD, Gluecklich B, Watson CW et al: An evaluation of electroencephalographic monitoring for carotid study. Surgery 78:787, 1975
35. Sundt TM Jr, Sharbrough FW, Anderson RE et al: Cerebral blood flow measurements and electroencephalograms during carotid endarterectomy. J Neurosurg 41:310, 1974
36. Larson CP: Personal communication.
37. Cucchiara RF, Sharbrough FW, Messick JM et al: An electroencephalographic filter-processor as an indicator of cerebral ischemia during carotid endarterectomy. Anesthesiology 51:77, 1979
38. Moore WS, Yee JM, Hall AD: Collateral cerebral blood pressure. An index of tolerance to temporary carotid occlusion. Arch Surg 106:520, 1973
39. Hays RJ, Levinson SA, Wylie EJ: Intraoperative measurement of carotid back pressure as a guide to operative management for carotid endarterectomy. Surg 72:953, 1972
40. McKay RD, Sundt TM, Michenfelder JD et al: Internal carotid artery stump pressure and cerebral blood flow during carotid endarterectomy. Anesthesiology 45:390, 1976
41. Matsumoto GH, Baker JD, Watson CW et al: EEG surveillance as a means of extending operability in high risk carotid endarterectomy. Stroke 7:554, 1976
42. Larson CP, Ehrenfeld WK, Wade JG et al: Jugular venous oxygen saturation as an index of adequacy of cerebral oxygenation. Surgery 62:31, 1967
43. Akl BF, Blakeley WR, Lewis CE et al: Carotid endarterectomy: is a shunt necessary? Am J Surg 130:760, 1975
44. Boysen G, Engell HC, Henriksen H: The effect of induced hypertension on internal carotid artery pressure and regional cerebral blood

flow during temporary carotid clamping for endarterectomy. Neurology 22:1133, 1972

45. Fourcade HE, Larson CP, Ehrenfeld WK et al: The effects of CO_2 and systemic hypertension on cerebral perfusion pressure during carotid endarterectomy. Anesthesiology 33:383, 1970

46. Edwards WT: Letter to the Editor: Preanesthetic management of the hypertensive patient. N Engl J Med 301:158, 1979

47. Fitch W: Anaesthesia for carotid artery surgery. Br J Anaesth 48:791, 1976

48. Eastcott HHG, Pickering GW, Rob CG: Reconstruction of internal carotid artery in a patient with intermittent attacks of hemiplegia. Lancet 2:994, 1954

49. Michenfelder JD: Personal communication

50. Wells BA, Keats AS, Cooley DA: Increased tolerance to cerebral ischemia produced by general anesthesia during temporary carotid occlusion. Surgery 54:216, 1963

51. Smith AL: Barbiturate protection in cerebral hypoxia. Anesthesiology 47:285, 1977

52. Smith AL, Hoff JT, Nielsen SL et al: Barbiturate protection in acute focal cerebral ischemia. Stroke 5:1, 1974

53. Michenfelder JD, Milde JH: Influence of anesthetics on metabolic, functional and pathological responses to regional cerebral ischemia. Stroke 6:405, 1975

POSTOPERATIVE CONCERNS

54. Wade JG, Larson CP, Hickey RF et al: Effect of carotid endarterectomy on carotid chemoreceptor and baroreceptor function in man. N Engl J Med 282:823, 1970

COMBINED CORONARY AND CAROTID ARTERIAL DISEASE

55. Mehigan FT, Buch WS, Pipkin RD et al: A planned approach to coexistent cerebrovascular disease in coronary artery bypass candidates. Arch Surg 112:1403, 1977

56. Bernhard VM, Johnson WD, Peterson JJ: Carotid artery stenosis: association with surgery for coronary artery disease. Arch Surg 105:837, 1972

57. Morris GC: Discussion: Ann Surg 187:657, 1978

58. Reis RL, Hannah H: Management of patients with severe, coexistent coronary artery and peripheral vascular disease. J Thorac Cardiovasc Surg 73:909, 1977

59. Hertzer NR, Loop FD, Taylor PC: Staged and combined surgical approach to simultaneous carotid and coronary artery vascular disease. Surgery 84:803, 1978

Part VII SPECIAL CONSIDERATIONS

24

Coagulation Evaluation and Management

NORIG ELLISON

INTRODUCTION

A working knowledge of the normal hemostatic mechanism and of the manifestations of bleeding, a system for evaluation of abnormal bleeding, and a rationale for selecting among the available forms of treatment are essential for the practicing anesthesiologist. While consultation with a hematologist experienced in the management of abnormal bleeding is desirable in complex cases, the initial steps in evaluation, ranging from recognition of abnormal bleeding to ordering the appropriate laboratory tests and the start of therapy, will commonly be carried out intraoperatively.

Bleeding represents a defect in hemostasis,

and abnormal bleeding represents blood loss in excess of that which could be expected in a given patient at that stage in the procedure. For example, during cardiopulmonary bypass, the hemostatic mechanism is essentially totally paralyzed by heparin, and that is to be expected. Following bypass termination and heparin reversal, total hemostatic paralysis is not to be expected, and would require evaluation and treatment before the chest could safely be closed. Because *hemostasis is a tripartite function depending on vascular integrity, platelet function, and coagulation factors,* complete evaluation of abnormal bleeding must include an examination of all three parts of the hemostatic mechanism.[1]

Figure 24–1 illustrates the sequence of the

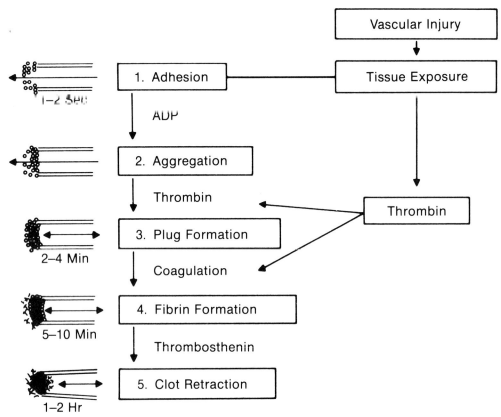

Fig. 24-1. Formation of the permanent hemostatic plug. The three parts of the hemostatic triangle are active in different steps. The contribution of platelet and vascular integrity occurs primarily in the first three steps which collectively represent primary hemostasis. During the last two steps, the coagulation mechanism, in part under the influence of platelets, produces a permanent hemostatic plug. (Harker LA: Hemostasis Manual. Seattle, University of Washington Press, 1970)

five events which occur and their time span following a blood vessel injury. Primary hemostasis, which is the result of the interaction between platelet and vessel, does not involve the coagulation mechanism and is represented by the first three steps. The release of vasoactive substances as platelets aggregate contributes further to the cessation of bleeding by decreasing the orifice. An adequate number of normally functioning platelets is, therefore, essential for primary hemostasis. The final two steps comprise the sequence of events in the formation of the definitive hemostatic plug. First, activation of the coagulation mechanism results in conversion of fibrinogen to a loose fibrin clot. Factor XIII activation by thrombin induces cross-polymerization of the fibrin, resulting in a firm, insoluble clot, which in turn retracts into a firm, definitive hemostatic plug under the influence of platelets. The entire sequence of events normally takes less than 2 hours.[2-4]

NORMAL HEMOSTASIS

VASCULAR INTEGRITY

Vascular integrity, which is defined as a state of unbroken or complete blood vessels, is routinely defective during every surgical procedure. While the spontaneous arrest of bleeding from ruptured vessels conveying blood under pressure involves autonomic mechanisms which are extremely complex in detail, the mechanical principles governing the loss of blood through such a defect are quite simple. Blood loss will continue as long as pressure within the vessel exceeds the pressure outside. The body defense mechanisms involved in the arrest of blood loss, through restoration of vascular integrity, comprise seven different principles:

1. A *hemostatic plug* will form, occluding the defect.
2. *Local vasoconstriction* will occur, decreasing the size of the defect.
3. *Anastamotic dilation* will occur, shunting blood away from the defect.

4. *Bleeding into tissues* will increase the extravascular pressure, decreasing the intra/extravascular gradient.
5. *Increased permeability of the microcirculation,* which results from tissue injury, will promote further increase in extravascular pressure as edema fluid escapes from the blood vessels.
6. *Hemoconcentration,* resulting from diminished plasma volume, will tend to slow circulation and further reduce intravascular pressure.
7. Continual blood loss without replacement will eventually produce *sufficient hypotension* to minimize or halt the blood loss. The technique of deliberate hypotension, which has long been used to minimize intraoperative blood loss, is based on this principle.

Figure 24–2 illustrates these defense mechanisms schematically.[5] The importance of each of these defense mechanisms in a given situation varies greatly. Vascular contraction to decrease the pressure differential is more important in arteries than in veins, which are comparatively nonelastic. Similarly, arteries are thicker than veins and thus more resistant to trauma. Thin-walled veins may rupture with only slight trauma, particularly in the legs because of the additional hydrostatic pressure.[6]

Finally, surgical ligation of the bleeding vessel will restore vascular integrity more quickly in many instances in which the above-listed mechanisms would ultimately work, and completely in instances in which these mechanisms would not suffice until irreparable harm had occurred (*e.g.,* in a patient with a ruptured abdominal aortic aneurysm).

PLATELETS

Platelets have been called the keystone of the hemostatic arch because of their involvement in all phases of hemostasis.[7] Not only are they the first nonvascular direct response of the body to bleeding, they are involved in activating the coagulation mechanism, and finally in initiating clot retraction.[8]

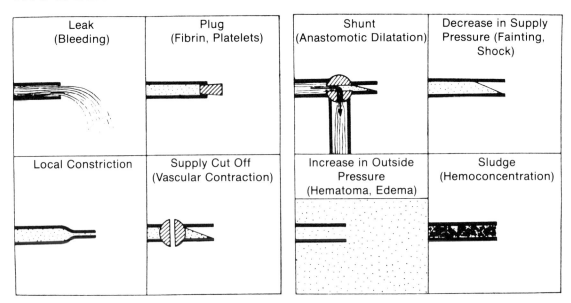

Fig. 24-2. Physical factors involved in spontaneous arrest of bleeding from injured blood vessel. These factors are compared to controlling water from a ruptured pipe. (MacFarlane RE (ed): The Haemostatic Mechanism in Man and Other Animals, London, Academic Press, 1970. Reproduced with permission of the Zoological Society of London)

The initial event in platelet activation is exposure of the platelet to an appropriate stimulus. *In vivo,* the stimulus is usually platelet contact with collagen-containing subendothelial basement membrane following damage to a vessel. The platelet reacts by undergoing a shape change, from its natural disc form to a spiny sphere. After completing the shape change, the activated platelets become "sticky" and form primary aggregates. Stickiness, more formally termed platelet adhesion, and primary aggregation appear to develop simultaneously. *Platelet adhesion* is the affinity of platelets for nonplatelet surfaces. *Primary aggregation* is a reversible process in which platelets develop an affinity for each other. One theory suggests the adhesion is initiated by platelet contact with collagen, and with primary aggregation is stimulated by low levels of adenosine diphosphate (ADP) released during the initial injury to the vessel.[9] Calcium and fibrinogen must be present for ADP-induced aggregation to occur.

This phase of platelet activation culminates with the release reaction, wherein the contents of cytoplasmic granules are released extracellularly. The released substances include ADP, serotonin, platelet Factor 4 (PF4), catecholamines, and factors that modify vascular permeability and integrity. ADP is a most potent aggregating agent, and its escape from platelets undergoing the release reaction causes more and more platelets to become activated. If the stimulus to platelet activation is minor and few platelets extrude their intragranular contents, then insufficient ADP will be released to cause self-sustaining aggregation. Platelets already aggregated will resume their native shape and return to the circulation. If, however, a threshold concentration of ADP is achieved, large numbers of platelets undergo the release reaction and aggregate irreversibly with each other. This is termed *secondary aggregation.* The released vasoactive substances stimulate the contraction of the open vessel.

Platelets not only form a plug as an initial

step in securing hemostasis, they also actively participate in several steps of the coagulation cascade, as indicated in Figure 24–3. Platelet Factor 3 (PF3) is essential for activation of Factor X by the complex of Factor IXa, Factor VIII, and calcium ion, and for conversion of prothrombin to thrombin by the complex of Factor Xa, Factor V, and calcium ion. PF3 is a property of lipoproteins within, and inseparable from, the platelet membrane. In contrast, PF4 can be recovered from the plasma after platelet aggregation. PF4, a protein present in the granular fraction of platelet homogenates, neutralizes heparin. The exact role of PF4 is not definitely established, but the inactivation of Factor Xa, which requires only minute amounts of heparin in circulating blood might be prevented by PF4.[9]

Platelets also have been shown to play a role in the activation of Factor XII in the presence of ADP, and possibly to provide an alternative route bypassing Factor XIIa by collagen-induced activation of Factor XI. This may explain why patients deficient in Factor XII, who have markedly abnormal coagulation profiles, do not bleed excessively.

Fibrinogen, originating from plasma and from thrombin-induced irreversible aggregation of platelets, is converted to fibrin, resulting in a network of fibrin surrounding and permeating the platelet mass or hemostatic plug. The final step in the sequence, clot retraction, is caused by another platelet protein, thrombosthenin.

COAGULATION MECHANISM

The majority of blood vessels are less than 1 mm in diameter and, in vessels of this caliber, platelets and coagulation factors play the major role in securing hemostasis.[10] Thus, an efficient coagulation mechanism is essential to prevent bleeding. Figure 24–3 outlines the currently accepted theory of the coagulation scheme, emphasizing the contribution of platelets. Table 24–1 lists the coagulation factors with just some of the synonyms. By common consent, the suffix *a* is used to designate the activated form and the numeral *VI* has not been assigned to another factor. Three factors (I, V, and VIII) do not exist in an enzymatically active form. With the exception of Factors III and IV, all of the factors are

Table 24-1. List of Coagulation Factors

FACTOR	SYNONYM	CLINICAL SYNDROME CAUSED BY DEFICIENCY
I	Fibrinogen	Yes
II	Prothrombin, prethrombin	Yes
III	Tissue factor, tissue thromboplastin	No
IV	Calcium	No
V	Labile factor, proaccelerin, plasma accelerator globulin (ac-G)	Yes
VI	NO FACTOR ASSIGNED TO THIS NUMERAL	
VII	Stable factor, proconvertin, autoprothrombin I, serum prothrombin conversion accleration (SPCA)	Yes
VIII	Antihemophilia globulin (AHG) Antihemophilic factor (AFG) Thromboplastinogen, platelet cofactor I, antihemophilia Factor A	Yes
IX	Plasma thromboplastin component (PTC), Christmas Factor, autothrombin II, antihemophilic Factor B, platelet cofactor II	Yes
X	Stuart–Prower factor, autoprothrombin C (or III)	Yes
XI	Plasma thromboplastin antecedent (PTA), Rosenthal syndrome, antihemophilic Factor C	Mild
XII	Hageman factor, glass factor	No
XIII	Fibrin stabilizing factor (FSF) Laki-Lorand factor, fibrinase serum factor, urea-insolubility factor	Yes

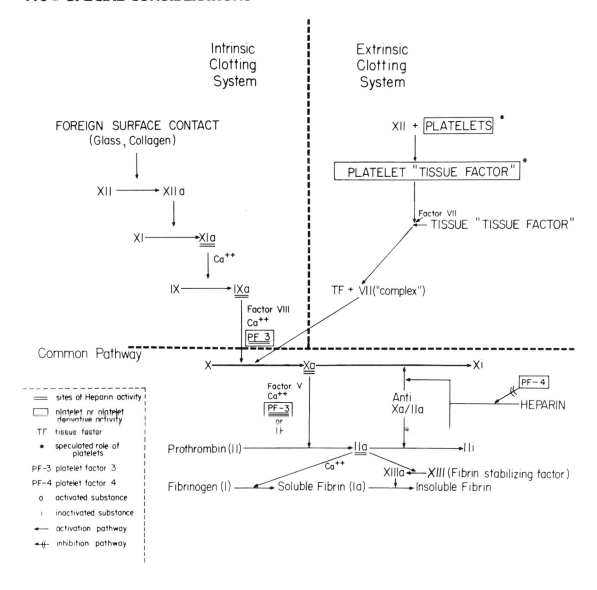

Fig. 24-3. The generally accepted scheme of the coagulation cascade is modified to emphasize the sites of platelet and heparin activity. *Upper left section* contains intrinsic clotting system, *upper right section* contains extrinsic clotting system, and *lower section contains* the final common pathway. Substances enclosed in *boxes* represent platelet or platelet derivative activity. *Underlined factors* illustrate sites of heparin activity. The *right portion* of the final common pathway illustrates the theoretical interaction of heparin with platelet Factor 4 (PF4), and its effect on the inactivation of Factors Xa and IIa. Heparin, in combination with circulating substances anti-Xa/IIa, facilitates inactivation of Xa and IIa. PF4 antagonizes this heparin activity. (Barrer MJ, Ellison N: Platelet function. Anesthesiology 46:202–211, 1977)

plasma proteins. The introduction in 1964 of a standard nomenclature for the coagulation Factors and the use of a Roman numeral to identify each factor brought a semblance of order to what had previously been a most chaotic field. Unfortunately, the Roman numerals were assigned to the factors in the order of the discovery of the factors rather than in the order of the sequence of reactions within the coagulation cascade.

Primary hemostasis, the formation of the platelet plug, is accompanied by the activation of the coagulation mechanism or cascade, the end result of which is formation of the definitive hemostatic plug. In the final common pathway, Factor X is activated by the end product of either the intrinsic or extrinsic system. The complex sequence of events which leads up to activation of Factor X serves as a biologic amplifier, so that only a small stimulus is needed to initiate fibrin formation from fibrinogen. With a molecular weight of 340,000, fibrinogen conversion proceeds in a stepwise fashion with (1) thrombin splitting off two fibrinopeptides, A and B, constituting about 3.0 percent of the fibrinogen molecule; (2) spontaneous polymerization of fibrin monomers into a loose fibrin net; and (3) under the stimulus of Factor XIIIa, conversion of the loose fibrin net by covalent bonds to a more firm meshwork. Finally platelets induce retraction of the clot to form the definitive hemostatic plug.[11]

The coagulation mechanism not only has the capacity to respond promptly to limit the loss of blood, it also has *several built-in checks to keep the fibrin formation localized,* and to prevent the coagulation process from continuing to the point of complete intravascular thrombosis. These include the following:

1. *Rapid blood flow* producing dilution of coagulation factors below threshold levels
2. *Clearance of activated coagulation factors* by the liver and reticuloendothelial systems
3. *Blocking action of naturally occurring inhibitory plasma proteins,* such as antithrombin III on the action of thrombin

The separation of the intrinsic and extrinsic systems in Figure 24–3 is somewhat artificial in that, *in vivo,* tissue factor probably triggers both systems. Clearly both systems are necessary for effective hemostasis because patients with isolated deficiencies in either system do present with clinical bleeding syndromes. Table 24–1 indicates which factors are associated with clinical bleeding syndromes. Table 24–2 demonstrates the minimum levels of coagulation factors (and platelets) necessary for adequate hemostasis. Factor XII deficiency, which is associated with markedly prolonged *in vitro* clotting, is not associated with a clinical syndrome, and that associated with Factor XI is usually quite mild. In contrast, deficiencies of the two other antihemophiliac globulins, Factors VIII and IX, may be associated with severe bleeding depending on the Factor level.[12]

FIBRINOLYSIS

In addition to the built-in checks on the coagulation mechanism previously listed, the plasminogen system digests fibrin to prevent thrombotic occlusion of a vessel. The plasminogen system contains, as does the coagulation system, inactive profactors, activators, and inhibitors. Fibrin formation is usually associated with the release of plasminogen activators, which are derived from endothelium and lysozomes, and convert plasminogen to plasmin, an event which tends to limit the extent of the fibrin formation. *Fibrinolysis, then, is a defense mechanism designed to localize fibrin deposition to the area of injury.* Recognized physiologic activators include vigorous exercise, anoxia, and stress, in addition to coagulation during which tissue damage, Factor XIIa, and thrombin all can activate plasminogen to plasmin. The activation of the fibrinolytic system in response to the intravascular deposition of fibrin is, therefore, a defense mechanism known as *secondary fibrinolysis.* This may occur in the extreme form in disseminated intravascular coagulation (DIC). Listed below are some of the many causes of DIC.[13]

Potential Causes of DIC Divided into Three Basic Mechanisms*

1. Cellular damage releasing into the bloodstream phospholipids, which are necessary for both the extrinsic and intrinsic systems of coagulation to function
   Examples: Hemolytic transfusion reaction, malaria, trauma, extracorporeal circulation, near drowning
2. Endothelial damage resulting in activation of the intrinsic clotting system through exposure of blood to collagen
   Examples: Viremia, heat stroke, meningococcemia, trauma, aortic aneurysm, shock, glomerulonephritis
3. Introduction of tissue factor into the blood stream resulting in activation of the extrinsic clotting system
   Examples: Neoplams, leukemia, trauma and tissue injury, obstetric defibrination syndromes, extracorporeal circulation, burns, transplant rejection

*The difficulty in dividing causes of DIC into different categories is illustrated by the listing of trauma in all three categories. Trauma can damage cells, injure blood vesels and expose collagen, and introduce tissue factor into the blood stream. (Modified from Minna JD, Robboy SJ, Colman RW: Disseminated Intravascular Coagulation in Man. Springfield, Ill, Charles C Thomas, 1974)

Within the past decade there has been increasing recognition of the importance of fibrinolysis as a body defense mechanism when DIC occurs. In such cases, plasmin circulates intravascularly and digests not only fibrin but also fibrinogen and Factors V and VIII. Ordinarily, *in vivo* plasmin acts primarily on fibrin, breaking it down into successively smaller fragments, fibrin split products, which possess anticoagulant properties of their own by inhibiting polymerization of fibrin monomers.

Primary fibrinolysis, an extremely rare condition which may occur for example, in patients with cirrhosis or posturologic surgery, must be differentiated from *secondary fibrinolysis.* Infusion of streptokinase or urokinase will also primarily activate the fibrinolytic system. This will be presented further during the discussion of the effects of cardiopulmonary bypass equipment on platelets and coagulation.[13]

Table 24-2. Minimum Levels of Coagulation Factors and Platelets Necessary for Effective Hemostasis; Distribution and Fate of Clotting Factors after Transfusion Therapy, and Schedules

FACTOR	MINIMAL LEVEL FOR SURGICAL HEMOSTASIS (PER CENT OF NORMAL)	APPARENT VOLUME OF DISTRIBUTION (× PLASMA VOLUME)	IN-VIVO HALF-LIFE (HOURS)	THERA-PEUTIC AGENT	DOSE (PER KG BODY WEIGHT)	
					Initial	Maintenance
I	50–100	2–5	72–144	Cryoprecipitate	Ppt from 100 ml	Ppt from 14–20 ml, qd
II	20–40	1.5–2	72–120	Plasma	10–15 ml	5–10 ml, qd
V	5–20	?	12–36	Fresh or frozen plasma	10–15 ml	10 ml, qd
VII	10–20	2–4	4–6	Plasma	5–10 ml	5 ml, qd
VIII	30	1–1.5	10–18	Cryoprecipitate	Ppt from 70 ml	Ppt from 35 ml, bld
von Willebrand's	30			Plasma	10 ml	10 ml q 2–3 d
IX	20–25	2–5	18–36	Plasma or II, VII, IX, X conc.	60 ml Variable	7 ml qd
X	10–20	1–2	24–60	Plasma	15 ml	10 ml, qd
XI	20–30	1–1.33	40–80	Plasma	10 ml	5 ml, qd
XII	0	?	?50–70	Plasma	5 ml	5 ml, qd
XIII	1–3	?	?72–120	Plasma	2–3 ml	None
Platelets	50,000–100,000/mm^3			Platelet concentrate	1–2 units per desired 10,000 increment in count	

TESTS OF HEMOSTASIS

GENERAL

The first step in laboratory analysis of hemostasis is *obtaining a blood specimen* and this must be done with the same attention to detail as performing the actual test. Although the use of siliconized needles and syringes has been advocated, disposable needles and plastic syringes are satisfactory.[14] The venopuncture should be accurate and atraumatic to avoid introducing tissue juice. One way to ensure this is to use a two-syringe technique in which the first syringe is discarded after collection of 2 mm and a second syringe is attached to the indwelling needle to collect the sample. The second syringe size and additives will vary depending on what tests are to be performed.

An alternate approach to obtaining a blood specimen is the use of indwelling arterial or central venous cannulae. These lines may contain heparin flush solutions, and the frequent contamination of samples of heparin has promoted many laboratories to proscribe samples for coagulation tests being obtained from such lines. This proscription is not necessary if samples are collected with the same attention to detail as with venopuncture collection. *Particularly important is the need to withdraw an adequate aliquot before collecting a sample.* In an arterial line with a deadspace of 2 ml between patient and sampling port, withdrawing 4 ml before collecting the sample will eliminate the chance of heparin contamination. This 4 ml aliquot may then either be discarded or returned aseptically and immediately to the patient.[15]

Additionally, the use of indwelling catheters around which hemostasis has been secured will obviate the need for venopuncture, with its attendant introduction of another defect in vascular integrity. This may be especially important in patients with a hemorrhagic diathesis who are already bleeding from previous venopuncture sites. In the event venopuncture is required in patients with bleeding diathesis, care must be taken to prevent continued bleeding by the application of an occlusive pressure dressing.

Quality control in the performance of each test is most important. Rigid attention to detail must be paid by all personnel to insure that results are comparable. Differences in normal values between labs may be explained by slight variations in actual performance of a given test. However, within a given lab, such variations must not exist.[16] All tests should be performed in duplicate, and a normal control sample should be tested at the same time.

An increasing number of *mechanical devices* are available to perform coagulation tests, with the endpoint being measured by electrical, magnetic, mechanical, or optical methods. While these machines all have the advantage of reducing human variability in a given test, they are more expensive, except in large-volume laboratories where their use has resulted in more efficient processing of samples and usually more rapidly available results. However, an automated activated coagulation time device and a machine for measuring thrombin time are being used in the operating room with success.[17, 18]

One of the limiting factors on the value of any test is how fast the results will be available. For this reason, tests which can be performed in the operating room appeal to many. Tests of hemostasis performed in the operating room should meet the following criteria:[19]

1. The anesthesiologist needs to perform only *simple maneuvers* to obtain reliable, reproducible results
2. *Minimum equipment,* which is compact, inexpensive, and operates quietly
3. *Results are available quickly,* even with abnormally prolonged times.
4. Preferably, the test can be *performed on whole blood,* rather than plasma.
5. *Test reagents must be stable* indefinitely.
6. The test *cannot divert prolonged attention* away from the anesthesiologist's usual duties.

An alternative approach to evaluation of hemostasis directly by the anesthetist is the use

Table 24-3. Tests of Hemostasis Useful in the Operating Room

TEST	NORMAL RANGE	COMMENT
Platelet Function		
1. Platelet count	150,000–300,000/mm^3	First step in any evaluation of platelet function. Care must be taken in collecting sample.
2. Bleeding time	3–8 min	Most widely accepted test of platelet function. Yields reproducible, reliable results if all variables are controlled. (Arms cannot be at side if this test is to be performed).
3. Clot retraction	Should be complete within 2 hours	Useful additional information obtained from the WBCT (see below)
Coagulation Mechanism		
4. Whole blood coagulation time, one tube	2.5–4.25 min	Useful test of hemostasis if all variables are controlled. Clot can be observed for retraction (platelet function) or dissolution (fibrinolysis).
5. Activated coagulation time		Valuable OR test with results available more quickly than WBCT and equally reproducible if attention to technique is rigid. Automated device especially valuable in view of minimal effort required.
Manual	75–90 sec	
Automated	94–104 sec	
Fibrinolysis		
6. Clot dissolution	Should not occur	Clot dissolution can be looked for after performing WBCT. Care must be taken not to confuse fragmentation of the weak, friable clot of hypofibrinogenemia from fibrinolysis. (A fibrinogen level will help here.)

of laboratory technicians in the operating room vicinity. Bull and coworkers using a manual ACT,[20] and Cohen and coworkers using a mechanical device to measure thrombin times,[18] have both used this approach. With the continued growth of clinical laboratories adjacent to, or within the confines of, operating suites, providing rapid arterial blood gas and electrolyte analysis, incorporation of basic tests of hemostasis into such clinical laboratories would be a desirable step forward.

The actual tests are now presented in detail. They are presented in this manner not to intimidate nor bore the reader, but to emphasize the complex and interfering problems in coagulation testing. Table 24–3 further demonstrates these tests for hemostasis.

TESTS OF PLATELET FUNCTION

Platelet Count

Because *most bleeding attributed to platelet problems is secondary to a reduction in number,* a platelet count is usually the first test to be performed. All platelet count techniques suf-

fer from the same potential pitfall inherent in handling platelets, which tend to clump, fragment, and adhere to the sides of collecting implements. For this reason, tissue damage and blood manipulation during collection must be minimized to reduce the influence of this inherent platelet characteristic on the result.[21, 22] The platelet count is a quantitative test only and does not measure platelet quality nor function.

Counts can be performed with either light or phase microscopy. Electronic counters seem to offer greatest accuracy. Low platelet counts may occur in a wide variety of systemic disorders: varying from aplastic anemia to septicemia or cardiopulmonary bypass, as well as in idiopathic thrombocytopenia, which has been called *immune thrombocytopenia.* Bleeding rarely occurs unless values, which normally range from 150,000 to 350,000/mm^3 acutely decrease to below 50 to 70,000/mm^3.

Bleeding Time, Ivy Forearm Method

The Ivy bleeding time is the *most widely accepted clinical test of platelet function.*[23] It measures both platelet quality and quantity. Inability to control many variables has made the Duke earlobe method obsolete. These variables include the length and depth of the incision, the venous pressure, and patient cooperation.[23, 24]

A blood pressure cuff is inflated to, and maintained throughout the test at, 40 torr to standardize venous and capillary pressures. A site free of superficial vein, hair, scar, or other lesions on the volar forearm surface is selected and cleansed with 70 percent alcohol. After the alcohol has dried, an incision is made, 10.0 mm long and 5.0 mm deep. Use of a template facilitates exactness in making the incision. The use of topical or injected anesthetic drugs at the testing area distorts and invalidates the results. Timing begins with the incision, and blood is blotted at 30-second intervals with filter paper, care being taken not to touch the wound directly and not to disturb the clot. The endpoint is reached when blood no longer appears on

the filter paper. Normal bleeding time is from 3 to 8 minutes. Children or uncooperative adults may not keep their arm still, invalidating the test.[21]

The bleeding time is prolonged in cases of thrombocytopenia (commonly seen after CPB and massive blood transfusion) (Fig. 24–4) and in defects of platelet functions such as Glanzmann's thrombasthenia. Classically, in untreated von Willebrand's disease, a prolonged bleeding time and a low Factor VIII level are both present, whereas in patients with other plasma deficiencies, the bleeding time is normal. After Factor VIII levels have been increased to normal levels in patients with von Willebrand's disease, clinical bleeding is not a problem even though a prolonged bleeding time may persist. In DIC, the depression in fibrinogen levels is accompanied by a decrease in the platelet count; the prolonged bleeding time often seen in DIC is caused by the latter.

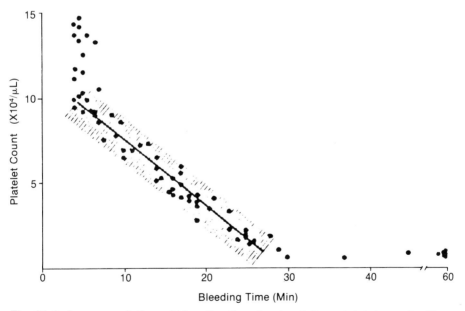

Fig. 24-4. Inverse relation of bleeding time to circulating platelet count with thrombocytopenia on the basis of impaired production when the concentration of platelets is between 10,000 and 100,000/mm³. The regression line is shown by the *solid line* and 95% confidence limts are indicated by the *shaded area.* (Harker LA, Slichter SJ: The bleeding time as a screening test for evaluation of platelet function. N Engl J Med 287:155–159, 1972. Reprinted by permission from the New England Journal of Medicine.)

Rumpel–Leed Tourniquet Test

A tourniquet is inflated to a point midway between systolic and distolic pressure for 5 minutes. The number of petechiae in a circle drawn 3 cm in diameter on the volar surface of the midforearm is counted 5 minutes after release of the tourniquet. A normal value is less than ten petechiae within the circle. However, when the test is positive, the number of petechiae often need not be counted because the forearm is covered with showers of petechiae. In the presence of an adequate number of normally functioning platelets, a positive test is attributed to alterations in capillary pressure and fragility and is called the *capillary fragility test* or *Gofflin index*.[21]

Positive test results are seen in certain primary disorders of platelet function such as von Willebrand's disease or Glanzmann's thrombasthenia as well as thrombocytopenia. Additionally, diseases of blood vessels and connective tissue such as scurvy or dysproteinemias, senile degeneration of connective tissue, and rheumatoid arthritis may be associated with positive results. The lack of specificity of this test makes interpretation most difficult.

Platelet Adhesiveness

Platelet adhesiveness has been measured by many different techniques. Bowie's method is the most widely used. Platelet counts are determined before and after a blood sample is infused over glass beads. The difference between the two counts divided by the original count is expressed as a percentage. The normal range is 37 to 84 percent. The term *platelet retention test* has been suggested to describe this test because aggregation of platelets to each other as well as adhesion of platelets to the glass beads determines the percent decrease. An *in vivo* variation of this test has been described in which serial platelet counts are performed on blood exuding from an incision made in the performance of a template bleeding time. Serial platelet counts are made at 2-minute intervals beginning at 1 minute and continuing until bleeding stops or the ninth minute. Platelet counts will decrease to very low levels as the bleeding diminishes because of the adherence of most of the platelets to surfaces of the cut tissues. In addition to the decrease in platelet retention seen in primary platelet function defects such as von Willebrand's disease, platelet function defects secondary to myelofibrosis or uremia will demonstrate decreased retention.[21]

Platelet Aggregation

The tendency of platelets to adhere to one another is termed *platelet aggregation*. The platelet aggregometer, designed to measure this platelet function spectrophotometrically, has provided much information about the physiology of platelets.[21, 25]

Platelet rich plasma (PRP) and platelet poor plasma (PPP) are prepared from citrated plasma, and used to standardize the aggregometer. PRP represents 0 percent light transmission, and PPP, 100 percent transmission. Aliquots of PRP, 0.5 ml, are placed in cuvettes and kept in a water bath at 37°C for 3 minutes. The warmed PRP cuvette is then placed in the aggregometer and stirred at 1000 rpm. After the recorder is started and checked for accuracy, 0.1 ml of reagent is added and the change in light transmission noted.

Figure 24–5 depicts a typical curve, showing the calibration of PPP and PRP followed by the addition of a reagent inducing primary aggregation, the release reaction, and secondary aggregation. While impairment of platelet aggregation does not always correlate with clinical bleeding, abnormal response with many aggregating agents has been noted in Glanzmann's thrombasthenia, in patients with von Willebrand's disease whose platelets will not aggregate in response to ristocetin, and in patients who have taken aspirin whose platelets will not undergo the release reaction for up to 10 days.

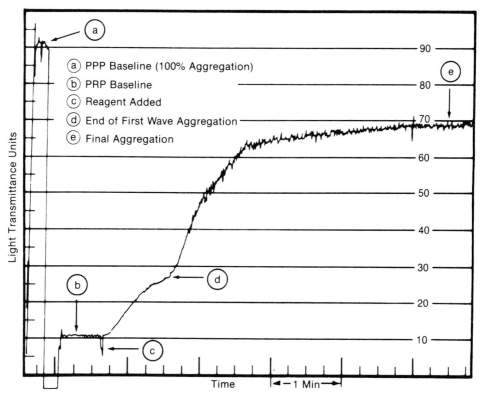

Fig. 24-5. Typical platelet aggregation curve in response to epinephrine. *a.* Baseline for 100% light transmission (zero % absorption) is set with platelet-poor plasma (PPP). *b.* Baseline for 0% light transmission (100% absorption) is set with platelet-rich plasma (PRP). *c.* Test reagent is added and initiates first wave or primary aggregation. *d.* If stimulus provided at *c* is sufficiently intense, platlets will undergo the release reaction and procede to complete, secondary, or final aggregation at *e.* One measure of the sensitivity of platelets is to determine the minimum stimulus necessary at *c* to produce *d* and *e.*

Clot Retraction

Clot retraction is another function of platelets which can be grossly measured. When maintained at 37°C, a clot should begin to retract within 2 to 4 hours. While efforts to quantitate the degree of retraction have been attempted (*e.g.,* measuring the amount of serum expressed by the clot after 4 hours), the test remains a qualitative positive or negative test (*i.e.,* the presence of any clot retraction is accepted as satisfactory. Clot retraction is a function of hematocrit, fibrinogen, platelets, and possibly viscosity.[21] Retraction may be delayed or incomplete in thrombocytopenia or primary platelet defects.

TESTS OF COAGULATION MECHANISM

Lee–White Whole Blood Coagulation Time (WBCT)

The Lee–White WBCT, probably the oldest test of coagulation, has been criticized as being insensitive. Failure to control many variables that can influence the result explains most of the criticism. These variables include size of test tube, quality of glass, temperature, volume of blood, number of test tubes (*i.e.*, one-, two-, three-tube test), definitions of endpoint, as well as frequency and vigor of tilting. When these variables are controlled, the test can give much valuable information and is especially helpful to the anesthesiologist in the operative setting, in view of the minimal equipment necessary.[26, 27]

One milliliter of venous blood is placed in each of either one, two, or three test tubes each maintained at 37°C. (The results with one tube are comparable to three, so that there is no need to perform the three-tube test).[27] At 30-second intervals, the tube is tilted 90° and back, permitting the liquid blood to run down the side to produce maximal surface activation. If more than one tube is used, the second tube is tilted in exactly the same manner when the first tube clots, and the third tube when the second has clotted. Normal values for one-tube WBCT are 2.5 to 4.25 minutes.

Deficiencies of factors in the intrinsic system or final common pathway may prolong the WBCT. However these deficiencies must be quite marked. Most commonly today the test is used to monitor heparin therapy.

Activated Coagulation Time (ACT)

The ACT is a modification of the WBCT, in which celite is added to promote maximal early activation of Factor XII. It thus measures abnormalities in the intrinsic system or final common pathway.

Two milliliters of blood are collected and placed in a test tube containing celite and the timer is started. The tube is inverted once per second for 30 seconds to mix the contents thoroughly, and then it is placed in a heat block held over a 40 watt light bulb and rocked slowly until clotting occurs. Normal values are 75 to 90 seconds.

This test has been widely used to monitor heparin therapy.[28] The results are available more quickly then with the WBCT, and they do not show as much variability. The development of an automated ACT device (Hemochron) has furthered the use of this test in the operating room.[29] Normal values for the

automated variation of the ACT are provided by the manufacturer, usually in the range of 90 to 120 seconds.

Partial Thromboplastin Time (PTT)

This test evaluates the intrinsic system and final common pathway, but eliminates the platelet variable by adding cephalin as a substitute for platelet Factor 3. The original test, where modified by the addition of kaolin to produce maximal contact activation, is called the activated PTT (aPTT).

Equal volumes of 0.1 ml of oxalated plasma and 0.5 percent kaolin suspension are incubated at 37°C for 5 minutes. Then 0.1 ml of 0.15 percent suspension of cephalin is added and mixed. Finally, 0.1 ml of 0.02M $CaCl_2$ is added and the timer is started. The tube is gently rolled until fibrin strands form, the timer being stopped at first fibrin formation. Normal aPTT values are less than 35 seconds.

This test will detect deficiencies of coagulation factors below 25 percent of normal levels, except Factors VII and XIII. The aPTT is also prolonged in the presence of heparin and circulating anticoagulants. In most coagulation labs today, this test is done by a machine.

Prothrombin Time (PT)

The PT is one of the oldest and most commonly performed tests of coagulation today because it is the test of choice to monitor coumarin anticoagulation. The PT tests the extrinsic system in the same way that the aPTT tests the intrinsic system.[30] Both the PT and aPTT, of course, test the final common pathway.

Equal volumes, 0.1 ml of platelet-rich oxalated plasma and thromboplastin are mixed in a test tube maintained at 37°C. Then 0.1 ml of 0.02M $CaCl_2$ is added and the timer started. The tube is rapidly and gently tilted until fibrin first forms. Elapsed time is the PT.

One of the principal determinants of the elapsed time will be the strength of the thromboplastin suspension, which may vary greatly. For this reason the use of a control plasma and reporting both values are recommended in lieu of *percent activity.*[30] Abnormal tests may be the result of a coagulation factor deficiency or a circulating anticoagulant. To differentiate these, the test is repeated with equal volumes of control plasma (0.1 ml) and patient's plasma (0.1 ml) being compared to a 9:1 patient (0.18 ml):control (0.02 ml) plasma. Continued prolongation of PT in the former suggests the presence of an inhibitor whereas shortening with the latter suggests a coagulation factor deficiency in the patient is more likely. Because Factor V is labile and necessary for this test, the test should be run as soon as possible after the blood is drawn or the separated plasma refrigerated if storage up to 4 hours is necessary.[31]

Thrombin Time (TT)

This test bypasses all but the final stage of fibrin formatoin. Thrombin solution is prepared and diluted until the TT of control oxalated plasma falls into the range of 20 to 35 seconds. Equal volumes, 0.2 ml, of the patient's oxalated plasma and thrombin solution are mixed and the timer started. The tube is continuously gently agitated in a water bath at 37°C until fibrin is formed. By diluting the thrombin suspension, this test can be made even more sensitive.

Prolonged TT is caused by (1) fibrinogen level less than 90 mg/dl, (2) heparin or heparin-like anticoagulants which inhibit antithrombin, or (3) an abnormal fibrinogen. If a mixture of patient's plasma with control plasma is closer to that of a patient's plasma

alone than to that of control plasma alone, an anticoagulant is present. If the patient is not on heparin, it is likely that fibrin split products are present.[31]

Reptilase Time

This test is a modification of the thrombin time in which Reptilase-R, a thrombin-like enzyme isolated from the venom of *Bothrops atrox*, is used. Reptilase-R is different from thrombin in that the latter splits off fibrinopeptides A, AP, and B whereas the former releases A and AP only. This difference explains why Reptilase-R is slightly or not at all influenced by fibrinogen split products or heparin or both.

To perform the test, mix 0.3 ml citrated human plasma with 0.1 ml reconstituted reagent at 37°C and start the timer. Normal value is 18 to 22 seconds.

Comparison of this time and the thrombin time gives valuable information as summarized in Table 24-4.

Specific Factor Assays or Mixing Tests

Plasma samples known to be deficient in a specific factor are used to identify the deficient factor. For example, an abnormal PT may be caused by deficiencies of Factors V, VII, and X in addition to prothrombin and fibrinogen. A PT assay using plasma deficient in Factor V, VII, or X is performed by serial diluting known, for example, Factor V-deficient plasma with buffered saline (10%, 25%, 50%, and 100% plasma) and performing a PT. The patient's plasma from the abnormal PT is then tested in the same manner, using 100

Table 24-4. Interpretation of Combined Thrombin and Reptilase Times

THROMBIN TIME	REPTILASE TIME	CAUSE	REMARKS
Prolonged	Equally prolonged	Hypo- or afibrinogenemia	Ascertain by determination of fibrinogen
Prolonged	Strongly prolonged	Dysfibrinogenemia	Congenital or acquired (hepatoma)
Prolonged	Normal	Heparin	Neutralize heparin then perform TT. If still prolonged: fibrinogen split products; If normalized: heparin
Prolonged	Slightly prolonged	Fibrin split products	

and 50 percent. By comparison to the known-deficient plasma, the concentration of Factor V in the patient's plasma can be calculated. If this level is normal, then the assay can be repeated using other factor-deficient plasma.

In a similar manner, PTT assay can be performed for Factors VIII, IX, XI, and XII.

TESTS OF FIBRINOLYSIS

WBCT Clot Dissolution

The clot produced during the WBCT (see above) should be observed while maintained at 37°C for dissolution. Normally, this will not occur in up to 48 hours. In the presence of fibrinolysis, this may occur in less than 1 hour. Care must be taken not to mistake fragmentation of the weak, friable clot, if hypofibrinogenemia, for fibrinolysis. A fibrinogen level will obviously help in distinguishing these two possibilities.

Lysis of Normal Clot

A confirmatory test of fibrinolysis is performed by mixing a clot from normal plasma with an equal volume of patient's plasma or serum. If the clot lyses within 24 hours, increased fibrinolytic active is present. This test may be falsely normal if the patient's plasma is plasminogen-depleted because of the active fibrinolysis.[32]

Euglobulin Lysis Time (ELT)

When plasma is diluted with water, the proteins that precipitate out are known as euglobulins. Plasminogen activator, plasminogen, plasmin, and fibrinogen are all euglobulins and can be separated from water soluble inhibitors.

Sampling is extremely important in this test because prolonged venostasis (*e.g.*, tourniquet on too long) and trauma (*e.g.*, excessive alcohol rub of the skin) stimulate the release of plasminogen activator. Samples should be maintained at 5°C and plasma separation should be completed within 30 minutes. To perform the test, mix 7.5 ml of

0.008% acetic acid and 0.5 ml of plasma and maintain near the freezing point. After mixing gently decant the supernatant and allow the tube to drain. Stir sediment, add 1.8 ml of buffered saline, and warm to 37°C. Add 20 units of thrombin and stir while maintaining at 37°C. Inspect tube regularly for lysis. Normal ELT is greater than 2 hours.[32]

In addition to errors in sampling technique which produce a shortened ELT, platelets prolong the ELT because of their antiplasmin activities, so PPP should be used in testing. Inadequate draining will leave residual antiplasmin which will also prolong the ELT. pH is critical with maximal lysis occurring with precipitation of globulins at pH 6.2.[33]

Fibrin(ogen) Split Products

In the presence of breakdown products of fibrinogen and fibrin, coagulase-positive *Staphyloccocus aureus* become adherent to one another and produce visible clumping. Serial dilutions of fibrinogen standards and patient serum are prepared and mixed with bacterial suspension. The bacteria will form a smooth suspension when no clumping has occurred. The lowest dilution where clumping is easily visualized is the endpoint. Comparison of the standard fibrinogen dilution endpoint gives the final answer, which is expressed in μg/ml fibrinogen equivalents, with values greater than 12 μg/ml indicating active fibrinolysis.

ROUTINE PREOPERATIVE EVALUATION

The best method for detection of a hemorrhagic diathesis is a *properly taken history.* One of the most important items to be checked in the history is the *hemostatic response to a prior surgical experience.* With respect to any bleeding episode, the history should establish severity, site, duration, and etiology as well as similar episodes, age at onset of symptoms, family history, and any related information the patient may think relevant. Especially important in the history is a *detailed record of drug ingestion.* While patients may volunteer that they are taking anticoagulants, they may neglect to mention that they are taking aspirin (or aspirin-containing compounds), a drug which exhibits a coumarin-like effect in high doses, and prolongs the bleeding time in low doses. There are many other drugs that may impair platelet function. Drug history should include details about occupation and exposure to toxic agents or ionizing radiation. The *age at onset* is an equally important clue with bleeding problems starting in infancy or early childhood, suggestive of a congenital defect.

Physical examination may detect evidence of a hemorrhagic diathesis. Petechiae or prolonged bleeding following superficial trauma are usually the result of vascular or platelet abnormalities. In contrast, the subcutaneous bleeding seen in deficiencies of coagulation factors is usually an ecchymosis as opposed to discrete petechiae seen with vascular or platelet abnormalities. Hemarthrosis, or deep bleeding into muscles, is more likely to be seen with a coagulation factor deficiency.

A *screening coagulation profile* on any patient scheduled for cardiovascular surgery, or any patient whose history suggests a hemorrhagic diathesis is essential. One such profile includes PT, aPTT, platelet count, fibrinogen

level, and bleeding time. In the operating room, a baseline whole blood coagulation or an automated ACT may be performed. While the yield from such a profile may be low, the advantage of not having to include a preexisting defect in the differential diagnosis of a bleeding disorder which occurs intraoperatively justifies the effort. With a negative history and a normal screening coagulation profile, this is a valid assumption.[34]

Figure 24–6 illustrates why no one test, nor pair of tests, is sufficient to make an accurate diagnosis of a bleeding disorder. While between them the aPTT and PT serve to test both the intrinsic and extrinsic systems and final common pathway, more refined mixing tests using plasma known to be deficient in, for example, Factor VIII, are necessary before a definitive diagnosis of hemophilia A can be made. For that reason, a history of excessive bleeding must be given serious consideration, and quantitative assays of at least the three hemophilia Factors (VIII, IX, and XI) should be performed in such a patient, in addition to the screening tests, to be certain that there is no preexisting bleeding diathesis.[34, 35]

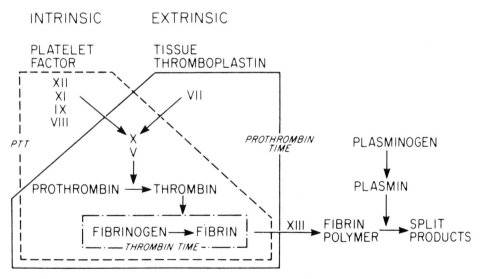

Fig. 24-6. Schematic representation of the coagulation mechanism as measured *in vitro*. Factors involved in the prothrombin time, partial thromboplastin time (PTT), and the thrombin time are noted. (Neerhout RC: Evaluation and management of surgical patients with complicating hematologic conditions. Pediatr Clin North Am 16:681–692, 1969)

ACQUIRED DEFICIENCIES IN CARDIAC SURGERY

PUMP EFFECTS

Platelets

A consistent finding in studies of hemostasis has been a decrease in the platelet count during cardiopulmonary bypass. The major portion of this decrease occurs during the first 2 to 5 minutes of bypass, and has been shown to be associated with a decrease in platelet adhesiveness.[36] This thrombocytopenia, which is the most dramatic and consistent change in hemostasis associated with cardiopulmonary bypass, may in part be caused by hemodilution.[37] However, platelet aggregation on foreign surfaces (mechanical equipment), platelet sequestration, or platelet destruction or all of these may also be factors contributing to a decrease.[38, 39] Platelets adhere to surface-bound proteins if fibrinogen or gammaglobulin are present. Earlier work, suggesting that albumin does not promote platelet adhesion, but may in fact impair platelet adhesion if the artificial surface is exposed to albumin before being exposed to plasma, has recently been confirmed in vitro.[38] Platelet counts remained stable at 95 percent of initial levels versus 18 percent in control animals, when the extracorporeal circuit was primed with 2.5 percent albumin before institution of bypass.

de Laval and coworkers reported that ^{51}Cr-tagged platelets are sequestered in the liver of splenectonized dogs during 2 hours of bypass, and that 80 percent of the platelets return to the circulation within 2 hours after bypass is terminated.[39] The direct blood-gas interfce of film oxygenators has been shown to cause extensive damage to blood cells, platelets, proteins, and lipids. The high energy surface between gas and blood, and the necessity of constantly creating and removing this surface during the oxygenating process are the principal causes of blood alterations observed in film oxygenators. Membrane oxygenators reduce, but do not eliminate this injury. Dutton and coworkers found fewer platelet aggregate emboli produced by membrane oxygenators in humans,[40] and Hill found that changes in formed blood elements caused by contact with foreign surfaces was reduced.[41] This reduction in blood trauma is probably the result of a reduction in surface energy at the membrane-blood interface, and also the result of providing a permanent surface that is not constantly created and removed.

In addition to the reduction in platelet count, studies have shown a change in platelet function in some patients. McKenna and coworkers, in a prospective study of hemostasis and extracorporeal circulation involving 512 patients, found inadequate surgical hemostasis to be the principal cause of excessive bleeding.[42] In the cases where there was a generalized hemostatic defect, they frequently found a qualitative platelet function defect, characterized by a decreased aggregation in response to high and low dose ADP, and decreased adhesiveness, as well as a prolonged bleeding time. This qualitative platelet defect did not correlate with length of bypass, decrease in platelet count, or concentration of circulating fibrin split products.[43]

Pharmacologic manipulation of platelets to prevent them from aggregating while on bypass is an area of promising research. Becker used dipyridamole to inhibit porcine platelets, and found increased platelets during and after bypass, as well as better platelet aggregation in response to ADP.[44] More recently prostaglandin E_1, a potent reversible platelet inhibitor, has been shown to preserve platelet function and number during bypass in monkeys.[45]

The management of patients in whom platelet quantity or quality may be contributing to excessive bleeding post-bypass requires the administration of *platelet concentrates*. However, the routine use of this blood product following open-heart surgery is both unnecessary and wasteful of a blood component in short supply.[46] In patients who have platelet counts less than 50,000 to 70,000/mm³, *and* in whom there is excessive bleeding, the use of platelet transfusion to raise the count is indicated. While the increment in platelet count per unit of platelets infused is extremely variable, an increase of 5 to 10,000 platelets/mm³ for each unit of platelet concentrated infused is a reasonable estimate.[47] Platelets stored at 22°C have been reported to survive longer after transfusion. However, platelets stored at 22°C do not function as well for the first few hours after infusion and, therefore, platelets stored at 4°C would appear to be indicated to treat patients who are bleeding because of a qualitative or quantitative platelet defect.[47]

Fibrinogen, Fibrinolysis, and DIC

Fibrinogen levels usually decrease to some degree during bypass, and this decrease is associated with an increase in fibrin split products. Together with the aforementioned decrease in platelets, this triad would suggest that at least limited DIC occurs, which may be caused by inadequate heparinization, inadequate perfusion, or other causes of DIC

(see above). Other potential causes involved in this triad may include (1) hemodilution with nonblood product primes, (2) mechanical destruction of platelets and clotting factors by the oxygenators and pumps, and (3) effects related to a primary fibrinolysis associated with cardiopulmonary bypass.

Many studies have demonstrated an *increase in fibrinolytic activity* in association with extracorporeal circulation, though not necessarily associated with pathologic bleeding, and some have advocated the use of ε-aminocaproic acid (EACA) in these cases.[48–51] Figure 24–7 illustrates where EACA acts to block plasminogen conversion to plasmin. If the case is one of primary fibrinolysis, the use of EACA is logical. However, if the case is one of secondary fibrinolysis, the use of EACA may result in a thromboembolic catastrophe.[52] *Because the incidence of primary fibrinolysis is very low, and that associated with extracorporeal circulation is infrequently associated with excessive bleeding, withholding EACA therapy is both logical and conservative.*[53]

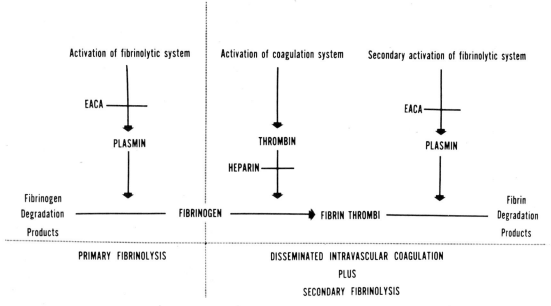

Fig. 24-7. Schematic representation of primary fibrinolysis and fibrinolysis secondary to disseminated intravascular coagulation (DIC). Although ε-aminocaproic acid (EACA) inhibits primary fibrinolysis, it also inhibits secondary fibrinolysis, one of the main defenses against DIC. (Miller RD: Complications of massive blood transfusion. Anesthesiology 39:82–93, 1973)

HEPARIN-PROTAMINE INTERACTION

The use of heparin to prevent blood from clotting on exposure to the foreign surface of the heart-lung machine is essential. Bull and coworkers clearly showed the value of individualizing heparin dosage when they demonstrated a threefold variation in patient sensitivity (i.e., the degree of prolongation of coagulation in response to a given dose of heparin) and a fourfold variation in heparin decay rates.[54] Figure 24–8 illustrates their method of administering heparin. After determining a baseline ACT, they administer a 200 unit/kg dose of heparin, and measure a second ACT to determine the patient's sensitivity. From these two points, the additional dose of heparin necessary to reach the therapeutic range is calculated and administered.[*55]

What constitutes the therapeutic range for cardiopulmonary bypass remains controversial. In long-term use of the extracorporeal membrane oxygenator (ECMO), for treatment of respiratory insufficiency, there is minimal introduction of damaged tissues or tissue juice into the circulation, and an ACT in the range of 180 to 200 seconds has proven to be a safe lower limit.[55] In routine cardiopulmonary bypass Bull and associates have found that with a manually performed ACT in excess of 300 seconds, blood does not form even small clots after the conclusion of bypass, and recommend 300 seconds as a safe lower limit. More recently, Young and coworkers advocated keeping the automated ACT above 400 seconds, using as their criteria the appearance of fibrin monomer. Monitoring the appearance of fibrin monomer was a more sensitive microscopic method for activation of the coagulation process than looking for formation of gross clots.[56] Heparin levels which prolong the ACT to greater than 300 to 400 seconds do not render the blood infinitely incoagulable, and care must be taken to ensure that heparin levels remain sufficiently elevated so that the exposure to the large foreign surface of bypass equipment does not produce life-threatening coagulation. The frequently reported rise in fibrin split products seen during cardiopulmonary bypass may be a reflection of the body's response to borderline (inadequate) heparinization or low levels of antithrombin III, resulting in minimal fibrin formation and secondarily activating fibrinolysis.

Among the factors which may effect heparin requirements, the confusion of milligrams versus units of heparin and temperature are perhaps the most common. A unit of heparin is defined as the amount required to prolong the coagulation of 1 ml whole blood for 3 minutes. Beef lung heparin contains not less than 120 units/mg. To minimize confusion, heparin doses should be expressed in terms of units, not milligrams. With respect to temperature, Cohen and coworkers have confirmed the suggestions of others that the half-life of heparin is prolonged with cooling and, in fact, with temperatures below 25°C, heparin decay is almost totally arrested.[57] For this reason, subsequent doses of heparin need not be administered as frequently, if at all, during total body hypothermia. Equally important, with rewarming, heparin levels must be monitored in some manner to ensure adequate heparin effect.

While much of the confusion surrounding heparin requirements was eliminated with demonstration of the need for individual variation of dose, protamine requirements remain a confused and controversial area. There are two principal areas of confusion. The first area deals with the failure, when giving heparin-protamine formulas, to specify how much heparin is to be neutralized: the intial dose, the initial plus any supplemental doses, the initial and supplemental, plus any heparin added to the pump prime.[58] The second area of confusion is the question of protamine's own anticoagulation properties. In vitro, protamine will retard clot formation. Following cardiopulmonary bypass

---

[*]The therapeutic range varies with the indication for heparin therapy. In minidose heparin administration for pulmonary embolus prophylaxis, no change in measurable coagulation parameters is desired. In treatment of acute thrombophlebitis or pulmonary embolism, prolongation of the aPTT to 2 to 2 1/2 times control value is desired. During cardiopulmonary bypass, considerably longer prolongation as outlined above is desired.

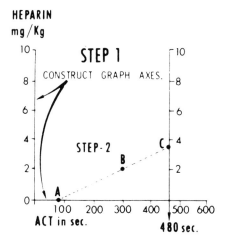

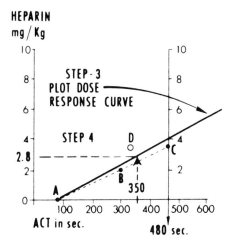

STEP 2

DETERMINE INITIAL ACT (A) AND ADMINISTER 2 mg/kg HEPARIN, THEN

MEASURE ACT (B) AND PLOT BOTH VALUES.

EXTRAPOLATE AN IMAGINARY LINE THROUGH "A" AND "B" TO INTERSECT WITH 480 second LINE TO FIND POINT "C".

EXAMPLE: 3.5 mg/kg HEPARIN IS NEEDED TO PRODUCE 480 sec. ACT OR 1.5 mg/kg IN ADDITION TO THE 2 mg/kg HEPARIN ALREADY GIVEN.

STEP 3

AFTER REQUIRED HEPARIN HAS BEEN GIVEN, MEASURE ACT, PLOT POINT "D".

IF POINT "D" DOES NOT SUPERIMPOSE ON POINT "C", THEN A DOSE RESPONSE CURVE IS DRAWN FROM "A" TO A POINT MIDWAY BETWEEN "C" AND "D".

STEP 4

AFTER 60 minutes, MEASURE THE ACT. DETERMINE AMOUNT OF HEPARIN IN PATIENT'S CIRCULATION FROM THE DOSE RESPONSE CURVE.

EXAMPLE: ASSUME AN ACT OF 350 sec.; THE HEPARIN LEVEL WOULD BE 2.8 mg/kg. TO RETURN TO 480 sec., 1.2 mg/kg OF HEPARIN IS NEEDED.

STEP 5

TO REVERSE ANTICOAGULATION, CIRCULATING HEPARIN LEVEL IS DETERMINED AS IN STEP 4. THE NEUTRALIZING DOSE OF PROTAMINE IS HEPARIN LEVEL mg/kg X 1.3.

EXAMPLE: ACT OF 325 seconds IS MEASURED. HEPARIN LEVEL IS 2.6 mg/kg, AND 3.4 mg/kg PROTAMINE IS REQUIRED.

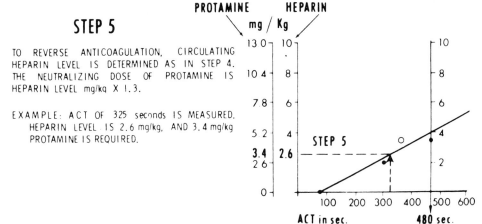

Fig. 24-8. Procedure for construction and use of a dose-response curve in heparin administration to a patient undergoing cardiopulmonary bypass surgery, utilizing the activated coagulation time (ACT). (Bull BS et al: Heparin therapy during extracorporeal circulation. J Thorac Cardiovasc Surg 69:685–689, 1975)

in patients, Guffin and coworkers have shown that using excessive doses of protamine produces increased chest bottle drainage, as well as prolonged closure time, the latter presumably being related to the increased oozing seen with excess protamine.[59] *In vitro*, protamine has been shown to impair platelet aggregation in response to ADP, and this may explain the bleeding problems seen following excessive doses of protamine.[60] Individualization of protamine doses is just as essential as individualization of heparin doses. Using a 1:1 heparin:protamine ratio based on the total dose of heparin administered to the patient, but not the pump prime, and then checking for heparin effect with either an ACT or protamine titration is an effective, conservative way of neutralizing heparin. If heparin effect is noted, additional protamine is adminstered and blood is again checked for heparin effect.

Should excessive bleeding, which is not caused by obvious inadequate surgical hemostasis, occur later in the closure, or in the ICU, blood should again be checked for heparin effect. Heparin rebound, which is defined as the recurrence of heparin effect in blood following laboratory-demonstrated adequate neutralization with protamine, has been described up to 24 hours following heparin neutralization, and is especially apt to occur in the first 4 to 6 hours after neutralization.[61] While the occurrence of heparin rebound is probably a relatively rare event in the usual clinical setting, the diagnosis is easily made by means of an ACT and a protamine titration, and specific, simple treatment with protamine is readily available.

BREAKS IN TECHNIQUE

The diagnosis of a break in technique may present a particularly difficult diagnostic problem in the first of what can become a series of cases. Diligent detective work may be necessary to identify the problem. Brooks and Bahnson reported an "epidemic of hemorrhage following cardiopulmonary bypass" in which six consecutive patients averaged 2852 ml blood loss versus an average of 562 ml for patients before and after the epidemic.

The epidemic ceased abruptly when soaking in 20 percent sodium hydroxide was added to the technique of cleaning a reusable pump oxygenator. While unable to identify precisely the etiology of the outbreak, they suggested that contamination with a sterile pyrogenic plasminogen activator may have been the cause.[62] Examples of other breaks in technique include the use of the wrong concentration of heparin and the wrong conversion factor for milligrams of heparin to units of heparin.

INADEQUATE SURGICAL HEMOSTASIS

The six *Ps* of hemostasis in patients following cardiopulmonary bypass in order of decreasing importance are: *prolene, protamine, platelets, plasma, pressure, and patience.*

If a patient has been adequately heparized during bypass to prevent consumption of coagulation factors and platelets necessary for hemostasis post-bypass, if the heparin has been adequately neutralized with protamine as measured by a protamine titration, and if a repeat coagulogram (aPTT, PT, platelet count, fibrinogen level, and bleeding time) is normal in the face of continued excessive bleeding, reexploration with the anticipation of finding a break in vascular integrity is indicated.[63, 64] The possibility of inadequate surgical hemostasis must not be ignored even when there are other reasons for abnormal hemostasis. It should be emphasized that in surgical bleeding, clots do form and may plug the chest tubes, leading to a hidden blood loss greatly in excess of the measured loss. However, even in the presence of normal coagulation tests, it is not rare for reexploration to fail to turn up a discrete bleeding vessel even in the face of moderate amounts of bleeding.

ACQUIRED DEFICIENCIES IN NONCARDIAC SURGERY

In contrast to congenital deficiencies (to be discussed later), which are usually limited to one factor, acquired deficiencies are usually multifactoral. Six common acquired deficiencies of hemostasis are caused by *(1) DIC, (2) hepatic disease, (3) massive blood transfusion, (4) anticoagulants, (5) thrombocytopenia,* and *(6) inadequate surgical hemostasis.* The fourth, in part, and the fifth and sixth deficiencies were covered in the preceding section.

DIC

DIC is a pathologic syndrome in which formation of fibrin thrombi, consumption of Factors V and VIII, loss of platelets, and activation of the fibrinolytic system suggest the presence of thrombin in the systemic circulation.[65] Just some of the potential causes of DIC were previously listed. Although coagulopathies associated with specific clinical entities such as a dead fetus or hemolytic transfusion reaction have long been recognized, appreciation of a common denominator and the term *disseminated intravascular coagulation,* are relatively recent developments. While DIC may be looked on as a "disease of medical progress" which is now being diagnosed more frequently because larger numbers of critically ill patients are surviving for longer periods, a more likely explanation is that the entity is now well-accepted and thus just being recognized more readily. The clinical findings of DIC may vary, with patients manifesting thrombotic, hemorrhagic, or mixed signs and symptoms. Furthermore, some patients with no clinical manifestations may have classic laboratory findings of DIC. This is especially true of patients who undergo surgery with cardiopulmonary bypass.

The hemorrhagic component of the DIC spectrum is readily appreciated, and has been characterized as a paradox, in that bleeding and thrombosis are occurring simultaneously, and are further complicated by another paradox in that one of the recommended forms of treatment of the hemorrhage is the administration of an anticoagulant—heparin.[66] The thrombotic component of the DIC spectrum, though obviously a necessary precursor to the hemorrhagic component, is less readily appreciated. There is no one pathognomonic laboratory test for DIC. As a practical matter, in a patient who presents with a typical clinical setting, and both

the platelet count and fibrinogen level are decreased, Hattersley has suggested that the diagnosis can be presumed until proven otherwise.[67]

Colman and Robboy have established the follwing criteria. In the absence of hepatic disease or blood transfusion, they use a screening triad of (1) PT greater than 15 seconds, (2) fibrinogen level less than 160 mg/dl, and (3) platelet count less than 150,000/mm^3. Abnormalities of all three indicate DIC. If results of two of these three tests are abnormal, then either the TT or fibrin split products must be abnormal to confirm the laboratory diagnosis of DIC.[68]

Again, the important differential diagnosis of *primary versus secondary fibrinolysis must be emphasized.* The conversion of plasminogen to plasmin, as a defense mechanism to the intravascular depositions of fibrin, will destroy fibrin or fibrinogen and Factors V and VIII. Both the consumption of platelets and coagulation factors, and the presence of fibrin split products which result from the plasmin degradation of fibrin or fibrinogen and which possess anticoagulant properties, will further aggravate the bleeding disorder. This is secondary fibrinolysis. In primary fibrinolysis, an extremely rare disorder in which the fibrinolytic system is activated wthout preexisting DIC, excessive plasminogen activator or plasmin is present and lyses clot or fibrin pathologically. Differentiation of primary from secondary fibrinolysis is vital because the treatments differ radically as outlined in the preceding section and illustrated in Figure 24–7.[66, 69–71]

DIC is never a primary disease state nor will every patient who receives, for example, an incompatible blood transfusion develop DIC. The body has several defense mechanisms which will eliminate any thrombin within the vascular tree. As mentioned previously, these include (1) rapid blood flow producing dilution of activated coagulation factors below clotting threshold levels, (2) liver and reticuloendothelial system clearance of activated coagulation factors, and (3) inhibition of thrombin produced by naturally occurring plasma proteins such as antithrombin III. Thus, in most cases of incompatible blood transfusion, the combination of rapid blood flow-dilution, hepatic-RES clearance, and naturally occurring inhibitors will prevent DIC. However, in cases of stagnant blood flow, such as shock; hepatic-RES impairment, such as hypoxemia; or where the insult is so overwhelming, such as massive transfusion of ABO-incompatible blood, DIC may develop.

The *initial treatment of DIC is not heparin.* Because DIC is never a primary disorder, the first goal of treatment should be correction of the primary disorder. This may be all that is necessary and DIC will be self-limited. However, in some patients with primary disorders such as septic shock or neoplasia, correction of the primary disorder may not be readily accomplished. While the administration of blood products sufficient to support oxygen-carrying capacity and to maintain intravascular volume is necessary in cases of continued bleeding, the infusion of fresh frozen plasma or platelet concentrates while the coagulopathy is ongoing may contribute to the bleeding by "adding fuel to the fire."[66, 72]

Heparin therapy in these patients is designed to stop clot formation and thus to inhibit the continued consumption of coagulation factors and platelets so that they can reach normal levels. Heparin doses of 40 to 80 units/kg are administered q4 to 6h, the object being to prolong the WBCT to 2 to 3 times the normal. Ideally, this should produce sufficient anticoagulation to prevent clot formation but not to produce bleeding. Monitoring heparin therapy with the WBCT is recommended instead of the aPTT because the latter is more sensitive to depleted coagulation factors and the anticoagulant effects of fibrin split products and cannot distinguish between them and the effect of heparin.[68]

Heparin therapy is by no means universally accepted in the treatment of DIC, and the decision to employ heparin is not to be taken lightly. There is some disagreement that heparin therapy at best merely replaces one cause of bleeding with another and that theoretical grounds are not sufficient to justify use of such a dangerous drug. I have been extremely reluctant to use heparin therapy in surgical patients especially in patients with severe hypofibrinogenemia (less than 50 mg/dl), an accompanying vasculitis, or local defect in the vasculature.[72]

A recent addition to the therapeutic regimen for DIC is cryoprecipitate. While this blood product was originally developed for treatment of hemophilia, a unit of cryoprecipitate contains one-third of the fibrinogen in the plasma from which it is derived. There is less risk of hepatitis with cryoprecipitate than with fibrinogen, (which is a pooled product that contains no Factor VIII). The use of cryoprecipitate will therefore increase levels of fibrinogen and Factor VIII, both of which are depressed in DIC.[67]

ANTICOAGULANTS

The two types of anticoagulants available, heparin and coumarin, are compared in Table 24-5. Heparin and its antidote, protamine, were covered in the preceding section.[73, 74]

Coumarin-like drugs inhibit production of prothrombin (Factor II) and Factors VII, IX, and X, which together are known as the prothrombin complex or vitamin K-dependent factors, while heparin inhibits the action of Factors IXa, Xa, and IIa (thrombin). Small doses of coumarin inhibit Factor VII, resulting in prolongation of the PT while the aPTT remains normal. In fact, when the PT of a patient on coumarin is in the therapeutic range because of Factor VII level depression, the prothrombin concentration is still normal. Larger doses of coumarin produce depressions of prothrombin and Factors IX and X in addition, resulting in prolongation of both PT and aPTT. Small doses of heparin inhibit Factor IXa initially, resulting in a prolonged aPTT and a normal PT. Larger doses affect Factors Xa and IIa, also resulting in a prolongation of both PT and aPTT.[74] The presence of heparin in the patient's blood can be confirmed by adding protamine to the patient's citrated plasma, and assessing whether this improves the aPTT.[75] Coumarin can also be measured in the patient's plasma, a technique especially valuable in suspected cases of surreptitious ingestion or "coumarin malingers."[73]

Surgery in patients whose blood is antico-

Table 24-5. Available Anticoagulants

	HEPARIN	COUMARIN
Route of Administration	Parenteral	Parenteral or oral
Peak Onset	Immediate	> 12 hours
Duration	< 6 hours	Up to 4–5 days
Action	Inhibit formation and action of thrombin	Depress prothrombin formation
Monitoring Test	WBCT, ACT, or aPTT	PT
Drug Interaction	Probably minimal	Maximal and variable
Antidote and onset	Protamine—immediate	Vitamin K—6 hours (with normal hepatic function) Plasma—immediate

agulated remains controversial. While the continuation of anticoagulants except for surgery of the eye, central nervous system, or large raw surfaces such as the liver bed has been advocated,[74] others recommend discontinuing anticoagulants for 12 hours. This can be accomplished by rapid reversal with parenteral vitamin K during the 24 hours prior to surgery if hepatic function is normal, and by beginning intravenous heparin 12 hours after operation.[76] In the event that reversal of the anticoagulant is elected, there is only one agent available to antagonize heparin. That agent is protamine, whose effect is immediate, and has been discussed previously.

Transfusion of blood or plasma, and vitamin K, are the two methods available to antagonize coumarin. While transfusion produces immediate results, there is no formula available to predict the volume of blood or plasma required because the degree of depression of the patient's coagulation factors for a given prothrombin time and the level of coagulation factors present in each unit of blood of plasma are extremely variable. Because the four vitamin K-dependent factors (II, VII, IX, and X) are all present in banked blood, fresh whole blood or fresh frozen plasma are not necessary. Vitamin K is the specific antidote for coumarin, but will take at least 3 to 6 hours for an effect in patients with normal liver function. Patients scheduled for open-heart surgery, particularly these with right-sided congestive heart failure (*e.g.*, patients with mitral valve disease who may well be on coumarin, especially if in atrial fibrillation), may not have normal hepatic function. Vitamin K_1 in doses of 2.5 to 50.0 mg, should be given orally or

parenterally depending on severity. Response to therapy should be monitored with serial prothrombin times to ensure a satisfactory response. Because the action of coumarin may last 4 to 5 days, it is advisable to follow the prothrombin time daily for that period. Concentrates of the prothrombin complex are no longer recommended as an antidote for coumarin because, as a pooled product, they have a high risk of hepatitis and also contain thrombogenic material or activated clotting factors which may initiate DIC.[73, 74]

LIVER DISEASE

Liver disease may produce bleeding because of defects in production of coagulation factors, thrombocytopenia on the basis of hypersplenism, excessive fibrinolysis, or on a mechanical basis as with esophageal varices. *In addition to the depression of the four vitamin K-dependent factors in the prothrombin complex, liver disease results in decreased production of Factors V and XI.* Therefore, vitamin K therapy alone, even in massive doses, will not correct the deficiency. Slight improvement following parental vitamin K may be seen because of malabsorption of vitamin K caused by lack of bile salts. This degree of improvement can be achieved with usual doses. Any improvement seen during vitamin K therapy results from improvement in the underlying liver pathology rather than from the administration of the vitamin *per se*.[77]

To distinguish between a bleeding disorder caused by vitamin K deficiency only and one resulting from advanced liver disease, a comparison of the PT of the patient's plasma mixed with fresh normal plasma (containing Factor V) and aged normal plasma (Factor V deficient), is performed. Correction of a prolonged PT with the fresh normal plasma only indicates the prolonged PT is caused by more than just a deficiency of the vitamin K-dependent factors. Alternatively, a therapeutic trial with vitamin K and measuring the PT response is performed. Improvement would suggest that the patient has mild liver disease because the four vitamin K-dependent factors are the first affected in liver disease or a deficiency of vitamin K resulting from malabsorption, inadequate diet, or coumarin administration.[78]

One iatrogenic cause of bleeding which may be seen in critical care patients is the *intestinal sterilization syndrome.* The intestinal flora are a major source of vitamin K in humans. Patients who have their gastrointestinal tracts sterilized with large doses of antibiotic preoperatively lose this source of vitamin K. If they are maintained on intravenous fluids or receive a restricted diet without vitamin K-containing foods, their vitamin K stores will be depleted in approximately one week. This syndrome is easily diagnosed on the basis of history, the finding of an isolated prolonged PT, and the prompt response to vitamin K administration.[78]

MASSIVE BLOOD TRANSFUSION

Factors V and VIII and platelets may be deficient in stored blood. The factor levels decrease 50 to 80 percent after 21 days of storage. However, the remaining levels, 20 to 50 percent, are well above the minimal hemostatic level for Factor V and usually for Factor VIII as outlined in Table 24-2. Thus, deficiencies of these two factors are rarely a primary cause of bleeding. An abnormal aPTT may suggest a deficiency of Factors V and VIII.[79, 80]

In contrast, the hemostatic effectiveness of stored platelets rapidly decays over 48 to 72 hours. In what amounted to a bioassay that clearly demonstrated this, Miller and coworkers infused 500 to 1000 ml of fresh frozen plasma (which contains Factors V and VIII but no platelets) into combat casualties who

were bleeding after receiving more than 20 units of blood.[81] They demonstrated return to normal of the activated partial thromboplastin and prothrombin times without correction of the bleeding disorders. Subsequent administration of fresh whole blood resulted in correction of these bleeding disorders.[81] Thus, dilutional thrombocytopenia can be corrected with either platelet concentrates or fresh whole blood or both. When dilutional thrombocytopenia is the cause of a bleeding disorder, deficiencies of Factor V and VIII, which are insufficient to produce bleeding on their own, may possibly aggravate the bleeding.

Rapid infusion of citrated blood will decrease ionized calcium. This decrease is transient and rapidly reversed as the infused citrate is metabolized. While there have been isolated case reports of bleeding as a result of depression of ionized calcium, most authorities agree that bleeding caused by ionized calcium depression is most unlikely. The myocardial depressant effects of a decrease in ionized calcium obviously occur long before the effects on the coagulation mechanism. Because the myocardial depression is treated with calcium chloride, the coagulation effects are not seen. Nevertheless, disorders of hemostasis remain one of the persistent problems in the area of massive transfusion. During acute massive hemorrhage, separating continued bleeding resulting from the precipitating cause from that caused by massive blood transfusion is always difficult. Clearly, the greatest problem in massive transfusion is logistical: having an adequate volume of compatible blood and blood products available at the right time.

CONGENITAL DEFICIENCIES

GENERAL PRINCIPLES OF TREATMENT

Historically, the existence of a given factor deficiency was first suspected from the clinical picture presented by a given patient. Factor VIII deficiency, classic hemophilia A, is the factor for which the kinetics of replacement therapy have been worked out best. The eight variables which will influence specific replacement of any factor are listed below.

1. Size of patient
2. Initial level of deficient factor
3. Hemostatic level of deficient factor
4. Potency of preparation
5. Extravascular distribution
6. Half-life
7. Metabolic rate
8. Magnitude of proposed surgical procedure

When a deficient factor is infused into a patient, the volume required depends on patient size, desired increment in level of deficient factor, and preparation potency. The *in vivo* survival of the transfused factor exhibits a characteristic double exponential curve, in which the early rapid disappearance represents equilibration with the extravascular space. The later slower disappearance represents the natural degradation, which is accelerated in febrile patients or in the presence of infection. Higher levels are required for longer periods of time, for example when a patient is going to have a major orthopedic procedure, rather than for dental extractions. The volume of deficient factor infused must take into consideration these eight variables to insure that the level remains above the minimal hemostatic level at all times. To accomplish this, the initial level produced is commonly considerably in excess of the minimal level sufficient to permit partial saturation of the extravascular stores, and to allow for intravascular decay with a reasonable booster schedule. Table 24-2 lists the therapeutic agents and commmonly accepted schedules of administration for the various coagulation factor deficiencies.[82, 83]

The effect of these eight variables may best be illustrated by the schedule of Factor VIII administration in a patient with hemophilia A. A 10 percent Factor VIII level will prevent spontaneous bleeding; 20 percent is necessary to ensure hemostasis in response to trauma; and a greater than 30 percent level is necessary to secure hemostasis following

major surgery. To ensure that Factor VIII levels do not decrease below 30 percent, it is common to infuse sufficent Factor VIII to raise the level to 80 to 100 percent and then give booster doses q12h. To calculate the dose of Factor VIII required, the following equation is used:

$$\text{Bags of cryoprecipitate} = (\% \text{ Factor VIII} \uparrow) (0.0001)(\text{Plasma Vol})$$

Where % Factor VIII ↑ is the difference between the patient's desired and present levels of Factor VIII, and 0.0001 is the conversion factor from % to units and from units to bags.

After the initial infusion, and a measure of Factor VIII levels has established that a satisfactory response was achieved, the patient should have a normal aPTT. The aPTT may then be measured serially following subsequent Factor VIII infusions, to be sure that the response remains satisfactory.

SPECIFIC FACTOR DEFICIENCIES

Factor I (hypo- or afibrinogenemia) deficiency is an extremely rare disorder which is transmitted by an autosomal recessive gene. This disorder may be even more rare than reported because some of the reported patients are suspected to have had DIC because of an associated reduction in platelet count. Severity is determined by the fibrinogen level, with those who are afibrinogenemic having the onset of bleeding starting with neonatal umbilical hemorrhage. Such severe cases rarely survive childhood.[84]

Factor II (hypoprothrombinemia) is a rare cause of prolonged PT. For isolated Factor II deficiency to cause a prolonged PT, the prothrombin concentration must be below 20 percent. Treatment is relatively easy with plasma in view of the long half-life of prothrombin.

Factor V (parahemophilia) deficiency, when first described in 1944, was the first new coagulation factor in 40 years since Morawitz's classic two stage theory of coagulation. Factor V is unstable on storage and, along with Factor VIII, requires fresh or frozen plasma for treatment. The disorder usually manifests itself in childhood and can be treated with plasma administered daily.

Factor VII. (pseudohemophilia) is the only coagulation factor whose deficiency is characterized by an abnormal PT and normal aPTT. Its clinical course varies from a very mild hemorrhagic, purpuric condition to severe bleeding. Treatment with plasma promptly corrects the deficiency.

Factor X deficiency produces a mild deficiency very clinically similar to that of Factor VII. Mucosal bleeding and hemarthrosis may occur later in life.

Factor XII deficiency is a laboratory curiosity. Despite markedly prolonged clotting *in vitro,* this deficiency does not affect clotting *in vivo.*

Factors VIII, IX, and XI deficiencies comprise the three hemophilias, A, B, and C. Factor XI deficiency, transmitted by a simple autosomal dominant gene, is a very mild condition which rarely produces bleeding problems except following surgery or trauma. Treatment with plasma daily readily corrects the deficiency in view of the long half-life. In contrast, Factor VIII and IX deficiencies, which are the most common deficiencies with estimated frequencies of 1:25,000 and 1:100,000 respectively, are associated with severe disabling bleeding, up to and including death.[85] Factors VIII and IX transmission are by a sex-linked recessive gene. In addition to a positive family history, these patients usually present with bleeding early in life, and this bleeding may be severe. Cryoprecipitate has been used effectively to treat hemophilia without the risk of fluid overload inherent in fresh frozen plasma.

One congenital bleeding disorder, *von Willebrand's disease,* merits special comment. When von Willebrand originally reported a familial bleeding disorder in 1926, he attributed the disorder to an abnormality of platelets and blood vessels. Subsequent investigation of the same patients 30 years later established that there was a reduction in Factor VIII levels also. Today it is agreed that a triad of prolonged bleeding time, reduced Factor VIII level, and altered platelet retention characterize the typical patient. Unfortunately, all three characteristics are not al-

ways present in each patient, nor even in the same patient all the time. This cyclical variability has resulted in confusion as to diagnosis. One pathogonomic test for von Willebrand's disease is the response to the infusion of plasma. In contrast to the patient with hemophilia whose Factor VIII level is maximal immediately after plasma or cryoprecipitate infusion, patients with von Willebrand's disease demonstrate the same immediate increase in Factor VIII levels, but then the level continues to increase for up to another 48 hours, indicating that the patient is producing Factor VIII. In other words, these patients seem to lack a factor that controls Factor VIII production, as opposed to lacking the ability to produce a rise in Factor VIII *per se.* Plasma infusion will produce an increase in Factor VIII levels, which is sustained for 20 to 30 hours. While the bleeding time will be corrected only for a few hours after infusion, clinical bleeding does not seem to be correlated with the bleeding time.

To date, successful surgery utilizing cardiopulmonary bypass has been reported in patients with deficiencies of Factors VIII and IX, as well as with von Willebrand's disease.[86-88] One measure of the magnitude of such an undertaking is that in 1972 the value of cryoprecipitate used to manage a patient with Factor VIII deficiency was over $80,000.00 for the operation. By 1981 this has escalated to well over $100,000.00.

AN APPROACH TO THE BLEEDING PATIENT

Diagnosis is directed initially toward the likely etiology, established by the clinical setting and associated pathologic abnormalities and utilizing appropriate tests of hemostasis where indicated. The tests outlined in Table 24-6 will facilitate a rapid evaluation and guide to therapy.

These tests can be performed quickly and reliably. The WBCT can be performed readily in the operating room or ICU, while blood is being transported to the laboratory for the other tests. No elaborate equipment or spe-

Table 24-6. Intraoperative Evaluations of the Patient with Hemostatic Deficiencies

TEST	COMMENT
1. Whole-blood coagulation time (WBCT) or activated coagulation time (ACT)	Can be done in OR; observe for clot retraction and lysis
2. Fibrinogen level	Depressed in DIC
3. Prothrombin time (PT)	Prolonged in hepatic disease, vitamin K deficiency, coumarin anticoagulation, DIC
4. Activated partial thromboplastin time (aPTT)	Prolonged in Factor V, VIII deficiencies (massive transfusion), the hemophilias, in the presence of heparin, or in the presence of fibrin split products
5. Platelet count	
6. Bleeding time	Platelet function

cial reagents are necessary for the WBCT, which can yield meaningful results if properly performed. The clot can then be observed for retraction (a rough measure of platelet function) or lysis. Care must be taken not to confuse the dissolution after vigorous shaking of a weak, friable clot caused by hypofibrinogenemia from true fibrinolysis. A fibrinogen level will obviously assist in making this distinction, as well as forming part of the triad of screening tests for DIC (along with the PT and platelet count). In addition to its value in screening for DIC, the PT is of value in diagnosing hepatic disease, vitamin K deficiency, or small doses of coumarin. As previously mentioned, the aPTT and PT will both be abnormal with higher doses of coumarin. Similarly, the aPTT will be prolonged with small doses of heparin, and both the PT and aPTT will be prolonged with higher doses of heparin. The bleeding time is especially valuable in these instances where the quality, rather than the quantity, of platelets is in question.

As with any laboratory determination, serial tests are of value in making a diagnosis and in assessing the response to therapy. This is especially true when initial screening test results were obtained in the preoperative or precritically ill state, and can serve as baseline values. Goal-directed therapy is dependent on accurate diagnosis. With the development of specific factor concentrates eliminating both the need for a shotgun approach with fresh frozen plasma and the danger of volume overload, the need for a spe-

cific diagnosis is essential. With the tests available today, such a specific diagnosis is almost always possible.

REFERENCES*

INTRODUCTION

1. Ellison N: Diagnosis and management of bleeding disorders. Anesthesiology 47:171–180, 1977
2. Harker LA: Hemostasis Manual. Seattle, University of Washington, 1970
3. Morrison FS: Hemorrhagic complications in surgery. In Artz and Hardy JD (eds): Management of Surgical Complications, pp 55-67. Philadelphia, WB Saunders, 1975
4. Biggs R: Human Blood Coagulation, Haemostasis, and Thrombosis. Philadelphia, FA Davis, 1972

NORMAL HEMOSTASIS

Vascular Integrity

5. MacFarlane RG (ed): Symposia Number 27 of the Zoological Society of London. The Haemostatic Mechanism in Man and Other Animals. London, Academic Press, 1970
6. Harker LA: Hemostasis Manual. Seattle, University of Washington, 1970

*At press time a new textbook on coagulation was published which provides a general source for this topic. The reader is referred to Fischbach DP, Fogdall RP: Coagulation: The Essentials. Baltimore, Williams & Wilkins, 1981

Platelets

7. Spaet T: The platelet in hemostasis. Ann NY Acad Sci 115:31–42, 1964
8. Barrer MJ, Ellison N: Platelet Function. Anesthesiology 46:202–211, 1977
9. Weiss HS: Platelet physiology and abnormalities of platelet function. N Engl J Med 293:531–541, 580–588, 1975

Coagulation Mechanism

10. MacFarlane RG: Hemorrhagic disease in surgery. Proceedings of the Royal Society of Medicine 58:25, 1964
11. Harker LA: Hemostasis Manual. Seattle, University of Washington, 1970
12. Ellison N: Diagnosis and management of bleeding disorders. Anesthesiology 47:171–180, 1977

Fibrinolysis

13. Minna JD, Robboy SJ, Colman RW: Disseminated Intravascular Coagulation, Springfield, ILL, Charles C Thomas, 1974

TESTS OF HEMOSTASIS

General

14. Bowie EJW, Thompson JH Jr., Didisheim P et al: Mayo Clinic Laboratory Manual of Hemostasis, Philadelphia, WB Saunders, 1971
15. Palermo LM, Andrews RA, Ellison N: Avoidance of heparin in contamination in coagulation studies drawn from indwelling lines. Anesth Analg (Cleve) 59:222–224, 1980
16. Erwin JC: Interpretation of laboratory tests in diagnosis of hemorrhagic disorders. Med Clin North Am 46:63–78, 1962
17. Hill JD, Dontigny L, de Laval MR et al: A simple method of heparin management during prolonged extracorporeal circulation. Ann Thorac Surg 17:129–134, 1974
18. Cohen JA, Frederickson EL, Kaplan J: Plasma heparin activity and antagonism during cardiopulmonary bypass with hypothermia. Anesth Analg (Cleve) 56:564–570, 1977
19. Jobes DR, Schwartz AJ, Ellison N et al: Monitoring heparin anticoagulation and its neutralization. Ann Thorac Surg 31:161–166, 1981
20. Bull BS, Korpman RA, Huse WM et al: Heparin therapy during extracorporeal circulation. I. Problems inherent in existing protocols. J Thorac Cardiovasc Surg 69:674–684, 1975

Tests of Platelet Function

21. Barrer MJ, Ellison N: Platelet Function. Anesthesiology 46:202–211, 1977
22. Bull BS, Korpman RA, Huse WM et al: Heparin therapy during extracorporeal circulation. I. Problems inherent in existing protocols. J Thorac Cardiovasc Surg 69:674–684, 1975
23. Levine PH: Platelet-function tests: Predictive value. New Engl J Med 292:1346–1347, 1975
24. Harker LA, Slichter SJ: The bleeding time as a screening test for evaluation of platelet function. New Engl J Med 287:155–159, 1972
25. Bowie EJW, Thompson JH Jr., Didisheim P et al: Mayo Clinic Laboratory Manual of Hemostasis, Philadelphia, WB Saunders, 1971

Tests of Coagulation Mechanism

26. Palermo LM, Andrews RA, Ellison N: Avoidance of heparin in contamination in coagulation studies drawn from indwelling lines. Anesth and Analg (Cleve) 59:222–224, 1980
27. Ellison N, Ominsky AJ, Wollman H: Is protamine a clinically important anticoagulant? A negative answer, Anesthesiology 35:621–629 1971
28. Bull BS, Korpman RA, Huse WM et al: Heparin therapy during extracorporeal circulation. I. Problems inherent in existing protocols. J Thorac Cardiovasc Surg 69:674–684, 1975
29. Jobes DR: Schwartz AJ, Ellison N et al: Monitoring heparin anticoagulation and its neutralization. Ann Thorac Surg 31:161–166, 1981
30. Ellison N, Ominsky AJ: Clinical considerations for the anesthesiologist whose patient is on autocoagulant therapy. Anesthesiology 39:328–336, 1973
31. Bowie EJW, Thompson JH Jr., Didisheim P et al: Mayo Clinic Laboratory Manual of Hemostasis, Philadelphia, WB Saunders, 1971

Tests of Fibrinolysis

32. Bowie EJW, Thompson JH Jr., Didisheim P et al: Mayo Clinic Laboratory Manual of Hemostasis, Philadelphia, WB Saunders, 1971
33. Sisson JA: Handbook of Clinical Pathology, Philadelphia, JB Lippincott Co, 1976

Routine Preoperative Evaluation

34. Ellison N: Diagnosis and management of bleeding disorders. Anesthesiology 47:171–180, 1977
35. Owen CA Jr., Bowie EJW, Didisheim P et al: The Diagnosis of Bleeding Disorders, Boston, Little, Brown and Co, 1969

ACQUIRED DEFICIENCIES IN CARDIAC SURGERY

Pump Effects

36. Salzman EW: Blood platelets and extracorporeal circulation. Transfusion 3:274–277, 1963
37. Laks H, Handin RI, Martin V et al: The effects of acute normovolemic hemodilution on coagulation and blood utilization in major surgery. J Surg Res 20: 225–231, 1976
38. Addonizio VP Jr., Macarak EJ, Nicolaou KC et al: Effects of prostacyclin and albumin on platelet loss during in vitro simulation of extracorporeal circulation. Blood, in press
39. de Laval MR, Hill JD, Mielke CH Jr et al: Blood platelets and extracorporeal circulation. Kinetic studies in dogs on cardiopulmonary bypass. J Thorac Cardiovasc Surg 69:144–154, 1975
40. Dutton RC, Edmunds LH Jr, Hutchinson JC et al: Platelet aggregate emboli produced in patients during cardiopulmonary bypass with membrane and bubble oxygenators and blood filters. J Thorac Cardiovasc Surg 67:258–265, 1974
41. Hill JD: Blood filtration during extracorporeal circulation. Ann Thorac Surg 15:313–316, 1973
42. Bachman F, McKenna R, Cole ER et al: The hemostatic mechanism after open-heart surgery. I. Studies on plasma coagulation factors after extracorporeal circulation. J Thorac Cardiovasc Surg 70:78–85, 1975
43. McKenna R, Bachman F, Whittaker B et al: The hemostatic mechanism after open-heart surgery. II. Frequency of abnormal platelet function during and after extracorporeal circulation. J Thorac Cardiovasc Surg 70:298–308, 1975
44. Becker RM, Smils ML, Dobell AR: Effect of platelet inhibition on platelet phenomena in cardiopulmonary bypass in pigs. Ann Surg 179:52–57, 1974
45. Addonizio VP Jr., Strauss JF III, Colman RW et al: Effects of prostaglandin E_1 on platelet loss during in vivo and in vitro extracorporeal circulation with a bubble oxygenator. J Thorac Cardiovasc Surg 77:119–126, 1979
46. Harding SA, Shakoor MA, Grindon AJ: Platelet support for cardiopulmonary bypass surgery. J Thorac Cardiovasc Surg 70:350–353, 1975
47. Barrer MJ, Ellison N: Platelet Function. Anesthesiology 46:202–211, 1977
48. Bick RL: Alterations of hemostasis associated with cardiopulmonary bypass: pathophysiology, prevention, diagnosis, and management. Semin Thromb Hemostas 3:59–97, 1976
49. Gans H, Castaneda AR: Problems in hemostasis during open heart surgery. VII. Changes in fibrinogen concentration during and after cardiopulmonary bypass with particular reference to the effect of heparin neutralization on fibrinogen. Arch Surg 165:551–556, 1967
50. McClure PD, Izsak J: The use of epsilon aminocaproic acid to reduce bleeding during cardiac bypass in children with congenital heart disease. Anesthesiology 40:604–608, 1974
51. Umlas J: Fibrinolysis and disseminated intravascular coagulation in open heart surgery. Transfusion 16:460–463, 1976
52. Miller RD: Problems in massive transfusion. Anesthesiology 39:82–93, 1973
53. Ellison N: Diagnosis and management of bleeding disorders. Anesthesiology 47:171–180, 1977

Heparin-Protamine Interaction

54. Bull BS, Korpman RA, Huse WM et al: Heparin therapy during extracorporeal circulation. I. Problems inherent in existing protocols. J Thorac Cardiovasc Surg 69:674–684, 1975
55. Bull BS, Huse WM, Brauer FS et al: Heparin therapy during extracorporeal circulation. II. The use of a dose-response curve to individualize heparin and protamine dosage. J Thorac Cardiovasc Surg 69:685–689, 1975
56. Young JA, Kisker CT, Doty DB: Adequate anticoagulation during cardiopulmonary bypass determined by activated clotting time and the appearance of fibin monomer. Ann Thorac Surg 26:231–240, 1978
57. Cohen JA, Frederickson EL, Kaplan J: Plasma heparin activity and antagonism during cardiopulmonary bypass with hypothermia. Anesth Analg (Cleve) 56:564–570, 1977

58. Ellison N, Ominsky AJ, Wollman H: Is protamine a clinically important anticoagulant? A negative answer. Anesthesiology 35:621–629, 1971

59. Guffin AY, Dunbar RW, Kaplan JA et al: Successful use of a reduced dose of protamine after cardiopulmonary bypass. Anesth Analg (Cleve) 55:110–113, 1976

60. Ellison N, Edmunds LH Jr, Colman RW: Platelet aggregation following heparin and protamine administration. Anesthesiology 48:65–68, 1978

61. Ellison N, Beatty CP, Blake DR et al: Heparin rebound. J Thorac Cardiovasc Surg 67:723–729, 1974

Breaks in Technique

62. Brooks DH, Bahnson HT: An outbreak of hemorrhage following cardiopulmonary bypass. J Thorac Cardiovasc Surg 61:449–452, 1972

Inadequate Surgical Hemostasis

63. Ellison N: Diagnosis and management of bleeding disorders. Anesthesiology 47:171–180, 1977

64. Bachman F, McKenna R, Cole ER et al: The hemostatic mechanism after open-heart surgery. I. Studies on plasma coagulation factors after extracorporeal circulation. J Thorac Cardiovasc Surg 70:78–85, 1975

ACQUIRED DEFICIENCIES IN NONCARDIAC SURGERY

DIC

65. Minna JD, Robboy SJ, Colman RW: Disseminated Intravascular Coagulation, Springfield, ILL, Charles C Thomas, 1974

66. Miller RD: Problems in massive transfusion. Anesthesiology 39:82–93, 1973

67. Hattersley PG, Kunkel M: Cryoprecipitates as a source of fibrinogen in treatment of disseminated intravascular coagulation. Transfusion 16:641–646, 1976

68. Colman RW & Robboy SS: Postoperative disseminated intravascular coagulation. Urol Clin North Am 3:107–112, 1974

69. Bick RL: Alterations of hemostasis associated with cardiopulmonary bypass: pathophysiology, prevention, diagnosis, and management. Semin Thromb Hemostas 3:59–97, 1976

70. McClure PD, Izsak J: The use of epsilon aminocaproic acid to reduce bleeding during cardiac bypass in children with congenital heart disease. Anesthesiology 40:604–608, 1974

71. Umlas J: Fibrinolysis and disseminated intravascular coagulation in open heart surgery. Transfusion 16:460–463, 1976

72. Ellison N: Diagnosis and mangement of bleeding disorders. Anesthesiology 47:171–180, 1977

Anticoagulants

73. Ellison N: Diagnosis and management of bleeding disorders. Anesthesiology 47:171–180, 1977

74. Ellison N, Ominsky AJ: Clinical considerations for the anesthesiologist whose patient is on autocoagulant therapy. Anesthesiology 39:328–336, 1973

75. Ellison N, Ominsky AJ, Wollman H: Is protamine a clinically important anticoagulant? A negative answer. Anesthesiology 35:621–629, 1971

76. Katholi RE, Nolan SP, McGuire LB: The management of anticoagulation during noncardiac operations in patients with prosthetic heart valves. Am Heart J 96:163–165, 1978

Liver Disease

77. Ellison N: Diagnosis and management of bleeding disorders. Anesthesiology 47:171–180, 1977

78. Owen CA Jr., Bowie EJW, Didisheim P et al: The Diagnosis of Bleeding Disorders, Boston, Little, Brown and Co, 1969

Massive Blood Transfusion

79. Bowie EJW, Thompson JH Jr., Didisheim P et al: Mayo Clinic Laboratory Manual of Hemostasis, Philadelphia, WB Saunders, 1971

80. Miller RD: Problems in massive transfusion. Anesthesiology 39:82–93, 1973

81. Miller RD, Robbins TO, Tong MJ et al: Coagulation defects associated with massive blood transfusion. Ann Surg 174:794–801, 1971

CONGENITAL DEFICIENCIES

General Principles of Treatment

82. Ellison N: Diagnosis and mangement of bleeding disorders. Anesthesiology 47:171–180, 1977
83. Britten AFH, Salzman EW: Surgery in congenital disorders of blood coagulation. Surg Gynecol Obstet 123:1333–1358, 1966

Specific Factor Deficiencies

84. Harker LA: Hemostasis Manual. Seattle, University of Washington, 1970

85. Britten AFH, Salzman EW: Surgery in congenital disorders of blood coagulation. Surg Gynecol Obstet 123:1333–1358, 1966
86. Brockman SK, Aprill SN, Robines FS: Aortic valve replacement in hemophilia. JAMA 222:660–661, 1972
87. Komp DM, Nolen SP, Carpenter SA: Open-heart surgery in patients with von Willebrand's disease. J Thorac Cardiovasc Surg 59:225–230, 1970
88. Lawson R, Pullman D, Brodeus et al: Tricuspid atresia with Christmas disease (hemophilia B). J Thorac Cardiovasc Surg 69:585–588, 1975

25

The Kidneys:
Function,
Failure, and
Protection in the
Perioperative
Period

MARK HILBERMAN

A successful outcome following cardiac surgery is dependent upon skillful management of the patient during anesthesia and cardiopulmonary bypass, successful operative repair, and the avoidance of major complications during the perioperative period. In this chapter, we briefly review renal function,[1-2] the concepts and calculations useful for quantifying renal function,[3-4] the relationship of cardiopulmonary bypass to renal function,[5] and the evolution of acute renal failure (ARF) following cardiac surgery.[6-9] Finally, we will discuss strategies for protecting the injured kidney or lessening the risk for developing acute renal failure secondary to depressed cardiac performance.[10-16]

QUANTIFYING RENAL FUNCTION

A BRIEF REVIEW OF RENAL FUNCTION

The kidneys function to eliminate certain soluble wastes from the body, and to maintain sodium, water, potassium, chloride, and acid base balance.[17-20] These basic tasks begin in the glomeruli where a protein-free ultrafiltrate of plasma is formed. The glomerular filtration rate (GFR) is determined by a Starling equilibrium:

$$GFR = K \times (\Delta P_{hydraulic} - \Delta P_{oncotic}) \quad (1)$$

where K is the glomerular permeability coefficient, $\Delta P_{hydraulic}$ represents the hydraulic pressure drop across the glomerular capillary wall (the difference between the blood pressure within the glomerular capillary and hydraulic—hydrostatic—pressure of the ultrafiltrate in Bowman's space, and $\Delta P_{oncotic}$ represents the oncotic pressure drop across the capillary wall. Equation (1) simplifies a dynamic relationship: as blood flows down the glomerular capillary, fluid is progressively lost by the formation of glomerular ultrafiltrate. With hemoconcentration, the oncotic pressure increases; ultrafiltration ceases as soon as $\Delta P_{hydraulic}$ and $\Delta P_{oncotic}$ are equal.[21] Elevation of $\Delta P_{oncotic}$ following administra-

tion of hyperoncotic serum albumin can diminish glomerular filtration.

Once the glomerular ultrafiltrate is formed, its contents are reshaped by the complex processes of tubular resorption of electrolytes and bicarbonate, the secretion of hydrogen ion, and variable tubular water permeability. Urinary concentrating ability depends upon intact tubular function, medullary blood flow, and the glomerular filtration rate. Normally these mechanisms achieve an enormous resorption of water and electrolytes: the volume of urine entering the bladder is approximately one percent of that entering Bowman's space.

The anesthesiologist and surgeon commonly encounter a depression of renal function related to renal hypoperfusion. Renal hypoperfusion causes a fall in the glomerular filtration rate, and, if not corrected, may lead to ARF. When the glomerular filtration rate is stable, the serum blood urea nitrogen (BUN) or serum creatinine provide useful information about the glomerular filtration rate. When acute changes in glomerular filtration rate occur however, these values take many days to reach equilibrium. Furthermore, oliguric renal failure in the postoperative period is associated with a rate of rise of serum BUN of 25 to 30 mg/dl/day.[22] In nonoliguric renal failure the rate for rise for BUN and creatinine averages 8 and 0.2 mg/dl/day, respectively with urine flows > 1 ml/min.[23] In addition to routine measurements (urinalysis, BUN, and creatinine), more detailed physiologic measurements are essential for monitoring potentially compromised renal function.

URINE FLOW

This basic measurement is the only one available immediately, and frequently must be used as a guide to the adequacy of fluid replacement. The frequent use of potent diuretics and the emergence of nonoliguric renal failure as the dominant form of renal failure[23, 24] necessitate additional measurements.

CLEARANCES

A clearance is a measurement of the rate of removal of a substance from the blood. Clearances of substances with special biologic properties provide important physiologic information.[25] The amount of the substance (x) which appears in the urine is equal to its clearance multiplied by its plasma concentration:

$$C_x \times P_x = U_x \times \dot{V} \tag{2}$$

where C is the clearance in ml/min, P the plasma concentration in mg/dl (or mosm/1), U the urinary concentration in the same units, and V the urine flow in ml/min. Rearranging,

$$C_x \text{ ml/min} = \frac{U_x \text{ mg/dl}}{P_x \text{ mg/dl}} \times \dot{V} \text{ ml/min} \tag{3}$$

The clearances of inulin or creatinine are used for estimation of the GFR, and the clearance of paraaminohippurate is used to measure the effective renal plasma flow. Clearances are normalized to average body surface area. A glomerular filtration rate of 130 ml/min/1.73m², normal in a young adult, falls to approximtely 100 ml/min/1.73m² at the age of 60, and 80 ml/min/1.73m² at the age of 80.[26]

ELECTROLYTE EXCRETION

Usually the stress of trauma or surgery results in sodium retention by the kidney. Patients with depressed cardiac function also exhibit sodium retention. The fractional excretion of sodium (FE_{Na}) is the best measurement of the ability of the renal tubule to conserve sodium,[27, 28] may be calculated from the clearances of sodium (C_{Na}) and creatinine (C_{cr}) or inulin:

$$\begin{aligned} FE_{Na} \% &= \frac{C_{Na}}{C_{Cr}} \times 100 \tag{4} \\ &= \frac{U_{Na} \times P_{Cr}}{U_{Cr} \times P_{Na}} \times 100 \end{aligned}$$

The fractional excretion of potassium is calculated in a similar fashion, and may be even more useful (see below). Diuretics markedly alter sodium excretion; their administration should be avoided for 4 hours before and during urine collection. The fractional excretion of sodium is usually less than 1 percent in the postoperative period, although during periods of sodium mobilization, higher values may be encountered.

URINARY CONCENTRATING ABILITY

The ability to concentrate or dilute urine is another characteristic of the normal kidney, which is lost when renal failure occurs. Concentrating ability is conveniently measured by the ratio of the urine: plasma osmolality. As with fractional electrolyte excretions, there are no absolute normal values; however, the postoperative patient normally retains salt and water, the urine is concentrated, and the urine: plasma osmolality ratio is greater than 1. Loss of concentrating, or diluting ability, is reflected by urine: plasma osmolality ratio fixed at 1.0 ± 0.1 (isosthenuria).

COMMENTS ON PERFORMING RENAL FUNCTION MEASUREMENTS

These critical measurements of renal function may be calculated by determining creatinine, sodium, potassium, and osmolality concentrations in a carefully timed, collected, and and measured urine specimen, and a simultaneous blood sample. Preoperative clearance measurements are warranted in patients with elevated BUNs or anticipated postoperative hemodynamic or renal problems. Twelve- to twenty-four-hour urine collections should be employed in patients without bladder catheters in place. However, note that urine flow ($\dot{V}$ in equation 3) is expressed in ml/min; 24-hour urine collections are not necessary. In catheterized postoperative patients, we prefer a 2-hour collection (lengthened to obtain a minimum urine volume of 100 ml, when necessary). At the start and end of the collection period, the bladder is emptied by manual compression, and all the tubing from an indwelling Foley catheter is drained of urine.

Intravenous pyelography, aortography,

and renal scans are valuable diagnostic tools which may be needed in the perioperative period, particularly when unilateral renal dysfunction is suspected, or previous renal or abdominal aortic surgery has been performed.

HEMODYNAMIC FUNCTION

Whenever more than transient difficulty is encountered (or anticipated) in restoring or maintaining normal circulatory and renal function in the surgical patient, intensive hemodynamic monitoring is essential. If renal dysfunction persists in the face of a normal or elevated central venous pressure (CVP) or if significant cardiac dysfunction exists, then a Swan–Ganz catheter should be used. The mean arterial pressure the CVP, the pulmonary capillary wedge (PCW) or pulmonary artery diastolic pressure, and careful cardiac output measurement all provide important information. Cardiac output should be normalized to cardiac index (CI) by dividing by the patient's body surface area (on admission). The left ventricular stroke work index is a useful measurement of myocardial function,[29, 30] which is particularly useful in monitoring patients with compromised cardiac function.[31, 32]

$$\text{LVSWI gm-m/m}^2 = \frac{\text{CI}}{\text{HR}} \times (\text{MAP} - \text{PCW}) \times 0.0136 \quad (5)$$

where *HR* is heart rate, in beats/min and pressures are measured in torr. (Approximate normal values are 2.8–4.2 l/min/m² for cardiac index and 30–110 g-m/m² for left ventricular stroke work index.) Normalized systemic and pulmonary vascular resistances may also be calculated:

$$\text{Systemic vascular resistance index} = \frac{\text{MAP} - \text{CVP}}{\text{CI}} \quad (6)$$

$$\text{Pulmonary vascular resistance index} = \frac{\text{PAM} - \text{PCW}}{\text{CI}} \quad (7)$$

where *PAM* is pulmonary artery mean pressure. The results may be left in Wood units (normal values are < 40 and < 7, respectively), or converted to the more usual dynes·sec·cm^{-5} by multiplying by 80. He-modynamic monitoring has been discussed in more detail in other chapters.

CARDIOPULMONARY BYPASS AND RENAL FUNCTION

Postoperative renal failure has been attributed primarily to the effects of cardiopulmonary bypass,[33–35] to postoperative cardiac dysfunction,[35–40] and to both.[41–43] While renal function has been shown to be severely depressed during cardiopulmonary bypass in humans, it appears to recover rapidly with restoration of cardiac function following bypass.[44, 45] Low flow, low pressure bypass is in use at Stanford University Medical Center, primarily to permit optimal hypothermic myocardial preservation (see Chap. 26). The magnitude and duration of systemic hypoperfusion which, with hemodilution, hypothermia, anesthesia, diuretics, and a hyperoncotic cardiopulmonary bypass priming solution, may be followed by return of normal postoperative renal function, has not been well defined. Hypothermia and hemodilution appear to provide important protection for the kidney, and are discussed in general terms elsewhere in this book (see Chaps. 14 and 26).

In 1960, Senning and coworkers reported a series of dog experiments which compared the renal effects of high-flow (100 ml/kg/min) to low-flow (40 ml/kg/min) bypass.[46] Nonpulsatile perfusion with a whole blood priming solution was used. Significant depression of renal function was evident in both flow groups, although it was more profound during low-flow bypass. The rate of recovery of renal function was not measured.

In another series of dog experiments, Jacobs and coworkers maintained bypass for 4 to 8 hours, and compared the effects of nonpulsatile and pulsatile perfusion on renal function.[47] A whole blood priming solution was used; bypass flow and arterial pressure were similar in the two groups. During pulsatile perfusion, peripheral resistance, serum lactate and urine flow remained near control levels, while creatinine clearance decreased to approximately 60 percent of control at the end of 4 hours. During nonpulsatile perfusion, a progressive rise in peripheral resistance and serum lactate was accompanied by a progressive decline in urine flow, and creatinine clearance fell below 25 percent of control at the end of 4 hours. Again, the recovery of renal function following bypass was not studied.

In general, renal functional data, which permit comparison between perfusion techniques are sparse. Furthermore, while pulsatile perfusion appears superior to nonpulsatile perfusion,[48-54] renal functional recovery following nonpulsatile perfusion is rapid when normal hemodynamics are restored.

THE DEVELOPMENT OF ACUTE RENAL FAILURE FOLLOWING CARDIAC OPERATION

Incidence, risk factor, pathophysiologic, and clinical data relating to the development of postoperative ARF in the patients at Stanford have been published.[55] These data permitted the following conclusions. Low-flow, low-pressure bypass usually provides satisfactory preservation of renal function during operative procedures. Severe depression of postoperative cardiac function with resultant renal ischemia is the critical common denominator present in patients who develop ARF. Finally, the pathogenesis of ARF is generally multifactorial, dependent upon superposition of additional insults upon ischemic kidneys.

INCIDENCE DATA AND RISK FACTOR ANALYSIS

These data are summarized in Columns 1 and 2 of Table 25–1. Two hundred and four patients underwent cardiac operation; one hundred and ninety-four patients were designated controls because they did not demonstrate postoperative renal dysfunction (5 patients) or acute renal failure (5 patients).

See Column 1. The incidence of ARF (2.5 %) was lower than previously reported.[56-63] Patients who developed acute renal failure or exhibited postoperative renal dysfunction were older, had a higher incidence of prior cardiac operation and active bacterial endocarditis, a higher average preoperative BUN, and a lower incidence of coronary artery bypass grafting as the sole cardiac surgical procedure than did the control population. Preoperative left ventricular dysfunction was greater in patients who developed postoperative renal dysfunction/failure. Presumably depressed preoperative left ventricular function presaged depressed postoperative left ventricular function, a critically important feature in the development of postoperative renal failure.[64-69] Fifty percent of the patients with impaired renal function died; by contrast, the mortality rate was below one percent in the control group.

THE ROLE OF CARDIOPULMONARY BYPASS

Of the bypass variables measured, mean arterial pressure did not appear important in determining renal outcome. However, the average duration of bypass was strikingly prolonged in the renal dysfunction/failure population, as has been reported a risk by others.[70-74] This reflects both a deleterious effect of prolonged bypass and an association between complex surgical procedures and depression of postoperative cardiac performance. The predictive importance of a history of prior cardiac operations, active bacterial endocarditis, and the lower incidence of coronary bypass operations also reflect this latter association.

Renal function was measured early in the postoperative period in patients with normal renal function. In prior studies, with apparently comparable patients, the postoperative glomerular filtration rate was depressed to 65 ml/min/1.73m^2,[75-77] and effective renal plasma flow was depressed to 220 to 300 ml/min/1.73m^2,[78-82], compared to 98 ± 30 and 382 ± 94 ml/min/1.73m^2, respectively, in this study.[83] Many differences in operative and

Table 25-1. Risk Factors Antecedent to ARF Following Cardiac Surgery

		1 6-MONTH CONTROL PERIOD Normal Controls	2 6-MONTH CONTROL PERIOD Renal Dysfunction/ ARF	3 18-MONTH STUDY PERIOD All Patients with Renal Dysfunction/ ARF
Number		194	10	32
Age	(Yr)	57 ± 12	62 ± 20	$64 \pm 13^*$
History of prior cardiac operation	(%)	7	20%	31%*
Active bacterial endocarditis	(%)	0.6	29%	26%*
Admission BUN	(mg/dl)	19 ± 8	34 ± 23	32 ± 20
Coronary, artery surgery only	(%)	52	20*	6*
Preoperative cardiac status				
Pulmonary capillary wedge pressure	(torr)	16 ± 9	$25 \pm 5^*$	$25 \pm 10^*$
Left ventricular end-diastolic pressure	(torr)	16 ± 7	24 ± 9	19 ± 9
Cardiac index	(l/min-m²)	$2.5 \pm .7$	$2.4 \pm .9$	$2.25 \pm .8$
Left ventricular dysfunction score	(0–9)	1.5 ± 2.3	$4.9 \pm 4^*$	$5.7 \pm 3.4^*$
Cardiopulmonary bypass data				
Flow	(ml/kg-min)	42 ± 7	$54 \pm 6^*$	$50 \pm 7^*$
Mean arterial pressure	(torr)	49 ± 7	49 ± 8	50 ± 8
Low mean arterial pressure	(min)	35 ± 19	33 ± 7	34 ± 7
Duration	(min)	110 ± 40	$156 \pm 46^*$	$159 \pm 62^*$
Aortic cross-clamp time	(min)	60 ± 22	73 ± 37	75 ± 31
Deaths	(%)	0.6%	60%*	50%*

Selected data related to the development and outcome of RD/ARF. These data illustrate important risk factor and CPB variables and are shown as mean ± SD, except when expressed as percentages. Asterisk (*) indicates data significantly different from controls in column 1 ($p < 0.05$). Columns 1 and 2 contain data from a 6-month control period; column 1 summarizes data from 194 patients who did not have renal failure or documented renal dysfunction, and column 2 summarizes data from the five patients who developed ARF and five additional patients from the control period who had detailed studies indicating severe renal dysfunction. Column 3 combines data from 29 RD/ARF patients studied in detail over an 18-month period, with three control period RD/ARF patients who were not studied in detail. This was done to provide a better sample for risk factor analysis.
(Hilberman M, Myers BD, Carrie BJ et al: Acute renal failure following cardiac surgery. J Thorac Cardiovasc Surg 77:880–889, 1979)

postoperative management preclude attributing the superior early postoperative renal function observed in these patients to low-flow, low-pressure cardiopulmonary bypass. Nevertheless, the data indicate that the emphasis placed upon maintenance of high bypass pressures and flows to preserve renal function cannot be universally substantiated.

CLINICAL EVENTS LEADING TO ACUTE RENAL FAILURE

Detailed correlation of physiologic and clinical data in 17 ARF patients led to the definition of four groups of patients: those in whom (A) ARF developed in the immediate preoperative or operative period; (B) ARF resulted from a progressive low cardiac output syndrome; (C) ARF followed withdrawal of mechanical or pharmacologic circulatory support; and, (D) ARF developed secondary to discrete hypotensive insult(s).[84]

Group A (4 patients, 1 survivor)

One septuagenarian had severe cardiac and renal dysfunction, and became anuric following preoperative angiography. The other three had preoperative septicemia. One of these patients sustained a cardiac arrest preoperatively and ARF ensued. Another developed renal dysfunction following preoperative streptomycin therapy, and ARF followed more than 5 hours of bypass. The fourth patient was moribund and in ARF at the time of operation, but demonstrated a dramatic recovery beginning on postoperative day 4.

Group B (3 patients, no survivors)

These patients evidenced a severe low-output syndrome which did not respond to therapy. In one, autopsy demonstrated that an acute aortic dissection from the site of intra-aortic balloon pump support insertion had occluded the renal arteries and complicated an already established renal dysfunction associated with extremely depressed cardiac function. In the second patient, a 3-hour bypass run and prophylactic gentamicin therapy added to the effects of extreme cardiac depression to cause ARF. In the third patient, a sustained low cardiac output state, following an extensive left ventricular aneurysmectomy, was the evident proximate cause of ARF.

Group C (7 patients, 3 survivors)

These seven patients appeared to progress to ARF following withdrawal of circulatory support and subsequent further hemodynamic depression. ARF developed on postoperative days 1, 4, 6, 7, 8, and 11. Two patients had low glomerular filtration rates and progressive azotemia, and were initially categorized in group B. In both, however, a glomerular filtration rate previously stable in the range of 20 to 30 ml/min/1.73m^2 decreased an additional 30 to 50 percent following removal of the intra-aortic balloon pump, at which time the fraction excretion of sodium also rose (initially less than 0.2%, increased to > 2%). One patient maintained mildly depressed renal function until withdrawal of intra-aortic balloon pump support was initiated, at which time ARF developed. One patient evidenced a drop in glomerular filtration rate to 17 ml/min/1.73m^2 on postoperative day 2, at which time the fractional sodium excretion was 0.05 percent. This patient's mean arterial pressure was increased by the addition of an epinephrine infusion at 22 ng/kg/min, and over the next 3 days the glomerular filtration rate increased steadily to 50 ml/min/1.73m^2. Following removal of the intra-aortic balloon pump, this patient sustained a cardiac arrest, and over the subsequent 48 hours developed ARF. Another patient had both septicemia and gentamicin therapy superimposed on withdrawal of circulatory support, with subsequent development of ARF. Still another patient who developed ARF following withdrawal of intra-aortic balloon pump recovered from his initial ARF, but demonstrated a secondary depression of renal function concurrent with gentamicin administration. One patient with preoperative renal dysfunction and severe left ventricular failure, underwent an uncomplicated operation, but ARF followed early withdrawal of inotropic support.

Group D (3 patients, 2 survivors)

These three patients had major hypotensive crises before the development of ARF. One patient sustained hypotension and oliguria for several hours before diagnosis and treatment of a silent hemorrhage into the left pleural space. This episode, late on postoperative day 2, was followed by ARF. The second patient developed dehiscence of the ventriculotomy suture line following left ventricular aneurysmectomy. After resuscitation and repair, the patient appeared to possess adequate renal function. Over the next two days, ARF developed in association with continued depression of hemodynamic status and concomitant high-dose epinephrine infusions. This episode of ARF resolved, but secondary and tertiary depressions of renal function followed gentamicin administration and recurrent sepsis, respectively. The last patient had recurrent bleeding, with two periods of hypovolemia and oliguria, following aortic and mitral valve replacement, tricuspid valvular annuloplasty, and reconstruction of the aortic root. The prolonged surgical procedure and two hypotensive insults seem sufficient to explain the subsequent ARF.

PATHOPHYSIOLOGICAL CHANGES CHARACTERIZING THE DEVELOPMENT OF ACUTE RENAL FAILURE

To define the sequential hemodynamic and renal function changes characteristic of the development of ARF, patients were classified by their lowest postoperation glomerular filtration rate.* Seven ARF patients were iden-

---

*Renal dysfunction was defined by a glomerular filtration rate between 20 ml/min/1.73m^2 and 1/2 the age adjusted normal value.[86] ARF was defined by a glomerular filtration rate below 15 ml/min/1.73m^2.

tified who, when studied within 24 hours of operation, demonstrated renal dysfunction, and then progressed to renal failure. In addition, seven renal dysfunction patients were identified who had complete physiologic data obtained at comparable times in the postoperative period. These 14 patients underwent complex surgical procedures, as evidenced by the operations performed, the prolongation of bypass duration, and the reduced survival (Table 25–2). Only one of the seven ARF patients survived, while all seven of the renal dysfunction patients survived.

The renal dysfunction patients demonstrated a significant, progressive increase in cardiac index and left ventricular stroke work

Table 25-2. Clinical Characteristics of ARF and Renal Dysfunction Patients*

AGE (YEARS)	DURATION OF CPB (MIN)	OPERATION	COMMENTS	OUTCOME
ARF Patients				
60	336	AVR, MVR, TAN, IABP	Prolonged CPB, low-output syndrome contributed to ARF, which developed following IABP removal (POD 7)	Died
69	213	CABG × 3, LVA (extensive) IABP	Prolonged low-output syndrome; ARF developed following IABP removal (POD 7)	Died
57	220	MVR (Reop), TVR, IABP	Only moderate depression of cardiac function; prolonged CPB, gentamicin therapy contributed to ARF (POD 3)	Lived
50	190	LVA; Reop LVA following PO rupture, IABP	High-dose catecholamine therapy, low-output syndrome and hypotensive crisis contributed to ARF (POD 4)	Died
62	187	CABG × 2, LVA × 2, MVR, IABP (transthoracic)	Prolonged CPB, low-output syndrome, gentamicin therapy contributed to ARF (POD 3)	Died
63	265	MVR, TAN, TVR, IABP	Low-output syndrome, high-dose catecholamine therapy contributed to ARF (POD 6); IABP support until death.	Died
75 62 ± 8	153 223 ± 60	LVA, IABP	Prolonged low-output syndrome resulted in ARF (POD 10); IABP support until death.	Died
Renal Dysfunction Patients				
66	112	CABG × 3, MVR, IABP	Prolonged IV vasoactive drug support	Lived
63	87	Reop MVR, IABP	Prolonged IV vasoactive drug support	Lived
54	140	CABG × 2, LVA, IABP	Prolonged IV vasoactive drug support	Lived
75	206	Reop CABG × 1, AVR, IABP	Cardiac recovery by POD 5	Lived
69	150	AVR, VSD, LVA, IABP	Patient taken to surgery anuric, obtunded, on IABP following acute myocardial infarction; Steady PO improvement	Lived
65	162	MVR, AVR	Early cardiac recovery, prolonged IV vasoactive drug support	Lived
67 66 ± 6	128 141 ± 38	LVA, CABG × 1, IABP	Prolonged IV vasoactive drug support	Lived

*The postoperative day shown in parenthesis is the day on which ARF was first present. ARF = acute renal failure; AVR = aortic valve replacement; CABG = coronary artery bypass graft; CPB = cardiopulmonary bypass; IABP = intra-aortic balloon pump; IV = intravenous; LVA = left ventricular aneurysmectomy; MVR = mitral valve replacement; PO = postoperative; POD = PO day; RD = renal dysfunction; Reop = A second or subsequent cardiac operation; TAN = tricuspid valvular annuloplasty; and TVR = tricuspid valve replacement. (Hilberman M, Myers BD, Derby G et al: J Thorac Cardiovasc Surg 79:838–846, 1980)

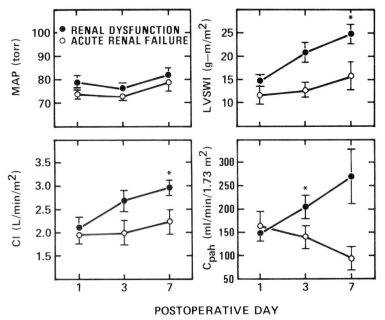

Fig. 25-1. Sequential changes in mean arterial pressure (*MAP*), cardiac index (*CI*), left ventricular stroke work index (*LVSWI*), and effective renal plasma flow (C_{pah}) in renal dysfunction and ARF patients during the first postoperative week. (Hilberman et al: J Thorac Cardiovasc Surg 79:838, 1980)

index during the first postoperative week (Fig. 25–1). This improvement was not reflected in the mean arterial pressure. Although depression of renal plasma flow was similar in the immediate postoperative period in renal dysfunction and ARF patients, renal plasma flow rose in renal dysfunction patients in parallel with hemodynamic improvement. ARF patients demonstrated similar initial depression of cardiac function, but failed to demonstrate hemodynamic improvement during the first postoperative week.

Failure of postoperative hemodynamic improvement was accompanied by postoperative renal functional deterioration in ARF patients (Figs. 25–2 and 25–3). ARF was nonoliguric and characterized by progressive azotemia and a declining glomerular filtration rate (Fig. 25–2). As a group, renal dysfunction patients showed no significant changes in these variables. A significant decline in concentrating ability was observed as ARF developed (U/P$_{osm}$ in Fig. 25–3). While on average renal dysfunction, patients retained concentrating ability, individual patients demonstrated transient isosthenuria. Both renal dysfunction and ARF patients manifested avid sodium retention in the immediate postoperative period (fractional excretion of sodium was less than 1 percent). ARF patients demonstrated a sharp increase in the fractional excretion sodium after ARF developed and a progressive rise in the fractional excretion of potassium, significant by midweek (see Fig. 25–3). Three renal dysfunction patients demonstrated elevation of FE$_{Na}$ to 3 to 6 percent during a period of weight loss and sodium excretion elevated the average fractional excretion of sodium on postoperative day 3. The average fractional excretion of potassium remained unchanged in renal dysfunction patients during the first postoperative week. Thus a fractional excretion of potassium greater than 100 percent emerged as a useful guide to acute renal failure.[85]

Progressive azotemia and oliguria remain classic criteria for ARF. However, this entity was nonoliguric in approximately 90 percent of the patients, in keeping with recent reports.[87–88] Transient oliguria was not infrequent; to maintain urine flow vasoactive drugs and diuretics were administered. In addition, aggressive intravenous crystalloid

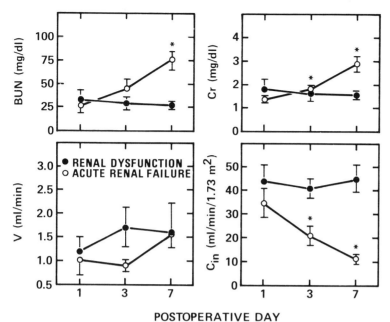

Fig. 25-2. Sequential changes in blood urea nitrogen (*BUN*), creatinine, (*Cr*), urine flow (*V*), and inulin clearance (C_{in}) in renal dysfunction and ARF patients during the first postoperative week. (Hilberman et al: J Thorac Cardiovasc Surg 79:838, 1980)

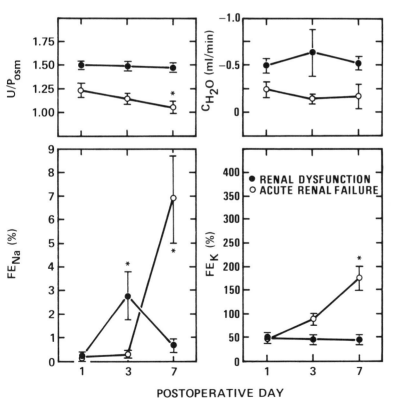

Fig. 25-3. Sequential changes in urine to plasma osmolality (U/P_{osm}), free water clearance (C_{H_2O}), fractional excretion of sodium (FE_{Na}), and fractional excretion of potassium (FE_K) in renal dysfunction and ARF patients during the first postoperative week. (Hilberman et al: J Thorac Cardiovasc Surg 79:838, 1980)

and colloid administration was used to achieve hemodynamic stability and maintain urine output, as evidenced by a weight gain of approximately 17 percent in both renal dysfunction and renal failure patients. The average rate of rise of creatinine in acute renal failure was 0.2 mg/dl/day, and BUN rose 8 mg/dl/day (compared to the BUN rise of 20–30 mg/kl/day reported previously in oliguric renal failure.[89] Both creatinine and BUN showed this slow rate of rise with a marked time delay before new plateau values were achieved. Depression of glomerular filtration rate and renal plasma flow was profound in renal dysfunction and renal failure patients in the early postoperative period. Renal failure patients demonstrated further deterioration in glomerular filtration rate which was frequently stable in renal dysfunction patients. The failure of glomerular filtration rate to improve may reflect filtration pressure dysequilibrium in these patients.

Sequential hemodynamic assessment was essential to understand the changes in renal function observed. With vigorous therapeutic support and few secondary hemodynamic insults, renal dysfunction patients recovered from postoperative cardiogenic shock, while renal failure patients did not. Cardiac index and left ventricular stroke work index were most sensitive in distinguishing the course of renal dysfunction from renal failure patients. Measurement of hemodynamic and renal function can quantify the effectiveness of mechanical or pharmacologic circulatory support. This information may help avert the progression from renal dysfunction to renal failure which appears to occur when secondary insults, which usually occurred in idiosyncratic combination, were superimposed upon extreme hemodynamic depression.

STRATEGIES FOR RENAL PROTECTION

OVERVIEW

Effective strategies for preventing or modifying ARF exist for the patient undergoing a cardiovascular operation. We would like to suggest a classification for protective regimens which the reader will find useful in analyzing this problem and developing a personalized plan for therapeutic intervention. Protection exists in two basic dimensions: bioenergetic and anaplerotic.

Bioenergetic Protection

Acute complete ischemia or chronic partial ischemia are the most common antecedents to ARF in these patients. Deprivation of oxygen or substrate supply to the tissue results in a bioenergetic deficit which may, in turn, result in tissue damage. The magnitude of the insult depends upon metabolic demand and upon the degree and duration of the ischemic insult. Bioenergetic protective regimens aim to minimize the potential supply/demand imbalance. Effective strategies include the use of hypothermia to decrease metabolic demands, rapid resuscitation following cardiac arrest or hemorrhagic hypotension, and efficient operative techniques which minimize the duration of renal ischemia. Patients with depressed cardiac performance have depressed renal blood flow which leads to renal failure directly (if sufficiently severe) or sensitizes the kidney to superimposed toxic or secondary hypoperfusion insults. Bioenergetic protection in these patients is best provided by manipulation of systemic hemodynamics using elevation of left atrial pressure, vasodilators, or inotropic agents.

Anaplerotic Protection

Anaplerosis is the repair or replacement of defective or injured parts. Tissue injury subsequent to a bioenergetic insult involves nonbioenergetic processes. That is, interruption of oxygen and substrate supply leads to depletion of high-energy phosphates, which is then followed by cell swelling, disruption of cellular membranes and organelles, abnormal uptake of calcium into mitochondria, and so on. These latter changes represent the injury process. Anaplerotic protective regimens aim to prevent these secondary changes or to permit the repair or replacement of injured cells and subcellular organelles or both, once injury has occurred. That effective anaplerotic protective regimens exist has been demonstrated most clearly with the use of diuretics to attenuate the acute renal failure which follow an ischemic insult, as detailed below. The demonstration by Siegel and coworkers[90] that postischemic infusion of adenine nucleotides and magnesium chloride into rats can attenuate the subsequent renal injury suggests that anaplerotic protective regimens can be developed that are more generally useful for organ protection than diuretics *per se.*

VASODILATORS

Sodium Nitroprusside

Sodium nitroprusside is frequently used to control hypertension or to improve systemic blood flow or both following cardiac operations.[91] Although nitroprusside causes renal vasodilatation when infused into isolated kidneys, the reported effects of nitroprusside on renal vascular resistance and blood flow in intact animals and humans have varied.[92–96] Several factors may alter the renal vascular response to nitroprusside administration. A decline in left atrial pressure may cause reflex renal vasoconstriction.[97, 98] A decline in renal perfusion pressure below the autoregulatory range will also decrease renal blood flow, despite a progressive decline in renal vascular resistance until perfusion pressure falls below 30 torr.[99–101] Renal vasodilators may abolish the autoregulation of renal blood flow;[102] once vasodilatation is maximal, renal blood flow and perfusion pressure will decline in parallel. Finally, with depression of left ventricular contractility nitroprusside is most effective in increasing cardiac output,[103] which should improve renal blood flow.[104] The previously conflicting reports of the renal effects of nitroprusside administration doubtless reflect the variable influences of these factors. As an example, Bastron and Kaloyonides reported that nitroprusside produced marked vasodilation and an increase in blood flow in the isolated prefused canine kidney;

however, in the intact animal, they found that a nitroprusside-induced reduction in arterial pressure caused a reduction in PAH clearance.[105]

A likely explanation for many of these conflicting reports lies in the failure to maintain left atrial pressure which, if allowed to decrease, may cause profound renal vasoconstriction. Kahl and coworkers reported the effects of diminished cardiac output on renal function in anesthetized dogs, using a model with two distinctively different levels of left atrial pressures. Superior vena caval obstruction decreased cardiac index, mean arterial and left atrial pressure, and resulted in profound renal vasoconstriction. Balloon inflation in the left atrium decreased cardiac index and arterial pressure, however, left atrial pressure was elevated and renal vascular resistance remained unchanged. Atrial hypotension is a potent stimulus for renal vasoconstriction,[106–108] however left atrial hypertension results in only weak renal vasodilation.[108] These reflexes can be abolished by vagotomy or by surgical denervation of the kidney.[108] In experimental animals, plasma renin activity varies inversely with atrial pressure,[107] thus humoral factors appear capable of contributing to renal vasoconstriction. Previous studies in which nitroprusside administration increased renal vascular resistance (or decreased renal blood flow) were performed under conditions likely to decrease atrial pressures to below-normal levels, however this variable was not measured.[108A–110] By contrast, in patients with congestive heart failure, left atrial pressure declined during nitroprusside infusion but remained in the high-to-normal range and renal blood flow improved significantly despite a decline in average mean arterial pressure to 72 torr (the left atrial pressure declined, but remained above normal).[111] An arterial pressure of 72 torr is similar to that in the clinical reports, which record a nitroprusside-induced decline in renal blood flow; therefore, it is doubtful that a decline in arterial pressure is the primary explanation for the discrepancies reported.

To define the effects of nitroprusside in

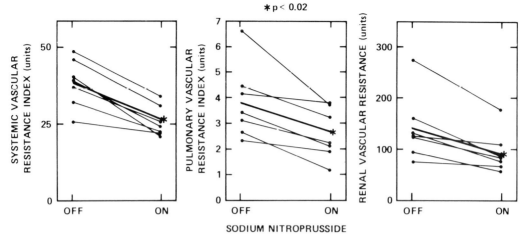

Fig. 25-4. Nitroprusside administration resulted in equivalent reduction in systemic, pulmonic, and renal vascular resistance when administered to postoperative cardiac surgical patients.

postoperative cardiac surgical patients, renal clearances and hemodynamics were measured in seven patients within 24 hours of coronary bypass grafting. Following baseline measurements (off nitroprusside), nitroprusside infusion was used to lower mean arterial pressure to 85 torr. Pulmonary wedge pressure was restored to baseline values by appropriate fluid therapy, and the measurements repeated 1 hour later. Nitroprusside administration resulted in equivalent decreases in renal (-33%), pulmonary (-29%), and systemic (-33%) vascular resistance (Fig. 25–4). Notwithstanding the decrease in arterial pressure, renal blood flow increased by 20 percent in direct proportion to the increase in cardiac index. No significant changes were observed in urine flow, sodium or potassium execution rates, and the urine:plasma osmolality ratio.[112]

Thus, in postoperative cardiac surgical patients, nitroprusside administration can be expected to improve renal blood flow, so long as left atrial hypotension is avoided, and the decline in systemic arterial pressure is not excessive. This improvement in renal blood flow achievable with nitroprusside may be critical for patients in whom severe depression of renal blood flow may occur as an antecedent to acute renal failure.

Convertive Enzyme Inhibition

Captopril has been recently reported to improve systemic and renal hemodynamics in patients with severe congestive heart failure.[113] The agent appears most effective in patients with high plasma renin levels, where its blockade or angiotensin formation and subsequent release of aldosterone appear important in decreasing both peripheral resistance and sodium retention. Unlike sodium nitroprusside, captopril increased renal plasma flow and caused a diuresis with sustained weight loss. Glomerular filtration rate was also increased in azotemic patients. Thus, this agent could be very useful in postoperative cardiac surgical patients.

INOTROPIC AGENTS

Dopamine is a naturally occurring catecholamine and a potent myocardial inotropic agent. The rapid growth in the usage of dopamine during the past decade was the result of its inotropic potency and its renal effects, which include vasodilation, diuresis, and natriuresis.[114-119] Newer inotropic agents are becoming available which may be more potent than dopamine in certain patients. In chronic cardiomyopathic heart failure dobutamine resulted in a greater, better sustained, increase in cardiac index than did dopamine.[118] Surprisingly, the improvement in renal function (urine flow, sodium excretion, and creatinine clearance) observed was statistically significant with dobutamine but not with dopamine.

We have recently compared the hemodynamic and renal function effects of these two agents. In postoperative cardiac surgical patients, doapmine appears to be the superior inotropic agent, particularly if used in combination with a readily controllable afterload reducing agent.[119, 120] Infusion rates were adjusted to achieve equal cardiac indices and renal and hemodynamic function were then measured. The infusion rate averaged 5.3 ± 1.4 µg/kg/min for dopamine and 3.2 ± 0.2 µg/kg/min for dobutamine. At equal cardiac indices, there was no difference in renal blood flow, mean arterial pressure, glomerular filtration rate, systemic vascular resistance index, and renal vascular resistance (Fig. 25–5).

Striking, in view of these similarities, was the diuresis which accompanied dopamine administration. Dopamine apparently inhibited both solute and water reabsorption as the increase in urine flow was accompanied by an increase in sodium and potassium excretion and by the production of a more dilute urine as measured by the urine:plasma inulin (or osmolality) ratio (Fig. 25–6). We interpreted these results to indicate that, in postoperative patients with depressed left ventricular performance, the effect of these inotropic agents on the systemic circulation will dominate any direct effect on the renal vasculature. Furthermore, dopamine appears to inhibit tubular solute and water reabsorption directly. This latter effect may be beneficial in and of itself (see below).

These data, the data on the effects of vasodilators on renal function and those on the sequential pathophysiology of ARF are convergent. They indicate the importance of depressed cardiac performance and the consequent depression of renal blood flow in the evolution of postoperative ARF. Furthermore, they indicate that the inotropic or va-

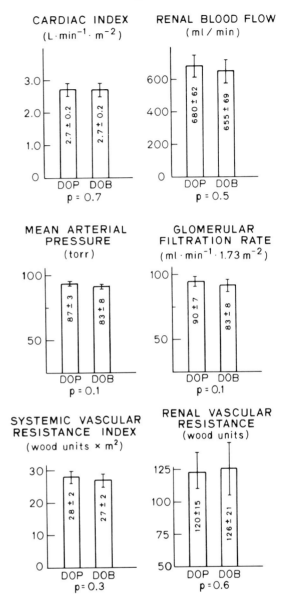

Fig. 25-5. Hemodynamic and renal function was studied in 12 postoperative patients with depressed left ventricular performance within 24 hours of cardiac operation. Infusion rates of dopamine (dop) and dobutamine (dob) were adjusted to achieve equal cardiac indices. Under the conditions renal blood flow, glomerular filtration rate, and renal vascular resistance were also the same. Date were analyzed by the student's t-test for paired data and are presented graphically as the mean ± SEM.

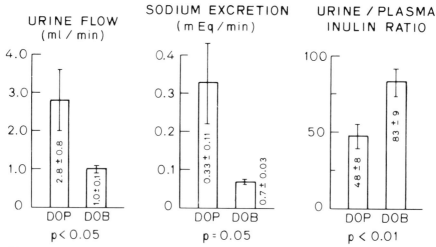

Fig. 25-6. At matched cardiac indices and equal renal blood flows, dopamine administration resulted in a significantly greater diuresis than did dobutamine. This appeared to result from a tubular inhibition of solute and water reabsorption as sodium and potassium excretions were increased and the urine was simultaneously more dilute (as measured by urine/plasma inulin and osmolality ratios).

sodilator drug, or combination of drugs, which most improves systemic hemodynamics will result in the greatest improvement in renal blood flow and renal function.

DIURETICS

Routine mannitol administration to prevent renal function deterioration during cardiovascular surgery became common during the 1960s. Barry and coworkers reported on the effectiveness of mannitol in maintaining renal function during and after aortic aneurysm surgery.[121] Porter and coworkers reported a sharp decrease in the incidence of renal failure following Starr–Edwards valve replacement subsequent to the introduction of routine mannitol administration during cardiopulmonary bypass.[122] The elegant experimental studies by Flores and associates demonstrated that the infusion of hypertonic mannitol during 60 to 120 min of total renal ischemia in rats, effectively blocked cell swelling upon reperfusion and interrupted a cyclic deterioration in renal function (Fig. 25–7).[123] Although cell swelling appears to be a transient postischemic phenomenon, evi-

dence continues to accumulate suggesting that hypertonic solutions do provide protection from the deleterious changes which follow ischemia.[124] Recently Schrier and Stein and their colleagues have demonstrated marked attenuation of the ARF induced by an ischemic insult in dogs.[125–129] Data available for several treatment regimens are presented in Table 25–3. Progressive sparing in the decline of glomerular filtration rate was provided by saline volume expansion (25% of the extracellular fluid volume), vasodilator pretreatment (acetylcholine), isotonic mannitol pretreatment, furosemide following insult, hypertonic mannitol pretreatment, and furosemide pretreatment. While glomerular structure was normal, severe tubular necrosis occurred in the kidneys of all treatment groups examined histologically. Preservation of glomerular filtration was attributed to mechanical maintenance of tubular patency by the induced diuresis (see Table 25–3 and Figs. 25–8 and 25–9). The data in Table 25–3 suggests that mannitol may be protective apart from its effect on solute excretion. At equal glomerular filtration rates (groups 5 and 6), urine flow and osmolar clearance appear lower in mannitol pretreated animals. Glomerular filtration rate fell more in the non-ischemic kidney in mannitol-treated animals than in furosemide-treated animals, it would appear that had the glomerular filtration rates been expressed as a percentage of the non-ischemic kidney, mannitol prophylaxis would have been superior. Subsequently,

glomerular filtration rate has been demonstrated to return to 80 percent of normal within 24 hours in mannitol pretreated animals.[130] Intrarenal infusion of bradykinin and prostaglandin E, renal vasodilators which also increase solute excretion, proved as effective as mannitol or furosemide.[128, 129] Thiazide diuretics, which increase renal vas-

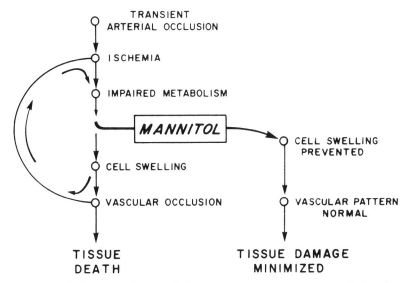

Fig. 25-7. Influence of mannitol upon the sequence of events leading to ARF. These authors suggested that cell swelling following ischemic injury was an important event in the development of ARF. (Flores et al: J Clin Invest 51: 118, 1972)

Table 25-3. Canine Renal Function After an Ischemic Insult

		C_{in} ML/MIN	V ML/MIN	C_{osm} ML/MIN
No treatment	1.3	0.02	0.03	
Saline volume expansion				
22.5 ml/kg, 0.9% saline		3.3	0.56	0.64
Acetylcholine				
20 μg/min into renal artery		5.9	0.83	0.84
Isotonic mannitol				
22.5 ml/kg, 5% mannitol		9.2	1.08	1.31
Furosemide postinsult				
10 mg/kg + 10 mg/kg/hr		15.4	7.55	7.13
Hypertonic mannitol				
6 ml/kg, 20% mannitol		16.6	2.8	3.55
Furosemide				
10 mg/kg + 10 mg/kg/hr		28.4	10.4	9.71

Unilateral renal function in dogs 3 hours after a 40-minute ischemic insult, data completed from Cronin RE, et al: Pathogenic mechanisms of early norepinephrine-induced acute renal failure: functional and histological correlates of protection. Kidney Int 14:115–125, 1978 and de Torrente A, et al: Effects of furosemide and acetylcholine in norepinephrine-induced acute renal failure. Am J Physiol 235:F131–F136, 1978. For details see original and text. These data substantiate the ability of diuretics to modify the renal function in acute renal failure.

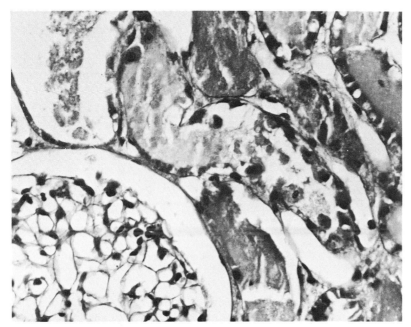

Fig. 25-8. Light micrograph demonstrating normal glomerular structure and extensive tubular necrosis with tubular obstruction 24 hours following ischemic insult (saline volume expansion, C_{in} = 4.0 ml/min). (Cronin et al: Kidney Int 14:122, 1978)

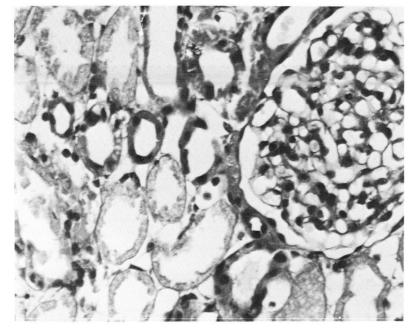

Fig. 25-9. Light micrograph demonstrating extensive cellular necrosis with patency of proximal tubular lumens 24 hrs following ischemic insult in animal protected by mannitol pretreatment (c_{in} = 21.3 ml/min). (Cronin et al: Kidney Int 14:122, 1978)

cular resistance and solute excretion, are not effective protective agents.[131] If the diuretic dosages used in dogs by Schrier's group were to be used in a 70 kg patient, the effective mannitol loading dose of 84 g (followed by approximately 300 g over 3.5 hrs) is reminiscent of the dose recommended by Barry and coworkers in noncrystalloid volume ex-

panded patients,[132] and appears more reasonable than furosemide dose (700 mg, followed by approximately 2,500 mg over 3.5 hrs).

With the appropriate reservation that animal and human ARF may differ, as may the renal response to therapy, these animal data appear relevant to humans. They are compatible with clinical reports,[132-135] and suggest that before or during an acute ischemic insult, a solute diuresis should be established, preferably with hyperoncotic mannitol. If pretreatment is not possible, prompt establishment of a diuresis following the insult is warranted. At Stanford, 12.5 g of 20 percent mannitol are added to the priming solution shortly after cardiopulmonary bypass is initiated and stabilized, and thereafter hourly. This appears to provide adequate routine protection. Patients with preoperative azotemia are at higher risk for developing ARF. In this event, we advocate establishing a mannitol diuresis before bypass, and to add 12.5 g of mannitol every half-hour during bypass. For aortic aneurysm and renal vascular surgery, where interruption of renal blood flow is anticipated, a brisk mannitol diuresis should be established with 1 to 2 g/kg of 20 percent mannitol administered intravenously before aortic cross-clamping; thereafter, 0.25 to 0.5 g/kg should be infused hourly until abdominal closure begins, and then gradually discontinued over the next few hours (the dosage should be reduced if the diuresis exceeds 2–3 ml/min). If, in the 15 minutes following discontinuation of bypass or removal of the aortic cross-clamp, postischemic oliguria exists (urine flow below 0.5 ml/min), we begin furosemide administration at 0.5 mg/kg. The dose is doubled every 10 to 15 minutes, up to 4 mg/kg or the establishment of a diuresis. If no response is obtained, a single dose of ethacrynic acid (0.5–1.0 mg/kg) is administered. Diuretic administration is not a substitute for hemodynamic optimization; care must be exercised to avoid increasing hemodynamic instability,[136] and urinary loss of fluids and electrolyte must be replaced.

SUMMARY

1. ARF follows cardiac surgery when severe hemodynamic depression results in persistent depression of renal blood flow. In some patients, the hemodynamic depres-

sion is sufficiently severe or prolonged to result in ARF. In the majority, this hemodynamic depression renders the kidneys vulnerable to additional hemodynamic or toxic insults, which would appear subtoxic to normal kidneys.

2. While the risk of developing ARF appears greatest in the immediate perioperative and postoperative period, certain patients with prolonged postoperative hemodynamic depression have a protracted period of risk. Meticulous hemodynamic management, including prolonged vasoactive drug support, appears capable of avoiding the progression to ARF in a significant percentage of these patients.

3. Cardiopulmonary bypass represents a hemodynamically marginal state which usually does not result in ARF if bypass flow is maintained and if the bypass is not excessively prolonged. However, in certain patients, particularly those with severe preoperative hemodynamic depression, cardiopulmonary bypass may result in ARF.

4. Measurement of cardiac index, left ventricular stroke work index, and the creatinine clearance provides essential data on systemic hemodynamics and renal function, not provided by measurement of cardiac preload and afterload. In addition, the measurement of the ratio of urine to plasma osmolality, and the fractional excretions of sodium and potassium provide important additional information on renal tubular integrity. Interpretation of these latter measurements requires knowledge of fluid and electrolyte balance and diuretic administration. These measurements appear particularly important in the overall assessment of renal function integrity because the creatinine clearance may remain at 25 to 50 percent of normal, even in the presence of histologic acute tubular necrosis.

5. Peripheral vasodilators, especially those causing significant arteriolar vasodilation, also cause renal vasodilation. So long as left atrial hypotension is avoided, a decrease in renal resistance and parallel in-

creases in renal and systemic blood flow may be achieved with these agents. It must be remembered that, once renal vasodilation is maximal, renal blood flow and renal perfusion pressure will decline in parallel.

6. Inotropic support with the most effective agent should result in the greatest improvement in renal blood flow. Dopamine's direct effects on the renal vasculature are dominated by its inotropic effectiveness in patients with depressed cardiac performance. Some of the increased urine flow observed with dopamine administration appears to be caused by a direct tubular effect of this drug.

7. Vigorous diuretic therapy, particularly if used before or during an acute period of depressed renal blood flow, appears capable of attenuating the renal response to an ischemic insult.

8. Intravenous fluid therapy should be used to achieve left atrial pressures that are normal or elevated (above 10 torr).

REFERENCES

GENERAL REFERENCES

1. Bastron RD, Deutsch S: Anesthesia and the Kidney, p 98. New York, Grune & Stratton, 1976. Excellent monograph.
2. Pitts RD: Physiology of the Kidney and Body Fluids, p 315. Chicago, Year Book Medical Publishers, 1974. Good basic physiology.
3. Espinel CH: The FE_{Na} test. JAMA 236:579–581, 1976
4. Miller TR, Anderson RJ, Linas SL et al: Urinary diagnostic indices in acute renal failure. Ann Intern Med 89:47–50, 1978. Excellent paper on renal functional measurement.
5. Lundberg S: Renal function during anesthesia and open-heart surgery in man. Acta Anaesth Scand [Suppl] 27:1–82, 1967
6. Hilberman M, Myers BD, Carrie BJ et al: Acute renal failure following cardiac surgery. J Thorac Cardiovasc Surg 77:880–889, 1979. Includes a detailed review and bibliography of prior works.

7. Bhat JG, Gluck M, Lowenstein J, Baldwin DS: Renal failure after open heart surgery. Ann Intern Med 84:677–682, 1976. Excellent recent paper emphasizing the role of cardiopulmonary bypass.
8. Hilberman M, Myers BD, Derby G et al: Sequential pathophysiological changes characterizing the progression from renal dysfunction to acute renal failure following cardiac surgery. J Thorac Cardiovasc Surg 79:838–846, 1980
9. Abel RM, Buckley MJ, Austen WG et al: Etiology, incidence and prognosis of renal failure following cardiac operations. J Thorac Cardiovasc Surg 71:323–333, 1976. Another recent paper, well documented and comprehensive.
10. Siegel NJ, Glazier W, Chaudry IH et al: Enhanced recovery from acute renal failure by the postischemic infusion of adenine nucleotides and magnesium chloride in rats. Kidney Int 17:338–349, 1980. Extremely interesting in its implications for tissue protection.
11. Kahl, FR, Flint JF, Szidon JP: Influence of left atrial distention on renal vasomotor tone. Am J Physiol 226:240–246, 1974
12. Maseda J, Hilberman M, Derby GD et al: The renal effects of sodium nitroprusside in postoperative cardiac surgical patients. Anesthesiology 54:284–288, 1981
13. Robie NW, Goldberg LI: Comparative systemic and regional hemodynamic effects of dopamine and dobutamine. Am Heart J 90:340–345, 1975
14. Hilberman M, Maseda J, Spencer RJ et al: The renal effects of dopamine and dobutamine. Anesthesiology 59:119, 1980
15. Flores J, DiBona DR, Beck CH, Leaf A: The role of cell swelling in ischemic renal damage and the protective effect of hypertonic solute. J Clin Invest 51:118–126, 1972
16. Cronin RE, de Torrente A, Miller PD et al: Pathogenic mechanisms of early norepinephrine-induced acute renal failure: functional and histological correlates of protection. Kidney Int 14:115–125, 1978

QUANTIFYING RENAL FUNCTION

17. Bastron RD, Deutsch S: Anesthesia and the Kidney, p 98. New York, Grune & Stratton, 1976. Excellent monograph.
18. Pitts RD: Physiology of the Kidney and Body

Fluids, p 315. Chicago, Year Book Medical Publishers, 1974. Good basic physiology.

19. Schrier RW (ed): Renal and Electrolyte Disorders, p 500. Boston, Little, Brown, & Co, 1976

20. Brenner BM, Rector FC (eds): The Kidney, p 1945. Philadelphia, WB Saunders, 1976. The definitive reference; second edition forthcoming

21. Brenner BM, Deen WM, Robertson CR: Glomerular filtration. In Brenner BM, Rector FC (eds): The Kidney, pp 251–271. Philadelphia, WB Saunders, 1976.

22. Porter GA, Kloster FE, Herr RJ et al: Renal complications associated with valve replacement surgery. J Thorac Cardiovasc Surg 53:145–152, 1967

23. Hilberman M, Myers BD, Derby G et al: Sequential pathophysiological changes characterizing the progression from renal dysfunction to acute renal failure following cardiac surgery. J Thorac Cardiovasc Surg 79:838–846, 1980

24. Anderson RJ, Linas SL, Berns AS et al: Nonoliguric acute renal failure. N Engl J Med 296:1134–1138, 1977

25. Levinsky NG, Levy M: Clearance Techniques. In Orloff J, Berliner RW, (eds): Handbook of Physiology, pp 103–118. Washington, D.C., American Physiological Society, 1973

26. Wesson LG: Physiology of the Human Kidney, p 99. New York, Grune & Stratton, 1969

27. Espinel CH: The FE_{Na} test. JAMA 236:579–581, 1976

28. Miller TR, Anderson RJ, Linas SL et al: Urinary diagnostic indices in acute renal failure. Ann Intern Med 89:47–50, 1978. Excellent paper on renal functional measurement.

29. Sarnoff SJ, Berglund E. Ventricular function. Circulation 9:706–718, 1954. Starling's law as we have learned it.

30. Chatterjee K, Swan HJC, Kanchik VS et al: Effects of vasodilator therapy for severe pump failure in acute myocardial infarction on short-term and late prognosis. Circulation 53:797–802, 1976

31. Hilberman M, Myers BD, Carrie BJ et al: Acute renal failure following cardiac surgery. J Thorac Cardiovasc Surg 77:880–889, 1979

32. Hilberman M, Myers BD, Derby G et al: Sequential pathophysiological changes characterizing the progression from renal dysfunction to acute renal failure following cardiac

surgery. J Thorac Cardiovasc Surg 79:838–846, 1980

CARDIOPULMONARY BYPASS AND RENAL FUNCTION

33. Bhat JG, Gluck M, Lowenstein J, Baldwin DS: Renal failure after open heart surgery. Ann Intern Med 84:677–682, 1976. Excellent recent paper, emphasizes role of cardiopulmonary bypass.

34. Abel RM, Buckley MJ, Austen WG et al: Etiology, incidence and prognosis of renal failure following cardiac operations. J Thorac Cardiovasc Surg 71:323–333, 1976. Another recent paper, well documented and comprehensive.

35. Krian A: Incidence, prevention and treatment of acute renal failure following cardiopulmonary bypass. Int Anesthesiol Clin 14:87–101, 1976

36. Hilberman M, Myers BD, Carrie BJ et al: Acute renal failure following cardiac surgery. J Thorac Cardiovasc Surg 77:880–889, 1979

37. Hilberman M, Myers BD, Derby G et al: Sequential pathophysiological changes characterizing the progression from renal dysfunction to acute renal failure following cardiac surgery. J Thorac Cardiovasc Surg 79:838–846, 1980

38. Dobernak RD, Reiser MP, Lillehie CW: Acute renal failure after open heart surgery utilizing extracorporeal circulation and total body perfusion. Analysis of 1000 patients. J Thorac Cardiovasc Surg 43:441–452, 1962

39. Mielke JE, Maher FT, Hunt JC, Kirklin JW: Renal performance in patients undergoing replacement of the aortic valve. Circulation 32:394–405, 1965

40. Porter GA, Koster FE, Herr RJ et al: Relationship between alterations in renal hemodynamics during cardiopulmonary bypass and postoperative renal function. Circulation 39:1005–1021, 1966

41. Hilberman M, Myers BD, Carrie BJ et al: Acute renal function following cardiac surgery. J Thorac Cardiovasc Surg 77:880–889, 1979. Includes a detailed review and bibliography of prior works.

42. Porter GA, Kloster FE, Herr RJ et al: Renal complications associated with valve replacement surgery. J Thorac Cardiovasc Surg 53:145–152, 1967

43. Hilberman M, Myers BD, Derby G et al: Sequential pathophysiological changes characterizing the progression from renal dysfunction to acute renal failure following cardiac surgery. J Thorac Cardiovasc Surg 79:838–846, 1980

44. Lundberg S: Renal function during anesthesia and open-heart surgery in man. Acta Anaesth Scand [Suppl] 27:1–82, 1967

45. Hilberman M, Myers BD, Carrie BJ et al: Acute renal failure following cardiac surgery. J Thorac Cardiovasc Surg 77:880–889, 1979

46. Senning A, Andres J, Bornstein P et al: Renal function during extracorporeal circulation at high and low flow rates. Ann Surg 151:63–70, 1960

47. Jacobs LA, Klopp EH, Seamme W et al: Improved organ function during cardiac bypass with a roller pump modified to deliver pulsatile flow. J Thorac Cardiovasc Surg 58:703–719, 1969

48. Mavroudis C: To pulse or not to pulse. Ann Thorac Surg 25:259–271, 1978

49. Wilkins H, Regelson W, Hoffmeister FS: The physiologic importance of pulsatile blood flow. N Engl J Med 267:443–446, 1962

50. Takeda J: Experimental study on peripheral circulation during extracorporeal circulation with a special reference to a comparison of pulsatile flow to non-pulsatile flow. Arch Chir Jap 29:1407–1430, 1960

51. Sanderson JM, Wright G, Sims FW: Brain damage in dogs immediately following pulsatile and nonpulsatile blood flows in extracorporeal circulation. Thorax 27:275–286, 1972

52. Taylor KM, Bain WH, Maxted KJ et al: Comparative studies of pulsatile and nonpulsatile flow during cardiopulmonary bypass. I. Pulsatile system employed and its hematologic effects. J Thorac Cardiovasc Surg 75:569–573, 1978

53. Taylor KM, Wright GS, Reid JM et al: Comparative studies of pulsatile and nonpulsatile flow during cardiopulmonary bypass. II. The effects of adrenal secretion of cortisol. J Thorac Cardiovasc Surg 75:574–578, 1978

54. Taylor KM, Wright GS, Bain WH et al: Comparative studies of pulsatile and nonpulsatile flow during cardiopulmonary bypass. III. Response of anterior pituitary gland to thyrotropin-releasing hormone. J Thorac Cardiovasc Surg 75:579–584, 1978

THE DEVELOPMENT OF ACUTE RENAL FAILURE FOLLOWING CARDIAC OPERATION

55. Hilberman M, Myers BD, Carrie BJ et al: Acute renal failure following cardiac surgery. J Thorac Cardiovasc Surg 77:880–889, 1979

56. Bhat JG, Gluck M, Lowenstein J, Baldwin DS: Renal failure after open heart surgery. Ann Intern Med 84:677–682, 1976. Excellent recent paper, emphasizes role of cardiopulmonary bypass.

57. Abel RM, Buckley MJ, Austen WG et al: Etiology, incidence and prognosis of renal failure following cardiac operations. J Thorac Cardiovasc Surg 71:323–333, 1976. Another recent paper, well documented and comprehensive.

58. Krian A: Incidence, prevention and treatment of acute renal failure following cardiopulmonary bypass. Int Anesthesiol Clin 14:87–101, 1976

59. Dobernak RD, Reiser MP, Lillehie CW: Acute renal failure after open heart surgery utilizing extracorporeal circulation and total body perfusion. Analysis of 1000 patients. J Thorac Cardiovasc Surg 43:441–452, 1962

60. Mielke JE, Maher FT, Hunt JC, Kirklin JW: Renal performance in patients undergoing replacement of the aortic valve. Circulation 32:394–405, 1965

61. Porter GA, Starr A: Management of postoperative renal failure following cardiovascular surgery. Surgery 65:390–398, 1968

62. Porter GA, Kloster FE, Herr RJ et al: Renal complications associated with valve replacement surgery. J Thorac Cardiovasc Surg 53:145–152, 1967

63. Yeboah ED, Petrie A, Pead JL: Acute renal failure and open heart surgery. Br Med J 1:415–418, 1972

64. Hilberman M, Myers BD, Derby G et al: Sequential pathophysiological changes characterizing the progression from renal dysfunction to acute renal failure following cardiac surgery. J Thorac Cardiovasc Surg 79:838–846, 1980

65. Dobernak RD, Reiser MP, Lillehie CW: Acute renal failure after open heart surgery utilizing extracorporeal circulation and total body perfusion. Analysis of 1000 patients. J Thorac Cardiovasc Surg 43:441–452, 1962

66. Mielke JE, Maher FT, Hunt JC, Kirklin JW: Renal performance in patients undergoing replacement of the aortic valve. Circulation 32:394–405, 1965

67. Porter GA, Kloster FE, Herr RJ et al: Relationship between alterations in renal hemodynamics during cardiopulmonary bypass and postoperative renal function. Circulation 39:1005–1021, 1966

68. Porter GA, Starr A: Management of postoperative renal failure following cardiovascular surgery. Surgery 65:390–398, 1968

69. Porter GA, Kloster FE, Herr RJ et al: Renal complications associated with valve replacement surgery. J Thorac Cardiovasc Surg 53:145–152, 1967

70. Bhat JG, Gluck M, Lowenstein J, Baldwin DS: Renal failure after open heart surgery. Ann Intern Med 84:677–682, 1976. Excellent recent paper, emphasizes role of cardiopulmonary bypass.

71. Abel RM, Buckley MJ, Austen WG et al: Etiology, incidence and prognosis of renal failure following cardiac operations. J Thorac Cardiovasc Surg 71:323–333, 1976. Another recent paper, well documented and comprehensive.

72. Krian A: Incidence, prevention and treatment of acute renal failure following cardiopulmonary bypass. Int Anesthesiol Clin 14:87–101, 1976

73. Porter GA, Starr A: Management of postoperative renal failure following cardiovascular surgery. Surgery 65:390–398, 1968

74. Porter GA, Kloster FE, Herr RJ et al: Renal complications associated with valve replacement surgery. J Thorac Cardiovasc Surg 53:145–152, 1967

75. Lundberg S: Renal function during anesthesia and open-heart surgery in man. Acta Anaesth Scan [Suppl] 27:1–82, 1967

76. Porter GA, Kloster FE, Herr RJ et al: Relationship between alterations in renal hemodynamics during cardiopulmonary bypass and postoperative renal function. Circulation 39:1005–1021, 1966

77. Porter GA, Kloster FE, Herr RJ et al: Renal complications associated with valve replacement surgery. J Thorac Cardiovasc Surg 53:145–152, 1967

78. Lundberg S: Renal function during anesthesia and open-heart surgery in man. Acta Anaesth Scand [Suppl] 27:1–82, 1967

79. Porter GA, Kloster FE, Herr RJ et al: Relationship between alterations in renal hemodynamics during cardiopulmonary bypass and postoperative renal function. Circulation 39:1005–1021, 1966

80. Porter GA, Starr A: Management of postoperative renal failure following cardiovascular surgery. Surgery 65:390–398, 1968

81. Porter GA, Kloster FE, Herr RJ et al: Renal complications associated with valve replacement surgery. J Thorac Cardiovasc Surg 53:145–152, 1967

82. Yeboah ED, Petrie A, Pead JL: Acute renal failure and open heart surgery. Br Med J 1:415–418, 1972

83. Hilberman M, Myers BD, Carrie BJ et al: Acute renal failure following cardiac surgery. J Thorac Cardiovasc Surg 77:880–889, 1979

84. Hilberman M, Myers BD, Carrie BJ et al: Acute renal failure following cardiac surgery. J Thorac Cardiovasc Surg 77:880–889, 1979

85. Hilberman M, Myers BD, Derby G et al: Sequential pathophysiological changes characterizing the progression from renal dysfunction to acute renal failure following cardiac surgery. J Thorac Cardiovasc Surg 79:838–846, 1980

85A. Bastron RD, Deutsch S: Anesthesia and the Kidney, p 98. New York, Grune & Stratton, 1976. Excellent monograph.

86. Wesson LG: Physiology of the Human Kidney, p 99. New York, Grune & Stratton, 1969

87. Miller TR, Anderson RJ, Linas SL et al: Urinary diagnostic indices in acute renal failure. Ann Intern Med 89:47–50, 1978. Excellent paper on renal functional measurement.

88. Anderson RJ, Linas SL, Berns AS et al: Nonoliguric acute renal failure. N Engl J Med 296:1134–1138, 1977

89. Porter GA, Kloster FE, Herr RJ et al: Renal complications associated with valve replacement surgery. J Thorac Cardiovasc Surg 53:145–152, 1967

STRATEGIES FOR RENAL PROTECTION

90. Siegel NJ, Glazier W, Chaudry IH et al: Enhanced recovery from acute renal failure by the postischemic infusion of adenine nucleotides and magnesium chloride in rats. Kidney Int 17:338–2349, 1980. Extremely interesting in its implications for tissue protection.

91. Tinker JH, Michenfelder JD: Sodium nitroprusside: pharmacology, toxicology and therapeutics. Anesthesiology 45:340–354, 1976

92. Page IH, Corcoran AC, Dustan HP et al: Cardiovascular actions of sodium nitroprusside in animals and hypertensive patients. Circulation 11:188–198, 1955

93. Bastron RD, Kaloyanides GJ: Effects of sodium nitroprusside on function in the isolated and intact dog kidney. J Pharmacol Exp Ther 181:244–249, 1972

94. Birch AA, Boyce WH: Changing renal blood flow following sodium nitroprusside in patients undergoing nephrolithotomy. Anesth Analg (Cleve) 56:102–109, 1977

95. Cogan J, Humphreys M, Carlson J et al: Afterload reduction increases renal blood flow and maintains glomerular filtration rate in patients with congestive heart failure. Circulation 61:316–323, 1980

96. Bagshaw RJ, Cox RH, Campbell KB: Sodium nitroprusside and regional arterial haemodynamics in the dog. Br J Anaesth 49:735–743, 1977

97. Kahl FR, Flint JF, Szidon JP: Influence of left atrial distention on renal vasomotor tone. Am J Physiol 226:240–246, 1974

98. Brosnihan KB, Bravo EL: Graded reductions of atrial pressure and renin release. Am J Physiol 235:H175–H181, 1978

99. Selkurt EE: The relation of renal blood flow to effective arterial pressure in the intact kidney of the dog. Am J Physiol 147:537–549, 1946

100. Shipley RE, Study RS: Changes in renal blood flow, extraction of inulin, glomerular filtration rate, tissue pressure and urine flow with acute alterations of renal artery blood pressure. Am J Physiol 167:676–688, 1951

101. Ritter ER: Pressure/flow relations in the kidney. Alleged effects of pulse pressure. Am J Physiol 168:480–489, 1952

102. Baer PG, Navar LG: Renal vasodilation and uncoupling of blood flow and filtration rate autoregulation. Kidney Int 4:12–21, 1973

103. Pouleur H, Covell JA, Ross J: Effects of nitroprusside on venous return and central blood volume in the absence and presence of acute heart failure. Circulation 61:328–337, 1980

104. Porter GA, Kloster FE, Bristow JD et al: Interrelationship of hemodynamic alterations of valvular heart disease and renal function: influences on renal sodium reabsorption. Am Heart J 84:189–202, 1972

105. Bastron RD, Kaloyanides GJ: Effects of sodium nitroprusside on function in the isolated and intact dog kidney. J Pharmacol Exp Ther 181:244–249, 1972

106. Kahl FR, Flint JF, Szidon JP: Influence of left atrial distention on renal vasomotor tone. Am J Physiol 226:240–246, 1974

107. Brosnihan KB, Bravo EL: Graded reductions of atrial pressure and renin release. AM J Physiol 235:H175–H181, 1978

108. Mason JM, Ledsome JR: Effects of obstruction of the mitral orifice or distension of the pulmonary vein-atrial junctions on renal and hind-limb vascular resistance in the dog. Circ Res 35:24–32, 1974

108A. Bastron RD, Kaloyanides GJ: Effects of sodium nitroprusside on function in the isolated and intact dog kidney. J Pharmacol Exp Ther 181:244–249, 1972

109. Birch AA, Boyce WH: Changing renal blood flow following sodium nitroprusside in patients undergoing nephrolithotomy. Anesth Analg (Cleve) 56:102–109, 1977

110. Bagshaw RJ, Cox RH, Campbell KB: Sodium nitroprusside and regional arterial haemodynamics in the dog. Br J Anaesth 49:735–743, 1977

111. Cogan J, Humphreys M, Carlson J et al: Afterload reduction increases renal blood flow and maintains glomerular filtration rate in patients with congestive heart failure. Circulation 61:316–323, 1980

112. Maseda J, Hilberman M, Derby GC: The renal effects of sodium nitroprusside in postoperative cardiac surgical patients. Anesthesiology 54:284–288, 1981

113. Creager MA, Halperin JL, Bernard DB et al: Acute regional circulatory and renal hemodynamic effects of converting-enzyme inhibition in patients with congestive heart failure. Circulation 64:483–489, 1981

114. Goldberg LI: Cardiovascular and renal actions of dopamine: Potential clinical applications. Pharmacol Rev 24:1–20, 1972

115. Goldberg LI, Hsieh YY, Rosnekov L: Newer catecholamines and treatment of heart failure and shock: an update on dopamine and a first look at dobutamine. Prog Cardiovasc Dis 19:327–339, 1977

116. Robie NW, Goldberg LI: Comparative systemic and regional hemodynamic effects of dopamine and dobutamine. Am Heart J 90:340–345, 1975

117. Tuttle RR, Mills J: Development of a new

catecholamine to selectively increase cardiac contractility. Circ Res 36:185–196, 1975

118. Leier CV, Heban PT, Huss P et al: Comparative systemic and regional hemodyanmic effects of dopamine and dobutamine in patients with cardiomyopathic heart failure. Circulation 58:466–475, 1978

119. Steen PA, Tinker JH, Pluth JR et al: Efficacy of dopamine, dobutamine, and epinephrine during emergence from cardiopulmonary bypass in man. Circulation 57:378–384, 1978

120. Hilberman M, Maseda J, Spencer RJ et al: The renal effects of dopamine and dobutamine. Anesthesiology 59:S119, 1980

121. Barry KG, Cohen A, Knochel JP et al: Mannitol infusion. II. The prevention of acute functional renal failure during resection of an aneurysm of the abdominal aorta. N Engl J Med 264:967–971, 1961

122. Bhat JG, Gluck M, Lowenstein J, Baldwin DS: Renal failure after open heart surgery. Ann Intern Med 84:677–682, 1976. Excellent recent paper emphasizing the role of cardiopulmonary bypass.

123. Flores J, DiBona DR, Beck CH, Leaf A: The role of cell swelling in ischemic renal damage and the protective effect of hypertonic solute. J Clin Invest 51:118–126, 1972

124. Frega NS, DiBona DR, Leaf A: Enhancement of recovery from experimental ischemic acute renal failure. In Leaf A et al (eds): Renal Pathophysiology, pp 203–212. New York, Raven Press, 1980. An excellent presentation.

125. Cronin RE, de Torrente A, Miller PD et al: Pathogenic mechanisms of early norepinephrine-induced acute renal failure: functional and histological correlates of protection. Kidney Int 14:115–125, 1978

126. de Torrente A, Miller PD, Cronin RE et al: Effects of furosemide and acetylcholine in norepinephrine-induced acute renal failure. Am J Physiol 235:F131–F136, 1978

127. Cronin RE, Erickson AM, de Torrente A

McDonald et al: Norepinephrine-induced acute renal failure: a reversible ischemic model of acute renal failure. Kidney Int 14:187–190, 1978

128. Mauk RH, Patak RV, Dadem SZ et al: Effect of prostaglandin E administration in a nephrotoxic and a vasoconstrictor model of acute renal failure. Kidney Int 12:122–130, 1970

129. Patak RV, Faden SZ, Lifschitz MD, Stein JH: Study of factors which modify the development of norepinephrine-induced acute renal failure in the dog. Kidney Int 15:227–237, 1979

130. Burke TS, Cronin RE, Duchin KL et al: Ischemia and tubule obstruction during acute renal failure in dogs. Role of mannitol in protection. Am J Physiol 238:F305–F314, 1980

131. Cogan J, Humphreys M, Carlson J et al: Afterload reduction increases renal blood flow and maintains glomerular filtration rate in patients with congestive heart failure. Circulation 61:316–323, 1980

132. Barry KG, Cohen A, Knochel FP et al: Mannitol infusion. II. The prevention of acute functional renal failure during resection of an aneurysm of the abdominal aorta. N Engl J Med 264:967–971, 1961

133. Porter GA, Kloster FE, Herr RJ et al: Renal complications associated with valve replacement surgery. J Thorac Cardiovasc Surg 53:145–152, 1967

134. Nuutinen W, Hollmen A: The effect or prophylactic use of furosemide on renal function during open heart surgery. Ann Chir Gynaecol 55:258–266, 1976

135. Stahl WM, Stone AM: Prophylactic diuresis with ethacrynic acid for prevention of postoperative renal failure. Ann Surg 172:361–368, 1970

136. Lucas CE, Zito JG, Carver KM et al: Questionable value of furosemide in preventing renal failure. Surgery 82:314–320, 1977

26

Uses of Hypothermia in Cardiovascular Surgery

BRUCE A. REITZ
ALLEN K. REAM

INTRODUCTION

It has been known since ancient times that cold will preserve body tissues and provide analgesia. Some of the first recorded systematic studies of the uses of hypothermia were done in the late 18th century by James Currie.[1] He examined the value of cooling patients with febrile illnesses and observed normal subjects cooled to a body temperature of 32°C. A major contribution of these early experiments was the development of a mercury thermometer for accurate verification of temperature.

No other specific uses for hypothermia were suggested until the 19th century, when several clinicians recognized the analgesic properties of cold, and devised applications.[2] Fay and Smith, in the 1930s, also demonstrated the analgesic effect of general body hypothermia when cooling patients with terminal cancer.[3] They established that patients could survive long periods (24–48 hours) of moderate hypothermia (30°C), and that hypothermia by itself could not arrest or cure malignancy.

Bigelow reported extensive experiments with dogs cooled below the generally accepted fibrillation threshold of 27°C in 1950.[4] He wished to develop a method for performing open-heart surgery. Anesthetized dogs were cooled by surface immersion in cold water baths to a body temperature of 25°C. After thoracotomy, circulatory arrest was maintained for 15 minutes. Fifteen percent of the animals survived with no apparent sequelae. Technique was a critical factor, in as much as Mohri in 1974, studied 12 dogs under analogous conditions cooled to 23°C, and reported 100 percent survival.[5]

Other groups, notably Swan[6] and Churchill–Davidson,[7] studied the hemodynamic and metabolic changes which occurred with surface cooling and rewarming, and variable periods of circulatory arrest. Lewis and Tauffic[8] reported the first successful clinical application, the closure of an atrial septal defect during a period of circulatory arrest lasting 5.5 minutes at 28°C in 1952. Many others applied this technique clinically in the early 1950s, but the procedure was cumbersome and provided limited time for intracardiac maneuvers so that only simple defects could be repaired.

Efforts during this same period led to successful equipment and techniques for cardiopulmonary bypass. The development of these machines is discussed in Chapter 14. However, the demonstration of preservation using hypothermia suggested that it could be combined with cardiopulmonary bypass to increase patient protection. Not only could bypass be used to provide rapid cooling (permitting a period of complete arrest), but the lowered body temperature permitted longer safe perfusions, decreased bypass flow, and reduced blood trauma.

Selective hypothermia of the heart during cardiopulmonary bypass was shown to enhance myocardial preservation while the aorta was occluded and coronary blood flow interrupted. These techniques were developed in the 1950s, and are reviewed in the section on myocardial preservation.

PHYSIOLOGY

OXYGEN REQUIREMENTS

The primary clinical value of hypothermia lies in the associated decreased rate of cellular oxygen-requiring enzymatic reactions. We first examine this principle and then the resulting effects on supply and biological regulation.

In isolated organs and cells, it has been demonstrated that a given enzymatically mediated reaction decreases by a fixed percentage for a fixed change in temperature over the biologic range. This is expressed as the Q_{10}, the ratio of decrease over a range of 10°C. For example, a Q_{10} of 2 means that oxygen consumption will fall 50 percent with 10°C fall in temperature. This concept appears to apply within the range of freezing water (0°C) to enzymatic disruption (approximately 42°C). The range of Q_{10} values for biologic processes varies, and usually is between 1 and 3. For example, the Q_{10} for diffusion is less than for oxygen consumption. Therefore, as temperature falls, the rate of oxygen consumption in general decreases more rapidly than cellular supply, and local stores are consumed more slowly. For this reason, hypothermia can protect cells from anoxia.

The measurement of total body oxygen consumption suggests that the Q_{10} rule also applies to intact animals. Figure 26–1 demonstrates this exponential relation for rat heart slices and for the dog. Note that because of this relation, the first 10°C reduction in body temperature provides a greater absolute reduction in oxygen consumption than the second 10°C.

OXYGEN AVAILABILITY

Oxygen availability is primarily determined by the adequacy of tissue perfusion. Perfusion depends on the flow, vascular resistance (as determined by the geometry of the vasculature), blood viscosity, partial pressure of oxygen, and the hemoglobin content. We may classify these effects as oxygen content, flow and the distribution of flow, and local exchange.

The oxygen content is determined by the partial pressure of oxygen at the alveolus, and the storage capacity of the blood at that partial pressure. (We ignore pulmonary shunting here.) At 37°C, adequacy of content depends on the hemoglobin concentration. But as temperature decreases, solubility of oxygen in plasma increases. With normal cardiac output, calculation suggests that dissolved oxygen alone may be adequate if the temperature is lowered sufficiently. This can be appreciated with a simple example. At normal cardiac output, the arteriovenous (A-V) difference is approximately 4 ml/dl. If the patient is breathing 100 percent oxygen, the dissolved oxygen is approximately 2 ml/dl. When the increase in solubility with hypothermia (50% more oxygen at 20°C)[9] and decreased demand are taken into account, it is apparent that with a 10°C decrease in temperature dissolved oxygen is theoretically adequate if local flow does not change.

However, flow is often a major consideration. Flow is reduced during bypass, to reduce blood trauma. Particularly when cooling with nonpulsatile cardiopulmonary bypass, there may be uneven distribution of flow, and therefore uneven cooling. Hence, surface cooling remains attractive for physiologic reasons, though technically more inconvenient. The same consideration suggests that controlled vasodilation during cooling can be protective by increasing the rate of equilibration.

The release of oxygen from hemoglobin is

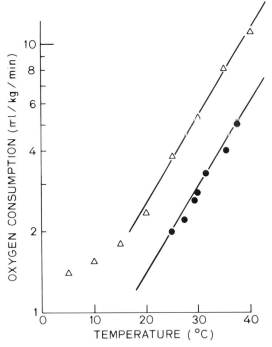

Fig. 26-1. Oxygen consumption versus temperature. The logarithm of oxygen consumption (QO_2) at various temperatures for both tissue culture slices of rat brain (*open triangles*) and the intact dog (*closed circles*). The slope of both, the Q_{10}, is 2.13. (Rat data modified from Field J: Effect of temperature on the oxygen consumption of brain tissue. J Neurophysiol 1:117–126, 1944; Canine whole animal data modified from Spurr GB, Hutt BK, Horvath SM: Responses of dogs to hypothermia. Am J Physiol 179:139–145, 1954)

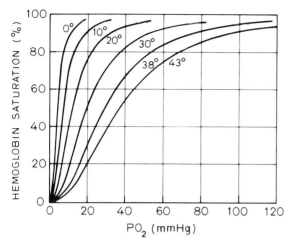

Fig. 26-2. Variation of hemoglobin saturation versus pO₂ with changing temperature. As temperature declines, the curves shift to the left, indicating that oxygen is more firmly bound to hemoglobin for a given value of pO₂ at lower temperature. (Modified from Brown WEL, Hill AV: The oxygen-dissociation curve of blood, and its thermodynamical basis. Proc R Soc Lond [Biol] 94:297–334, 1923)

suggests an increase in total body oxygen consumption with elevated carbon dioxide tension, but benefit in terms of enhanced tissue preservation has not been demonstrated (see Chap. 2). The benefits of hypocarbia appear to be enhanced by hypothermia.[10] Numerous animal and clinical studies of hypothermia have failed to demonstrate that tissue anoxia is a significant problem when flow is adequate during cooling and warming.

Of greater importance is the increased blood viscosity, particularly at low flow.[11] The resistance to resuming flow increases dramatically as the hematocrit rises above 50,[12] and is associated with sludging (capillary stasis). Both because of the reduced hemoglobin requirement for transport, and the undesirable increase in viscosity with decreasing temperature, hemodilution is preferred. With cardiopulmonary bypass, the require-

another significant consideration when hypothermia is used. The hemoglobin saturation curve is sensitive to temperature, as shown in Figure 26–2. With decreasing temperature, the curve shifts to the left so that for a given partial pressure, more oxygen remains bound to hemoglobin. The practical result is that the diffusion gradient to the intracellular site of oxidation is reduced. However, this concern appears largely theoretical because a partial pressure of less than 2 torr is adequate at the mitochondrial level. While diffusion is slowed by the reduction in gradient and temperature, local storage is increased by increased solubility and reduced demand. Should anaerobic metabolism occur, the dissociation curve shifts to the right, improving the release of oxygen from hemoglobin, as shown in Figure 26–3.

Increasing the partial pressure of carbon dioxide also shifts the curve to the right, largely through the effect on pH. However, this does not appear to be a clinically useful maneuver because acidosis adversely affects cellular metabolism. Experimental evidence

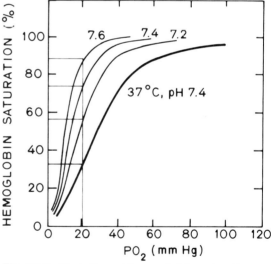

Fig. 26-3. Variation of hemoglobin saturation versus pO₂ with changing pH. Temperature is constant at 16°C. As the pH decreases, the curve shifts to the right, indicating that oxygen is less firmly bound to hemoglobin for a given value of pO₂ with increasing acidosis. (Modified from Severinghaus JW, Stupfel M: Respiratory physiologic studies during hypothermia. In The Physiology of Induced Hypothermia. National Academy of Science, National Research Council, Publication 451, pp 52-57, 1958)

ment for hemodilution permits the use of a nonblood prime.

The effect of hypothermia on homeostatic mechanisms is complex, and is not yet fully understood. The protective effect of hypothermia appears directly related to the associated decrease in rate of oxygen consumption. However, not all of the effects on regulatory mechanisms are beneficial and some are very sensitive to management technique. This impression is reinforced by the fact that increasing the depth and duration of hypothermia increases the patient risk unless supportive measures become more com-

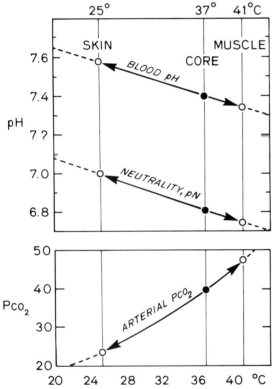

Fig. 26-4. Changes in arterial pH and pCO₂ in humans as 37°C blood arrives at the skin or exercising muscle at temperatures of 25 and 41°C, respectively. Neutrality of water, pN, changes in parallel with the changes in blood pH. Thus the relative alkalinity of the blood or the ratio between [OH⁻] and [H⁺] ion remains constant. (Modified from Rahn H: In Carbon Dioxide and Metabolic Regulation. Berlin, Springer–Verlag, 1974)

plex and aggressive. And a limit clearly remains, given present knowledge.

Several areas are only partially defined. Coagulation is impaired with hypothermia, and recovery is incomplete on warming. The mechanisms are poorly understood, but appear to center on inactivation, reduced rate of reaction, and depletion of labile factors. Blood gas solubilities and pH both change with temperature, and discussion continues as to the most appropriate balance with hypothermia.

THE APPROPRIATE pH AND pCO₂

The traditional presumption has been that the optimal value of blood pH at a body temperature of 37°C is also the optimal pH at a lower body temperature. In practical terms, because most instruments warm the blood to 37°C to make a determination, this laboratory value must be *corrected* to the blood gas the pH values at body temperature. The value of pH at body temperature, using this approach, should always be approximately 7.4?

More recently, however, it has been noted that the proper reference value may be electrochemical neutrality, where pH equals pOH.[13, 14] It may then be hypothesized that it is the normal offset of physiologic pH at 37°C (0.6 units alkaline of the neutral point at pH = 6.8) which should be maintained. With cooling, the pH of the neutral point rises, with warming it falls; hence, blood pH should also.

Several observations support this hypothesis. With exercise in warm muscle and at the skin with cooling, the changes in pH maintain this 0.6 unit offset of the neutral point in humans (Fig. 26–4). Study of many other vertebrate species with acclimation to different body temperatures shows the same variation in blood pH (Fig. 26–5).[15, 16] This conclusion is reinforced by the fact that while HCO₃⁻ content varied somewhat with the 35 species of vertebrates examined, HCO₃⁻ content was essentially constant with changing temperature in each species.[13]

An interesting byproduct of these observations is the corresponding change in pCO_2. The pH is maintained in the proper range by keeping HCO_3^- constant. Because of the blood buffer system behavior (presumably caused primarily by the presence of imidazole of peptide-histidine buffer), a constant HCO_3^- results when total blood CO_2 content is constant, despite changing temperature. Hence, alveolar ventilation relative to oxygen consumption should increase with decreasing temperature because a lower pCO_2 will compensate for rising solubility.

The net result is that a minute ventilation should not markedly decrease with decreasing body temperature. This appears to be the actual response in poikilotherms, the group thought most likely to exhibit appropriate respiratory control responses with changing body temperature. The suggested practical rule is for every 10°C decrease in body temperature, the blood pCO_2 should decrease about 35 percent.[14]

As can readily be appreciated from examination of Figure 26–4, this approach suggests that the blood pH should be kept such that when the blood is warmed to 37°C, the pH is approximately 7.42. In other words, *uncorrected* pH and pCO_2, with the laboratory measurements made at 37°C, should be used.

It is also possible to manage patients by this approach using end tidal pCO_2 measurements. However, estimation is more difficult during cooling or warming, when body temperature is not uniform. The temperature of the blood in the lungs should be used to estimate the value of end tidal pCO_2, which is most desirable. This temperature can be markedly different from rectal or skin temperature, and is probably best estimated from esophageal or deep airway temperature. An additional correction may also be necessary if the temperature of the gas at the site of measurement is significantly different from the presumed lung temperature. The usual offset of -1 to -3 torr from arterial to end tidal values may also vary with temperature and surgical manipulation. For these reasons, it is desirable to periodically check HCO_3^- content by direct blood gas determinations.

Rahn's hypothesis, that the most desirable

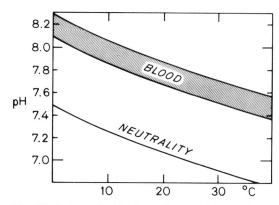

Fig. 26-5. Blood pH of exotherms, homeotherms, and the pH of neutral water as a function of body temperature. (Modified from Rahn H: In Carbon Dioxide and Metabolic Regulation. Berlin, Springer–Verlag, 1974)

pH is referenced to neutrality, is not yet fully accepted by the clinical community. However, the presumption that it is correct is reinforced by both clinical impression and the failure to identify clearly contradictory findings. A recent study by Becker and colleagues is particularly interesting.[17, 18] In puppies studied after cardiac arrest for one hour at 16°C, the seven animals with pH varied as in poikilotherms exhibited normal cardiac performance (as measured by the relation between stroke work index and left atrial pressure) post-bypass; however, in the seven held at a pH of 7.4 throughout, there was a 50 percent depression in cardiac performance post-bypass. Moreover, cerebral blood flow was improved by poikilothermic regulation such that decreasing pCO_2 to 10 torr doubled cerebral blood flow. More recent work strongly supports this position.[18a, 18b, 18c]

LEVELS OF HYPOTHERMIA

Because of the evident ethical and experimental constraints, clinical concepts are largely empiric. Terminology has developed which describes the temperature levels differing in practice. These are shown, together with the approximate safe limits of circulatory arrest, in Table 26–1. This data is derived from reported experience with infants and

Table 26-1. Definition of Levels of Hypothermia and the Approximate Safe Periods of Total Circulatory Arrest in Humans at Those Levels

LEVELS OF HYPOTHERMIA	TEMPERATURE (°C)	SAFE CIRCULATORY OCCLUSION (MINS)
Mild	37–32	4–10
Moderate	32–28	10–16
Deep	28–18	16–60
Profound	18–4	60–90

adults. The safe limit refers to survival of the cells of the cerebral cortex; these are thought to be the most susceptible to anoxic or hypoxic injury. The heart and other organs seem to tolerate significantly longer periods of ischemia at each temperature level.

Mild and moderate hypothermia can be achieved solely by surface cooling and rewarming without mechanical support of the circulation. Deep hypothermia achieved through surface cooling has also been employed in infants. However, deep and profound hypothermia is usually accomplished with cardiopulmonary bypass. While the safe period of circulatory arrest is prolonged by lowering body temperature, the length of time the perfused patient can be maintained decreases with the temperature. Mild hypothermia can be tolerated for several days, but profound hypothermia is tolerated for only a few hours.

PHARMACOLOGY

Two aspects of drug pharamacology must be considered in relation to hypothermia. First, special drug requirements are created by the physiologic response to hypothermia. Second, hypothermia alters drug action and metabolism.

A great advantage of homeothermic regulation is the ability to increase heat production in response of a cold stimulus by shivering. However, in this instance the mechanism is undesirable. The best pharmacologic therapy is the use of specific, centrally acting blocking agents, such as the narcotics or phenothiazines. Among the latter, chlorpromazine is effective in intravenous milligram doses, and also produces vasodilation. Muscle relaxants also block shivering, but are less effective because the centrally mediated cardiovascular responses must be separately treated. Least desirable is deep anesthesia because unwanted anesthetic depression is produced after hypothermia has occurred, at a time when removal of the agent is quite difficult.

A major risk of the transition phases of cooling and rewarming is the development of large thermal gradients in body tissue, implying slow heat transfer and increasing the risk of an imbalance between metabolite supply and demand. Pharmacologic vasodilation is essential during this time. Middle artery-level blocking agents appear most appropriate (see Chap. 2), but nitroprusside is also quite valuable for blood pressure control, and because of its rapid response time.

Because hypothermia itself is anesthetic, drug requirements are reduced. Shivering disappears spontaneously below approximately 32°C. Drug requirements are also reduced because hypothermia decreases the rate of elimination. When these considerations are coupled with the desire for prompt postoperative emergence, it is clear that anesthetic agents must be given in moderation, and long-acting drugs should ordinarily be avoided. We believe that the effect of a long-acting premedication can be seen postoperatively, and for this reason, usually use a short-acting narcotic for premedication.

The transport and rate of tissue equilibration of drugs is also slowed by the reduction and variable distribution of blood flow. Major inhalation agents are particularly undesirable for this reason because they must be used near normal levels at induction, but then cannot be eliminated effectively at lower temperatures when their depressant effects are undesirable.

These condsiderations seem obvious, but the principal technical difficulty is force of habit. The anesthesiologist must constantly reassess habits appropriate in other situations, to be sure that they are valid during hypothermia.

WHOLE-BODY HYPOTHERMIA

MODERATE HYPOTHERMIA

Most experience has been with moderate cooling. A reduced perfusion temperature permits lower flow, reducing blood trauma, lengthening the safe period of bypass, and reducing the amount and temperature of the blood returning to the heart. This latter effect improves operating conditions and maintains myocardial hypothermia. In the event of a catastrophic accident to the bypass machine or cannulae, circulatory arrest can be extended while the defect is corrected. More profound hypothermia in routine clinical uses seems unwarranted, prolonging operation for the time necessary for rewarming and introducing unnecessary complications.

Moderate hypothermia can be achieved by either active cooling of the bypass prime, or more slowly, by leaving the prime at room temperature until rewarming to normothermia begins. Aggressive warming begins approximately 10 minutes before release of the aortic clamp in order to be close to 37 degrees when bypass is discontinued.

This is the most common hypothermia technique,[19] and is described in more detail in Chapters 14 and 22.

Moderate hypothermia by surface cooling has also been applied in neurosurgery with controlled hypotension and temperature ranging down to 30°C. This technique has also been used postoperatively, in patients recovering from head trauma, and after a period of ischemia following cardiac arrest. Drowning victims have been kept hypo-

thermic by surface cooling for up to 48 hours, to decrease oxygen consumption during the period of cerebral edema.[20] In all of these situations, prospective controlled studies have been difficult to conduct, but many clinicians feel the technique is beneficial.

DEEP HYPOTHERMIA WITH CIRCULATORY ARREST: INFANTS

Although pump oxygenators have become synonymous with routine cardiac surgery, there are particular instances where the advantages of deep hypothermia with circulatory arrest are desirable. Approximately 1 percent of all newborn infants have congenital abnormalities and one-half of these will die during the first year of life if untreated. The first attempts were palliative, but the trend in recent years has been toward more definitive repair in infancy. However, a high mortality rate has been previously associated with conventional bypass techniques in some centers. This is especially true for infants less than 8 kg and less than 1 year of age. Hikasa reported a series of 78 infants treated before 1964 using hypothermia with circulatory arrest.[21] The excellent results reported stimulated others to explore the technique.

Advocates of this technique believe that the postoperative respiratory insufficiency seen after conventional cardiopulmonary bypass is virtually eliminated. Furthermore, the heart is empty and relaxed, facilitating repair. Cooling and rewarming may be accomplished by bypass, with a greater assurance of metabolic support and cardiac resuscitation. A major benefit of the technique is the ability to extend the period of arrest by interposing periods of perfusion.

Other workers believe that bypass can be avoided altogether, obviating complications associated with the pump, oxygenator, heparinization, and cannulation.[22] Although manual cardiac massage is required for short periods, this is not believed to be detrimental, and surface methods are used for both cooling and rewarming.

DEEP HYPOTHERMIA WITH CIRCULATORY ARREST: ADULTS

Circulatory arrest in adults has been advocated for a number of applications involving complicated cardiovascular pathology. In a series of 33 patients with difficult cardiac problems treated by hypothermic arrest, Lillehei reported a 21 percent hospital mortality.[23] When the technique was applied to replacement of the aortic arch, mortality was less than with conventional perfusion techniques.[24, 25]

Modification of this technique has been used in severe metabolic illnesses. Klebanoff reported in 1972 on the treatment of patients with stage IV hepatic coma by total body washout using an asanguinous hypothermia perfusate.[26] The theoretical basis of the maneuver is that washout of poisonous toxins will allow liver regeneration. The patient is perfused with a cold, asanguinous electrolyte solution, lowering body temperature to 20°C. He is then transfused with donor blood, and warmed to normal temperature. In the first six patients, two survived with normal liver function after stage IV coma. Four others showed improvement in liver function, but died of complications of their primary disease.

The use of hypothermia and circulatory arrest for the resection of cerebral artery aneurysms was undertaken in the early 1960s at the Mayo Clinic.[27] Initially, central cannulation with an open chest was performed, but better patient survival was obtained after the introduction of a closed-chest technique, using femoral artery and vein cannulation. In 1966, Uihlein reported the treatment of 67 intracranial aneurysms in 66 patients by induced deep hypothermia with extracorporeal circulation and arrest.[28] Fifteen died, approximately half of the deaths related to the extracorporeal perfusion technique. The temperature was usually reduced to 18 to 20°C, but the duration of arrest was not specified.

Recent neurosurgical advances include the development of better anesthetic techniques and the use of the operating microscope. But, while many aneurysms previously thought to be unresectable can be removed using these techniques, some giant aneurysms, tumors, and vascular malformations still require circulatory arrest. We have applied this modality recently with excellent results.[29]

TECHNIQUES

As outlined above, there are two cooling techniques used in order to achieve deep hypothermia: surface cooling and core cooling. *Surface cooling* consists of removing heat from the body surface and cooling at a slower and more uniform rate from the outside to the interior. This method depends on circulation maintained by the patient's own cardiovascular system. The second method is core cooling by use of cardiopulmonary bypass. *Core cooling* is usually much more rapid than surface cooling but allows the development of greater temperature gradients. When either method is used, however, the initial phase of cooling is facilitated by anesthetic paralysis of the shivering and vasospastic responses. In the application of hypothermia to surgery on infants, both techniques have been used to advantage; on theoretical grounds, the predominant use of surface cooling and core warming is more attractive.[30]

Because descriptions in the literature are incomplete, this section first describes a unified approach to adult hypothermia in detail. We then discuss modified attitudes at other centers and application to infants.

Preparation

The major hazard of deep hypothermia appears to be the complexity of the procedure. Preparation is essential. A written protocol should be circulated, and all special requirements should be arranged in advance. Surface cooling of adults is adequate without immersion if all modalities are used, including perfused cooling blankets, vasodilation, transfusion of chilled electrolyte solution, ventilation with dry gas (open circle), and maintaining low room temperature. We have tested a cooling suit, similar to that employed by astronauts, but find only a small advantage over cooling blankets. Premedication should be short acting, because of the lingering postoperative depressant effects of hypothermia.

Intravascular catheters are placed while the patient is in the operating room. The patient should be warm until anesthetized in order to avoid hypertension, shivering, and other stress. A narcotic premedication is helpful to reduce the likelihood of shivering, and any pain associated with catheter placement.

Induction

Agents disposing to elevated intracranial pressure should be avoided. Controlled ventilation should be maintained to assure low pCO_2. An end tidal CO_2 monitor should be employed as arterial blood gas samples involve too much delay. Cold is anesthetic, hence little agent is required later. We prefer narcotic, in modest dose, with minimal long-acting premedication, to facilitate postoperative emergence, and routinely use thiopental because of its presumed protective effects. Approximately 2 g/70kg is administered as an infusion over about 1 hour after induction.

Cooling Before Bypass

Surface cooling should be initiated as soon as the patient is unresponsive. We commonly administer small doses (1 mg) of chlorpromazine to block shivering while the patient is light, and to facilitate vasodilation. Because patients can be unstable while cooling, nitroprusside is helpful because of its rapid action, but less effective alone because it does not dilate middle artery vessels as effectively. Regitine and other agents with an inotropic component should be avoided. With effort, core temperature can be reduced to 30 to 27°C by the time of bypass, the desirable lower limit.

Carbon dioxide solubility rises and production falls with temperature. Hypercarbia may increase the risk of arrhythmias and cardiac arrest with cooling[31] and the appropriate hypothermic pH is greater than at 37°C. As previously noted, adequate management is achieved by maintaining minute ventilation at initial values until adjustment proves necessary to keep *uncorrected* arterial pH at the normal value of 7.42.

We remove blood during the cooling phase, retaining it in the room (not chilled) in CPD bags. A reasonable goal is a PCV on bypass of 18 (for a target temperature of 20°C). This can be reached in a 70 kg patient with normal preoperative hematocrit by removing three units of blood, and adding 1 unit of packed cells to 2 liters of bypass prime. Replacement is normal saline, with 6 mEq/l potassium added. Infusion is matched to blood withdrawal to stabilize heart filling pressures; typically 1 l/unit of blood removed is given during the first hour. The serum potassium should be checked several times. Occasionally, depressed heart rate and/or contractility can be reversed by administration of $CaCl_2$ 0.5 to 1.0 g IV.

If the purpose is a noncardiac procedure, the vascular surgeon will cannulate through the groin, and the chest is prepped, but not opened. The cannulation technique is illustrated in Figure 26–6. A large catheter is passed through the right femoral vein to the region of the right atrium and through the left femoral vein to the bifurcation of the iliac veins. Arterial return is provided into the right femoral artery and the left femoral artery is clamped before occlusion of the left femoral vein by the insertion of the cannula. With this cannulation, flow rates of between 2.5 and 3.5 l/min can be maintained in adults and effective core cooling and rewarming accomplished. The addition of pulsatile flow to the bypass circuit has been shown to speed both cooling and rewarming when used in infants undergoing cardiac surgery,[32] and also appears helpful in adults.

Cooling During Bypass

The bypass setup should be reviewed with the perfusionist before starting. A supplementary heat exchanger is always required (particularly for rewarming) and must be in-

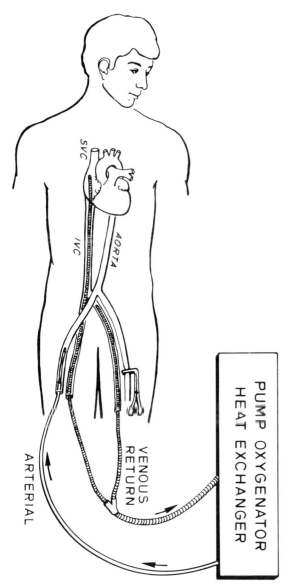

Fig. 26-6. Femoral cannulation employed for cardiopulmonary bypass to induce hypothermia and circulatory arrest. Both femoral veins are cannulated to assure sufficient venous return to the pump-oxygenator; a single femoral artery is cannulated for arterial return, with the alternate femoral artery clamped to prevent vascular engorgement of the leg because the femoral vein is obstructed by the venous cannula.

stalled in the countercurrent mode. Water to the heat exchanger should *never* exceed 41°C (42°C will denature blood, even if the bulk temperature is much lower). All routines must be reviewed because many assumptions are not reliable out of the usual temperature range. For example, at 20°C, anoxic blood is cherry red. Decreasing ventilation with temperature may unacceptably decrease pH. (See earlier discussion of pH and temperature; we recommend *uncorrected* values.) The external heat exchanger must be upstream of the oxygenator (in the venous return side), so that gas emboli are not transmitted to the patient during rewarming, because of decreased gas solubility in blood as the temperature rises.

The perfusionist will cool below the target temperature initially, then warm to the target temperature as the patient approaches it. The anesthetist should paralyze the patient fully before arrest because cellular hypoxia can produce movement and it is impossible to administer drugs during circulatory arrest.

Warming

Warming is technically much more difficult than cooling because the permissible gradient between the warm blood and the target of 37°C should be a maximum of 10°C. Thus, every effort must be made to assure uniform, effective transfer to, and preservation of, body heat. The warming-blanket bath should be warmed during arrest and connected to the blanket as soon as warming begins.

If the patient's chest has not been opened, defibrillation should be attempted when the heart temperature is estimated to be at 27°C (*not* the rectal temperature). With a healthy heart, defibrillation is often spontaneous. If the heart has not been subjected to prolonged ischemia during the surgery, such as with aortic cross-clamping, filling pressures should be returned to high normal as quickly as the patient will tolerate them, in order to boost cardiac output, and hasten rewarming. (Note the omission of the "loafing time" dis-

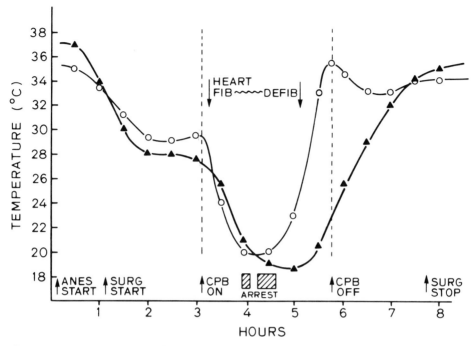

Fig. 26-7. Temperatures of a patient undergoing cardiopulmonary bypass to induce hypothermia and circulatory arrest in order to repair a giant cerebral artery aneurysm. The rectal temperature is shown by *closed triangles* and the nasopharyngeal temperature by *open circles*. The time at which the heart spontaneously fibrillates during cooling and defibrillates during rewarming is shown, as is the interval of complete circulatory arrest.

cussed in Chap. 14). Aggressive use of vasodilators is essential to assure warming of peripheral tissues.

We and others have observed improved warming with pulsatile perfusion prior to restoring normal cardiac output, provided either by the patient's own heart or by pulsatile bypass.[32-34]

A temperature record representative of a patient undergoing hypothermia and arrest for a neurosurgical procedure is shown in Figure 26–7. The temperature record demonstrates that the patient will cool again after bypass is discontinued, as the cool periphery continues to equilibrate with the more highly perfused core. Bypass may be discontinued when patient temperature is 34 to 36°C and further rewarming provided by surface means and the patient's own mechanisms for maintaining temperature.

Heparin reversal and transfusion require care. We prefer giving protamine first, then fresh frozen plasma, factor IX and the previously removed patient blood. Overly rapid administration can produce lethal cardiac depression. Fresh (less than 2 hours old, unchilled) whole blood is ideal and may avert the need for factor therapy. Calcium administration is often helpful. However, a more common tendency is to use the standard coagulation tests, and under-correct the coagulopathy. For reasons not well understood, these patients often continue to bleed after administration of frozen plasma and platelets, despite nearly normal coagulation studies, but stop bleeding with Factor IX complex and cryoprecipitate. Our bias is that early aggressive therapy is associated with a lower total postoperative transfusion requirement. For many of these patients, postoperative bleeding is a potentially lethal complication.

Transport and Intensive Care

The intensive care unit should be instructed to continue rapid but uniform warming, using perfusion blankets above and below the patient. The coagulopathy will often completely disappear a few hours after return to 37°C, and the patient can be safely extubated if short-acting anesthetic agents have been used. Significant memory deficits normally persist for several days.

Other Examples

Examples from two other centers illustrate variations on this approach. The University of Washington enhances surface cooling by the application of ice bags and administers dextran for hemodilution and reduction of viscosity. Rewarming is accomplished with a bath and heating lamp. With infants, this approach does not require cardiopulmonary bypass.[35] Barratt–Boyes, in New Zealand, employs surface cooling to 25°C and brief cardiopulmonary bypass.[36] The technique is similar to that described in detail above.

Other centers have also reported these techniques, or modifications of them.[37] Most use some type of bypass support for the terminal cooling and for rewarming as described by Barratt–Boyes. The results reported seem to be an improvement over the results obtained previously with perfusion alone in small infants. However, these series are small, and include a wide spectrum of congenital lesions. Suffice it to say that hypothermia can be used with excellent results when undertaken by an experienced team, committed to its application.

Teams at Stanford University have continued to use standard cardiopulmonary bypass at low flow (50–75 ml/kg-min) in infants as small as 2.6 kg with satisfactory results. It is extremely difficult to make an accurate comparison between the various groups of cardiac lesions which have been reported. The difficulties are compounded when operative variables are added to patient variables. Both conventional bypass and deep hypothermia can be used successfully. Mortality rates should be lowered in the future as patients are more accurately characterized preoperatively and management errors are eliminated.

COMPLICATIONS

Specific complications associated with hypothermia include acid-base disturbances, thermal damage, coagulation disturbances, and arrhythmias.

Lactic acidosis is seldom seen when tissue perfusion has been adequate during the induction of hypothermia. When circulatory arrest is included, the degree of acidosis depends on the duration of and the temperature during arrest. It appears that intervening periods of perfusion are most effective when flow is adequate to support fully aerobic metabolism. Some speculate that anoxia may be preferable during arrest to hypoxia (with very low perfusion), on the basis that continued cellular metabolism may hasten the development of irreversible injury.

Thermal damage is an important consideration. Injury occurs when a local increase in oxygen demand exceeds supply or when there is direct thermal injury to tissue. Thermal blankets should not be more than 10°C warmer than the patient's body temperature, and not more than 40°C maximum.[38] This concern applies also to cardiopulmonary bypass, but with less force, because the supply temperature is then warmer than the temperature of the perfused tissue. As noted previously, the maximum temperature is that applied to the blood, not the bulk temperature of the blood, and should not exceed 41°C.

Hypothermia is associated with coagulopathies. Below 34°C the enzymatic steps leading to blood coagulation are increasingly slowed. In fact, some groups using surface cooling and rewarming in infants do not use heparin for cardiac operations.[39] These investigators have shown return to normal clotting studies following cooling, arrest, and rewarming. They feel that bleeding is less in their patients than when standard cardiopulmonary bypass is employed. Their data would indicate that cooling and rewarming *per se* are not responsible for loss of clotting factors or platelets, but that the addition of the heart-lung machine (particularly the bubble oxygenator) is the primary reason for coagulation disturbances. There is evidence that the gas-blood interface in bubble oxygenators denatures proteins, and that hypothermia exaggerates this effect.

When adults are cooled and rewarmed, with long perfusion times, a large defect in coagulation results which may not be fully documented by the usual laborabory tests. Empirically, it can be reversed by the administration of fresh frozen plasma, platelets, and additional specific factors. Conventionally applied coagulation tests (excluding the bleeding time) after arrest and partial rewarming (>34°C), may indicate adequate recovery of clotting function, despite continued bleeding responsive to factor therapy.

A complication associated with hypothermia of less than 30°C has been ventricular fibrillation. Arrhythmias seldom occur above 30°C unless there is underlying myocardial anoxia as a result of any cause, or underlying cardiac disease. When oxygenation is well-maintained and pH is controlled by adequate ventilatory support, arrhythmias including fibrillation have been extremely rare, even in children with cardiac defects. Hypercarbia ($pCO_2 > 40$ torr) also appears to predispose to arrhythmias leading to cardiac arrest in the 27 to 30°C range. While easily reversed with countershock, a pCO_2 of 30 to 36 torr at a blood temperature of 37°C, or 26 torr at a blood temperature of 28°C is preferable, and can be assured with adequate end tidal monitoring.

When perfusion cooling is used, ventricular fibrillation occurs quickly when the perfusate temperature is below 23°C. This is of no consequence, however, because the circulation is maintained through bypass. Atrial fibrillation is common during rewarming, in the 28 to 32°C range, but almost always returns to normal sinus rhythm on return to normothermia. Of note is the rare case of accidental exposure to cold in which patients have been hypothermic to 6°C, and recovered without ventricular defibrillation.[40] The available evidence suggests that slow cooling is considerably safer if steps to minimize thermal gradients are *not* taken.

MYOCARDIAL PRESERVATION

BACKGROUND

During the first decade of open-heart surgery, postoperative low cardiac output was usually believed to be secondary to the preoperative status of the patient. However by 1970, three observations were accepted: (1) inadequate myocardial protection during surgery was implicated as a major cause of postoperative low cardiac output;[41] (2) inadequate myocardial protection was associated with the late development of cardiomyopathy, after successful valve replacement or defect repair;[42] and (3) a rare and exreme form of intraoperative damage, *stone heart*, was recognized to be secondary to poor intraoperative myocardial protection of the severely hypertrophied heart.[43]

Myocardial injury is usually caused by a discrepancy between oxygen supply and demand, rather than by absolute demand. In the beating heart, the subendocardium of the left ventricle is most susceptible to ischemic injury because it receives blood only during diastole. Coronary vessels traverse the myocardium from the epicardial supply vessels to the endocardium. These feeding vessels are squeezed shut during systole, leaving the endocardium with less perfusion reserve. Left ventricular hypertrophy enhances this effect, further diminishing reserve.

The endocardial viability ratio (EVR) is an expression of the ratio of available supply to actual demand, and is the ratio of diastolic perfusion index to tension time index. It does not take into account changes in basal oxygen demand or inotropic state, but is still clinically useful. Unlike the rate-pressure product, the numeric threshold associated with ischemia is relatively consistent from patient to patient. The reader is referred to Chapter 2 for a complete discussion.

In recent years, reliable monitoring of systolic arterial pressure and pulmonary capillary wedge pressure in patients with high risk has greatly decreased the incidence of ischemic events during induction and the prebypass interval. The concept of the EVR provides a useful means of applying this monitoring information.

OLDER METHODS

Cardiopulmonary bypass permits open-heart surgery. However, occlusion of the aorta with consequent interruption of coronary flow is necessary for optimal operating conditions. This iatrogenic myocardial ischemia leads to irreversible injury, unless protective measures are taken. There are three traditional measures which have been widely accepted: (1) continuous coronary artery perfusion, (2) ischemic arrest at normothermia or with moderate whole-body hypothermia, and (3) the use of ischemic arrest with profound local hypothermia of the heart. All of these methods were used extensively from 1960 to 1975, and continue to be used in many centers at the present time. Recently a fourth technique, cardioplegia, has been widely applied.

Coronary Artery Perfusion

The first widely used method was coronary artery perfusion. The delivery of adequately oxygenated blood from the bypass circuit to the coronary arteries seemed to be the most effective alternative for myocardial protection. However, this required extensive technical alterations, especially when the aortic root was opened and the coronary arteries had to be directly cannulated. A major disadvantage was the resulting trauma (including dissection) associated with perfusion apparatus which supplied a fixed flow, irrespective of the resulting perfusion pressure. Also, it often was not possible to perfuse the entire heart, because of variant coronary anatomy, or other technical difficulties.

In theory, the heart continues to beat. But in practice, fibrillation frequently occurred, with a resulting maldistribution of blood flow.[44]

The presence of blood within the heart and the moving and turgid myocardium increased the difficulty of surgery. The flow rates and cannulae employed also resulted in damage to blood elements. However, despite these problems, this method was the most widely used in clinical practice until very recently, and good results have been reported.[45]

Ischemic Arrest with Moderate Whole-body Hypothermia

Arrest during mild or moderate whole-body hypothermia seemed to provide greatly improved operating conditions and relative safety for many intracardiac procedures. The maximum safe period of ischemia was short—about 15 to 25 minutes. Because of this short interval, intermittent reperfusion was often advocated, but this may have aggravated ischemic damage.[46] This method was most often associated with the syndrome of stone heart and the method is now almost universally abandoned.

Ischemic Arrest with Profound Local Hypothermia

With this method, the aorta is occluded and the heart is selectively cooled during the ischemic interval. The rationale is that myocardial oxygen demand is greatly reduced.

Among the first investigators to suggest this technique were Berne and Cross.[47] They suggested the use of perfusion of the aortic root with cold blood after cross-clamping. Others used a single application of ice or slush within the pericardial well,[48] and Shumway and Lower reported the use of a continuous cold saline drip into the pericardial well in order to provide local hypothermia.[49] Both experimentally and clinically, local hypothermia extended the interval of safety while maintaining the technical advantages of ischemia.[50] The heart becomes still, flaccid, and easy to manipulate, when ischemia is established. The technique provided excellent results when used by many surgeons. The technical advantages inherent in this technique, and its rationale, are now widely appreciated.

COLD CARDIOPLEGIA

This technique was introduced in 1955 by Melrose.[51] He injected a solution of potassium citrate into the aortic root, resulting in immediate flaccid electromechanical arrest. His solution appeared to cause myocardial necrosis, caused by an extremely high osmolarity and potassium concentration[52] and, for this reason, cardioplegia fell into disrepute until the advent of safe methods in the 1970s. Several investigators continued the study of cardioplegia during the 1960s, particularly Bretschneider in Germany,[53] but it was not until the work of Gay and Ebert that attention was again focused on this technique.[54] Their work and that of many subsequent investigators has shown additive benefit when complete electromechanical arrest is combined with cardiac hypothermia. Morphologic and functional preservation of the myocardium during induced ischemia have been well documented, experimentally and clinically.[55, 56] The method most frequently used for inducing cardioplegia is the introduction of a solution containing increased potassium (blood *or* asanguinous) into the aortic root or coronary arteries. Many formulations of the solution have been recommended, and no clear advantage to any is presently known. The solution composition for clinical use at Stanford Medical Center is shown in Table 26–2. The important principle appears to be the rapid induction of electromechanical arrest soon after the interval of ischemia is initiated. Complete and rapid arrest with concomitant hypothermia reduces oxygen demand to low levels, a substrate for anaerobic metabolism is provided, and the high osmolality of the solution provides additional metabolic protection. All of these assumptions are supported by detailed studies.[56]

Table 26-2. Stanford Cardioplegic Solution Composition and Physical Characteristics

Potassium	mEq/l	30
Sodium	mEq/l	25
Chloride	mEq/l	30
Bicarbonate	mEq/l	25
Dextrose	g/l	50
Mannitol	g/l	12.5
Osmolality	mg	440
pH (@ 4°C)	units	8.1–8.4

Immediate Electromechanical Arrest

Immediate arrest avoids needless expenditure of tissue energy stores. If obligatory tissue metabolic requirements are low enough, the very small energy output of anaerobic metabolism can support cell membrane integrity.

Many chemical additives have been suggested for producing immediate arrest. Potassium is the predominant intracellar cation, and a logical means of reducing transmembrane polarization, so that hyperkalemic solutions have been most often used. Diastolic arrest, through membrane depolarization, persists so long as extracellular potassium is sufficiently elevated. However, a potassium concentration above 40 mEq/l may be deleterious, and should not be employed.[57] Hypothermia reduces the potassium concentration needed to produce cardioplegia, permitting an increased safety margin.

Cardioplegia can also be produced by elevated extracellular magnesium. The mechanism appears to be the blockage of calcium entry into the cell by occupation of calcium receptor sites on the cell membrane. Isolated heart studies suggest that a magnesium concentration of 15 mEq/l, the normal intracellular concentration, may provide additional myocardial protection.[58]

Extracellular hypocalcemia will produce cardioplegia by eventually limiting the amount of ionic calcium available to trigger myocardial contraction. Isolated heart studies suggest that complete absence of calcium for a significant period results in severe damage to the sarcolemmic membrane, although this may have no clinical importance because of noncoronary collateral flow (see below).[59]

The calcium antagonists, verapamil and nifedipine, have shown promise for enhancing myocardial protection during ischemic arrest.[60] These agents appear to block the initial flooding of calcium into cells upon reperfusion, maintaining the concentration of ionic calcium low during the initial phase of reoxygenation. Although their exact mode of action is unknown, they appear to be highly beneficial in myocardial protection. See Chapter 3.

Finally, cardioplegia has been induced with several anesthetic agents, such as procaine.[61] Apparently procaine stabilizes the cell membrane, but the exact mechanism is unknown. Procaine alone produces myocardial protection during induced ischemia, but not significantly greater than that produced by any other method of induced cardioplegia. A major clinical disadvantage is its continued effect after reperfusion, which is slowly reversed; reperfusion may continue for 20 to 30 minutes before a satisfactory rhythm returns.

Hypothermia

Studies to compare the relative affect of electromechanical arrest versus hypothermia are conflicting.[61] However, the majority support the concept that hypothermia is more important than arrest in providing myocardial protection. At 22°C, the arrested heart requires only 0.31 ml oxygen/100g/min, and at 15°C, only 0.27 ml/100g/min. The effect of extremely low temperatures, below 10°C, are unknown, and are difficult to achieve clinically.

Topical hypothermia can be combined effectively with cold cardioplegia.[62] A pericardial well is fashioned by incising the pericardium and suturing the cut edges to the surgical drapes to form a bowl around the heart. A small plastic catheter (#18 French nasogastric tube) is connected to two liter containers of 4°C saline, as shown in Figure 26–8. After cardiac arrest and application of the aortic cross-clamp, cold cardioplegia is begun through a #18 intravenous catheter in the aortic root, and external cooling is initiated by a continous flow of cold saline. When the heart is opened, lavage of the interior is also performed. The external catheter and suitably placed suction maintain the level of continually replaced cold saline over the entire surface of the heart.

Important adjuncts to the technique are the use of moderate whole-body hypothermia (28–30°C), relatively low bypass flow (40–60 ml/kg/min), and positioning of the operating table by tilting it slightly to the left and elevating the head approximately 20°C. It is useful to remove the bronchial venous return by venting through the pulmonary artery with a sump vent. If the heart is not opened, the aortic root catheter can be used as an adequate left ventricular vent if low-flow perfusion is employed. However, blood then passes throught the left ventricle, causing some endocardial warming.

Metabolic Substrate

It may be important to provide substrates for potential anaerobic metabolism during ischemia. Many cardioplegic formulations have incorporated dextrose; some incorporate blood to transfer additional oxygen. In studies of isolated hearts, the addition of substrate does not apparently improve myocardial protection, probably because of the accumulation of anaerobic metabolites which impair glycolysis.[63] In the clinical setting, noncoronary collateral flow or intermittent cardioplegic reinfusion may wash away these metabolites, and permit an increase in anaerobic metabolism.

Because an anoxic heart relies upon anaerobic glycolysis, intracellular lactic acid accumulates, lowering pH and impeding enzymatic function. Buffering prolongs the period of anaerobic metabolism. Available evidence suggests that the optimal pH with decreasing temperature becomes more alkaline. Buckberg believes that cardioplegic solutions should be buffered to a high pH if the temperature is below 28°C, and suggests a pH of 7.8 at 20°C.[64] Lactate should not be used as the buffer because of its poor buffering ca-

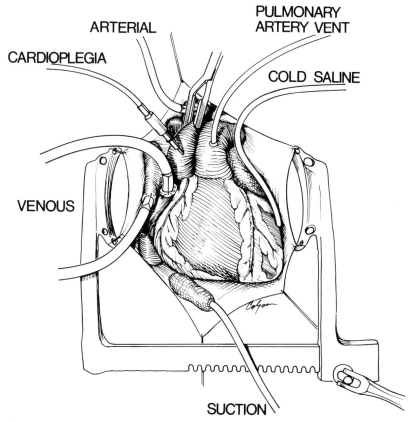

Fig. 26-8. Appearance of the heart during aortic occlusion. A 14-gauge needle in the proximal ascending aorta delivers cold cardioplegia solution. Topical hypothermia is produced by continuous lavage of the pericardial well by saline solution at 4°C. Decompression of the heart is accomplished by gentle aspiration of a 14-French sump vent placed in the main pulmonary artery.

pacity with lowered temperature and its inhibiting effect on anaerobic metabolism.

Noncoronary Collateral Flow

Aortic cross-clamping interrupts the coronary circulation but does not eliminate all blood flow to the heart. Noncoronary collateral channels come from mediastinal and bronchial vessels which course through pericardial attachments and the posterior atrial wall to the myocardium.[65] These collaterals are seen during cardiac transplantation when the heart is excised at the midatrial level, and a number of small vessels bleed from the cut atrial surface. These channels provide a variable flow, greatest in association with ventricular hypertrophy and ischemic coronary disease. In animals, measured flow is 0.5 to 10 ml/100g/min.[65]

This flow has the effect of diluting the cardioplegic solution. Not only are the desirable pharmacologic effects reversed or eliminated, but rewarming occurs. This may result in fibrillation or normal electromechanical activity, reducing myocardial protection. Studies suggest that these effects can be avoided by multidose cardioplegia.[66] Another attractive alternative is the combination of continuous topical local hypothermia with initial cardioplegia as described above. This may be preferable if the risk of injury from cardioplegia solution constituents cannot be eliminated. With this combination, the myocardial temperature can be consistently maintained below 20°C, and flaccid arrest continues despite reversal of potassium-induced cardioplegia. Because the amount of noncoronary collateral flow depends on systemic perfusion pressure, it can be reduced by low bypass flows and systemic hypothermia.

As Buckberg has emphasized, the presence of noncoronary collateral flow will minimize the effects of both harmful and beneficial solutions.[67] At present, no single solution formulation has been shown to be distinctly superior for providing myocardial protection. We prefer the combination of a single cardioplegic infusion with continuous profound local hypothermia for myocardial protection.

SUMMARY

The history of the medical use of hypothermia is a fascinating subject, complicated by confusion between the deleterious effects of hypothermia itself and the derangements produced during warming and cooling. The technique was explored early in the history of open-heart surgery, then neglected as simpler bypass techniques were developed, and is now achieving new recognition as more aggressive surgical therapy comes into use.

The principal advantage of hypothermia is the reduction in obligatory metabolic oxygen demand. Most complications appear related to the derangements produced as temperature is altered at the beginning or end of the procedure. Gaps between supply and demand can easily develop, and the complexity of the procedure permits errors (*e.g.,* inadequate monitoring or gas embolization).

The ideal metabolic and regulatory status during hypothermia remains to be defined, but it seems clear that respiratory alkalosis at body temperature, relative to a pH of 7.42, and minimal anesthetic depression with aggressive vasodilation, are protective. Recent careful work suggests that *uncorrected* blood gas values for pH and pCO_2 should be used. Hypothermia-induced coagulopathy is a ma

jor problem with deep hypothermia, but can be managed effectively with modern component therapy.

Surface cooling and core warming appear to be most attractive in reference to theoretical concerns about tissue preservation. In practice, the techniques are usually combined to hasten temperature changes, improve control, and reduce tissue temperature gradients. The greatest risk associated with profound hypothermia appears to be uncontrolled temperature gradients which accelerate the development of tissue hypoxia.

Aggressive application of the principles of local cooling with induced myocardial ischemia has been particularly beneficial in the evolution of techniques in open-heart surgery. The complexity of the procedure and patient risk are ameliorated by topical hypothermia, with only moderate whole-body hypothermia.

Yet the value of profound hypothermia for specialized procedures has increased as new applications have developed. Recent history suggests the increasing use of profound hypothermia, with specific indications, but only in centers equipped and trained for this complex undertaking.

REFERENCES

INTRODUCTION

1. Currie J: Medical Reports on the Effect of Water, Cold and Warm, as a Remedy in Fever and Other Disease. Liverpool, Codell and Davies, 1797.
2. Swan H: Clinical hypothermia: a lady with a past and some promise for the future. Surgery 73:736–758, 1973
3. Smith LW, Fay T: Observations on human beings with cancer: maintenance at reduced temperatures of 75–90°F. Am J Clin Pathol 10:1–11, 1940
4. Bigelow WG, Callaghan JC, Hoppes JA: General hypothermia for experimental intracardiac surgery: the use of electrophrenic respirations, an artificial pacemaker for cardiac standstill and radio frequency rewarming in general hypothermia. Ann Surg 132:531–539, 1950

5. Mohri H, Martin WE, Sato S et al: Oxygen utilization during surface-induced deep hypothermia. Ann Thorac Surg 18:494–503, 1974
6. Swan H, Zeavin I, Blount SG Jr et al: Surgery by direct vision in the open heart during hypothermia. JAMA 153:1081–1085, 1953
7. Churchill–Davidson HC, McMillan IKR, Melrose DG: Hypothermia: An experimental study of surface cooling. Lancet 2:1011–1013, 1953
8. Lewis FJ, Tauffic M: Closure of atrial septal defects with the aid of hypothermia; experimental accomplishments and the report of one successful case. Surgery 33:52–59, 1953

PHYSIOLOGY

Oxygen Availability

9. Hervey GR: Physiological changes encountered in hypothermia. Proc R Soc Med 66:1053–1058, 1973
10. Ohmura A, Wong KC, Westenskow DR, et al: Effects of hypocarbia and normocarbia on cardiovascular dynamics and regional circulation in the hypothermic dog. Anesthesiology 50:293–298, 1979
11. Merrill EW, Gilliland ER, Cokelet G et al: Rheology of human blood, near and at zero flow: effects of temperature and hematocrit level. Biophysical J 3:199–213, 1963
12. Marty AT, Eraklis AJ, Pelletier GA et al: The rheologic effects of hypothermia on blood with high hematocrit values. J Thorac Cardiovasc Surg 61:735–738, 1971

THE APPROPRIATE pH AND pCO₂

13. Rahn, H: Body temperature and acid-base regulation (review article). Pneumonologie 151:87–94, 1974
14. Rahn, H: pCO₂, pH and body temperature. In Nahas G, and Schaefer KE (eds): Carbon Dioxide and Metabolic Regulation, pp 152–162. Berlin Springer–Verlag, 1974
15. Howell BJ, Baumgardner FW, Bondi K et al: Acid-base balance in cold blooded vertebrates as a function of body temperature. Am J Physiol 218:600–606, 1970
16. Rahn H: Acid-base regulation and temperature in the evolution of vertebrates. Proc International Union Physiological Science 8:91–92, 1971

17. Becker H, Vinten–Johansen J, Maloney JV Jr et al: Effect of pH adjustment in deep hypothermia and circulatory arrest. Chirurgische Forum Fur Experimentelle und Kleinische Forschung 80:291–294, 1980
18. McConnel DH, White F, Nelson R et al: Importance of alkalosis in maintenance of ideal blood pH during hypothermia. Surg Forum 26:263–265, 1975
18a. Ream AK, Reitz BA, Silverberg GD: Temperature correction of PCO₂ and pH in estimating acid–base status: An example of the emperor's new clothes? Anesthesiology 56(1):41–44, 1982
18b. Becker H, Vinten–Johansen J, Buckberg GD et al: Myocardial damage caused by keeping pH 7.40 during systemic deep hypothermia. J Thorac Cardiovasc Surg 82:810–820, 1981
18c. White FN: A comparative physiological approach to hypothermia. J Thorac Cardiovasc Surg 82:821–831, 1981

WHOLE BODY HYPOTHERMIA

Moderate Hypothermia

19. MacDonald DJ: Current practice of hypothermia in British Cardiac Surgery. Br J Anaesth 47:1011–1017, 1975
20. Madden FR, Stemler FW, Hiestand WA: Effect of certain chemical agents and physical conditions on the body temperature of mice and the relationship of temperature to drowning survivals. Am J Physiol 180:121–123, 1955

Deep Hypothermia with Circulatory Arrest: Infants

21. Horiuchi T, Koyamada K, Matano I et al: Radical operations for ventricular septal defect in infancy. J Thorac Cardiovasc Surg 46:180–190, 1963
22. Mohri H, Dillard DH, Crawford EW: Method of surface-induced deep hypothermia for open-heart surgery in infants. J Thorac Cardiovasc Surg 58:262–270, 1969

Deep Hypothermia with Circulatory Arrest: Adults

23. Lillehei CW, Todd DB, Levy MJ et al: Partial cardiopulmonary bypass, hypothermia, and total circulatory arrest. J Thorac Cardiovasc Surg 58:530–543, 1969

24. Griepp RB, Stinson EB, Hollingsworth JF et al: Prosthetic replacement of the aortic arch. J Thorac Cardiovasc Surg 70:1051–1063, 1975

25. Ott DA, Frazier OH, Cooley DA: Resection of the aortic arch using deep hypothermia and temporary circulatory arrest. Circulation [Suppl I] 58:227–231, 1978

26. Klebanoff G: Total body washout for liver coma. Contemp Surg 2:13–16, 1973

27. Michenfelder JD, Kirklin FW, Uihlein A et al: Clinical experience with a closed-chest method of producing profound hypothermia and total circulatory arrest in neurosurgery. Ann Surg 159:125–131, 1964

28. Uihlein A, MacCarty CS, Michenfelder JD et al: Deep hypothermia and surgical treatment of intracranial aneurysms. JAMA 195:639–641, 1966

29. Silverberg GD, Reitz BA and Ream AK: Hypothermia and cardiac arrest in the treatment of giant cerebral aneurysm and medullary hemangioblastoma. J Neurosurg 55:337–346, 1981

Techniques

30. Hikasa Y, Shirotani H, Satomura K et al: Open heart surgery in infants with an aid of hypothermic anaesthesia. Arch Jap Chir 36:495, 1967

31. Prakash O, Jonson B, Bos E et al: Cardiorespiratory and metabolic effects of profound hypothermia. Crit Care Med 6:165–171, 1978

32. Williams GD, Seifen AB, Lawson NW et al: Pulsatile perfusion versus conventional high-flow nonpulsatile perfusion for rapid core cooling and rewarming of infants for circulatory arrest in cardiac operation. J Thorac Cardiovasc Surg 78:667–677, 1979

33. Sasaki Y: Perfusion cooling by pulsatile flow. Jpn J Surg 7:96–104, 1977

34. Toledo–Pereyra LH, Chee M, Lillehei RC: Effects of pulsatile perfusion pressure and storage on hearts preserved for 24 hours under hypothermia, for transplantation. Ann Thorac Surg 27:24–31, 1978

35. Mohri H, Dillard DH, Crawford EW: Method of surface-induced deep hypothermia for open-heart surgery in infants. J Thorac Cardiovasc Surg 58:262–270, 1969

36. Barratt–Boyes BG, Simpson M, Neutze JM: Intracardiac surgery in neonates and infants using deep hypothermia with surface cooling and limited cardiopulmonary bypass. Circulation [Suppl I] 43:25–30, 1971

37. Rittenhouse EA, Mohri H, Dillard DH et al: Deep hypothermia in cardiovascular surgery. Ann Thorac Surg 17:63–98, 1974

Complications

38. Rill MR: Safety and Performance of Hypothermia Devices, pp 1–46. Washington, DC, Food and Drug Administration, 1978

39. Mohri H, Dillard DH, Crawford EW: Method of surface-induced deep hypothermia for open-heart surgery in infants. J Thorac Cardiovasc Surg 58:262–270, 1969

40. Fruchan AF: Accidental hypothermia: report of eight cases of subnormal body temperature due to exposure. Arch Intern Med 106:218–229, 1960

MYOCARDIAL PRESERVATION

Background

41. Taber RE, Morales AR, Fine G: Myocardial necrosis and the postoperative low cardiac output syndrome. Ann Thorac Surg 4:12–28, 1967

42. Michelis LL: Intraoperative protection of the myocardium. Ann Thorac Surg 20:3–6, 1975

43. Cooley DA, Reul GJ and Wukasch DC: Ischemic contracture of the heart: "stone heart." Am J Cardiol 29:575–577, 1972

Older Methods

44. Buckberg GD, Hottenrott CE: Ventricular fibrillation: Its effect on myocardial flow, distribution, and performance. Ann Thorac Surg 20:76–85, 1975

45. Michelis LL: Coronary artery perfusion. Ann Thorac Surg 20:72–75, 1975

46. Levitsky S, Wright RN, Rao KS et al: Does intermittent coronary perfusion offer greater myocardial protection than continuous aortic cross-clamping? Surgery 82:51–59, 1977

47. Cross FS, Jones RD, Berne RM: Localized cardiac hypothermia as an adjunct to elective cardiac arrest. Surg Forum 8:355–359, 1957

48. Urschel HC, Greenberg JS, Hufnagel CA: Elective cardioplegia by local cardiac hypothermia. New Engl J Med 261:1330–1332, 1959

49. Shumway NE, Lower RR: Topical cardiac hypothermia for extended periods of anoxic arrest. Surg Forum 10:563–566, 1959

50. Brody WR, Reitz BA: Topical hypothermia

protection of the myocardium. Ann Thorac Surg 20:66–69, 1975

Cold Cardioplegia

51. Melrose DG, Drewer B, Bentall HH, et al: Elective cardiac arrest. Lancet 2:21–22, 1955
52. Tyers GFO, Todd GJ, Niebauer IM et al: The mechanism of myocardial damage following potassium citrate (Melrose) cardioplegia. Surgery 78:45–53, 1975
53. Bretschneider H Jr, Hubner G, Knoll D: Myocardial resistance and tolerance to ischemia: physiological and biochemical basis. J Cardiovasc Surg 16:241–260, 1975
54. Gay WA Jr, Ebert PA: Functional, metabolic and morphological effects of potassium-induced cardioplegia. Surgery 74:284–290, 1973
55. Kirklin JW, Conti VR, Blackstone EH: Prevention of myocardial damage during cardiac operations. New Engl J Med 301:135–141, 1979
56. Buckberg GD: A proposed "solution" to the cardioplegia controversy. J Thorac Cardiovasc Surg 77:803–815, 1979
57. Gharagozloo F, Bulkley BH, Hutchins GM et al: Potassium-induced cardioplegia during normothermic cardiac arrest. J Thorac Cardiovasc Surg 77:602–607, 1979
58. Hearse DJ, Steward DA, Braimbridge MV: Myocardial protection during ischemic cardiac arrest. Importance of magnesium in cardioplegic infusates. J Thorac Cardiovasc Surg 75:875–877, 1978
59. Jynge P, Hearse DJ, Braimbridge MV et al: Myocardial protection during ischemic cardiac arrest. J Thorac Cardiovasc Surg 73:848–855, 1977
60. Clark RE, Ferguson TB, West PN et al: Pharmacologic preservation of the ischemic heart. Ann Thorac Surg 24:307–314, 1977
61. Buckberg GD: A proposed "solution" to the cardioplegia controversy. J Thorac Cardiovasc Surg 77:803–815, 1979
62. Nelson RL, Goldstein SM, McConnel DH et al: Improved myocardial performance after aortic cross-clamping by combining pharmacologic arrest with topical hypothermia. Circulation [Suppl III] 54:III12–16, 1975
63. Hearse DH, Steward DA, Braimbridge MV: Myocardial protection during ischemic cardiac arrest. Possible deleterious effects of glucose and mannitol in coronary infusates. J Thorac Cardiovasc Surg 76:16–23, 1978
64. White F, Nelson RL, Goldstein SM et al: The importance of alkalosis in maintenance of "ideal" blood pH during hypothermia. Surg Forum 26:263–265, 1975
65. Brazier J, Hottenrott C, Buckberg GD: Noncoronary collateral myocardial blood flow. Ann Thorac Surg 19:426–435, 1975
66. Follette D, Fey K, Mulder D et al: Prolonged safe aortic clamping by combining membrane stabilization, multidose cardioplegia, and appropriate pH reperfusion. J Thorac Cardiovasc Surg 74:682–690, 1977
67. Buckberg GD: A proposed "solution" to the cardioplegia controversy. J Thorac Cardiovasc Surg 77:803–815, 1979

27

Cardiac Assist Devices and the Artificial Heart

ALLEN K. REAM
PEER M. PORTNER

INTRODUCTION

With the exception of short-term cardiopulmonary bypass, cardiac assist devices have not been important to the anesthesiologist until very recently. Originally a laboratory concept, they are now entering widespread clinical use. Because the field is changing so rapidly, we discuss the concept as a complete entity, without attempting to precisely define the evolving interests and responsibilities of those working in anesthesia. It seems likely, however, that all of the selected material is professionally relevant.

The concept of the cardiac assist device is simply stated: to support systemic perfusion by adding to or replacing the output of the natural heart and to support the heart by reducing oxygen demand or increasing oxygen supply. These goals underlie all of the presumed benefits of the devices that have been developed. While the most challenging goal is complete heart replacement, most efforts have been directed toward augmenting natural function. The artificial heart is the final goal in the progression of technical developments, and is much discussed because technical difficulty and subjective reactions make it a fascinating and controversial concept.

In the discussion which follows, we trace the evolution of assist devices, emphasizing those in clinical use (particularly the intraaortic balloon), and concluding with an overview of problems, prospects, and controversies. While this chapter can be read alone, the reader may find it profitable to review the chapters on cardiopulmonary bypass (Chap. 14) and myocardial and hemodynamic function (Chap. 2). Several references are also suggested for further background reading.[1-6]

Early developments were essential to the success of cardiopulmonary bypass. These developments are discussed in Chapter 14, and include techniques for pumping blood, gas exchange, asepsis, and anticoagulation.

The next phase of development began with successful cardiopulmonary bypass in the early 1950s. Attempts were made to assist the beating heart. This effort required better control systems in order to synchronize with the natural system, and better techniques, because extended support was necessary. As these devices improved, more of the system became implantable. Today, we have totally implantable electrically powered devices at an advanced stage of animal testing, with periods of circulatory support extending to 6 months.

The final step, to total artificial circulatory support, now appears close. Human-sized animals have been kept alive on a total artificial heart for months, and trials in humans appear to be only a few years away. Unfortunately, nearly all of these experimental devices have been pneumatically powered, an approach which has no possibility of being suitable for general clinical use. The technical problems yet to be overcome are severe, including increased efficiency to permit *in vivo* energy storage, improved reliability, and improved blood-materials compatibility. The most probable means of solution of these problems is the application of technology developed for permanent left ventricular assist devices.

DEVICES

Because of the large number of technical problems and the enormous variety of alternatives available, it is most convenient to classify first by function, rather than by chronology. Three major functional categories are presented in Table 27-1: direct cardiac assistance, series devices, and parallel devices. Although parallel devices represent the ear-

Table 27-1. Classification of Circulatory Assist Devices

DIRECT ASSIST
1. Cardiac massage
2. Artificial myocardium
3. Ventricular balloon

SERIES ASSIST
1. Valved series pumps
2. Invasive counterpulsation
   a. Arterial-arterial bypass
   b. Arterial compression
   c. Valveless bladder sewn in aorta
   d. Intraaortic balloon
3. External counterpulsation
   a. Airway
   b. BASH
   c. External body compression

PARALLEL ASSIST
1. External peripheral
   a. Venovenous with oxygenation
   b. Venoarterial without oxygenation
   c. Venoarterial with oxygenation
2. External central
   a. Left atrium to femoral artery, no thoracotomy (Dennis)
   b. Left atrium to axillary artery, pulsatile (DeBakey)
   c. Left atrium to aorta (Litwak)
   d. Left ventricle (through aortic valve) to aorta (Zwart)
   e. Left ventricle (through apex) to aorta, with filter (Peters)
3. Implanted pump (LVAD) (Bernhard)
   a. Left ventricle
   b. Biventricular

liest efforts, they are considered last because they also define the path to total heart replacement.

DIRECT ASSIST

Cardiac compression is an obvious approach, and has been attempted by several groups, beginning in 1956.[7-9] The first attempt inflated and deflated the pericardial sac with air. Later versions used a nondistensible cup surrounding the heart, with an inner, inflatable bladder, sometimes with suction to avoid ejecting the heart during compression. Problems include myocardial trauma (which can be severe), inadequate right-sided filling with transmitted left-sided pressure, loss of the wringing motion of contraction (with disrupted intracardiac flow patterns), and injury to the coronary arteries near the rim of the cup. American interest in this device has lapsed, but development efforts continue in the Soviet Union. The primary application now appears to be temporary support of a prospective donor of noncardiac organs.

Direct replacement of nonfunctional myocardium with a permanent pulsatile prosthesis has been attempted,[10] but the benefits are no greater than with the intraaortic balloon (discussed below), while cost and risk are substantially increased.

Synchronous balloon pulsation within the ventricle has also been attempted, with temporary improvement in systemic perfusion.[11, 12] However, this technique appears to have little to recommend it because the improvement is at the expense of a considerable increase in systolic myocardial tension and hence increased oxygen demand and risk of rupture.

SERIES ASSIST (OR COUNTERPULSATION)

The conceptual basis for this approach is the presumption that reducing the pressure into which the heart pumps both reduces myocardial oxygen demand (by reducing systolic wall tension) and increases stroke volume (by decreasing end systolic volume). Although the first logical attempt might be to add a pump just downstream of the left ventricle, virtually all serious attempts have avoided this approach because of the anatomic difficulty of surgically implanting such a pump, and the associated problem of compromised coronary perfusion. Instead, the same effect is accomplished by cyclically varying either the blood volume or vascular volume of the systemic arterial tree, so that any pressure decrease during systole is offset by a pressure increase during diastole.

The original counterpulsation technique was developed in 1957 by Birtwell.[13] The first study was presented in 1958, and published in 1961.[14] One or both femoral arteries were cannulated, and attached to a valveless, pneumatically operated actuator. A volume of blood (30–70 ml in humans) was alternately withdrawn and returned with each cardiac cycle. At least one other version was

developed,[15] and pumping was also attempted using the subclavian artery.[16] The major problems with this approach were associated with the femoral cannulae. The desired flow rate required excessive flow velocity, causing hemolysis and vascular injury. For these reasons, the pumping volume was usually not adequate.

In 1958, Birtwell produced counterpulsation with a saline-filled balloon in the aorta, cycled using the previous actuator. This work was reported in 1962,[17] the same year that Moulopoulos reported the first gas-filled intraaortic balloon (IAB).[18] The gas-filled IAB has since become the dominant clinical device for therapy utilizing counterpulsation.

Effort also continued on a surgically implanted counterpulsation device. In 1958, Kantrowitz used periaortic circumferential diaphragmatic muscle strips stimulated through the phrenic nerve.[19] Subsequently, Kantrowitz, Nose, and Akutsu tested a series, valveless, pulsatile chamber, usually implanted in the ascending aorta.[20] The dynamic aortic patch, the most recent effort, is essentially an IAB sewn into the aortic wall.[21, 22] While the drive line may be larger because it is extravascular, increased implantation time has been associated with infection, and the technique has not been copied. Recently, Phillips has reported a valveless pumping chamber connecting the aortic arch and distal thoracic aorta, which appears functionally similar.[23] However, in comparison with recent parallel assist devices, this approach no longer appears attractive.

In 1963, Dennis,[24] Osborn,[25] and Birtwell[26] independently reported success in applying counterpulsation externally. Positive pressure applied to the legs compresses the vascular bed, expelling both arterial and venous blood. The arterial effect mimics invasive counterpulsation. Venous return is increased, increasing filling pressure and cardiac output. This result may require therapeutic measures in a patient who cannot tolerate increased filling pressure. Birtwell's original system utilized rigid tubes, with an inner hydraulically driven bladder which surrounded the legs. Newer systems use a nondistensible but flexible outer fabric tube. It is claimed that effective support can be provided up to a heart rate of 200. The practical aspects of the design are subtle and important. As an example, the first machine tended to gradually eject the patient with each positive pressure cycle.

While initially greeted with skepticism, external counterpulsation is gradually being accepted, and appears capable of providing effective circulatory assistance. Clinical results are similar to those with the IAB reported below,[27, 28] and the device can be quickly applied without surgery. However, this approach is less effective because the pulse pressure must be generated from the periphery and is therefore smaller centrally. It limits access to the patient. And there is some concern about injury to the venous valves in the legs. A collaborative clinical trial is presently underway in the United States, and the device is recommended for ambulance use in the Soviet Union.

Other external modes of counterpulsation have been tested, but not proven particularly effective. An early effort was airway counterpulsation.[29] More dramatic was *body acceleration synchronous with heartbeat* (BASH). This system consisted of a horizontal table, capable of accelerations of up to 1.5 g. The intent was to cyclically move the column of blood in the ascending thoracic aorta, essentially mimicking the effects of counterpulsation.[30] The concept is of historical interest only because it is likely to damage mesenteric attachments, unpleasant in use, and only modestly effective.

Of all these techniques, the most widely successful are external counterpulsation, usually encasing only the legs, and the IAB. The IAB is favored because it is more effective, and once in use, less likely to compromise general patient care. The only apparent advantage of external counterpulsation is that it is noninvasive. In the following discussion, we use the IAB to illustrate the practical aspects of counterpulsation. A more detailed discussion is provided by Weber.[31]

The balloon is normally introduced through the femoral artery, and positioned just below the aortic arch. It is then cyclically inflated and deflated so that average pressure during systole is maximally decreased, and average pressure during diastole is maximally increased (Fig. 27-1). The presumed benefits are three: to reduce myocardial oxygen demand by reducing afterload, to increase myocardial oxygen availability by increasing mean diastolic pressure (the period when coronary flow occurs), and to increase stroke volume by reducing afterload (and hence end systolic ventricular volume). Because of coronary autoregulation, early studies which examined coronary blood flow gave variable results (IAB support sometimes reduces coronary flow, when demand also appears reduced). However, the endocardial viability ratio (see Chap. 2) is improved.[32]

It appears that the first clinical trials of the IAB were conducted by Kantrowitz.[33] As with the following studies by Bregman[34] and Buckley,[35] they reported improvement or correction of the shock state following myocardial infarction. While alterations in mean systolic and diastolic pressure were modest (10–20%), this appeared sufficient to offer measurable clinical benefit.

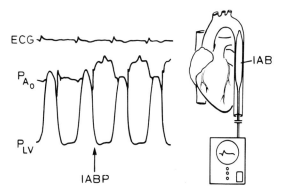

Fig. 27-1. Principles of intraaortic balloon (*IAB*) counterpulsation. The IAB is positioned in the thoracic aorta and driven in synchrony with the ECG by an external console. Shown is the influence of intraaortic balloon pumping (IABP) on aortic root (PA_0) and left ventricular (PLV) pressures (*i.e.*, the respective augmentation of aortic diastolic pressure and reduction in ventricular systolic pressure). (Weber KT, Janicki JS: Ann Thorac Surg 17:603, 1974)

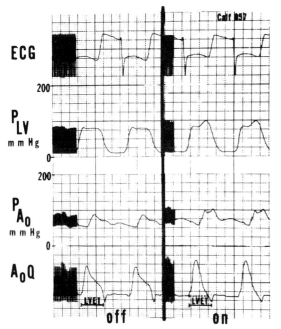

Fig. 27-2. The experimental results of premature IAB inflation before aortic valve closure are shown for a conscious calf preparation following left circumflex coronary artery occlusion. Aortic (P_{A_0}) and ventricular (P_{LV}) pressures and aortic root flow (AoQ) are shown for the basal (*off*) and IAB (*on*) states. Note the late rise in P_{LV}, the diminished diastolic augmentation in P_{A_0}, and the reduction in stroke volume and abbreviation in ventricular ejection time (LVET). The *solid* and *dotted lines* in the *right-handed panel* represent the duration of ejection during basal and IAB states, respectively. Note that Weber's notation is not consistent with terminology in this book. (Weber KT, Janicki JS: Ann Thorac Surg 17:603, 1974)

Because of the physical constraints, however, the balloon is marginally effective unless all the accessible parameters are optimized. A larger balloon size improves pumping, but the diameter must be slightly less than that of the aorta for maximum efficiency. The volume is also limited by the possible size of the catheter, and consequent rate of gas flow. A typical upper limit for a 70 kg adult is approximately 35 ml.[36] The balloon size is also constrained by the diameter of the femoral artery. A new balloon, which elimi-

nates the catheter inside the balloon, promises to relieve this constraint.[37, 38]

Arguments persist about the best gas with which to fill the balloon. Helium is preferred because it has the lowest practically obtainable viscosity, permitting very rapid balloon response. With a very fast timing circuit, the balloon can be deflated after detection of each QRS complex, fast enough to assure a reduction in afterload. Carbon dioxide is too slow for this maneuver, and requires a timing circuit which, after a delay, inflates the balloon for a limited period. In effect, with helium it is possible to time the balloon for each heartbeat. With carbon dioxide the timing signal from one heart beat controls the balloon during the following heartbeat, sacrificing the ability to appropriately respond to a single premature ventricular contraction. The advantage of carbon dioxide is that the volume of gas necessary to produce injury, should the balloon leak, is considerably higher.

Balloon timing is a crucial factor. Kantrowitz reported a very high incidence of myocardial rupture in his first series, which was first thought to be associated with poor timing, leading to occasional very high systolic pressure, perhaps associated with ectopic beats. Many now suspect that rupture was a consequence of myocardial necrosis, made more evident because the IAB prolonged patient survival. However, a more likely problem is simply the failure to provide significant augmentation. The criteria for ideal timing are still under discussion, but most agree that the optimal adjustment is sensitive to heart rate, usually quite narrow in tolerance, and very sensitive to arrhythmias. (Fig. 27-2).

Minor complications of IAB therapy are probably common, though difficult to demonstrate if the patient recovers. In a series of patients coming to necropsy, the most common complication was aortic dissection, followed in diminishing incidence by arterial thrombi, arterial emboli, limb ischemia, and local infection.[39] It would appear that most complications are associated with insertion, rather than subsequent operation. Two instances of rupture with helium have been reported, one of which was fatal.[40] All of the present commercial devices use a safety chamber to limit the amount of gas that can be ejected after rupture to roughly one stroke volume.

Clinical results suggest that in patients in cardiogenic shock who are treated with the IAB, evident hemodynamic improvement occurs within a few hours if use of the device is associated with an altered course. In successful cases, the balloon is usually removed within 2 days, but may be used longer. A significant percentage of improving patients are stable on the balloon, but require other therapy (such as surgery) before weaning can successfully occur.[41] Thus, an emerging application is acute postoperative support following open-heart surgery, or other situations in which the patient can be expected to improve, if supported over the short term. It has been suggested that the early use of the IAB can reduce the size of a myocardial infarction, but conflicting results are reported.[42] The balloon is not very effective at high heart rates, with arrhythmias, or with very low arterial pressure.[43] In such cases, a parallel device may be necessary.

PARALLEL ASSIST

Circulatory assistance can also be effected by supplanting the pumping work of the heart, using a mechanical device in parallel. In this case, the assist device takes over the work of the heart, as the degree of assistance increases, until total support, when the contribution of the biologic heart becomes superfluous. This is the goal of the total artificial heart.

External, Peripheral

The simplest form of parallel assistance is to approach the patient through the femoral vessels, using a roller pump with cannulae. Venoarterial bypass without oxygenation provides some assistance, but must be limited to a modest fraction of cardiac output. Similarly, venovenous bypass with oxygenation pro-

vides only limited support. Venoarterial bypass with oxygenation is promising, but limited by the associated blood trauma with present oxygenators. For support for more than 6 to 8 hours, as noted in Chapter 14, clinical successes presently reported utilize not more than 70 percent bypass flow.

External, Central

A significant problem with the femoral approach is the maximum flow achievable because of vessel size. The first significant approach to central cannulation was reported by Dennis, who passed a cannula into the left atrium, through a jugular vein and the atrial septum.[44] The technique did not require thoracotomy, and was successful in a clinical attempt.

DeBakey, using an air-driven pulsatile pump connected from the left atrium to the axillary artery, attempted support in 1971.[45] However, the clinical trials were not successful, because blood return was inadequate, and the pump also slowly filled with clot. A more recent design has not yet been clinically evaluated.[46] Litwak attempted a more conservative approach, pumping from the left atrium to ascending aorta through a roller pump.[47, 48] In the most recent study, 13 of 19 patients were successfully weaned, with 7 of 19 discharged from the hospital[49] (Fig. 27-3). Both procedures require thoracotomy. Both were attractive, however, because the pump could be removed without surgery, leaving the truncated or obturated lines for removal at a later, safer time.

However, withdrawing blood from the atrium provided only a modest improvement in blood supply to the assist device. While the potential flow is higher, normal atrial filling pressures are too low to overcome the resistance of a long cannula, and suction quickly collapses the atrium, further increasing flow resistance. Direct comparison of atrial and ventricular withdrawal in dogs supports these conclusions.[50]

The first serious attempt to atrialize the ventricle was made by Zwart, by inserting a

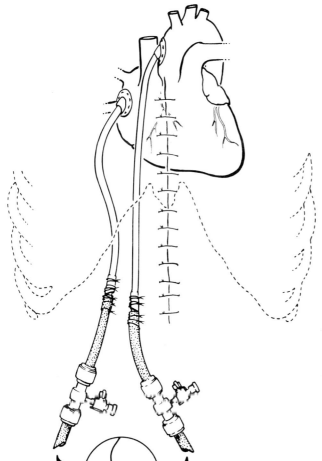

Fig. 27-3. Left heart support by pumping from left atrium to ascending aorta, using a roller pump. (Litwack RS et al: Ann Thorac Surg 21:191, 1976)

LA OUTFLOW   ROLLER PUMP   AORTIC INFLOW

cannula in the ventricle through the carotid or axillary artery and the aortic valve, returning blood through the femoral artery.[51] A thoracotomy was not required. Animal studies showed a flow of 2 to 4 l/min, with an average of 30 percent reduction with ventricular fibrillation. More recently, Golding was able to exceed 5.5 l/min, using a transaortic valve cannula, and centrifugal pump.[52] Pulsations were added using an external IAB. Peters pumped blood through a roller pump and filter from the left ventricular apex to the femoral artery.[53] Preliminary clinical trials are encouraging, but the value of the filter remains to be demonstrated. The lack of automatic flow control appears to be a significant pa-

tient hazard. Taguchi has also provided extended clinical support by left apical bypass, using local infusion of heparin to reduce dose requirements.[54] Both Peters and Taguchi have provided biventricular support, using this technique. The significant early designs undergoing clinical trial are summarized in Figure 27-4.

Implanted Pump

The need to improve filling and the goal of long-term assistance both lead to an implantable device. However, as previously noted, the first attempts were with series devices and were not successful. The first device to achieve broader acceptance and multicenter clinical trials, has been the left ventricular assist device (LVAD), shown in Figure 27-5. First developed by a collaborative effort between Bernhard and the Thermo-Electron Corporation,[55] it was initially supported by the NIH as an interim device, primarily useful for testing of pump design. However, it gradually became evident that the design has useful clinical properties, and it became a central concept. Studies now include over 1000 animals of adult human size, and over 45 clinical trials with the original design and minor variations,[56-60] and considerable additional work with designs stimulated by the original concept.[61-63]

The function of all devices described in the literature, under the acronym LVAD, is pumping from the left ventricular apex to the aorta through a valved, pulsatile pump. In the original design and in all clinical trials to date, the pump consists of an outer, rigid shell, and inner bladder, with ejection following the introduction of gas between the shell and bladder. The pump was intended to operate synchronously, ejecting after each heartbeat and then accepting blood from the next contraction. In this way, the peak systolic pressure generated in the left ventricle can be kept quite low, if cardiac stroke volume is less than assist pump volume.

However, in the pneumatic version of the

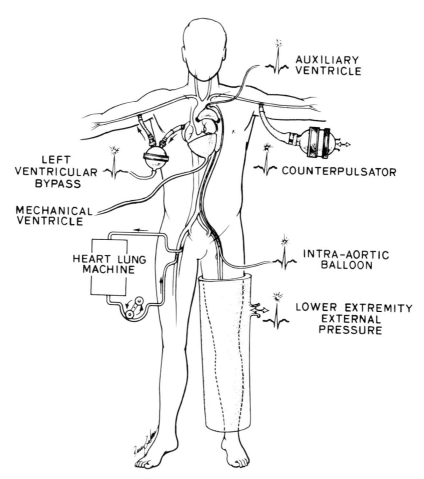

Fig. 27-4. A composite illustration of early circulatory assist devices which have received clinical trial. (Kennedy JH, Bricker DL: Am J Cardiol 27:33, 1971)

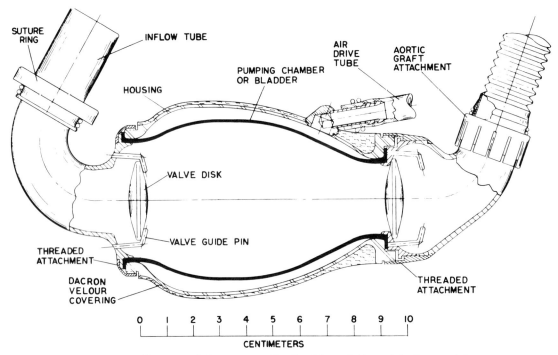

Fig. 27-5. A schematic diagram of the pneumatically driven left ventricular assist device (LVAD). (Bernhard W, LaFarge G: In Artificial Heart Program Conference, p. 565. Washington, D.C., U.S. Government Printing Office, 1969)

pump, timing is accompanied by the ECG and control of the pneumatic drive system. In practice, most drive systems do not track well because the delays inherent in this approach, as with carbon dioxide in the IAB, are significant. Thus, in most of the studies of long-term support reported, pump timing has been asynchronous to the natural heart for a significant period of time. Some suggest that synchronous timing adds little, because the effect on individual parameters is small. However, as shown in Figure 2-20, the improvement in the endocardial viability ratio is roughly doubled with synchronous pumping. Figure 27-6 shows the results of pumping synchronously, asynchronously, and turning the pump off in a calf of human size.

It is difficult to find quickly the optimal phase delay in a given situation. In the original studies, investigators operated the pump at each synchronous setting until the patient was hemodynamically stable, and then se-

lected the optimal state. While effective, the method was slow. Branch and Ream suggested that initial synchronization could be rapidly obtained by setting the pump to run at a fixed frequency, slightly different from that of the supported heart.[64] With a frequency difference of 1 to 3 beats/min, the timing for maximum support could be quickly determined. Minor adjustments were then necessary to account for physiologic adaptation. This approach appears suitable for automation with the new control systems just now appearing (see Fig. 27-6).

Norman has suggested that asynchronous operation may be preferable in the presence of severe arrhythmias;[65] it appears that this problem is most severe for the pneumatic systems. Mechanical systems now under development can trigger directly on left ventricular ejection,[66] and these systems are preferable because they can be completely implanted (Fig. 27-7).

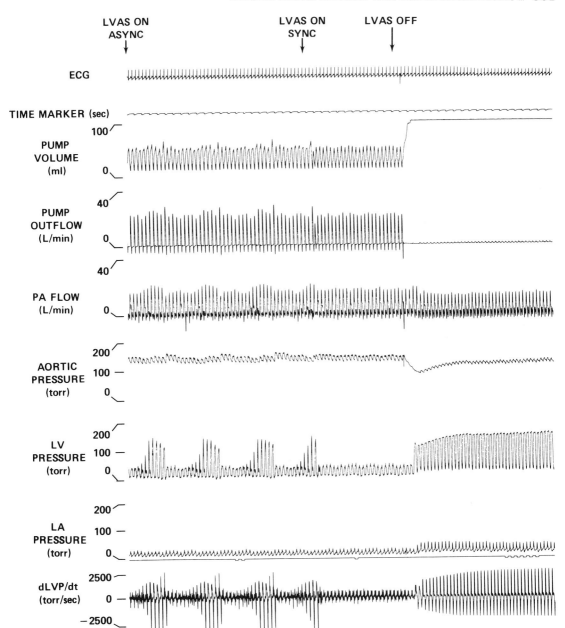

Fig. 27-6. Hemodynamic data collected during *in vivo* **implantation of a left ventricular assist system (LVAS).** *Far right:* LVAS off. *Center:* LVAS on, running synchronously, with optimal phasing with the heart. Peak left ventricular pressure is very low; the aortic valve does not open. *Left:* LVAS running asynchronously at a rate slightly different from that of the heart, such that there is a difference of approximately 3.5 beats during the displayed interval. Peak ventricular pressure is very low when phasing is optimal, and rises to near off-values when phasing is approximately one-half cardiac cycle later (see also Chap. 2). *dLVP/dt* = first derivative of left ventricular pressure; *LA* = left atrium; *LV* = left ventricle; *PA* = pulmonary artery. (Oyer PE et al: Development of a totally implantable, electrically actuated left ventricular assist system. Am J Surg 140:17–25, 1980)

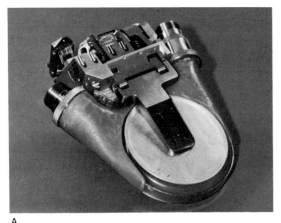

A

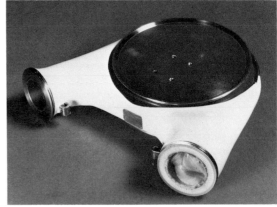

B

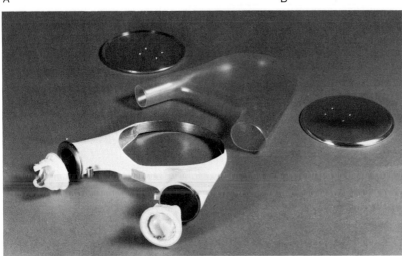

C

Fig. 27-7. A prototype left ventricular assist system (LVAS), with an implantable drive system. *A.* An exploded view of the pump, showing the heterograft valves, housing, pump bladder, and pusher plates. *B.* The assembled system, with the electrical to mechanical energy converter in place. (Andros Incorporated and Stanford University)

Another significant problem is determining optimal control is widespread uncertainty about the optimal physiologic result.[67-68] When the device is initially implanted, maximum support seems warranted to assure systemic perfusion, and to put the heart to rest. But if this is effective and continued, it appears likely that the heart will not be stressed sufficiently to (1) develop the capability to support the circulation without the device in the case of temporary assistance or (2) to prevent atrophy sufficient to compromise function of the atrialized ventricle, in the case of permanent assistance. An early approach for temporary assistance was to permit the heart to eject on occasional beats. But this is a substantial increase in work load,

and with a failing heart, may produce progressive dilation and injury.

Under normal conditions, the oxygen consumption (and work) of the heart is related to systolic pressure (afterload). In this situation, even if the aortic valve does not open, the same result applies.[69] However, the approach is technically difficult, because the assist device must be controlled with unusual precision to assure control of left ventricular systolic pressure. Most control systems used with the LVAD lack this precision.

While it is difficult to interpret with precision the results of early clinical trials in patients in cardiogenic shock following cardiotomy, several conclusions appear reasonable. The LVAD does provide more effective support of the circulation than the IAB, in that it can take over completely for the left ventricle. While present clinical results are very modest (of 42 patients, the LVAD was removable in 12, and 4 ultimately survived),[70] patients are admitted to LVAD therapy only after all other measures have failed, and they have been in cardiogenic shock for a significant period. In a number of the patients who did not survive, the device provided effective support, but cardiac function was inadequate when it was turned off. The study criteria are gradually broadening to permit earlier intervention, and it appears likely the incidence of survival will increase, as was noted in the early IAB studies. Also, as previously noted, the control systems used in present clinical studies do not permit a graded approach to weaning. It appears highly probable that a graded, controlled, and gradual increase in work load during the weaning process will increase the probability of recovery in marginal patients.

The primary limitation of this approach is that the right ventricle is not supported. While inflow from the left ventricle provides better return than inflow from the left atrium,

the pump cannot fill adequately if right failure is severe.[71] In some instances, right assist may be sufficient when the left ventricular component of failure is insignificant.[72] However, this clinical situation may require biventricular support, a step closer to total heart replacement (Fig. 27-8).[73] The reader should also be aware that left ventricular support (with an LVAD) in the event of biventricular failure can appear to be successful over a few hours, if blood volume is sufficient to permit adequate return to the left heart. However, right-sided circulatory pressures rise markedly, producing cardiac and pulmonary injuries which assure the patient's ultimate demise. While questions have been raised regarding possible pulmonary injury secondary to right-heart bypass, it appears that assuring the appropriate pressure and flow is sufficient to avoid injury.[74]

FUTURE APPLICATION AND THE TOTAL ARTIFICIAL HEART

The logical progression from the LVAD is to biventricular support, and then total heart replacement. In this section we briefly outline

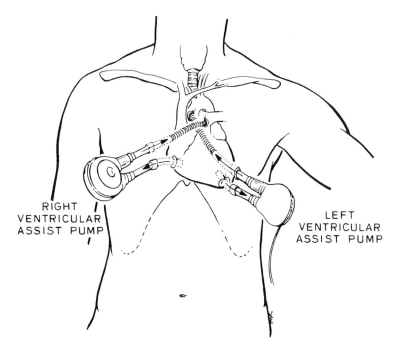

RIGHT VENTRICULAR ASSIST PUMP

LEFT VENTRICULAR ASSIST PUMP

Fig. 27-8. Clinical application of biventricular mechanical circulatory assistance. The left ventricular assist pump inlet tube is positioned within the left ventricular chamber, but the right pump inlet tube is positioned in the right atrium. This chamber is readily accessible, and permits unobstructed filling of the right pump. The right pump return cannula is anastomosed to the main pulmonary artery. Most clinical trials with this device involved only left-side support. A few patients have been supported bilaterally, and one patient has received right side support. (Pierce WS: American Society of Artificial Internal Organs Journal 2:1, 1979)

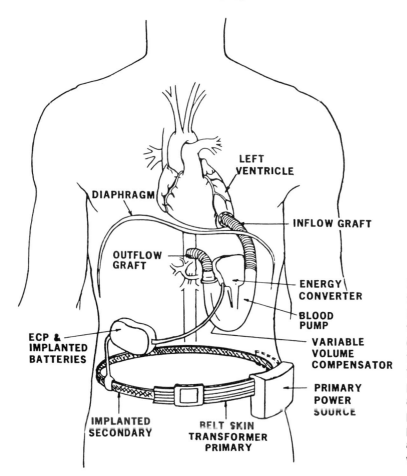

Fig. 27-9. A possible configuration for a permanently implanted left ventricular assist system (LVAS). Power is transmitted through unbroken skin to storage batteries and the pump drive system. This approach permits a staged procedure, with later implantation of the batteries and transmission system if weaning is unsuccessful.

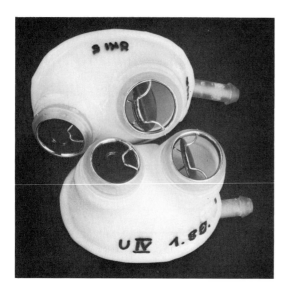

Fig. 27-10. An example of one of the more promising pneumatically driven artificial hearts. (Photograph courtesy of Dr. Felix Unger).

progress, the discussion is continued in the following discussion of problems.

Developments have followed two converging courses. The first and oldest has been continued attempts at direct total heart replacement. Most of these devices, and all current designs, have been pneumatically powered. The second, an evolutionary approach from assist to full support and replacement has provided useful information. It appears likely that technology developed for permanent left ventricular assist devices will determine the ultimate design (Fig. 27-9). But space in the chest is limited, and total support is compromised in the present of the natural heart. The duration of successful total heart replacement in animals has gradually increased. At this writing, animals of adult human size have been maintained solely on an artificial heart for more than 6 months.

Typically a total heart is roughly of natural

size, exclusive of the drive system, and is implanted by anastomosis to the natural atrial remnants. An example of a pneumatically driven device is shown in Figure 27-10. The reader is referred to Akutsu (Texas Heart Institute),[75] Atsumi (Japan),[76] Bucherl (Germany),[77] Jarvik and Kolff (Salt Lake City),[78] Nose (Cleveland Clinic),[79] Pierce (Hershey),[80] and Unger (Austria)[81] for extensive discussion. The critical problems and limitations are discussed in the next section.

PROBLEMS

THE BLOOD INTERFACE

A major technical problem has been the lack of a material which does not stimulate thrombus formation when exposed to blood. Many approaches have been tried; each offered some advantage but was less than ideal.[82] Ablative materials such as magnesium have been tried. Unfortunately, while the surface remains clean, the ablated material is often biologically active. Because highly charged molecules, such as heparin, often interfere with clotting, charged surfaces have been created. The only moderately successful technique involves heparin binding, and is now commercially available. Low surface-free energy appears to reduce interaction, but the correlation with individual materials is uncertain, and often unreliable. Hydrogels have been investigated. Binding water, they present a largely aqueous surface to the blood, but lack mechanical integrity. And, while the surface remains clean, it is at the expense of continued microembolization.

A second approach is to form a surface which is a suitable substrate for development of a living interface. An early effort was to floc the surface with fibers of uniform size and length. Fibrin formed in this mesh, forming a pseudointima. If the mesh were too long, the intima could grow, leaving the base too far from nutrients and resulting in necrosis of the deeper layers, and the surface would then embolize. Or it would continue to grow until the vascular space was filled. Microporous texturing sometimes reduced

the thickness of the pseudointima, but did not always result in a stable surface. The Cleveland group coats the surface with treated protein to provide a substrate for a permanent biologic intima.[83] Others have seeded the surface with autologous cells to develop a living intima.[84] But this approach requires preparation weeks before surgical implantation. Some surfaces, such as graphite-impregnated urethane,[85] pyrolytic carbon, and silicone have proved excellent for reasons which are obscure.

Perhaps the most frustrating aspect of this effort is the fact that, although considerable effort has been expended at an international level, there are still no reliable *in vitro* tests to predict *in vivo* performance. Long-term animal implantation is mandatory to prove a new approach.

It is possible to reduce the thrombus formation by creating a very smooth surface, reducing the opportunity for adhesion, disturbed flow, and perhaps surface-free energy. But while an excellent solution over the artificial surface, this leads to one of the major technical problems remaining: pannus formation at the interface with the natural intima. When the boundary is created, the intima proliferates and grows outward because it will not adhere to the smooth surface, often producing an obstruction or emboli.

Anticoagulation, such as occurs with heparin, aspirin, or warfarin, can reduce the incidence of thrombus formation. But the normal clotting system is otherwise an advantage, and should be preserved. Anticoagulation may now be reasonably avoided in many instances because of improved techniques and materials.[86]

Also complicating the situation is the requirement that some materials (such as in a balloon or bladder) must be flexible. Flexible materials which are also blood compatible usually have compromised mechanical properties.

A second major consideration is the flow pattern. Hemolysis has been a common phenomenon in these devices.[87] It is usually a function of the shear stress (controlled by the flow contour) and the material in contact with the blood. Reducing shear partially compensates for a less than ideal material. Turbulent flow increases the risk of thrombus formation by creating eddys and high local shear. Valves are a particular problem in this regard. Interestingly, pulsatile flow reduces these undesirable effects by inhibiting particle aggregation. In general, modern devices represent empirical improvements in the relation between flow and material.

Finally, calcification has been a major problem in experimental animals.[88] While these are often calves which are in a rapid growth phase, the problem may still carry over to humans, and it increases substantially the difficulty of interpreting the results of long-term animal experiments. Some evidence suggests that calcification may be accelerated by mechanical stress.[89] This has been particularly vexing in the use of heterograft valves (usually from the pig).

CONTROL

Device control is a problem in both the assist device and the artificial heart, but the constraints are different. For the assist device, the control system must match the remaining physiologic control systems. In the artificial heart, it must replace them. This has led to considerable difficulty in designing control systems for the total heart, because much of the successful work in assist devices depends on sensing signals (such as heart rate), which are no longer available after total replacement.

The first presumption was that a device which followed the practical result of the Starling principle (see Chap. 2), increasing output with increasing filling pressure, would be adequate. While sufficient in short-term experiments, this approach alone lacks sufficient responsiveness.[90] Small changes in parameters can result in a severe imbalance in right- and left-sided blood volume, an apparent cause of the high incidence of pulmonary edema in early artificial heart implantation.[91] And as heart transplant studies have amply demonstrated, relying solely on the Starling mechanism leads to a dangerous delay in the circulatory response to exercise,

and a concomitant increase in circulating blood volume, further increasing the risk of tissue injury.

The most promising control system known at present appears to be that of Pierce, in which control proceeds in a serial manner.[92] The left heart is controlled by sensing systemic arterial pressure and varying heart rate to vary output with a fixed stroke volume. The right heart, which is enslaved to this heart rate, is controlled by sensing left atrial pressure and varying the rate of ejection to vary stroke volume. Preliminary results are very encouraging.[93, 94] Practical considerations are the need to define the control pressures and a stable technique for pressure measurement. The anesthesiologist would do well to ponder the implications for control of the natural heart in a compromised patient; it is a different and useful way of thinking about the problem.

Finally, there appears to be general agreement that tissue monitoring should also be part of an ideal control loop. A possible measurement is mixed venous oxygen tension.[95]

PULSATILE FLOW

The merits of pulsatile flow have beeen discussed with reference to cardiopulmonary bypass. We consider here the problems associated with prolonged support. Because the references are not repeated, the reader is encouraged to review the discussion in Chapter 14.

While the data suggests that pulsatile flow is superior, doubt remains as to the degree. Some differences, such as in hemolysis, seem related to pump design.[96] While the increase in urine output with pulsatile flow under bypass conditions seems significant,[97, 98] it may relate to the adequacy of perfusion.[99] In the present state of oxygenator technology, there is good reason to keep perfusion as low as is acceptable. An artificial heart must provide a reasonable perfusion reserve. This tentative conclusion is reinforced by the evidence that pulseless flow increases systemic vascular resistance about 10 to 15 percent.[100–102] A higher perfusion pressure is required if this does not reflect tissue requirements. Further, the apparent protective effect of pulsatile flow on the fibrillating myocardium is not relevant to an artificial heart replacement.[103] And finally, reports of negative findings with the Bregman device (discussed in Chap. 14) under typical applications are beginning to appear,[104-106] although it may have special application in warming.

While some data are available to show short-term changes in hormone levels,[107] the sparse data in long-term animal studies do not clearly indicate that this is a problem.[108]

Another consideration has influenced the discussion. Centrifugal pumps have been developed which have minimal blood damage with nonpulsatile flow.[109, 110] However, these pumps are relatively inefficient, and seem to have no relevance to the implantable circulatory support device (see Chap. 14).

In the nuclear heart designs, heat dissipation is an important factor. Pulsatile flow improves heat exchange. However, at present, the successful application of this technology to the artificial heart seems unlikely.

Finally, recent mechanical designs have led to the question of left-right heart synchronization. Desynchronization does not appear to reduce efficiency or cause physiologic injury.[111] On the right side, the relationship to the respiratory phase appears more important.

TECHNICAL AND MECHANICAL CONSTRAINTS

Not surprisingly, a major technical problem has been developing agreement on system specifications. The original, conservative approach led to liberal functional specifications and devices which were too large and required too much energy with current technology to be successful. A large part of the cost of technology is the refinement of a particular design. Much of this effort can be wasted if the design goals are changed. We suggest that a useful initial goal is a device which can pump 7 l/min, into a mean pressure up to 100 torr for 16 hours without outside energy input.

Pump power sources have evolved in three major phases.[112, 113] The early designs were pneumatic because of the ease and simplicity of implementation. But in long-term use, the large drive lines required for adequate gas flow substantially increase the risk of infection. Also, because of the inherent size and inefficiency of pneumatic drive systems, and the impossibility of avoiding gas loss over long periods, it is generally agreed that these systems are not fully implantable.[114]

A second major effort was to develop systems which derive their power from thermal energy. Surprisingly, thermal storage efficiency has been achieved which is significantly better than with the best rechargable batteries. But the only logical primary source of heat is nuclear energy. Electrical conversion to mechanical energy is more efficient than thermal, removing the incentive for an electrical heat source. The combination of radiation hazard, extreme chemical toxicity of plutonium (the most likely source), and the large heat load which must be dissipated because of low conversion efficiency suggests that this approach is unlikely to be successful. Further, the hazard of this technology to others appears to be considerable.[115]

The remaining practical option is an electrical drive. Systems of high electrical to mechanical energy conversion efficiency (more than 65% as opposed to 14% for thermal) have been constructed,[116] leading to overall realizable efficiencies (source to energy imparted to moving blood) which may exceed 50 percent. Adequate miniaturization appears practical, with the exception of energy storage. With the presently achievable electrical storage density, a totally implanted system can run for perhaps 1 hour unsupported. Work on improved batteries and fuel cells continues; for the present, power is supplied by percutaneous transmission. It appears that 24-hour storage is a fully acceptable goal: the patient can recharge while sleeping.

Finally, development is entering the period where durability, quietness, ease of repair, and fail-safe behavior are becoming major goals. A significant but subtle result of these considerations is that designs are often becoming simpler as they become more effective. Control systems are simpler and external sensors are often no longer required. Simplicity improves reliability. While improvements in pumping chamber design reflect painfully acquired information about flow, recent developments also reflect the need to physically integrate the pump and power source to minimize size and weight. While reducing design flexibility, this also reduces complexity.

OTHER PHYSIOLOGIC CONSTRAINTS

A major practical problem is determining the optimal configuration and location for the device. In the case of an assist device, any needed space is an additional requirement. In the case of the total artificial heart, the pump logically replaces the heart. However, in most current designs, the drive system is large enough to suggest implanting it elsewhere in the thorax or abdomen. A nontrival aspect is the means of suspension; sustained pressure at too high a level results in tissue absorption and loss of support, even with bone. Thus the size, shape, weight, and specific gravity are all important considerations.[117]

A second problem is venting. In the natural heart, size changes with pumping are naturally accommodated by the lungs and mediastinum. In the case of the device, tissue encapsulation gradually reduces system compliance, leading to filling problems. At present, no fully adequate solutions exist, and more work must be done.

Valve design remains a major limitation. Heterograft valves have limited life, and often fail because of calcification. Blood damage and mechanical failure remain concerns.

Percutaneous energy transmission represents a biologic insult. When the line is brought through the skin, an avenue of infection results. Embedding the line in a thin fenestrated collar of tissue-compatible material (which is parallel to the surface of the skin) permits the early development of connective tissue investment of the collar, giving a mechanically strong connection. Fixation

also reduces the likelihood of developing a separation plane which can transmit infection. But in present designs, extension of epithelial tissue from the surface of the skin along the surface of the collar leads to extrusion after several months.

Electromagnetic transmission through unbroken skin appears most promising, but problems remain. The coil alignment must be adequate, secondary heating minimized, and the implanted portion must be aesthetically and functionally acceptable to the patient.[118]

In addition to the effects already discussed, some others appear to be possible problems. Infection continues to terminate many experiments, though long-term experience with pacemakers and vascular prostheses suggests that this is largely a matter of technique. Hepatic and pulmonary injury appear related to known causes (hemolysis and abnormal perfusion pressures) but continue to terminate animal experiments. Catecholamine levels remain elevated after artificial heart implantation in animals, though recovery from this initial abnormality appears likely.[119, 120] However, sham surgery suggests that many of the complications specifically suggested to be secondary to the use of the artificial heart are related to the surgical procedure and are controllable.[121]

APPLICATION: POPULATION AND ETHICAL CONCERNS

An emotional reluctance to consider the application of advanced circulatory support devices and the artificial heart appears founded on justifiable concerns. It is feared that the devices will be used to terminally extend life in nonproductive ways, that quality of life will be sacrificed to survival, and that the costs of this technology will divert resources (dollars and skills) from other significant medical benefits. All of these are legitimate concerns, and must be considered. Also, some physicians fear the increased nonmedical interference in medical practice which comes with high technology. As in the case of the tomographic scanner, such concerns may be justified, but must be separated from the scientific evaluation. It may be useful for those who share such fears to read the account of nursing care for one such patient.[122]

Another concern, supported by experience with drug evaluation, is that clinical trials be ethical and responsible. We agree with Cooper, who suggests that the question, "Can a physician run a controlled study on a patient, and still fulfill his obligation to him?" should be replaced by the question, "Can a physician treat his patient with any unproven therapy . . . outside of a study that will establish efficacy, and still fulfill his obligation to him?"[123]

A major fear of proponents of the artificial heart is that early clinical trials may be inappropriately discouraging. Their fears merit some consideration in view of early experience with the IAB. Initial clinical results were extremely discouraging because the device was used in patients who proved to be beyond salvage by any known technique, and with lesions which did not improve during prolonged support.

The major goals of devices are three: (1) to sustain life temporarily until the patient recovers, (2) to sustain life until definitive therapy can be provided, and (3) to sustain life permanently. As Cooper has pointed out, hostility has resulted from situations in which a temporary assist device has been adequate to sustain life, but neither goals (1) nor (2) could be satisfied. Future trials must include a clear definition of appropriate devices,[123] the appropriate patient population,[124, 125] and the appropriate time to terminate support.[126]

The left ventricular assist device may be useful for all three categories.[127, 128] Postsurgical support may assure recovery with only supportive therapy in some patients. In others, it may provide systemic support while the information and resources for definitive therapy (such as surgical correction) is obtained.[129] And because univentricular failure is most common, it appears likely to be effective as a permanent assist device when technologically adequate.

The total artificial heart may be useful for temporary support before cardiac transplan-tation.[130, 131] Its suitability for permanent replacement depends on the ethical concerns already listed.[132] Although not an early goal of significance, its value in pharmacologic[133] and physiologic[134] studies may be considerable.

The question of informed consent has worried some physicians. In the only legal question raised in reference to this procedure, the courts upheld the concept that the usual requirements were sufficient.[135]

SUMMARY

While all of these considerations may appear overwhelming, it is noteworthy that the first patient to receive a cardiac pacemaker (1958) is living at the time of this writing, with more than 22 replacements. The pioneers in new therapies never fare as well as those who follow, but the most relevant question is how they fared relative to the available alternatives. It is clear that assist devices have become a permanent part of medical therapy, and it appears likely that replacement devices will follow. We must prepare for that day.

REFERENCES

INTRODUCTION

1. Sanders CA, Buckley MJ, Leinback RC et al: Mechanical circulatory assistance. Circulation 45:1292–1313, 1972
2. Kolff WJ, Lawson J: Status of the artificial heart and cardiac assist devices in the United States. Trans Am Soc Artif Intern Organs 21:620–638, 1975
3. Akutsu T: Artificial Heart: Total Replacement and Partial Support. Tokyo, Igaku Shoin, 1975
4. Kantrowitz A: The development of mechanical assistance to the failing human heart. Med Instrum 10:224–227, 1976
5. Kolff WJ: Artificial organs and transplantation. Transplant Proc 9:53–63, 1977
6. Kennedy JH, Bricker DL: Criteria for selection of patients for mechanical circulatory support. Am J Cardiol 27:33–40, 1971

DEVICES

Direct Assist

7. Bencini A, Parolo LP: The pneumomassage of the heart. Surgery 39:375–384, 1976
8. Kolobow T, Bowman RL: Biventricular cardiac assistance energized by suction actuated coil of a single constricting rubber ventricle. Trans Am Soc Artif Intern Organs 11:57–64, 1965
9. Anstadt GL, Schiff P, Baue AE: Prolonged circulatory support by direct mechanical ventricular assistance. Trans Am Soc Artif Intern Organs 12:72–79, 1966
10. Freed PS, Imamura H, von Recum A et al: A prosthetic myocardium: hemodynamic results with a new tilting arm model. Trans Am Soc Artif Intern Organs 24:84–92, 1978
11. Bregman D, Parodi EN, Malm JR: Left ventricular and unidirectional intra-aortic balloon pumping. J Thorac Cardiovasc Surg 68:677–686, 1974
12. Donald DE, McGoon DC: Circulatory support by a left ventricular balloon pump. Circulation (Suppl I) 43:I96–I100, 1971

Series Assist (or Counterpulsation)

13. Birtwell WC, Clauss RH, Dennis C et al: The evolution of counterpulsation techniques. Med Instrum 10:217–223, 1976
14. Clauss RH, Birtwell WC, Albertal G et al: Assisted circulation. I. Arterial counterpulsator. J Thorac Cardiovasc Surg 41:447–458, 1961
15. Watkins DH, Callaghan PB: Postsystolic myocardial augmentation. Arch Surg 90:544–553, 1965
16. Jacoby JA, Craddock LD, Wolf PS et al: Clinical experience with counterpulsation in coronary artery disease. J Thorac Cardiovasc Surg 56:846–857, 1968
17. Clauss RH, Missier, P, Reed GE et al: Assisted circulation by counterpulsation with intra-aortic balloon: methods and effects. Presented at Annual Conference on Engineering in Medicine and Biology, Chicago, 1962
18. Moulopoulos SC, Topaz S, Kolff WL: Diastolic balloon pumping (with carbon dioxide) in aorta: Mechanical assistance to the failing circulation. Am Heart J 63:669–675, 1962
19. Kantrowitz A, McKinnon WMP: Experimental use of diaphragm as auxiliary myocardium. Surg Forum 9:266–268, 1958

20. Cournand A, Ranges HA: Catheterization of the right auricle in man. Proc Soc Exp Biol Med 46:462–466, 1941
21. Sujansky E, Tjonneland S, Freed PS et al: A dynamic aortic patch as a permanent mechanical auxiliary ventricle: experimental studies. Surgery 66:875–882, 1969
22. Kantrowitz A, Krakauer J, Rubenfire M et al: Initial clinical experience with a new permanent mechanical auxiliary ventricle: the dynamic aortic patch. Trans Am Soc Artif Organs 18:159–167, 1972
23. Phillips SJ, Kongtahworn C, Zeff RH et al: A new left ventricular assist device: clinical experience in two patients. Trans Am Soc Artif Intern Organs 25:186–191, 1979
24. Dennis C, Moreno R, Hall DP et al: Studies on external counterpulsation as a potential measure for acute left heart failure. Trans Am Soc Artif Intern Org 9:186–191, 1963
25. Osborn J, Main J, Beachley F et al: Circulatory support by leg or airway pulses in experimental myocardial insufficiency. Circulation 28:781–782, 1963
26. Birtwell W, Giron F, Soroff H et al: Support of the systemic circulation and left ventricular assist by synchronous pulsation of extramural pressure. Trans Am Soc Artif Intern Org 11:43–51, 1965
27. Soroff HS, Cloutier CT, Birtwell WC et al: External counterpulsation. JAMA 229:1441–1450, 1974
28. Amsterdam EA, Banas J, Criley JM et al: Clinical assessment of external pressure circulatory assistance in acute myocardial infarction. Am J Cardiology 45:349–356, 1980
29. Birtwell, WC, Soroff HS, Sachs BF et al: Assisted circulation. V. The use of the lungs as pump. A method for assisting pulmonary blood flow by varying airway pressure synchronously with the EKG. Trans Am Soc Artif Intern Organs 9:192–201, 1963
30. Arntzenius AC, Keeps J, Rodrigo FA et al: Circulatory effects of body acceleration given synchronously with the heart beat (BASH). Bibl Cardiol 26:180–187, 1970
31. Weber KT, Janicki JS: Intraaortic balloon counterpulsation: a review of physiological principles, clinical results, and device safety. Ann Thorac Surg 17:603–636, 1974
32. Philips PA, Bregman D: Intraoperative application of intraaortic balloon counterpulsation determined by clinical monitoring of the endocardial viability ratio. Ann Thorac Surg 23:45–51, 1977

33. Kantrowitz A, Tjonneland S, Freed PS: Initial clinical experience with intraaortic balloon pumping in cardiogenic shock. JAMA 203:113–118, 1968

34. Bregman D, Kripke DC, Goetz RH: The effect of synchronous unidirectional intraaortic balloon pumping on hemodynamics and coronary blood flow in cardiogenic shock. Trans Am Soc Artif Intern Organs 16:439–449, 1970

35. Buckley MJ, Leinback RC, Kastor JA et al: Hemodynamic evaluation of intra-aortic balloon pumping in man. Circulation 46 (Suppl II):130–136, 1970

36. Sturm JT, McGee MG, Fuhrman TM, et al: Treatment of postoperative low output syndrome with intraaortic balloon pumping: experience with 419 patients. Am J Cardiol 45:1033–1036, 1980

37. Subramanian VA, Goldstein JE, Sos TA et al: Preliminary clinical experience with percutaneous intraaortic balloon pumping. Circulation (Suppl I) 62:I123–I129, 1980

38. Bregman D, Casarella WJ: Percutaneous intraaortic balloon pumping: initial clinical experience. Ann Thorac Surg 29:153–155, 1980

39. Isner JM, Cohen SR, Virmani R et al: Complications of the intraaortic balloon counterpulsation device: clinical and morphologic observations in 45 necropsy patients. Am J Cardiol 45:260–268, 1980

40. Rajani R, Keo WJ, Bedard P: Rupture of an intraaortic balloon. J Thorac Cardiovasc Surg 79:301–302, 1980

41. Sturm JT, Fuhr an TM, Igo SR et al: Quantitative indices of intra-aortic balloon pump dependence during post infarction cardiogenic shock. Artif Organs 4:8–12, 1980

42. Laas J, Campbell CD, Takanashi Y et al: Failure of intra-aortic balloon pumping to reduce experimental myocardial infarct size in swine. J Thorac Cardiovasc Surg 80:85–93, 1980

43. Bregman D, Parodi EN, Malm JR: Left ventricular and unidirectional intra-aortic balloon pumping. J Thorac Cardiovasc Surg 68:677–686, 1974

Parallel Assist

44. Dennis C, Hall DP, Moreno JR et al: Left atrial cannulation without thoracotomy for total left heart bypass. Acta Chir Scand 123:267–279, 1962

45. DeBakey ME: Left ventricular bypass pump for cardiac assistance. Am J Cardiol 27:3–11, 1971

46. Chimoskey JE, O'Bannon W, Cant JR et al: Recent experience with the Baylor left ventricular bypass pump. Biomater Med Devices Artif Organs 5:361–377, 1977

47. Litwak RS, Koffsky RM, Lukban SB et al: Implanted heart assist device after intracardiac surgery. New Engl J Med 291:1341–1343, 1974

48. Litwak RS, Koffsky RM, Jurado RA et al: Use of a left heart assist device after intracardiac surgery: technique and clinical experience. Ann Thorac Surg 21:191–202, 1976

49. Koffsky RM, Litwak RS, Mitchell BL et al: A simple left heart assist device for use after intracardiac surgery: development, deployment and clinical experience. Artif Organs 2:257–262, 1978

50. Pennock JL, Pae WE, Pierce WS et al: Reduction of myocardial infarct size: Comparison between left atrial and left ventricular bypass. Circulation 59:275–279, 1979

51. Zwart HH, Kralios AC, Eastwood N et al: Effects of partial and complete unloading of the failing left ventricle by transarterial left heart bypass. J Thorac Cardiovasc Surg 63:865–872, 1972

52. Golding LR, Groves LK, Peter M et al: Initial clinical experience with a new temporary left ventricular assist device. Ann Thorac Surg 29:66–69, 1980

53. Peters JL, McRea JC, Fukumasu H et al: Transapical left ventricular bypass: A method for partial or total circulatory support. Artif Organs 2:263–267, 1978

54. Taguchi K, Mochizuki T, Miyoshi N et al: Flow control in prologed ventricular bypass and clinical application in 15 patients. Trans Am Soc Artif Intern Organs 24:104–112, 1978

55. Bernhard W, LaFarge G: Development and evaluation of a left ventricular–aortic assist device. In Hastings FW, Harmison LT (eds): Artificial Heart Program Conference, pp 559–579. Washington, DC, U.S. Government Printing Office, 1969

56. Norman JC, Bregman D: Mechanical circulatory support: evolving perspectives. Trans Am Soc Artif Intern Organs 24:782–787

57. Norman JC: Partial artificial hearts: mechanical cloning of the ventricle. Artif Organs 2:235–243, 1978

58. Berger RL, McCormick JR, Stetz JD et al: Successful use of a paracorporeal left ventricular assist device in man. JAMA 243:46–49, 1980

59. Holub DA, Hibbs CW, Sturm JT et al: Clinical trials of an abdominal left ventricular assist device: progress report. Trans Am Soc Artif Intern Organs 25:197–204, 1979

60. Bernhard WF, Poirier V, LaFarge CG et al: A new method for temporary left ventricular bypass. J Thorac Cardiovasc Surg 70:880–895, 1975

61. Pierce WS, Donachy JH, Landis DL et al: Prolonged mechanical support of the left ventricle. Circulation (Suppl I) 58:I133–I146, 1978

62. Turina MT, Bosio R, Senning A: Paracorporeal artificial heart in postoperative heart failure. Artif Organs 2:273–276, 1978

63. Wolner E, Thoma H, Deutsch M, et al: Das forschungprojekt "Kunstliches Herz." Wiener Klinische Wochenschrift 91:74–81, 1979

64. Branch CE, Ream AK: A synchronous control system for a totally implanted circulatory assist device. Am J Cardiol 27:20–32, 1971

65. Naifeh JG, Thompson PA, Johnson MD et al: Performance of an abdominal left ventricular assist device during induced tachycardias and dysrhythmias. J Thorac Cardiovasc Surg 72:175–181, 1976

66. Portner PM, Oyer PE, Miller PI et al: Evolution of the solenoid actuated left ventricular assist system. Artif Organs 2:402–412, 1978

67. Kennedy JH: Sub-total versus partial circulatory bypass of the left heart: a critical review. Biomater Med Devices Artif Organs 4:367–383, 1976

68. Peters JL, McRea JC, Fukumasu H et al: Transapical left ventricular bypass: A method for partial or total circulatory support. Artif Organs 2:263–267, 1978

69. Laas J, Campbell CD, Takanashi Y et al: Oxygen consumptoin of the left ventricle during transapical left ventricular bypass. J Thorac Cardiovasc Surg 80:280–288, 1980

70. Bernhard W, LaFarge G: Development and evaluation of a left ventricular–aortic assist device. In Hastings FW, Harmison LT (eds): Artificial Heart Program Conference, pp 559–579. Washington, DC, U.S. Government Printing Office, 1969

71. Pierce WS: Clinical left ventricular bypass: Problems of pump inflow obstruction and right ventricular failure. American Society Artificial Internal Organs Journal 2:1–9, 1979

72. Parr GVS, Pierce WS, Rosenberg G et al: Right ventricular failure after repair of left ventricular aneurysm. J Thorac Cardiovasc Surg 80:79–84, 1980

73. Olsen EK, Pierce WS, Donachy JH et al: A two and one half year clinical experience with a mechanical left ventricular assist pump in the treatment of profound postoperative heart failure. Int J Artif Organs 2:197–206, 1979

74. LaFarge CG, Bankole M, Bernhard WF: Physiologic evaluation of chronic right ventricular bypass. Circulation (Suppl I) 43:I90–I95, 1971

Future Applications and the Total Artificial Heart

75. Akutsu T: Artificial Heart: Total Replacement and Partial Support. Tokyo, Igaku Shoin, 1975

76. Atsumi K: Current status of artificial heart in Japan. Int J Artif Organs 3:161–167, 1980

77. Bucherl ES: The artificial heart—progress, problems, and further development. Med Prog Technol 4:61–70, 1976

78. Jarvik RK, Lawson JH, Olsen DB et al: The beat goes on: status of the artificial heart 1977. Int J Artif Organs 1:21–27, 1978

79. Kasai S, Koshino I, Washizu T et al: Survival for 145 days with a total artificial heart. J Thorac Cardiovasc Surg 73:637–646, 1977

80. Pierce WS, Brighton JA, Donachy JH et al: The artificial heart. Arch Surg 12:1430–1438, 1977

81. Unger F, Deutsch M, Fasching W et al: Eine neue konstruktion fur ein total Kunstliches herz: das ellipsoidherz. Wiener Klinische Wochenschrift 88:447–449, 1976

PROBLEMS

The Blood Interface

82. Bernhard WF, LaFarge CG, Liss RH et al: An appraisal of blood trauma and the blood-prosthetic interface during left ventricular bypass in the calf and humans. Ann Thorac Surg 26:427–437, 1978

83. Hayashi K, Snow J, Washizu T et al: Biolized intrathoracic left ventricular assist device. Med Instrum 11:202–207, 1977

84. Bernhard WF, Colo NA, Wesolowski BS et al: Development of collagenous linings on impermeable prosthetic surfaces. J Thorac Cardiovasc Surg 79:522–564, 1980

85. Wakabayashi A, Connolly JE, Stemmer EA et al: Heparinless left heart bypass for resection of thoracic aortic aneurysms. Am J Surg 130:212–218, 1975

86. Wakabayashi A, Connolly JE, Stemmer EA et al: Clinical experience with heparinless veno-arterial bypass without oxygenation for the treatment of acute cardiogenic shock. J Thorac Cardiovasc Surg 68:687–695, 1974

87. Kasai S, Koshino I, Washizu T et al: Is progressive anemia inherent to total artificial heart recipients? Trans Am Soc Artif Intern Organs 22:489–496, 1976

88. Pierce WS, Donachy JH, Rosenberg G: Calcification inside artificial hearts: inhibition by Warfarin-Sodium. Science 208:601–603, 1980

89. Whalen RH, Snow JL. Harasaki H et al: Mechanical strain and calcification in blood pumps. Trans Am Soc Artif Intern Organs 26:487–492, 1980

Control

90. Bucherl ES, Affeld K, Baer P et al: Total artificial heart replacement. Int J Artif Organs 2:141–152, 1979

91. Murakami T, Ozawa K, Harasaki H et al: Transient and permanent problems associated with the total artificial heart implantation. Trans Am Soc Artif Intern Organs 25:239–247

92. Pierce WS, Landis D, O'Bannon et al: Automatic control of the artificial heart. Trans Am Soc Artif Intern Organs 22:347–356, 1976

93. Landis DL, Pierce WS, Rosenberg G et al: Long-term *in vivo* automatic electronic control of the artificial heart. Trans Am Soc Artif Intern Organs 23:519–525, 1977

94. Kasai S, Koshino I, Washian T et al: Survival for 145 days with a total artificial heart. J Thorac Cardiovasc Surg 73:637–646, 1977

95. Stanley TH, Volder J, Kolff WJ; Extrinsic artificial heart control via mixed venous blood gas tension analysis. Trans Am Soc Artif Intern Organs 19:258–261, 1973

Pulsatile Flow

96. Bivona JC, Stanczewski B, Pasupathy C et al: *In vivo* evaluation of pulsatile ventricle pump by perfusion via left heart bypass technique. J Thorac Cardiovasc Surg 67:571–578, 1974

97. Goodman TA, Gerard DF, Berstein EF et al: The effects of pulseless perfusion on the distribution of renal cortical blood flow and on renin release. Surgery 80:31–39, 1976

98. Boucher JK, Rudy LW, Edmunds LH: Organ blood flow during pulsatile cardiopulmonary bypass. J Appl Physiol 36:86–90, 1974

99. Sink JD, Chitwood WR, Hill RC et al: Comparison of nonpulsatile and pulsatile extracorporeal circulation on renal cortical blood flow. Ann Thorac Surg 29:57–62, 1980

100. Mandelbaum I, Berry J, Silbert M et al: Regional blood flow during pulsatile and nonpulsatile perfusion. Arch Surg 91:771–812, 1965

101. Giron F, Birtwell WC, Soroff HS et al: Hemodynamic effects of pulsatile and nonpulsatile flow. Arch Surg 93:802–810, 1966

102. Dunn J, Kirsh MM, Harness J et al: Hemodynamic, metabolic and hematologic effects of pulsatile cardiopulmonary bypass. J Thorac Cardiovasc Surg 68:138–147, 1974

103. Habal SM, Weiss MB, Spotnitz HM et al: Effects of pulsatile and nonpulsatile coronary perfusion on performance of the canine left ventricle. J Thorac Cardiovasc Surg 72:742–755, 1976

104. Grover FL, Fewel JG, Vinas J et al: Effects of aortic balloon pumping during cardiopulmonary bypass on myocardial perfusion, metabolism, and contractility. Chest 75:37–44, 1979

105. Zumbro GL, Shearer G, Fishback ME et al: A prospective evaluation of the pulsatile assist device. Ann Thorac Surg 28:269–273, 1979

106. Frater RWM, Wakayama S, Oka Y et al: Pulsatile cardiopulmonary bypass: Failure to influence hemodynamics or hormones. Circulation (Suppl I) 62:I19–I25, 1980

107. Taylor KM, Bain WH, Maxted KJ et al: Comparative studies of pulsatile and nonpulsatile flow during cardiopulmonary bypass. J Thorac Cardiovasc Surg 75:569–584, 1978

108. Moores WY, Hannon JP, Crum J et al: Coronary flow distribution and dynamics during continuous and pulsatile extracorporeal circulation in the pig. Ann Thorac Surg 24:582–590, 1977

109. Johnston GG, Hammill F, Marzec U et al: Prolonged pulseless perfusion in unanesthetized calves. Arch Surg 111:1225–1230, 1976

110. Golding LR, Harasaki H, Loop FD et al: Use of a centrifugal pump for temporary left ventricular assist system. Trans Am Soc Artif Intern Organs 24:93–97, 1978

111. Peters JL, Volder J, Kessler T et al: use of the artificial heart for basic cardiovascular research. Chest 67:199–206, 1975

Technical and Mechanical Constraints

112. Dennis C: Present and future of the artificial heart. Biomater Med Devices Artif Organs 3:155–160, 1975
113. Portner PM: Driving systems for total artificial hearts. Proceedings of the World Symposium Artificial Heart Berlin, Springer–Verlag, in press.
114. Jarvik RK, Smith LM, Lawson JH et al: Comparison of pneumatic and electrically powered total artificial hearts in vivo. Trans Am Soc Artif Intern Organs 24:593–599, 1978
115. Dong E, and Andreopoulos S: Heartbeat. New York, Coward, McCann & Geoghegan, 1978
116. Portner P: An efficient electromechanical left ventricular assist system. In F Unger (ed): Assisted Circulation, pp 147–160. Berlin, Springer–Verlag, 1979

Other Physiologic Constraints

117. Urzua J, Sudilovsky O, Panke T et al: Anatomic constraints for the implantation of an artificial heart. J Surg Res 17:262–268, 1974
118. Portner PM, Laforge DH, Ptzele S: Transcutaneous energy for an implanted electrical circulatory support system using distributed inductive coupling. Proc European Soc Artif Organs 6:109–112, 1979
119. Stanley TH, Liu W, Gentry S et al: Blood and urine catecholamine concentrations after implantation of artificial heart. J Thorac Cardiovasc Surg 71:704–710, 1976
120. Lunn JK, Liu WS, Stanley TH et al: Effects of treadmill exercise on cardiovascular and respiratory dynamics before and after artificial heart implantation. Trans Am Soc Artif Intern Organs 22:315–322, 1976
121. Chimoskey JE, Lynch EC, Cant JR et al: Forty-one variables following thoracotomy in calves. Biomat Med Dev Art Org 6:245–272, 1978

Application: Population and Ethical Concerns

122. Nelson R, Smith J, Drummond R et al: Care of a man with a partial artificial heart. Am J Nurs 73:1580–1584, 1973
123. Cooper T, Harmison LT: Cardiopulmonary support systems: problems in clinical applications. Transplantat Proc 3:1497–1501, 1971
124. Jarvik RK, Olsen DB, Kessler TR et al: Criteria for human total artificial heart implantation based on steady state animal data. Trans Am Soc Artif Intern Organs 23:535–541, 1977
125. Gunnar RM, Loeb HS, Johnson SA et al: Cardiovascular assist devices in cardiogenic shock. JAMA 236:1619–1621, 1976
126. Kennedy JH, Bricker DL: Criteria for selection of patients for mechanical circulatory support. Am J Cardiol 27:33–40, 1971
127. Nose Y, Golding LR, Loop FD: Role of left ventricular assist devices in clinical heart transplantation. Transplant Proc 11:313–316, 1979
128. Norman JC: ALVAD 1979: Precedence, potentials, prospects and problems. Cardiovasc Dis Bull Texas Heart Institute 6:384–389, 1979
129. Hardy MA, Dobelle W, Bregman D et al: Cardiac transplantation following mechanical circulatory support. Trans Am Soc Artif Intern Organs 25:182–185, 1979
130. Cooley DA: Transplantation versus prosthetic replacement of the heart. Biomater Med Devices Artif Organs 3:481–488, 1975
131. Losman JG: Human technology after cardiac epigenesis. S Afr Med J 52:570–572, 1977
132. Kolff WJ, Lawson J: Perspectives for the total artificial heart. Transplant Proc 11:317–324, 1979
133. Stanley TH, English JB, Lunn JK et al: Use of the Bovine with an artificial heart as an experimental pharmacologic model. Artif Organs 2:310–313, 1978
134. Honda T, Fuque JM, Edmonds CH et al: Applications of total artificial heart for studies of circulatory physiology: measurement of resistance to venous return in postoperative awake calves. Ann Biomed Eng 4:271–279, 1976
135. Curran WJ: The first mechanical heart transplant: informed consent and experimentation. New Engl J Med 291:1015–1016, 1974

Part VIII EDUCATION

28

Education and Training of the Cardiac Anesthesiologist

MICHAEL A. FLYNN
RICHARD P. FOGDALL

The cornerstone of a good educational program is a good teaching staff, comprising knowledgeable clinicians and scientists who bring to their work an enthusiasm and commitment the student can emulate.[1]

A cardiac anesthesia training period offers an ideal situation for a successful educational exercise. It provides the combination of a highly motivated postgraduate physician, in an operative apprenticeship with personalized teaching, and small group learning in the lecture room. This is an excellent opportunity to mold personality, habits, and performance in an environment which encourages communication and interaction between teacher and resident. It must be remembered that the triad of patient care, teaching, and research may occur simultaneously if the program is correctly designed.

Material concerning research into, and objective analysis of, cardiac resident and faculty education is difficult to find in the literature. Many written comments are based on individual bias and opinions. Among some important questions which are not addressed are the following:

1. Do good programs turn out superior practitioners of cardiac anesthesia? How do we assess this?
2. What impact does board certification have on the practice of cardiac anesthesia? Should certification be obligatory? Should subspecialty cardiac certification be mandatory?
3. How many operative patients should a resident anesthetize in order to produce an optimally trained person? What effect does a greater or lesser number of patients have on the quality of the final product?
4. How important is it to successfully pass an advanced cardiac life support course?
5. What do we expect from our finished product (the fully trained resident or fellow), and how do we each achieve the ideal in our own situation?

These questions, and others, will be explored in this chapter. We will also utilize some comparisons offered from an informal survey of some of our colleagues in 18 major centers of anesthesia in North America.[2]

THE LEARNING PROCESS

Before we discuss the details of a training program in cardiac anesthesia, we should consider the general process of learning. This chapter will not be a treatise on education and learning processes, so the reader will need to consult textbooks on education for these specifics. The reader is also referred to three thought-provoking articles dealing with medical education.[3-5] We have assumed, for most of our discussion, that the person in the student role is motivated, intelligent, behaves reasonably, and has acquired good basic learning skills. Are these assumptions accurate?

Motivation is reasonably easy to evaluate. Behavior is also, and a behavioral problem may disrupt learning or patient care, and thus ultimately doom the process. Intelligence may be more difficult to evaluate in some circumstances, yet we can usually agree upon a minimum degree of intelligence required for residency. If a physician arrives at a residency training program, he or she must have graduated from college, medical school, and internship, passed several national examinations, and is therefore presumed to be a good learner. Correct? Not at all. Good basic learning skills cannot be taken for granted. Some residents have never developed an optimal approach to learning. And unfortunately, occasionally some are even in the wrong profession.

An exceptional look at some aspects of basic learning is seen in the classical work of Holt.[6] He describes two classes of students, those who are thinkers and those who are guessers. The thinkers can *reason, analyze* situations, and are *problem-centered* people. They ask why and how, and can translate information learned from one situation to a similar one. Such students have a greater chance of dealing with many of the problems facing medicine (including anesthesia) and medical education today,[3-5] than the guessers. A thinker gains maximally in a training program, and can become a safe, competent, and knowledgeable cardiac anesthesiologist.

The guessers are students who are *answer-centered*. They take a wild grab at an answer, the instant right answer, in order to take the pressure off the questioning. "Right answers pay off—they please the teacher."[6] Many students, and residents, are successful at this game; they have practiced it over many years, and can read their teachers well. Selection of college students for medical school favors the answer grabber, who takes all the right courses to get *A* grades.[7] This student rarely takes philosophy, history, humanities, and the like, but may excel at factual information in biology. The pass/fail system of (non)grading in medical school ironically may have assisted in the decline of quality residents for some programs.[8, 9] Grading assessments may be necessary in order for some students to evaluate performance or to encourage improvement. Yet the results of grading may be painful. "Failure in a success-oriented culture is hard to take."[6] The cardiac anesthesia resident who is an answer-grabber will have difficulty analyzing critical situations, solving complex patient-care problems, and may grab at the *wrong* answer in an emergency.

How do we know if a resident is *really learning?* Below are listed some criteria (modified from Holt[6]) for evaluation of real learning. In essence, if a topic or problem has been understood and qualifies as new learning, the resident must have thoroughly digested, grasped, reasoned with, and applied the information.

Why is real learning so important? Real learning is crucial to the attainment of knowledge which will lead to optimal performance. Optimal performance of clinical care should produce, in turn, maximum benefit to the patient.

CARDIAC ANESTHESIA TRAINING OBJECTIVES

How do we define the objectives and goals necessary for excellent training in cardiac anesthesia? Let us look at one program's objectives. The Institut de Cardiologé de Montreal expects a resident in cardiac anesthesia to be able to meet the following criteria at the end of a 3-month rotation:

1. Assess the anesthetic risk of cardiac patients.
2. Premedicate and prepare the cardiac patient for cardiac and general surgery.
3. Safely anesthetize cardiac patients for cardiac and general surgery.
4. Cooperate actively with surgical colleagues in the postoperative care of cardiac patients.
5. Cannulate the radial artery and the internal jugular vein, and install Swan–Ganz catheters. The resident should be aware of the complications of these techniques, and of the preventive measures involved, and management of, complications.[2]

To this we would add the following requirements:

6. Should be unruffled by stress and fatigue, able to maintain good clinical judgment under stressful situations, and able to act quickly and accurately in diagnosis, interpretation, and treatment (a "thinker")
7. Should have detailed knowledge of the anatomy, physiology and pharmacology of the following systems: cardiac, respiratory, coagulation, hematologic, neurologic, renal, hepatic, neuromuscular, and be able to utilize clinically this knowledge
8. Should know, understand, and be able

Criteria for "Real Learning"

The anesthesia resident must be able to:

State the problem in his own words
Give examples of it, if applicable
Recognize its various forms
See connections between it and other facts or ideas
Make use of it or create something entirely new out of it
Foresee some of its consequences
State its opposite, or converse, if applicable

to apply correctly appropriate monitoring techniques

9. Should have mature clinical judgment; should pay scrupulous attention to detail, and have the ability to observe and interpret clinical signs

10. Should have equal adaptability with pediatric, as well as adult, cardiovascular and related diseases

11. Should develop the technical skills specifically required for cardiovascular anesthesia, as well as mastering those skills which mark an all-around anesthesia specialist

12. Should work as a team member, and leader, with residents, fellows, surgeons and nurses

13. Should establish the talent, training and scholarship necessary for obtaining and applying new knowledge, and have a firm basis for continuing education

14. Along with the development in scholarship, should be encouraged to develop an interest in research in cardiac anesthesia

15. Should effectively transmit knowledge to others, both verbally and in writing; the development of teaching habits and communication with other departments and personnel will assist in spreading knowledge and interest.

Table 28-1. Cardiac Anesthesia Resident: Overall Training Objectives

KNOWLEDGE DEVELOPMENT
  Attitude and character
  Scholarship
  Continuing education

SKILL ACQUISITION
  Disciplines of medical field
  Technical skills and correct use
  Monitoring capabilities
  Pediatric and adult care capabilities

DELIVERY OF CARE
  Judgment
  Risk evaluation and assessment
  Planning and execution
  Follow-up

EXTENSION OF BASICS
  Research
  Teaching and writing
  Community health objectives

These criteria can equally be applied to training at any stage of development of the cardiac anesthesiologist: resident, fellow, community practitioner, or teacher. The overall training objectives are summarized in Table 28-1.

DEVELOPMENT OF THE CARDIAC ANESTHESIOLOGIST

Cardiovascular anesthesia and standard anesthesia are quite different. As mentioned in Chapter 1, this is not "sit-down" anesthesia. What happens on the "other side of the screen" affects what the anesthesiologist does or must do. The pace is fast and decisions are critical. There is much opportunity for misadventure. Clearly the anesthesiologist should be "geared up"—watching, anticipating, and preventing misadventure.

> Most of us have our engines running at about ten percent of their power. Why no more? And how do some people manage to keep revved up to twenty percent or thirty percent of their full power—or even more?[10]

This thirty-plus percent person is our ideal cardiac anesthesiologist. How might such a physician be developed?

BACKGROUND TRAINING

At the student level, a knowledge of basic anatomy, physiology, and pharmacology is required, as well as an ability to apply this to the cardiac patient. Respiratory physiology and pharmacology with particular stress on pulmonary circulation and gas exchange, various abnormalities and the effects of pharmacologic agents are necessary. A knowledge of renal and hepatic physiology, and the effects of hemodynamic and pharmacologic agents on their function, as well as neurophysiology, pharmacology, and physiology of blood and coagulation, must be achieved.

During internship, a rotation including general medicine and cardiology is desirable. Introductory rotations through intensive care, anesthesia, surgery, obstetrics, and pediatrics may be of additional value.

For residents, 1 year of general anesthesia rotation is desirable before entering cardiac anesthesiology training. In 12 programs with over 800 cardiopulmonary bypass cases per year, which responded to our survey,[11] 66 percent of the programs started the cardiac rotation during the second year, and the majority thought the second or third year most appropriate for the rotation. Half of the programs had residents who had rotated through general, thoracic, and major vascular anesthesia before cardiac anesthesia. Cardiology, adult, and pediatric intensive care rotations may be of great assistance to the resident, though some programs preferred to rotate their residents through the intensive care unit after the initial cardiac anesthesia experience.

Achievement of general anesthesia knowledge and skills on healthier patients, before attempting to enter the stressful situation of cardiac anesthesia, is obviously preferable. Mundane anesthetic concerns must not be distractions in the cardiac suite. At Stanford, we delay the cardiac rotation if a resident seems unsuitable, according to evaluations in other rotations. In an ideal training experience, a rotation through the cardiac catheterization laboratory including detailed interpretation of cardiac catheterization data, could precede or be combined with cardiac anesthesia rotations. Additional experiences in echocardiography and interpretation of ECGs would be of value.

There are no objective data on which to determine the timing of the cardiac anesthesia rotation. However, commencement of the rotation during the second year of residency appears logical for the average resident and the average program.

PROGRAM DESIGN

At present, there is no clearly identifiable, ideal cardiac anesthesia training program. Of course, we all have our biases, mostly in favor of our own programs. If we attempt to define an ideal program, we might find use-ful information, and be able to contrast it with our own experiences.

Curriculum Design

Before designing a curriculum and teaching program there must be specific program goals, which should generally cover all of the program objectives outlined in Table 28-1.

1. As previously mentioned, the necessary character involves a combination of good clinician and technician, who is able to act in harmony as a team member in times of stress and fatigue. The cardiac anesthesiologist must be able to provide rapid, simultaneous diagnosis and treatment. All education begins with imitation,[12] and this is especially true in attitude and character development. This requires an appropriate faculty model.

2. A curriculum should state in detail the specific skill requirements for competence as a cardiac anesthesiologist. This should be summarized in a resident handout, and translated into specific goal requirements.

3. The resident should have a complete, detailed list of theoretical knowledge requirements necessary to complement developing skills.

4. A guide for sources of information and method of study should be outlined, including instructional methods and materials. Of the programs we surveyed,[11] over 75 percent handed out a notebook or reading list, and many had specific texts and reprints reserved for the rotation. Extremely elaborate and current collections of articles and reviews are available in some departments.

5. The resident should know what is expected after the period of training, to maintain and further develop skills and knowledge.

6. A program should be organized so that its members can analyze both the program and the program products (the residents and fellows) in an objective manner.[13] In doing so, anesthesiologists can use the advice of education specialists in designing course requirements.[13-16]

7. A test series should be developed (or an existing one used) to test each objective. This would obviously be an enormous task unless limited to the main objectives. Without testing there is no way of knowing if objectives have been achieved or whether the resident is performing as expected. One of the functions of the ABA/ASA Joint Council on In-training is to give feedback of deficiencies to residents and program directors. The Board examination after completion of training is not the appropriate place for initial feedback on performance and achievements.

Instructional Methods

We will now briefly outline possibilities for instructional methods. We refer the specially interested reader to an edition of International Anesthesiology Clinics for a more complete discussion by educators and curricula designers.[13-16]

Lecture Series. A well developed series of systematic lectures should provide the resident with a clear idea of the necessary breadth and depth of study. This fairly economical method of instruction involves hours of preparation by each lecturer, and minimal expenditure of the trainee's time, probably accounting for its popularity. A lecture should assist the resident in meeting course objectives, and stimulate enough interest and awareness to encourage further study. This is not an easy task! In fact, if a lecture achieves these objectives, it should be recorded (on videotape) and reviewed by others who wish to learn the subject. A test developed from the lecture objectives may tell the teacher and student what each has achieved. Lecture assessments assist in evaluating the effectiveness of the lecture, and in revising or reviewing for future presentations (Fig. 28-1).

Of the programs we surveyed, 75 percent had a lecture either weekly or biweekly for cardiac anesthesia residents. Two programs had blocks of several weeks during which time all residents (and faculty) were exposed to cardiac anesthesia topics presented by their own and visiting faculty. A block system combined with weekly lectures by faculty and fellows would seem optimal.

The Seminar or Small Group Discussion. This type of activity presents an opportunity to draw out knowledge and to discuss its application. It is particularly useful in a program with several residents simultaneously rotating through cardiac anesthesia. The aim should be to teach the student to prepare, think, and communicate with the group.

Individual Instruction. The faculty member may act as a stimulating influence or guide, allowing the resident to self-evaluate the training progress, and then select materials to be covered at the next session. We shall deal with the apprenticeship situation in the clinical setting.

Programmed or Computer-assisted Instruction. These procedures are more sophisticated, progressive training techniques, dealt with fully in the reference cited.[16] Their application to cardiac anesthesia has not yet been fully realized. Expense and the lack of appropriate equipment have been limiting factors.

Instructional Materials

Instructional materials range from printed texts and monographs, to sophisticated video and computer-assisted instructional equipment. In an analysis of the acquisition and application of new medical knowledge by a wide range of anesthesiologists, Fineberg found that published papers and colleagues were more important sources of information than continuing medical education courses.[17] Published papers were listed as an influential source of information for a higher portion of Board Certified than nonBoard Certified anesthesiologists.

Textbooks. A well-written textbook should supply an overall picture of a subject with history and background information. It

Fig. 28-1. Lecture assessment.

1st Yr Res _____   2nd Yr Res _____   Fellow _____   Intern _____   Med. Student ____

You attended a lecture given by Dr. _____. We would appreciate your evaluation of this lecture.

EXCELLENT   SATISFACTORY   UNSATISFACTORY

Content

   Has command of the subject. _____

   Presents material in an analytic way. _____

   Contrasts various points of view. _____
   Discusses current developments, and
     relates topics to other areas of
     knowledge. _____

Delivery

   States objectives. _____

   Summarizes major points. _____
   Presents material in an organized
     manner and provides emphasis. _____
   Uses slides effectively in terms
     of clarity. _____

   Appropriateness and easy readability. _____

Interest in Audience
   Is sensitive to the response of the
     audience. _____
   Encourages participation and
     welcomes questions and discussion. _____

   Enjoys teaching. _____

   Is enthusiastic about the subject. _____
   Makes the lecture interesting and
     has self-confidence. _____

Summary
a. Considering both the limitation and possibilities of the subject matter, course and time, how would you rate the overall teaching effectiveness of this faculty member?

Ineffective: _____   Moderately effective: _____   Extremely effective: _____

b. Specific comments for feedback purposes: (four categories: content, delivery, audience interaction, and miscellaneous).

Thank you for your time and assistance in assessing this teaching endeavor.

Table 28-2. Textbooks of Current and Special Interest to the Cardiovascular Anesthesiologist

	AUTHOR/EDITOR	TITLE	PUBLISHER
General	Ream and Fogdall (eds)	Acute Cardiovascular Management: Anesthesia and Intensive Care	JB Lippincott
	Rubenstein and Federman (eds)	Scientific American Medicine	Scientific American
	Fischbach and Fogdall	Coagulation: The Essentials	Williams & Wilkins
	Dubin	Rapid Interpretation of EKG	Cover Publishing
	Marriott	Practical Electrocardiography	Williams & Wilkins
	Saidman/Smith	Monitoring in Anesthesia	John Wiley and Sons
	Gravenstein/Newbower/Ream/ Smith/Borden (eds)	Monitoring Surgical Patients in the Operating Room	Charles C Thomas
	Hurst/Logue/Schlant/Wenger (eds)	The Heart	McGraw-Hill
	Editors, American Heart Association	Examination of the Heart (Five Booklets)	American Heart Association
	Weil/Henning (eds)	The Handbook of Critical Care Medicine	EM Books
Physiology	Berne/Levy	Cardiovascular Physiology	CV Mosby
	Rackley/Russell (eds)	Coronary Artery Disease: Recognition and Management	Futura Publishing
	Braunwald (ed)	The Myocardium: Failure and Infarction	HP Publishing
	Fishman	Heart Failure	McGraw-Hill
	Nunn	Applied Respiratory Physiology	Butterworths
	West	Respiratory Physiology	Williams & Wilkins
	West	Pulmonary Pathophysiology	Williams & Wilkins
	Hedley–Whyte/Burgess/Feeley/ Miller	Applied Physiology of Respiratory Care	Little, Brown & Co
Pharmacology	Editors, The New England Journal of Medicine	Drug Therapy, vols 1–6	Massachusetts Medical Society
	Eger	Anesthetic Uptake and Action	Williams & Wilkins
Equipment	Reed/Clark	Cardiopulmonary Perfusion	Texas Medical Press
	Ionescu/Woolor (eds)	Current Techniques in Extracorporeal Circulation	Butterworths
	Macintosh/Mushin/Epstein	Physics for the Anaesthetist	FA Davis (Blackwell)
	Dorsch/Dorsch	Understanding Anesthesia Equipment	Williams & Wilkins
Specialized and Miscellaneous	Eliot/Wolf/Forker (eds)	Cardiac Emergencies	Futura Publishing
	Goldberger/Wheat	Treatment of Cardiac Emergencies	CV Mosby
	Yang/Bentivoglio/Maranhao/ Goldberg	From Cardiac Catheterization Data to Hemodynamic Parameters	FA Davis
	Grossman	Cardiac Catheterization and Angiography	Lea & Febiger
	Ellestad	Stress Testing	FA Davis
	Miller	The Practice of Coronary Artery Bypass Surgery	Plenum Medical Book Co
	Lefrak/Starr	Cardiac Valve Prostheses	Appleton–Century– Crofts
	Fink	Congenital Cardiovascular Disease	Year Book Medical Publishers
	deJong	Physiology and Pharmacology of Local Anesthesia	Charles C Thomas
	Shnider	Obstetrical Anesthesia	Williams & Wilkins
History	Johnson	The History of Cardiac Surgery, 1896–1955	The Johns Hopkins Press
	Harvey, William (Translation by Whitteridge)	An Anatomical Disputation Covering the Movement of the Heart and Blood in Living Creatures	JB Lippincott (Blackwell)

This is only a starting list for personal reading. These texts are the choices of the two editors at the time of manuscript submission. It is obvious that additional works will become available while this manuscript is in press. We also realize that other editors might select other textbooks for inclusion in this list.

should attempt to place the subject in perspective, and give continuity with other works. A textbook should also be able to develop concepts from basic thoughts.

One of the inevitable problems of textbooks is making the information current, particularly in a subject area in which new innovations continually are occurring. Analysis of vintage of bibliography has been used to illustrate this point (it must also be emphasized that currency of information is certainly not the only criteria of excellence).[18] The teacher obviously has an important role in updating the bibliography for the resident or fellow, as well as reviewing or preparing new textbooks. A list of textbooks of current and special interest to the cardiac anesthesiologist is found in Table 28-2. It lists approximately 35 texts we believe contain essential material in this area.

Other Instructional Material. In addition to lectures and textbooks, all of the groups surveyed included journals, lectures, cardiac and general anesthesia meetings, and review articles as sources of information. We have prepared a list of applicable journals in Table 28-3. Half of the programs surveyed also included research seminars (though only three claimed regular research seminars within their own facilities).[11] An American Society of Anesthesiologists' multiple choice, self-assessment examination was used by many of the responding centers for faculty self-evaluation.

Meetings. Among the anesthesia meetings, the American Society of Anesthesiologists Annual Meeting, the public presentations of the Association of Cardiac Anesthesiologists, and The American Heart Association meetings were cited as sources of information for faculty.[11] The American Society of Anesthesiologsts Refresher Courses was cited as a source for residents and faculty.[11] General anesthesia, cardiovascular anesthesia, thoracic and cardiovascular surgery, pediatric, and subspecialty society meetings were also mentioned. Periodic symposia on cardiovascular anesthesia, electrocardiography, moni-

Table 28-3. Journals of Current and Special Interest to the Cardiovascular Anesthesiologist

GENERAL
  The New England Journal of Medicine
  Critical Care Medicine
  Clinical Pharmacology and Therapeutics
ANESTHESIA
  Anesthesiology
SURGICAL
  Journal of Thoracic and Cardiovascular Surgery
  The Journal of Extracorporeal Technology
CARDIOLOGY
  Circulation
  American Journal of Cardiology

toring, and critical care, sponsored by the American Society of Anesthesiologists and component societies, are also of value. In addition, timely meetings on special topics are offered by various university centers.

Audiovisual Aids. Apart from slides, audiovisual aids were mentioned only by two of the groups reviewed.[11] Tapes of roentgenograph interpretation, internal jugular vein cannulation, and respiratory flow-volume curves are available. Audiovisual aids are very amenable to training in cardiac anesthesia, and underutilized. Taping quality lectures and procedures such as catheter placement, anesthesia induction, tracheal intubation, epidural,[19, 20] and spinal anesthesia, and so on can be used to give feedback to both teacher and resident. At Stanford University, induction sequences and spinal anesthesia techniques by new residents have been recorded on videotape and reviewed, with encouraging results. The process is objective, the teaching value subjective.

TESTING OBJECTIVES

Testing has always been controversial. The thinking resident will be able to do well, and the answer-grabber will be unveiled, if testing is performed properly. If a subject is not objectively tested, then the teacher never knows if information has been learned or taught correctly, and thus valuable instruction time may be wasted.[14] Test devices may be self-assessment programs, multiple choice examinations, check lists for operative performance, oral examinations, and so on. All of these provide feedback to the teacher. Evaluations of teacher performance, in teaching practical skills or giving tutorials and lectures, will be covered later.

Of the programs reviewed,[11] the majority used an evaluation form and discussion among faculty in assessing resident performance. Very few admitted to using objective checklists and examinations. A meaningful way of using an examination would be to test a resident entering into the rotation, and then retest the resident after completion of the rotation, to assess progress. The exact questions used in written or oral examinations

will change continually. However, we have provided an outline containing those items, or areas, which deserve attention for inclusion in the curriculum and in testing processes in cardiovascular anesthesia (Table 28-4). The resident's performance can also be tested at the end of each day or month's rotation, which we will discuss later. If testing of basic knowledge is performed, by whatever means, a *process* for the testing should be followed, and understood by the resident. A suggested process is seen in Figure 28-2. This process is a proposed plan for objectivity assessing acquisition of the basic knowledge as background necessary for safe and competent cardiac patient care. We have successfully used this process at Stanford.

Table 28-4. Suggested Areas of Importance for Inclusion in the Curriculum and Testing Processes in Cardiovascular Anesthesia

GENERAL
History of cardiac anesthesia and surgery
Patient population, and associated diseases
Natural history of cardiovascular disease
Hemodynamics— cellular, organ, and system
Cardiac catheterization and echocardiography
Surgical selection and considerations
Physical diagnosis and patient history
Equipment, uses, and complications

PHYSIOLOGY
Cardiovascular
Respiratory
Central nervous system
Renal
Hepatic
Endocrine
Hematologic (esp. hemoglobin)

MONITORING
Electrocardiography
Electroencephalography
Arterial pressures
Ventricular filling pressures
Calculations: output/resistances, and the like
Arterial blood gasses
Temperature
Indications/contraindications
Techniques and equipment
Complications

PHARMACOLOGY
Anesthetic drugs (inhalation, IV, IM)
Muscle relaxants
Glycosides/inotropic agents/catecholamines
Vasodilators/antihypertensive drugs
Vasopressors
Antiarrhythmic drugs
Electrolyte effects

ADULT CARDIOVASCULAR SURGERY: IMPORTANT CONSIDERATIONS
Coronary artery disease
Vascular heart disease
Cardiomyopathy
Diseases of the aorta and major branches
Congenital cardiovascular disease in the adult

PEDIATRIC CARDIOVASCULAR SURGERY
Nomenclature
Basic hemodynamic problems
Palliative procedures
Anesthetic considerations and problems
Differences from standard adult care

COAGULATION
Basics
Drugs
Testing
Analysis and treatment
Complications

CARDIOPULMONARY BYPASS AND ASSIST DEVICES
Principles
Hypothermia/myocardial preservation
Equipment/primes/hemodilution
Intraaortic counterpulsation balloon assist
Pacemakers
Temporary cardiac replacement
Complications

CARDIAC TRANSPLANTATION
Physiology/pharmacology
Operative selection and expectation
Isolated heart function
Special operative considerations
Complications

POSTOPERATIVE CARE
Fluid/electrolyte management
Cardiovascular/respiratory management
Complications

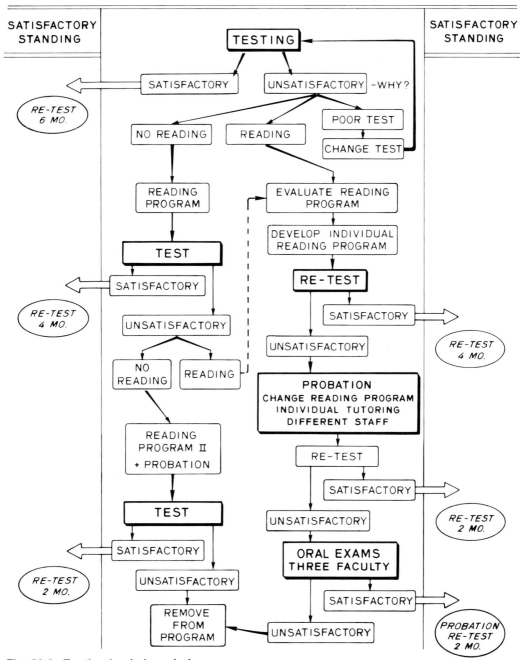

Fig. 28-2. Testing basic knowledge.

CLINICAL RESIDENT TRAINING

PREOPERATIVE TRAINING

The anesthesiologist's role in the care of the cardiovascular patient begins with preoperative assessment of the patient, and discussion of investigations. A group meeting consisting of cardiologists, surgeons, and anesthesiologists allows review of clinical findings, angiograms and other investigations, as well as discussion of other pertinent information.

This kind of meeting can be highly instructional for the resident, allowing insight into the criteria for patient selection, surgical planning, and possible anesthesia-related problems.

The actual preoperative evaluation has already been discussed in the Prebypass Chapter. At Stanford, the cardiovascular anesthesia handbook clearly establishes the preoperative objectives and information required, leaving no doubts in the mind of the resident. This preoperative visit also offers an excellent opportunity for faculty teaching and improving clinical skills at the bedside, in patients who often have remarkable physical findings. Above all, it is correct and humane for the patient to meet all members of the team responsible for operative and post-operative care.

OPERATIVE TRAINING

How many patients requiring cardiopulmonary bypass should a resident anesthetize each day? How many patients should a resident anesthetize during cardiac anesthesia training? How long should the training period be?

In approximately 70 percent of the programs surveyed,[21] the residents are involved with one patient per day. These programs believe that this is optimal for the training process. The majority of programs rotate residents for only 2 months, and most of that majority thought that satisfactory, though aproximately half of all the programs surveyed thought a 3-month rotation ideal. In one program with 1600 cardiopulmonary bypass operations yearly, a total of four months in the two-year residency is spent in cardiac anesthesia. At another, with 4,400 operations yearly, the faculty believes strongly that the number of patients per day should be high, and thus each resident provides anesthesia for three patients per day during the 2-month rotation.

The responsibility of only one patient per day should allow the resident time to provide follow-up visits and participate actively in postoperative care, although in many programs an intensive care rotation is covered separately. The amount of information absorbed routinely during the care of two patients per day is probably maximal; a saturation point must surely be reached sometime during the second case.

All the programs agree that one faculty member per resident is desirable, although in the program with the largest number of operations, a policy of graded responsibility leads to one faculty member supervising two residents. Some programs very strongly believe that it is to the patient's and resident's benefit to have individual 1:1 coverage. Certainly it would seem optimal for maximum teaching achievement. The fact that faculty are available at any time, as well as present during crucial moments, gives the resident a sense of security, without which initial learning would be difficult. Graded responsibility, at a later stage, helps to develop the ability to make decisions and act on them, a skill which will be only too necessary at the end of the standard American 2-year (after internship) residency program.

An important objective during the cardiac anesthesia rotation is that of development and improvement in monitoring skills, both invasive and noninvasive. This is an ideal time to teach the principles of who, when, and how to monitor. The resident should be taught how to assess the results of monitoring, and to be able to correlate findings with clinical observations. These principles are outlined in our monitoring chapters.

Exposure to varying techniques of anesthesia for the cardiac patient may be rather confusing or frustrating initially (especially if the resident is involved with more than one faculty per day). The opinion of those we surveyed was that as graduate students, the initial confusion is replaced later by enlightenment and benefit. The resident is then able to choose a preferred technique during the latter stages of, or after, training, while avoiding premature commitment to a particular technique solely because it is "familiar."

OPERATIVE TRAINING AND PATIENT WELFARE

Drui and coworkers analyzed the time spent by the anesthesiologist in directing attention to the patient and surgical field.[22] They made the startling observation that, during surgery involving cardiopulmonary bypass, the anesthesiologist's attention was distracted from the field 46 percent of the time, and that such distractions occurred in 42 percent of all operations studied. Lambert found similar results.[23] To combat these distractions, a regular scanning pattern is actively taught, encouraged, and tested at Stanford. During times of rapid change, Lambert observed that very short, functional or technical types of teaching could be pursued (*e.g.*, correction of residents' techniques or demonstration of a new skill).[23] During steady-state anesthesia, more intensive teaching may be pursued (so long as the scanning pattern of patient, instruments, IVs, and so on is not interrupted). Correct positioning of the tutor, so that the resident is able to monitor anesthesia, and the tutor the student, has been stressed by Paget,[24] and we strongly concur.

Paget states that teaching in the operating room is only desirable if it does not entail distraction from patient care.[24] Fisk argues that if essential skills can only be taught during clinical management, and if the teaching of these skills distracts from patient care, then it may be necessary to accept a certain amount of distraction in order that essential teaching objectives may be achieved.[25] The amount of distraction possible is obviously up to the mature judgment of the tutor, and to be kept to a minimum.

Continuous assessment of knowledge, clinical skills, and resident patient care performance is obviously essential. Figure 28-3 demonstrates the daily check list evaluation used by one of us (RPF) at Stanford, with immediate feedback to the resident upon safe transport of the patient to the intensive care unit. Such an intense evaluation is of immediate interest and assistance to the resident, and important information is not forgotten because of any time lag. In addition, at Stanford, all faculty involved in cardiac teaching combine to produce a monthly evaluation of the resident's performance, at the end of each rotation month (Fig. 28-4).

How should faculty evaluations of resident patient care performance proceed? This will be dictated by the general makeup of the program, the faculty, and the individual resident. One outline we suggest is found in Figure 28-5, it provides for multiple points at which the process can be used to give maximum opportunities for an accurate and fair assessment of cardiac anesthesia resident performance.

POSTOPERATIVE TRAINING

All of the institutions we surveyed were involved in postoperative intensive care, and the majority considered it an essential part of their training program.[21] Critical care involvement is a prime attraction to the specialty, and the clinical judgment and skills acquired in cardiac anesthesia are essential to intensive care work. The organization of intensive care units and critical care teaching has almost uniformly gravitated to anesthesia-trained faculty, who are uniquely educated to provide this direction. Such a program is immensely valuable in the total educational processes of cardiac anesthesia.

Some of the frustrations of postoperative intensive care are outlined by Safar and Grenvik.[26] We have listed some of these problems below. Many of the problems are solved by

---

Problems in Intensive Care Unit Teaching

Admitting physician education
Admitting physician availability
Primary responsibility for patient care
Fragmentation of patient care
Delegation of responsibility
High volume of critically-ill patients
Inexperienced residents working with experienced critical care nurses
Varying specialty resident backgrounds
Research occurring with limited patient responsibility
Research procedures thrust upon ICU nurses without consultation, nor credit for assistance given

---

Fig. 28-3. Resident/fellow evaluation—daily checklist.

Cardiovascular Anesthesia Service   Name of Trainee: _____

Stanford University School of Medicine   Date: _____

Training Status: R$_1$ [   ], R$_2$ [   ], F [   ], Other [   ] _____

Case Type and Age: _____

	Sat.	Unsat.	Comments
Preoperative:			
Evaluation			
Presentation			
Preparation			
Notes			
Line Placement:			
Preparation			
Rapport with Patient			
Technical Skills			
Management			
Prebypass:			
OR Preparation			
Induction			
Intubation			
Management			
Pre-CPB Preparations			
Bypass:			
Transition			
Management			
Evaluations (lab, etc.)			
Infusion Drug Preparations			
Blood/Coag Preparations			
Post-CPB:			
Transition			
Management: Cardiovascular			
Respiratory			
Volume			
Blood/Coag			
Preparations for ICU			
ICU:			
Transporation			
Change Over			
Patient Status			
Postop Note			
General:			
Anesthesia Record			
"Style"			
Understanding Concepts			
Working with Attending			
Working with Surgeons			
Working with Nurses			
Complications			

Comments and/or Recommendations:

R.P.F.

Fig. 28-4. Resident/fellow evaluation—monthly.

Stanford Cardiovascular Anesthesia Service
Stanford University School of Medicine

Resident: _____
Rotation Date: _____

Check where appropriate:	Oustanding	Adequate	Inadequate
A. Patient care areas:			
1. Preoperative evaluation of patient, cath data, lab			
2. Planning anesthesia technique			
3. Line placement			
4. Induction/intubation sequence			
5. Attention to operative field			
6. All-knowing ("Scan Pattern")			
7. Record keeping/neatness			
8. Postoperative visits			
9. Performed as per handout			
B. Knowledge areas:			
1. Reading CV literature			
2. Reading CV handout			
3. Understands basic CV physiology			
4. Understands pharmacology & use of CV drugs			
5. Able to integrate new material			
C. Personal Qualities:			
1. Rapport with patient			
2. Communication with surgeons			
3. Communication with nurses			
4. Rapport with Anes. faculty			
5. Endurance/stamina			
6. Inquisitiveness/creativity			
7. Response to O.R. stress			
8. Response to workload			

D. List one area in which this resident may be truly outstanding:

E. List two areas in which this resident could improve:

F. Results of rotation examination:

G. Additional comments:

H. Rank resident
☐ top 10%
☐ top 25%
☐ middle 50%
☐ bottom 25%

Completed by: Individual _____ , Group meeting _____

Signed: _____

Date: _____

R.P.F.

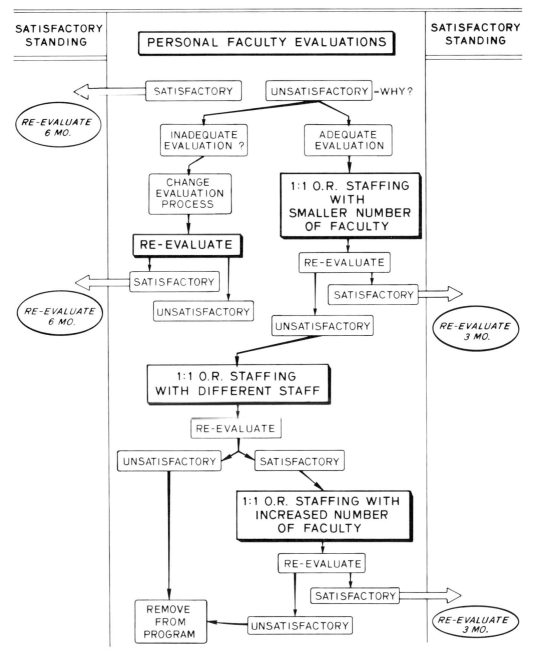

Fig. 28-5. Performance evaluation.

the intensive care unit director or coordinator taking responsibility for the patient. We are all either familiar with, or can imagine, the problems that arise when the admitting physician insists on sole responsibility. These problems are further accentuated if the ad-mitting physician has no training in critical care medicine, or is unavailable during long days in the operating room or office. Lack of overall coordination of the various subspecialties may lead to fragmentation of care and department territorialism. The combination of these factors along with the presence of highly-trained and intelligent nurses, working with inexperienced house officers, can lead to extreme tension in the intensive care unit.

Delegation of responsibility to anesthesia or intensive care unit junior house staff, while experienced staff are reluctant or unable to participate, can lead to poor patient care. The intensive care unit director must make allowances for the varying background training of each of the residents who rotates through the unit. Each specialty should contribute to and gain knowledge from the other. Clinical research and the introduction of innovative care cannot be initiated easily in an intensive care unit unless the director is solely responsible for the unit and overall patient care.

These obstacles must be controlled if the cardiac anesthesia resident is to have a meaningful learning experience in postoperative intensive care. For practical purposes, it is impossible for any resident to give full-time care to the postoperative cardiac patient, when involved in simultaneous administration of operative anesthesia. For this reason the intensive care and operative rotations should be separate. Ideally the operative rotation should precede the intensive care unit rotation.

The intensive care unit has an essential role in establishing good habits for the cardiac anesthesia resident. After taking care of patients who are cold, vasoconstricted, and unstable, the resident will be more sensitive to postoperative concerns on return to the operating room. In addition, the resident should be taught to give a detailed history of clinical findings, pertinent preoperative data, operative findings, and procedure to those requiring this information. Combined with this, anesthetic technique, complications, fluid balance, post-bypass status and other relevant data should be accurately summarized for the intensive care unit staff. Finally, the patient should be stabilized by both the anesthesia resident responsible for the anesthesia, and the colleague rotating through the intensive care unit. Further discussion of the details of intensive care unit training are beyond the scope of this chapter.

FELLOWSHIP TRAINING

Replies to our survey show tremendous differences in organization of cardiac anesthesia fellowship programs.[27] Fellowships vary from the extremes of purely laboratory research, to full-time clinical activities. Programs also offer both clinical and research activities in differing proportions, according to the overall activities of the institution. Of the larger institutes of cardiac anesthesia replying to our survey, 90 percent had fellowship programs; whereas in smaller programs, with 100 to 400 total operative cases per year, only 40 percent had fellowships. Regionalization appears to have taken place naturally. Thus, programs give different emphasis to the aims of fellowship training, according to their resources and initiatives.

Several programs agree that rotation through an intensive care unit, cardiology, and the catheterization laboratory would be optimal, if time allowed, during a clinically oriented fellowship. Very few programs allow fellows the responsibility for supervision of operative anesthesia during the fellowship year, though this would seem a logical extension of the management of complex clinical cases. Legal and fiscal problems appear to be most important obstacles. However, a fellowship year is a valuable time to learn teaching skills, both in the operating room and in the lecture room. Public speaking courses used concomitantly with videotape evaluations and critiques by experts, greatly enhance lecture performances. This period also offers an opportunity for institutions to choose and groom new faculty. While many fellows in cardiac anesthesia are indeed being prepared for a teaching career, the resident anticipating private practice will still gain immensely from a fellowship period. Such a period may clearly place him or her above peers in private practice—a standing which leads to improved patient care in the community. We

---

Cardiovascular Anesthesia Fellowship Training Goals

Management of complex clinical problems.
Increased patient responsibility
Beginning teaching responsibility
Research project planning and execution
Learning writing skills
Learning to read critically
Preparation of grant proposals
Presentations at scientific meetings
Grooming for an academic position

---

have seen many examples of this phenomenon in our own graduates.

A transfer of specialized concepts from faculty to fellow should be the goal of the year. Close monitoring of, and assistance with, research projects should be an integral part of fellowship. The fellow should have an opportunity to learn to critically read, write, and present specific papers, under the supervision of experienced faculty. Time spent during this year, or a second fellowship year, learning the intricacies of grant proposal preparations may prove invaluable at a later stage. We have summarized some of the goals of fellowship training above.

CONTINUING POSTGRADUATE EDUCATION

The purpose of a liberal arts education is to expand to the limit the individual's capacity, and desire, for self-education, for seeking and finding meaning, truth, and enjoyment in everything he does. A. Whitney Griswold (in Holt[28])

While this flowery-sounding statement seems eloquent, does it pertain to the cardiac anesthesiologist or to the general anesthesiologist in private practice? Certainly it must. All physicians complete residency or fellowship training with a sigh of relief (at last school is over!). But actually, the process of continued training and education is just beginning. The term *commencement*, used for undergraduate education termination, is an

appropriate term for the start of practice or faculty appointment as well.

MOTIVATION

There are no data demonstrating clearly at what point many physicians, and other critical care professionals, decline in the pursuit of knowledge. Some stop reading, some stop listening, and some unfortunately stop learning. Others, who often are remembered as stars during residency, continue to read, attend conferences, share their knowledge with colleagues, and continually improve their patient care. It is amazing however, how some anesthesiologists can be well behind the state-of-the-art 7 or 8 years after formal residency training. This is not as important during anesthesia for an appendectomy, but certainly will be for cardiac anesthesia. Knowledge and technique in this area are expanding weekly.

We have many biases, and some data, relating to regionalization of care for the critically ill (which will be discussed later).[29–33] We also have biases related as to which anesthesiologists should be caring for patients undergoing cardiovascular surgery. We will not, however, risk the emotional, legal, or legislative consequences of additional comment in this area. Suffice that at some point in practice, an anesthesiologist caring for such patients will probably desire, or need, updating in all of the aspects of cardiac anesthesia. Some of the motivations for seeking a specific program of continuing education in cardiac anesthesia are listed below.

Cardiovascular Anesthesia: Motivation for Continuing Education

Personal improvement
Enhancement of noncardiac patients' care
Recognition desired as a subspecialist in cardiovascular anesthesia
Preparation for board examinations or recertification
Desire to prepare for higher income—generating cases (with higher reimbursement values)
Requested or demanded by a third party (surgeon, anesthesia colleague, hospital board, legal authority, and so on)

PROBLEMS

One problem in designing formal programs for continuing cardiac anesthesia education is manpower pressures in the major cardiac anesthesia centers. Active cardiac anesthesia faculty are overworked and "time-squeezed" as it is.[34, 35] A nationwide shortage of anesthesia faculty presently exists, and will not improve in the near future.[34, 35] The time required to develop programs, and then provide the actual personalized instruction is a massive undertaking. Inherent also is the possibility that resident or fellow training will suffer with the divergence and dilution of faculty attention toward the continuing education programs. Clearly under these circumstances, such a faculty shortage will limit the availability of continuing education programs.

Regionalization of patient care for certain disease entities may reduce such pressures because smaller hospitals will not be caring for such patients, and retraining needs in certain disciplines *may* therefore decline. This hypothesis requires time for testing.

SELECTION

The selection of anesthesiologists for inclusion in a formal program of continuing cardiac anesthesia education is difficult. Certain basic criteria will need to be met, these are outlined below. In addition, the needs of the anesthesiologist will be highly variable. Some concerns are the amount of time which has passed since formal residency training, degree of ongoing reading and self-education, level of present knowledge and skills, level of sophistication of colleagues and hospital environment, ability to transmit acquired information to colleagues, motivation, and expectations of the prospective trainee.

Present involvement in the care of the critically ill (neuroanesthesia, intensive care, emergency room care, and so on) will assist the anesthesiologist to absorb new information quickly. Physicians presently using newer drugs, techniques, and skills will find a formal program in cardiac anesthesia much

Suggested Criteria/Requirements for Admission to a Formal Continuing Education Program in Cardiovascular Anesthesia

License to practice medicine in state
VQE or FLEX if foreign medical school graduate
Letter from candidate's hospital, confirming the physician's status
Current curriculum vitae
Recommendations from two of the candidate's physician colleagues
Letter from applicant requesting personalized continuing education, and the physician's expectations
Personal visit and interview

easier, and perhaps more rewarding. The amount of training time will vary with the individual, and the program will require an intense *personalized* approach to reach the eventual goal of improved patient care.

At Stanford, we have provided such an intense, personalized programs for several years. The results are greatly encouraging, and feedback from recipients of such programs is both enlightening and delightful. The faculty time commitment for such programs, however, has been high, and negative impact upon other faculty activities is obvious. The only hope for relief, to accomplish widespread continuing education in this area, is a substantial enlargement of cardiac anesthesia faculties.

CURRICULUM

There also are no data to assist in the development of a uniform curriculum content for continued education in cardiac anesthesia. Because such programs require a personalized approach to each applicant, only an estimate of a "bare-bones" curriculum is possible. We have hesitated to spell out some basic thoughts in this area, because of the obvious possibilities that legal entities and others might seize upon the information as a standard. *There is no standard!* In our *experience*, a *rough approximation* of the time which might be required to accomplish such a formal program can be *estimated* as in Table 28-5. Some physicians may need more or less time than suggested. These are only *starting points* to assist in the establishment of a program. Table 28-6 provides more detail regarding a possible breakdown of time spent in various activities. We have listed two categories of time, one for the anesthesiologist who currently cares for the critically ill patient of a noncardiac anesthesia nature, and one who has no recent exposure to any of the techniques, drugs, or procedures. These *estimates* are for routine, adult cardiac anesthesia, and are highly variable. The exact time will be determined by the end product.

Table 28-5. Continuing Education in Cardiovascular Anesthesia a Suggested Basic Initial Curriculum

Introductory basic lectures
  Anatomy
  Physiology
  Pharmacology
  Monitoring
  Coagulation
  Cardiac catheterization and evaluation
  Surgical considerations
  Cardiopulmonary bypass
  Anesthesia considerations
  Practical pointers
	12 hours

Advanced cardiac life support	16 hours
Operative observation	15–20 hours
Operative direct care	45–120 hours
Examinations (written and oral)	8 hours
Postoperative intensive care unit care (optional, but suggested)	40–80 hours

Proposed Criteria for Satisfactory Completion of a Formal Continuing Education Program in Cardiovascular Anesthesia

Read material assigned
Fulfill proposed activity schedule
Perform satisfactorily all cases assigned
Receive ACLS certificate
Pass written or oral examinations (or both) as assigned
Receive "satisfactory" ratings by three-fourths of the faculty working with the applicant (skills, attitude, poise, basics, ability to integrate information with patient care, and so on)
Pass American Society of Anesthesiologists Cardiovascular Anesthesia self-evaluation examination
Obvious steps to obtain American Board of Anesthesiology certification (if nonBoard certified)

ASSESSMENT

Some assessment of success or failure must be made after a period of time in formal continuing education in cardiac anesthesia. The best assessment is direct evaluation of patient care at the bedside (operating room), coupled with acquisition of the basic skills and knowledge required to accomplish high-quality patient care. The body of knowledge required by an average resident and presented in Table 28-4 is a starting point for assessment. In addition, the suggested basic criteria for completion of such a program are outlined above. (Some of the points are intended to provoke questions and comments from the reader.)

FACULTY ACTIVITY AND EDUCATION

CONTINUING EDUCATION

Much of what we have said previously regarding formal postgraduate education relates to the private practitioner of anesthesia. The academic anesthesiologist who is not continually exposed to critically ill patients also may seek continuing education in cardiac anesthesia. However, most of the faculty in academic anesthesia centers are continuously involved in the care of referred patients with severe cardiovascular disease. These patients may be referred for cardiovascular procedures, or for noncardiovascular surgery. Therefore, most faculty are familiar with sophisticated monitoring new drugs, new techniques, and so on. In many academic anesthesia centers, faculty rotate their teaching functions in such a way as to provide continuing balance and input among various disciplines. They are also involved in other academic pursuits which assist in keeping their skills and knowledge up-to-date.

Having secured excellent faculty, some occasionally from one's own residency or fellowship programs (where they can be observed and assessed closely), the problem then is one of retaining excellence, particu-

Table 28-6. Continuing Education in Cardiovascular Anesthesia: Suggested Initial Perioperative Activity

Activity	MINIMUM TIME SPENT (HOURS)	
	Current Critical Care Experience	No Current Critical Care Experience
Lectures	12	12
ACLS	16	16
Reading: Handout/notebook	4	4
Major text(s)	20	30
Allied texts	4	20
Observation of cardiovascular anesthesia, monitoring, postoperative care	15	20
Personal review of H & P, angiograms, cardiac catheterization, and so on	4	4
Personally provided anesthesia care to patients	90	180

No pediatric cardiac cases
No "special" cases (e.g., mapping, aortic arch, IHSS)
See text for further comments.

larly in continuing education. Journals, meetings, and discussions combined with texts and review courses are common means of faculty continuing education programs. Peer review of research papers, lectures, articles, book chapters, and textbooks serve as useful, if not occasionally painful, sources of education and insight. Comments from colleagues at Board examinations, which can often be recalled with amazing clarity, may also fall into this category. The American Society of Anesthesiologists self-assessment examinations were frequently cited as important sources of self-evaluation in our survey.[36] The fact that almost all continuing education seminars are taught by academic anesthesia faculty demonstrates the general level of faculty continuing education.

ASSESSMENT OF TEACHING

New faculty tend to be observed and assessed over a 3- to 6-month period, before full commitment in many institutions.[36] At Stanford, feedback from residents, fellows, and other departments is used to help all faculty in assessing their own teaching skills and effectiveness, and hopefully in correcting deficiencies or bad habits. The assessment of lectures has already been mentioned (see Fig. 28-1). Overall teaching assessment is also

performed at Stanford, and demonstrated in Figure 28-6.

The University of Pennsylvania has instituted resident evaluation of faculty teaching, which was reported at the 1979 American Society of Anesthesiologist Annual Scientific Meeting.[37] They claim an objective system for collecting residents' opinions of faculty performance as teachers of clinical anesthesia. There are five major categories: availability, personal attributes, case-related teaching ability, didactic teaching, and overall contribution to your learning. These are scored from *outstanding* through *good* and *adequate* to *inadequate*. There is also a category for comments, and a score available for *no contact* with the particular faculty member.

Their results have shown that

Full professors were less available, but their teaching performance was superior to that of the associate professor, which in turn was superior to that of the assistant professors. (PA) [personal attributes] ratings, were similar for full and associate professors but lower for assistant professors. (CRT) [case-related teaching], (DT) [didactic teaching], (OC) [overall contribution to your learning] ratings increased with rank. Confidence in the system increased when the chairman of the department associated correctly 95% of the faculty with the *un*identified evaluations.[37]

Fig. 28-6. Evaluation of faculty by residents.

Department of Anesthesia
Stanford University School of Medicine

Faculty Name: _____   Date of Evaluation: _____

Resident Name: _____   1st   2nd   3rd   4th   5th year (circle)
    (optional)

Period of Contact (one month, two months, etc.): _____
Frequency

Daily _____	Rating Code: 4 = Outstanding
3 or more/week _____	3 = Good
once/week _____	2 = Fair
1 to 3/month _____	1 = Poor
	0 = No information/not applicable

PARAMETER	RATING	COMMENTS & RECOMMENDATIONS
1. Ability to gather information and evaluate patient.		
2. Technical skills.		
3. Quality of judgment and advice in patient management.		
4. Knowledge of literature.		
5. Perceptivity and sensitivity in dealing with patient and professional personnel.		
6. Organization of thought and clarity of expression.		
7. Ability to stimulate your reading.		
8. Motivation, interest in teaching and accessability.		
9. Contributions at rounds and conferences.		
10. As a teacher of basic science, in this specialty.		

Fig. 28-6. (Continued)

PARAMETER	RATING	COMMENTS & RECOMMENDATIONS
11. Personal rapport with house-staff; i.e., openness to new ideas and criticism; sensitivity to you as an individual with individual needs.		
12. How adequate was the feedback as to your performance?		
13. Overall evaluation.		
14. Comparative ranking: 4 = top 25% 3 = top 50% 2 = bottom 50% 1 = bottom 25%		

What specific suggestions would you offer this faculty member in the way of improving teaching performance?

They further claim that

the procedure for evaluating anesthesia teaching offers several advantages: all residents are willing to participate; data are inherently consistent and reliable by statistical tests; characterizations of faculty teaching performance agree well with recognized performance as judged by academic rank and the chairman's opinion; and objective data document teaching ability and allow the chairman to counsel those who should improve. Annual repetition will examine changing opinions of graduate residents and document improved staff teaching for academic management decisions.[37]

CLINICAL AND RESEARCH ENDEAVORS

Faculty commitment to clinical activity and research depends upon the individual, the academic appointment, and the availability of research opportunities. In our survey, it was revealed that during clinical time, cardiac anesthesia faculty were involved in the care of two patients per day in 50 percent of the programs responding.[36] In one institution, faculty were responsible for up to six patients per day. The speed of surgery and efficiency of operating room turnover, as well as number of residents covered simultaneously, are obviously important factors in determining daily workload. Operating activity occupies the majority of the total time for almost all academic anesthesiologists.[38]

The remainder of an academic cardiac anesthesiologist's time, sometimes preciously little, must be spent on all other academic endeavors: preparing, executing, and writing research; writing textbooks, book chapters, and reviews; giving talks and continuing education courses; working with nursing and paramedical groups; personal reading; hospital, medical center, and university committee assignments; testing and choosing new equipment; informal activities with residents and fellows; serving as an academic advisor for undergraduate and postgraduate students; and more. In some departments, even many mundane chores also fall to the faculty members (*e.g.,* copying, secretarial-type work). Clearly, the opportunities for high-volume, time-consuming research endeavors are very limited, and not comparable to the opportunities of a medicine colleague who performs periodic clinical rounds and consultations. The mission of most cardiac anesthesiologists is teaching and service oriented, and quite skewed toward the lower academic ranks.

INTERDEPARTMENTAL ACTIVITIES

Faculty cardiac anesthesiologists are in a unique position to lecture in other departments, in all areas of cardiac physiology, pharmacology, anesthesia and monitoring, and particularly in advanced cardiac life support. The combination of technical skills and theoretical knowledge allows essential and rewarding interactions with many departments. The image of anesthesia as a consultative specialty, and its responsibility for dissemination of knowledge in many disciplines, both in the medical school and community, rests on the academic anesthesiologist.

Among the institutions we surveyed, all had some interaction, usually in the form of lectures, with departments such as cardiac surgery, cardiology, physiology, pharmacology, pediatrics, advanced cardiac life-support programs, nursing programs, and medical students. Many contribute substantially to the educational programs of national and international meetings.

Advanced cardiac life support (ACLS) programs have exposed surprising gaps in knowledge and skills among anesthesiologists (the very people who should be the experts).[39, 40] This topic has generated much controversy. In our questionnaire, several hospitals claimed they required a basic CPR review course to be completed by their residents, but only one (Stanford) insists on an ACLS course. Surely cardiac anesthesia residents should complete the course during or before the cardiac anesthesia rotation. The cardiac faculty should not only complete the course themselves, but take a very active role in teaching and setting standards. ACLS also

offers an ideal opportunity for teaching impact upon other departments. At Stanford, *all* new anesthesia, surgical, and medical residents must pass a two-day American Heart Association course in ACLS. Anesthesia faculty, including the cardiac subgroup, are very involved in teaching and maintaining standards. Stanford medical students have the opportunity of taking a much longer ACLS course. An added bonus to our specialty in teaching such a medical student course is the excellent opportunity to expose the "cream" of the future physicians to anesthesia.

PROBLEMS, RECOMMENDATIONS, AND SUMMARY

Nationwide, what are the two or three areas of cardiac anesthesia which are taught least well? Of all the institutions questioned,[41] the most frequent answer (33%) was pediatric cardiac anesthesia—particularly congenital cardiac anomalies. This response occurred mainly from programs performing 150 to 400 cardiopulmonary bypass operations per year, and is presumably because of the small number of cases available outside children's hospitals. Postoperative cardiac intensive care was mentioned by 25 percent, then a potpourri including research and statistics, coagulation, cardiac catheterization data, monitoring, and noncardiac surgery for cardiac patients. The institution with the *most* operations replied that an inadequate number of operations led to the greatest weakness in a program.

How do we improve our programs? According to our survey, two institutions claim they improve their respective programs by setting the standards for others! Most claim that discussion and interaction among faculty serves as the focus for improvement, presumably as a result of facts learned at meetings and lectures, as well as personal research and observation.

Should cardiac anesthesia be regionalized? Of the institutions performing 700 to 4400 cardiopulmonary bypass operations per year,

60 percent replied "yes," and some had very strong views on promoting regionalization, particularly for pediatric cardiac surgery and anesthesia. Of the institutions with a lesser caseload (150–400), the large majority were also in favor of regionalization, although some fear the danger of producing a "surgical mill" which might depersonalize the patient. As Luft and coworkers have demonstrated,[42] previous recommendations for regionalization of cardiopulmonary bypass surgery, including minimum numbers of procedures for a given institution, have relied on the opinion of experts.[43–45] Luft and colleagues show objectively a decrease in mortality in open-heart surgery, coronary artery bypass grafts, vascular surgery (and transurethral resection of the prostate) in hospitals in which 200 or more of these operations were performed annually.[42] Morbidity was not examined. Their survey was taken from hospitals participating in the Professional Activities Study (PAS) data system.

To an extent, partial regionalization has already occurred. However, it probably would be politically impractical to implement further regionalization, particularly in private practice. *In addition, academic medicine has not come to grips with the problem of pushing regionalization, while simultaneously graduating high-quality physicians into the community.*[46] *A game of academic suicide may be in the making.*

There is a very strong argument for regionalization of pediatric cardiac anesthesia patients, particularly those with congenital and neonatal problems. It is essential to provide anesthesia, surgical, and postoperative nursing personnel who are very familiar with neonatal and pediatric patients. It is then possible to rotate a senior resident or fellow through such a institution, if he or she has a particular interest in pediatric cardiac anesthesia. A presently highly organized and successful system for transport of critically ill neonatal and pediatric patients in California serves to help to regionalize care for those patients.[47]

In summary, we will again quote Safar and Grenvik "The design of any training program requires interrelated steps: 1) the develop-

ment of objectives which define the desired end-product in measurable terms, 2) the development of the program related to these objectives, and 3) development and implementation of evaluation."[48] Programs which provide the successful use of these three steps should provide the medical community with exceptional cardiac anesthesiologists. Successful cardiac anesthesia programs should thus increase the level of critical care directly, and indirectly, in the community.

In our introduction, we asked five questions. To some, we have no correct answer presently, only educated guesses. To others, especially with respect to setting objectives, accomplishing objectives, developing curricula, organizing programs for continuing reeducation, student assessment, and improving patient care, we have provided some suggestions. We hope we have stimulated thought, and encouraged further exploration in the education of the cardiac anesthesiologist.

REFERENCES

INTRODUCTION

1. Safar P, Grenvik A: Organization and physician education in critical care medicine, Anesthesiology 47:82–95, 1977
2. Flynn MA, Fogdall RP, Ream AK: Personal communication. Survey of 18 major institutions of cardiovascular anesthesia in North America, 1979

THE LEARNING PROCESS

3. Tosteson DC: Learning in medicine. N Engl J Med 301:690–694, 1979
4. Moy RH: Critical values in medical education. N Engl J Med 301:694–697, 1979
5. Kennedy D: Creative tension: FDA and medicine. N Engl J Med 298:846–850, 1978
6. Holt J: How Children Fail. New York, Pitman Publishing, 1964
7. Wolf SG: "I can't afford a 'B'." N Engl J Med 299:949–950, 1978

8. Moss TJ, Deland EC, Maloney JV Jr: Selection of medical students for graduate training: pass/Fail versus grades. N Engl J Med 299:25–27, 1978

9. Federman DD: Will Pass/Fail pass? N Engl J Med 299:43–44, 1978

DEVELOPMENT OF THE CARDIAC ANESTHESIOLOGIST

10. Holt J: How Children Fail. New York, Pitman Publishing, 1964

11. Flynn MA, Fogdall RP, Ream AK: Personal communication. Survey of 18 major institutions of cardiovascular anesthesia in North America, 1979

12. Safar P, Grenvik A: Organization and physician education in critical care medicine. Anesthsiology 47:82–95, 1977

13. Vaughn JJ Jr: Systematic anesthesia training: the way it could be. In Djokovic: Int Anesthesiol Clin 14:111–121, 1976

14. Vanderschmidt HF, Bullock DH: The evaluation process in curriculum design. In Djokovic: Int Anesthesiol Clin 14:15–32, 1976

15. Vaughn JJ Jr: Anesthesia residency training in the United States: the way it is. In Djokovic: Int Anesthesiol Clin 14:95–111, 1976

16. McArdle PJ: Instructional methods and materials. In Djokovic: Int Anesthesiol Clin 14:33–57, 1976

17. Fineburg HV, Gabel RA, Sosman MB: Acquisition and application of new medical knowledge by the anesthesiologist: three recent examples. Anesthesiology 48:130–136, 1978

18. Pittinger CB: How up-to-date are current anesthesia and related textbooks? Anesthesiology 49:278–281, 1978

19. Sivarajan M, Lane P, Miller EV et al: Continuous lumbar epidural anesthesia skill test. Anesthesiologyy S51:S342, 1979

20. Lane PE, Sivarajan M, Millerr E et al: Common errors during resident performance of continuous lumbar epidural analgesia. Anesthesiology S51:S343, 1979

CLINICAL RESIDENT TRAINING

21. Flynn MA, Fogdall RP, Ream AK: Personal communication. Survey of 18 major institutions of cardiovascular anesthesia in North America, 1979

22. Drui AB, Behm RJ, Martin WE: Predesign investigation of the anesthesia operational environment. Anesth Analg (Cleve) 52:584–591, 1973

23. Lambert TF, Paget NS: Teaching and learning in the operating theatre. Anaesth Intensive Care 4:304–307, 1976

24. Paget NS, Lambert TF: Tutor-student interaction in the operating theatre. Anaesth Intensive Care 4:301–303, 1976

25. Fisk GC: Teaching in the operating theatre. Anaesth Intensive Care 4:196–197, 1977

26. Safar P, Grenvik A: Organization and physician education in critical care medicine. Anesthesiology 47:82–95, 1977

FELLOWSHIP TRAINING

27. Flynn MA, Fogdall RP, Ream AK: personal communication. Survey of 18 major institutions of cardiovascular anesthesia in North America, 1979

CONTINUING POSTGRADUATE EDUCATION

28. Holt J: How Children Fail. New York, Pitman Publishing, 1964

29. Luft HS, Bunker JP, Enthoven AC: Should operations be regionalized: the empirical relation between surgical volume and mortality. N Engl J Med 301:1364–1369, 1979

30. Longmire WP, Millinkoff SM: Regionalization of operations. N Engl J Med 301:1393–1394, 1979

31. Scannell JG, Brown GE, Buckley MJ: Report of the Inter-society Commission for Heart Disease Resources: optimal resources for cardiac surgery: guideline for program planning and evaluation. Circulation 52:A23–A37, 1975

32. Cardiovascular Committee of the American College of Surgeons: guidelines for minimal standards in cardiovascular surgery. Ann Thorac Surg 15:243–248, 1973

33. U.S. President's Commission on Heart Disease, Cancer and Stroke: Report to the President: A national program to conquer heart disease, cancer and stroke, vol 2. Washington, DC, Government Printing Office, 1965

34. Steinhaus JE, Epstein RM, Hamilton WK et al (ASA Subcommittee on Academic Anesthesia Manpower): A survey of academic anesthesiology. Anesthesiology 47:53–61, 1977

35. Modell JH: A case for more faculty in anesthesia. Anesthesiology 47:4–5, 1977

FACULTY ACTIVITY AND EDUCATION

36. Flynn MA, Fogdall RP, Ream AK: Personal communication. Survey of 18 major institutions of cardiovascular anesthesia in North America, 1979
37. Lecky JM, Murphy FL, Greenhow DE et al: Resident evaluation of staff teaching. Anesthesiology S51:S339, 1979
38. Steinhaus JE, Epstein RM, Hamilton WK et al: (ASA Subcommittee on Academic Anesthesia Manpower): A survey of academic anesthesiology. Anesthesiology 47:53–61, 1977
39. Garman JK: Editorial: Are anesthesiologists experts in cardiopulmonary resuscitation? Anesthesiology 50:182–184, 1979
40. Schwartz AJ, Orkin FK, Ellison N: Anesthesiologists' training and knowledge of basic life support. Anesthesiology 50:191–194, 1979

PROBLEMS, RECOMMENDATIONS, AND SUMMARY

41. Flynn MA, Fogdall RP, Ream AK: Personal communication. Survey of 18 major institutions of cardiovascular anesthesia in North America, 1979

42. Luft HS, Bunker JP, Enthoven AC: Should operations be regionalized: the empirical relation between surgical volume and mortality. N Engl J Med 301:1364–1369, 1979
43. Scannell JG, Brown GE, Buckley MJ: Report of the Inter-society Commission for Heart Disease Resources: optimal resources for cardiac surgery: guideline for program planning and evaluation. Circulation 52:A23–A37, 1975
44. Cardiovascular Committee of the American College of Surgeons: guidelines for minimal standards in cardiovascular surgery. Ann Thorac Surg 15:243–248, 1973
45. U. S. President's Commission on Heart Disease, Cancer and Stroke: Report to the President: A national program to conquer heart disease, cancer and stroke, vol 2. Washington DC, Government Printing Office, 1965
46. Greene HR: Where have all the fellows gone? Hospital Physician 15:54–55, 1979
47. Hackel A: Regionalization and the Northern California Infant Medical Dispatch Center. In Graven SN (eds): Newborn Air Transport Conference. Denver, Mead Johnson Nutritional Division, 1978
48. Safar P, Grenvik A: Organization and physician education in critical care medicine, Anesthesiology 47:82–95, 1977

INDEX

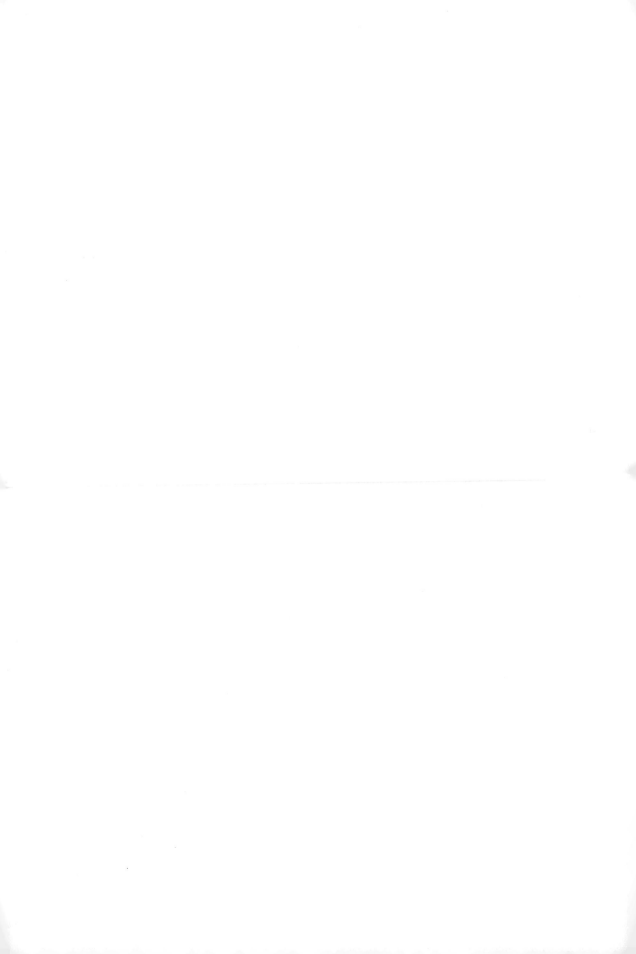